BAILEY & LOVE'S SHORT PRACTICE OF SURGERY

TWENTIETH EDITION

Revised by

A.J. HARDING RAINS

CBE, MS (Lond), FRCS (Eng)

Formerly Professor of Surgery, University of London at Charing Cross Hospital Medical School; Vice-President and Member of Council, Royal College of Surgeons of England; Hon. Consultant Surgeon, Charing Cross Hospital; Hon. Consultant Surgeon to the Army; Dean, Institute of Basic Medical Science; Dean and Assistant Director, British Postgraduate Medical Federation (University of London) in the South-West Thames Metropolitan Region; Examiner, Universities of London, Birmingham, Oxford (MCh), Belfast, Newcastle upon Tyne, Baghdad, Singapore (MMed) and Riyadh; Examiner for the Primary FRCS (Eng) and Member of the Court of Examiners, Royal College of Surgeons of England; Examiner, Professional and Linguistics Assessment Board GMC and for the GDC; President, The National Association of Theatre Nurses; Examiner for the Faculty of Anaesthetists, Royal College of Surgeons of England; Editor, Annals of the Royal College of Surgeons. Editor, Journal of The Royal Society of Medicine.

AND

CHARLES V. MANN

BM, BCh, MA, MCh (Oxon), FRCS (Eng)

Consultant Surgeon, The London Hospital; Consultant Surgeon, St Mark's Hospital, London; Examiner in Surgery, University of London; Formerly Chairman, Court of Examiners, Royal College of Surgeons of England; President, Section of Colo-Proctology, Royal Society of Medicine; Postgraduate Dean, London Hospital Medical College.

WITH 36 SPECIALIST CONTRIBUTORS

1355 illustrations (236 coloured)

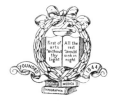

LONDON
H. K. LEWIS & Co. Ltd.
1988

First Edition 1932
Second Edition 1935
Reprinted 1935
Third Edition 1936
Reprinted 1937
Fourth Edition 1938
Reprinted 1940
Fifth Edition 1941
Reprinted 1942
Sixth Edition 1943
Reprinted 1944
Seventh Edition 1946
Reprinted 1948
Eighth Edition 1948–9
Ninth Edition 1952
Italian Edition 1952
Turkish Edition 1955
Tenth Edition 1956
Reprinted 1957
Eleventh Edition 1959
Reprinted 1960
Twelfth Edition 1962
Reprinted 1964
Spanish Edition 1965
Thirteenth Edition 1965
Fourteenth Edition 1968
Reprinted 1969
Fifteenth Edition 1971
Reprinted 1972
Sixteenth Edition 1975
Reprinted 1976
Seventeenth Edition 1977
Reprinted 1978
Eighteenth Edition 1981
Nineteenth Edition 1984
Twentieth Edition 1988

H. K. Lewis & Co. Ltd.
1959, 1962, 1965, 1968, 1971, 1975, 1977, 1981, 1984, 1988

I.S.B. No. 07186 0501 2

PRINTED IN GREAT BRITAIN
FOR H. K. LEWIS AND CO LTD, 136 GOWER STREET, LONDON
BY HAZELL WATSON AND VINEY LIMITED, AYLESBURY, BUCKS

PREFACE TO THE TWENTIETH EDITION

The practice of surgery has been changed spectacularly by rapid advances in basic and applied sciences. Biological advances have led to complete new fields of oncological and immunological treatments, with transplantation now a major area of surgical interest. Pharmaceutical research has introduced powerful new drugs and has altered completely the control of inflammation and infectious disease. New bio-engineering techniques have brought progress in the treatment of fractures, joint replacement methods and the latest hardware used in intensive care and rehabilitation units.

Continued advances in electronic technology assist surgeons of all countries to offer considerable benefits to patients. Ultrasonic, computed tomographic and magnetic resonance imaging can facilitate accurate diagnosis, assist treatment and enhance follow-up, affording increased comfort and safety to the patient through the advantages of non-invasive techniques.

This edition of 'Short Practice' incorporates these advances. The student is first led through the essential principles of surgery and then into the organ-related chapters which display the whole range of modern surgery. Specialist contributors have again assisted the editors in providing balanced and authoritative surveys of the latest information required for attaining a satisfactory standard for qualifying and post-graduate examinations, and establishing a sound basis for surgical practice.

The editors gratefully acknowledge all those who have contributed to this extensive revision with new material, and those who have proffered suggestions from all parts of the world. We continue the tradition of recognising wherever possible the sources of contributions which add so greatly to the value of the text and illustrations.

January 1988

A. J. HARDING RAINS
CHARLES V. MANN

SPECIALIST CONTRIBUTORS

Fractures, Orthopaedics, Neurosurgery

PAUL J. GREGG, MD, FRCS, *Professor of Orthopaedic Surgery, University of Leicester, Hon. Consultant Orthopaedic Surgeon, Leicester Royal Infirmary and Glenfield General Hospital, Leicester.* (Chapters 15–24)

BRIAN McKIBBIN, MS (Ill.), MD, FRCS, *Professor of Traumatic and Orthopaedic Surgery, University of Wales College of Medicine, Consultant Orthopaedic Surgeon, South Glamorgan Health Authority.* (Chapters 25, 27, 28)

JOHN GARFIELD, MA, MChir, FRCP, FRCS, *Consultant Neurosurgeon, Wessex Neurological Centre, Southampton, Hon. Clinical Teacher in Neurosurgery, University of Southampton.* (Chapters 26, 27, 28)

Urology and Transplantation

R. C. TIPTAFT, BSc, FRCS, *Consultant Urological Surgeon, St Thomas's Hospital, London.* (Chapters 56–61)

A. DAVID MEE, FRCS, *Consultant Urological Surgeon, Charing Cross Hospital, London.* (Chapter 62)

Cardiothoracic Surgery

T. A. H. ENGLISH, MA, BSc, FRCS, *Consultant Cardiothoracic Surgeon, Papworth and Addenbrooke's Hospitals, Cambridge.* (Chapter 41)

RAYMOND L. HURT, FRCS, *Consultant Thoracic Surgeon, North Middlesex and St Bartholomew's Hospitals, London.* (Chapters 40, 43)

F. C. WELLS, MS, FRCS, *Consultant Cardiothoracic Surgeon, Papworth Hospital, Cambridge.* (Chapters 41, 43)

Gastrointestinal Surgery

ROBERT SHIELDS, MD, FRCS, *Professor of Surgery, University of Liverpool.* (Chapter 45)

CHRISTOPHER WASTELL, MS, FRCS, *Professor and Hon. Consultant Surgeon, Charing Cross and Westminster Medical Schools, and Westminster and St Stephen's Hospitals, London.* (Chapter 44)

ALAN G. JOHNSON, MChir, FRCS, *Professor of Surgery, University of Sheffield.* (Chapter 45)

H. H. THOMPSON, MS, FRCS, *Senior Lecturer in Surgery and Hon. Consultant Surgeon, The London Hospital.* (Chapter 47)

T. G. ALLEN-MERSH, MD, FRCS, *Senior Lecturer and Hon. Consultant Surgeon, Charing Cross and Westminster Medical School, London.* (Chapters 46, 48)

CHARLES V. MANN, MCh, FRCS, *Consultant Surgeon, The London and St Mark's Hospitals, London.* (Chapters 49–54)

R. D. ROSIN, MS, FRCS, *Consultant Surgeon, St Mary's Hospital, London.* (Chapter 42)

Endocrine Surgery

GERALD WESTBURY, FRCS, FRCP, *Professor of Surgery, Institute of Cancer Research, Hon. Consultant Surgeon, Royal Marsden Hospital, Consultant Surgeon, Westminster Hospital, London.* (Chapters 10, 39)

MALCOLM H. WHEELER, MD, FRCS, *Consultant Surgeon, University Hospital of Wales and the Royal Infirmary, Cardiff.* (Chapter 37)

ANTHONY W. GOODE, MD, FRCS, *Assistant Director, Surgical Unit and Hon. Consultant Surgeon, The London Hospital.* (Chapter 38)

Oral and Ear, Nose and Throat Surgery

G. R. SEWARD, MDS, FDSRCS, *Professor of Oral Surgery, The London Hospital Medical College. Dean, Faculty of Dental Surgery, Royal College of Surgeons of England.* (Chapters 30–33)

H. B. HOLDEN, FRCS, *Consultant ENT Surgeon, Charing Cross Hospital, London.* (Chapters 33–35)

A. D. CHEESEMAN, BSc, FRCS, *Consultant Otolaryngologist, Charing Cross and Royal National Ear, Nose and Throat Hospitals, London.* (Chapters 33–35)

A. E. S. RICHARDS, FRCS, *Consultant ENT Surgeon, Charing Cross Hospital, London.* (Chapters 33–35)

Ophthalmic Surgery

BRUCE MATHALONE, FRCS, *Consultant Ophthalmic Surgeon, Westminster and Charing Cross Hospitals, London and The Royal Eye Unit, Kingston-upon-Thames.* (Chapter 29)

Vascular and Lymphatic Surgery

R. A. P. SCOTT, MCh, FRCS, *Consultant Surgeon and Consultant in Vascular Surgery, Royal West Sussex (St Richard's) Hospital, Chichester.* (Chapters 13, 14)

J. McIVOR, FDSRCS, FRCR, *Consultant Radiologist, Charing Cross Hospital, London.* (Chapter 9)

CONTENTS

PAGE

Preface   V

CHAPTER

1. THE HEALING AND MANAGEMENT OF WOUNDS   I
2. BULLET, BOMB AND BLAST INJURIES   12
3. WOUND INFECTION   19
4. SPECIAL INFECTIONS. VIRUSES. AIDS. IMMUNOLOGY   33
5. HAEMORRHAGE. SHOCK. BLOOD TRANSFUSION. ANALGESIA   56
6. FLUID, ELECTROLYTE AND ACID-BASE BALANCE   77
7. NUTRITION   91
8. TUMOURS. CYSTS. ULCERS. SINUSES   101
9. LYMPHATICS AND LYMPH NODES   118
10. SKIN. BURNS   132
11. THE HAND   157
12. THE FOOT   171
13. VASCULAR DISEASE—VEINS   182
14. VASCULAR DISEASE—ARTERIES   193
15. FRACTURES AND DISLOCATIONS—GENERAL PRINCIPLES   235
16. FRACTURES AND DISLOCATIONS. UPPER LIMB   269
17. FRACTURES AND DISLOCATIONS. LOWER LIMB AND PELVIS   301
18. INFECTIONS OF BONES AND JOINTS   344
19. THE RHEUMATIC DISEASES   357
20. TUMOURS OF BONES AND JOINTS   372
21. CONGENITAL DISEASES OF BONES AND JOINTS   380
22. DISORDERS OF THE GROWING SKELETON   396
23. GENERALISED DISEASES OF BONE   410
24. DISEASES OF MUSCLES, TENDONS AND FASCIAE   415
25. NEUROLOGICAL DISORDERS AFFECTING THE MUSCULO-SKELETAL SYSTEM   423
26. THE HEAD (SCALP, SKULL AND BRAIN)   433
27. THE SPINE, THE VERTEBRAL COLUMN AND SPINAL CORD   489
28. NERVES   510
29. THE EYE AND ORBIT   530

CHAPTER | PAGE

30. FACE, PALATE, LIPS, MAXILLO-FACIAL INJURIES 539
31. THE SALIVARY GLANDS 559
32. THE MOUTH. THE CHEEK. THE TONGUE 574
33. THE TEETH AND GUMS, JAWS, NOSE, EAR 596
34. THE PHARYNX 625
35. THE LARYNX 639
36. THE NECK 648
37. THE THYROID GLAND AND THE THYROGLOSSAL TRACT 660
38. THE PARATHYROID AND ADRENAL GLANDS 694
39. THE BREAST 712
40. THE THORAX 740
41. THE HEART AND PERICARDIUM 787
42. ANASTOMOSES 814
43. THE OESOPHAGUS 827
44. THE STOMACH AND DUODENUM 855
45. THE LIVER 903
46. THE SPLEEN 937
47. THE GALLBLADDER AND BILE DUCTS 953
48. THE PANCREAS 980
49. THE PERITONEUM. OMENTUM. MESENTERY
    AND RETROPERITONEAL SPACE 1003
50. THE SMALL AND LARGE INTESTINES 1027
51. INTESTINAL OBSTRUCTION 1065
52. THE VERMIFORM APPENDIX 1090
53. THE RECTUM 1110
54. THE ANUS AND ANAL CANAL 1131
55. HERNIAS. UMBILICUS. ABDOMINAL WALL 1165
56. URINARY SYMPTOMS. INVESTIGATION OF THE
    URINARY TRACT. ANURIA 1193
57. THE KIDNEYS AND URETERS 1208
58. THE URINARY BLADDER 1254
59. THE PROSTATE AND SEMINAL VESICLES 1298
60. THE URETHRA AND PENIS 1320
61. THE TESTES AND THE SCROTUM 1352
62. ORGAN TRANSPLANTATION 1376
63. THE SURGICAL PATIENT 1388
    INDEX 1391

SAYINGS OF THE GREAT

Both Hamilton Bailey and McNeill Love, when medical students, served as clerks to Sir Robert Hutchison, 1871–1960, who was Consulting Physician to the London Hospital and President of the Royal College of Physicians. They never tired of quoting his 'Medical Litany' which is appropriate for all clinicians, and, perhaps especially, to those who are surgically minded.

> 'From inability to leave well alone;
> From too much zeal for what is new and
>   contempt for what is old;
> From putting knowledge before wisdom,
>   science before art, cleverness before
>   common sense;
> From treating patients as cases; and
> From making the cure of a disease more
>   grievous than its endurance,
> Good Lord, deliver us.'

to which may be added:

'The patient is the centre of the medical universe around which all our works revolve and towards which all our efforts trend.' J. B. Murphy, 1857–1916, Professor of Surgery, Northwestern University, Chicago, U.S.A.

'To study the phenomenon of disease without books is to sail an uncharted sea, while to study books without patients is not to go to sea at all.' Sir William Osler, 1849–1919, Professor of Medicine, Oxford, England.

'A knowledge of healthy and diseased actions is not less necessary to be understood than the principles of other sciences. By an acquaintance with principles we learn the cause of disease. Without this knowledge a man cannot be a surgeon . . . The last part of surgery, namely operations, is a reflection on the healing art; it is a tacit acknowledgement of the insufficiency of surgery. It is like an armed savage who attempts to get that by force which a civilised man would by stratagem.' John Hunter, 1728–1793, Surgeon, St. George's Hospital, London. The founder of the modern surgeon.

'In investigating Nature you will do well to bear ever in mind that in every question there is the truth, whatever our notions may be. This seems perhaps a very simple consideration, yet it is strange how often it seems to be disregarded. If we had nothing but pecuniary rewards and worldly honours to look to, our profession would not be one to be desired. But in its practice you will find it to be attended with peculiar privileges; second to none in intense interest and pure pleasures. It is our proud office to tend the fleshy tabernacle of the immortal spirit, and our path, if rightly followed, will be guided by unfettered truth and love unfeigned. In the pursuit of this noble and holy calling I wish you all God-speed.' 'Promoter's address, Graduation in Medicine, University of Edinburgh, August, 1876' by Lord Lister, the Founder of Modern Surgery.

A SHORT PRACTICE OF SURGERY

CHAPTER I

THE HEALING AND MANAGEMENT OF WOUNDS

'A wise physician skilled our wounds to heal is more than armies for the common weal[1]'.—Homer
'Skin is the best dressing'.—Lister

The healing of wounds caused by accident, assault, warfare and surgical operations has always been a central consideration in surgical practice because any breach in the surfaces of the body—the skin and mucous membrane—exposes the deeper tissues to the danger of infection (Chapter 3). Therefore, it is necessary to assist the healing process of the body to restore an intact surface as soon as possible. Immediate closure of a wound (*primary suture*) using sutures,[2] clips, staples and adhesive materials favours healing with minimal scarring (*Healing by First Intention*) (figs 1, 2, 3, 4, 5.).

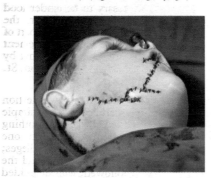

FIG. 1.—Accurate primary suture for healing by first intention.
(the late Rainsford Mowlem, FRCS).

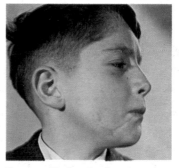

FIG. 2.—Healing by first intention. See figs 1 and 3.

Other methods of providing skin cover—in the presence of devitalised tissue, swelling tension and skin loss—include *delayed primary suture* (p. 7), *skin grafting* (p. 8 and Chapter 10) and *secondary suture* (p. 9).

---

[1] Weal = the general good, the welfare of a country.
[2] Suture (Latin) = Sewing together (a stitch). A seam. Ligature (Latin) = Anything that binds together.

Homer, *date of birth uncertain between 1050 and 850 B.C., somewhere in Greece. Still regarded as the great epic poet and author of the 'Iliad' and the 'Odyssey'.*
Joseph Lister (Lord Lister), *1827–1912. Professor of Surgery, Glasgow, Scotland (1860–1869), Edinburgh (1869–1877), and King's College Hospital, London (1877–1892).*

Healing by Second Intention takes place: when the wound edges are not brought together, when there is irreparable skin loss, and when the wound becomes infected, breaks apart or has to be laid open. An ulcer (fig. 6) heals in the same way. The process is slower than healing by first intention, and there is more scar tissue (p. 5). The topical (local) methods employed to encourage healing are similar to those used for ulcers (Chapter 8).

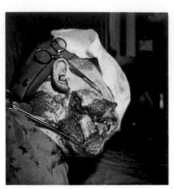

Fig. 3.—Severe facio-maxillary injury—see figs 1 and 2.
(the late Rainsford Mowlem FRCS)

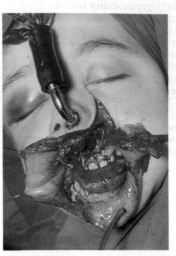

Fig. 4.—Split-open face from a road traffic accident.
(the late Rainsford Mowlem, FRCS)

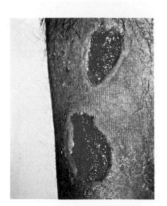

Fig. 6.—Ulcers of the leg healing by second intention. Note the red granulation tissue.

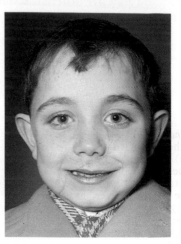

Fig. 5.—Healing by first intention after primary suture of split-open face (above).
(the late Rainsford Mowlem, FRCS)

The Biological Process of Healing.—There are three phases of healing beginning with the phase of inflammation[1] (days 1–4) and merging into phase two, which is the phase of

---

[1] 'Inflammation'. It should be remembered that this word does not imply bacterial infection, but the first phase of the healing process.

proliferation (granulation tissue) (days 5–20), and then into phase three, the phase of differentiation (scar tissue) from day 20 onward.

Phase 1. Inflammation.—Immediately on wounding there is a change in tissue tension which causes a change in the charge on the collagen molecule. The constituents of the blood flowing into the wound come into contact with collagen and clotting is induced, with activation of kinin and complement cascades. Platelets become adherent and with the clotting factors form a haemostatic plug. The blood vessels undergo brief constriction followed by vasodilatation under the influence of histamine from platelets and mast cells. Capillary permeability increases; serotonin, the kinins and prostaglandins (the chemical mediators of the inflammatory response) maintain capillary engorgement. Red and white blood cells escape through the vessel walls and a network of fibrin forms over the wound, which within 3 hours is surrounded by a few lymphocytes and an increasing number of polymorph neutrophils. These neutrophils have a predominantly lytic function because of their lysosome content. Monocytes begin to appear in increasing numbers and become the dominant cell type by the fifth day. They are phagocytic and ingest cellular debris. Depression of this macrophage function will delay wound healing (see Immunology section Chapter 4). By the end of the first phase new capillaries bud from endothelial cells in capillaries near the wound edge while in the connective tissue surrounding the vessels, mesenchymal cells differentiate to become fibroblasts.

Clinically, this phase is manifest by the classical features of inflammation namely: *heat, redness, tenderness, swelling* and *loss of function* (fig. 7).

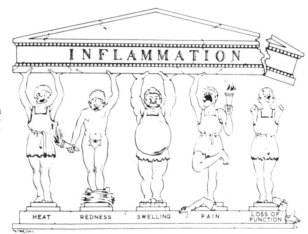

FIG. 7.—The Greeks had a word for it! *(With permission of Professors W. G. Spector and D. A. Willoughby. Artist, Mr. P. Cull.)*

Phase 2. Granulation tissue.—By day 5 significant numbers of fibroblasts have begun to synthesise (a) *collagen* and (b) *ground substance.*

(a) *Collagen* is the extracellular fibrous framework that gives strength and form to tissues. There are several types of collagen which differ in the aminoacid sequence of the constituent chains, although proline, hydroxyproline and glycine are predominant. Type 1 collagen is found in skin, tendon, bone and ligament. Type 2 occurs in cartilage and type 3 is found in fetal dermis and is replaced by type 1 collagen at birth. Granulation tissue gives rise predominantly to type 1 collagen. Hydroxylation of immature proto-collagen requires oxygen, ferrous ions and ascorbic acid. Further maturation involving glycosylation produces more stable tropocollagen. Tropocollagen is held together by weak electrostatic forces and is soluble in weak salt solutions. It is thus extruded from the fibroblast, but disappears quickly as it matures by cross linkage to other collagen molecules resulting in stronger less soluble collagen. This collagen, though stable, is not inert, and it undergoes constant turnover under the influence of tissue collagenases. Thicker collagen fibres soon abound and are laid down haphazardly.

(b) *Ground substance* is the amorphous matrix of connective tissue and contains water, electrolytes, mucopolysaccharides and glycoproteins. Ground substance is a thin gel, but in cartilage it is elastic. It is produced by fibroblasts and is involved in the formation and maturation of extra-cellular collagen. It exists as a water rich phase and in equilibrium with a colloid phase. Complexes occur between proteins and polysaccharides that bestow particular properties on ground substance. The types of mucopolysaccharides, include chondroitin, chondroitin-4-sulphate, chondroitin-6-sulphate, dermatin sulphate, keratin sulphate and hyaluronic acid.

Phase 3. Scar tissue.—There is no clear demarcation between proliferation and differentiation. The latter starts in the proliferating granulation tissue and continues indefinitely. There is a rationalisation of the copious new blood vessels, and notably a remodelling of the haphazard arrangement of the collagen fibres. New collagen is synthesised in a more orderly fashion along the lines of tension in the scar. Collagen turnover and remodelling in the scar never stops. Indeed, the turnover of collagen in scar tissue is faster than in other tissues. (For the healing of bone, see Chapter 15.)

Repair of the epithelial surface.—The epithelial defect in an incised wound is initially plugged with fibrin coagulum and the epidermis turns downwards over the edge of the underlying dermis. At 24 hours, basal cells are mobilising on the undersurface of the epidermis and by 48 hours the advancing epithelial edge has undergone cellular hypertrophy and mitosis. The epithelium migrates but stops when it meets the opposite advancing epithelium.

When there has been superficial skin loss, dermal pits which are left behind act as islands for regenerating epithelium. However, once lost there is no regeneration of hair follicles, sweat or sebaceous glands in the new epidermis.

Factors Influencing Wound Healing

Blood supply. Wounds of the face and hands, however horrifying on first appearance (fig. 3) heal well because of an excellent blood supply. Wounds below the knees, over the shin and calf—notably in the elderly—heal badly because of a relatively poor blood supply.

Tension of the tissues inhibits local blood supply and leads to wound failure. Local swelling and therefore tension builds up automatically during the first 48 hours after injury as part of the phenomenon of inflammation. *Haematoma*, *venous stasis* (e.g. in a dependant limb), and *infection* also increase tension.

Age.—Protein turnover reduces with age and this is reflected by a slow rate of healing.

Rest.—Granulation tissue has a delicate blood supply that is easily damaged by movement and shearing forces. With early mobilisation being desirable after surgery, the surgeon must carefully consider his advice to the individual patient to avoid both the hazards of prolonged rest and the discomfort of premature mobilisation.

Infection.—Once infection is established the fibroblast must compete with bacteria and inflammatory cells for oxygen and nutrients. Thus, overall collagen synthesis is inevitably reduced and collagen breakdown enhanced by collagenolytic enzyme activity. Infection is a major factor in the failure of wounds to heal.

Malnutrition.—Malnutrition has been associated with the defective synthesis of both collagen and ground substance. Severe protein calorie malnutrition has long been implicated in the failure of wounds to heal, while similarly lesser degrees of malnutrition depress healing. Vitamin C is necessary for synthesis of ground substance and maturation of collagen. Vitamin D is essential for new bone formation and Vitamin A for epithelialisation. Calcium, zinc, copper and manganese are essential minerals and patients with burns and intestinal fistulas, in particular, become zinc depleted and require supplementation.

Uraemia.—Experimentally the addition of urea to tissue cultures of fibroblasts inhibits their growth. Clinically uraemia is implicated in the retardation of wound healing in patients.

Jaundice.—Jaundice is associated with a reduction in wound strength. The appearance of fibroblasts and the formation of new blood vessels are both delayed. Biopsies of skin in jaundiced patients show a reduction of the enzyme prolyl-hydroxylase involved in collagen maturation.

Steroids.—An inflammatory response is essential for wound healing to proceed normally. Steroids depress wound healing by their anti-inflammatory action. New vessels are abnormal and sparse, as are fibroblasts. If steroids are given after the inflammatory phase of wound healing, there is little overall effect on healing.

Radiation.—Radiation causes cell death by both damaging DNA and disrupting intracellular metabolism.

SUMMARY OF ADVERSE FACTORS

General Factors	Local Factors
Age	Tissue tension
Malnutrition	Haematoma formation
Vitamin deficiency	Necrotic tissue
Trace metal deficiency (Chapter 7)	Local infection
Anaemia	Foreign body present
Malignant disease	A poor blood supply due to vascular disease or
Uraemia	trauma
Jaundice	Faulty technique of wound closure
Diabetes	Recurrent trauma
Generalised infection	Local x-irradiation
Cytotoxic drugs and steroids	

SCARS

The stages through which a scar passes are: *Stage 1.* (0–4 weeks) The scar is fine, soft, not contracted, not strong. *Stage 2.* (4–12 weeks). The scar becomes red, hard, thick and strong. It tends to contract. *Stage 3.* (12–40 weeks) The scar gradually becomes soft, supple, white and tends to relax.

The rate and extent to which these changes occur vary with (*a*) the position of the scar on the body, (*b*) the direction of the scar with regard to the lines of skin tension, (*c*) the age of the patient, (*d*) the ethnic group.

(*a*) *Position on the Body.*—The worst position on the body for scars is over the sternum. Scars in this area very regularly become severely hypertrophic and even truly keloidal (fig. 8). The region over the shoulder is also a poor one for making scars, as is the back.

(*b*) *Direction with regard to lines of skin tension.*—See incisions (below).

(*c*) *Age.*—The best scars are obtained in very old people with fine wrinkled skin and by 9 months after operation may be almost invisible. Another favourable age is the first year of life. The worst period for scars likely to contract is in older children.

(*d*) *Ethnic Group.*—The more highly pigmented the person the worse the scars will be.

Hypertrophic Scars.—This type of scar is common in young people and particularly after injuries such as burns (fig. 9). It is so common as to be considered the normal pattern of scar formation. Both the intensity and the duration of the active phase of scar formation are increased. However, even in cases where severe hypertrophy occurs the scar does not become worse after 12 weeks. By this time, the scar is very thick, red and often itchy, and this condition then persists in this severe state for a further 3 to 6 months. After this time, it gradually regresses. *Compression treatment.*—Fashioned elastic appliances are particularly useful in flattening and maturing these scars. Stockings, armlets, gloves, body pieces, and face and neck helmets can be made[1] (Chapter 10).

Keloid[2] (figs. 8 and 9).—True keloid in white-skinned people is a rare condition, and the only common site is over the sternum. It is said that the true keloid spreads into normal tissue not affected by the original injury or operation. However, in many scars this is difficult to determine, and the certain distinction between the true keloid and the hypertrophic scar is found not in the appearance, but in the time scale. The hypertrophic scar never gets worse after 6 months, but a true keloid continues to get worse even after a year, and some may even progress for 5 to 10 years. It would appear that the maturation and stabilisation of the collagen fibrils is inhibited (p. 3). Treatment is extremely difficult. Excision and resuture are certain to be followed by recurrence and although x-ray treatment was used in the hope that this would prevent recurrence the results of this are uncertain. Improved results have been obtained by shaving away the excess tissue, taking care not to carry the incision into normal tissue at any point and then resurfacing the area by a thin skin graft. Some excellent results have been obtained by the injection of steroid preparations.

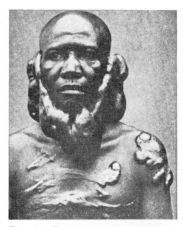

FIG. 8.—Extensive keloid in a West African.
(C. Bowesman, FRCS, Kumasi, Ghana.)

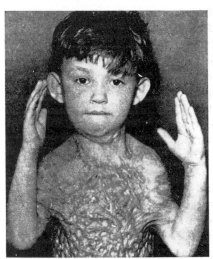

FIG. 9.—Hypertrophic scars and contractures following burns.
(The late Patrick Clarkson, FRCS)

INCISIONS

The object of a surgical incision is to expose the part operated on to best advantage, and this should be combined with a desire to finish with a scar which is as good and as inconspicuous as possible. The creases and wrinkles in the skin are parallel with the lines of skin tension and it is in accordance with these lines that incisions should be made.

---

[1] Tubigrip pressure garments by Seton®, Tubiton House, Oldham, England, or Jobst anti burnscar™ supports by Jobst®, Toledo, Ohio, U.S.A.

[2] Keloid = Like a claw.

Incisions should not be made directly across skin creases unless there is some over-riding reason as the resulting scar will become hypertrophic. In no circumstances should an incision be made directly across the crease in the flexor surface of a joint. Adequate exposure can be obtained by making incisions 'S' or 'Z' shaped if a single straight incision will not suffice.

Confusion has arisen in the past because of the interpretation of the significance of Langer's lines. These lines which were worked out by Langer in 1862, are associated with the distribution of the collagen and elastic fibres in the skin, and are not of importance with regard to skin incisions.

Types of Wound and their Closure

Incised Wounds = Primary Suture.—The majority of incised wounds are caused by a sharp knife or glass and are relatively clean. Structures will be damaged only along the track of penetration with minimal injury to tissues on either side. After suitable exploration these wounds may be closed by *primary suture*, if possible, within six hours of injury. Damaged tendons, nerves and major blood vessels should be repaired at the time of primary surgery. Microsurgical techniques have extended the scope of the repair of nerves, small blood vessels and therefore limb salvage procedures.

Penetrating wounds. Beware the innocent-looking stab wound of the abdomen! Not infrequently the long stiletto knife blade has traversed several intraperitoneal viscera. All such wounds must be explored layer by layer and with a view to laparotomy, even in the initial absence of peritonism. Wounds in the thigh are common, especially in the meat trade (butcher's thigh[1]).

Lacerated Wounds = Wound Excision and Primary Suture of Skin.— Wounds with jagged edges, commonly seen following road traffic accidents, are frequently dirty and contaminated with organic matter. In the presence of devitalised tissue, especially muscle, the risk of infection is increased. Within six hours of injury, the key to success lies in the meticulous removal of all dead tissue, the removal of organic matter such as clothing and irrigation of the raw area prior to a layered closure of the wound. The object is to convert the lacerated wound into one that approximates to an incised wound (see figs. 3, 4 and 5). Complicated repair of tendons and nerves is not recommended at the time of initial surgery because of the risk of infection and normally must wait for 4–6 weeks when good superficial cover has been assured.

Crushed and Devitalised Wounds = Wound Excision and Delayed Primary Suture.—*Industrial and severe road traffic accidents* account for the majority of these wounds. *War injuries* also fall into this group, but as the mechanism of wounding is slightly different they are considered separately (Chapter 2).

The area and depth of devitalised tissue depends upon the area and weight of the crushing force and on the duration and velocity of impact. Severe crushing injury may have a profound general as well as local effect especially if pressure is unrelieved (Crush syndrome Chapter 5).

---

[1] Butcher's thigh. Accidental division of the femoral artery caused by the slipping of the boning knife during the preparation of joints of meat (see Chapter 1

Karl Langer, 1819–1887. Professor of Anatomy, Vienna.

Three difficulties exist in dealing with this type of wound:

1. One cannot with certainty distinguish between viable and non-viable tissue.

2. The inflammatory oedema and therefore the tissue tension will, if attempts are made to close the wound by primary suture, rise to dangerously high levels resulting in local ischaemia[1] and local death in tissues which were previously viable. Dead muscle is the ideal environment for the development of infection (gas-gangrene) (Chapter 4).

3. The wound may be heavily contaminated by bacteria.

The key to the management of these wounds is the excision of all dead tissue and the prevention of tissue tension. All necrotic muscle must be moved along with indriven organic matter. Tension beneath the deep fascia must be relieved by a long fasciotomy incision. After irrigation the wound should be left open and dressed. The wound is re-examined 4–6 days later. If it is found that all remaining tissue is viable and the oedema has subsided sufficiently to allow the wound to be sutured without tension, *delayed primary suture* can be performed.

N.B.—if there is any doubt about the advisability of suture—DON'T SUTURE.

Wounds with Skin Loss (figs. 10, 11 and 12).—Healing of the skin is of importance as a barrier to infection, and because the healing of deeper structures, such as the tendons and bones, can only take place satisfactorily in the presence of an intact skin cover.

The longer any exposed surface remains raw the greater will be the scarring, the deformity and the disability. The procedures should be:

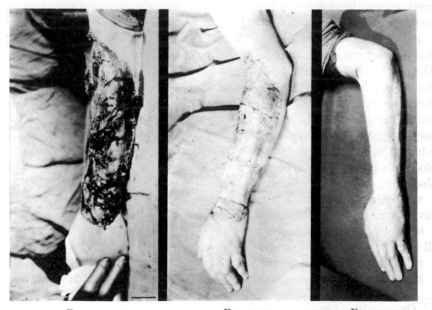

FIG. 10   FIG. 11   FIG. 12

FIGS. 10,11 and 12.—Wound excision and primary skin grafting.

[1] Ischaemia (Greek) = A lack of blood flow.

1. Clean incised wounds with skin loss—Primary grafting.
2. Lacerated wounds with skin loss—Wound excision and primary grafting.
3. Crushed and devitalised wounds with skin loss—Wound excision and delayed primary, or occasionally secondary skin grafting.

Secondary Suture, by freeing skin at the edge of a granulating wound is rarely used. It is easier and safer to perform secondary skin grafting and to carry out any reconstructive surgery later.

PRACTICAL MANAGEMENT OF THE SEVERELY INJURED

It is probably true to say that simple first-aid principles account for the saving of more lives than heroic surgery.[1]

1. *Secure the casualty from further injury in the danger zone.* This is particularly applicable on motorways.

2. *Airway.* Ensure an adequate airway, removing blood and debris from the victim's mouth and throat. The use of a good light and mechanical suction are important aids. Maintain and protect the airway by placing the victim in the lateral position, head down, using an oropharyngeal airway if available. In the hands of skilled personnel endotracheal intubation has several advantages in major trauma victims: the airway is secured and protected in addition to providing the facility for artificial ventilation and tracheobronchial suction. The deeply unconscious patient and the severe chest injury associated with a large flail segment benefit greatly by intubation and assisted ventilation. Tracheostomy and cricothyroidostomy are reserved for those cases that cannot be intubated.

3. *Stop haemorrhage* (Chapter 5). Bleeding can usually be controlled by the application of local pressure using a padded dressing. A tourniquet can be life-saving in traumatic amputation of a limb (see Chapter 5, tourniquet abuse).

4. *Secure an intravenous line.* The body compensates so well for blood loss that its response can lull the resuscitation officer into a false sense of security. The estimation of loss of blood is sometimes difficult. A large bore cannula should be inserted into a vein before it collapses due to shock. Perfusion of tissues by an adequate circulation volume is the aim of early resuscitation. Initially a crystalloid solution (*e.g.* Hartmann's compound sodium lactate), may be given i.v., followed by such plasma expanders as 3·5–4% gelatin solution (*e.g.* Haemaccel ®) or Dextran 70[2] while waiting for cross-matched blood. Only rarely, in the severely exsanguinated, is universal donor O-negative blood infused.

5. *Oxygen administration.* It has been shown that the inhalation of oxygen is of advantage to the major trauma victim.

6. *Splint fractures.* To prevent pain and further damage to soft tissue structures all fractures of the limbs should be splinted.

7. *Relieve intrapleural or intrapericardial tension.* (Chapters 2, 40 and 41).

8. *Relief of intragastric tension.* A nasogastric tube may be necessary.

---

[1] The essentials of *First Aid*—attention to the three B's—'Breathing' (airway), 'Bleeding' (Chapter 5) and 'Breaks' (fractures). Beware of and prevent *the second accident,* namely loss of life due to lack of sustained first aid during transport and until handing over to a proper resuscitation team. In a war arena the watchword is ABE (Airway, Bleeding, Evacuation).

[2] A sample of blood for crossmatching should be taken before giving Dextran.

Points in the Examination of the Wounded

1. Examine the patient for other injuries. Is the patient shocked?

2. Examine the wound. Bleeding and pain often make inspection difficult. Much useful information can be obtained from a brief superficial look at the wound.

3. Have any deep structures been divided by the injury? More complications occur simply because the observer has failed to think about what structures might have been involved than because of any technical short-comings in the operation. Limbs—has a major blood vessel been injured? Examine the peripheral pulse. Has a tendon been involved? Test movement. Has a nerve been involved? Test movement and sensation. Examine for fractures. The abdomen—has a viscus been involved? If so, which viscus? Examine the urine after catheterisation if necessary. The head—has the skull been damaged or the dura breached with injury to the brain, eye or the ear? (See Head Injuries, Chapter 26.)

Procedure in Operative Surgery.—Dirty wounds are initially cleaned with a detergent antiseptic solution, *i.e.* Cetavlon ® or Povidone iodine. Once the temporary dressing is removed the wound may bleed profusely. A brief inspection of the large wounds enables one to plan surgery before operation. Tattered skin should be trimmed but viable skin must not be excised. If necessary the wound must be extended, preferably in a longitudinal direction, to obtain a good view of underlying tissue. The deep fascia must be freely excised in the presence of tension or haematoma beneath in order to open up the muscle compartments. Damaged muscle must be excised until the muscle bleeds freely and contracts when cut. Bone is often viable and any fragment should be replaced in position. Foreign bodies should be located and removed. Tendons, nerves, and major blood vessels crossing the wound should be carefully examined to determine if they have been injured. Wounds of the abdomen, chest, and head have to be explored, layer by layer (fig. 13). The guidelines already given regarding repair must be followed (also see Chapter 2). Any necessary splintage should be applied both to immobilise the fracture and to rest the soft tissues, *even* in the absence of a broken bone.

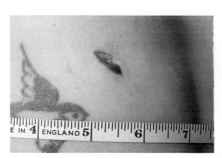

Fig. 13.—Stab wound of the chest wall which required thoracotomy.

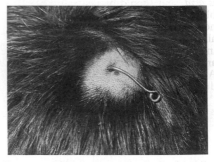

Fig. 14.—This patient was hooked while swimming underwater.
(*Dr M. P. Solanki, MS, Bombay, India.*)

Foreign Bodies in the Tissues. In every case of suspected foreign body which is opaque to x-rays, a radiograph must be taken in at least two planes. When removal is attempted, a good light, ample time, proper anaesthesia and a bloodless field are all invaluable together with the use of x-rays in the localisation of the object by means of metal skin markers, needles and, if available, an x-ray image intensifier with a T.V. display screen.

Domestic needles commonly become impacted between the small bones of the hand or foot and unless a small fragment is lodged deeply, removal is advisable. Startling cases are on record in which a needle has entered the venous circulation and become embedded in the heart muscle.

Sewing-machine needles occasionally transfix the terminal phalanx and nail, and then break. The finger should be forcibly pressed on to a hard surface, so that the fragment retraces its path and it is removed with forceps.

Fish hooks, and similar articles which possess barbs, are removed by pushing the hook onwards in such a direction that it emerges through the skin at the nearest point. The barb is nipped off, and the hook withdrawn (fig. 14).

Gravel is often driven into the subcutaneous tissues of the face, hands, or knees. Ugly scars are the penalty for incomplete removal—a particularly distressing sequel if occurring on the face—'tattoo marks'. An anaesthetic and meticulous removal are indicated. A nailbrush may be useful here.

Glass splinters. Contrary to popular belief, most glass is radio-opaque in soft tissues. Every lacerated or punctured wound caused by glass must be examined radiographically, as it is surprising how often fragments of glass are otherwise missed. In the majority of cases removal is indicated.

Pieces of clothing may be found (see above and Chapter 2).

Bites and Stings

Human bites, potentially serious, are discussed in Chapter 11.

Bites of animals such as the horse, cat, and dog require the usual treatment of wounds. Where there is the slightest suspicion that the animal is suffering from rabies, the bite should be freely excised. If possible, the responsible animal should be kept under observation, or, if it has been killed, Negri bodies should be sought in the brain. Prophylactic treatment can be obtained only at a special institute.

Snake Bites.—In England the only poisonous reptile is the adder, or viper (*Vipera berus*), but a fatal result is unlikely. First-aid measures consist of the application of a tourniquet, and within the first few minutes sucking the wound may remove some of the venom. Antihistamine drugs are given. Excision of the wound causes unnecessary trauma. Antivenom serum is not used in England because of the risk of serum anaphylaxis and serum sickness.

Scorpion stings, well known in the deserts, cause intense pain for many hours and constitutional upset. Local hydrocortisone injection may give relief.

Bees and Wasps.—Most bees, as distinct from wasps, suffer avulsion of their sting and poison gland, which is left protruding from the wound. Pressure on the gland squeezes poison into the tissues, so the gland and sting should be removed by scraping. *Bee venom is acid*, and should be neutralised by the application of ammonia, soda, or methylene-blue. *Wasp venom is alkaline*, and requires an acid, such as vinegar or lemon juice, for its neutralisation.[1] Antihistamine drugs are given orally, and local application is of value in allaying local irritation. If an anaphylactic reaction occurs, adrenaline (1:1000) 0·5 ml, is injected intramuscularly every 10 minutes until the patient recovers. Stings on the tongue are serious and the oedema so caused may involve the laryngeal glottis (Chapter 35). Anaphylaxis can be more likely to occur in those receiving non-steroidal anti-inflammatory drugs.

Antibiotics in the Treatment of Wounds (See Chapter 3).

---

[1] Bicarbonate for Bee, Vinegar for Vasp!

Adelchi Negri, 1876–1912. Professor of Bacteriology, Pavia, Italy. Discovered deeply staining inclusion bodies in the cells of the central nervous system in cases of rabies in 1903.

CHAPTER 2

BULLET, BOMB AND BLAST INJURIES

War wounds are often caused by bullets or by fragments from exploding mines, bombs and shells. In penetrating wounds the bullet or fragment (the missile) is lodged in the body. In perforating wounds, usually due to high velocity rifle and automatic machine gun bullets, the missile passes completely through the head, trunk or limbs.

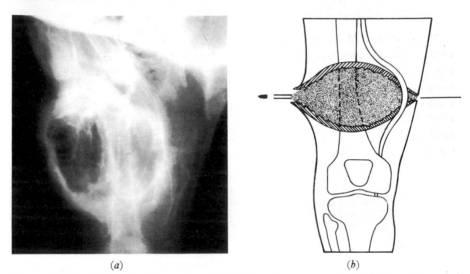

(a)   (b)

FIG. 15.—High velocity missile (experimental). (a) X-ray taken 30 msec after the bullet had traversed the limb. The cavity is collapsing. (b) Cavitational destructive effect due to the energy of the high velocity missile. The arteries and nerves are often temporarily displaced by such an insult.

MISSILE INJURIES

Mechanism of Missile Injuries.—As the missile traverses the tissues it gives up energy calculated from the formula $KE = \frac{1}{2} M (V_1{}^2 - V_2{}^2)$ where M = mass, V_1 = velocity at entry and V_2 = velocity at exit.

The low velocity missile, such as a bullet from a pistol, travelling below 400 metres per second, lacerates and crushes the tissues along the missile track.

The high velocity missile, *e.g.* the rifle bullet, travelling about 1000 metres per second, or the bomb fragment at 2000 metres per second, may give up much more energy to cause in addition a phenomenon known as temporary cavitation (fig. 15). The extent of cavitation depends upon the density and elasticity of the target organ and it is associated with tissue injury many centimetres around the missile track. Within the closed skull there is in addition a rapid high pressure shock wave causing injury at a distance. Thus, vital centres at the base of the brain may be injured in a wound of the cranium, the liver may be shattered by a perforating missile but comparatively little damage may be seen in a 'through and through' wound of a lung. In the limbs blood vessels, nerves and bone may also be damaged at a distance from the wound track and fragments of bone may act as secondary missiles. Devitalization of muscle surrounding the missile track in the depths of a wound provides a perfect culture medium for the growth of pathogenic bacteria, which are sucked in from the entrance and exit wounds due to the pulsatile nature of the temporary cavity.

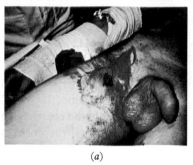
(a)

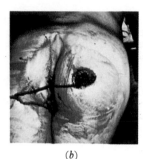
(b)

FIG. 16.—High velocity missile wound. (a) Entrance wound. (b) Exit wound.

Management of Missile Injuries.—The entrance and exit wounds do not indicate the considerable damage that may have occurred to the deeper structures (fig. 16). This can only be determined by full exploration. In limb wounds exploration is followed by thorough wound excision, after which, with very few exceptions, the wound is left open. Delayed primary closure follows within 4–10 days after injury. The patient must be completely undressed and examined prior to operation but it is wise to retain any pressure dressing over a wound until the operation is due to begin:

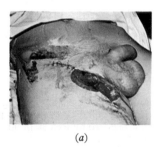
(a)

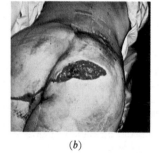
(b)

FIG. 17.—High velocity missile wound. (a) Extensive exploration of the entrance wound in the groin was required in order to adequately complete wound debridement and gain proximal control of the femoral artery should this have been damaged. The extent of the skin incision is clearly demonstrated, which was partially restored at initial operation after exploration of the large vessels. (b) The exit wound in the buttock is shown here at the end of wound debridement prior to delayed primary closure.

1. *After cleaning with an antiseptic*, generous longitudinal incisions are made through the skin in order to examine thoroughly the deeper structures and to facilitate subsequent extension of the exposure, should this be required. A minimal amount of skin edge (i.e., only that which has been contaminated) is excised around the entrance and exit wounds, because damage to the elastic skin only extends a few millimetres beyond the wound.

2. *The deep fascia is exposed*, and must be incised in a longitudinal direction in order to allow adequate inspection of the necrotic area and to decompress the underlying muscle which will swell subsequently (Débridement).[1]

---

[1] Note on 'Debridement' (Débridement = unleashing).—This term was introduced by Dominique Jean Larrey, 1766–1842, the famous French surgeon in Napoleon's army. He used it to describe the removal of bullets, bits of cloth, loose bits of bone and soft tissue—a much less extensive procedure than the thorough wound excision which is now practised.

3. *Neurovascular bundles in the wound track are identified* (fig. 17) but nerves should not be dissected out at this stage.

4. *Dead muscle* that does not bleed, does not contract, and has an unhealthy colour must be excised. Where there is doubt about the viability of bruised muscle it should be excised.

5. *Foreign matter* should be removed from the wound. Pieces of clothing are looked for especially, both in the missile track and in the tissue planes on either side. It is not necessary to remove every piece of metal seen on an x-ray. Multiple very small penetrating steel fragments from mines, shells, bombs and grenades may be difficult to retrieve from the limbs.

6. *Tendon repair* should not be performed at this initial operation. Tattered ends should be trimmed.

7. *Severed nerves* are marked with sutures but repair should not be attempted at this stage. It is important to examine the patient for nerve injury prior to the operation and to record in the operation notes the type of nerve injury (Chapter 28). The majority of nerve injuries of the limbs are neuropraxias which recover.

SUMMARY—DO'S AND DON'TS OF MISSILE INJURIES

DO	DON'T
INCISE THE SKIN GENEROUSLY	EXCISE TOO MUCH SKIN FROM
INCISE THE DEEP FASCIA WIDELY	WOUND MARGIN
IDENTIFY NEUROVASCULAR	PRACTISE KEYHOLE SURGERY
BUNDLES	STITCH TENDONS OR NERVES
EXCISE ALL DEAD MUSCLE	REMOVE BONE
REMOVE ALL INDRIVEN CLOTHING	CLOSE THE WOUND
LEAVE WOUND OPEN AT END OF	PACK THE WOUND TIGHTLY BUT
OPERATION	ALLOW FREE DRAINAGE, USING
RECORD THE EXTENT OF DAMAGE	LIGHTLY FLUFFED GAUZE
IN OPERATION NOTES	

8. *Bone* may be shattered by a high velocity missile, yet at operation most of the fragments will be found still to have an attachment to periosteum or muscle. On no account should the fragments be discarded, because loss of bone results in loss of limb length or in non-union. Any contaminated bone is cleaned as well as possible by using that useful instrument of military surgery, the Volkmann's spoon or curette. Internal fixation is not employed at the time of initial surgery, except in some cases of multiple fractures in the hand or foot. External fixation is permitted and is especially useful where there is a large area of skin loss. In most cases the padded plaster of Paris cast will suffice.

9. *Major artery or vein damage* should be repaired if time permits. The ends of the vessel are trimmed and sutured. If any tension is likely a reversed vein graft may be inserted to bridge the arterial gap (Chapter 13), and the repair must be covered by muscle. The rest of the wound is left open for delayed primary closure. Synthetic grafts must not be used.

10. *Joints* injured need thorough inspection, and cleaning with copious irrigation with saline to remove organic matter. Any exposed articular cartilage should be covered by at least one layer of tissue, preferably synovium, otherwise muscle or skin should be used.

11. *At the end of the operation* the wound is irrigated thoroughly with saline to remove remaining debris. Haemostasis is secured with the aid of hot packs and the wound is left open without closure of either the fascial layer or the skin, even in the presence of exposed bone. A lightly fluffed gause dressing is placed over the wound to allow free drainage.

12. Immobilisation in a well-padded plaster of Paris splint aids rest to the soft tissues, whether or not there is an accompanying fracture.

13. Antibiotic cover with benzylpenicillin is advised for all wounds, and broad spectrum antibiotics are added in those that involve bones and joints and also in all cases of abdominal injuries which receive metronidazole in addition (Chapter 3).

Richard von Volkmann, 1830–1889. Professor of Surgery, Halle, Germany.

Delayed Primary Closure.—All wounds treated by wound excision and left open are inspected under a general anaesthetic on about the 4th to 6th day after injury. Provided the wound looks healthy delayed primary suture is performed.

Traumatic amputations are tidied up, completed at the lowest level possible and left open for delayed primary closure. If there is much skin loss or if a limb is very swollen, split skin grafting may be used to effect wound closure in order to avoid skin tension. If, at the time of delayed primary closure dead muscle is found, which is not uncommon in traumatic amputation due to land mines, the muscle is excised and the wound left open for a further period before closure.

Gunshot Wounds of the Abdomen.—Every penetrating gunshot wound of the abdomen should be explored by laparotomy. Prior to surgery a catheter must be passed into the bladder. The rectum should be examined. The patient should be resuscitated and blood should be available.

A midline incision is used. It has the advantage of facilitating rapid access and extension when required. Blood usually comes from mesenteric vessels but major haemorrhage may come from the liver or the major vessels. Haemorrhage must be controlled and careful examination is then made of all the abdominal contents.

In all wounds of the stomach the lesser sac must be opened in order to inspect the posterior gastric wall. Retroperitoneal haematoma in the region of the duodenum requires inspection of the posterior wall by Kocher's method (Chapter 44). Haematoma surrounding the retroperitoneal parts of the ascending and descending colon may also necessitate exploration but non-expanding retroperitoneal haematomas over the kidneys are best left undisturbed.

Small intestinal perforations are either excised and closed transversely, or the damaged section is resected if there are multiple holes in a short length. Mesenteric tears may necessitate bowel resection (Chapter 49).

Colonic and rectal wounds require a colostomy (Chapter 50). On the right side if the colon injury is minor, there is no contamination of the peritoneal cavity, and the patient is seen soon after injury, the damaged bowel may be excised and an anastomosis performed. Major wounds of the caecum and ascending colon require resection of the damaged segment and a vented ileo-transverse anastomosis or the bringing of the two ends to the surface, the proximal as a colostomy or ileostomy and the distal as a mucous fistula. On the left side the injured colon is resected, the proximal end brought out as a colostomy and the distal end as a mucous fistula. If the distal end cannot be brought to the surface, as in rectal injuries, it may be closed off as in a Hartmann procedure (Chapter 53). In all cases drains should be placed down to the injured area.

Renal injury is treated conservatively. Immediate nephrectomy is seldom indicated. A divided ureter may be brought to the surface or may be repaired over a 'pigtail' stent.

The control of haemorrhage in pelvic injuries may be very difficult and may require the ligature of an internal iliac artery. It is better to control bleeding from the extra peritoneal rectum by excision and suture of the rectal injury and the establishment of a defunctioning colostomy and mucous fistula. Adequate drainage must be established by excising the coccyx and placing drains in the presacral area.

Bladder and urethral injuries are treated by suprapubic cystotomy with placement of a retropubic drain after wound excision.

Liver injuries in the majority of cases require only placement of an adequate external drain. In a few cases suture of liver substance is required to secure haemostasis. Sutures should be placed deeply into the liver parenchyma to eliminate dead space. In a very few cases resection of devitalised tissue by finger fracture is required (Chapter 45).

Damage to the spleen and tail of the pancreas is treated by resection. Missile injury of the head of the pancreas is seldom seen in the operating room because damage to it and the surrounding structures is usually fatal. In a very few cases it may be possible to apply a loop of jejunum to create an internal fistula.

Peritoneal toilet using saline or weak antiseptic is important to assist in the removal of spilled bowel contents and blood clot. Intraperitoneal drainage should always be employed whenever bowel has been breached.

The laparotomy wound is closed in the normal manner. The entrance and exit wound

Emil Theodor Kocher, 1841–1917. Professor of Surgery, Berne, Switzerland.
Henri Albert Charles Antoine Hartmann, 1860–1952. Professor of Surgery, Paris, France.

should be debrided and the peritoneum closed. The rest of the missile wound of the abdominal wall can be left open for subsequent late closure.

Gunshot Wounds of the Chest (See also Chapter 40).—It is important to secure an airtight seal of a sucking wound of the chest. Such a wound, if left open, will collapse the lung on the affected side with alteration of the ventilation/perfusion ratio and in addition will decrease both the quality and the quantity of air entering the uninjured lung. As dyspnoea increases due to anoxia the mediastinum shifts on respiration and decreases the venous return to the heart. This disturbance of cardiopulmonary function can be prevented by the simple first-aid measure of sealing the hole in the chest wall.

All penetrating wounds of the pleura and lung require adequate venting of the pleural cavity in order to prevent and deal with the embarrassment to respiration caused by the accumulation of blood (haemothorax) and occasionally of air under tension (tension pneumothorax). It may be necessary to insert chest drains before a chest x-ray can be done.

Once pulmonary function is stabilised the operation of wound excision is carried out. During the excision of large chest wall wounds the pleural cavity is often entered and an opportunity should be taken to remove any retained foreign material, arrest haemorrhage (usually from an intercostal or internal mammary vessel), and to oversew holes in the lung. Correct placement of the chest tubes is then confirmed. The pleura is closed and the wound left open for subsequent delayed primary closure.

In war, 90% of chest wounds can be treated by drainage of the pleural cavity and excision of the wounds in the chest wall. Formal thoracotomy is most urgently indicated for: (1) Continuing haemorrhage from a venting tube and more rarely for (2) suspected mediastinal injury and (3) persistent air leak. It is most commonly indicated for retained foreign body of more than 1·5 cm diameter in the lung. In thoraco-abdominal injuries the thoracic part of the injury is treated by tube drainage and the abdominal part by laparotomy through a midline incision.

Gunshot Wounds of the Head.—The penetrating high velocity missile wound of the brain is lethal. The management of low velocity penetrating and tangential wounds depends initially on the maintenance of a satisfactory airway and restoration of blood volume in order to maintain adequate oxygenation of the brain. Good x-rays are mandatory to localise indriven bone fragments. Wound excision is carried out using gentle irrigation and suction to remove necrotic brain and bony fragments. Every effort, including the use of a piece of temporalis fascia, is made to close the dura.

It has been shown that the application of intermittent positive pressure ventilation (pCO_2 4–4·7 kPa) assists in the reduction of intracranial pressure by reducing brain swelling. Intracranial transducers inserted through burr holes may be employed to monitor intracranial pressure.

Shotgun Injuries.—Accidents from 12-bore shotguns are common and often lethal. It is never possible to retrieve all the shot and indeed to do so would result in too much damage to the body. Wound excision should be carried out on the major wound, particularly looking for indriven clothing. Laparotomy is essential if it is thought that any of the shot has traversed an abdominal viscus. The retention of lead shot in the body can result in a dangerously high lead concentration which should be monitored. After a time this concentration will fall due to encapsulation of the lead pellets by fibrous tissue.

BLAST INJURIES

Mechanism of Explosive Blast Injury.—The explosive pressure that accompanies the bursting of bombs or shells ruptures their casing and imparts a high velocity to the resulting fragments. These fragments cause even more devastating damage to the tissues than bullets as they are unstable in flight and tear through the tissues at great speed in a tumbling fashion. In addition, all explosions are accompanied by a *complex blast wave*. The two main components of this wave are a *blast pressure wave*, with a positive and negative phase, and the *mass movement of air*.

The positive pressure phase of the blast wave lasts only a few milliseconds, but close to an explosion it may rise to over 1000 pounds per square inch (6894 kN/m²). As the tympanic membrane ruptures at about 20 pounds per square inch (138 kM/m²), it is evident that the effects on the human body of such an explosion can be devastating, especially in confined areas. Like sound waves, the blast pressure waves flow over and around an obstruction and affect anyone sheltering behind a wall. The pressure affecting such a person is known as the *incident pressure* (defined as the pressure level at 90° to direction of travel of the blast shock front). Also any person standing in front of a wall facing an explosion is subjected to the added effect of *reflected pressure*.

The negative phase of a pressure wave is of less amplitude but lasts longer than the positive phase.

A *mass movement of air* results from the rapidly expanding gases at the heart of an explosion which displace air at high velocity. This mass movement of air causes a *blast wind* which may result in total disintegration of the body and, at lesser levels, traumatic amputation. A person standing behind a wall will be protected from the blast wind unless, of course, the object or building collapses and causes a crushing injury.

Blast waves travel more rapidly and further in water being a more dense medium than air. Blast injuries in water are therefore more severe for a given distance than they are in air.

In the body, when the 'front' of pressure travels from one medium to another of less density, fragmentation of tissue occurs. The pulmonary alveoli and the gas-filled intestinal viscera, both structures with fluid/air interfaces, are particularly susceptible to damage by blast waves.

Management of Blast Injuries.—The most vulnerable organs to the blast wave are the ear drums; lungs and gastrointestinal tract. Casualties may present in a dramatic form with traumatic amputation, the haemorrhage from which can only be controlled by a tourniquet. The deafness of the victims of blast, due to rupture of the tympanic membrane, makes communication with them difficult. They must be carefully examined for many have multiple wounds. The management of these wounds is in no way different from that of missile injuries. Very often the soft tissues are heavily contaminated with organic debris due to the force of the explosion opening up tissue planes and driving in foreign bodies at some distance from the wound. Some cases are associated with multiple small wounds affecting a limb. It is not always practical to explore fully every wound. The deeper wounds should have priority of management due to the more serious consequences of infection. In many blast injuries one cannot be sure of complete wound excision and therefore it becomes imperative that all blast wounds should be left open at the end of the initial operation and delayed primary suture performed four to seven days later.

Blast Injury to the Auditory System.—Blast damages the hearing in three ways. There may be rupture of the tympanic membrane, dislocation of the ossicles or damage to the inner ear. The last is sometimes accompanied by permanent deafness.

Blast Injury to the Lung.—The rapid inward movement of the chest wall propelled by the blast wave may cause bruising of the lung but leave no outward sign. Minor bruising is maybe symptomless and diagnosed only by x-ray. Major bruising is associated with blood in the alveoli and in the lung tissue. Oedema develops within a few hours and its onset may be precipitated by over transfusion with electrolyte solutions. In the severe case the patient develops a cough with frothy blood stained sputum, dyspnoea and a feeling of general apprehension. Blood gas analysis will show arterial hypoxia and a raised pCO_2. Chest x-ray in the initial stages may show bruising mainly on one side (fig. 18) but as oedema develops may show an opaque, fluffy appearance around the hilum of each lung.

Management.—All victims of blast should be carefully monitored, especially if the eardrums are damaged, and chest x-ray repeated during the initial forty-eight hours. Oxygen is administered and fluid overload avoided. Steroids are valuable if toxic gases have been inhaled. Blood gas analysis may indicate the need for assisted positive pressure ventilation with a positive expiratory end-pressure.

Blast Injury of the Gastrointestinal System.—Injury to the gas-filled viscera is more

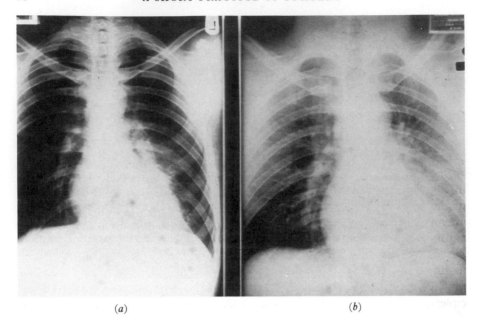

(a) (b)

FIG. 18.—(a) Chest x-ray of soldier admitted immediately after sustaining minor burns, lacerations and bruises from a terrorist booby-trap bomb. (b) Chest x-ray three hours later showing pulmonary contusion. No treatment required. Spontaneous resolution.
(Royal Army Medical College)

common in underwater explosions than air blasts. Perforation of stomach or caecum may occur. The clinical presentation is one of increasing abdominal pain accompanied by signs of peritonism and often gas under the diaphragm. Urgent laparotomy is indicated.

Blast Wounds to the Eye.—So often one fails to notice damage to an eye at the time of initial examination. It is important to appreciate that the conjunctival haemorrhage, accompanying a blast injury, may herald a more serious underlying problem of penetration of the globe by foreign bodies. The pupil must be carefully examined and any distortion of the iris investigated.

Other factors which increase the morbidity and mortality following bomb-blast injuries are the associated chemical and thermal burns, and the inhalation of toxic gases and smoke.

CHAPTER 3

WOUND INFECTION

INFECTION AND SEPSIS[1]

Background.—Louis Pasteur first described fermentation by micro-organisms in 1857 and later showed the effect of heat upon them, the way in which they might be grown by sub-culture, the way in which virulent strains might be attenuated to create vaccines and, eventually, the value of isolation in preventing natural spread (of natural infection) from an infected to a non-infected subject. Based on this work, Lister introduced active and successful *antiseptic* techniques to surgery (1867), and he established the guiding principle for good surgical practice upon which the present day specialties are based (the antisepsis principle[2]). His technical approach (destruction of infective organisms by physico-chemical means) nowadays is complemented by the *aseptic* approach of employing many different measures to reduce the risk of colonising wounds to a minimum.

Since World War I (1914–1918) it has been recognised that despite aseptic techniques wounds can become infected by (*a*) initial contamination, for example by skin clostridia and Gram-positive organisms (fig. 19), and (*b*) hospital ward infections spreading from other infected wounds (cross infection). Fatal infections with *Staph. aureus*, haemolytic Streptococci (pyogenes) and *Pseudomonas aeruginosa*, particularly affecting patients in burns and trauma units, continue to occur.

Following the introduction of antibiotics (1940's) the infections acquired during or after surgery changed from being *Gram-positive* i.e. Staphylococcal in

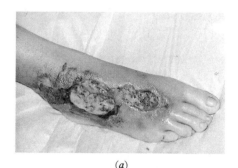
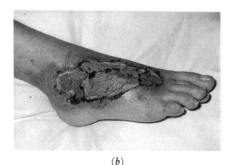

(a)   (b)

Fig. 19.—A near fatal infection by initial contamination (streptococcus). (*a*) Sloughing of the dorsum of the foot. (*b*) Skin grafting on recovery.

---

[1] Sepsis is the term used to describe the real effect of infection, a process of decomposition (literally rotting), putrefaction and poisoning which, if unchecked, can lead to a fatal outcome.

[2] For this work he is called 'the father of modern surgery'. The meaning of his principle, which he struggled to point out and get adopted is that safe surgery depends on an unremitting battle against the causes of sepsis = ANTI SEPSIS.

Joseph Lister (see p. 1).
Louis Pasteur, 1822–1895. French Chemist and Bacteriologist. Founder of the Pasteur Institute, Paris.

origin to those that are predominantly *Gram-negative*: *Eschericia coli*, *Klebsiella* and *Proteus mirabilis*, *Pseudomonas aeruginosa*. These became endemic in surgical wards. In recent years the re-emergence of multi-resistant Staphyloccal infection in the busy surgical units of urban general hospitals has shown the opportunism of bacteria to survive in a hostile antibiotic environment by genetic adaptations such as constitutional change (mutation) or plasmid acquisition ('infectious resistance').

Anaerobic Infections (Table C)

Anaerobic bacteria usually become established in damaged and/or ischaemic tissue following which bacteraemia may occur and blood cultures will become positive. The normal anaerobic bacterial flora are:

1. Oral cavity: Anaerobic cocci, bacteroides (not usually fragilis), fusiforms (actinomycetes and spirochaetes in small numbers) and veillonella (anaerobic Gram-negative cocci).

2. Lower female genital tract: Bacteroides melanogenicum, *B. fragilis*, 'fusiforms', anaerobic cocci and *Cl. welchii*.[1]

3. Skin: Anaerobic diphtheroids (propionobacteria) and cocci.

4. Colon and rectum: All bacteroides species including fragilis, fusiforms and clostridia. Anaerobic streptococci.

Anaerobic cocci, (peptococci and peptostreptococci).—These Gram-positive organisms are found in the skin, perioral, respiratory and soft tissue infections. The rapidly spreading 'synergistic infective gangrene' (Chapter 14) is caused by *Staphylococcus aureus* and anaerobic streptococci; the β-lactamase of the former protects the latter from the effects of penicillin and for proper treatment requires metronidazole together with an antistaphylococcal antibiotic.

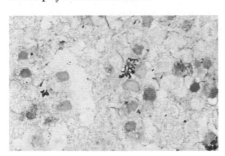

FIG. 20.—Staphylococcal pus.

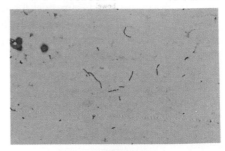

FIG. 21.—Streptococci.

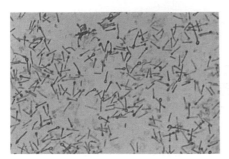

FIG. 22.—*Clostridium tetani* (drum-stick spores).

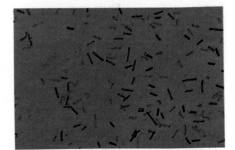

FIG. 23.—*Clostridium difficile.*

[1] *William Henry Welch, 1850–1934. Professor of Pathology, Johns Hopkins University, Baltimore, Maryland, USA.*

PRINCIPAL ORGANISMS OF SEPSIS

A. GRAM-POSITIVE COCCI

	Site and spread	Principal Infections	Antibiotic Sensitivity
Staph. aureus (fig. 20)	Lives in nostrils of 50% population; sometimes on skin. Present in infected discharges. *Spread* by contact, on hands etc. Airborne spread by skin squames and garment dust.	Boils, styes, septic hands, breast abscess, wound infection, osteomyelitis, septicaemia, post-operative pneumonia.	*Outside hospital* most strains now form penicillinase and are Penicillin-resistant. *In hospital*, many are resistant also to several other drugs. Most are still sensitive to Flucloxacillin if not, Vancomycin may be needed.
Staph. epidermidis (Staph. albus) and other coagulase-negative staphylococci, normally non-pathogenic; opportunistic pathogens.	Nasal and skin carriers are very common. *Spread* same as *Staph. aureus*, but more numerous in air of rooms.	Minor skin sepsis or stitch abscess; cause dangerous infection of prosthetic heart valves and orthopaedic prosthetic operations. Colonises intravenous cannula sites and may cause bacteraemia.	As *Staph. aureus*. Multi-resistant strains are common. Sensitivity testing is the only guide to therapy.
Staph. saprophyticus	Found on skin though not common.	Urinary tract infection in young women.	Usually sensitive to trimethoprim sulphonamide, ampicillin.
Str. pyogenes (Group A)	Live in pharynx of 5–10% of population. *Spread* by contact, and airborne from respiratory tract and wound discharges.	Tonsillitis, otitis, scarlet fever. Dangerous in wounds, cellulitis, septicaemia. Infections tend to spread rapidly in tissues.	Sensitive to Penicillin and erythromycin. Resistant to aminoglycosides and often to tetracycline.
Str. pneumoniae (Pneumococcus) A capsulated diplococcus.	Lives in nasopharynx of many normal people.	Post-operative and other pneumonia, otitis media and sinusitis, septicaemia. In young girls, occasionally peritonitis perhaps entering via the Fallopian tube.	As *Str. pyogenes*, but penicillin resistance has appeared in some countries, though still rare in Great Britain.
Str. faecalis.	Large bowel	Abdominal sepsis, usually mixed with other organisms.	*Str. faecalis* is usually sensitive to ampicillin or mezlocillin. Enterococci in general are not sensitive to Cephalosporins.

B. GRAM-NEGATIVE BACILLI

	Site and Spread	Principal Infections	Antibiotic Sensitivity
Escherichia coli	Normal inhabitant of large bowel	Wounds, especially abdominal; intra-abdominal sepsis cholangitis etc. The commonest cause of urinary infection.	Usually sensitive to Cephalosporins. Some are sensitive to Ampicillin or Trimethoprim. Most are sensitive to Gentamicin. Hospital strains can become resistant to many drugs.
Klebsiella	As *E. coli*	As *E. coli*	As *E. coli*, but Ampicillin resistant.
Proteus	Large Bowel	As *E. coli*. Splits urea into NH_3 making urine alkaline causing phosphate deposits	Similar to *E. coli*.
Pseudomonas aeruginosa	Large bowel. Often colonises moist lesions, its principal habitat. Also found in contaminated lotions, sinks etc.	An opportunist that attacks damaged tissues, burns, tracheostomy wounds, urinary tract.	Sensitive to Gentamicin, Azlocillin and some cephalosporins (Ceftazadime) and Ciprofloxacin.
Haemophilus influenza	Nasopharynx and upper respiratory tract.	Paranasal sinus infection. Respiratory tract infections (especially post-operative) broncho-pneumonia).	Ampicillin (some may be resistant). Co-trimoxazole and Ceftazadime.

C. ANAEROBIC ORGANISMS

Anaerobic bacteria	Site and Spread	Principal Infections	Antibiotic Sensitivity
Gram-positive cocci Peptococci Streptococci	Colon, vagina, oropharynx and skin.	Abdominal, oral and female sepsis. Cerebral abscesses.	Metronidazole, Penicillin.
Gram-negative bacilli *Bacteroides fragilis Bacteroides melanogenicum*	Colon, rectum, vagina, oro-pharynx.	Intra-abdominal sepsis. Pelvic sepsis, gingivitis, subphrenic and pelvic abscess.	Metronidazole (some also to Cefotaxime).
Gram-positive bacilli. *Actinomycosis*	Colon and rectum.	Actinomycosis gut, jaw, uterus.	Penicillin, Metronidazole.
Surgically important Clostridia: *Cl. perfringens* 'A'	Large bowel of animals and man. Skin of the perineum and perianal region, (and parts contaminated by faeces).	Gas-gangrene especially following trauma, open fractures and large muscle mass injury.	Penicillin, Metronidazole.
Cl. tetani (fig. 22)		Tetanus	Penicillin, Metronidazole
Cl. difficile (fig. 23)	Large bowel	Pseudomembranous colitis, and antibiotic associated colitis caused by cytotoxins. Any antibiotic may result in super infection with this organism which can spread among post-operative patients.	Oral Metronidazole Oral Vancomycin.

respiratory tract infection. Respiratory support machines in anaesthesia, intensive post-operative care, and the need for endotracheal intubation or tracheostomy post-operatively in some patients exposes them to the risk of instrument-
spread infection. If, for example, humidifiers or ventilators are allowed to become
colonised by Pseudomonas and other hydrophilic Gram-negative bacteria, infection can be transferred from patient to patient by this apparatus.

Opportunistic Infection

Opportunities for one or more opportunist organisms, normally of low patho-
genicity, are favoured by (a) reduced host defence (immune deficiency) and (b)
maintained therapeutic invasive procedures.

(a) *Reduced Host Defence (Immune Deficiency).*—Serious, atypical, and often
fatal infection is increasingly seen in patients following renal (or other organ)
transplantation on immunosuppressive therapy, in those receiving cytotoxic therapy and radiotherapy for neoplasia, and also those on steroid therapy. Severe
burns and anaesthesia are in themselves immunosuppressive. Starvation is
another factor. Some powerful broad spectrum antibiotics can depress the
immune response. Immune deficiency is also a feature in the very old and in the
very young, especially the premature baby. AIDS[1] (HIV[2] infection) is another
consideration (Chapter 4).

(b) *Maintained Therapeutic Invasive Procedures.*—These include intravenous
cannulation, intravesical catheterisation, tracheostomy with pulmonary ventilation or any surgical procedure which permits the body defences to admit skin
organisms to invade the tissues. The use of disinfectant skin dressings, disinfectant prophylaxis such as bladder irrigation with chlorhexidine or neomycin poly-
myxin solution and aseptic techniques will in many cases reduce the risk of
opportunist infections becoming established.

The commonest surgical opportunists are gram-negative organisms of which
the most frequent are *E. coli*, pseudomonas species, klebsiella sp, proteus sp,
acinetobacter and serratia. These infections originate either from the patient's
own alimentary tract or by cross-infection from other patients within the hospital,
and they are spread by the hands of attendants. The oncology, intensive care,
organ graft, burns and neurosurgical units have a high incidence of this type of
opportunist infection and the isolates found in these units are often multi-resistant to antibiotics. Indeed, this resistance may be transferred to other species
causing the emergence of virtually untreatable bacilli as a significant part of the
microbial flora within the units. Such infections are not only difficult to treat but
result in the infected patient becoming a reservoir from which the hands of staff,
equipment, instruments (such as catheters and endoscopes) and the intestinal
tracts of other patients can become colonised.

Of the Gram-positive opportunist infections *Staphylococcus epidermidis* is most
frequently found and is usually derived from the skin of the patient. A local
infection or bacteraemia is often associated with intravenous and central venous
lines, prosthetic grafts to heart or joints, ventriculo-peritoneal shunts and upper

---

[1] AIDS = acquired immune deficiency syndrome.
[2] HIV = human immuno-virus.

renal tract catheterisation. Following splenectomy, *Streptococcus pneumoniae* is specifically associated with fatal bacteraemia.

Pseudomonas aeruginosa, Staph. epidermidis and *Candida* species may produce bacteraemias and disseminated lesions while mycobacterial disease with *M. tuberculosis* and BCG may spread atypically. Viruses, (particulary Herpes virus, Cytomegalovirus and Varicella zoster) can produce severe disease with fatal pneumonitis, haemorrhagic skin lesions or progressive mucocutaneous disease. Fungal infections include *Yeasts, Aspergillus fumigatus* and protozoal infestations (cryptosporidial diarrhoea or pneumocystis carinii pneumonia).

Diagnosis and treatment.—Cultures from the sites of the procedures, or swabs from body orifices will help in establishing which bacteria are present and which are antibiotic resistant. Frequently the patients are febrile following surgery and immunosuppression and whilst culturing continues treatment will be required. This should be a combination of a broad spectrum penicillin with an aminoglycoside, giving the widest cover for Gram-positive and Gram-negative organisms (e.g. mezlocillin infusion and gentamicin); these combined with metronidazole will produce a response in the majority of patients. In surgical units a multiple resistant pseudomonas or klebsiella species can become 'resident opprtunists'; these are combatted by a strict rotation of antibiotic chemotherapy, constant vigilance in aseptic techniques and meticulous 'one patient' nursing care in order to prevent the organisms overwhelming the antiseptic procedures and being spread to all the patients on the unit. Some infections may prove difficult to eradicate despite the apparent sensitivity of the organisms, e.g. aorto-iliac grafts may become persistently infected by *Staph. epidermidis*.

SPREAD OF INFECTION

Cellulitis

Cellulitis is inflammation spreading along the subcutaneous or a fascial plane often as the result of infection with *Streptcoccus pyogenes* which has entered the tissue through an accidental wound, graze, or scratch, or following surgical incision. Unchecked this may lead to septicaemia after a rapid spread within the tissues. Initially red and itchy at the site of the innoculation, the skin swells and becomes tender, frequently being shiny. There may be local gangrene (fig. 193). Rest, elevation of the part, and the appropriate antibiotic should lead to resolution, but any underlying condition (e.g. diabetes) should be treated.

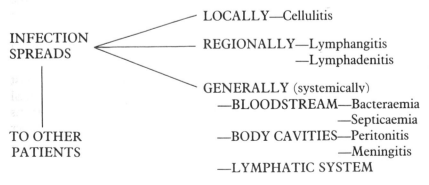

INFECTION SPREADS

LOCALLY—Cellulitis

REGIONALLY—Lymphangitis
—Lymphadenitis

GENERALLY (systemically)
—BLOODSTREAM—Bacteraemia
—Septicaemia
—BODY CAVITIES—Peritonitis
—Meningitis
—LYMPHATIC SYSTEM

TO OTHER PATIENTS

vegetations upon a cardiac valve by echocardiography can be decisively diagnostic of endocarditis.

Computed tomography (CT) scans are usually necessary for localising brain lesions and abscesses although isotope scans can demonstrate these also.

PREVENTING INFECTION

Antibiotic Prophylaxis is used to prevent bacteraemia and wound infection when instrumentation or surgery is performed upon a site with normal flora or where infection already exists (*e.g.* cystoscopy when bladder infection is known to be present). It should be maintained for a short period, seldom using more than three doses, the maximum duration being 48 hours. Prophylaxis should cover and control the known or likely pathogens. Prophylaxis may conveniently be given intravenously as a bolus after induction of anaesthesia or, if intra-muscular antibiotics are to be used, may be given one hour before surgery. Aminoglycosides such as gentamicin require that serum levels be monitored if they are used for more than 36 hours. If renal function is known to be satisfactory three doses only of 80–120 mg given at 8 hour intervals may be used for a normal adult.

Metronidazole may be given as one gram *per rectum* (suppository) with resulting excellent blood levels; the first suppository should be given 1½ hours pre-operatively. Topical antibiotics should be reserved for use in eye or ear surgery; skin antibiotics are seldom if ever indicated and can lead to severe antibiotic resistant infections.

Antibiotic impregnated 'cement' or 'beads' for use in orthopaedic prosthetic operations are gaining favour; they act as a local reservoir giving slow release to the site of operation. Alternative regimes are based on single doses of cephalosporins, *e.g.* prior to the open reduction of fractures.

Care should be taken with diabetics (superadded candida and multi-resistant Gram-negative infections) and patients who are immuno-deficient or immuno-suppressed, *e.g.* receiving steroid therapy or receiving radiotherapy. Penicillin prophylaxis for up to one week is mandatory for the prevention of Clostridial gas gangrene at the time of lower limb amputation through the thigh in those patients who have diabetic or severe peripheral vascular disease.

PREVENTING INFECTION IN SURGICAL PROCEDURES

Abdominal procedures	Colorectal surgery	Ampicillin 500 mg I.V. 8 hourly × 3* + Metronidazole
	Appendicectomy	Metronidazole 1 gram rectally
	Peritonitis	Ampicillin 500 mg Gentamicin 120 mg followed by 80 mg twice at 8 hour intervals with Metronidazole
	Biliary	Ampicillin or a cephalosporin
	Urinary tract Instrumentation or surgery	Amoxycillin 3 g or single dose of Gentamicin 120 mg if previously infected
Obstetric surgery	Vaginal hysterectomy, termination of pregnancy with history of pelvic inflammatory disease or abdominal caesarean	Ampicillin 500 mg I.M. Metronidazole 1 g rectally once only

Orthopaedic	Compound fractures	Ampicillin 500 mg 8 hourly with Flucloxacillin 500 mg 6 hourly (or Erythromycin 500 mg 6 hourly if Penicillin hypersensitive)
	Elective or prosthetic surgery	48 hours only Ampicillin 500 mg 8 hourly and Flucloxacillin 500 mg 8 hourly
	Lower limb amputation	Penicillin 2 mega units at induction and thereafter 4 mega units daily for 5–7 days
Patients with known valvular disease, prosthetic grafts of the cardio-vascular system (e.g. aortic or aortic valve), history of rheumatic fever	1. Dental surgery 2. Urethral catheterisation 3. Operations under general anaesthesia	Amoxycillin 3 g orally and Probenecid 1 g orally (if allergic to Penicillin, Erythromycin 1·5 g orally followed by 0·5 g 6 hours later). If general anaesthesia or gastrointestinal investigation is being performed a single dose of Gentamicin 1·5 mg per kg of body weight I.M. must be added

* × 3 means for three doses only

Preventing Infection at Operation.—The open wound is at risk of contamination from airborne dust which carries bacteria derived from skin organisms of attendants and operating room personnel. Positive pressure, filtered ventilation of the operating theatre prevents bacteria gaining entry with the air. Ultra-clean ventilation (laminar flow and fine filters) has been shown to reduce wound infection rate by two-fold. Body exhaust suits carrying away the infected skin particles of the surgeons and assistants clearly reduces the number of infected particles near the wound and has been shown to reduce the wound infection rate by seven-fold.

The patients own skin is a source of infection especially at abdominal operations and can be treated by pre-operative bathing, and skin preparation with alcoholic povidone iodine solution or 5% chlorhexidine in 70% alcohol. Povidone iodine compresses applied to the thigh for one hour prior to hip arthroplasty reduce the risk of self infection. At the time of operation, the use of a plastic adhesive film (Opsite®) through which the incision is made helps to prevent contamination during the operation itself. Surgical hand washing with hexachlorophane, chlorhexidine, or povidone iodine and the use of gloves, mask and change of clothes all contribute to reducing the risk of surgeon transmitted infection.

Instruments.—Central hospital and theatre sterile supply departments use high temperature autoclaves (132°C) for sterilising instruments, whilst equipment made of heat sensitive material may be sterilised at 80°C in sub-atmospheric pressures ('low temperature steam') with or without a formalin injection cycle (*e.g.* for cystoscopes). Some endoscopes (*e.g.* colonoscopes) may require special procedures for disinfection; liquid gluteraldehyde is often useful for disinfection of cleaned instruments. Where viral infections (Hepatitis B) are implicated hypochlorites or steam disinfection are used while in operating theatres the infection control policy will clearly lay down guidelines for the disinfection of blood contaminated instruments before cleaning if possible. The exercise of proper professional care will usually prevent self-inflicted injuries with instruments that may be at risk of spreading Hepatitis B virus or HIV virus (AIDS Chapter 4) by blood contamination.

Controlling Surgical Infection—Control of Infection Team.—Vigilance, education and definition of policies for controlling infection in surgical wards is best placed in the hands of a Control of Infection team consisting of a control of infection nurse of considerable seniority, a medical microbiologist and a surgeon. Not only is it necessary to monitor the type of infections and the resistance and distribution of the bacteria, but the in-service education on the principles of wound care, catheter toilet, aseptic dressing techniques can best be managed by such a team. Isolation of high risk patients, modification of antibiotic regimes, and the prevention of spread of any resistant infections will all require the combined speciality interest for the advice to be authoritative, acceptable and effective.

PRINCIPLES OF ANTIMICROBIAL TREATMENT

Antimicrobials may be used to prevent (see prophylaxis above) or treat established infection. The use of antibiotics in established infection in surgical practice requires the isolation of the bacterium and a determination of its sensitivity; this is the over-riding first requirement for after antibiotics are administered the clinical picture may be confused, the patient no better, and the opportunity to make a precise diagnosis has been lost.

Presented with pus the microbiologist will isolate the causative organism and this can then guide therapy. There are two approaches to therapy:

(a) *The use of a quite narrow spectrum antibiotic* to treat a known sensitive infection; *e.g.*, a multi-resistant staphylococcus sensitive to flucloxacillin (or if not, vancomycin), isolated from pus may be treated solely with this specific Gram-positive antibiotic.

(b) *The use of broad-spectrum antibiotic combinations* where the organism is not known or where it is suspected that there may be one, two or more, generally gut-derived bacteria responsible for the infection. Thus, following emergency surgery within the abdomen or requiring the opening of bowel where any of the gut organisms may be responsible for subsequent peritoneal or bacteraemic infection, then a combination of broad-spectrum penicillin such as ampicillin or mezlocillin with an aminoglycoside (e.g. gentamicin) and metronidazole may be used post-operatively to support the patients own body defences.

In surgical units with multiple resistant pseudomonas or other Gram-negative species (such as klebsiella) which have become 'resident opportunists', there may become a need for a rotation of anti-pseudomonal and anti-Gram-negative chemotherapy between the broad-spectrum penicillins, *e.g.* azlocillin 2 g i.v. 8 hourly and cephalosporins, *e.g.* ceftazidime 50–100 mg per kg per day, or cefotaxime 2 g 8 hourly. The use of these routines, the monitoring of subsequent wound infection and the alternation of combinations of chemotherapy should be monitored by the control of infection team. It should never be forgotten in treating post-operative pyrexial infection that a failure to respond to a very broad-spectrum of these combined antibiotics requires a very critical bedside review to exclude collections of pus and other causes of a raised temperature.

New antibiotics should be used with caution[1] and sensitivities wherever possible should have been obtained. There are certain general rules from which the choice of antibiotics may be based originally; thus it is unusual for *Pseudomonas aeruginosa* ever to be found as a primary infecting organism unless the patient has had surgical or hospital treatment. Local antibiotic sensitivity patterns vary from centre to centre and from country to country and the sensitivity patterns of common pathogens will be known to the hospital microbiologist.

Antimicrobial Chemotherapy

Antimicrobials may be produced by living organisms (antibiotics) or synthetically. Some are bactericidal (*e.g.* penicillins, aminoglycosides) and others bacteriostatic (tetracycline and erythromycin). In general, penicillins act upon the cell wall and are most effective against bacteria that are multiplying and synthesizing new cell wall materials. The bacteriocides act at ribosomal level, preventing or distorting the production of proteins required to maintain the integrity of the enzymes in the bacterial cell.

Penicillin.—Used after Florey and Chain produced the first therapeutic preparation in 1941, Benzyl-penicillin has proved most effective against gram-positive pathogens including the Group A, B, G *Strep. haemolyticus*, *Strep. pneumoniae*, the Clostridia and some of the Staphylococci which do not produce β-lactamase. It is still effective against syphilis, and actinomycosis and may be used to treat streptococcal infections specifically even if other antibiotics are required as part of therapy of a mixed infection.

Flucloxacillin/Methicillin.—These are β-lactamase resistant penicillins and are therefore of use in treating staphylococcal β-lactamase producing organisms. This is the only reason for using them and flucloxacillin has poor activity against other pathogens.

Ampicillin/Amoxycillin.—β-lactam penicillins absorbed orally or may be given parenterally. Amoxycillin serum levels are usually twice those of ampicillin and pharmacodynamically amoxycillin is superior. Both are effective against enterobacteriacae, against *Strep. faecalis* and the majority of group D streptococci, but not klebsiella or pseudomonas. They are effective against *H. influenzae* if it is not a β-lactamase producer. Either may be used as a first line broad spectrum penicillin effective in urinary and respiratory tract infections.

Mezlocillin/Azlocillin.—These are ureido-penicillins with good activity against citrobacter, enterobacter and klebsiella. Azlocillin is particularly effective against pseudomonas. Each has some activity against bacteroides and enterococci but each is susceptible to β-lactamase. Combined with an aminoglycoside mezlocillin is a valuable treatment for severe mixed infections, particularly gram-negative organisms in the immuno-compromised patient. Klebsiella strains are best treated with mezlocillin, pseudomonas strains with azlocillin.

Clavulanic acid.—Clavulanic acid is available combined with amoxycillin for oral treatment. This anti-β-lactamase protects the amoxycillin from inactivation by β-lactamase producing bacteria. It is of considerable value for treating klebsiella and β-lactamase producing *E. coli* infections, but of no value against pseudomonas. Sometimes it is used for localised cellulitis or superficial staphylococcal infection. It is available for oral or intravenous therapy.

Cephalosporins.—There are many β-lactamase-susceptible (not further considered here) and β-lactamase-stable cephalosporins available. There are two which find a place in surgical practice; cefotaxime and ceftazidime; the former is most effective in intra-abdominal skin and soft tissue infections being active against *Staph. aureus*, most enterobacteria as well as *N. meningitidis*, *Strep. pneumoniae* and *H. influenzae*.

As a group the enterococci (*Strep. faecalis*) are not sensitive to any of the cephalosporins. Ceftazidime whilst being active against the Gram-negative organisms and to a lesser extent *Staph. aureus* is most effective against *Pseudomonas aeruginosa*. Both these cephalosporins may be combined with an aminoglycoside such as gentamicin.

---

[1] Sir Robert Hutchinson, 1871–1960, Physician, London Hospital, used to warn 'that it is always well before handing the cup of knowledge to the young, to wait until the froth has settled'.

Lord Howard Walter Florey, 1898–1968, Professor of Pathology, Oxford, England, 1935–1962.
Sir Ernest Boris Chain, 1906–1978, Professor of Biochemistry, Imperial College, London University.

Aminoglycosides.—Gentamicin and tobramycin have similar activity and are particularly effective against the Gram-negative enterobacteriacae. Gentamicin is effective against many strains of pseudomonas, although resistance develops rapidly but all aminoglycosides are inactive against anaerobes and streptococci. Serum levels immediately before and one hour after intra-muscular injection must be taken 48 hours after the start of therapy and dosage should be modified such that the trough level remains at or below 2·5 mg per litre and the peak level should not rise above 10 mg per litre. Ototoxicity including acoustic and labyrinth-like damage can follow the sustained high toxic levels and the cooperation of the microbiological assay department must be obtained when any patient is started on gentamicin.

Tetracyclines.—These broad spectrum bacteriostatic antibiotics should never be used in pregnancy or in children. They are indicated only in cases of typhus, for the treatment of brucellosis, mycoplasma infection, or chlamydia infection.

Chloramphenicol.—Chloramphenicol is a useful drug which is bacteriocidal when used against haemophilus influenzae. Also it is best reserved for meningitis or severe cases of typhoid, but it may be used in the severely ill with good effect, *e.g.* pulmonary infections of the elderly.

Fusidic Acid.—Fusidic acid is a synthetic antistaphylococcal drug to which resistance rapidly develops. The use of topical fucidin ointment should be resisted and the drug should be reserved for combined therapy with erythromycin or flucloxacillin.

Erythromycin is of value against Gram-positive bacteria particularly the Gram-positive cocci. It is effective against legionella and is used prophylactically for surgery and invasive investigations (such as cystoscopy) in patients who are at high risk of bacteraemia and who have been shown to be hypersensitive to penicillin.

Trimethoprim.—Trimethoprim is often used with sulphamethoxazole as co-trimoxazole but is in its own right an effective antibiotic against *E. coli* and klebsiella. Fewer than 10% of these strains are resistant to trimethoprim at present, although infectious (plasmid-mediated) resistance has been described. Side effects of the combination with sulphonamide are nearly always the result of sulphonamide induced hypersensitive reactions.

Rifampicin.—Rifampicin is effective against gram-positive staphylococci and streptococci as well as being an effective treatment for tuberculosis. Staphylococci rapidly become resistant and it should therefore be used in combination with other antibiotics but has proved most effective in surgical wound infections with multi-resistant staphylococci.

Vancomycin.—Vancomycin is most active against Gram-positive bacteria. It is toxic for the 8th cranial nerve and is also nephrotoxic. Serum levels should always be monitored but this antibiotic has proved most effective against multi-resistant staphylococcal infection, and when given orally it is effective against *Cl. difficile* in cases of pseudomembranous colitis.

Metronidazole.—Metronidazole is active against all (and only truly) anaerobic bacteria. It is particularly safe, attains high levels in secretions including saliva, CSF and cellular fluids, and may be administered orally (up to 600 mg 8 hourly), rectally (up to 1 g suppository 8 hourly) or intravenously. Infections with anaerobic cocci, bacteroides and clostridia are effectively treated—or prevented—by its use. Metronidazole (or its analogue tinidazole) is responsible for the reduction of severe anaerobic infection in abdominal, colorectal, and pelvic surgery over the last decade.

CHAPTER 4

SPECIAL INFECTIONS. VIRUSES. AIDS. IMMUNOLOGY

THE CLOSTRIDIA

Tetanus

It has been estimated that every year between 300,000 and 500,000 cases of tetanus occur worldwide with an overall mortality of 40–45%. In the U.K., 200 cases occur annually, and the condition is also relatively uncommon elsewhere in Europe, in the U.S.S.R. and in N. America. The burden of this agonising infection falls on those in the other countries of the world, particularly on the children, the neonates (tetanus neonatorum), and on the elderly. An education programme to have universal active immunisation can and will lead to a reduction of the number of cases and, significantly, the mortality.[1]

Clostridium tetani, the causal organism, is a gram-positive anaerobic rod with terminal spores (drum stick appearance (fig. 22)). Found in manure and soil (notably in market garden areas) it will invade any wound. It multiplies and produces a powerful toxin in any deep contused wound in the presence of dead tissue, foreign bodies and other bacteria. Penetrating injury from the hoof of an animal can be associated with this infection, while the prick from a rose thorn in a well manured rose garden can be the sting of death to an elderly assiduous horticulturalist. The exotoxin produced in the innoculation site inhibits the cholinesterase at the motor end plates, resulting in an excess of acetylcholine locally and therefore a sustained state of tonic muscle spasm. The exotoxin also travels along the nerves to the central nervous system and causes extreme hyperexcitability of motor neurones in the anterior horn cells, thereby evoking explosive and widespread reflex spasms of muscle in reponse to sensory stimuli. Once fixed in the nerve tissue the toxin can no longer be neutralised by antitoxin.

Period of Onset.—The shorter the interval between the first symptom and the first reflex spasm the poorer is the prognosis.[2] If the interval is less than 48 hours death is likely. It should be remembered that wounds containing tetanus organisms may have healed and been forgotten for months or years before some (unknown) change produces the right conditions for the organism to multiply and produce toxin (*latent tetanus*).

Symptoms and Signs.—Dysphagia, jaw stiffness and severe pains in the neck, back and abdomen precede the tonic muscle spasms. The sardonic smile of

---

[1] Tetanus toxoid (now known as Tetanus Vaccine) practically eliminated tetanus in the armies during World War II (1939–45). Today, if active immunity is properly initiated and maintained in an individual, death is unlikely even in the presence of clinical tetanus.

[2] Hippocrates, *circa* 460–377 B.C., is believed to have been the first to recognise this fact.

tetanus (Risus sardonicus) is evidence of the onset of tonic muscle spasm. Respiration and swallowing become progressively more difficult, and reflex convulsions occur affecting all muscles and causing great pain, opisthotonus[1] and even muscle rupture. The spasms are spontaneous, but can be induced by trivial stimuli such as noise or movement, and when severe will prevent respiration and produce cyanosis. Between the reflex convulsions the tonic muscular spasm remains, thus distinguishing tetanus from strychnine poisoning. The temperature is elevated, the pulse is rapid, and respiratory failure and death during a cyanotic attack will usually follow if treatment is not initiated.

At an early stage, the symptoms and signs of tetanus might be mistaken for tonsillitis, 'flu, backstrain, or an acute upper abdominal condition. Therefore careful examination of the patient for a wound is of paramount importance.

Treatment.—Isolation, quietness and comfort, drainage of pus and wound toilet will be needed. *Human anti-tetanus globulin* (e.g. Humotet) is given i.m. to limit the effects of free toxin and should be used in doses of 250–500 units to give cover throughout the period of establishing active immunity by giving toxoid (Tetanus Vaccine, Adsorbed) i.m. Antibiotics, including penicillin and metronidazole are indicated along with measures to protect the lungs.

Stage 1 Case.—A *mild case* where there is tonic rigidity alone will require initial sedation, relaxation by drugs such as promazine up to 200 mg i.m. and a barbiturate or diazepam (5–50 mg i.v.). These drugs will be needed approximately 4 times during any 24 hour period.

Stage 2 Case.—A *seriously ill case* with dysphagia and reflex spasm will need to have a nasogastric tube passed and sedation continued. The diet, the need for intravenous nutrition, the maintenance of balanced protein intake, and of renal function and cardiac function will be priorities. A tracheostomy should be considered if the patient has any difficulty in breathing. The meticulous care of the tracheostomy tube includes suction and humidification (Chapter 35).

Stage 3—Dangerously Ill.—A major cyanotic convulsion will require curarisation (e.g. up to 40 mg tubocurarine i.v. initially and afterwards i.m. to maintain relaxation).[2] Intermittent positive pressure respiration should be provided, and intensive nursing care with increasing sedation would be needed because it has been estimated that a case at this stage will require at least 350 individual acts of nursing each day. The objective is to reduce the risk of death from spasms or pneumonia wherever possible whilst realising that a lethal amount of toxin has already caused severe damage to the motorneurones and the brain with concomitant myocarditis and vascular failure. If recovery takes place, the patient can be weaned from the ventilator (after about 14 days so long as convulsions do not recur when the effects of the relaxants wear off).

Results.—With the proper attention to nursing care, prophylactic antibiotic therapy, active and passive immunisation against tetanus and where indicated tracheostomy, curarisation, and assisted respiration the death rate can be reduced

---

[1] Opisthotonus = drawn backwards. Spasm of the extensors of the neck, back and legs to form a backward curvature.

[2] It should be remembered that the curarised patient though unresponsive is conscious and sensitive and can hear everything that is being said.

to approximately 15%. The results in the very young and very old nevertheless are still poor.

Gas Gangrene

Wounds allowing the patients own faecal flora, or Clostridial spores in the soil, to enter the tissues can give rise to anaerobic gas producing infections. Surgery around the hip joint, and leg amputations are high risk from this postoperative complication, as are the wounds of warfare (Chapter 2). *Clostridium perfringens* (*Welchii*) is usually the cause, but other Clostridia including *Cl. oedematiens* and *Cl. septicum* may be causal. *Cl. welchii* is found in the stools and therefore is also found in the perineum and occasionally as normal flora in the vagina.

Clostridial invasion of a traumatised muscle affects the whole of that muscle from origin to insertion, producing a foul smelling necrosis of the bundles which lose contractibility and become dull red, green and black in appearance. If septicaemia occurs, gas is produced in many organs, notably the liver (which at necropsy drips with frothy blood—the 'foaming liver').

Subcutaneous tissues alone can be infected, the foul smelling necrosis, often spreading extensively can begin in the margin of an abdominal or thoracic wound.

Clinical Features.—The wound is under tension and between the sutures the pouting edges exude a brownish and foul smelling fluid. The skin becomes discoloured—a khaki colour—due to associated haemolysis. Crepitus[1] can usually be detected. An x-ray will show the gas in the muscles or under the skin. The patient, though toxic and pale, with raised pulse, misleadingly appears mentally clear.

Treatment, to be effective, requires immediate action, namely:
(1) Maximum doses of penicillin (up to 2 grams 4 hourly)
(2) Blood transfusion.
(3) Either exposure of all the affected muscle groups by long incisions or, in the subcutaneous infections, multiple subcutaneous drainage and slough extraction by incisions into the subcutaneous tissue.
(4) The use of antiserum, up to 3 ampoules of polyvalent serum being given immediately and repeated 6 hours later.
(5) The use of hyperbaric oxygen where this is available. It is said to be helpful in the post-operative period.

Clostridial Pseudomembranous Colitis

This is an acute, profuse antibiotic-associated diarrhoea which produces characteristic changes of the colon, recognisable sigmoidoscopically by a pseudomembrane and subsequently by sloughing of the colonic mucosa. The organism responsible, *Cl. difficile*, produces a toxin which cross reacts with *Cl. sordellii* antitoxin to produce a serious, sometimes fatal, colitis. The bacterium is readily found in culture and the toxin easily demonstrated in the faeces. The treatment is by oral vancomycin or metronidazole. The condition is no respector of age or sex.

---

[1] Crepitus, to the examining hand, feels like an old hair mattress.

William Henry Welch, 1850–1934. Professor of Pathology, Johns Hopkins University, Baltimore, Maryland, U.S.A. Discovered the causative organism of gas gangrene in 1892.

THE SALMONELLA

Salmonella typhi, para-typhi.—These are enteric pathogens which cause enteric fevers with bacteraemia, osteitis and sometimes perforation of ileal ulcers. Persistence of the bacteria in the gallbladder may lead to the carrier state and subsequently person to person spread in the community (Chapter 47). Chloramphenicol is the antibiotic of choice for *S. typhi* infection as some strains are resistant to broad spectrum β-lactam antibiotics.

The other salmonellas are associated with food poisoning, diarrhoea and (therefore) dehydration. Control of the symptoms only is usually required and the use of antimicrobials is not usually helpful for thereby resistant strains are encouraged, excretion can be prolonged and in any case the intestinal symptoms are self limiting. In the unusual event of systemic spread and bacteraemia it will be necessary to use the antibiotics to which the isolate is sensitive. If treatment is started before the organism is isolated a broad spectrum penicillin combined with an aminoglycoside may then be required. The commonest non-typhoid salmonellas are *S. typhimurium*, *S. enteritidis* and *S. virchow*. They are found in cattle, calves, poultry, turkeys and domestic animals and infection in man is by direct spread from contaminated food. These organisms can spread within a hospital if patients (or staff) with diarrhoea are not recognised as a risk; close contacts of excreta must be properly protected by apron and gloves to reduce the likelihood of the infection being spread by unwashed hands which have become contaminated with faeces.

THE MYCOBACTERIA

Tuberculosis

Mycobacterium tuberculosis.—This acid-fast bacillus is spread by airborne infection (or from infected cows in the case of bovine tuberculosis). There are three routes of primary infection:

(*a*) Direct spread to lungs.

(*b*) From tonsils to the lymph nodes of the neck where an abscess may form and track round the edge of the sternomastoid muscle producing a collar stud abscess.

(*c*) From lower ileal infection to the lymph nodes of the ileocaecal angle.

The bacterium which produces no pigment grows well at 37°C and may be seen, if there are very many organisms, in the Ziehl-Nielsen stained smear. Growth of the bacteria takes six weeks, thus sensitivities to the anti-tuberculous drugs will be delayed.

For the accounts of the manifestations of this disease in various organs as applied to the practice of surgery, the reader is referred to the appropriate chapters of this book.

Guidelines for Treatment.—(1) Nutrition and hygienic living conditions are still crucially important in preventing the spread of this infection.

(2) Treatment with triple therapy consisting of rifampicin 600 mg isoniazid 300 mg and ethambutol 25 mg per kg body weight per day given orally for at least 2 to 3 months is the standard chemotherapy at present. Sensitivity testing is usually available at the end of the first period of triple therapy and if the source of the infection is with an organism that is resistant to one of these drugs appropriate changes can then be made. In cases of pulmonary tuberculosis the sputum should be examined to assess progress every month until the smears are negative, but should the number of acid fast bacilli increase or the cultures remain positive the development of resistance or non compliance of the patient with treatment should be considered. Genito-urinary and orthopaedic tuberculosis is usually effectively treated by the standard 9 month course but the use of

Daniel Elmer Salmon, 1850–1914, Pathologist, U.S.A.

pyrazinamide with rifampicin and isoniazid may be required. All these anti-tuberculous drugs have side effects which may require repeated careful assessment and control; isoniazid causes a peripheral neuritis, ethambutol produces visual impairment and rifampicin is hepatotoxic.

It should be remembered that it is nigh impossible to eradicate every tubercle bacillus from the body. Lying dormant and enveloped in fibrous tissue any remaining bacilli are still able to cause a flare-up of the disease, particularly after trauma, after gastrointestinal operations resulting in nutritional deficiency, and in old age.

Opportunist mycobacteria.—'Slow growing' opportunist mycobacteriae may be found producing lesions similar to *M. tuberculosis* in susceptible patients. Thus *M. kansasii* is a slow growing opportunist mycobacterium which may cause pulmonary lesions. *M. chelonei* and *M. fortuitum* occasionally cause subcutaneous abscesses following skin trauma. This group should always be remembered in the differential diagnosis of subcutaneous abscesses associated with skin traumas or injections (e.g. tetanus immunisation). Skin granulomas in swimmers may be caused by *M. marinum* while the surgically important Buruli ulcer occurring in East Africa affects the exposed surface of the limbs, is caused by *M. ulcerans* and presents as a spreading granulomatous nodule which subsequently breaks down and forms an ulcer. Incision of the nodule at an early stage and treatment with rifampcin may prevent an ulcer forming, but secondary infection of a Buruli ulcer may result in fibrosis and considerable deformities of a limb as a result. All the opportunist mycobacteria should be cultured in order to assess their sensitivity to the anti-mycobacterial drugs.

Leprosy (Hansen's Disease[1])

There are probably from ten to fifteen million leprosy sufferers in the world today.

Leprosy is an infectious disease widely spread throughout the tropical and sub-tropical areas of the world. It is caused by *Mycobacterium leprae*, an acid-fast bacillus morphologically like the tubercle bacillus. It is mainly, but not entirely, contracted in childhood and late adolescence. While the mode of transmission regarding the portal of entry of *M. leprae* is not known, the source of infection is mainly from the nasal secretions of patients with lepromatous leprosy and not from their skin. Leprosy is no longer endemic in Northern Europe, as it was in the Middle Ages and in Norway until the late 19th century; neither is it now spread by immigrants in Europe. These facts suggest that leprosy requires for its transmission some factors associated with poverty or lack of hygiene that is common in the areas where it is still endemic. A vast change in the outlook for this disease has occurred in the last 30 years. The condition was formerly regarded as hopeless, but in spite of the fact that it is now curable only 25% of the cases of this widely spread disease are under treatment. It is probably true to say that leprosy causes more paralysis, deformity, and misery than any other disease, but that in many cases these could now be prevented by modern therapy, given an adequate service for early diagnosis.

Although leprosy is a systemic infection, it presents predominantly as an infection of the skin, upper respiratory tract and dermal and peripheral nerves. Leprosy must always be considered in a patient presenting with a combination of skin *and* neural disorder,

---

[1] After Hansen who first showed leprosy was a bacterial infection caused by *M. leprae*. Because of the stigma attached to leprosy, Dr. R. G. Cochrane and others recommended that it should be referred to as Hansen's disease.

Robert Koch, 1843–1910. Professor of Hygiene and Bacteria, Pathology, Berlin (1885–1910). Discovered mycobacterium tuberculosis whilst working in the Imperial Health Office, Berlin in 1882.
Gerhard Henrik Armauer Hansen, 1841–1912. Physician in Charge of a Leper Hospital near Bergen, Norway.
Robert Greenhill Cochrane, Contemporary. Formerly Medical Superintendent, Kola Ndoto Leprosarium, Shinyange, Tanzania.

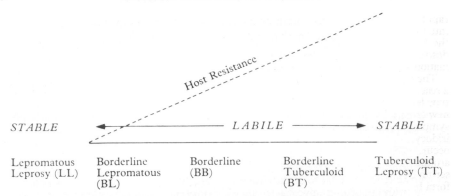

FIG. 24.—Ridley-Jopling classification of leprosy based on immunity of host.

particularly because of the variation in the preponderance of these two manifestations and the tremendous variation in the appearance and histopathology of the dermal lesions, among individual patients with leprosy. These diverse manifestations led to a plethora of classification systems until Ridley and Jopling found that there was a spectrum of disease in leprosy determined by the resistance of the host (fig. 24). The spectrum ranges from polar lepromatous (LL) to polar tuberculoid (TT) leprosy, denoting patients with minimal and maximal irreversible capacities to mount an immunological response against *M. leprae*. The majority of patients are more labile in having some residual immunological capacity against *M. leprae*, and thus are represented as borderline (BB), or borderline-lepromatous (BL) or borderline-tuberculoid (BT), if they veer more towards lepromatous or tuberculoid leprosy. If left untreated, patients anywhere within the borderline spectrum can deteriorate towards lepromatous leprosy, whereas under treatment they will shift towards polar tuberculoid leprosy.

Lepromatous Leprosy

There is little or no resistance, the bacilli multiply with little cellular response, until the subcutaneous tissues may be loaded with masses of bacilli, many of them distending macrophages as large 'globi'. The cellular infiltrate is mainly of macrophages with a few lymphocytes.

Tuberculoid Leprosy

There is a strong tissue response, the bacilli are not numerous and are seldom seen except by special concentration methods. The histology consists of an epitheloid granuloma, many lymphocytes and a few giant cells.

Characteristically *tuberculoid* leprosy causes sharply localised lesions often affecting only one part of the body, while *lepromatous* leprosy is symmetrical and extensive. Since the damage in leprosy is mainly due to the response of the host cells, *tuberculoid* leprosy causes early, severe but localised deformity, while *lepromatous* leprosy causes deformity late, and more mildly and widely spread. The most severely deformed patients are those affected by some of the border-line forms where the disease may be both widespread through the body and also rather violent in its reactions.

A unique feature of the disease is not only its predilection for the surface of the body, but also for the cool part of the surface. Warm areas like the axilla and gluteal cleft are spared, while the parts of the upper respiratory tract, like the lining of the nose, are severely involved. The testis is affected, while the ovary, and other deeply placed glands and organs, are unaffected. Since leprosy does not affect the vital organs of the body, it rarely causes death, and patients do not even feel ill for most of the time they have the disease.

During treatment, many patients manifest acute episodes which are referred to as 'reactions' of which there are two distinct types:

The 'lepra or Type 1 reaction' occurs in the borderline form of leprosy (BT, BB and BL), in which the skin lesions become erythematous, warm to touch and may break down, and the nerves swell and become painful and tender to touch. It is usually caused by a

William Henry Jopling, Contemporary. Formerly Consultant Leprologist, Hospital for Tropical Diseases, London.
Dennis Snow Ridley, Contemporary. Consultant Pathologist, Hospital for Tropical Diseases, London.

rapid increase in cell-mediated immunity by the host with an outpouring of lymphocytes into the lesions giving rise to acute inflammation with associated oedema. For this reason, the lesions have been referred to as 'reversal reactions', advantageous by resulting in destruction of *M. leprae*, but causing irreversible destruction of axons when the inflammation and oedema occur in nerves.

The other type of reaction is referred to as erythema nodosum leprosum (ENL or Type 2 reaction), usually occurring during treatment but confined to patients with lepromatous type leprosy (BL, LL). Here there are no changes in the established leprosy lesions, but new crops of very small erythematous lesions in the skin appear associated with systemic symptoms such as malaise, fever and nerve and joint pain. Occasionally, rhinitis, acute iridocyclitis, swollen and tender lymph glands, acute epididymo-orchitis and proteinuria occur. This is an Arthus type reaction, due to the deposition of immune complexes in and around blood vessels, locally or generalised thoughout the body, and more akin to chronic serum sickness. This reaction may come and go or be persistent, and can in its severest form be fatal.

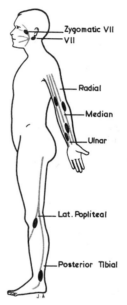

Fig. 25.—Sites of motor paralysis in leprosy.

(1) Ulnar nerve just above elbow joint or wrist joint.
(2) Median nerve just above wrist joint.
(3) Lateral popliteal at knee joint.
(4) Posterior tibial above ankle joint.
(5) Facial nerve in the bony canal or the zygomatic branch.
(6) Radial nerve at the elbow (rarely).

(After Paul Brand, F.R.C.S.)

One of the most characteristic features of leprosy is its effect on nerves (fig. 25). Histologically, the cellular infiltrate may be seen localised around nerve fibres in and under the skin and, on clinical examination, superficial nerves such as the ulnar and posterior auricular may be observed to be swollen and tender. The anaesthesia that results from nerve involvement is an important point in diagnosis, and is also a cause of secondary damage and deformity. Much of the loss and disfigurement of hands and feet which has always been associated with leprosy is now known to be due not to leprosy itself, but to the damage and misuse which follows loss of pain sensation.

Medical Treatment.—Diaminodiphenylsulphone (Dapsone, DDS) (50–100 mg/ daily) is now the standard treatment for all forms of leprosy. It is a bacteriostatic drug and experience has shown that in leprosy it has to be given for a long time—at least 3 years for all forms of tuberculoid leprosy and probably for life for all forms of lepromatous leprosy—for even when it is given to lepromatous patients until they become bacteriologically negative (5–10 years), they can still relapse when treatment is stopped. For many years it was considered that reactional episodes occurred more commonly when the full dose of DDS was given from the beginning of treatment and that reactions, once developed, persisted if dapsone treatment was continued. Both these ideas have now been proved to be fallacious.

DDS Resistance.—Since 1964 resistance has been recognised, in ever increasing frequency throughout the world, among patients with lepromatous leprosy, and that it occurs much more commonly in those patients who have received smaller doses of DDS in the past or have had their treatment interrupted. Since DDS resistance oocurs only among patients with lepromatous type leprosy, it is now recommended that new patients with lepromatous leprosy must be initiated with DDS plus two other drugs (in line with the successful use of combined therapy for the prevention of drug resistance in tuberculosis). The other antileprosy drugs of proven value are rifampicin, clofazimine and ethionamide/prothionamide. Rifampicin, the first bactericidal drug against *M. leprae*, has been shown to act more rapidly than any of the other antileprosy drugs, although much more expensive. Fortunately, rifampicin is effective in a dose of 600 mg once monthly. Therefore, the combined regimen recommended by WHO is: DDS (100 mg) and clofazimine (50 mg) daily with supervised doses of rifampicin (600 mg) and clofazimine (300 mg) monthly for two years minimum for all new lepromatous patients. Clofazimine produces a red coloration of the skin, which in some lighter skin patients may be unacceptable. Such patients should be given ethionamide/prothionamide (250 mg) daily as an alternative to clofazimine. This same regimen is also recommended for lepromatous patients with suspected DDS resistance. Where possible treatment for all these patients should be continued to skin negativity, rather than only two years.

For reactions, symptomatic treatment should be given for the milder cases, including analgesics and tranquillisers. For the more severe reactions various proprietary antimonial drugs, such as Stibophen and Fouadin, *etc.*, have proved beneficial as has chloroquine. For a still more persistent and severe lepra and ENL reactions it may be absolutely essential to give steroids to tide the patients over and particularly to protect the nerves. For patients with the most severe ENL reactions, but not lepra reactions, Thalidomide has proved to be as beneficial as steroids. If Thalidomide is available it *must be confined* to male patients or females outside the child-bearing age. Clofazimine in high doses can suppress all but the most severe ENL reactions.

Surgery.—The Deformities of Leprosy are divided into *primary*—those which are caused directly by leprosy and its reactions, and *secondary*—those which result from anaesthesia and consequent misuse. The stigma of leprosy is the stigma of deformity, and a wide-open field awaits the plastic surgeon in this disease.

The Face.—*Primary deformity*: the skin of the face becomes thickened and sometimes nodular in lepromatous leprosy (fig. 26); the forehead, cheeks, nose, and ears are especially affected. The result in the acute phase is referred to as 'leonine facies'. This infiltration subsides under medical treatment, but may leave the skin wrinkled and without its normal support, producing, in a younger person, a caricature of old age. The hair of the eyebrows falls out and the lateral cartilages and septum of the nose may be destroyed leaving collapse of the centre of the nose and lifting of the tip towards the bridge (fig. 27). The upper branches of the facial nerve may be paralysed, giving rise to lagophthalmos; the lower branches are sometimes partially paralysed.

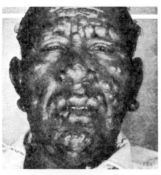

Fig. 26.—Nodular lepromatous leprosy.

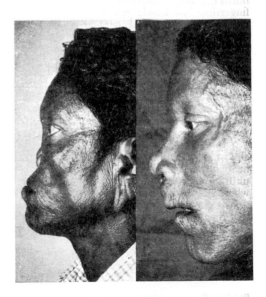

Fig. 27.—(*Left*) Extreme case of nasal collapse. (*Right*) After post-nasal epithelial inlay.
(N.H. Antia, F.R.C.S.) (*By permission from the Annals of the Royal College of Surgeons of England.*)

The patient with the above deformities usually finds it quite impossible to return to normal social relationships even though his leprosy may be cured. Plastic surgery can completely transform such a face using a post-nasal inlay to the nose (fig. 27), and an 'island flap' for the eyebrows. A temporalis muscle segment reactivates the eyelids and a face-lift may restore more normal contours to the skin.

Eyes.—Some of the blindness of leprosy is simply due to exposure following paralysis of the eyelids. This is correctable by plastic surgery. Other causes of loss of vision are lepromatous infiltration of the anterior segment of the eye and acute allergic changes of the tissues associated with reaction. Acute plastic irido-cyclitis is one of the commonest manifestations of this allergic reaction. Any redness of the eye or loss of visual acuity in leprosy demands full examination and prompt treatment if the sight is to be saved.

Hands (fig. 28).[1]—*Primary Deformity.*—In the upper limbs, leprosy causes paralysis frequently in the ulnar nerve at the elbow and in the median nerve at the wrist (fig. 25) but rarely in the motor part of the radial nerve (1%).

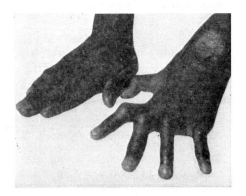

FIG. 28.—Clawed left hand in leprosy. The patient commonly loses the use of all the small muscles of the hand, but few forearm muscles. The fingers are clawed and the thumb lies completely unopposed.
(*Dr. R. G. Cochrane, London.*)

Treatment.—The extensor carpi radialis brevis muscle is extended into the hand with free grafts which run along the lines of the lumbrical tendons to correct the clawing of the fingers. The flexor sublimis tendon to the ring finger is withdrawn in the forearm and rerouted to oppose the thumb along the line of the abductor brevis. In this way the fingers and thumb may be balanced and function almost normally. Before attempting operation it is important to make sure that the fingers are made mobile by massage and exercise.

Secondary Deformity.—Since the hand is often totally anaesthetic the patient frequently burns himself, or damages himself by the uninhibited strength which he uses through his fingertips. His hands become scarred and progressively absorbed until only stumps remain. It takes patience and perseverance to teach every patient that his hands can be preserved only by constant alertness to foresee possible dangers, and constant gentleness to his own tissues which are not protected by pain. Once he is convinced that it is not leprosy that is destroying his fingers he may be willing to accept the discipline of caring for himself.

Feet.—*Primary Deformity.*—In the lower limbs the posterior tibial nerve is often involved at the ankle, giving rise to 'clawing' of the toes and anaesthesia of the sole of the foot. The lateral popliteal nerve may also be destroyed, giving rise to foot-drop. The medial popliteal nerve is never involved, so the tibialis posterior muscle can be safely used to correct foot-drop.

Secondary Deformity.—The anaesthesia of the sole of the foot is very serious because almost every patient with insensitive feet sooner or later develops trophic ulceration. If he then continues to walk on his ulcers, the condition progresses and the infection spreads until, after a few years, the foot is contracted and distorted, and destroyed to the point where amputation must be advised.

It is important for the patient to understand the pathology of his ulcers and to realise that they are not due directly to leprosy. These ulcers heal readily with rest in a plaster cast and their recurrence can be prevented by the regular use of special footwear designed to spread the weight evenly over the whole foot.

---

[1] The work on reconstruction of the hand in Hansen's disease was started by Professor Paul Brand.

Paul Wilson Brand, Contemporary. Chief of the Rehabilitation Branch, U.S. Public Health Service Hospital, Carville, Louisiana, U.S.A.

THE TREPONEMAS

Syphilis.[1] For a detailed description of venereal syphilis reference should be made to a text book on venereal disease.

Acquired Syphilis

Acquired syphilis is a venereal infection caused by *Treponema pallidum* (fig. 29), a delicate spiral organism (spirochaete), 6–15 µm in length. A dramatic decline in incidence after the introduction of penicillin has been followed by a gradual but significant increase throughout the world.

Transmission is by direct contact with a surface lesion containing treponemes which penetrate the skin or mucosa at the point of contact. Since treponemes are present only in the surface lesions of EARLY syphilis, i.e. primary, secondary and the first two years of latency, syphilis is only infective during that period. After 2 years, acquired syphilis is rarely communicable and the ulcerative cutaneous lesions of tertiary syphilis are not infective as they contain few, if any, treponemes. The organism dies rapidly on drying, hence infective early lesions are predominantly sited on moist areas, e.g. genitals, mouth and anus, so that infection almost always occurs during intercourse including oro-genital contact and—of great importance now—homosexual practices involving the anus and rectum.

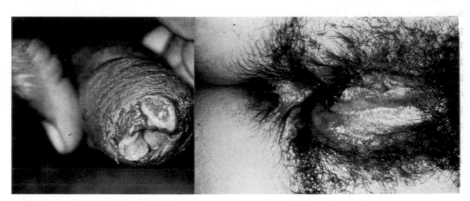

FIG. 29.—Penile primary chancres.   FIG. 30.—Vulval chancre in a female.

Clinical Features.—The disease is divided into 4 stages:

Primary Syphilis.—A primary sore or chancre (figs 29 and 30) develops at the site of entry of the treponemes in about 3-4 weeks. It may resolve at any stage of its development and thus be quite atypical. It may simulate other penile or vulval lesions, traumatic lesions such as splits or tears, chancroid, herpes genitalis, burns, furuncles and carcinoma as well as balanoposthitis and lymphogranuloma venereum (Chapter 60).

---

[1] Syphilis derives its name from a poem by a Physician, Girolamo Fracastoro (1478–1553), published in Venice in 1530. The poem tells of the shepherd, Syphilus, who was struck down by the disease as a punishment for insulting Apollo.

On his return from Haiti in 1493, Christopher Columbus (1451–1506) brought back syphilis, parrots and rare plants. The King and Queen of Spain received him with highest honours.

Starting as an indurated papule, it becomes eroded and when fully developed will present the following signs of a classical Hunterian chancre: a shallow, indurated, painless, non-bleeding ulcer, usually single, oval or round, with a raised hyperaemic margin, often extending into a dusky red oedema. A painless, discrete and rubbery enlargement of the associated lymph nodes occurs. The prepuce of the penis *must* always be fully retracted as otherwise tiny sores in the coronal sulcus may be missed. As there are no constitutional symptoms a female patient will be unaware of the presence of a cervical chancre, a lesion which accounts for about 45% of all sores in that sex. Extragenital chancres of the lip,[1] tongue, nipple, etc. are now rare, but rectal and perianal primaries are common in homosexuals and are usually atypical, frequently resembling painful anal fissures which occasionally get excised in error. Spasm of the anal sphincter is usually less with true sores and a typical (lateral) inguinal lymphadenitis may be present.

Diagnosis is by finding *Treponema pallidum* in the clear exudate from the lesion by dark-field microscopy. The serum tests do not become positive for ten to ninety days (usually 3–5 weeks) after the appearance of the chancre, hence initial negative results must never be interpreted as excluding primary syphilis. This is because the tests identify a gradually developing antibody response. The tests should be repeated for up to 3 months where doubt persists.

Secondary Syphilis.—Signs usually appear in 6–12 weeks, extremes being 3 weeks to 6 months. The commonest sign is a dull red or coppery rash, which is generalised, symmetrical, indolent and non-irritant. Often inconspicuous, sometimes absent (in 25% of cases), the rash is characteristically pleomorphic, being roseolar or macular at first, with papular, papulo-squamous or other elements appearing later. Papules on contiguous moist sites, e.g. vulva, perineum, may enlarge to form condylomata lata, fleshy, wart-like growths teeming with treponemes. Small, round, superficial erosions may occur in the mouth where they may coalesce to form the so-called snail-track ulcers. The rash can resemble that of any known rash producing condition in the whole of medicine. A generalised, painless lymphadenopathy often occurs and less common symptoms include sore throat, hoarseness, 'moth-eaten' alopecia, hepatitis, iritis, bone and joint pains. Bone or osteoscopic pains may be severe and prolonged for several weeks without any other supporting signs and the diagnosis is often missed. Acute meningitis or cranial nerve or spinal root palsies due to an irregular pachymeningitis occur. Constitutional effects, malaise, headache, backache and pyrexia normally mild, are occasionally of prostrating severity. Secondary syphilis is also a cause of pyrexia of unascertained origin (PUO).

Full spontaneous recovery always occurs.

Latent Syphilis.—Follows the untreated secondary stage and lasts from 2 years to a lifetime. There are no signs, but the serum tests are positive.

Late Syphilis.—(*Syn.* Tertiary Syphilis). Syphilis in all its stages is essentially a vascular disease. In each stage, treponemes cause inflammatory reactions in the perivascular lymphatics with plasma cell cuffing of terminal vessels. In the ter-

---

[1] Primary sores on the lips usually result from kissing, and a case is recorded in which a gentleman with secondary ulceration of the mouth infected five young ladies at a dance, each of whom developed a chancre on the lip.

John Hunter, 1728–1793. Surgeon, St George's Hospital, London. To further his knowledge of venereal disease he either inoculated himself or another with syphilis in 1767.

tiary stage only there is subsequent obliterative endarteritis, tissue necrosis and fibrosis. Since almost any structure may be involved, the signs can be extraordinarily variable and will be referable to the site or system involved. Only about 35% of untreated syphilitics will develop tertiary syphilis. About 5–15 years after infection, 10% will develop *neurosyphilis*, 10–12% *cardiovascular syphilis* and after six months up to many years later, 10–15% will develop *late benign syphilis* involving less vital structures. The three types are not mutually exclusive. The typical lesion of late benign syphilis is the localised *gumma* (fig. 31) or diffuse gummatous infiltration. The gumma is a syphilitic hypersensitivity reaction consisting of granulation tissue with central necrosis. Sloughing of a subcutaneous gumma may produce the typical, painless, punched-out gummatous ulcer with a 'washleather' base (fig. 32). On healing, it leaves a silvery 'tissue-paper' scar. Alterna-

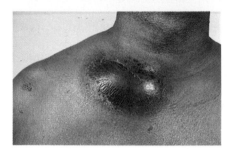

FIG. 31.—Gumma overlying the sternoclavicular joint. A classical site.

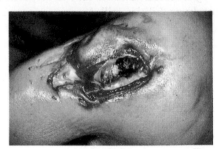

FIG. 32.—Punched-out gumma of the shoulder. This lesion was characteristically painless.

tively, the gummatous process may be nodular or infiltrative without ulceration and slow peripheral spread occurs with central healing. The individual lesions are round and indurated and grouped lesions are circinate in outline with sharply defined, hyperpigmented margins.

Serological Tests for Treponemal Diseases are of two types:

(1) *Non-specific (syn. Reagin, Non-treponemal, Lipoidal antigen tests)*.—Examples are the Cardiolipin Wasserman (C/WR), Kahn, Meinicke, Ven.Dis.Ref.Lab slide test. The last is the best. These test the presence of any antibody reagin in the serum of patients with treponemal infections, but biologic false positives (B.F.P.) arise from reagin present in non-treponemal conditions, e.g. malaria, vaccinia, glandular fever, and also after any kind of vaccination. Stronger and persistent reactions may occur in leprosy, sarcoidosis, collagen diseases and chronic liver disorders. A diagnosis of syphilis requires confirmation from one or more of the specific tests.

(2) *Group specific tests (Treponemal antigen tests)*.—Examples are: Reiter's Protein Complement Fixation Test (RPCFT), Treponema pallidum Haemagglutination Assay (TPHA), Absorbed Fluorescent Antibody Test (FTA. Abs), Treponema Pallidum Immobilisation Test (TPI).

The first is obsolescent (in the U.K.) and the last rarely required. The routine practice is to perform the VDRL and TPHA adding the FTA if either is positive or the clinical findings justify it. In primary syphilis, the usual order of conversion is FTA, VDRL with rising titre and TPHA, though this sequence is not invariable. After treatment, the VDRL usually reverts to negative in up to six months, the FTA in seventy per cent, but the TPHA hardly ever of which facts the patients must be told—'a little scar in the blood' is usually adequate. Persistence of Treponemal antibodies, if it is known that adequate treatment has been given, is not a cause for concern but if there is any doubt, confirmed reactions on repetition should be treated as for latent infection.

The Treatment of Syphilis.—No local treatment except isotonic saline should be applied to a suspected chancre until dark-field examinations have proved negative on 3 successive days. No treponemicidal antibiotics should be prescribed until syphilis is confirmed or excluded, but if there is secondary infection a course of sulphonamides may help. Penicillin has supplanted all other forms of treatment. A high cure rate is achieved in early syphilis with intramuscular Procaine Penicillin G 600,000 units daily for 15 days. This dosage is prolonged to 21–30 days for late syphilis. Clinical and serological observation should be continued for two years after treatment. For penicillin-sensitive patients, tetracycline, erythromycin and cephaloridine are all treponemicidal but experience with them is limited. The best treatment is doxycycline 100 mg thrice daily for the equivalent period.

Jarisch Herxheimer Reaction.—About 6 hours after the first injection 60% of early syphilitics will develop pyrexia, malaise and possible rigors lasting a few hours only. Patients must be warned about this. The reaction is infrequent in late syphilis, but may be more serious. In late cases only, prednisone 10 mg four times daily for three days before the main treatment should prevent it.

Prognosis is excellent after standard treatment for early syphilis. In late syphilis, particularly of the cardiovascular system, cure of the underlying disease may not significantly improve the condition of the patient.

Congenital Syphilis

Transmission.—Infection occurs when treponemes from an infected expectant mother cross the placental barrier to the fetal circulation. The more recent the mother's infection, the more likely is this to occur and the more serious the effects on the child. The results of fetal infection vary from death in late fetal life or early infancy, or the birth and normal development of an apparently healthy child who nevertheless has latent congenital syphilis.

Early Congenital Syphilis.—Signs in the newborn, which may be delayed for a few weeks, include a generalised rash, mucous erosions as in secondary syphilis, and the 'snuffles', a syphilitic rhinitis with nasal discharge which interferes with suckling causing loss of weight, epiphysitis, periostitis, osteochondritis, hepatosplenomegaly and basal meningitis. Signs may be so slight as to escape notice or so severe as to cause death in early infancy usually due to syphilitic 'pneumonia alba'.

Late Congenital Syphilis.—The extraordinary variety of clinical manifestations which can occur in acquired tertiary syphilis can also occur in childhood or puberty in late congenital syphilis; e.g. congenital neurosyphilis, cutaneous, visceral or skeletal gummata, but congenital cardiovascular syphilis is practically unknown. In addition, some manifestations, the *Stigmata*, occur in congenital, but never in acquired syphilis.

The stigmata of late congenital syphilis (Hutchinson's classic triad) consist of:

(1) *Interstital Keratitis.*—The most frequent of the stigmata, is a syphilitic hypersensitivity reaction with onset between 5–15 years. The cornea becomes inflamed causing pain, lacrimation and photophobia. It tends to be bilateral and recurrent. Prolonged severe recurrent attacks result in a hazy 'ground glass' appearance of the cornea, with yellowish-red corneal patches in severe cases (salmon patches)[1]. It is uninfluenced by anti-syphilitic treatment but can be controlled by local cortisone treatment.

(2) *8th Nerve Deafness.*—A progressive, bilateral, perceptive deafness, onset about puberty, but occasionally delayed until later and uninfluenced by treatment.

(3) *Hutchinson's Teeth.*—A peg or band-shaped deformity of the upper central incisors, second dentition. Moon's Molars (mulberry molars): the 6-year molars erupt with dwarfed cusps. Other classical signs include saddle nose (fig. 33), perforation of the palate (fig. 34), sabre tibia, Clutton's joints (painless effusions, commonly in the knee joint) and parietal bossing.

---

[1] Not to be confused with the salmon-patch birthmark.

Karl Herxheimer, 1861–1944, Dermatologist, Frankfurt, Germany.
Sir Jonathan Hutchinson, 1828–1913. Surgeon, The London Hospital (1859–1883). Described Hutchinson's teeth and the triad in 1858.
Henry Moon, 1845–1892. Dental Surgeon, Guy's Hospital, London (1870–1887). Described Moon's Molars in 1876.
Henry Hugh Clutton, 1850–1909. Surgeon, St. Thomas's Hospital, London. Described these joints in 1886.

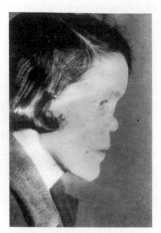

FIG. 33.—Saddle nose of congenital syphilis.

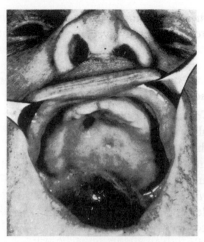

FIG. 34.—Perforation of palate.

Prevention and Treatment of Congenital Syphilis.—Six hundred thousand units of Procaine Penicillin G given to the mother for 15 days as early as possible in pregnancy will not only protect her from the ravages of late syphilis but will prevent infection of the fetus, or may even cure it *in utero*, if already infected. An infected neonate whose mother received no treatment during pregnancy should be treated as for late acquired syphilis with the dosage adjusted to weight.

Neonatal Serology.—An expectant mother who has received no treatment during pregnancy, or who is an untreated latent syphilitic may produce a child free from syphilis but seropositive due to passive transfer of maternal IgG antibodies. This serological problem can be solved by performing tests on the IgG and IgM fractions of the infant's serum but not on the cord blood. In the case of passive transfer the IgG tests will be positive and the IgM tests negative. Positive IgM tests indicate active disease in the child since the IgM fraction of the maternal serum proteins does not cross the barrier of the normal placenta. Exceptions occur if the placenta has been damaged from other causes. In all cases, careful clinical and serological follow-up of mother and child is essential. The virtual disappearance of congenital syphilis from the United Kingdom and similar countries is one of the great triumphs of modern medicine. In England, only four cases under two years old were reported in 1984.

Syphilis Contacts.—At all stages of the disease the known contacts must be followed up. This applies to late and congenital cases when other members of the patient's family are often found to have untreated latent syphilis.

Yaws[1] (Framboesia)

Yaws is an endemic disease of rural areas in tropical countries of high humidity. The causative organisms, *Treponema pertenue*, appears indistinguishable from *Tr. pallidum* and produces identical serological reactions. Direct contact with an early lesion is the usual mode of transmission. It is not sexually transmitted. The primary lesion is most frequently seen on the legs of children. About one month after infection a papule appears at the site of entry of the treponeme, this ulcerates giving the lesion a pink, raised, raspberry-like (framboesia[2]) appearance. Secondary lesions, usually papillomatous, appear some weeks later. After 5 or more years of latency a minority of patients develop late gummatous-like lesions of soft

---

[1] The possible answer to 'What's Yaws?' is 'Syphilis'.
[2] Framboise (Fr.) = Raspberry.

tissue or bone similar to those of tertiary syphilis. The cardiovascular and nervous systems are not involved and congenital yaws does not occur. Treat as for syphilis.

OTHER INFECTIONS (NON-VIRAL)

Candidiasis

Candida albicans (formerly called *Monilia*) is a yeast, frequently present in small numbers in the healthy bowel and mouth. It may cause primary infection in the newborn, or superinfection when flora are disturbed by antibiotic treatment. In *Thrush* (candidal stomatitis) white patches are seen in the mouth; it may occur in infants, in post-operative patients, and with ill-fitting dental plates. *Vaginitis* is common in pregnancy and diabetes. Candida may infect moist skin under breasts, and the nail folds and cause severe intertrigo.

Administration of broad-spectrum antibiotics often results in proliferation of candida in the respiratory tract and bowel, and may be responsible for digestive upsets. Systemic candidiasis with invasion of lung and blood-stream is a complication of immuno-suppression in transplantation surgery and in the chemotherapy of malignant disease. Oral thrush also occurs in AIDS.

Candida infections are treated by the topical antibiotic nystatin or by gentian violet. Treatments for vaginal candidiasis include pessary treatment with clotrimazole (Canesten), miconazole nitrate (Gyno-daktarin), econazole (Ecostatin), isoconazole nitrate (Travogyn) from one to six days or nystatin for fourteen days. Ketaconazole 200 mg b.d. for 5 days is a recent oral treatment. In all cases of treatment failure, the male partner should be investigated for balanoposthitis, easily cured with clotrimazole or nystatin ointments locally. In very severe cases, particularly in pregnancy, prior local treatment with gentian violet may be indicated.

Chancroid (Soft Sore)

This infection is rare in western countries.

It is caused by the Gram-negative strepto-bacillus Ducrey (*Haemophillus ducreyi*). Two to five days after infection sores, often multiple, appear on the genitals. They become pustular and ulcerate, forming rounded, painful, soft, readily bleeding ulcers with undermined edges. Inguinal adenitis follows, the swollen nodes being hard and tender causing a feeling of stiffess in the groin. Resolution may occur at this stage, but suppuration may follow, the nodes becoming matted together forming a fluctuant unilocular abscess (bubo) with red overlying skin, in one or both groins. The bubo should never be incised since healing is very slow. Aspiration is correct. Phagedaena[1] sometimes occurs.

Treatment.—Any antibiotic which may prevent the identification of *T. pallidum* in a case of concomitant syphilitic infection, or when the aetiology of the lesion is in doubt, is contraindicated. Sulphonamide 4 g daily for 7–10 days is the treatment of choice or cotrimoxazole two tablets twice daily for the same period and only isotonic 0·9% saline locally.

Gonorrhoea.—This veneral disease is discussed in relation to the Genitourinary system, Chapters 60 and 61.

Lympho-granuloma Venereum is described in Chapter 60.

Granuloma Inguinale is described in Chapter 60.

---

[1] Phagedaena—A rapidly spreading destructive ulceration.

Augusto Ducrey, 1860–1940. Professor of Dermatology, Pisa, Italy. Described the causative organism of chancroid in 1889.

Erysipelas

Erysipelas a spreading inflammation of the skin and subcutaneous tissues due to an infection by *Strep. pyogenes* (*Streptococcus haemolyticus* of Lancefields group A). Poor hygienic living conditions, recurrent upper respiratory tract infections, debilitating illness, and extremes of life are predisposing causes and the lesion develops around a scratch or abrasion which is the site of inoculation of the streptococcus. A rapid toxaemia associated with the local infection and a rose pink rash extending over the adjacent skin rapidly develops. The rash has a very clear edge and considerable oedema occurs (fig. 35) over some tissues when infected, *e.g.* orbit or scrotum. Following the fading of the rash, a brown discolouration of the skin remains. The *Strep. pyogenes* remains fully sensitive to penicillin.

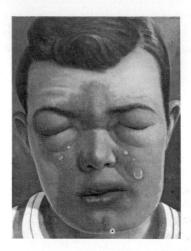

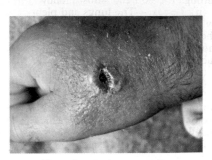

FIG. 35.—Erysipelas with lymphatic oedema of face and eyelids. The patient was unable to open his eyes.

FIG. 36.—Anthrax pustule.
(*Dr. W. D. Paterson, Carlisle.*)

Anthrax

B. anthracis is a large Gram-positive aerobic spore-forming rod. It is very resistant to heat and antiseptics. The disease is found in cattle and is likely to appear in people who handle carcases, wool, hides, hair, and bone-meal.

The **cutaneous type** is the commonest human variety; the incubation period is from three to four days. The lesion usually commences on an exposed portion of the body, such as the hands, forearms, or face. An itching papule (fig. 36) occurs, around which a patch of induration soon becomes evident. The papule suppurates and is replaced by a black slough, and a ring of vesicles appears on the surrounding indurated area. This stage comprises the typical 'malignant pustule'. A brawny, congested area of induration develops around the site of infection. The regional lymph nodes are involved. Toxaemia is always in evidence. A smear of vesicle fluid is used to confirm the diagnosis by culture and animal inoculation.

Treatment—Penicillin is the treatment of choice.

Prevention.—Must include precautions to sterilise potentially infected animal products and wool from countries where the disease is endemic.

Differential Diagnosis.—The condition is easily mistaken for a severe furuncle (Chapter 30).

Other forms of anthrax are rarely, if ever, now seen, *e.g.* **Woolsorter's Disease**, a pneumonia due to inhalation of spores and an **Alimentary Type**, following ingestion of spores.

Actinomycosis

This disease is caused by *Actinomyces israelii*, an anaerobic Gram-positive branching filamentous organism which sometimes lives as a harmless parasite in the tonsillar crypts and dental cavities of the otherwise normal mouth. It is popularly supposed that it occurs in corn and grasses, but the pathogenic organism does not do so. If the organism invades tissue, it causes a subacute pyogenic inflammation with considerable induration and sinus formation. Trauma and the presence of carious teeth are important predisposing factors in the development of lesions in the mouth. *Diagnosis* depends on finding the organism in pus or in tissue section. Pus should be collected in a sterile tube (a swab is usually insufficient) and inspected in a good light for the presence of pin-head sized 'sulphur granules'. On microscopy the granules are seen to consist of Gram-positive mycelia. The peripheral filaments radiate[1] from the central part of the granule and may be surrounded by Gram-negative tissue clubs.

Culture.—The presence of secondary organisms often makes this difficult.

The lesions are characterised by the formation of a firm, indurated mass, the edges of which are indefinite. Lymph nodes are not affected, but if a vein is invaded, pyaemia is likely.

There are four main clinical forms of actinomycosis:

(i) *Facio-cervical* is the commonest. The lower jaw is more frequently affected, often adjacent to a carious tooth. The gum becomes so indurated that it simulates a bony swelling. Nodules appear, which soften and burst, the overlying skin of the face and neck becomes indurated and bluish in colour, softening occurs in patches. Abscesses burst through the skin and sinuses follow.

(ii) *Thorax.*—The lungs and pleura are infected either by aspiration of the fungus or by direct spread from the pharynx or neck, or even upwards through the diaphragm. The chest wall, in the late stages, becomes riddled with sinuses. An empyema is not uncommon, and the infection can easily spread through the diaphragm to the liver and the subphrenic spaces.

(iii) *Right iliac fossa* (Chapter 50).

(iv) *Liver* (Chapter 45).

Treatment.—Actinomyces is usually sensitive to penicillin, tetracycline and some other antibiotics (*e.g.* Lincomycin), but the sensitivity should be checked in the laboratory. A prolonged intensive course of penicillin (10 mega units reducing to 4 mega units daily) is usually the best treatment until all signs of the disease have disappeared.

Madura Foot (and Hand).—See Chapters 12, 11.

PARASITIC DISEASES

Filariasis.—see Chapter 9.
Hydatid Disease.—see Chapter 45.
Bilharziasis.—see Chapter 58.
Amoebiasis.—see Chapter 50.
Dracunculs mediensis.—see Chapter 8.

VIRUSES

Hepatitis A Virus (HAV).—see Chapter 45.

Hepatitis B Virus (HBV)

This may follow blood transfusion, plasma infusion and, rarely, the administration of sera, infection resembling infective hepatitis except that incubation is about twelve weeks. Transmission by plasma has been reduced by avoiding the pooling of plasma from a large number of donors. Transmission by syringes is prevented if all syringes are disposable. It occurs amongst those who are drug addicts and possibly after tattooing or ear piercing. There is an extremely high rate amongst certain homosexual communities, particularly in Europe and the United States. In certain centres in London and similarly abroad, more than 50% of the male homosexual patients have antibody which affords complete protection and about 5% have the disease. In Athens, a group of prostitutes was found to have a rate twenty times that of married pregnant women, presumably due to more frequent coitus near the period or to other sexually transmitted diseases, producing bleeding that transmits the infection.

Infection with hepatitis B virus is associated with the appearance in the serum of one or more antigens, *viz*: hepatitis B surface antigen (HB_sAg), hepatitis B core antigen (HB_cAg), the Dane particle (probably the complete virus) and DNA polymerase activity. Under electron microscopy, particles can be seen in the sera of these patients and are associated with the virus. These particles are antigenic. Such patients usually suffer the

---

[1] Actinomyces = Ray fungus.

severest form of hepatitis. The antigen is the scourge of renal dialysis and transplantation units, and hospital staff must avoid contact with blood from such patients.

Hepatitis non-A non-B is a variant, with an incubation period similar to HBV, but with milder clinical features.

Human Immunodeficiency Viruses (HIV I and II)—Acquired Immune Deficiency Syndrome (AIDS)

AIDS is caused by retroviruses of the order Lentivirinae discovered in 1983 originally named lymphadenopathy associated virus (LAV) or human T-cell lymphoma virus III (HTLV III) (fig. 37). The syndrome is defined for epidemiological purposes to be a profound cellular immune deficiency causing a variety of opportunistic infections and neoplasias, but is only part of a range of manifestations of infection by the virus. It preferentially infects the T-helper lymphocytes, causing immune depression, and also infects monocytes, lung and nerve cells, the latter leading to acute meningitis/encephalopathy or a variety of chronic syndromes of dementia, ataxia, spinal cord degeneration or peripheral neuropathy. Infection is persistent, probably for life, but many carriers of the virus have no symptoms and may never progress to AIDS.

Spread of Infection.—The virus is present in most body fluids but most importantly in

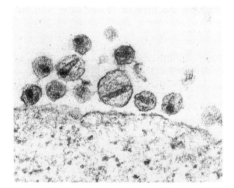

FIG. 37.—The Virus of AIDS.
(Abraham Karpas, Cambridge)

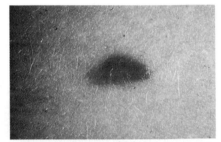

FIG. 38.—A skin lesion of Kaposi's sarcoma.
(John K. Oates, London)

blood and semen. Thus spread is almost entirely by sexual contact, particularly homosexual anal-receptive intercourse, transfusion of infected blood or blood products, and sharing of unsterilised needles and syringes. The fetus of a mother carrying the virus can be infected.

Clinical Features of HIV Infection.—*General.* Infection with the virus causes malaise, weight loss and fevers in up to 30% of individuals, although single or multiple opportunistic infections may also contribute. There is frequently persistent lymphadenopathy and splenomegaly: affected lymph nodes show reactive hyperplasia, but lymphomas are also found. There may be thrombocytopenia. *The chest.* Pneumonia due to *Pneumocystis carinii* is the commonest presentation of AIDS, but Cytomegalovirus and Mycobacteria may be responsible and transbronchial lung biopsy is needed to make a firm diagnosis. *The skin.* Kaposi's sarcoma is the other frequent manifestation of AIDS (fig. 38). It appears as purplish or brown non-pruritic nodules or macules anywhere on the skin or hard palate and is frequently invasive; biopsy shows spindle cells and vascular elements. AIDS can also present with severe necrotizing Herpes simplex. A number of other non-specific skin complaints are common among infected patients, including intertrigo, folliculitis, and eczema. *The gastrointestinal tract.* Persistent diarrhoea can be due to HIV infection alone but Cryptosporidium, Salmonella, Cytomegalovirus and other organisms may be the cause in AIDS. Oral and oesophageal candidiasis may occur. *The nervous system.* In addition to the direct effects of the virus, meningitis may be caused by Cryptococcus and mycobacteria, and parenchymal infection by Toxoplasma, fungi, and Herpes simplex. Cerebral lymphoma and some infections may present as space occupying lesions so CT scanning is advisable before lumbar puncture.

Detection of HIV Infection.—As most carriers are asymptomatic the diagnosis should be considered and actively excluded if the patient is in a risk group (patient or sexual partner homosexual, haemophiliac, intravenous drug abuser, or recently in Central Africa). Antibodies to the virus can be detected by tests of high sensitivity and specificity but no clinically feasible antigen test is available and a negative antibody test may be misleading if taken before seroconversion occurs (usually about 3 weeks after infection but occasionally much longer).

Prevention of Spread.—Surgery in carriers of the virus should be done with precautions suitable for Hepatitis B. Spillages of blood should be cleaned up with dilute hypochlorite, which rapidly inactivates the virus, and contaminated waste disposed of safely. Blood should be taken by experienced staff wearing gloves and using disposable equipment which must be safely discarded. Blood for transfusion should be screened for antibody and persons from risk groups discouraged from donating blood or organs. All specimens must be appropriately labelled to alert all handlers of the material. If these precautions are observed, the risk of infection to health care workers and others seems extremely small, and there is no justification for refusing to operate on such patients.

Treatment of AIDS Sufferers.—Opportunistic infections should be given prompt effective chemotherapy wherever possible, the most successful being cotrimoxazole for Pneumocystis pneumonia. Cytotoxic therapy for tumours has largely been abandoned because of an increased incidence of opportunistic infections. Attempts to reconstitute the immune system have produced only partial and temporary success, and no therapy has been found to control the virus. Therefore until a vaccine has been developed (indeed, vaccines according to type), prevention is all-important.

BASIC IMMUNOLOGY

The Nature of the Immune Response

Micro-organisms invading a normal individual usually pose little or no problem; indeed, the microflora colonising the new-born infant are not even considered as an infection as the event has no pathogenic consequences. This balance between the body and the infectious environment is crucially dependent upon those intangibles we group together as a 'good state of health', including, in this context, the ability to mount a vigorous and effective immune response.

Several factors may influence the vigor or effectiveness of the immune response. The deliberate and generalised immunosuppression used to prevent rejection of foreign organ grafts is probably the most familiar example of a profoundly reduced immune response which can result not only in an increased incidence of infection but also an increased incidence of tumours, in particular, lymphomas. Similarly, severe malnourishment, lymphoproliferative diseases or infection of some patients with HIV I and II (the causative agent of acquired immune deficiency syndrome—AIDS) can also result in severe immunodepression (see above).

It is essential to realise, however, that the sheer complexity of the immune response brings with it in-built homeostatic mechanisms which can often compensate for variations in immune performance. Thus whereas stress, anaesthesia or major surgery can result in a disturbance of immune function, the magnitude or duration of the changes are such that the compensation mechanisms render them unimportant. This is in direct contrast to the factors identified above, which frequently result in severe, life threatening conditions.

Cells in the Immune Response.—Lymphocytes and macrophages form the two basic cellular types which are essential to the many different forms of the immune response identified to date. Although they have profoundly different functions, both cells are equally necessary if the immune response is to be effective.

NORMAL PATHWAYS FOR LYMPHOCYTE DIFFERENTIATION

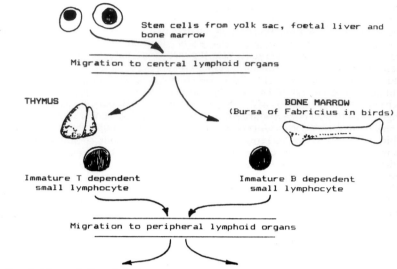

FAILURE OF LYMPHOCYTE DIFFERENTIATION IN IMMUNODEFICIENCY

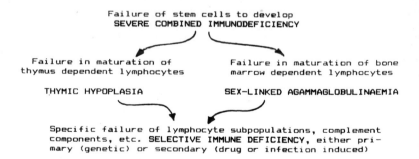

FIG. 39.—Lymphocyte differentiation. The normal pathways for lymphocyte differentiation during ontogeny are well understood, particularly in avian species where there is a separate primary lymphoid organ for T (thymus dependent) and B (bursa dependent) lymphocyte differentiation. In mammals, including man, thymus function is distinct but there is no separate organ for B cell development. This function has been taken over by the bone marrow, which therefore supplies both stem cells and the environment for their differentiation.

A genetic failure early in one of these pathways can result in profound immune deficiency affecting several parts of the immune system. Alternatively, a failure in a later pathway can produce a relatively inconsequential selective deficiency which is well tolerated because of the 'belt and braces' back-up in the immune system. Although cases of primary immune deficiency are relatively rare, secondary immune deficiency (e.g. AIDS) is becoming increasingly common.

Macrophages.—Macrophages and blood monocytes together form the mononuclear phagocyte system which plays a major role in the phagocytosis and destruction of invading micro-organisms. Other macrophages have less well developed microbicidal killing systems and are responsible for antigen presentation to T and B lymphocytes.

Lymphocytes arise from haemopoetic stem cells which grow in the thymus or bone marrow during the perinatal period. Although at this stage the lymphocytes are immature and unable to support an immune response, they soon mature as they migrate via the blood to the peripheral lymphoid organs (spleen, lymph nodes, gut associated lymphoid tissue, etc.). The mature lymphoid system consists of an enormous number of lymphocytes (about 10^{12}), many of which spend their time endlessly circulating from blood to spleen, to lymph nodes or into non-lymphoid extra vascular spaces and then back into the blood via the lymph channels. These lymphocytes have a morphology which closely resembles that seen in a typical blood film; they are small, non-dividing mononuclear cells which apparently spend most of their time doing nothing. However, this whole impression changes dramatically once a lymphocyte contacts its specific antigen.

Antigens and lymphocytes.—An antigen may be considered as any foreign molecule which can bind to a lymphocyte and cause it to respond by expressing its predetermined function. This will happen even if the same antigen is part of a micro-organism in a natural infection, in a dead or attenuated vaccine or even a totally synthetic molecule produced, for example, by genetic engineering. Provided the antigen can bind to its *specific* lymphocyte, the end result is the same.

We each have the ability to recognise up to about 10^8 different antigens, which is apparently enough to cope effectively with our antigenic universe as evidenced by our survival. Considering the total number of lymphocytes (about 10^{12}) it will be obvious that we each start with about 10,000 lymphocytes for each *different* antigenic determinant. Contact with foreign antigens, for example in the form of a measles vaccine or infection, will specifically select those pre-existing lymphocytes to which the measles antigens bind, causing them to divide and change their function. The increased frequency of measles-specific lymphocytes produced by cell division means that the immune system is then better able to cope upon a second contact with the same infection or antigen. By this means lymphocyte based immune responses have a capacity for specific memory.

Two types of lymphocytes.—Lymphocytes which grow up in the thymus (*thymus dependent or T lymphocytes*) are functionally distinct from those which grow up in the bone marrow (*bone marrow dependent or B lymphocytes*). These differentiation pathways are shown in fig. 39.

Upon contact with antigen, small B lymphocytes change to dividing blast-like cells which then either (*a*) revert to small lymphocytes and are responsible for memory or (*b*) change further to become plasma cells, which then produce and secrete antibody into the blood and body fluids. Significantly, the secreted antibody binds to exactly the same antigens responsible for stimulating the original set of B lymphocytes.

Antibody molecules all share the same general protein structure and so are grouped together under the chemical name of immunoglobulin (Ig as standard abbreviation). There are different classes of immunoglobulin, which are found in different parts of the body and have very different biological roles (summarized in the Table with fig. 40).

The production of antibody is the first step in the expression of humoral immunity. Thereafter, depending on the type and location of the antigen, other secondary effects of antigen-antibody binding may be activated. IgM and IgG combined with antigen are especially effective at 'fixing' complement leading to cytolysis if the antigen is cell associated or promotion of phagocytosis in the case of antigens on micro-organisms.

T lymphocytes never produce antibody. Instead they produce their specific immune effect by direct contact between cell and antigen. Antigenic stimulation of T lymphocytes also results in the accumulation of memory cells, thus accounting for the accelerated rejection of a second allograft provided it has similar antigenic characteristics to those of an earlier graft.

Functional types of T lymphocytes.—T lymphocytes have a dual role in the immune response as they serve both to control the pace of response (immune regulation) as well as providing their own specialised effector functions (fig. 41). For example, the fine tuning of B lymphocyte stimulation by antigen is provided by T helper lymphocytes (Th) which act to increase the efficacy of stimulation, whereas a separate subset of T suppressor lymphocytes (Ts) can act to turn off the response to the same antigen. The effector functions of T lymphocytes, expressed during cell mediated immunity, are mediated by cytotoxic T lymphocytes (Tc) which are able to kill allogeneic or virus infected cells and other T lymphocytes which secrete biologically active molecules (lymphokines) which modulate the function of both lymphocytes and phagocytic cells.

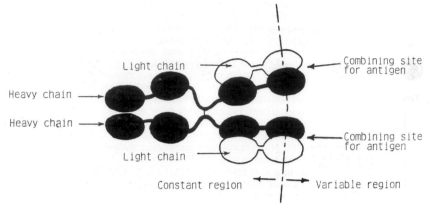

FIG. 40.—Generalised structure of an immunoglobulin subunit.

The variable regions of the light and heavy chains determine the shape of the combining site for antigen, whereas the constant region determines the biological role of the immunoglobulin (Ig) class, *e.g.* ability to fix complement, cross the placenta, etc.

TABLE.—Immunoglobulin classes—structure and function.

IgM	Large molecule of 5 basic subunits. Efficient at combating intravascular micro-organisms either by neutralisation or by promotion of phagocytosis after complement fixation. Monomeric form in B lymphocyte membrane serves as antigen receptor
IgG	Small molecule of single subunit, which penetrates tissues efficiently. Is only Ig class to cross placenta to protect the neonate. Promotes phagocytosis of micro-organisms.
IgA	Major immunoglobulin in sero-mucous secretions, thus has important role in protecting body surfaces against 'attack' by micro-organisms. Molecule consists of 2 subunits stabilised by a secretory piece which protects against proteolytic enzymes in secretions.
IgD	Little free in serum. Membrane bound on B lymphocytes where it probably acts as a receptor for antigen.
IgE	Binds strongly to receptor sites on mast cells and basophils. Combination with antigen results in cell degranulation, thus causing symptoms of atopic allergy. Probably important in immunity to intestinal helminths.

Consequences of immunosuppression.—Accumulating evidence suggests that several viral infections can be immunosuppressive, most dramatically following HIV infection where the Th lymphocytes are almost absent in AIDS victims. Although exotic or opportunistic infections are common in these patients, the same is not true of transplant recipients given immunosuppressive therapy. Immediately post operation severe opportunistic infection is virtually unknown, the major problems being restricted to surgical wounds and post-operative lung infections. Thereafter cytomegalovirus (CMV) is the most important infectious agent complicating the course of recovery. Kidney transplant centres report figures of between 60 and 90% of their patients showing the broad range of clinical effects attributable to the virus. Furthermore, it is clear that CMV infection predisposes to bacterial, fungal and protozoal superinfection. Therefore, it is important to monitor continuously the level of immunosuppressive therapy in order to strike a balance between graft rejection and total immunological paralysis.

FUNCTIONAL SUB-SETS OF LYMPHOCYTES

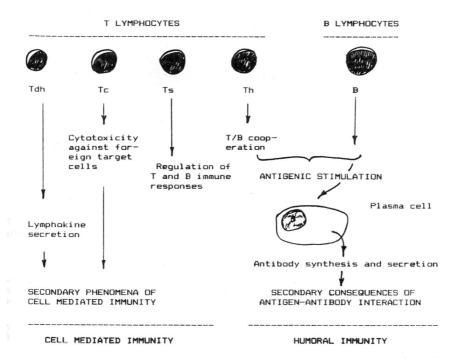

FIG. 41.—Lymphocytes in the immune response. Several of the functional sub-populations of T lymphocytes can be mediated by cells in the same lineage and expressing the cell surface phenotype as detected by monoclonal antibody markers. B lymphocytes also comprise at least 5 functional sub-sets, based on the 5 classes of immunoglobulin.

Amyloid Disease

Amyloid Disease primary or secondary[1]. The primary form is either idiopathic or a complication of multiple myelomatosis. The secondary form may be seen in cases of chronic osteomyelitis, bronchiectasis, tuberculosis, rheumatoid arthritis and lepromatous leprosy. Abnormal protein, related to immunoglobulins and lymphocytes, is deposited in the walls of the arterioles and later in the larger vessels. Microscopically, congo-red stains the infiltrated tissues. The kidneys, intestine, liver, and spleen are specially affected. Polyuria occurs due to infiltration of the glomeruli of the kidneys. Diarrhoea ensues owing to infiltration of the mucosal villi. The spleen and liver become enlarged and palpable. The diagnosis can be made on rectal biopsy—a simple, safe and reliable method. If the source of the infection can be eradicated, early amyloid will resolve. Amyloid material is also found in the medullary carcinoma of the thyroid (Chapter 37).

---

[1] It is most important to bear in mind that this degeneration is a possibility in anyone who has prolonged suppuration from whatever cause.

CHAPTER 5

HAEMORRHAGE. SHOCK. BLOOD TRANSFUSION. ANALGESIA

HAEMORRHAGE

Classification of Haemorrhage

1. **Arterial haemorrhage** is recognised as bright red blood, spurting as a jet which rises and falls in time with the pulse. In protracted bleeding, and when quantities of intravenous fluids other than blood are given, it can become watery in appearance.

2. **Venous haemorrhage** is a darker red, a steady and copious flow. The colour darkens still further from excessive oxygen desaturation when blood loss is severe, or in respiratory depression or obstruction.[1] Blood loss is particularly rapid when large veins are opened (*e.g.* common femoral, jugular).

Venous bleeding can be under increased pressure as in asphyxia, or from ruptured varicose veins (Chapter 13). Also portal vein pressures (Chapter 41) are high enough to cause rapid blood loss, especially in portal hypertension with oesophageal varices. Pulmonary artery haemorrhage is dark red (venous blood) at around 30 mmHg[2] ($\approx$ 4kPa), whereas bleeding from the pulmonary veins is bright red.

3. **Capillary haemorrhage** is a bright red, often rapid ooze. If continuing for many hours blood loss can become serious (as in haemophilia, p. 74).

4. **Primary haemorrhage** is that which occurs at the time of injury or operation.

5. **Reactionary haemorrhage** may follow primary haemorrhage within 24 hours (usually 4–6 hours) and is mainly due to rolling ('slipping') of a ligature, dislodgement of a clot, or cessation of reflex vasospasm. The precipitating circumstances are (a) the rise of blood pressure and the refilling of the venous system on recovery from shock, (b) restlessness, coughing and vomiting which raise the venous pressure (*e.g.* reactionary venous haemorrhage within a few hours of thyroidectomy).

Venous haemorrhage, whether primary or reactionary, can tax the skill of even an experienced surgeon for it may be exceedingly difficult to bring under control (Chapter 13). Penetrating wounds involving main veins in the thigh or groin are potentially fatal, as exsanguination may follow the removal of a first-aid dressing which has apparently controlled the bleeding (butcher's thigh, Chapter 14). Such a wound should never be treated in a perfunctory manner; it requires careful examination and closure in an operating theatre.

6. **Secondary haemorrhage** occurs after 7–14 days, and is due to infection and sloughing of part of the wall of an artery. Predisposing factors are pressure

---

[1] Occasionally dark blood is due to the presence of sulph- or met-haemoglobin.
[2] 1 mmHg $\approx$ 133 Pascals in the S.I. system.

of a drainage tube, a fragment of bone, a ligature in an infected area, or cancer. It is also a complication of arterial surgery and amputations. It is heralded by 'warning' haemorrhages, which are bright red stains on the dressing, followed by a sudden severe haemorrhage which may be fatal. A warning haematemesis may occur in the case of a peptic ulcer and is a danger signal which it is imprudent to ignore. In advanced cancer the erosion of a main vessel (*e.g.* carotid, uterine) by a locally ulcerating growth becomes the way of a swift and merciful termination to the patient's suffering. Secondary haemorrhage is prone to occur with ano-rectal wounds, e.g. after haemorrhoidectomy.

7. **External haemorrhage** is visible, *revealed haemorrhage.*

8. **Internal haemorrhage** is invisible, *concealed haemorrhage.* Internal bleeding may be *concealed* as in ruptured spleen or liver, fractured femur, ruptured ectopic gestation, or in cerebral haemorrhage. Concealed haemorrhage may become *revealed* as in haematemesis or melaena from a bleeding peptic ulcer, as in haematuria from a ruptured kidney, or via the vagina in accidental uterine haemorrhage of pregnancy.

Clinical features and Measurement of Acute Blood Loss

Beside visible blood loss the signs of continuing acute blood loss include *increasing pallor, increasing pulse rate, restlessness*, and in protracted bleeding, deep sighing respirations (*air hunger*). These signs are accompanied by a cold and clammy skin, empty veins, and later, by thirst, tinnitus and blindness (see also shock (p. 61) pathophysiology (p. 63) and fig. 42).

The Pulse Rate, the Blood Pressure and the Pulse Pressure.—Record keeping is essential, and is made at ¼ or ½ hourly intervals during an emergency and thereafter 4-hourly. It must be remembered that a *falling blood pressure* is not necessarily a feature of acute blood loss. A normal or slightly raised pressure can be recorded in otherwise fit individuals in the face of the signs of haemorrhage, and reliance on the reading can lead to a sense of false security, for collapse and death can occur suddenly.[1] *The pulse pressure* (systolic minus the diastolic pressure) is a measure of the stroke volume of the left heart. For example, if the pulse rate is not increased and the pulse pressure is low, the cardiac output is reduced. Measuring the pulse pressure is a good way of expressing numerically what a trained observer can feel in the pulse (using terms like 'thready pulse', 'low volume pulse').

Urine Output.—The measurement and recording of urine output is always mandatory in the management of all patients suffering from haemorrhage and shock (see Pathophysiology p. 63, and Clinical monitoring of shock p. 65).

Measuring Blood Loss.—(*a*) *Blood Clot.*—Blood clot the size of a clenched fist is roughly equal to 500 ml.

(*b*) *Swelling in Closed Fractures.*—Moderate swelling in closed fracture of the tibia equals 500–1500 ml blood loss. Moderate swelling in a fractured shaft of femur equals 500–2000 ml blood loss (Ruscoe Clarke).

(*c*) *Swab Weighing.*—In the operating theatre, blood loss can be measured by

---

[1] This phenomenon was reported during research at the front in World War I (1914–1918).

Alan Ruscoe Clarke, 1908–1959. Surgeon, Birmingham Accident Hospital, Birmingham, England.

weighing the swabs before and after use and adding the total so obtained
1 g = 1 ml) to the volume of blood collected in the suction or drainage bottles.
In extensive wounds and operations, the blood loss estimated in this way is much
less than the total amount of blood, plasma and water actually lost from the
vascular system because of 'loss' into the tissues, by evaporation of sweat from
the skin, water via the lungs and from the wound itself, accounting for at least
an additional 20%. Indeed, for operations such as radical mastectomy or partial
gastrectomy it is necessary to multiply the swab weighing total by a factor 1½.[1]
For larger wounds, as in abdominothoracic or abdominoperineal operations, the
total measured should be multiplied by 2.

Haemoglobin level.—This is estimated in g/100 ml (g/dl), normal values being
12–16 g/100 ml (12–16 g/dl). There is no immediate change in haemorrhage, but
within the space of a few hours the level is lowered by the haemodilution caused
by the movement of tissue fluid into the vascular compartment in order to restore
the blood volume. The degree of dilution can be gauged by the haematocrit
reading (P.C.V.) (fig. 42).

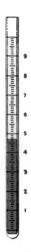

FIG. 42.—A haematrocrit is a stout glass tube 110 mm long with a 2·5–3·00 mm bore
and it is graduated 0–100. It is filled up to the 100 mark with a small quantity (about
0·8 ml) of oxalated or heparinised freshly drawn blood, and centrifuged at 2000–2300 g
for 15–20 minutes. The packed cell volume (P.C.V.) is read from the millimetre
reading gradations. The normal range for venous blood is: men, 40–56%; women,
35–48%; children, 32–44%. The P.C.V. can also be measured on capillary blood, using
very small amounts, in the microhaematocrit centrifuge. Some hours after the start of
haemorrhage, the P.C.V. will be lowered by haemodilution. In dehydration states and
the plasma loss in burns, the P.C.V. will be increased (haemoconcentration).

Blood Volume Determinations.—Either the volume of circulating plasma, or the volume occupied by the red cells, must be measured first. The haematocit reading will give
the ratio of plasma to red cells, and thus the total blood volume can be arrived at. The
normal blood volume is 70–85 ml of whole blood per kilogram body weight, or 35–50 ml
plasma/kg. Thus it varies between a few hundred ml in a neonate, up to 5–6 litres in an
adult (more in certain pathological conditions, *e.g.* high output cardiac failure from
chronic anaemia or arteriovenous fistula).

Measurement of Central Venous Pressure (CVP) see p. 66 and figs 44, 45
and 46. This has replaced clinical observations in many procedures involving
severe blood loss, e.g. cardiac or arterial operations.

The Treatment of Haemorrhage

 1. Stop the blood loss by (a) Pressure and Packing. (b) Position and Rest.
    (c) Procedure (Ligation, Repair, Excision).

---

[1] These important factors (Rains factors) were established in a series comparing swab-weighing
with the measurement of blood volume.

2. Restore blood volume by—Blood Transfusion (page 69). Albumin 4·5% (page 71). SAG-M blood (page 71). Saline, Gelatin, Dextran, Plasma Infusions (pages 71 and 75).

1(a) **Pressure and Packing.**—*The first-aid* treatment of haemorrhage from a wound is a pressure dressing made from anything handy which is soft and clean (linen) (even a rolled up forage cap stuffed into a wound has been effective in battle (Drummond)). The dressing or pack should be bound on tightly.

Other examples of pressure used to control haemorrhage include digital pressure, *e.g.*, the use of forefinger and thumb or a clothes-peg for epistaxis (Chapter 33). The use of a double balloon in the oesophagus and the stomach to control the bleeding from oesophageal varices (Chapter 45) is another example of pressure being applied.

Packing by means of rolls of wide gauze is an important standby in operative surgery. If several rolls are used the ends must be tied together to ensure complete removal later.

N.B.—If on removal of pressure or packing, bleeding appears to have ceased completely, one should not assume that all is well, especially when dealing with deep wounds involving large veins. Continued close observation is required and rapid operative action may be called for.

Tourniquets are to be avoided in *first aid*. They can only be used around the thigh or upper arm; they are difficult to apply tightly enough to interrupt arterial blood flow, and may only cause venous congestion and increased blood loss. There have been many examples of tourniquets of some kind being used for ruptured varicose veins causing exsanguination by only occluding venous return. (For example, a policeman was brought into a casualty department with seven tourniquets in place. The venous bleeding ceased as soon as they were removed!—such examples are still being encountered.) Tourniquets tight enough to obstruct arterial flow may cause contusion of the artery wall and thrombosis, especially if atheroma is present. Nerve conduction can also be seriously impaired, while to leave a tourniquet on for over an hour is to invite muscle death and the risk of renal failure (crush syndrome, p. 69). To sum up, it can be said that tourniquets are potentially dangerous because they may be applied too loosely, too tightly, or for too long.

In the operating theatre tourniquets are used (a) to control haemorrhage temporarily while exploration and repair are being carried out: (b) for some amputations (not for atherosclerotic gangrene); (c) in order to obtain a bloodless field for orthopaedic and soft tissue operations (cartilage, tendon, nerves, ganglia of tendon sheaths). The sphygmomanometer cuff is satisfactory as a pneumatic tourniquet, the cuff being inflated after elevation of the limb for five minues to reduce the vascularity. Alternatively, a bloodless operation field can be obtained by an Esmarch bandage applied spirally to the elevated limb commencing distally, and then wound on tightly. The distal spirals are unwound to expose the limb for operation.

Removal of a Tourniquet.—When a tourniquet is in place the time of application must be written large on the theatre blackboard and deleted only when it is removed. It is a wise precaution to attach the tourniquet to the operating table, so that it cannot be overlooked when the patient is lifted on to the trolley.

Venous Tourniquet.—A light rubber or a pneumatic tourniquet is applied to the upper arm prior to intravenous injections and sampling. It is also used in the diagnosis of varicose veins (Chapter 13).

1(b) **Position and Rest.**—*Elevation of limbs e.g.* in ruptured varicose veins, employs gravity to reduce bleeding. Elevation also causes helpful vasoconstriction (Lister). *A bed elevator* is often used to raise the foot of the bed as an aid to vasoconstriction for reducing the size of the vascular compartment, so facilitating blood flow to the brain and the restoration of a satisfactory blood pressure.

Sir William Alexander Duncan Drummond, Contemporary. Formerly Director-General, Army Medical Service (1956–1961).
Johann Friedrich August von Esmarch, 1823–1908. Professor of Surgery, Kiel, Germany (1857–1899). Developed the 'Esmarch Bandage' whilst working as a Military Surgeon during the Franco-Prussian War (1870–1871), and reported on its use in 1873.
Joseph Lister (Lord Lister), 1827–1912 (see footnote, p. 1).

Gravity is also used in certain operations, as in thyroidectomy when the patient is tilted feet downwards (anti-Trendelenburg position) or as in stripping of varicose veins when a head-down tilt is used (Trendelenburg).

In the ward as well as in the theatre, Esmarch bandages may be applied temporarily to the limbs in order to reduce the vascular compartment in shock.

Absolute rest is vital. This means nursing the patient in a comfortable recumbent position, and he should be relieved of unnecessary exertion. He does not wash or feed himself, and assistance is given for turning in bed, which must be at least two-hourly to prevent pressure sores.

Analgesia facilitates rest. Morphine (10–20 mg) relieves pain, calms restlessness, and aids coronary and cerebral blood flow. Its use is contraindicated where there is respiratory depression (as in head injuries) and in the very young and very old, when pethidine may be preferred. Morphine is best given intramuscularly, or intravenously in haemorrhage and shock. A subcutaneous dose is not easily absorbed because of vasoconstriction, and if repeated doses are given in this way an excessive amount is liable to be absorbed when the circulation improves. Morphine does not in itself produce sleep, and the patient, though relieved of pain, may remain wakeful and anxious. To induce sleep temazepam, a short acting 'non-hangover' benzodiazepam, may be used, otherwise chloral hydrate.

1(c) **Examples of Operative Techniques in Haemorrhage.**—Artery forceps ('haemostats') and clips are mechanical means of controlling bleeding by pressure. The clamped vessel can be ligated with catgut, cotton, thread or silk, or it can be coagulated with diathermy. When an incision is made through the scalp for craniotomy, the profuse bleeding is not easily arrested by direct forcipressure, so the cranial aponeurosis is picked up by a series of forceps which are everted together, thus exerting pressure. Silver clips (Cushing) may be applied to cerebral vessels.

Suturing may be employed. The vessel can be underrun or transfixed by needle and suture and then ligated, while if the continuty of a main vessel is to be restored, 4/0 silk or polypropylene is used (Chapter 14) on a 20 mm atraumatic needle.

Pressure by packing, using rolls of wide gauze has been previously mentioned, but temporary light pressure with a 'peanut' of gauze held by forceps aids the sealing of an arterial suture line after reconstruction following trauma, embolectomy, or in artery grafting. About five minutes is required for the platelets to seal the join.

Patches of vein or Dacron mesh may be used to repair a vascular defect. A patch of muscle, lightly hammered, provides thrombokinase to stop a troublesome ooze.

Other topical applications for oozing include gauze or sponge which is absorbed by the body. 'Oxycel' or gelatin sponge provides a network upon which fibrin and platelets can be deposited. This is the modern counterpart of the use of cobwebs by our forefathers, or sphagnum moss by our neolithic ancestors. Gauze soaked in adrenalin soln. (1:1000) or, for the person with a normal haemostatic mechanism, 'Stypven' (Russell viper venom) can be applied. Bone wax (Horsley) is used for oozing bone.

The whole or part of a bleeding viscus may have to be excised, *e.g.* splenectomy, partial hepatectomy. A ruptured kidney is treated conservatively if possible (Chapter 57).

2. **Restoration of Blood Volume.**—Blood Transfusion see p. 69, Infusions see p. 75.

Natural Blood Volume and Red Cell Recovery.—The recovery of blood volume begins immediately by the withdrawal of fluid from the tissues into the circulation. There is haemodilution. Plasma proteins are replaced by the liver. Red cell recovery takes some five to six weeks. The iron content will be less than normal if stores are depleted or absorption is impaired (*e.g.* after gastrectomy, Chapter 44).

Chronic Haemorrhage.—Examples of causes in surgical practice are bleeding haemorrhoids, fibroids, carcinoma of the caecum, peptic ulcer. There is no diminution of the

Friedrich Trendelenburg, 1844–1924. Professor of Surgery, Rostock (1875–1882), Bonn (1882–1895), and Leipzig (1895–1911). The Trendelenburg Position was first described in 1885.
Harvey Williams Cushing, 1869–1939. Professor of Surgery, Johns Hopkins University, Baltimore, Maryland, U.S.A. (1903–1912), and Harvard Medical School, Boston, Massachusetts U.S.A. (1912–1932).
Patrick Russell, 1727–1805. Physician who practised for a time at Aleppo, Syria, and later became naturalist to the East India Company. He produced a memoir on Poisonous Snakes in 1787.
Sir Victor Alexander Haden Horsley, 1857–1916. Surgeon, University College Hospital, London. Horsley's Wax consists of seven parts of Beeswax to one part of Almond Oil. (Died of heatstroke or paratyphoid fever in Mesopotamia. One of the original Authors (McN. L.) attended his funeral.)

blood volume as there is time for plasma replacement, but red cell replacement lags behind (microcytic hypocromic anaemia) resulting in a state of anaemic hypoxia, requiring an increased cardiac output. These patients develop high-output cardiac failure; they must not be transfused with normal blood, but require packed cells instead. Acute haemorrhage in such cases is poorly compensated, as oxygen carriage is already depleted.

SHOCK

Shock is a life-threatening situation. In most cases it is due to poor tissue perfusion with impaired cellular metabolism, manifested in turn by serious pathophysiological abnormalities.

Types of Shock

While there is some practical wisdom in the saying 'shock means haemorrhage, and haemorrhage means shock', there are other causes of shock with different features:

Vasovagal Shock is brought about by pooling of blood in larger vascular reservoirs (limb muscles) and by dilatation of the splanchnic arteriolar bed, causing reduced venous return to the heart, low cardiac output and bradycardia. Consequently the reduced cerebral perfusion causes cerebral hypoxia and unconsciousness, but prostration and reflex vasoconstriction so increases the venous return and cardiac output as to restore cerebral perfusion and consciousness. It must be remembered that if the patient is maintained in an upright or sitting position (*e.g.* in a dental chair) permanent cerebral damage will occur.

Psychogenic Shock immediately follows a sudden fright (bad news), or accompanies severe pain (a blow to the testes) and the effect varies in intensity from a slight faint to sudden death. The expression 'I nearly died of fright' is not necessarily hyperbolical.

Neurogenic Shock is caused by traumatic or pharmacological blockade of the sympathetic nervous system, producing dilatation of resistance arterioles and capacitance veins (see below) leading to relative hypovolaemia and hypotension. There is a low blood pressure, a normal or increased cardiac output, a normal pulse rate and a warm dry skin. Trauma to the spinal cord and spinal anaesthesia lead to a systolic pressure of around 70 mmHg which may be corrected by putting the patient in the Trendelenburg position, the rapid administration of fluids and/or a vasopressor drug.

Hypovolaemic Shock is due to loss of intravascular volume by haemorrhage, dehydration, vomiting and diarrhoea (cholera, acute enterocolitis). Until 10–15% blood volume is lost, the cardiac output is maintained by tachycardia and vasoconstriction. Fluid moves into the intravascular space from the interstitial space—a 'transcapillary refill' which may exceed 1 litre in an hour in injured but otherwise fit patients. Also the venous capacitance vessels constrict, pushing blood into the arterial system and therefore compensating for the volume deficit without hypotension.

Traumatic Shock is due primarily to hypovolaemia from bleeding externally (open wounds), from bleeding internally (torn vessels in the mediastinal or peritoneal cavities, ruptured organs such as liver and spleen, fractured bones), or by fluid loss into contused tissue or into distended bowel. Also contusion to the heart itself may cause pump failure and shock, while damage to the nervous system or to the respiratory system results in hypoxia.

Burns Shock occurs as a result of rapid plasma loss from the damaged tissues, causing hypovolaemia. When 25% or more of the body surface area is burnt a generalised capillary leakage may result in gross hypovolaemia in the first 24 hours. Endotoxaemia due to infection makes matters worse and large volumes of colloidal and crystalloid fluids are required for resuscitation (p. 75).

Cardiogenic Shock occurs when more than 50% of the wall of the left ventricle is damaged by infarction. Fluid overload, particularly when using colloids can lead to overdistension of the left ventricle with pump failure. The resultant high filling pressures exerted by the right ventricle make fluid leak out of the pulmonary capillaries thereby causing pulmonary oedema and hypoxia. And should arrhythmias occur, they will also reduce the pumping efficiency of the heart, while hypovolaemia from excess sweating, vomiting, diarrhoea will further diminish cardiac output.

Acute Massive Pulmonary Embolism from a thrombus originating in a deep vein, or an air embolus (more than 50 ml), if obstructing more than 50% of the pulmonary vasculature will cause acute right ventricular failure. This greatly reduces venous return to the left ventricle and cardiac output falls catastrophically causing sudden death or severe shock.

Septic (Endotoxic) Shock.—(*a*) *Hyperdynamic (Warm) Septic Shock* occurs in serious gram-negative infections (Chapter 3), *e.g.* from strangulated intestine, peritonitis, leaking oesophageal or intestinal anastomoses, suppurative biliary conditions. At first the patient has a normal or increased cardiac output with tachycardia and a warm dry skin, but the blood is shunted past the tissue cells which become damaged by anaerobic metabolism (lactic acidosis). The capillary membranes start to leak and endotoxin is absorbed into the blood stream leading to a generalised systemic inflammatory state. The immediate and ready treatment of the cause including the drainage of pus is vital to the recovery of the patient at this stage (in strangulated hernia 'the danger is in the delay, not in the operation').

(*b*) *Hypovolaemic Hypodynamic (Cold) Septic Shock* follows if severe sepsis or endotoxaemia is allowed to persist. Generalised capillary leakage and other fluid losses lead to severe hypovolaemia with reduced cardiac output, tachycardia and vasoconstriction. The systemic infection induces cardiac depression, pulmonary hypertension, pulmonary oedema and hypoxia which in turn reduces cardiac output still further. The patient becomes cold, clammy, drowsy, and tachypnoeic, but still can be converted to hyperdynamic (warm) shock by the administration of several litres of plasma or other colloidal solution. The similar use of crystalloid solutions may give rise to systemic and pulmonary oedema with hypoxia but is better than nothing.

Anaphylactic Shock. Penicillin administration is amongst the common causes of anaphylaxis. Other causes include anaesthetics, dextrans, serum injections stings and the consumption of shellfish. The antigen combines with IgE on the mast cells and basophils, releasing large amounts of histamine and SRS-A (Slow Release Substance-Anaphylaxis). These compounds cause bronchospasm, laryngeal oedema, and respiratory distress with hypoxia, massive vasodilatation, hypotension and shock. The mortality is around 10%.

Notes on terms used

Resistance arterioles are the small calibre vessels 0·02–0·05 mm diameter containing abundant smooth muscle in their walls, the tone of which is controlled by local humoral factors and the sympathetic nerve fibres. The calibre of these small vessels gives rise to the peripheral vascular resistance, controlling blood pressure and blood flow through the capillary beds. The larger arteries merely serve to supply the arterioles with blood.

Capacitance veins comprise the entire venous network from the post-capillary venules to the large calibre veins in limbs, abdomen and thorax and which normally contain 70% of the circulating blood volume. Although thin-walled with relatively little smooth muscle, sympathetic nerve stimulation contracts them, reducing their diameter and emptying the blood into the arterial side of the circulation.

A colloidal solution is one in which the majority of solute particles have a molecular weight greater than 30,000. The term includes all plasma solutions (p. 71), including Human Plasma Protein Fraction (HPPF), dextrans, gelatin (*e.g.* Haemaccel®), and hydroxyethyl starch. Blood is not usually included in this term.

Minute volume ventilation is the volume of air (or oxygen) which enters the patient's lungs in one (each) minute, and is the product of respiratory rate and tidal volume.

Hyperventilation occurs when the patient is 'overbreathing' due to pain, anxiety or shock, such that the arterial carbon dioxide tension ($PaCO_2$) is lowered from the normal 40 mmHg (5·5 kPa).

Aspects of the Pathophysiology of Haemorrhage and Shock

Low cardiac output is an early feature in shock, except warm septic shock and neurogenic shock. Vasoconstriction occurs in an attempt to maintain perfusion pressures to the vital organs such as the brain, liver and kidneys as well as the heart muscle itself. Venoconstriction pushes more blood into the dynamic circulation whilst tachycardia helps to maintain a flagging cardiac output. The minute ventilation rises 1½–2 times and the respiratory rate 2–3 times maintaining oxygenation (except in cardiogenic shock with pulmonary oedema). The renal blood flow is reduced with consequent reduction of glomerular filtration and urine output. The renin/angiotensin mechanism is activated with further vasoconstriction and aldosterone release, causing salt and water retention. Release of antidiuretic hormone (ADH) decreases the volume and increases the concentration of urine. However in early sepsis the patient though hypovolaemic may produce inappropriately large amounts of dilute urine (see below).

As cardiac output falls, the hypotension and tachycardia cause poor perfusion of the coronary arteries, and this, in conjunction with hypoxia, metabolic acidosis and the release of specific cardiac depressants (endotoxaemia, pancreatitis) causes yet further cardiac depression and pump failure, a vicious circle indeed.

The cells become starved of oxygen and anaerobic metabolism leads to lactic acidosis. Eventually the cell membranes cannot pump sodium out of the cells; sodium enters the cells and potassium leaks out (an old axiom—'sodium stays, potassium flees'). Thus the serum potassium is elevated. Calcium, however, leaks into the cells, lowering the serum calcium. Furthermore, the intracellular lysosomes break down and release powerful enzymes causing further damage. The cells are sick = '*the sick cell syndrome*'.

The platelets are activated in shock due to the stagnation of blood in the capillaries. Blood sludging with red cell aggregation may progress to the formation of small clots and indeed to disseminated intravascular coagulation (DIC) (p. 74). Several coagulation factors are consumed (platelets, fibrinogen, factor V, factor VIII, prothrombin), and troublesome bleeding may occur from needle puncture sites, wound edges and mucosal surfaces.

Diagnostic Difficulties

The prognosis of a shocked patient is related to the *duration* and *degree* of the shocked state,[1] therefore prompt diagnosis of the type of shock is essential. But

---

[1]For example, acute renal failure can occur immediately following a shortlived episode of profound shock.

because of a thready and irregular pulse, the measurement of the blood pressure with a standard sphygmomanometer can be inaccurate and misleading. Doppler pressure monitoring may be adopted, and, if skilled hands are available, intra-arterial pressure monitoring should be considered. The E.C.G. should be monitored, and it will help to differentiate cardiogenic shock from other types, and will reveal the nature of the many arrhythmias that may occur. A chest x-ray may differentiate between pulmonary embolism, mediastinal trauma and tamponade.

The measurement of Central Venous Pressure (CVP) (p. 66) and its response to a small fluid challenge (200 ml) may assist in distinguishing between cardiogenic shock and hypovolaemic shock, but it must be emphasised that in the seriously ill patient the CVP is not a reliable indicator of left ventricular function because of the wide disparity that can exist between the left and the right ventricular functions.

The Pulmonary Capillary Wedge Pressure (PCWP). A better indicator of both circulating blood volume and left ventricular function is the Pulmonary Capillary Wedge Pressure (PCWP) obtained by a pulmonary artery flotation balloon catheter (fig. 43) (Swan Ganz®). This can be used to differentiate between left and right ventricular failure, pulmonary embolus, septic shock and ruptured mitral valve, and can also be an accurate guide to therapy with fluids, inotropic agents and vasodilators. It may also be used to measure cardiac output by a thermodilution technique simply at the bedside.

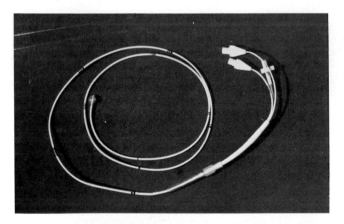

Fig. 43.—Swan Ganz triple channel catheter. Beside the lumen for balloon inflation, with locking 'gate' to prevent deflation, this type includes an extra channel for proximal pressure monitoring. Another type includes a thermistor wire for computing cardiac output. Marks are at 10 cm intervals from the tip.

Pulmonary Capillary Wedge Pressure measurement.—This is a specialised procedure requiring supervised training, practice, patience and experience in interpreting the values measured and waveforms indicated. The complications may include arrhythmias, pulmonary infarction, pulmonary artery rupture, balloon rupture and catheter knotting, in addition to the complications from central venous cannulation. The catheter should not be left *in situ* for more than 72 hours; if further haemodynamic monitoring is required, a new catheter should be inserted.

Method.—Strict aseptic central venous cannulation is performed (*e.g.* via Rt internal jugular vein, p. 66) and using the appropriate introducers, cannula and guide wire, the catheter, flushed with and wiped with heparin saline, is introduced into the right atrium. The balloon, inflated with 1·5 ml air is advanced slowly via the right ventricle into the pulmonary artery, checked by x-ray, and monitored by pressure tracing which becomes characteristically flat when the balloon wedges in a small branch, to give the capillary

H. J. C. Swan M.D. Contemporary. Professor of Medicine, UCLA School of Medicine, Director of Cardiology, Cedars Sinai Medical Center.
William Ganz, M.D. Contemporary. Professor of Medicine, UCLA School of Medicine, Senior Research Scientist, Cedars Sinai Medical Center, Los Angeles, U.S.A.

pressure (indicating left atrial pressure). With the balloon deflated the pulmonary artery pressure is obtained. The balloon must *never* be reinflated in the absence of a normal pulmonary artery wave-form as this means that the tip alone is wedged and reinflation might therefore rupture the pulmonary artery. Withdrawal 2–3 cm is mandatory until the wave form reappears and reinflation can be permitted.

The transducer should be placed at the mid-axillary point (zero reference point); the normal P.C.W.P. is between 8 and 12 mmHg ($10 \cdot 5$ and $15 \cdot 5$ cm H_2O) and normal pulmonary artery pressure is 25 mmHg systolic and 10 mmHg diastolic.

Clinical Decision.—With intra-abdominal catastrophies it should be stressed again that the surgeon cannot escape the responsibility of performing an exploratory laparotomy for suspected peritonitis or intra-abdominal bleeding, because after any appropriate and adequate operative treatment the intravenous therapy, hitherto ineffective will have its desired effect and the patient begin to recover. Indeed it can be stated that the act of laparotomy on an anaesthetised patient from an intensive therapy unit (ITU) is less of a hazard than leaving the patient to continue in his predicament. Intra-peritoneal lavage which tests for the presence of blood may help to confirm the need to operate.

Clinical monitoring[1] (figs. 44, 45)

Once the word 'shock' is mentioned, the medical staff should be galvanised into action, and the observation and the treatment of the patient intensified.

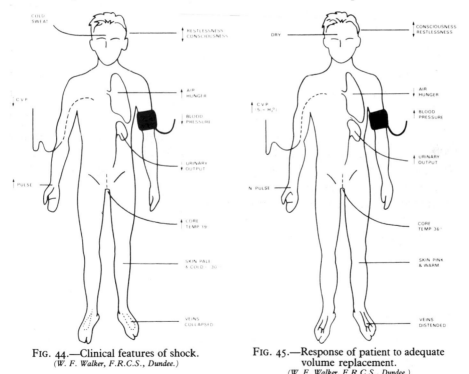

FIG. 44.—Clinical features of shock.
(*W. F. Walker, F.R.C.S., Dundee.*)

FIG. 45.—Response of patient to adequate volume replacement.
(*W. F. Walker, F.R.C.S., Dundee.*)

[1]It is implicit that clinical monitoring takes in the observation and assessment of the whole person including appearance, behaviour, warmth of skin and in a good light the colour of nail beds and mucous membranes. In shock restlessness, coldness, clamminess and cyanosis tell of trouble, whereas alertness, warmth and pinkness usually proclaim problems overcome.

Assessments of degrees of haemodynamic impairment have to be made as rapidly as possible.

The measurement of blood pressure can help in early shock. As already stated (haemorrhage, p. 57) *the pulse pressure* gives a good indication of stroke volume and therefore cardiac output. The *diastolic pressure* gives an indication of the degree of vasoconstriction, and the *systolic pressure* the rigidity of the main vessels in combination with vasoconstriction and stroke volume. Thus, when the blood pressure changes from 100/60 to 90/70 mmHg, the stroke volume will probably be reduced by 50%. In late shock, the sphygmomanometer cuff pressure may be unobtainable due to vasoconstriction and reduced stroke volume, making the Korotkoff sounds inaudible, and, as suggested above, an intra-arterial cannula is of great value. The arterial pressure can be measured with an extra tall (150 cm) manometer if a pressure transducer is not available.

Respiration.—The rate and depth of respiration is an important indicator of shock. Initial hyperventilation is a normal response to trauma, sepsis, and early shock. Indeed, if the patient is not hyperventilating there may well be central nervous or respiratory system damage, but on the other hand persistent hyperventilation indicates that the shock state is not being corrected adequately and is a compensatory mechanism to drop the $PaCO_2$ so as to correct the metabolic acidosis.

Urine.—The urine output is an indicator of renal blood flow, which is determined by the cardiac output. In severe sepsis a paradox can occur in which the patient may pass 100–200 ml per hour in spite of being hypovolaemic, often oedematous, and with a high CVP and with pulmonary oedema. If fluids are restricted at this stage the blood pressure and urine output may fall suddenly; this greatly increases the mortality. The key to the paradox is found in the urine for it has a low sodium concentration and therefore fluids, particularly colloidal solutions, should be given to restore blood volume.

CVP. The central venous pressure should be monitored (fig. 46) but, as already indicated, it can be misleading in patients with cardiac dysfunction or pulmonary damage who may well require measurements of the Pulmonary Capillary Wedge Pressure (PCWP).

In summary, patient monitoring in shock should include:

1. Blood pressure (recording systolic and diastolic pressure, the pulse pressure, using an intra-arterial line if necessary)
2. Heart rate and rhythm (cardioscope)
3. Respiratory rate and depth
4. CVP
5. PCWP in severe shock or when the diagnosis is in doubt
6. Urine output
7. Serial blood gases and serum electrolyte measurements (Chapter 6).

Method.—A commercially available intravenous catheter, made to proper standards and of requisite length (20 cm), is passed into the right internal jugular vein. The surface marking of the vein is a line drawn between the lobe of the ear and the medial end of the clavicle. With the patient in the head-down position, and using full aseptic precautions, the catheter needle, mounted on a syringe, is either inserted (a) downwards in the line of the vein after entrance through the skin some 3–4 finger breadths above the sternoclavicular joint, usually through the anterior fibres of the sternomastoid muscle, or (b) through

Nicholai Korotkoff, 1874–?. Russian physician. Described the sounds heard on auscultation after release of pneumatic cuff.

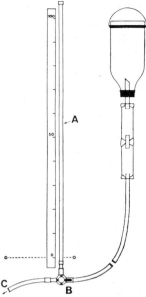

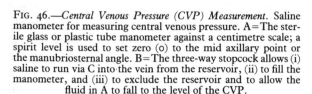

FIG. 46.—*Central Venous Pressure (CVP) Measurement.* Saline manometer for measuring central venous pressure. A=The sterile glass or plastic tube manometer against a centimetre scale; a spirit level is used to set zero (o) to the mid axillary point or the manubriosternal angle. B=The three-way stopcock allows (i) saline to run via C into the vein from the reservoir, (ii) to fill the manometer, and (iii) to exclude the reservoir and to allow the fluid in A to fall to the level of the CVP.

a skin puncture 3 cm above the medial end of the clavicle in the hollow between the two heads of the sternomastoid muscle and beneath which lies the lower bulb of the vein, the needle being first aimed in the direction of the suprasternal notch. The head-down position is used to distend the vein and to prevent air being sucked in (air embolism Chapter 14). Insertion (a) is best avoided in the unanaesthetised patient.

The catheter tip should be positioned in the superior vena cava (confirmed radiologically at the first opportunity). Preceding every measurement the patency of the catheter is confirmed by lowering the saline reservoir briefly to check the free reflux of blood in the connecting tubing (fig. 46C). It must be emphasised that the use of this method requires supervised training, skill, practice and patience, also reference to the special manuals, because the complications can be serious (*e.g.,* pneumothorax, haemothorax, brachial plexus and major artery damage). The catheter must be removed when not required for CVP measurement, and should not be kept in position as a matter of convenience for electrolyte or parenteral infusions (the latter entering the pleural cavity or the mediastinum can be lethal).

The infra-clavicular route tends to be reserved for parenteral nutrition (Chapter 7).

An alternative, though perhaps less accurate method, is the insertion of a longer catheter (60 cm) via the median basilic vein in the antecubital fossa. It may be difficult to position the tip so as to be certain that central pressure is being measured.

The catheter is connected to the saline manometer (fig. 46). Readings with the zero reference point at the mid axillary point are 0–5 cm=low, 15+=high, alternatively at the manubriosternal angle (angle of Louis) they are 0–2 cm=low, 10+=high. Therefore, if the CVP is low the venous return should be supplemented by intravenous infusion, but not if the pressure is high.

Treatment of shock

The management of all types of shock requires vigorous aggressive treatment. The objectives are to increase the cardiac output and to improve tissue perfusion, especially in the coronary, cerebral, renal and mesenteric vascular beds. The plan of action should be based on (1) the primary problem—arrest of haemorrhage, draining pus *etc.*, (ii) improving ventricular filling by giving adequate fluid replacement—using plasma protein fraction or plasma in sepsis and burns,

Antoine Louis, 1723–1792. Surgeon, Paris.

(iii) improving myocardial contractility with inotropic agents—dopamine, dobutamine, adrenaline infusions, and (iv) correcting acid-base disturbances—using molar sodium bicarbonate when the pH is less than 7·2—, and electrolyte abnormalities—especially potassium and calcium.

In endotoxic shock, once the haemodynamic status has been improved, full doses of the currently favoured broad-spectrum antibiotics (Chapter 3) are given in support of the appropriate treatment of the causal lesion. A stepwise increase in the number of types of antibiotics employed is preferable to a massive injection of an array which can cause floodings of the body with bacterial membrane debris, thus increasing the severity of the insult to the patient. In many centres, large doses of steroids (methylprednisolone 30 mg/kg) are given 8 hourly for 1 to 2 days. This is said to improve perfusion, reduce capillary leakage and systemic inflammatory effects.

Diabetic patients in endotoxic shock are in a precarious position. Careful monitoring and control of their nutrition and insulin requirements are necessary under, if available, the instruction of a clinician with a special interest in diabetes.

Vasodilators (hydralazine, phentolamine, glyceryl trinitrate infusions, chlorpromazine boluses) may be given provided the blood volume has been corrected and cardiac depression treated such that the systolic blood pressure is 90 mmHg or more. The indication is persistent vasoconstriction with oliguria, high CVP or PCWP and pulmonary oedema. Such therapy will improve cardiac output and tissue perfusion and reduce the work done by the heart. But it must be emphasised that vasodilators can *only be used with extreme caution* and full haemodynamic monitoring, because the sudden production of vasodilation in a hypovolaemic or dehydrated patient can be followed by a catastrophic fall in arterial blood pressure. These drugs should be given only in small intravenous doses or infusions and only until the extremities become warm and pink and the veins are dilated and well filled.

OXYGEN THERAPY

Indications in Surgery.—In shock its value has been disputed, but it is of special value in chest injuries, in severe haemorrhage, in toxic haemolysis, *e.g.* gas gangrene, in coal gas poisoning and in over-morphinisation. It may also be used in pulmonary embolism, fat embolism, spontaneous pneumothorax, acute pulmonary oedema, and cardiac infarction, and in cases of acute bronchitis, pneumonia, and anoxic cor pulmonale. The usual method employs a disposable polythene mask, delivering 4–6 litres per minute. For patients with chronic bronchitis and emphysema there is a risk of a high concentration of oxygen reducing the carbon dioxide drive for respiration, so causing carbon dioxide narcosis. The safe concentration (Campbell) is about 27% oxygen delivered by a Venturi or disposable Ventimask in which a jet of oxygen at 4 litres per minute strikes the side walls of the air intake aperture and sucks in about 50 litres of air per minute thus giving the necessary mixture.

Endotracheal intubation and positive pressure ventilation is indicated if there is inadequate tidal volume or minute ventilation, or if the PaO_2 is less than about 70% saturation. A higher concentration of oxygen may be administered in this way, but the procedure will reduce venous return through the thorax and may further reduce cardiac output if the patient is hypovolaemic. In cardiogenic shock with high filling pressures, however, this is the treatment of choice.

Edward James Moran Campbell, Contemporary. Professor of Medicine, McMaster University, Hamilton, Ontario, Canada.

Oxygen tents may also be used if a high concentration of oxygen is required. Children should be reassured, as they are likely to be frightened by confinement in an enclosed space, and, if possible, nervous patients should be accustomed to a tent before the necessity arises. Sedation is used. Nurses are warned against the risk of explosion, and naked lights and smoking are forbidden in the proximity of the tent.

Hyperbaric Oxygen. Oxygen Drenching.—Oxygen, when it is administered at 1 or 2 atmospheres above atmospheric pressure in a compression chamber will at least double the arterial plasma of oxygen saturation and so the oxygen perfusion of tissues can be increased. When such a chamber is available it can supplant the use of carbogen (oxygen with 5 or 7% carbon dioxide) in the treatment of carbon monoxide poisoning, and may be used for the treatment of anaerobic infections, *e.g.* tetanus and gas gangrene, bedsores and frostbite. Oxygen is also a radio-sensitiser in the treatment of cancer. Drenching has been used to treat paralytic ileus and meteorism, for since the gas in the distended bowel is nitrogen, breathing pure oxygen so reduces the partial pressure of nitrogen in the lungs and plasma that reabsorption from the bowel takes place.

Topical Oxygen Therapy.—Hydrogen peroxide 5 or 10 volumes, and 2% zinc peroxide, giving off nascent oxygen are used locally on wounds infected with anaerobic or microaerophilic organisms, *e.g.* spreading symbiotic gangrene of the abdominal wall (Chapter 55). It is also used to free the sloughs of ulcers.

CRUSH SYNDROME

This syndrome is commonly associated with earthquakes, air-raids and with mining and other accidents. As a result of massive crushing of muscles, oligaemic shock occurs, due mainly to extravasation of blood into adjacent muscles. Myohaemoglobin enters the circulation and acute renal tubular necrosis is likely to result. The degree of shock has no relation to the development of the syndrome. A similar effect may follow the application of a tourniquet for too long a period (p. 59)!

First-aid treatment may necessitate the application of a tourniquet to the affected limb, which is gradually released so that deleterious substances are admitted to the circulation in small quantities. The crushed muscle often swells considerably, and being confined within unyielding deep fascia, tension develops, impeding the circulation and increasing the extent of ischaemic damage. The limb feels tense and pain is severe. Tension should be relieved by parallel incisions, through which the swollen muscle protrudes. The patient may appear to be comparatively well for two or three days following the accident, but excretion of urine is scanty. Apathy, restlessness, and possibly mild delirium indicate deficient renal function, and uraemia supervenes. If oliguria develops, the fluid intake must be restricted to 'x' plus 400 ml, 'x' being the urinary output for the previous twenty-four hours. The urine should be rendered alkaline by the administration of sodium citrate and sodium bicarbonate. *Rheomacrodex* (p. 75) is useful, by clearing blood sludging and myohaemoglobin, or *mannitol*. Dialysis may be life-saving.

Mannitol, a sugar of low molecular weight, is used to prevent acute renal failure in shock, in the crush syndrome, and to reduce the mortality after operations for obstructive jaundice (Dawson). It promotes an osmotic diuresis. Dose.—Up to 1 g/kg body weight i.v. in 12 hr as a 20% solution (*e.g.* three infusions of 100 ml during and after operation). Test doses may be used in cases of diminished urine output to determine whether hydration therapy or the strictly-limited-fluid regimen (Chapter 56) is to be adopted. Catheterisation (indwelling) is helpful to prevent retention due to rapid overfilling of the bladder and to provide means of accurate recording of the response to therapy.

BLOOD TRANSFUSION

The indications for transfusion in surgical practice are as follows:

1. Following traumatic incidents where there has been severe blood loss, or haemorrhage from pathological lesions, *e.g.* from gastrointestinal tract.

2. During major operative procedures where a certain amount of blood loss is inevitable, *e.g.* abdomino-perineal or cardiovascular surgery.

3. Following severe burns where, despite initial fluid and protein replacement, there may be associated haemolysis.

John Leonard Dawson, Contemporary. Surgeon, King's College Hospital, London.

4. Post-operatively in a patient who has become severely debilitated and anaemic as the result of infection, septicaemia, *etc.*

5. Pre-operatively (usually in the form of packed cells given slowly—see Blood Fractions (below) and Complications (p. 73)) in cases of chronic anaemia where surgery is indicated urgently, *i.e.* where there is inadequate time for iron or other replacement therapy, or where the anaemia is unresponsive to therapy, *e.g.* aplastic anaemia.

6. To arrest haemorrhage or as a prophylactic measure prior to surgery, in a patient with a haemorrhagic state such as thrombocytopenia, haemophilia or liver disease. (See Blood Fractions below.)

Preparation of Blood Products for Transfusion.—It is important that blood donors should be fit and with no history of serious disease, in particular hepatitis and HIV I and II infection (AIDS) which are transmitted in donor blood.

Blood is collected into a sterile commercially prepared plastic bag with needle and plastic tube attached in a complete, closed sterile unit.

With the donor lying on a couch, a sphygmomanometer cuff is applied to the upper arm and inflated to a pressure of 70 mmHg (9·3 kPa) or 80 mmHg (10·6 kPa). After introducing 0.5 ml of local anaesthetic, the 15 gauge needle is introduced into the median cubital vein and 410 ml of blood allowed to run into the bag containing 75 ml of anticoagulant solution (CPD).[1]

During collection the blood is constantly mixed with the anticoagulant to prevent clotting and at the end of the procedure the tube is clamped and the needle removed. Specimens for use in blood grouping and cross-matching procedures may be obtained by clamping off small sections of the plastic tubing containing the donor blood.

Blood Storage.—All blood for transfusion must be stored in special blood bank refrigerators controlled at 4°C±2°C. Blood allowed to stand at higher temperatures for more than 2 hours is in danger of transmitting infection.

CPD blood has a shelf-life of 3 weeks (CPDA-1—5 weeks). The red blood cells, or erythrocytes, suffer a temporary reduction (24–72 hours) in their ability to release oxygen to the tissues of the recipient, so if a patient requires an urgent and massive transfusion it is wise to give one or two units of blood which are less than 7 days old.

White blood cells are rapidly destroyed in stored blood.

Platelets.—At 4°C the survival of platelets is considerably reduced, and few are functionally useful after 24 hours. Platelets which are separated (see 3 below) show good survival even after 72 hours.

Clotting Factors.—Like platelets, clotting factors VIII and V are labile and their levels fall quickly.

Blood Fractions.—Whole blood may be divided into various fractions. This is not only more economical of blood donors but certain fractions are more appropriate than whole blood transfusion for certain clinical conditions. Fractionation procedures are relatively safe and simple, using sealed sterile plastic bag units.

1. *Packed red cells* are especially advisable in patients with chronic anaemia, in the elderly, in small children, and in patients in whom introduction of large volumes of fluid may cause cardiac failure. Packed red cells are suitable for most forms of transfusion therapy including major surgery especially in association with clear fluids. Good packing can be obtained by letting the blood sediment and removing the plasma, or by centrifugation of whole blood at 2000–2300 g for 15–20 minutes.

2. *Platelet rich plasma* is suitable for transfusions to patients with thrombocytopenia who are either bleeding or require surgery. It is prepared by centrifugation of freshly donated blood at 150–200 g for 15–20 minutes.

3. *Platelet concentrate* for transfusion to patients with thrombocytopenia is prepared by centrifugation of platelet-rich plasma at 1200–1500 g for 15–20 minutes.

---

[1]At most blood transfusion centres a citrate-phosphate-dextrose solution (CPD) is the anticoagulant favoured. Oxygen availability is improved. Before long citrate-phosphate-dextrose-adenosine (CPDA-1) will be widely used in the U.K.; the addition of adenosine increases the shelf life to 5 weeks. CPD is constituted as follows: Trisodium citrate (dihydrate) 26·3 g, citric acid (monohydrate) 3·27 g, sodium dihydrogen phosphate (monohydrate) 2·51 g, dextrose 23·2 g, water to 1 litre. 63 ml of the solution (pH 5·6–5·8) are mixed with 450 ml blood.

4. *Plasma.*—This is removed after centrifugation of whole blood at 2000–2300 g for 15–20 minutes and it may be further processed or fractionated in various ways.

(*a*) *Human albumin 4·5%.*—Repeated fractionation of plasma by organic liquids followed by heat treatment results in this plasma fraction which is rich in protein but free from the danger of transmission of serum hepatitis. This may be stored for several months in liquid form at 4°C and is suitable for replacement of protein, *e.g.* following severe burns.

(*b*) *Fresh frozen plasma.*—Plasma removed from fresh blood obtained within 4 hours is rapidly frozen by immersing in solid carbon dioxide and ethyl alcohol mixture. This is stored at –40°C and is a good source of all the coagulation factors. It is the treatment of choice when considering surgery in patients with abnormal coagulation due to severe liver failure. It may also be given in any of the congenital clotting factor deficiency diseases especially *Christmas disease*[1] (Factor IX deficiency) or haemophilia (Factor VIII deficiency).

(*c*) *Cryoprecipitate.*—When fresh frozen plasma is allowed to thaw at 4°C a white glutinous precipitate remains and if the supernatant plasma is removed, this cryoprecipitate is a very rich source of Factor VIII. It is stored at –40°C and immediately available for treatment of patients with haemophilia (Factor VIII deficiency). The advantage of cryoprecipitate treatment in haemophilia is the simplicity of administering large quantities of Factor VIII in relatively small volumes by intravenous injection. It is also a rich source of fibrinogen, of value in hypofibrinogenaemic states.

(*d*) *Fibrinogen* is prepared by organic liquid fractionation of plasma and stored in the dried form. When reconstituted with distilled water it is used in patients with severe depletion of fibrinogen, *e.g.* disseminated intravascular coagulation or congenital afibrinogenaemia. It does, however, carry a high risk of hepatitis.

SAG-M (SAG-Mannitol) Blood.—Because of the need for blood products, there will be an increasing use of 'SAG-M' blood. A proportion of blood donations will have all the plasma removed, which will be replaced with 100 ml of a crystalloid solution containing:

Sodium chloride	877 mg
Adenine	16·9 mg
Glucose anhydrous	818 mg
Mannitol	525 mg

This allows good viability of the cells, but there is practically no protein (albumin) present. For top-up transfusions for anaemia, this will not constitute a problem.

For healthy adults the plasma albumin level will not be compromised by a replacement transfusion of up to 4 units of SAG-M blood, after which whole blood should be used. If this is not available, more SAG-M blood may be given, supplemented by 1 unit (400 ml) of 4·5% Human Albumin Solution B.P. for every 2 units of SAG-M blood. After 8 units of SAG-M red cells have been transfused, the need for fresh frozen plasma and platelets should be considered, after first checking the coagulation status and platelet count.

Blood Grouping and Cross-Matching

Human red cells have on the cell surface many different antigens. For practical purposes, there are two groups of antigens which are of major importance in surgical practice:

(1) **Antigens of the ABO Blood Groups.**—These are strongly antigenic and are associated with naturally occurring antibodies in the serum. Individuals show four different ABO cell groups viz:

Red cell group	*Serum contains*
A	Anti B antibody
B	Anti A antibody
AB	No ABO antibody
O	Anti A and Anti B antibody

---

[1]So-called after the name of the first patient in whom the disease was discovered.

(2) **Antigens of the Rhesus Blood Groups.**—The antigen of major importance in this group is Rh(D) which is strongly antigenic and is present in approximately 85% of the population in the United Kingdom. Antibodies to the D antigen are not naturally present in the serum of the remaining 15% of individuals but their formation may be stimulated by the transfusion of Rh-positive blood. Such acquired antibodies are capable, during pregnancy, of crossing the placenta and if present in a Rh-negative mother may cause severe haemolytic anaemia and even death (hydrops fetalis) in a Rhesus-positive fetus *in utero*. The other minor blood group antigens may be associated with naturally occurring antibodies or may stimulate the formation of antibodies on relatively rare occasions.

Incompatibility.—If antibodies present in the recipient's serum are incompatible with the donors cells a transfusion reaction will result. This is the result of agglutination and haemolysis of the donated cells leading in severe cases to acute renal tubular necrosis and renal failure. For this reason therefore, it is essential that all transfusions should be preceded by:

(1) *ABO and Rhesus grouping* of the recipient's and donor's cells so that only ABO and Rh(D) compatible blood is given.

(2) Direct matching of the recipient's serum with the donor's cells to confirm ABO compatibility and to test for Rhesus and any other blood group antibody present in the serum of the recipient.

Blood grouping and cross-matching require full laboratory procedures, requiring 1 hour. In emergencies it may be necessary to reduce this time but the risk of doing this must be weighed against the danger to the patient by the delay in transfusion entailed by the full procedures. In such emergencies it may be advisable to restore the patient's blood volume by saline, gelatin (*e.g.* Haemaccel®), dextran,[1] or human albumin 4·5% until blood has been made available. Alternatively donor blood, group O-negative, which is compatible with the majority of individuals should be given and this should always be available in acute emergency situations.

Giving Blood.—Blood transfusion is commenced by:

(*a*) selection and preparation of the site (Chapter 6).

(*b*) careful checking of the donor blood:—this should bear a compatibility label stating the patient's name, hospital reference number, ward and blood group.

(*c*) Insertion of the needle or cannula:—the latter may be valuable if intravenous therapy is required for any length of time.

(*d*) Giving detailed written instructions as to the rate of flow (*e.g.* 40 drops per minute allows one 540 ml unit of blood to be transfused in 4 hours).

In acute emergencies it may be necessary to increase the rate of flow and it is possible to give 1–2 units in 30 minutes by a pressure cuff around a plastic bag of blood.

Warming Blood.—During cardiopulmonary operations the blood may be warmed before reaching the patient by passing it through a blood warming unit thus reducing the risk of cardiac arrest from large volumes of cold blood direct from the refrigerator.

Filtering Blood.—A filter (Pall®[2]) with an absolute filtration rating of 40 μm will filter off platelet aggregates and leucocyte membranes in stored blood.

Autotransfusion.—This is an old, well-tried method of immediately restoring a patient's blood volume, transfusion with his or her own blood. In an emergency, for example, in a case of ruptured ectopic gestation, the blood is collected from the peritoneal

---

[1]After collection of a cross-match sample.
[2]Pall Biomedical Ltd., Portsmouth, England.

cavity and put into a sterile container suitable for connecting to transfusion tubing. The classical method of filtration of this blood to prevent the transfusion of any small clots is to place a piece of sterile gauze within the container. Nowadays special autotransfusion apparatus is being marketed. For major elective procedures the patient may 'donate' his or her own blood, withdrawal and storage taking place up to three weeks (see p. 70 and footnote p. 70) before it is required. Natural blood volume and most of the red cell recovery will have taken place in that time.

Complications of Blood Transfusion

(1) **Congestive Cardiac Failure.**—This is especially liable to occur in the elderly or where there is cardiovascular insufficiency and may result from too rapid infusion of large volumes of blood. It is advisable in the individual with chronic anaemia to give packed red cells and at the same time give diuretic drugs. The transfusion should be given slowly, *i.e.* 1 unit over 4–6 hours and if necessary on 2 separate occasions.

(2) **'Transfusion Reactions.'**—These may be the result of:

(*i*) *Incompatibility.*—This should be avoided if the correct procedures of grouping and cross-matching have been adopted but in fact it is nearly always due to human error in the collection, labelling or checking of the specimens and donor bags. The patient develops a rigor, temperature, pain in the loins and may become extremely alarmed. The transfusion should be stopped immediately and a fresh specimen of venous blood and urine from the patient sent together with the residue of *all* the used units of donor blood to the laboratory for checking.

A close watch should be kept on the patient's pulse, blood pressure and urinary output. Frusemide 80–120 mg i.v. is given to provoke a diuresis, and repeated if the urine output falls below 30 ml per hour (see Anuria, Chapter 56).

(*ii*) *Simple pyrexial reactions* in which the patient develops pyrexia, rigor and some increase in pulse rate. These are the result of 'pyrogens' in the donor apparatus and are largely avoided by the use of plastic disposable giving sets.

(iii) *Allergic reactions* in which the patient develops mild tachycardia and an urticarial rash; rarely an acute anaphylactic reaction may occur. This is the result of allergic reaction to plasma products in the donor blood. The reaction is treated by stopping the transfusion and giving an antihistamine drug (chlorpheniramine, 10 mg, or diphenhydrazine, 25 mg).

(iv) *Sensitisation to leucocytes and platelets.*—This is not uncommon in those patients who have received many transfusions in the past, *e.g.* for thalassaemia, refractory anaemia or aplastic anaemia. The individual develops antibodies to donated white cells or platelets which cause reactions with each transfusion. They may be minimised by giving packed red cells from which plasma and 'buffy coat layers' have been removed or by 'washing' of donor cells. Aspirin, antihistamines or steroids may also be given to the recipient if necessary.

(v) *Immunological sensitisation.*—Only the ABO and Rh(D) groups are considered for blood transfusion. Immune antibodies may be stimulated by transfusion, and may give rise to difficulties with compatibility tests or to haemolytic transfusion reactions.

(3) **Infections.**—There are three main reasons for blood transfusion causing infection in the recipient.

(i) *Serum hepatitis virus* may be transmitted from the donor and is usually a severe hepatitis arising approximately 3 months after the transfusion. It should be avoided by adequate verbal screening of the blood donor and by testing for the presence of the hepatitis associated antigen in the blood prior to transfusion.

(ii) *HIV infection* can be transmitted by blood and blood products. All donors must be screened (see AIDS Chapter 4). Haemophiliacs are at special risk.

(iii) *Bacterial infection* as the result of faulty storage. This arises most commonly from the donor blood being left in a warm room for some hours before the transfusion is commenced. This allows proliferation of any bacteria and transfusion of such infected blood may result in severe septicaemia in the recipient and rapid death.

(4) **Thrombophlebitis** (Chapter 13).

(5) **Air Embolism** (Chapter 14).

(6) **Coagulation Failure** due to (*a*) *Dilution of clotting factors/platelets* due to large volumes of stored blood being used to replace losses as stored blood is low in platelets, Factor VIII and Factor V. (*b*) *Disseminated intravascular coagulation* (DIC)[1] following an incompatible blood transfusion particularly ABO incompatibility. The further haemorrhage may be treated by replacement of the deficient factors (usually fibrinogen, Factors VIII, V and II, and platelets), with fresh frozen plasma, cryoprecipitate and platelet concentrates. Paradoxically, heparin may be used for DIC.

Haemophilia and the Congenital Haemorrhagic Diseases

Haemophilia (haemophilia A) is a haemorrhagic diathesis caused by the congenital deficiency in the blood of Factor VIII (antihaemophilic globulin AHG). It is a sex-linked characteristic, transmitted by the asymptomatic female carriers, and manifest only in males.

The levels of Factor VIII in the blood of severe haemophiliacs may be less than 1% of the average normal level. In the case of spontaneous haemorrhage, *e.g.* into joints, treatment should aim at raising the level to at least 20%. Should surgery be anticipated in the haemophiliac, the level should be raised to 50–100%.

Factor VIII concentrates are superceding cryoprecipitates. The amount of either preparation depends on the problem and the level required for haemostasis, *i.e.*, more for surgery than for a haemarthrosis! Frequent monitoring of the Factor VIII level will be necessary in cases involving major surgery.

Alternative forms of therapy include fresh blood, if necessary for blood loss, fresh frozen plasma, or, more rarely, dried concentrates of animal AHG (and see AIDS).

Christmas Disease (haemophilia B) is a congenital disease resulting from the deficiency of Factor IX (Christmas factor). Clinically the manifestations of the disease are similar to haemophilia, but treatment is less predictable. Factor IX is replaced by the transfusion of fresh-frozen plasma, or by reconstituted dried concentrates of human factor IX.

Haemophilic Joints.—In both haemophilia and Christmas disease haemorrhage into joints is very common, and persistent and recurrent haemarthrosis may result in permanent damage to the articular surfaces and disorganisation of the joint. The most important feature of treatment is that it should be prompt. Replacement of the clotting factor should be instituted immediately and before severe tension is allowed to build up in the joint.

Von Willebrand's Disease, with bizarre episodic bleeding manifestations is a type of Factor VIII haemorrhagic disease, with low plasma levels of both Factor VIII complement and Factor VIII related antigen, and platelet abnormalities.

Sickle cell disorders can be a serious problem in surgery, especially children. All patients of the negroid ethnic type should be screened for the presence of sickle haemo-

---

[1]Other acute causes of disseminated intravascular coagulation include: major trauma, burns, lung and prostate operations, cardiac arrest, pulmonary embolism, amniotic fluid embolism in ruptured placenta, acute liver failure. Disseminated malignant disease, and a retained dead fetus are chronic causes.

E. A. Von Willebrand, 1870–1949. Finnish Physician who described the clinical features in 1926.

globin. In *Sickle cell trait* (HbA+S), care to avoid hypoxia during anaesthesia is important. In *Sickle cell anaemia*, a preoperative partial exchange transfusion of packed cells to reduce the haemoglobin S level to less than 30% may be required, depending on the procedure and the length of the operation. Oxygen is needed as well as the prevention of hypoxia, hypothermia, and dehydration. Spinal anaesthesia and tourniquets are contraindicated. Pigment gallstone formation is common; rarely splenomegaly may be a problem.

Blood Substitutes—Albumin, Dextran, Gelatin

One of the most urgent requirements in a patient suffering from acute blood loss is the re-establishment of a normal blood volume. This may be achieved satisfactorily with a number of plasma substitutes.

Human Albumin 4·5% has superseded the use of dried plasma and can be used whilst cross-matching is being performed. Two to three units (1·2 L) are given i.v. in half an hour. It is valuable in patients with burns where there has been severe loss of protein. There is no risk of transmitting hepatitis.

Dextrans are polysaccharide polymers of varying molecular weight producing an osmotic pressure similar to that of plasma. They have the disadvantage of inducing rouleaux of the red cells and this interferes with bloodgrouping and cross-matching procedures, hence the need for a blood sample beforehand. Dextrans interfere with platelet function and may be associated with abnormal bleeding, and for this reason it is recommended that the total volume of Dextran should not exceed 1000 ml.

Low molecular weight dextran (40,000) (Dextran 40, Rheomacrodex®) has an immediate effect in restoring plasma volume, but it is transitory because the small molecules are readily excreted by the kidney. It may be useful in preventing sludging of red cells in small blood vessels, *e.g.* of the kidney, and thus preventing the renal shutdown associated with severe hypotension. It is less likely to induce rouleaux formation than the high molecular weight compounds.

The high molecular weight dextrans (110,000 and 70,000) (Dextran 110 and Dextran 70) are less effective in the early phase of hypovolaemia but are longer-acting since they are retained for some time within the circulation.

Gelatin in a degraded form (mol. wt around 30,000) is used increasingly as a plasma expander. Up to 1000 ml of a 3·4–4% solution (containing anions and cations) is given i.v. (*e.g.* Haemaccel®, Gelafusine®).

POST-OPERATIVE ANALGESIA

Many patients, including doctors, testify to the inadequacy of the relief of post-operative pain. Several factors, such as the site of the operation, the drugs used in the premedication and during the anaesthetic, concomitant regional techniques and the emotional state of the patient, cause great variation between patients in the dose and frequency of medication used.

When post-operative pain is inadequately treated, the suffering of the patient increases the stress of the whole procedure, and can delay recovery. The inability to cough and breathe deeply leads to retention of secretions, pulmonary atelectasis and pneumonia. Immobility leads to venous stasis, deep vein thrombosis and pulmonary embolisation.

The signs of pain include restlessness, tachycardia, sweating, pallor and hypertension; if the pain is severe, hypotension may occur.

Systemic Narcotic Analgesia.—The most widely used analgesic agents are the opiates, such as morphine and pethidine given intramuscularly every 4–6 hours. This technique partially relieves pain in most patients, but the efficacy varies widely. It is a safe technique, and economical in medical and nursing time. However, the time interval between doses varies enormously, the absorption of the drug may be delayed by vasoconstriction, and opiates can induce nausea. The nursing staff must make an objective assessment of the patient's pain level, and often they are concerned about the dangers of overdose, leading to respiratory depression, and addiction. As a result, patients are frequently under-treated.

If the patient is maintained on assisted ventilation larger doses of opiates can be administered.

The administration of small intravenous boluses of opiate may be more satisfactory, but requires a specially trained nurse or a doctor to stay with the patient to titrate the dose against the patient's pain. However, it is a standard technique on intensive and coronary care units, and in theatre recovery.

When the patient is fully awake, he may be allowed to administer his own analgesic drug intravenously for example by using a Cardiff Palliator.[1] This has been found to be an efficacious, acceptable and safe technique; further, it has been shown that patients give themselves the same or a smaller total dose of drug than when the nursing staff treat them; this is probably the result of the pain being kept more consistently under control. The patient must be the best judge of his own pain.

New analgesics have been developed with partial agonist and antagonist actions, in an attempt to reduce the incidence of respiratory depression. These include buprenorphine and meptazinol, administered intramuscularly or intravenously.

Oral analgesics.[2]—For milder pain it is to be remembered that oral non-narcotic or non-addictive narcotic analgesics can be most effective. Aspirin, paracetamol, codeine and dehydrocodeine tartrate prescribed with due regard to the contraindications and side-effects listed in a formularly are worthy of first consideration.

Peripheral Nerve Blockade.—A field block of the cutaneous nerves supplying sensation to the skin area surrounding the wound, using local anaesthetic agents, may be performed towards the end of the operation. However, the duration of action will be 4 hours at the most. The intercostal nerves at thoracotomy may be dissected and frozen using a crypoprobe at operation, giving analgesia for several weeks with normal sensation returning at the end of that time.

Epidural (Extradural) Blockade.—Injection of a local anaesthetic agent into the extradural space in the thoracic or lumbar spine gives excellent analgesia during and after an operation on the lower half of the body. The stress reaction to the operation, and the incidence of deep vein thrombosis, will be reduced when this technique is used. If a catheter is inserted into the extradural space, local anaesthetic agents may be injected repeatedly, giving post-operative pain relief, allowing coughing, deep breathing and early mobilisation.

N.B. The procedure is not without risk and should not be attempted unless the blood pressure is monitored with each 'top-up', and always competent medical staff with full resuscitation equipment immediately available, because hypotension, total spinal anaesthesia and convulsions can sometimes occur. A continuous infusion by pump of local anaesthetic into an extradural catheter may increase safety, but constant supervision by the specially trained is absolutely essential.

Similar constraints apply to the injections of small doses of morphine (2 mg) in 10 ml preservative-free solution, and to even smaller intrathecal doses (1 mg) in patients supervised in recovery and intensive care units. Analgesia without the disadvantages of motor weakness or hypotension can be achieved, but there is a risk of respiratory depression which may be somewhat reduced by keeping the patient in the semi-reclining rather than in the supine position, but requiring naloxone for reversal. Should this be ineffective the patient may need ventilatory assistance.

Inhalation.—Entonox®, comprising 50% nitrous oxide and 50% oxygen, may be used intermittently prior to physiotherapy to reduce the pain of coughing and chest percussion. But this should not be used continuously for long periods (over 24 hours), however, because of the possibility of marrow suppression.

---

[1]Graseby Dynamics Ltd., Watford, Herts, England.
[2]The editors and contributors deprecate the insidious and increasing use of the word 'painkiller' for an oral analgesic tablet.

CHAPTER 6

FLUID, ELECTROLYTE AND ACID-BASE BALANCE

DAILY WATER BALANCE OF A HEALTHY ADULT (70kg)

Intake		Output	
Water from beverage	1200 ml	1500 ml	Urine
Water from 'solid food'	1000 ml	900 ml	Insensible loss from skin and lungs
Water from oxidation	300 ml	100 ml	Faeces

The Intake is derived from two sources (a) exogenous, and (b) endogenous.

Exogenous water is either drunk or ingested in solid food. The quantities vary within wide limits, but average 2 to 3 litres per twenty-four hours, of which nearly half is contained in solid food.

Taking into consideration their body-weight, the water requirements of infants and children are relatively greater than those of adults because of (a) the larger surface area per unit of body-weight; (b) the greater metabolic activity due to growth; (c) the comparatively poor concentrating ability of the immature kidneys of the neonate.

Endogenous water is released during the oxidation of ingested food and the amount is less than 500 ml per twenty-four hours. During starvation this amount is supplemented by water released from the breakdown of body tissues.

The Output.—Water is lost from the body by four routes;

1. *By the Lungs.*—About 400 ml of water is lost in expired air each twenty-four hours. In a dry atmosphere, and when the respiratory rate is increased, the loss is correspondingly greater.

2. *By the Skin.*—When the body becomes overheated there is visible perspiration, but throughout life invisible perspiration is always proceeding. The cutaneous fluid loss varies within wide limits in accordance with the atmospheric temperature and humidity, muscular activity, and body temperature. In a temperate climate the average loss is between 600 and 1000 ml per twenty-four hours.

3. *Faeces.*—Between 60 and 150 ml of water are lost by this route daily. In diarrhoea this amount is multiplied not only by the number of stools, but according to their fluidity and size.

4. *Urine.*—The output of urine is under the control of a secretion of the posterior lobe of the pituitary gland (the anti-diuretic hormone) which controls the tonicity of the body fluids, a function that it performs by stimulating the reabsorption of water from the renal tubules, thus varying the amount excreted after the requirements of the first three routes have been met. The normal urinary output is 1500 ml per twenty-four hours, and provided the kidneys are healthy,

the specific gravity of the urine bears a direct relationship to the volume. A minimum urinary output of 400 ml per 24 hours is required to excrete the end products of protein metabolism.

Water Depletion.—*Pure water depletion* is usually due to diminished intake. This may be due to difficulty or inability to swallow because of painful conditions of the mouth and pharynx or obstruction in the oesophagus. Exhaustion and paresis of the pharyngeal muscles will produce a similar picture. Pure water depletion may also follow the increased loss from the lungs after tracheostomy. This loss may be as much as 500 ml in excess of the normal insensible loss. After tracheostomy humidification of the inspired air is an important preventive measure.

Clinical Features.—The main symptoms are weakness and intense thirst. The urinary output is diminished and its specific gravity increased. The increased serum osmotic pressure causes water to leave the cells (intracellular dehydration) and thus prevents peripheral circulatory failure. Investigations would show an elevated haematocrit, serum sodium and urea.

Treatment.—The intake of water must be increased initially. If swallowing is possible, the nursing staff must ensure a regular half hourly or hourly intake. Intravenous 5% dextrose or dextrose saline is given if swallowing is impossible (water is not isotonic and would haemolyse blood). Careful charting of intake and output is essential. A diuresis signals that enough has been given, and thereafter care must be taken not to overload and cause water intoxication.

Relative water depletion is seen following excessive loss of water from the kidneys in diabetes insipidus, occasionally following head injury, during the diuretic phase following acute renal failure, too rapid relief of lower urinary tract obstruction and following renal transplantation. These patients are best managed by giving 0.45% saline and with frequent estimation of the serum and urinary sodium.

Water Intoxication can occur when excessive amounts of 5% dextrose, water or hypotonic solutions are given orally, intravenously, subcutaneously or rectally. Colo-rectal washouts with plain water or sodium free solutions in patients with Hirschsprung's disease have caused water intoxication in children (Chapter 50). A similar problem has occurred when water has been inadvertently used instead of saline during total bowel wash-through prior to colonic surgery.

Other causes of water intoxication include excessive uptake of water from irrigation fluid during transurethral resection of the prostate, lung conditions such as lobar pneumonia and empyema, A.D.H.—secreting tumours such as oat-cell carcinoma of bronchus.

Clinical Features.—These include drowsiness, weakness, sometimes convulsions and coma. The patient appears to be in shock—which is incorrect, because the blood-pressure is not low and the pulse is not unduly rapid until the patient is moribund. Nausea and vomiting of clear fluid are common, and usually the patient passes a considerable amount of dilute urine. Laboratory investigations would show low haematocrit and a high mean corpuscular volume (M.C.V.). The serum sodium and other electrolyte concentrations may be low with normal or low urea.

Treatment.—The intake of water having been stopped, the best course is masterly inactivity. If after several days the water-logged patient is still stuporous (due, no doubt, to renal inactivity), it is permissible to infuse *very slowly* not more than 200 ml of hypertonic (5.85%) saline solution intravenously (1 ml contains 1 mmol Na). If this brings about improvement and a diuresis begins the infusion should be stopped forthwith, otherwise circulatory failure from overloading (due to the sudden shift of fluid from cells and tissue spaces) or cardiac arrest is liable to ensue.

ELECTROLYTE BALANCE

When inorganic salts are in solution, as in the extracellular or intracellular fluids of the body, they dissociate into ions. Ions are of two kinds (a) *Cations*, which are electropositive and (b) *Anions*, which are electronegative: collectively these are the electrolytes. The most accurate way of describing the chemical concentration, reactivity, and osmotic power of these ions is in S.I. units as milli-moles per litre (mmol/l).[1] The cations include sodium, potassium, calcium, and magnesium; the anions chloride, phosphate, bicarbonate, and sulphate. The distribution of the salts within the fluid compartments of the body controls the passage of water through the cell walls and maintains acid-base equilibrium.

Sodium Balance

Sodium is the principal cation content of the extracellular fluid. The total body sodium amounts to approximately 5000 mmol, of which 44% is in the extracellular fluid, 9% in the intracellular fluid, the remaining 47% being in bone. The sodium housed in bone merits special notice: a little more than half of it is osmotically inactive, and requires acid for its solution; the remainder is water-soluble and exchangeable. Thus there is a large storehouse of sodium ready to compensate abnormal loss from the body. The daily intake of sodium is inconstant. On an average it is 80–100 mmol sodium chloride or 570 ml of isotonic 0.9% saline solution. An equivalent amount is excreted daily, mainly in the urine, also a little in the faeces. The loss in perspiration normally is negligible; however, in persons not acclimatised to tropical heat prolonged profuse sweating results in a considerable loss of sodium—as much as 85 mmol per hour (J. Nash). If water alone is given to counterbalance the fluid loss, serious sodium depletion can occur from excessive sweating. (See also mucoviscidosis, Chapter 48.)

Control by Adrenal Corticoids.—The output of sodium, governed by the variation in the avidity with which the renal tubules reabsorb sodium from the glomerular filtrate and the amount of sodium excreted by the sweat glands, is under the control of the adrenal corticoids, the most powerful conservator of sodium being *aldosterone*. When the adrenal glands have been destroyed by disease or extirpated, there is an unbridled loss of sodium in the urine.

The Sodium Excretion Shut-down of Trauma.—Following trauma of any kind (including operation trauma) there is a spell, the length of which varies directly with the degree of tissue damage, of almost non-excretion of sodium. During this period the output of sodium, reduced to not more than 10 mmol *per diem*, cannot be increased by a supplemented intake of sodium. For this reason it is most inadvisable to administer large quantities of isotonic (0.9%) saline solution soon after an operation. The period of sodium excretion shut-down lasts for at least forty-eight hours and is due to increased adrenocortical activity.

Sodium Depletion (syn. Hyponatraemia).—The most frequent cause of sodium depletion seen in surgical practice is obstruction of the small intestine, with its rapid loss of gastric, biliary, pancreatic, and intestinal secretions by antiperistalsis and ejection, whether by vomiting or aspiration. Duodenal, total biliary, pancreatic, and high intestinal external fistulae also are all notorious for bringing about early and profound hyponatraemia. Severe diarrhoea due to

---

[1] In S.I. units, mEq/l is replaced by mmol/l. Thus comparing the total of anions with the total of cations is no longer possible. However for monovalent ions (sodium, potassium, chloride and bicarbonate) 1 mEq=1 mmol, so numerically at least the additions are possible.

Michael Faraday, 1791–1867. Pioneer of electro-magnetism, introduced the words 'electrolyte', 'cation', 'anion'.
Joseph Nash, 1902–1945. Assistant Professor of Surgery, New York College of Medicine, New York, U.S.A. Died in Germany on active service while Surgical Chief of the Ninetieth General Hospital, U.S. Army.

dysentery, cholera, ulcerative colitis, or pseudomembranous colitis will cause hyponatraemia with acidosis. The finding of hyponatraemia with elevated potassium would suggest adrenocortical insufficiency. Hyponatraemia is also seen in the syndrome of inappropriate secretion of antidiuretic hormone as in bronchial carcinoma.

There is one other less obvious, and surreptitious, means whereby the patient is robbed of sodium, and that is by gastric aspiration combined with allowing the patient to drink as he pleases and promptly aspirating the fluid swallowed. The act of drinking excites the flow of gastric juice, and this is also aspirated. During this form of therapy, should the patient be receiving intravenous dextrose solution, as opposed to dextrose-saline solution, to maintain fluid balance, he will soon become a victim of hyponatraemia.

Clinical features of hyponatraemia with salt and water depletion are due to extracellular dehydration. In established cases the eyes are sunken and the face is drawn. In infants the anterior fontanelle is depressed. The tongue is coated and dry; in advanced cases it is brown in colour. Unlike the dehydration produced by loss of water only, in water + salt depletion thirst is not particularly in evidence. The skin is dry and often wrinkled, making the patient look older than his years. The subcutaneous tissue feels lax. Peripheral veins are contracted and contain dark blood. The arterial blood-pressure is likely to be below normal. The urine is scanty, dark in colour, of a high specific gravity, and except in cases of salt-losing nephritis contains little or no chloride.

Presuming that the haemoglobin level before the dehydration commenced was normal, the haematocrit reading (P.C.V.) provides an index of the degree of haemoconcentration. On the other hand, haemoconcentration can be masked by pre-existing anaemia (Chapter 5). Laboratory investigations would show normal or slightly reduced serum sodium with low urinary output and low urinary sodium.

Treatment.—The sodium deficit is replaced by an intravenous infusion of 0.5 to 2 litres of isotonic saline or Ringer's solution, depending on the severity of the hyponatraemia. It is important to watch the plasma protein levels in order to avoid overdosage, thus causing hypoproteinaemia and oedema. In severe cases the first step is to restore the circulating blood volume by a rapid infusion of plasma or plasma substitute (Chapter 5).

Post-operative Hyponatraemia.—Hyponatraemia with a normal or increased extracellular fluid volume arises as a result of too prolonged administration of a sodium-free solution (5% dextrose) intravenously. Symptoms seldom present until such treatment has been in progress for more than forty-eight hours (cf. Water Intoxication, p. 78). Early symptoms are headache and giddiness. Hyponatraemia causes pylorospasm and the resulting vomiting adds to the sodium deficit. Should renal function be impaired there will be an associated low level of urinary chlorides.

Treatment.—See water intoxication, p. 78.

Syndrome of inappropriate anti-diuretic hormone secretion (S.I.A.D.H.) may be seen in elderly surgical patients exposed to acute surgical stress such as pain, trauma or operation. Other causes include head injury, tumours producing A.D.H.-like hormone (bronchus) and as a side effect of numerous medications. The excess A.D.H. causes water retention and an increase in the extra cellular fluid volume. This causes a shut off in the secretion of aldosterone resulting a high urinary sodium loss and low serum sodium.

Clinical features would include lassitude and depression, convulsions and coma.

Investigation would show a low serum sodium and low serum osmolality and a high urinary sodium and osmolality.

Treatment.—Restrict fluid intake. See water intoxication (p. 78).

Sodium excess (syn. Hypernatraemia) is likely to arise if a patient is given an excessive amount of 0.9% saline solution intravenously during early post-operative period when, as has been described, some degree of sodium retention is to be expected. The result is an overloading of the circulation with salt and its accompanying water. Even a sub-clinical degree of sodium excess is harmful, for it results in oedema of intestinal and other suture lines. In addition there is danger of pulmonary oedema.

Clinical Features.—Slight puffiness of the face is the only early sign. The patient himself makes no complaint. Pitting oedema should be sought, especially in the sacral region, but for pitting oedema to be present at least 4·5 litres excess fluid must have accumulated in the tissue spaces (Marriott). The patient's weight increases *pari passu* with the water-logging, and the aid of bed-scales should be sought. Signs of overhydration in infancy (infants are very susceptible) are increased tension in the anterior fontanelle, increased weight, increase in the number of urinations, and oedema.

Treatment.—The infusion must be stopped. In established cases with distended jugular veins and pulmonary oedema, treatment should follow the lines suggested in Chapter 40.

Potassium Balance

Potassium is almost entirely intracellular. No less than 98% is intracellular, and only 2% is present in the extracellular fluid. Three-quarters of the total body potassium (approximately 3500 mmol) is found in skeletal muscles. When the body needs endogenous protein as a source of energy, potassium, as well as nitrogen, is mobilised. The mobilised potassium passes to the extracellular fluid, but the surplus over and above the normal content is so rapidly excreted by healthy kidneys that the concentration of potassium in the serum remains unaltered. Each day a normal adult ingests 52–78 mmol of potassium in food; fruit and milk and honey are rich in this cation. Except for a very small quantity in formed faeces and a still smaller quantity in sweat, an amount corresponding to the intake is excreted in the urine.

Potassium Depletion

The Augmented Potassium Excretion of Trauma.—Following trauma, including operation trauma, there is a spell, varying directly with the degree of tissue damage, of increased excretion of potassium by the kidneys. This loss is greatest during the first twenty-four hours and lasts, for example in the case of partial gastrectomy, about three or four days. It will be noticed that the behaviour of the body's potassium in the post-trauma phase is the exact opposite to that of sodium—the potassium flees; the sodium stays. So great are the body's reserves of potassium that, unless the patient was severely depleted at the time of the operation, the therapeutic administration of potassium (always a responsible undertaking) does not arise until the third day of intravenous alimentation.

Hugh Leslie Marriott, 1900–1982. Physician, Middlesex Hospital, London.

Hypokalaemia can occur suddenly or gradually.

Sudden hypokalaemia is unlikely to be encountered in surgical practice. It occurs most frequently in diabetic coma treated by insulin and prolonged infusion of saline solution.

Gradual hypokalaemia is the type met with in surgical practice. The diarrhoea from ulcerative colitis, villous tumours of the rectum (Chapter 53) and the loss from external fistulae of the alimentary tract are common causes (*e.g.* duodenal fistula, ileostomy); the potassium content of the discharge from some of these fistulae is twice that of the plasma potassium concentration. Another frequent cause of hypokalaemia is prolonged gastroduodenal aspiration with fluid replacement by intravenous isotonic saline solution. It is also prone to occur in the postoperative period following extensive resections for carcinoma of the alimentary tract, because often the operation has to be undertaken after months of weightloss and potassium depletion.

Clinical Features.—The patient lies listlessly in bed. Speech is slurred and slow; often the patient fails to complete a sentence. Intense drowsiness soon follows and all the patient desires is to be left in tranquillity to sleep. Muscular hypotonia is the outstanding physical sign. Reflexes are lost and incontinence of urine is common. Abdominal distension amounting to paralytic ileus is a constant accompaniment, and in all cases of paralytic ileus the serum potassium value should be investigated.

Weakness of the respiratory muscles frequently occurs and results in rapid, shallow, gasping respirations; these are conducive to post-operative pulmonary complications. The diastolic blood pressure is low, but there is usually a bounding pulse and a presystolic murmur. The diagnosis should be confirmed by electrocardiography, which may show a prolonged QT interval, depression of the ST segment, and a lowering or inversion of the T wave (fig. 47).

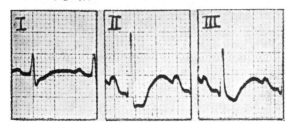

FIG. 47. — Electrocardiographic changes in severe hypokalaemia. The serum potassium estimation was 1.6 mmol/l.
(W. F. Walker, FRCS, Dundee.)

Treatment

Oral Potassium.—Potassium is usually given in the form of milk, meat extracts, fruit juices and honey. Potassium chloride, 2 g effervescent tablets, is given by mouth six-hourly.

Intravenous Potassium.—Should ingestion be inadequate or contraindicated, this route must be used. It is not without the danger of giving too much too quickly (especially when renal function is impaired), thus raising the serum concentration to a dangerous level and causing cardiac arrest. Administration should be properly controlled; the level of potassium should be checked daily; the urine output must be adequate (1000 ml per twenty-four hours—40 ml per hour). *When there is no associated alkalosis*, the potassium deficit can be restored by adding up to 20 mmol potassium chloride to a litre of 5% dextrose or 0.9% saline solution, which is given over eight hours.

Hypokalaemic alkalosis, see p. 88.

Estimation of Electrolyte Balance

Sodium.—Sodium, with its equivalent anions, accounts for about 90% of the osmotic pressure of the plasma. Changes in the sodium content coincide with changes in the osmolality of all the body fluids. The serum sodium value is normally between 137 and 147 mmol per litre. Whenever possible the *serum chloride* and *bicarbonate* should be estimated simultaneously, since variations in the one may be accompanied by opposite changes in the other. The normal level of chloride is 95 to 105 mmol/l, and of bicarbonate 25 to 30 mmol/l; the sum of the two remains roughly constant at 120 to 135 mmol/l.

Potassium.—Potassium deficiency is present if the serum potassium value is less than 3·5 mmol/l. The normal range is 3·5–5·0 mmol/l. It must be remembered that intracellular potassium deficiency may be present although the plasma concentration is normal, and that deficiency is to be expected if oral feeding has been withheld for more than four days. Estimation of potassium in the urine or aspirated gastro-intestinal contents serve as a guide to the rate of depletion and the replacement necessary (W. J. Griffiths). Electrocardiography may also be used (fig. 47).

Calcium.—Calcium is an extracellular cation with a plasma concentration of 2·2–2·5 mmol/l. It exists in three forms: bound to protein, free non-ionised and free ionised, the last form being the component necessary for blood coagulation and affecting neuromuscular excitability. The ionised proportion falls with increasing pH; thus in respiratory alkalosis due to hyperventilation there may be tetany—with an apparently normal total serum calcium level. In the urine the ionisation and the solubility of calcium is similarly depressed if the pH is elevated, thus promoting stone formation. The serum level of calcium is likely to be modified by any factor promoting or inhibiting its absorption from the bowel, its storage in bone or its elimination by the kidneys: such factors include vitamin D and phytic acid, parathormone and calcitonin (Chapter 38), and the state of renal and small bowel function.

The management of abnormal calcium blood levels depends, where possible, on removal of the cause, *e.g.* removal of a parathyroid tumour (Chapter 38). In hypocalcaemia with tetany (Chapter 38) or in the coagulation disorder due to massive transfusion of blood containing acid citrate dextrose (ACD, Chapter 5), 10 ml of 10% calcium gluconate may be injected slowly intravenously. If oral administration is possible, calcium aspirin is useful (Chapter 38). On a long-term basis the diet should be adjusted to provide a high calcium and a low phosphate intake.

Magnesium.—Magnesium is an intracellular cation which shares some of the properties of potassium and some of calcium. The normal magnesium concentration is 0.7–0.9 mmol per litre. The average daily intake is approximately 10 mmol. Magnesium deficiency may occur when there is prolonged loss of gastro-intestinal secretions due to fistulae or ulcerative colitis, very prolonged administration of intravenous fluids without magnesium supplements, following massive small bowel resections, and in some cases of cirrhosis of the liver or disease of the parathyroids. The clinical picture of magnesium deficiency is marked by central nervous system irritability, E.C.G. changes, lowered blood pressure and lowered protein synthesis. The best method of diagnosing magnesium deficiency is the measurement of urinary magnesium after an intravenous loading dose. Normally 90% of the loading dose is promptly excreted in the urine.

Treatment.—In severe depletion 40 mmol as magnesium sulphate can be given in 5% dextrose or isotonic saline over a 24-hour period. Magnesium supplements are essential in hyperalimentation.

PARENTERAL FLUID THERAPY

To overload the circulation is a grievous fault, and grievously does the patient pay for it.

The administration of fluid by any route other than the alimentary canal, *i.e.* intravenous, intramuscular, subcutaneous, or into the bone marrow, is known as parenteral administration.[1]

---

[1] Parenteral = Greek, para + enteron = beside intestine.

William James Griffiths, Contemporary. Formerly Chemical Pathologist, St. Thomas's Hospital, London.

The sterility of a solution for parenteral use must be assured. Furthermore, the solution must be free from dead bacteria and other particulate matter, as also must be the delivery tube.

Solutions mainly in use:

1. **Plasma, Albumin 4.5%** (Chapter 5).

2. **Dextrose 5%** is an isotonic solution that supplies calories without electrolytes. It is useful mainly in the very early post-operative period when sodium excretion is reduced. It is also valuable when the salt requirements of a patient needing much fluid have been satisfied on a particular day. Prolonged administration of 5% dextrose solution is liable to result in hyponatraemia, and may cause thrombosis of the vein used.[1]

3. **Isotonic (0.9%) saline solution** is needed in the following conditions: when a large amount of sodium has been lost by vomiting, or by gastric, duodenal, or intestinal aspiration or through an alimentary fistula. Possibly, on occasions, excessive sweating may justify its use.

These two solutions meet all the requirements in 95% of cases.

4. **Dextrose 4.3% with saline 0.18%** (one fifth normal saline).—This solution is isotonic. Usually it is referred to as dextrose-saline. *It must not be confused with 5% Dextrose in saline which is hypertonic.*

5. **Ringer's Lactate solution** contains sodium, potassium and chloride in almost the same concentrations as they are in the plasma. It also contains some calcium and some lactate. This solution can be used in hypovolaemic shock while awaiting blood. It is also suitable for replacing lost intestinal secretions.

6. **Darrow's solution** contains sufficient potassium to combat hypokalaemia and in surgical practice it is a safe and convenient method of supplying this cation provided alkalosis is not present. The rate of infusion should not exceed 60 drops a minute.

COMPOSITION OF PLASMA AND INTRAVENOUS FLUIDS (mmol/l)

	Na	K	Cl	HCO$_3$	Lactate
Plasma	137–147	4–5·5	95–105	22–25	—
Isotonic[2] Saline	153	—	153	—	—
1/5 Isotonic Saline 4·3% Dextrose	30·6	—	30·6	—	—
Ringer's Lactate	130	4	110	—	28
Darrow's	124	36	104	—	56

A Suggested Routine Post-operative Fluid Regime.—From the above information we know the average patient requires (1) 2000/3000 ml of water daily; (2) At least 100 mmol of Na daily; (3) about 60 mmol of K daily. These requirements are altered by the metabolic response to trauma. In the first 24 hours after surgery there is an increased secretion of anti-diuretic hormone and aldosterone. The patient will require no salt and less water than normal in this 24-hour period. Two litres of 5% dextrose is sufficient intravenous fluid when all abnormal operative loss has been replaced. During the second and subsequent 24-

---

[1] Compared with dextran, saline solutions also are more thrombogenic (Janvrin), but dextran has its own disadvantages and limitations (p. 75).

[2] It is inadvisable to use the term 'normal' saline because chemically normal saline contains 5·8 g/100 ml.

Sydney Ringer, 1835–1910. Physician, University College Hospital, London.
Daniel Cady Darrow, 1895–1965. Professor of Pediatrics, Duke University School of Medicine, Durham, North Carolina, U.S.A.
Simon Benest Janvrin, Contemporary. Surgeon, Crawley Hospital, England.

hour periods the metabolic response to trauma diminishes and the patient needs 2 litres of 5% dextrose and 1 litre of isotonic saline per 24 hours. On the 3rd post-operative day and thereafter 20 mmol of potassium is added to each litre to give a total of 60 mmol per 24 hours.

An alternative regime is to give 3 litres of isotonic solution 4·3% dextrose 0·18% saline daily and add 20 mmol of potassium chloride to each litre on the 3rd post-operative day.

Continuous Intravenous Infusion (Venoclysis).—Because of the certainty with which the fluid enters the circulation without the necessity of being absorbed, this is by far the most usual method of parenteral administration. If a suitable vein can be rendered prominent by the application of a light tourniquet, it can be entered by a hollow needle (venepuncture) (fig. 48). The limb is then immobilised by placing it on a light splint, or if a vein of the forearm is used, with a few strips of adhesive plaster.

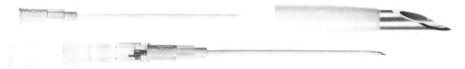

FIG. 48.—Intravenous cannula (ABBOCATH).[1] The cannula is made of teflon and is radiopaque.

Site.—As a routine measure, a vein on the forearm, or on the back of the hand is chosen. In women, young children, and even some men, especially when the venous pressure is low, a visible or palpable vein may not be found in the arm; consequently another site must be used. The external jugular vein, internal jugular vein, subclavian vein, or cephalic vein in the deltopectoral groove, can be selected. Because of the risks of thrombo-phlebitis and pulmonary embolism, a vein of the leg (*e.g.* the long saphenous vein in front of the medial malleolus) should not be selected if it can reasonably be avoided. This injunction does not hold good for infants and small children, who are singularly immune to thrombophlebitis.

Contraindications to Intravenous Therapy

1. *The Failing Heart.*—A history of dyspnoea on exertion, uncompensated valvular disease, or any possibility of myocardial insufficiency should call for hesitation in increasing the bulk of circulating fluid.

2. *Pulmonary Congestion.*—Where there are signs of oedema of the bases of the lungs the method should be absolutely forbidden.

Clinical Guide to Fluid Requirements.—When a patient is admitted in a dehydrated condition it is of course impossible to measure the loss of fluid and electrolytes he has sustained, but a detailed history of the nature and quantity of the fluid lost (usually, in surgical practice, by vomiting), and particularly the appearance of the patient (p. 87), are the means by which the amount of electrolytic solution he should receive is estimated.

---

[1] Abbocath, Abbott. A manufacturer's instructions concerning the insertion and fixation of any plastic catheter must be followed carefully, as fracture of the tube and disappearance of part of it up a vein has occurred. If difficulty is encountered, both needle and catheter should be withdrawn at the same time.

The haematocrit reading (Chapter 5) may help. If large quantities of fluid are necessary, the monitoring of central venous pressure, pulmonary wedge pressure (Chapter 5) and urinary output are needed to determine the optimum rate and volume of the infusion (Chapter 5). The replacement is commenced by giving isotonic (0·9%) saline solution intravenously. When the bulk of the loss has been made up in this way, the *maintenance* of fluid balance is effected with dextrose-saline solution. In cases of extreme dehydration, where peripheral circulatory impairment (shock) is in evidence, it is necessary to commence by supplementing the volume of circulating fluid by dextran or plasma infusion (Chapter 5), and to follow this by substituting isotonic saline solution. When the fluid loss is considered to be rectified and fluid by mouth is contraindicated, it is again advisable to supply the maintenance fluid requirements in the form of dextrose-saline solution.

In infants with dehydration, the amount of fluid required will be approximately the same as the weight loss, *i.e.* the difference between the estimated and actual weight (1 g equals 1 ml).

Rate of Flow.—Using a plastic transfusion set, 15 drops of fluid are approximately equal to 1 ml. At a rate of 30 drops per minute 1 litre will be given in eight hours, at 45 drops per minute it will take six hours, and at 60 drops some four hours. In severely dehydrated patients the rate of the first hour can be accelerated to well over 100 drops per minute, after which it should be cut to 50 or 60 drops. The maintenance dose rate is about 30 drops (3 litres in twenty-four hours).

The programme of rates to be used should be written down on the treatment card or fluid balance chart, and without further instructions the nursing staff should not exceed this rate.

Injection of Drugs and other Additives.—These may be given either via diaphragm of the connector close to the cannula, or by using a Y connection to another infusion bottle. In like manner an infusion pump can be used to administer small volumes of a drug accurately and continuously, *e.g.* heparin (Chapter 14).

I.V. Filtration/Air Elimination.—A filter will exclude microbial contaminants and reduce the incidence of thrombophlebitis, as well as venting entrained air.

Continuous rectal infusion (proctoclysis) was introduced by the celebrated J. B. Murphy, of Chicago, yet today it is seldom employed. The administration of fluid via the rectum has the advantage of simplicity. It requires but little apparatus, and neither asepsis nor isotonicity. Dilute saline given per rectum avoids the absorption of an excessive quantity of water that may well result in hydraemia (1 pint (568 ml) of isotonic solution is added to 4 pints (2·3 litres) of *tap water*). Via a catheter in the rectum, the fluid is given by the drip method according to the needs of the patient. The rate of administration should not be greater than 50 drops a minute.

Charting Fluid Intake and Output (fig. 49).—It is essential that the amount of fluid the patient receives is recorded. It is equally important that all urine passed in each twenty-four hours is measured and recorded. To this figure is added fluid recovered by gastro-intestinal aspiration, and that lost from an intestinal, urinary, biliary, or pancreatic fistula plus 1000 ml for insensible loss from

John Benjamin Murphy, 1857–1916. Professor of Surgery, Northwestern University, Chicago, Illinois, U.S.A. Introduced Continuous Rectal Infusion in 1908.

| HOUR ENDING | ORAL | | INTRAVENOUS | | URINE | ASPIRATION OR VOMIT | OTHER |
	AMOUNT	TYPE	PUT UP	GIVEN			
24 hour TOTALS							

Fig. 49.—Fluid balance chart. There is no column for insensible loss because the nurse is unable to measure this. Insensible loss is taken into consideration by the Medical Officer when he writes up orders for the ensuing twenty-four hours.

the lungs and skin. If the patient has been sweating, the last figure is increased.

Other Aids to Maintaining Correct Fluid Balance.—In addition to the fluid balance chart, the following also are important:

1. **Clinical.**—Much information can be gleaned at the bedside.

If the fluid balance is correct, a warm, dry, pink, elastic skin denotes a good circulation and a satisfactory blood volume. The tongue is moist.

Circulatory overloading requires constant watchfulness, for the initial symptoms are nil and the signs non-proclamatory. A raised jugular venous pressure indicates that the patient has received too much fluid, or too much salt.

2. **Blood Indices.**—Serum electrolyte estimations, as well as those of the haemoglobin, haematocrit and the plasma-proteins, are all helpful in ascertaining that the amount of fluid the patient is receiving is adequate, yet not excessive.

3. **Weight.**—Daily weighing is extremely useful in assessing that the amount of fluid given is correct. In patients subsisting entirely on parenteral fluid there should be a daily *loss* of weight of 150 g.

4. **Blood Volume Estimations** (Chapter 5).

Vitamin Requirements (see also Chapter 7).—Antibiotics produce vitamin deficiency, notably of complex B. Therefore it is best to err on the side of safety and assume that a liberal amount of vitamin B will be required. Vitamin C should be given in large doses, to ensure saturation.

Twin ampoules of Parentrovite[1] are recommended once or twice a week. They are mixed before being injected intramuscularly or via the intravenous drip.

ACID-BASE BALANCE

In health the reaction of the blood lies within the range pH 7·36 to 7·44. The terms acidosis and alkalosis in clinical practice indicate a change or a tendency to a change in the pH of the blood in a particular direction. In acidosis there is an accumulation of acid or a loss of a base causing a fall or a tendency to a fall in the pH. The converse occurs in alkalosis. The pH of the blood is regulated and controlled by various buffering systems essentially consisting of weak acids and bases, of which the most important is the bicarbonate-carbonic acid ratio $HCO_3:H_2CO_3$. It is also regulated by the removal of CO_2 by the lungs and by the excretion of both acids and bases by the kidneys.

---

[1] Contains large doses of vitamin B complex and ascorbic acid (Vitamins Ltd.).

The ratio of bicarbonate to carbonic acid is normally 20:1. Alteration in this ratio alters the pH regardless of the absolute values of the bicarbonate and carbonic acid. A decrease in the ratio leads to increased acidity, and vice versa.

The bicarbonate level can be altered by metabolic factors, while the carbonic acid level is subject to alteration by respiratory factors. Alteration of one is followed automatically by a compensatory alteration in the other so that the ratio (HCO_3:H_2CO_3) and therefore the pH of the blood remains constant.

Measurement of Acid-base Disturbances.—These measurements are 'normally made on arterial or arterialised capillary' blood. PCO_2 is a measurement of the tension or partial pressure of carbon dioxide in the blood. The normal arterial PCO_2 is 31–42 mmHg (4·1–5·6 kPa). PO_2 is a measurement of the tension or partial pressure of oxygen in the blood. The normal arterial PO_2 is 80–110 mmHg (10·5–14·5 kPa).

Standard bicarbonate is the concentration of the serum bicarbonate after *fully oxygenated* blood has been equilibrated with CO_2 at 40 mmHg (5·3 kPa) at 38°C. This eliminates respiratory causes and respiratory compensation for altered bicarbonate levels. Normal 22–25 mmol/l.

Base excess or deficit expresses in mmol the total of buffer anions present in the blood in excess or deficit of normal. (Normal base excess or deficit + 2·5.) Base excess or deficit multiplied by 0·3 times the body weight in kg gives the total extracellular excess or deficit of base in mmol (Mellemgaard and Astrup). Metabolic causes of acid base disturbances are indicated by changes in the standard bicarbonate level and base excess or deficit. Respiratory causes of acid base disturbances are indicated by changes in the PCO_2 and PO_2.

ALKALOSIS

Metabolic alkalosis (a condition of base excess or a deficit of any acid other than H_2CO_3) can be caused by:

(*a*) Excessive ingestion of absorbable alkali. Such is not uncommon in patients who take proprietary indigestion remedies without medical supervision.

(*b*) Loss of acid from the stomach by repeated vomiting or aspiration.

(*c*) Cortisone excess, usually the result of over-administration of adrenal corticoids, but occasionally due to Cushing's syndrome (Chapter 38).

Compensation is effected by (i) retention of carbon dioxide by the lungs and (ii) excretion of bicarbonate base by the kidneys (alkaline urine).

Alkalosis due to loss of acid from the stomach is by far the most common and most important. In its most typical form it is seen in patients with pyloric stenosis in whom the loss of acid by repeated vomiting is often accentuated by the taking of medicines containing sodium bicarbonate. The most striking feature of severe alkalosis is Cheyne-Stokes' respiration with periods of apnoea lasting from five to thirty seconds. Tetany sometimes occurs. Latent tetany is more common, and can be unveiled by Trousseau's sign (Chapter 38). Regarding other signs, the dual phenomenon of severe alkalosis and hypokalaemia are so interwoven that their clinical separation is well-nigh impossible. Subclinical degrees of alkalosis are recognisable only by a raised standard bicarbonate concentration and a positive base excess. Severe alkalosis may result in renal epithelial damage, and consequent renal insufficiency.

Treatment.—Metabolic alkalosis without hypokalaemia seldom requires direct treatment. The cause of the alkalosis should be removed where possible and a high urinary output encouraged.

Hypokalaemic alkalosis is seen in patients who have lost potassium and acid due to repeated vomiting from pyloric stenosis. The low serum potassium causes potassium to leave the cell and be replaced by Na$^+$ and H$^+$ ion. The shift of H$^+$ ion into the cell causes

K. Mellemgaard, Contemporary. *Physician, Rigshospitalet, Copenhagen.*
Poul Astrup, Contemporary. *Clinical Chemist, Rigshospitalet, Copenhagen.*
John Cheyne, *1777–1836. Physician, Meath Hospital, Dublin (1811–1831). First Professor of Medicine, Royal College of Surgeons in Ireland (1813–1828), and Physician General to the Forces in Ireland (1820–1831). Described this type of Periodic Respiration in 1818.*
William Stokes, *1804–1878. Physician, Meath Hospital, Dublin (1826–1875), and Regius Professor of Medicine, Dublin (1845–1878). In an account of Periodic Breathing in 1846, he acknowledged Cheyne's observation.*

intracellular acidosis and increases the extracellular alkalosis. The kidneys continue to excrete K^+ and acid urine due to intracellular acidosis of the kidney cells themselves.

Treatment.—An ampoule of 20 mmol of potassium chloride is added to 500 ml 5% dextrose solution and given intravenously.

Respiratory alkalosis a condition where the CO_2 tension in the arterial blood (PCO_2) is below the normal range of 31–42 mmHg (4·1–5·6 kPa), is caused most commonly in surgical practice by excessive pulmonary ventilation carried out upon an anaesthetised patient who has been given a muscle relaxant. Other causes are hyperventilation occasioned by high altitudes, hyperpyrexia, a lesion of the hypothalamus, and hysteria. Compensation, which depends on increased renal excretion of bicarbonate, usually is inadequate. During anaesthesia alkalosis is accompanied by pallor and a fall of blood-pressure. In severe cases respiratory arrest follows.

Treatment.—Respiratory suppression due to alkalosis is rectified by insufflation of carbon dioxide.

ACIDOSIS

Metabolic acidosis (a condition where there is a deficit of base or an excess of any acid other than H_2CO_3) occurs as a result of:

(*a*) *Loss of bases* such as occurs in sustained diarrhoea, ulcerative colitis, gastro-colic fistula, a high intestinal fistula, or prolonged *intestinal* aspiration.

(*b*) *Increase in fixed acids* due to the formation of ketone bodies as in diabetes or starvation, the retention of metabolites in renal insufficiency, and the rapid increase of lactic and pyruvic acids by anaerobic tissue metabolism due to shock, following cardiac arrest (Chapter 41), or the release of the clamped aorta in the surgery of abdominal aneurysm (Chapter 14). Acute acidosis with pH levels of 7·1 are frequently encountered in such cases.

Clinical Features.—In severe acidosis the leading sign is rapid, deep, noisy respirations which are unremittent save, perhaps, momentarily while the patient endeavours unsuccessfully to moisten his dry lips with his parched tongue. The hyperpnoea is due to over-stimulation of the respiratory centre by the reduction of pH of the blood, and the physiological purpose of over-breathing is to eliminate as much as possible of the acid substance H_2CO_3. Except in renal acidosis, the pulse-rate and the blood-pressure are raised. The urine is strongly acid. The standard bicarbonate level is lowered and there is a base deficit (p. 88 acid-base measurements).

Treatment.—Cases belonging to class (*a*) are readily rectified by the administration of Ringer's lactate solution or slow infusion of dilute sodium bicarbonate solution. When dehydration is in evidence the prelude to treatment with sodium bicarbonate solution should be rapid infusion of sufficient isotonic saline solution to restore the extracellular fluid volume. The treatment of acidosis due to renal failure is discussed in Chapter 56.

The acute acidosis after releasing a cross-clamped aorta or in cardiac arrest requires the infusion of 50–150 mmol of 8·4% sodium bicarbonate solution (see base excess, p. 88).

Acidosis due to transplantation of the ureters into the colon is discussed in Chapter 57.

Respiratory acidosis (a condition where the PCO_2 is above the normal range) is caused by impaired alveolar ventilation.

In practice this problem most commonly occurs when there is inadequate ventilation of the anaesthetised patient, or when the effects of muscle relaxants have not worn off or been fully reversed at the end of the anaesthetic. There is also a risk of respiratory acidosis when the patient undergoing surgery already has pre-existing pulmonary disease (*e.g.* chronic bronchitis or emphysema), and this is accentuated by thoracic and upper abdominal incisions.

The Anion Gap.—This is a calculated estimation of the undetermined or unmeasured anions in the blood. It is sometimes used to establish the cause of a metabolic acidosis. Anion gap = $(Na + K) - (HCO_3 + Cl)$. The normal anion gap is 10–16 mmol/litre. An increased anion gap is seen in metabolic acidosis due to ketoacidosis, lactic acidosis, poisoning (salicylates) and renal failure. A normal anion gap is seen in metabolic acidosis due to renal tubular acidosis and loss of alkali due to diarrhoea, intestinal obstruction or intestinal fistula and in the hyperchloraemia of ureterocolic anastomosis.

CHAPTER 7

NUTRITION

Malnutrition.—In surgical practice malnutrition is common, being present before or occurring after operation in about 50 per cent of patients, possibly more in some parts of the world.

Preoperative Malnutrition may be due to starvation or to a failure of digestion. Starvation is caused by (i) difficulty in obtaining food (poverty), (ii) difficulty in swallowing food (dysphagia), (iii) difficulty in retaining swallowed food (vomiting), and (iv) self neglect (e.g. in the elderly and in alcoholics). Failure of proper digestion may, for example, be due to pancreatic or biliary disease (carcinoma, jaundice due to stones), and duodenal and jejunal conditions (fistula, blind loop syndrome).

Postoperative (Post-traumatic) Malnutrition is hopefully in most cases of a transient nature consequent upon a short period of starvation and the stress reaction to trauma. Recovery from any nitrogen deficit due to protein catabolism will follow on the return of normal feeding. Any delay in return to a normal diet such as may be imposed by the dictates of the operation (oesophagectomy), or a complication (paralytic ileus from peritonitis), means that severe malnourishment is likely to occur.

Hypercatabolic State.—Severe sepsis (subphrenic abscess), severe trauma (burns) and other severe disturbances of major viscera (pancreatitis), are accompanied by an accelerated and profound breakdown of tissue proteins.

TYPICAL DAILY POSTOPERATIVE NITROGEN LOSS

	Nitrogen Loss g	Muscle Loss g
Herniotomy	3	80
Appendicectomy	6	200
Cholecystectomy	12	320
Fractured Femur	15	400
Oesophagectomy	90	2500
Peritonitis	18	570
Sepsis	23	730

In starvation the metabolic changes are directed to minimising tissue loss and in some circumstances a man can survive for about 120 days. Glucose reserves are available only for 24 hours and thereafter are derived principally from muscle, so that catabolism begins almost immediately after food deprivation. In the first 72 hours there is a rapid weight loss due to loss of sodium and water, then the resting metabolic expenditure falls and daily nitrogen losses over two weeks fall from about 10 g to 3–4 g. Progressively fat provides most of the energy requirements yielding 9 cal/g, while carbohydrate derived by gluconeogenesis in the liver from amino acids is utilised by brain, adrenal glands and red cells—

all obligatory glucose users. After about 21 days the central nervous system adapts to using ketones derived from fat. The gluconeogenesis and ketosis of starvation may be easily inhibited by glucose intake.

After injury or surgical operation there is an increased oxygen and calorie consumption and a negative nitrogen balance (Cuthbertson). The increase in resting metabolic expenditure ranges from minimal after uncomplicated surgery to 30% with multiple fractures, 45% in peritonitis and up to 100% in burns. An increase in metabolic rate and protein catabolism of more than 25% is regarded as a hypercatabolic state.

The endocrine profile, activated by fear, apprehension and nervous stimuli from damaged tissues is altered after stress with an increase in secretion of most hormones in turn resulting in changes in substrate handling by the body.

Glycogen breakdown in muscle and liver is accelerated principally by adrenaline and glucagon leading to increased blood glucose levels, while increased cortisol and glucagon induces gluconeogenesis from amino acids. Lipolysis—fat breakdown—is increased by growth hormone, glucagon and noradrenaline. Thus control of glucose levels is impaired, and, together with depressed peripheral clearance, results in 'the diabetes of injury'.

The stimulated protein breakdown in the postoperative period is associated with a change in synthesis rate in the body cell mass and this results in a negative nitrogen balance indicating loss of protein derived from muscle and viscera. Larger losses are seen in muscular athletic men and the smallest losses in wasted patients. Epidural anaesthesia inhibits the normal postoperative increases in cortisol, adrenaline, aldosterone and growth hormone, and so may reduce the negative nitrogen balance. Nitrogen balance may be improved during enteral or parenteral feeding if the patient can be mobilised.

The Effects of Malnutrition include poor wound healing manifest as wound dehiscence (Chapter 1) and leaking anastomoses of bowel, delayed callus formation, disordered coagulation, reduced enzyme synthesis, impaired oxidative metabolism of drugs by the liver, immunological depression with increasing susceptibility to infection, decreased tolerance to radiotherapy and cytotoxic chemotherapy, all with the severe mental apathy and physical exhaustion of the patient.

SOME CLINICAL INDICATIONS FOR NUTRITIONAL SUPPORT

1. Preoperative Nutritional Depletion	6. Anorexia Nervosa
2. Postoperative Complications	7. Intractible Vomiting
a. Ileus more than 4 days	8. Maxillo-facial Trauma
b. Sepsis	9. Traumatic Coma
c. Fistula formation	10. Multiple Trauma
3. Intestinal Fistula	11. Burns
4. Massive Bowel Resection	12. Malignant Disease
5. Management of	13. Renal Failure
a. Pancreatitis	14. Liver Disease
b. Malabsorption Syndromes	15. Cardiac Valve Disease
c. Ulcerative Colitis	
d. Radiation Enteritis	
e. Pyloric Stenosis	

Assessment and Management

Thus it is essential for the clinician to be aware of the need (a) to assess the state of nutrition of a patient, and if malnutrition is present or threatens (b) to consider the nutritional requirements and then (c) to use methods of sustaining normality or rectifying any deficiency.

(*a*) **Assessment.**—A malnourished patient has a characteristic appearance, lean and hungry in most cases of starvation, lean and apathetic in post-traumatic depletion, with a superimposed hectic flush around sunken cheeks and pinched

Sir David Cuthbertson, C.B.E., Contemporary. Honorary Consultant in Clinical Biochemistry, Glasgow Royal Infirmary, Scotland.

nose in a hypercatabolic state. The clinician as he places his comforting hand on the patient's shoulder discerns the bony scapula bereft of almost all its muscle. However, these clinical observations only detect gross malnutrition and therefore measurement of the nutritional status is essential (Goode). The parameters include:

(i) *Body weight.*—Careful weighing on a bed weighing machine is the obvious way of detecting the progress or otherwise of the patient. The desirable weight of the patient can be checked by reference to the appropriate tables, or by applying the body mass index (B.M.I.) $= \dfrac{\text{Wt (kg)}}{\text{Height}^2 \text{ (m)}}$. A woman should have an index of 20, 21, or 23, and a man 20·5, 22, 23·5 according to size of frame (small, medium, large).

(ii) *Upper arm circumference.*—Feeding is indicated if less than 23 cm in females, and 25 cm in males.

(iii) *Triceps skin fold thickness.*—Using a skin fold caliper, the minimum is 13 mm in females and 10 mm in males.

(iv) *Serum albumin* should not be less than 35 g/l.

(v) *Lymphocyte count.*—Less than 1500/mm³ indicates an impaired cellular defence mechanism.

(vi) *Candida skin test.*—A negative reaction also means defective cell mediated immunity.

(vii) *Nitrogen balance studies.*—The total nitrogen intake is compared with the loss from all sources, such as urine, fistula drainage and nasogastric aspirate (1 litre=1 g nitrogen). A greater loss than intake indicates a negative balance and tissue breakdown. A positive balance means anabolism-tissue synthesis.

DAILY CALORIE AND NITROGEN REQUIREMENTS
(after Ivan D. A. Johnston)

	Postoperative	*Hypercatabolic States*
Water ml/kg	35	40–45
Kcal/kg	35	45–55
Kcal/g Nitrogen	180	200–280
Nitrogen g/kg	0·2	0·25–0·30

Other measurements include those determining the rate of muscle breakdown, such as urinary creatinine excretion, or 3-methyl histidine excretion. Today body potassium and nitrogen are used to assess the absolute size of the body cell mass. ¹⁴C leucine incorporation is a measure of the synthesis rate, while serum transferrin is used as a measure of visceral protein synthesis (needs to be more than 1·5 g/l).

(*b*) **Nutritional requirements** include carbohydrate, fat, protein, vitamins, minerals and trace elements.

Calories are provided by carbohydrate and fat. A healthy adult at rest requires 1500–2000 non-protein calories per day for energy. Carbohydrate provides 4·1 kcal/g (16·8 kJ/g) and fat 9·1 kcal/g (37·8 kJ/g). The number of non-protein

Anthony William Goode, Contemporary. Assistant Director, The Surgical Unit, The London Hospital, London.
Ivan David Alexander Johnston, Contemporary. Professor of Surgery, University of Newcastle-upon-Tyne.

calories given should bear a definite relationship to the nitrogen intake. A typical regime would feature 2000 kcals: 13g N (about 150:1).

Nitrogen requirements.—The minimum for dynamic tissue turnover and so to keep a healthy adult in positive nitrogen balance is about 35–40 g of protein or 5·5–6·5 g of nitrogen per day. The hypercatabolic patient requiring hyperalimentation may need three or four times this amount of protein. A daily negative nitrogen balance of 10 g N is not unusual and is equivalent to a loss of 62·5 g of protein of 300 g of muscle tissue.

Vitamins.—Whatever the method of feeding, vitamins are necessary as supplements, as they are essential for the maintenance of normal metabolic function and cannot be synthesised by the body.

The water-soluble vitamins B and C act as coenzymes in collagen formation and wound healing. Postoperatively the vitamin C requirement increases to 60–80 mg/day. Preoperative depletion is exacerbated by anorexia, smoking, aspirin and barbiturate therapy. Vitamin B_{12} is given 500 μg i.m. weekly particularly to those with initial low levels (coeliac disease, Crohn's disease, ileal resection or bypass, blind loop syndrome, tapeworm infestation, reduced pancreatic secretion, tropical sprue, excess alcohol intake, anti-convulsant therapy, and after gastric surgery). As the serum folate falls, especially in those on parenteral nutrition, folinic acid is required daily in doses of 3–6 mg i.m.

The fat-soluble vitamins A, D, E, and K are reduced in steatorrhoea and the absence of bile. Vitamin A, 5000 units per week, is required after surgery, and when appropriate it enhances the antitumour effect of cyclophosphamide. Vitamin K 5–10 mg i.m. weekly reduces any bleeding tendency. If commercially available vitamin additives are put into an infusion, the container should be protected from the light.

Minerals and trace elements.—Sodium, potassium, iron, calcium and magnesium deficiencies must be identified and made good (p. 82). Zinc deficiency is manifest as a rash on the face and perineum which does not respond to antifungal therapy, stomatitis which causes disturbance of taste (dysgeusia), and alopecia. Copper deficiency results in leucopaenia and anaemia, while lack of chromium may give rise to glucose intolerance. In the 14 trace elements that are considered essential for normal enzyme activities within the body are also included manganese, cobalt, molybdenum and vanadium. It is to be remembered that long term parenteral nutrition can result in depletion.

(*c*) **Methods of Feeding.**—These are predominantly enteral and less commonly parenteral.

Enteral Nutrition

(1) **By mouth.**—Obviously, as this is the natural way it should always be attempted. Only when it is known that this route cannot be used or is ineffective are other methods considered.

Feeding by mouth demands *common sense, cleanliness and compassion* on the part of the medical attendants. It is *common sense* to ensure that an adequate, palatable and varied diet, including all the nutritional requirements, is provided at regular intervals, more frequently than regular meal times if necessary. It is common sense to begin with a liquid diet as soon as bowel sounds return after an abdominal operation, and not, for example, to allow a plate of fish and chips to be put in front of a patient the day after his gangrenous appendix has been removed. Promotion to semi-solid (light) and then to more solid food (full diet) follows in steps of 3–7 days according to progress. *Cleanliness* in the preparation and serving of food and of the utensils used is of paramount importance in avoiding gastrointestinal infection causing vomiting and diarrhoea. A salmonella infection amongst elderly patients and children may be a mortal blow. *Compassion* is needed to ensure that the patient actually receives and ingests the proffered food. Food must be placed within reach of an enfeebled patient. Assistance is often required and should be freely given. Dental care may be necessary to facilitate oral intake, and false teeth may need consideration.

(2) **By tube.**—A nasogastric tube which has been passed to allow regular gastric aspiration to be performed may also be used for feeding liquidised diets. Fine bore tubing can be used instead, being favourably received by most patients as not so irritating as the larger tube. It is invaluable when passed with the aid of an endoscope through an oesophageal stricture into the stomach, enabling thereby the effects of starvation to be reversed.

EXAMPLES[1] OF ENTERAL DIETS[2]

A) Liquids

Constituents per litre (as applied)

	Nitrogen (g)	Fat (g)	CHO (g)	kJ/kcal	Osmolality (mOsm)
Clinifeed Favour	6·0	33·1	140·0	4200/1003	335
Isocal	5·1	42·0	126·0	4240/1013	290
Nutrauxil	6·1	34·0	138·0	4200/1003	300

B) Powders

Constituents per 100 g

	Nitrogen (g)	Fat (g)	CHO (g)	kJ/kcal
Ensure	2·2	31·5	54·5	1831/437
Flexical	1·6	15·0	66·9	1856/443
Vivonex HN (high nitrogen)	2·5	0·3	79·0	1570/370

Technique of Fine Bore Tube Insertion and Usage.—The patient may be sitting or lying, preferably the former. The introducer wire is lubricated with water and inserted into the fine bore tube. The tube is passed through the nose via the nasopharynx and oesophagus into the stomach. Withdraw the wire and tape the tube to the patient. Check the position of the tube by x-ray as passage into a bronchus can occur quite easily. Alternatively a quick check can be made by injecting 5 ml of air down the tube and listening for its bubbling entry into the stomach through a stethoscope.

Administration of the feeds is either by gravity or by means of an infusion pump.

[1] The table is only representative of the range available. Dieticians and pharmacists should be involved in the prescribing of enteral feeding regimes in much the same way as they are involved in parenteral feeding.
[2] Suppliers: Clinifeed—Roussel Laboratories Ltd, Uxbridge, Middlesex
      Isocal & Flexical—Bristol-Myers Pharmaceuticals, Slough, Bucks
      Nutrauxil—KabiVitrum Ltd, Uxbridge, Middlesex
      Ensure—Abbot Laboratories Ltd, Queenborough, Kent
      Vivonex—Norwich Eaton Ltd, Gosforth, Tyne & Wear.

Notes on Problems of Tube Feeding.—Gastric emptying should be normal. In ill patients ensure that the stomach empties by injecting 60 ml water down a nasogastric tube and aspirate 4 hourly. If after 24 hours fluid is passing through the stomach, commence feeding for the first day and aspirate intermittently to ensure that the stomach empties. Then remove the tube and introduce the fine-bore tube.

Blockage of a 1 mm bore tube is cleared by flushing through with 2 ml water—do not add effervescent potassium to the feed as curdling will follow.

Most fine-bore tubes incorporate a male 'luer' lock connector making the nasogastric drip system incompatible with intravenous lines.

Check the drip rate hourly.

All feeds should be stored at 4°C until use, not exposed to room temperature for more than eight hours, and discarded if not used after twelve hours. As diet kitchens may be a source of klebsiella infection the bacteriological monitoring of feeds is desirable.

Unwanted effects.—Nausea, vomiting and pulmonary aspiration are avoided by regulation of the infusion rate and ensuring initial gastric emptying. Diabetes and hyperosmolar states are related to high carbohydrate intake with particular hazard for the established diabetic. *Diarrhoea* is common and the pathogenesis is not fully understood, but fluid and electrolytes are secreted into the bowel in response to a high osmotic load. Also the use of broad spectrum antibiotics is associated with diarrhoea. Commence with half strength feed and increase slowly to standard concentration over days given at a slow constant rate, avoiding milk because of possible lactose intolerance, and a high fat content giving steatorrhoea. Mild disturbances of liver function can be associated with both enteral and parenteral feeding, due to intrahepatic cholestasis. Metronidazole 500 mg b.d. may prevent overgrowth of the anaerobic bacteria responsible.

(3) **Gastrostomy** may be performed at the end of an operation which is likely to be followed by a period of malnutrition (*e.g.* peritonitis with bowel resection). To begin with it is used for gastric drainage and avoids the use of a nasogastric tube, and as soon as bowel sounds return it is used for feeding. A simple rubber or plastic tube (8–10 mm diam) with an additional hole made near the tip is passed through a separate 'stab' incision through the upper left rectus muscle. On other elective occasions a short muscle-splitting incision is made (even under local anaesthesia). The tube is inserted through a 'stab' incision in the anterior wall of the stomach for about 10 cm and fixed to the wall by catgut. Using two rows of purse-string sutures tube and stomach are pushed in to form an ink-well (Kader-Senn). The stomach is tacked to the anterior parietes. The tube should be directed towards the fundus of the stomach as paradoxically it seems to function better in this direction. The tube is secured to the skin by tunnelling within an adhesive plaster dressing and connected to a bag (or the feed) using wide bore connections to avoid blockage by curds, mucus etc. The use of catgut enables the tube to be removed when desired after about ten days.

(4) **Jejunostomy** may be performed instead of a gastrostomy if the use of the stomach is contraindicated, e.g. after an extended gastrectomy.

Parenteral Nutrition

Parenteral nutrition by intravenous feeding is used in less than 4–5 per cent of all hospital admissions, either when enteral feeding is not possible, or to supplement deficient enteral feeding. Contraindications include cardiac failure, severe liver disease, disorders of fat metabolism, uncontrolled diabetes, shock and severe blood dyscrasias. It must be remembered that total parenteral nutrition is not to be undertaken lightly. It is potentially hazardous and can be dangerous in inexperienced hands. The recent trend towards the formation of

Bronislaw Kader, 1863–1937. Surgeon, Poland.
Nicholas Senn, 1844–1908. Surgeon, U.S.A.

multidiscipline nutritional care teams including dieticians and pharmacists is a major advance and their advice should be sought.

When planning an intravenous feeding regimen, first weigh the patient and calculate the fluid needs for the next 24 hours. Calorie and nitrogen intake should be calculated on a body weight basis remembering that daily needs may change. Daily biochemical patient monitoring is essential.

MONITORING FEEDING REGIMENS

Daily	Body weight
	Fluid balance
	Full blood count, urea and electrolytes
	Blood glucose
	Urine and plasma osmolality
	Electrolyte and nitrogen analysis of urine and gastrointestinal losses
	Acid base status
Thrice Weekly	Serum calcium, magnesium and phosphate
	Plasma proteins
	Liver function tests
	Clotting studies
Ten Days	Serum B12, folate, iron, lactate and triglycerides
	Trace elements

Most feeding teams decide on the nitrogen and calorie requirements of their patients and tailor-make the feeds from the wide variety of amino acid solutions with and without electrolytes and the various concentrations of dextrose and fat available. Typically these are mixed under laminar flow sterile conditions in the pharmacy into 3 litre bags giving sufficient for 24 hours or, better still, supplied to specifications by one of the companies involved in the manufacture of I.V. solutions. 20% glucose is equivalent to 770 kcal/l/(3200 kJ/l) and 20% Intralipid (KabiVitrum) is equivalent to 2000 kcal/ (8400 kJ/l).

SOME AVAILABLE SOLUTIONS FOR I.V. FEEDING

	Non-protein Calories per litre	N g/litre	Na (mmol/litre)	K	Mg	PO_4	Ca
Vamin 9 Glucose	400	9·4	50	20	1·5	—	2·5
Synthamin 14	—	14·3	73	60	5	30	—
Aminoplex 14	—	13·4	35	30	—	—	—
Intralipid 20%	2000	—	—	—	—	15	—

As most glucose solutions are hypertonic and irritant they are usually given through central veins, the cannulation of which requires technical finesse. In the short term the nutritional requirements in aseptic patients can be adequately met with mixtures of amino acids, fat and glucose given peripherally. Fat buffers the vein wall and sometimes sub-therapeutic doses of heparin and hydrocortisone are given to act locally in the prevention of thrombophlebitis. The energy requirements of surgical patients have often been overestimated; few will require more than 2000 kcal (8400 kJ) per day (Macfie).

J.Macfie, Contemporary, Senior Surgical Registrar, Leeds.

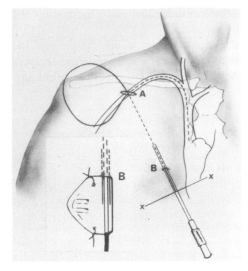

FIG. 50.—Subclavian catheterisation with a skin tunnel. Note: The sedated patient is placed in the head down position. The procedure is carried out in a clean room using strict aseptic technique. Insert: the plastic clip which grips the emerging catheter at B and sleeve, suitably anchored with sutures (*after J. Powell-Tuck*).

Technique for Central Venous Catheter Insertion with a Skin Tunnel (fig. 50).—Percutaneous catheter insertion requires expertise to prevent the *complications* which may occur in one in five attempts. These are air embolism, pneumothorax and injury to the subclavian artery or brachial plexus because of significant variation in relationship of the subclavian vein to the clavicle and first rib. A subclavian vein cutdown technique may be employed to allow cannulation of the vein under direct vision. A silicone rubber catheter of 1 mm diam (Vygon[1]) is inserted by infraclavicular approach, the introducer inserted under local anaesthetic through a 1 cm skin incision (A) 2 cm below the midclavicular point. The position of the catheter is checked radiologically ensuring the tip is in the superior vena cava or right atrium. The catheter hub is removed and the introducer withdrawn. The introducer is now inserted through the skin puncture at (B) about 7 cm below and medial to (A); it is passed through the subcutaneous tissue to emerge at (A) and the catheter threaded through the introducer at (A) until it is seen within the transparent introducer at (B). The introducer is partially withdrawn and cut at X—X so that 2 cm remains in the tunnel and 2 cm protrudes, and the catheter pushed fully through the 4 cm sleeve avoiding kinks at (A). (A) and (B) are cleaned with chlorhexidine in alcohol and sprayed with povidone iodine powder. Incision (A) is closed with a stitch and covered with a sterile dressing. *Caution.*—It is possible for the catheter tip to perforate the vein wall. If this occurs in the pleural cavity a pneumothorax can be caused. Before the infusion is started, it is essential to confirm by a free back-flow of blood that the catheter remains in the lumen of the vessel.

Commence using half strength solution and increase to the desired daily intake over days. Additives to solutions should be avoided and given through a separate line, although central mixing in pharmacy allows addition under sterile conditions into a 3 litre bag delivery system.

Catheter-related sepsis may occur in up to one third of patients fed parenterally. Skin flora are important in the pathogenesis of this sepsis and the skin at the site of the catheter insertion should be swabbed on alternate days. Bacteriological skin culture shows a strong association between microbial growth, usually *Staphylococcus epidermidis*, and the development of catheter-related infection. Factors known to increase the risk of infection include variation from the strict nursing protocol for care of the catheter, the age of the patient, and the duration of hospital stay before the institution of parenteral nutrition.

Home Parenteral Nutrition

Chronic intestinal failure results in a failure of adequate nutrient absorption from the gut to maintain body weight. This may follow extensive bowel resection, multiple high output fistulas, motility disorders and extensive Crohn's disease. Such patients require

[1] 'Vygon' U.K. Ltd., Uxbridge, England.

Jeremy Powell-Tuck, Contemporary. Senior Registrar, Charing Cross Hospital, London.

prolonged nutritional management by a skilled and experienced team. Long-term home parenteral nutrition depends upon suitable case selection and extensive patient training by experienced nurses together with a comprehensive hospital pharmaceutical service: the patient will live at home and manage his own parenteral feeding. With successful treatment, many patients are able to return to work or care for the home and family unaided or with minimum help.

Notes on Solutions.—Fructose, sorbital or alcohol solutions are potentially disadvantageous due to an associated lactic acidosis or hepatocellular damage. Fat, isotonic preparations of vegetable oils in water with an emulsification agent, or purified egg phospholipid in intralipid (to stabilise the mixture) should not be used 12 hours before blood sampling as they interfere with analysis. The rate of clearance of intravenous fat is increased after surgery or when energy demands are high (Feggetter).

The nitrogen sources are either casein hydrolysates, or laevorotatory isomers of amino acids. In such solutions all essential amino acids should be present with a broad spectrum of the non-essential amino acids. No single amino acid should predominate since if its utilisation is inefficient this will interfere with the utilisation of the others (Tweedle). In sepsis, renal failure and hepatic failure the use of solutions containing only essential amino acids, isoleucine, leucine, valine, phenylalanine, lysine and tyrosine is under investigation.

Complications.—The initial complications of parenteral feeding arise from *malposition of the catheter tip*, and x-ray confirmation of the site of the catheter tip is mandatory before infusion. *Infection*, particularly septicaemia, arises from continuous direct vascular access and immune depression in malnourished patients, together with the solutions being ideal bacterial and fungal culture media. Catheter insertion with strict asepsis, daily care of the entry site cleaned with 1–2% tincture of iodine and alcohol solutions and the strict use of the line only for nutrient solutions all contribute to prevention. However, if a patient develops an unexplained fever, hypotension, vomiting, diarrhoea, confusion or seizures, a full clinical examination with appropriate radiology and bacteriological culture of blood, sputum, urine and swabs of the catheter site are indicated. If a source of infection is

BIOCHEMICAL COMPLICATIONS DURING PARENTERAL NUTRITION AND THEIR CORRECTION

Complication	Clinical Presentation	Cause	Correction
Hyponatraemia	Confusion Apathy	Water intoxication G.I. or renal loss	Reduce water intake Increase Na^+ intake
Hypokalaemia	Apathy Cardiac irregularity	Inadequate K^+ intake G.I. or renal loss	Increase K^+ intake
Hypomagnesaemia	Weakness Vertigo Convulsions	Inadequate Mg^{++} intake G.I. or renal loss	Increase Mg^{++} intake
Hypophosphataemia	Apathy, confusion, Panesthesis, RBC oxygen dissociation	Inadequate inorganic phosphate intake	Increase PO_4 intake
Azotaemia	Apathy	Dehydration Calorie: Nitrogen imbalance	Increase water intake Increase Calorie: Nitrogen ratio to 185:1
Hyperammonaemia	Apathy, seizures, coma	Hepatic dysfunction Amino acid deficiency	Reduce infusion rate or stop
Hyperglycaemia	Increased blood sugar	Unsuspected diabetes Underlying sepsis Excess infusion of carbohydrate	Treat underlying cause Treat underlying cause Reduce infusion rate
Hypoglycaemia	Lethargy Vasoconstriction	Interrupted infusion	Give dextrose
Hyperosmolar dehydration	Hyperglycaemia Dehydration Increased serum sodium and osmolality Apathy Coma	Hyperglycaemia	Correct hyperglycaemia and give half strength saline

Jeremy George Weightman Feggetter, Contemporary. Surgeon, Ashington and Freeman Hospitals, Newcastle-upon-tyne.
David Ernest Frederick Tweedle, Contemporary. Senior Lecturer in Surgery, University of Manchester.

discovered it is treated, but if no source is found and the fever persists for 24 hours remove the catheter and send the tip for bacteriological and fungal culture, candida albicans, staphylococci or klebsiella frequently being isolated. Recommence the parenteral regimen using a new catheter at a fresh site.

Prolonged use of amino acids and glucose alone will result in essential fatty acid deficiency, with *dermatitis*, *anaemia and increased capillary permeability*, a complication avoided by the use of intravenous fat solutions or essential fatty acids rubbed into the skin weekly. Similarly *hypophosphataemia* is seen with such regimens and accentuated by the use of insulin, resulting in enzyme defects, ATP deficiency and a shift to the left in the oxygen dissociation curve, is prevented by a daily intake of 13 mmol of potassium dihydrogen phosphate. *Jaundice* occurring during parenteral nutrition is cholestatic, perhaps the result of sepsis, malnutrition and hypoxia and feeding should be temporarily discontinued. *Metabolic acidosis*, much less common if fructose and alcohol are avoided, may arise from infusion of available hydrogen ions in amino acid solutions and is simply corrected with sodium bicarbonate solution.

Steroids.—Anabolic steroids (*e.g.* Durabolin 25 mg i.m. weekly) may be used to improve nitrogen balance, but the effect may not be observed for some days.

CHAPTER 8

TUMOURS. CYSTS. ULCERS. SINUSES

TUMOURS

A tumour is a new formation of cells of independent growth which fulfils no useful function. The term 'tumour' should be reserved for new growths; its loose application to inflammatory swellings, such as Pott's puffy 'tumour' (Chapter 26), or to enlargement of an organ due to hypertrophy, should be abandoned.

Causation.—Over 300 years ago it was stated that 'any kind of external irritation, whether from motion, heat, or acrimony, may cause cancer'. Natives of Kashmir are prone to cancer of the skin of the thighs and lower abdomen. This is due to their habit of keeping warm by squatting and hugging earthenware pots containing glowing charcoal (the pot being termed a *kangri*), with the result that the adjacent skin is irritated by heat and fumes. 'Chimney-sweeps" cancer (Chapter 61), and 'countryman's lip' (Chapter 30), and tar workers' cancer (fig. 51) are other examples of carcinoma due to chronic irritation.

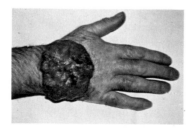

FIG. 51.—Squamous-celled carcinoma on the back of the hand of a tar worker.

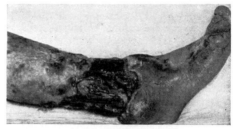

FIG. 52.—Squamous-celled carcinoma in a varicose ulcer (note everted edge).

Regeneration of tissue, with possibly the awakening of erstwhile dormant embryonic cells, may encourage malignant changes. Primary carcinoma of the liver is sometimes seen in cases of cirrhosis, and arises from the liver cells which are endeavouring to regenerate. Similarly, squamous-celled carcinoma occasionally occurs in a chronic ulcer (fig. 52), also Marjolin's ulcer in a scar (Chapter 10). A fibrosarcoma arising in a scar is not uncommon.

Viruses cause nucleal instability and are therefore implicated in some tumour origins, e.g. Burkitt's lymphoma, Kapozi's sarcoma (Chapter 9). A wart is the commonest example of a virus causing a tumour.

DEFINITIONS

Metaplasia.—The epithelium from which the tumour grows has already changed its characteristics, *e.g.* bladder transitional epithelium to squamous epithelium, gallbladder columnar to squamous epithelium, bronchial columnar to squamous epithelium, even gastric columnar epithelial pattern to intestinal epithelial pattern.

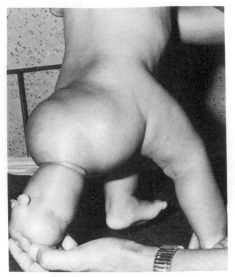

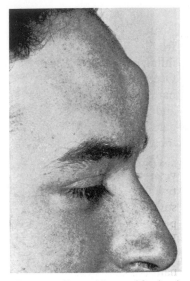

FIG. 53.—This sacrococcygeal teratoma had taken the shape of a leg (a third leg!) It had rudimentary toes and nails. It was successfully operated on.

(A. C. Bose, MS, FACS, Senior Consultant (Surgery) Armed Forces, India.)

FIG. 54.—Dermoid cyst of forehead.

Anaplasia.—Tumours produce cells which resemble those from which they arise, but with rapid growth the resemblance is less obvious (anaplastic change).

Teratomas arise from 'totipotent' cells, containing representative cells from all three embryonic layers: ectoderm, endoderm, mesoderm. Teratomatous 'dermoids', for example, contain hair, teeth, muscle, gland tissue. An unusual type is the sacrococcygeal teratoma (fig. 53) which can be considered as *foetus in foetu* (an 'included' foetus).

Blastomas develop from unipotent cells, and arise from any one of the three embryonic layers (*e.g.* neuroblastoma).

Dermoid Cysts.—'Dermoid' is a loose term given to cysts lined by squamous epithelium occurring in various parts of the body. Sebaceous cysts are lined by superficial squamous cells and should more accurately be called 'epidermoids'.

(i) *Teratomatous dermoids* (see above) are found in the ovary, testis, retroperitoneum, superior mediastinum, and the presacral area. Malignant change (carcinomatous or sarcomatous) can occur.

(ii) *Sequestration dermoids* (see Cysts) are not teratomas but are formed by the inclusion of epithelium beneath the surface at places where lines of developing skin meet and join (forehead (fig. 54), external angular process, Chapter 33, root of nose, Chapter 33, branchial cysts, Chapter 36).

(iii) *Implantation dermoids* (see Cysts) may follow puncture wounds, commonly of the fingers.

Innocent or Malignant.—An **innocent or benign tumour** is usually encapsulated, and does not disseminate nor recur after removal. Symptoms and effects, which can be harmful, are due to its size, position, and pressure. Certain adenomas secrete a *hormone* which may affect bodily functions. Innocent tumours are often multiple.

Malignant Tumours.—The characteristics of malignancy are: (*a*) Invasion of surrounding tissues, (*b*) pleomorphism (variable shapes) of cells, (*c*) rapid growth, (*d*) the tendency to spread to other parts of the body by the lymphatics and the blood-stream, (*e*) general weight loss.

It has been suggested that the division of tumours into these two major groups imposes a concept which is too rigid (Walter). A third group of intermediate tumours exists which includes carcinoid tumours, 'adenoma' of the bronchus, 'mixed' salivary tumours, basal cell carcinoma, *etc.* These intermediate types invade locally, but are much less inclined to lymphatic or especially vascular dissemination.

John B. Walter, Contemporary, Associate Professor of Pathology, University of Toronto, Canada.

BENIGN TUMOURS

Adenoma.—Adenomas arise in secretory glands, and resemble the structure from which they arise. They are encapsulated, and sometimes they profoundly influence metabolism, as in the case of the thyroid, parathyroid and pancreas. Occasionally an adenoma contains a large proportion of fibrous tissue, *e.g.* the hard fibro-adenoma in the breast, while in other situations, notably the pancreas and thyroid gland, cystic degeneration is common. Those arising from secretory glands of mucous membrane are liable to pedunculation, as in the case of rectal 'polypus'.

Papilloma.—A papilloma consists of a central axis of connective tissue, blood-vessels, and lymphatics; the surface is covered by epithelium, either squamous, transitional, cuboidal or columnar, according to the site of the tumour. The surface may be merely roughened, or composed of innumerable delicate villous processes, as in the case of those occurring in the kidney, bladder and rectum. In these situations papillomas resemble malignant tumours, as secondary growths arise by implantation, and, sooner or later, the tumour becomes frankly malignant (Chapter 58). Other common sites for papillomas are the skin, the colon, the tongue and lip, the vocal cords and the walls of cysts, particularly those in connection with the breast and ovary.

Fibroma.—A true fibroma (containing only fibrous connective tissue) is rare. Most fibromas are combined with other mesodermal tissues such as muscle (fibromyoma), fat (fibrolipoma), and nerve sheaths (neurofibroma), *etc.* Multiple tumours are not uncommon, as, for example, in neurofibromatosis (von Recklinghausen's disease).

Fibromas are either *hard* or *soft*, depending on the proportion of fibrous to the other cellular tissue. Soft fibromas are common in the subcutaneous tissue of the face, and appear as soft brown swellings.[1]

Desmoid.—This unusual type of fibroma occurs in the abdominal wall (Chapter 55).
Keloid (fig. 8). In patients with familial polyposis they occur also intra-abdominally (Chapter 50).

Lipoma.—A lipoma is a slowly growing tumour composed of fat cells of adult type. Lipomas may be encapsulated or diffuse. They occur anywhere in the body where fat is found and earn the titles of the 'universal tumour' or the 'ubiquitous tumour'. The head and neck area, abdominal wall, and the thighs are particularly favoured sites.

Encapsulated lipomas are among the commonest of tumours. The characteristic features are the presence of a definite edge and lobulation. A sense of fluctuation may be obtained. As would be expected, a lipoma deeply situated is liable to be mistaken for other swellings. Most lipomas are painless, but some give rise to an aching sensation which may radiate.

Multiple lipomas are not uncommon. The tumours remain small or moderate in size, and are sometimes painful, in which case the condition is probably one of *neurolipomatosis. Dercum's disease (adiposis dolorosa)*, characterised by tender deposits of fat, especially on the trunk, is an associated condition.

---

[1] Oliver Cromwell (1599-1658), Lord Protector of England from 1653 until his death, was disfigured by one of these tumours which he called a wart. He insisted that his portraits should show him 'wart and all'.

Francis Xavier Dercum, 1856-1931. Neurologist, Jefferson Medical College, Philadelphia, Pennsylvania, U.S.A. Described Adiposis Dolorosa in 1888.

Should the lipoma contain an excessive amount of fibrous tissue it is termed a *fibrolipoma*. In other cases considerable vascularity is present, often with telangiectasis of the overlying skin, in which case the tumour is a *naevolipoma*. Large lipomas of the thigh (fig. 55), the shoulder (fig. 56) and the retroperitoneum occasionally undergo *sarcomatous changes*. *Myxomatous degeneration, saponification* and *calcification* sometimes occur in lipomas of long duration.

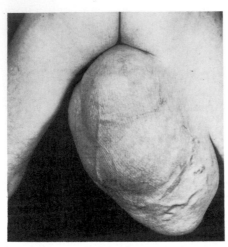

FIG. 55.—Giant lipoma of the thigh.

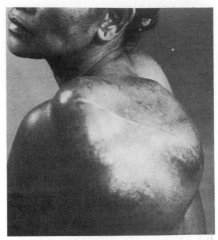

FIG. 56.—Liposarcoma. Note incision of previous operation.
(*Dr. R. S. Naik, Durg, India.*)

Clinically, circumscribed lipomas are classified according to their situation:

(i) *Subcutaneous*.—Commonly found on the shoulders or the back, although no part of the body is immune. A lipoma may be present over the site of a spina bifida. Subcutaneous lipomas occasionally become pedunculated (lipoma arborescens).

(ii) *Subfascial*.—Occurring under the palmar or plantar fascia, they are liable to be mistaken for tuberculous tenosynovitis, as the tough, overlying fascia masks the definite edge and lobulation of the tumour. Difficulty is encountered in complete removal as pressure encourages the tumour to ramify. Subfascial lipomas also occur in the areolar layer under the epicranial aponeurosis, and if of long duration they erode the underlying bone, so that a depression is palpable on pushing the tumour to one side.

(iii) *Subsynovial*.—From the fatty padding around joints, especially the knee. They are apt to be mistaken for Baker's cysts (Chapter 24) but are easily distinguished as, in distinction to a cyst or bursa, their consistency is constant whether the joint is in extension or flexion.

(iv) *Intra-articular*.

(v) *Intermuscular*.—Mainly in the thigh or around the shoulder. Owing to transmitted pressure the tumour becomes firmer when the adjacent muscles are contracted. Weakness or aching results, owing to mechanical interference with muscular action. The condition is often difficult to distinguish from a fibrosarcoma.

(vi) *Parosteal* occasionally occur under the periosteum of a bone.

(vii) *Subserous* are sometimes found beneath the pleura, where they constitute one variety of innocent thoracic tumour. A retroperitoneal lipoma may grow to enormous dimensions, and simulate a hydronephrosis or pancreatic cyst.

(viii) *Submucous* occur under the mucous membrane of the respiratory or alimentary tracts. Rarely a submucous lipoma in the larynx causes respiratory obstruction. A submucous lipoma can occur in the tongue (Chapter 32). One situated in the intestine is likely to cause an intussusception, which is the first indication of its presence.

(ix) *Extradural*.—A lipoma is a rare variety of spinal tumour. Owing to the absence of fat within the skull intracranial lipomas do not occur.

(x) *Intraglandular*.—Lipomas have been found occasionally in the pancreas, under the renal capsule and in the breast (see Chapter 39).

Treatment.—If a lipoma is causing trouble on account of its site, size, appearance, or the presence of pain, removal is indicated.

During operation, any finger-like projections of the tumour into the surrounding tissue must also be removed. Although the tumour is relatively avascular, care is needed to obtain complete haemostasis in the resulting cavity—drainage often is necessary—otherwise a haematoma is common, which may be followed by infection and delay in wound healing.

Diffuse lipoma occasionally occurs in the subcutaneous tissue of the neck, from which it spreads on to the preauricular region of the face. The tumour is not obviously encapsulated, and gives rise to no trouble beyond being unsightly.

Neuroma.—True neuromas are rare tumours, and occur in connection with the sympathetic system. They comprise the following types:

(*a*) *Ganglioneuroma* (Chapter 38), which consist of ganglion cells and nerve fibres. It arises in connection with the sympathetic cord, and therefore is found in the retroperitoneal tissue, or in the neck or thorax.

(*b*) *Neuroblastoma*, which is less differentiated than the ganglioneuroma, the cells being of an embryonic type. The tumour somewhat resembles a round-celled sarcoma, and disseminates by the blood-stream. It occurs in infants and young children. It may occasionally undergo spontaneous remission.

(*c*) *Myelinic neuroma* is very rare, being composed only of nerve fibres, as the ganglion cells are absent. They arise in connection with the spinal cord or pia mater.

Neurilemmoma (*syn.* Schwannoma).—These lobulated and encapsulated tumours arise from the neurilemmal cells. They are soft and whitish in appearance. They displace the nerve from which they arise and can be removed (fig. 57).

Neurofibroma arise from the connective tissue of the nerve sheath. The following varieties are described.

Local.—A single neurofibroma is usually found in the subcutaneous tissue. The 'painful subcutaneous nodule' forms a smooth firm swelling which may be moved in a lateral direction, but is otherwise fixed by the nerve from which it arises. Paraesthesia or pain is likely to occur from the pressure of the tumour on the nerve fibres which are spread over its surface. Cystic degeneration or sarcomatous changes occasionally occur.

Neurofibromas may also grow from the sheath of a peripheral nerve or a cranial

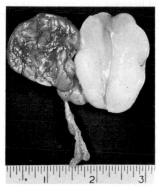

Fig. 57.—Neurilemmoma of the lingual nerve attached to submandibular salivary gland.

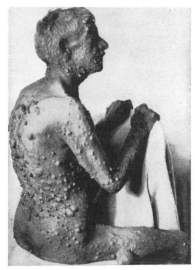

Fig. 58.—Neurofibromatosis.

nerve (*e.g.* the acoustic tumour, Chapter 26). As the nerve fibres are 'part and parcel' of the tumour they are difficult to remove without removal of the nerve itself. In major nerves recurrence is known, also malignant (sarcomatous) change.

Generalised Neurofibromatosis (*syn.* von Recklinghausen's Disease of Nerves).— In this inherited (autosomal dominant) disease, any cranial, spinal or peripheral nerve may be diffusely or nodularly thickened (fig. 58). The over-growth occurs in connection with the endoneurium. Associated pigmentation of the skin is common, and sarcomatous changes may occur.

Plexiform Neurofibromatosis.—This rare condition usually occurs in connection with branches of the fifth cranial nerve (fig. 59), although it may occur in the extremities (fig. 60). The affected nerves become enormously thickened as a result of myxofibromatous degeneration of the endoneurium.

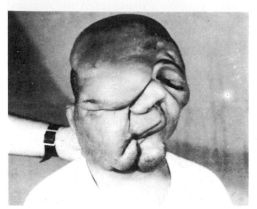

FIG. 59.—Plexiform neurofibromatosis of the 5th cranial nerve. If occurring in the scalp, the underlying skull may be eroded, and in other situations the involved skin sometimes hangs down in pendulous folds with grotesque effects (*cf.* Treves' elephant man).

(*Dr. P. Nayak, MS, Bombay.*)

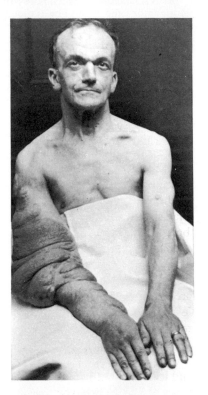

FIG. 60.—Plexiform neurofibromatosis affecting the right arm.

Elephantiasis Neuromatosa is a rare and congenital condition. The skin is coarse, dry, and thickened, resembling an elephant's hide, and the subcutaneous tissues become greatly thickened. If a leg is affected, the patient finds walking increasingly difficult.

False Neuroma—Arises from the connective tissue of the nerve sheath after injury to a nerve (lacerations or amputation). These swellings consist of fibrous tissue and coiled nerve fibres.

Haemangiomas are described in Chapter 10.

Glomangioma (*syn.* **Glomus Tumour.**)—These tumours arise from a cutaneous glomus composed of a tortuous arteriole which communicates directly with a venule, the vessels being surrounded with a network of small nerves. These specialised organs regulate the temperature of the skin, and are found in the limbs, especially the nail-beds. The tumour is compressible. The associated pain is out of all proportion to the size of the tumour,

Friedrich Daniel von Recklinghausen, 1833-1910. Professor of Pathology, Strasbourg, France (1872-1906). Described Generalised Neurofibromatosis in 1882.
Sir Frederick Treves, 1853-1923. Surgeon, The London Hospital.

which may be only a few millimetres in diameter. The pain is burning in nature and radiates peripherally, and is more often noticeable when the limb is exposed to sudden changes of temperature.

On section the tumour consists of a mixture of blood spaces, nerve tissue and muscle fibres derived from the wall of the arteriole (angiomyoneuroma). Large cuboidal cells are frequently seen (glomal cells). Cutaneous glomus tumours grow very slowly, and do not become malignant. They should be excised.

Hamartoma.—The term hamartoma is roughly translated from the Greek[1] as a 'fault' or 'misfire' or 'error' tumour, and its original meaning was 'missing the mark in spear throwing'. It is a developmental malformation consisting of a tumour-like overgrowth of tissue or tissues proper to the part. The possible range therefore is very wide, and the lesions are often multiple. Common lesions that are hamartomas are benign pigmented moles, and the majority of angiomas and neurofibromas. On rare occasions a malignant change occurs in a hamartoma, but for practical purposes the lesion is benign (Peters).

MALIGNANT TUMOURS

CARCINOMA AND SARCOMA

Carcinomas arise from cells which are ectodermal or endodermal in origin, and accordingly they are classified squamous, basal-celled, or glandular. Sarcomas occur in connection with structures of mesoblastic origin; hence fibrosarcoma, osteosarcoma.

Carcinoma

(i) **Squamous** arises from surfaces covered by squamous epithelium, particularly as a result of chronic irritation. Also chronic irritation of transitional cells (*e.g.* by a stone in the renal pelvis) or columnar cells (*e.g.* the gall bladder) will cause a change in these cells to a squamous type (*squamous metaplasia*) and so lead on to carcinoma. The regional lymph nodes are likely to be invaded, and may also be infected from the sepsis attendant upon the primary growth. Blood-borne metastases occur, but rarely from skin carcinoma.

Macroscopically, squamous-celled carcinomas are either proliferative or ulcerative. On section solid masses of polyhedral cells are seen, which invade the deeper structures. 'Cell-nests' are usually apparent in slowly growing cases, and are due to deeper cells becoming flattened and undergoing keratinisation. 'Prickle' (acanthotic) cells are characteristic, and resemble those present in the epidermis.

(ii) **Basal-celled** (*syn.* Rodent Ulcer, Chapter 10).

(iii) **Glandular** commonly occurs in the alimentary tract, breast and uterus, and less frequently in the kidney, prostate, gall-bladder, and thyroid. The three types of glandular carcinoma are as follows:

(*a*) *Carcinoma simplex*, in which the cells are arranged in circumscribed groups, no glandular structure being recognisable. This type commonly occurs in the breast, and the majority of cells are spheroidal or polygonal in shape.

(*b*) *Adenocarcinoma*, so called from the tendency of the cells to form acini, which resemble those of the gland from which they are derived. The alveoli are ductless, and the walls are composed of layers of cells which invade the surrounding tissues. The cells of the primary growth, and even of the metastases, sometimes retain secretory powers.

---

[1] Hamartano (Greek) = I miss.

Philip Michael Peters, 1916–1977. Pathologist, Royal Northern Hospital, London.

(*c*) *Colloid* (mucoid) is a degenerative process which develops in tumours arising from mucin-seeking cells. The mucin permeates the stroma of the growth, which appears as a gelatinous mass and is typically seen in the colon and stomach. stomach.

Glandular carcinoma is also subdivided into various types, *e.g.* encephaloid, scirrhus and atrophic scirrhus. These distinctions depend clinically on their rate of growth, and pathologically on the relative proportions of fibrous tissue and gland elements. Examples occur in the breast (Chapter 39).

Methods of Spread.—(i) **Direct spread (local extension)**. Invasion takes place readily along connective tissue planes, but no structures are resistant. Veins are invaded before arteries.

(ii) **Blood-stream.** Cancer cells may be detected in the venous blood draining an organ involved by carcinoma. A carcinoma of the kidney may invade the renal vein and grow inside the lumen into the vena cava. Malignant emboli may be arrested in the lungs (secondary deposits—metastases), but bizarre blood-borne deposits are not infrequently observed.

(iii) **Lymphatics** by permeation and by embolism.

Lymphatic Permeation.—The malignant cells grow along the lymphatic vessels from the primary growth. This may even occur in a retrograde direction. The cancer cells stimulate perilymphatic fibrosis, but this does not stop the advance of the disease. In some instances, notably malignant melanoma (Chapter 10), groups of cells may so overcome the surrounding fibrosis, as to give rise to intermediate deposits between the primary growth and the lymph nodes.

Lymphatic Embolism.—Cancer cells invade a lymphatic vessel and are carried by the lymph circulation to a regional node, so that nodes comparatively distant from the tumour may be involved in the early stages.

(iv) **Seeding.**—Implantation of carcinoma has been observed in situations where skin or mucous membrane is closely in contact with a primary growth. Examples of this '*kiss cancer*' are carcinoma of the lower lip affecting the upper, and carcinoma of the labium majus giving rise to a similar growth on the opposite side of the vulva. Recurrence after operation is occasionally due to *implantation* of malignant cells in the wound. Examples of this mischance are the appearance of a malignant deposit in the bladder scar after suprapubic removal of a primary growth, and nodules of carcinoma in the scar of the incision after mastectomy. When the peritoneum is involved, cells from a carcinoma may spread like snowflakes all over its serous surface. This *transcoelomic spread* is specially notable when cells from a colloid carcinoma of the stomach gravitate on to an active ovary and give rise to malignant ovarian tumours (Krukenberg's tumour, Chapter 44), which may be the first manifestation of gastric malignancy.

Grading and Staging.—Grading and staging are used to assess the degree of malignancy of the tumour as an indication of the prognosis, and may be used as a guide to determine the type and the extent of the treatment which is required.

TNM Classification.[1]—This is a detailed clinical staging which is arrived at simply by the clinician ascertaining the following points during his examination of the patient: What is the extent of the primary **T**umour? Are any lymph **N**odes affected? Are there any

---

[1] Adopted by the International Union against Cancer. TNM Classification has been extended to many sites of cancer.

Metastases? The information so obtained is scored, *for example in carcinoma of the breast*, as follows:

Tumour	Nodes	Metastasis
T_1 = 2 cm or less. No skin fixation.	N_0 = No nodes.	M_0 = No metastasis.
T_2 = More than 2 cm, but less than 5 cm. Skin tethered or dimpled. No pectoral fixation.	N_1 = Axillary nodes movable (*a*) not significant, (*b*) significant.	M_1 = Metastases are present including involvement of skin beyond breast, and contralateral nodes.
T_3 = More than 5 cm, but less than 10 cm. Skin infiltrated or ulcerated. Pectoral fixation.	N_2 = Axillary nodes fixed. N_3 = Supraclavicular nodes. Oedema of arm.	
T_4 = More than 10 cm. Skin involved but not beyond breast. Chest-wall fixation.		

Thus, for example, one patient may have a carcinoma which is $T_1N_0M_0$, while in another the extent of the disease may be $T_2N_2M_1$. This scoring can be applied easily to the commonly used method of *clinical stage grouping* of carcinoma of the breast (described in Chapter 39). Metastases present is equivalent to Stage IV.

Dukes' Staging.—This is a method of classifying the spread of carcinoma of the rectum and is described in Chapter 53.

Sarcomas

Sarcomas differ from carcinomas, not only in their derivation, but in their age incidence, as they are most common during the first and second decades. Sarcomas often grow with rapidity, and dissemination occurs mainly by the bloodstream ('cannon-ball' secondary deposits in the lung).

The macroscopic appearance of a sarcoma varies considerably. As the word implies, most tumours appear as a fleshy mass, but their consistency depends on the relative proportion of fibrous and vascular tissue. Haemorrhage commonly occurs owing to the very thin walls of the veins, which in some places are represented merely by venous spaces.

Sarcomatous cells may reproduce tissue similar to that from which the tumour originated, *e.g.* osteosarcoma or chondrosarcoma. Sometimes a sarcoma develops in pre-existing benign tumours, such as fibroma or a uterine fibroid, and also in bones which are affected by osteitis deformans (Chapter 23).

Fibrosarcoma is composed of spindle cells of varying lengths (the rounder they are the more malignant they are), and occurs in muscle sheaths, scars and as a fibrous epulis (Chapter 33). A fibrosarcoma of a muscle sheath presents as an elastic or firm and slowly growing swelling. Dilated veins over the tumour suggest malignancy, and if not obvious they may be demonstrated by infra-red photography. On palpation the tumour often feels warm and pulsation may even be detected.

Recurrent Fibroid.—Fibrosarcomas not uncommonly arise in scar tissue, sometimes many years after the scar developed.[1]

Treatment of Fibrosarcoma.—The spread of a sarcoma is hastened by incomplete removal. *The moral is that wide excision with surrounding healthy tissues should*

---

[1] Sir James Paget, 1814-1899, Surgeon, St. Bartholomew's Hospital, London, described this type as a 'recurrent fibroid'.

Cuthbert Esquire Dukes, 1890-1977. Consulting Pathologist, St. Mark's Hospital, London.

be practised in all cases. This may mean amputation in the case of a limb. If wide local excision is unsuccessful, or if untreated, a fibrosarcoma eventually fungates through the skin. Metastases are widely scattered, and, unfortunately, radiotherapy has but little effect on either the primary growth or on the secondary deposits.

Lymphomas arise in lymph nodes, tonsils, Peyer's patches or lymph nodules in the intestines. Lymph nodes of the neck or mediastinum are most commonly affected (Chapter 9).

Synovioma.—This rather uncommon tumour may arise in any synovial joint or tendon sheath, especially those of the hand. It appears as a soft, painless swelling, and sarcomatous changes can occur. The diagnosis can only be established by excision and biopsy of the tumour.

Naevus and Melanoma are described in Chapter 10.

Endothelioma. Mesothelioma.[1]—The endothelial linings of blood-vessels, lymphatic spaces and serous membranes occasionally give rise to neoplasms. They can be malignant. They arise from the pleura (Chapter 40) and rarely from the pericardium or peritoneum. The original cells are flattened, but they become spheroidal or cuboidal when neoplastic changes occur. The 'endothelioma' (meningioma) of the dura mater is thought to arise from the arachnoid membrane, which is *not* an endothelial structure (Chapter 26).

Peritheliomas are tumours arising in the endothelial lining of small blood-vessels or lymphatics. Carotid body tumours are probably of this nature (Chapter 36).

BENIGN → MALIGNANT

Certain innocent neoplasms are prone to undergo malignant changes, and it is important, both for treatment and prognosis, to realise when this occurs. Some or all of the following changes may be recognised:

(i) *Increase in size*—comparatively rapid enlargement is always suspicious, *e.g.* a neurofibroma which is becoming sarcomatous.

(ii) *Increased vasularity*—dilated cutaneous veins, ulceration and bleeding in the case of a superficial growth (*e.g.* melanoma).

(iii) *Fixity*—due to invasion of surrounding structures.

(iv) *Involvement of adjacent structures*—Facial palsy suggests a malignant change in an otherwise longstanding parotid pleomorphic adenoma.

(v) *Dissemination*—discovery of secondary deposits is occasionally the clue to the development of malignancy.

CYSTS

The word 'cyst' is derived from the Greek word meaning 'bladder'. The pathological term 'cyst' means a swelling consisting of a collection of fluid in a sac which is lined by epithelium or endothelium.

True cysts are usually lined by epithelium or endothelium. If infection supervenes, the lining may be composed of granulation tissue. The fluid is usually serous or mucoid and varies from brown-staining by altered blood to almost colourless. In epidermoid, dermoid, and branchial cysts the contents are like porridge or toothpaste, as a result of the secretion of desquamated cells. Cholesterol crystals are often found in the fluid.

False Cysts.—Certain collections of fluid are not regarded as true cysts. They are usually exudation and degeneration cysts. A pseudo-cyst of the pancreas is an encysted collection of fluid in the lesser sac. In tuberculous peritonitis fluid

---

[1] 'Blue' asbestos fibres have been shown to be a cause.

Johann Conrad Peyer, 1653-1712.

may be walled off in cystic form by adherent coils of intestine. Fluid may collect in the centre of a tumour (cystic degeneration), due to haemorrhage or colliquative necrosis. This can also happen in the brain as a result of ischaemia, and an 'apoplectic cyst' is formed.

A Classification of Cysts:

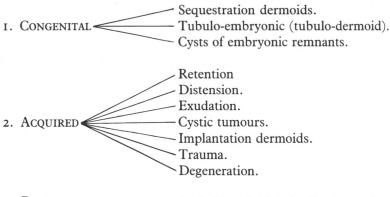

1. CONGENITAL
   - Sequestration dermoids.
   - Tubulo-embryonic (tubulo-dermoid).
   - Cysts of embryonic remnants.

2. ACQUIRED
   - Retention
   - Distension.
   - Exudation.
   - Cystic tumours.
   - Implantation dermoids.
   - Trauma.
   - Degeneration.

3. PARASITIC   Hydatid. Trichiniasis. Cysticercosis.

Congenital Cysts.—*The sequestration dermoid* is due to dermal cells being buried along the lines of closure of embryonic clefts and sinuses by skin fusion. The cyst is therefore lined by epidermis and contains paste-like desquamated material. The usual sites are (*a*) the midline of the body—especially in the neck, (*b*) above the outer canthus (external angular dermoid) (Chapter 31), (*c*) in the anterior triangle of the neck (branchial cyst, Chapter 36).

Tubulo-embryonic (tubulo-dermoid) cysts occur in the track of an ectodermal tube used in development, *e.g.* a thyroglossal cyst from the thyroglossal duct; a post-anal dermoid from the post-anal gut. In the brain, ependymal cysts arise from the sequestration of cells of the infolding neurectoderm.

Cysts of Embryonic Remnants.[1]—These arise from embryonic tubules and ducts which normally disappear or are only present as remnants. There are many examples in the urogenital system, *e.g.* in the male from remnants of the paramesonephric duct (Müllerian)—the hydatid of Morgagni, or from the mesonephric body and duct (Wolffian) (Chapter 57). Cysts of the urachus, and the vitello-intestinal duct are other examples of cysts and embryonic remnants.

Acquired Cysts.—*Retention cysts* are due to the accumulated secretion of a gland following obstruction of a duct. Examples are seen in the pancreas, the parotid, the breast, the epididymis, and Bartholin's gland. A sebaceous cyst starts with the obstruction of a sebaceous gland, but this is followed by the downgrowth and the accumulation of desquamated epidermal cells, thus turning it into an epidermoid cyst.

Distension cysts occur in the thyroid from dilation of the acini, or in the ovary from a follicle. Lymphatic cysts and cystic hygromas are distension cysts. *Exudation cysts* occur when fluid exudes into an anatomical space already lined by

---

[1] These cysts are not to be confused with teratomatous cysts (*e.g.* Dermoid).

Johannes Peter Müller, 1801-1858. Professor of Anatomy and Physiology, Berlin.
Giovanni Battista Morgagni, 1682-1771. Professor of Anatomy, Pudua, Italy.
Kaspar Friedrich Wolff, 1733-1794. Professor of Anatomy and Physiology, St. Petersburg (now Leningrad), U.S.S.R.
Caspar Bartholin, Secundus, 1655-1738. Professor of Medicine, Anatomy, and Physics, Copenhagen, Denmark.

endothelium, *e.g.* hydrocele, a bursa, or when a collection of exudate becomes encysted. These are false cysts.

Cystic Tumours.—Examples are cystic teratomas (dermoid cyst of the ovary) and cystadenomas (pseudomucinous, and serous cystadenoma of the ovary).

Ganglia (see Chapter 24).

Implantation dermoids arise from squamous epithelium which has been driven beneath the skin by a penetrating wound. They are classically found in the fingers of women who sew assiduously (fig. 61).

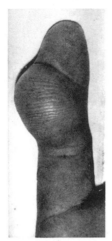

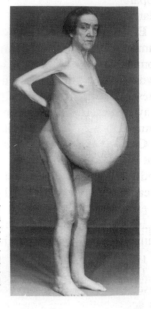

FIG. 61.—Implantation dermoid. The contents are desquamated cell-debris which may undergo mucoid degeneration.

FIG. 62.—Cachexia ovarica. The patient successfully underwent an operation for a giant ovarian cyst containing 15 litres of fluid. The site, size and weight of the cyst combined to cause the classical appearance of cachexia, lordosis, oedema of the legs, and an anxious expression.

Trauma.—A haematoma may resolve into a cyst. This sometimes happens to haematomas of muscle masses in the loin and antero-lateral aspects of the thigh or the shin. They are located between muscle, fascial, or subcutaneous planes and contain straw- or brown-coloured fluid containing cholesterol crystals. They become lined by endothelium and calcium salts may be laid down. Aspiration is only of temporary value, and a cure depends upon complete excision of the lining.

Degeneration Cysts.—These have already been discussed under false cysts.

Parasitic Cysts.—These are encysted forms in the life-cycle of various worms.

Hydatid Cyst of the *Taenia Echinococcus.*—This is described later according to the organ involved, *e.g.* liver, Chapter 45; lung, Chapter 40.

Trichiniasis.—Cysts of the *Trichina spiralis*, affecting muscle.

Cysticercosis.—Cysts of *Taenia solium*. A disease of the pig, man being rarely affected. Eosinophilia is present. The cysts occur in any organ. They calcify and may cause clinical effects according to their situation, especially in the brain. Only those cysts which are actually causing symptoms should be excised.

Clinical Features of a Cyst.—The swelling usually has a smooth spherical appearance. Fluctuation depends upon the pressure of fluid within; a tense cyst feels like a solid tumour, though careful palpation between two fingers may elicit a characteristic elasticity. In addition, a solid tumour is most hard at the centre; a cyst is least hard at the centre. If fluctuation is present, a cyst may be confused with a cold abscess or a lipoma. A cold abscess usually has a peculiar rim of thickening surrounding the soft centre. A lipoma may well test clinical acumen. *Transillumination*, while brilliantly clear in cysts containing serous fluid, does not really distinguish between a lipoma and a dermoid or branchial cyst. There is even an old axiom that 'when in doubt hedge on fat'. According to circumstances, ultrasonography, a test aspiration or excision reveals the true nature of the swelling.

Cysts may be painful, especially when infection or haemorrhage causes a sudden increase in the intracystic tension. Sometimes they change in size for no apparent reason. Occasionally they diminish due to rupture through a fascial plane.

Effects of a Cyst.—These are according to site and size. As with benign tumours, a cyst may compress ducts and blood-vessels. For example, the common bile duct may be obstructed by a choledochal cyst, a renal cyst, or a hydatid cyst. The pelvic veins may be obstructed by an ovarian cyst, the patient presenting for treatment of her varicose veins. The sheer size of an ovarian cyst may so increase intra-abdominal tension as to bring the patient to hospital with symptoms of a hiatus hernia.

Complications.—*Infection.*—The cyst becomes tense and painful, and adherent to surrounding tissues. An abscess may form and discharge on the surface and result in an ulcer or a sinus (viz. Cock's peculiar tumour, Chapter 10). Healing will not occur until the whole lining of the cyst or the embryonic track is excised.

Haemorrhage.—Sudden haemorrhage, as may occur in a thyroid cyst, causes a painful increase in size. In this particular case breathing may be difficult because of pressure on the trachea.

Torsion may occur in cysts which are attached to neighbouring structures by a vascular pedicle. Ovarian dermoids are sometimes brought to notice in this way as acute abdominal emergencies. The cyst (or cysts—they may be bilateral), turns to a purple or black colour as the venous and then the arterial supply is cut off.

Calcification follows haemorrhage, or infection, and may be the result of reaction to a parasite, *e.g.* hydatid cyst.

Cachexia Ovarica.—Enormous cysts are rarely seen nowadays (fig. 62).

ULCERS

An ulcer is a discontinuity of an epithelial surface. There is usually progressive destruction of surface tissue, cell by cell, as distinct from death of macroscopic portions (*e.g.* gangrene or necrosis). Ulcers are classified as *non-specific, specific* (*e.g.* tuberculous or syphilitic), or *malignant*.

Non-specific ulcers are due to infection of wounds, or physical or chemical agents. Local irritation, as in the case of a dental ulcer, or interference with the circulation, *e.g.* varicose veins are predisposing causes.

Trophic Ulcers[1] are due to an impairment of the nutrition of the tissues, which depends upon an adequate blood supply and also a properly functioning nerve supply. Ischaemia and anaesthesia will therefore cause these ulcers. Thus, in the

---

[1] Trophē (Greek) = Nutrition.

arm, chronic vasospasm, and syringomyelia, will cause ulceration of the tips of the fingers (respectively painful and painless). In the leg, painful ischaemic ulcers occur around the ankle or on the dorsum of the foot. Ulcers due to anaesthesia (diabetic neuritis, spina bifida, tabes dorsalis, leprosy, or a peripheral nerve injury) are often called *perforating ulcers* (fig. 63). Starting in a corn or bunion, they penetrate the foot, and the suppuration may involve the bones and joints and spread along fascial planes upwards, even involving the calf.

The life-history of an ulcer consists of three phases: (i) extension, (ii) transition, and (iii) repair. During the *stage of extension* the floor is covered with exudate and sloughs, while the base is indurated. The discharge is purulent and even blood-stained. (ii) The *transition stage* prepares for healing. The floor becomes cleaner, the sloughs separate, induration of the base diminishes, and the discharge becomes more serous. Small reddish areas of granulation tissue appear on the floor, and these link up until the whole surface is covered (fig. 6). (iii) The *stage of repair* consists of the transformation of granulation to fibrous tissue, which gradually contracts to form a scar. The epithelium gradually extends from the, now shelving, edge to cover the floor (at a rate of 1 mm per day). This healing edge consists of three zones—the outer of epithelium, which appears white, the middle one bluish in colour (where granulation tissue is covered by a few layers of epithelium), and the inner reddish zone of granulation tissue covered by a single layer of epithelial cells.

Local (Topical) Treatment of Non-specific Ulcers.—Any underlying cause is treated (*e.g.* varicose veins (Chapter 13), diabetes, arterial disease). Many lotions and non-adhesive applications are used to aid the separation of sloughs, hasten granulation, and stimulate epithelialisation. Hypochlorite solution (*e.g.* Eusol[1]) and 0·5% silver nitrate are popular in the early stages, and later 1% zinc sulphate solution (*e.g.* Lotio rubra). Ointments and creams used include zinc oxide and 1% hydrocortisone. Household vinegar (1:6) is very efficacious against pyocyaneus. Excessive granulation, commonly known as 'proud flesh', needs to be discouraged by excision, curettage, or by the application of a caustic, such as silver nitrate. Tetracycline (10%) in propylene glycol solution will clean an ulcer prior to skin grafting. Chronic or indolent ulcers often respond to infra-red radiation, short-wave therapy, or ultra-violet light.

Large ulcers in the healing phase should be covered by a free split skin graft as soon as the granulations are healthy. Healthy granulations are flat, are below the level of the surrounding skin, are pink in colour, and do not discharge pus.

Amnion has returned to fashion as an effective application to promote healing. Fresh from the delivery room, it is cleaned thoroughly by sterile gauze or brush, washed in a suitable hypochlorite solution, cut to size and applied like a skin graft. The rough chorion side helps to stimulate granulations, the smooth amnion side epithelialisation. Excess amnion is stored at 4°C in saline and used when replacement is necessary every 2 to 5 days (usually determined by infection). *Silver foil* is another type of cover used to promote healing.

CLINICAL EXAMINATION OF AN ULCER

This should be conducted in a systematic manner. The following are, with brief examples, the points which should be noted:

Site, *e.g.* 95% of rodent ulcers occur on the upper part of the face. Carcinoma typically affects the lower lip, while a primary chancre of syphilis is usually on the upper.

---

[1] Eusol = *E*dinburgh *U*niversity *SOL*ution.

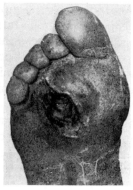

FIG. 63.—Perforating ulcer in a diabetic.

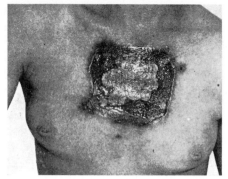

FIG. 64.—Dermatitis artefacta. This condition is due to self-mutilation, *e.g.* by the application of irritants, such as corrosives. The patient usually has a hysterical temperament, or litigation may be involved.

Size, particularly in relation to the length of history, *e.g.* a carcinoma extends more rapidly than a rodent ulcer, but more slowly than an inflammatory ulcer.

Shape, *e.g.* a rodent ulcer is usually circular. A gummatous ulcer, now a great rarity, is typically circular or serpiginous, due to the fusion of multiple circles: An ulcer with a square area or straight edge is suggestive of 'dermatitis artefacta' (fig. 64).

Edge (fig. 65).—A healing non-specific ulcer has a shelving edge. It is rolled or rampart if a rodent ulcer, and raised and everted if malignant (*e.g.* epithelioma), undermined and often bluish if tuberculous, vertically punched-out if syphilitic.

FIG. 65.—1. Healing ulcer.   2. Tuberculous ulcer.   3. Rodent ulcer.   4. Epithelioma.

Floor.—The floor is that which is seen by an observer, *e.g.* watery or apple-jelly granulations in a tuberculous ulcer, a wash-leather slough in a gummatous ulcer.

Base.—The base is what can be palpated. It may be indurated as in a carcinoma or attached to deep structures, *e.g.* a varicose ulcer to the tibia.

Discharge.—A purulent discharge indicates active infection. A blue-green coloration suggests infection with *Pseudomonas pyocyaneus*. A watery discharge is typical of tuberculosis. It is blood-stained in the extension phase of a non-specific ulcer. *Bacteriological examination* may reveal colonisation by coagulase positive staphylococci. Spirochaetes are found in a primary chancre (Chapter 3).

Lymph nodes are not enlarged in the case of a rodent ulcer, unless due to secondary infection. In the case of carcinoma, they may be enlarged, hard, and even fixed. The inguinal nodes draining a syphilitic chancre of the penis are firm and 'shotty', but contrarily the submandibular nodes draining a chancre of the lip are greatly enlarged.

Pain.—Non-specific ulcers in the extension and transition stages are painful (except the anaesthetic trophic type). Tuberculous ulcers vary, that of the tongue being very painful. Syphilitic ulcers are usually painless, but the anal chancre of the homosexual may be painful (*cf.* anal fissure, Chapter 54).

General Examination.—Evidence of debility, cardiac failure, all types of anaemia, including sickle cell anaemia, or diabetes must be sought.

Pathological examinations, *e.g.* biopsy, may confirm carcinoma. The serological and Mantoux tests may be of value.

Marjolin's Ulcer. (See Chapter 10).

ORIENTAL SORE (*syn.* DELHI BOIL, BAGHDAD SORE, ETC.)

This disease is due to infection by a protozoal parasite, *Leishmania tropica*, and is a common condition in Eastern countries which is occasionally imported to Western zones. An indurated papule appears on an exposed surface, usually the face. If untreated this breaks down to form an indolent ulcer, which eventually leaves an ugly, pigmented scar. The condition readily responds to intravenous injections of antimony tartrate, but very small lesions can be treated by carbon dioxide snow, and also currettage.

Bazin's disease (*syn.* erythema induratum) is due to localised areas of fat necrosis and particularly affects adolescent girls. Symmetrical purplish nodules appear, especially on the calves, and gradually break down to form indolent ulcers, which leave in their wake pigmented scars. Tuberculosis may be a cause in many instances, the ulcers responding to antituberculous drugs (Chapter 3). Sympathectomy also may be curative.

SINUSES AND FISTULAS

A *sinus*[1] is a blind track lined with granulations leading from an epithelial surface into the surrounding tissues. A *fistula*[2] is an abnormal communication between the lumen of one viscus and the lumen of another, or the body surface, or between vessels. Sinuses and fistulae may be congenital or acquired. Forms which have a congenital origin include pre-auricular sinuses (Chapter 30), branchial fistulas (Chapter 36), and tracheo-oesophageal fistulas (Chapter 43) arteriovenous fistulas (Chapter 14). The acquired forms often follow inadequate drainage of an abscess. Thus a perianal abscess may burst on the surface and lead to a sinus (erroneously termed a blind external 'fistula'). In other cases the abscess opens both into the anal canal and on to the surface, resulting in a true fistula-in-ano (Chapter 54). Acquired arteriovenous fistula are caused by trauma or operation (for renal dialysis).

Persistence of a Sinus or Fistula.—The reason for this will be found amongst the following:

(1) A foreign body or necrotic tissue is present (*e.g.* a suture, sequestrum, a faecolith or even a worm (see below)).

(2) Inefficient or non-dependent drainage.

(3) Unrelieved obstruction of the lumen of a viscus or tube distal to the fistula. Irritating discharges, such as urine or faeces, maintain continuous inflammation.

(4) Absence of rest, such as occurs in fistula-in-ano due to the normal contractions of the sphincter which also force faecal material into the internal opening.

(5) The walls have become lined with epithelium or endothelium (A-V fistula).

(6) Dense fibrosis prevents contraction and healing.

---

[1] Sinus (Latin) = A hollow; a bay or gulf.
[2] Fistula (Latin) = A pipe or tube.

Charles Mantoux, 1877-1947. Physician, Le Cannet, France.
Sir William Leishman, 1865-1926. Professor of Pathology, Royal Army Medical College.
Pierre Antoine Ernest Bazin, 1807-1878. Dermatologist, Hôpitol St. Louis, Paris.

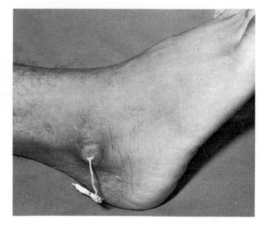

FIG. 66.—?Ulcer ?Sinus—presenting in a U.K. outpatient department! The 30 cm female Guinea worm is carefully extricated by being wound on a matchstick, a few turns a day to prevent breakage and retraction.

(7) Type of infection, *e.g.* tuberculosis or actinomycosis.

(8) The presence of malignant disease.

Treatment.—The remedy depends upon the removal or specific treatment of the cause (see appropriate pages).

Guinea Worm. (*Syn.* Dragon worm, *Dracunculus mediensis*) (fig. 66). The larval form enters through the wall of the stomach or duodenum in drinking water contaminated by a tiny cyclops crustacean which has consumed the larvae. Settling in the abdominal connective tissue the male and female mate, the pregnancy lasting about a year, and the female wanders in the subcutaneous tissues to select for egg laying a part of the anatomy likely to be submerged in water (containing the cyclops), usually the lower leg. Cellulitis, abscesses, ulcers and sinuses follow, through which the embryos are discharged, hopefully to be eaten by the cyclops. Baid travelled the interior of India and in 500 cases discerned a syndrome of the infestation, presenting with conjunctivitis (allergic) in 11%, fibrous contracture of joints in 19%, periostitis with oesteomyelitis in 21% and acute arthritis in 65%.

J. C. Baid, Contemporary. Surgeon, Jodhpur, India.

CHAPTER 9

LYMPHATICS AND LYMPH NODES

Acute lymphangitis occurs when infection, commonly by *Streptococcus pyogenes*, spreads beyond a point of infection to the group of lymph nodes draining that area, where an abscess may form. Occasionally the infection bypasses the group to affect another at a higher level. For example, if the point of infection is in the foot an abscess may form in the external iliac group of nodes rather than the superficial (lower) and deep inguinal groups and, because the point of infection may have healed and been forgotten, by the time the mass appears it may be mistaken for an appendix abscess.

Acute lymphangitis is seen as red blushes and streaks in the skin, corresponding to the inflamed lymphatics (fig. 67).

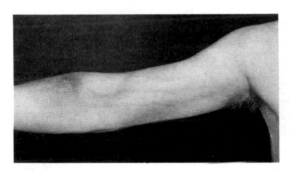

FIG. 67.—Acute lymphangitis of the arm. Red streaks extend from the infection on the forearm up to the enlarged and tender axillary lymph nodes. Toxaemia is often severe and is greater the more the infection has extended proximally.

Treatment consists of bed rest, with the affected limb comfortably elevated, and giving cloxacillin, which usually causes rapid resolution. *Only* when there are definite signs of pus should an incision be made.

Post lymphatic oedema.—Permanent lymphatic obstruction can follow in the wake of acute lymphangitis, leading to persistent oedema.

Chronic lymphangitis may follow repeated attacks of acute lymphangitis (see acquired, secondary, lymphoedema).

LYMPHANGIOGRAPHY

Lymphangiography is widely used to diagnose lymphoedema and to demonstrate the nature of lymphatic abnormality. The procedure is also used to detect malignant disease in the iliac and para-aortic lymph nodes, but is being gradually replaced by CT scanning and high resolution ultrasound as these techniques become more generally available.

Technique.—Pedal lymphangiogram. Blue dye is injected subcutaneously between the toes to outline the lymphatic vessels. A small incision is made on the dorsum of each foot and a 30G needle is passed into a vessel. Using an infusion pump, oily contrast medium

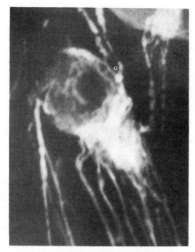

FIG. 68.—Lymphangiogram showing filling defect in an inguinal node caused by metastatic melanoma.

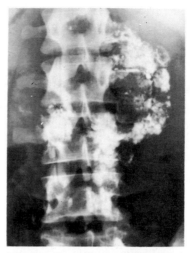

FIG. 69.—Lymphangiogram showing enlarged para-aortic nodes due to metastases from a testicular teratoma.

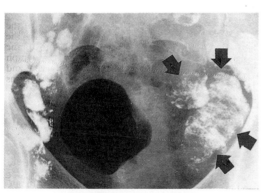

FIG. 70.—Lymphangiogram showing generalised enlargement of the left iliac lymph nodes (arrowed) due to Hodgkin's lymphoma.

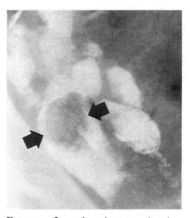

FIG. 71.—Lymphangiogram showing small filling defect in a right external iliac node (arrowed) due to metastatic carcinoma of the ovary. The CT scan was normal.

(ultra-fluid lipoidol) is injected slowly and subsequently lodges in the sinuses of the pelvic and abdominal lymph nodes.

Small metastatic deposits in the nodes cause filling defects due to obliteration of the lymph node sinuses (fig. 68) and large metastatic deposits produce larger filling defects and generalised enlargement of the affected lymph nodes (fig. 69). Malignant lymphoma produces generalised enlargement of the affected nodes with a 'foamy' or 'reticular' pattern of opacification (fig. 70).

Lymphangiography occasionally demonstrates small metastases in para-aortic and iliac lymph nodes which appear normal on CT scanning (fig. 71) but, in general, CT scanning is more accurate.

LYMPHOEDEMA

Lymphoedema is caused by the accumulation of fluid in the extracellular, extravascular fluid compartment and in the limbs it accumulates mainly in the subcutaneous tissues.[1] Lymphoedema can be congenital or acquired.

Congenital Lymphoedema

The clinical classification of congenital lymphoedema (Milroy's disease) depends on the age of onset; *lymphoedema congenita* being present at birth, *lymphoedema praecox* presenting at puberty and *lymphoedema tarda*[2] in adult life, but the condition is now commonly classified according to the findings at lymphangiography:

1. **Hypoplasia and aplasia** are the commonest congenital abnormalities which result in lymphoedema. The number of lymph vessels and nodes draining the affected limb is reduced, usually in the thigh where one or two vessels opacify instead of the usual five or more (fig. 72). Hypoplasia sometimes affects the para-aortic and pelvic lymph vessels and nodes, but this is less common (fig. 73). Lymphatic hypoplasia can be an incidental finding in patients being examined by pedal lymphangiography to stage malignant disease and is probably much more common than actual clinical lymphoedema.

Hypoplasia can be confidently diagnosed if a lymphatic vessel is cannulated and these abnormalities demonstrated, but it is sometimes impossible to find a lymphatic vessel in the subcutaneous tissues of the affected limb and these patients are usually diagnosed as suffering from 'lymphatic aplasia'.

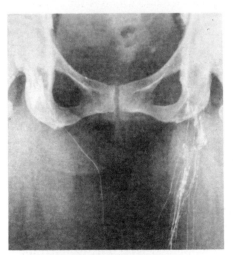

FIG. 72.—Congenital lymphoedema of right leg due to lymphatic hypoplasia.

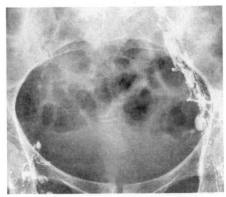

FIG. 73.—Bi-pedal lymphangiogram showing aplasia of the right iliac nodes and vessels in a patient with lymphoedema of the right leg. The vessels below the inguinal ligament were normal.

---

[1] *The Physical Sign of Pitting* on pressure over the lower part of the tibia is present in *early* lymphoedema just as it is in oedema due to back pressure (venous oedema) or as a result of factors associated with right ventricular failure and also the several causes of low plasma proteins. With the passing of time lymphoedema characteristically becomes *non-pitting oedema*, the subcutaneous thickening with fibrous tissue being worsened by recurring low grade lymphangitis and cellulitis.

[2] tarda = tardy = slow to come on.

William Forsyth Milroy, 1855–1942. Professor of Clinical Medicine, University of Nebraska, Omaha, Nebraska, U.S.A. Described hereditary oedema of the legs in 1892.

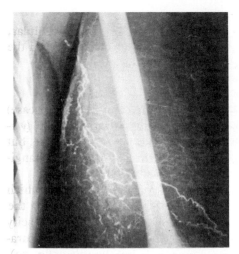

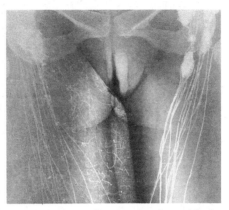

FIG. 74.—Obstructive lymphoedema of the left arm secondary to radical mastectomy plus radio-therapy.

FIG. 75.—Obstructive lymphoedema of the right leg following radiotherapy and a Wertheim's hysterectomy for carcinoma of the cervix.

Retrograde obliteration.—In patients with longstanding lymphoedema of pre-sumed congenital origin, lymphangiography may show that the main vessels are obstructed in the lower part of the limb and this phenomenon is attributed to 'retrograde obliteration' or 'die-back' of overloaded lymph vessels. This process probably contributes to the gradual increase in swelling which is such a common feature of lymphoedema.

2. **Varicose lymphatics** are a rare cause of congenital lymphoedema. The lymph vessels are dilated and tortuous and the condition is often associated with congenital arteriovenous fistulae.

Acquired lymphoedema (secondary lymphoedema)

This form of lymphoedema is usually due to obstruction and in such cases lymphangiography shows obstruction to the main lymphatic vessels with 'dermal back flow' into the subcutaneous lymph vessels (figs. 74 & 75). The causes of obstructive lymphoedema are: 1. Trauma, e.g. removal of axillary lymphatics in radical mastectomy. 2. Repeated acute infection, as in those who go about bare-foot. 3. Chronic infection, e.g. Tuberculosis, fungus infection, and also chronic infection of the cervix, even uterus. 4. Advanced malignant disease. Again, pro-longed lymphatic obstruction usually results in 'die-back' of the affected vessels, so that the site of the obstruction moves distally and this may account for the progressive nature of obstructive lymphoedema. The process is accelerated by soft tissue infection and lymphangitis. In some patients with mild congenital lymphatic hypoplasia, lymphoedema is precipitated as a result of lymphangitis.

FILARIASIS

Filariasis is a disease widely spread through tropical and sub-tropical countries.[1] It is due to a nematode worm, *Filaria sanguinis hominis* which is transmitted by a mosquito (*Culex fatigans*). Once in the human body, the female worm finds its way to the lymphatics and lymph nodes (especially the inguinal group). It attains sexual maturity in six to eighteen months and produces vast numbers of microfilariae, so that there may be 50 millions in the blood at one time. These can be discovered microscopically in a *nocturnal* blood smear. Obstruction of the lymph vessels ensues and this is manifested in: (1) varicosities of the lymphatic vessels producing chylous ascites and hydroceles and, sometimes, chyluria and chylous fistulae on the scrotum and groins. (2) Solid oedema (elephantiasis) (fig. 77) often affecting the legs, scrotum and arms, though it may occur anywhere. The oedema does not seem to be obstructive in origin, as lymphangiography in these patients shows that the main vessels in the lower limbs are patent and that the para-aortic vessels are dilated (fig. 78). The dilatation itself may be responsible for lymphoedema and chylous reflux by rendering the lymphatic valves incompetent (as with varicose veins) and allowing reflux from the main para-aortic vessels into the smaller vessels draining the subcutaneous and retroperitoneal tissues.

Treatment. The best method of treatment known at present is Hetrazan (diethylcarbamazine-citrate), which appears to sterilise or kill the adult female worm. Prevention by anti-mosquito measures is, of course, vitally important. Elephantiasis may require surgery (see below).

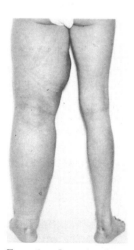

FIG. 76.— Lymphoedema of the left leg due to compression of the left common iliac vein.

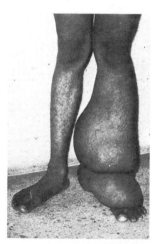

FIG. 77. — Lymphoedema (elephantiasis) due to filariasis.
(*R. S. Naik, Durg, India*)

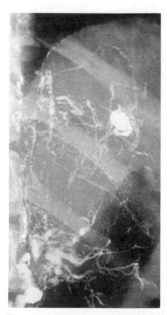

FIG. 78.—Reflux from dilated non-obstructed para-aortic vessels into the left kidney in a patient with chyluria due to filariasis.

---

[1] Sir Patrick Manson, 1844–1922, discovered elephantiasis was caused by filaria in 1877 while working in China.

Differential Diagnosis of Lymphoedema.—*Bilateral* oedema of the legs always requires an examination to exclude cardiac, renal and metabolic (hypoproteinaemia) causes. *Unilateral* lymphoedema may be confused with that caused by deep vein thrombosis, compression, or stricture, particularly of the common iliac vein on the left side (fig. 76) (Cockett). Operations to mobilise the aortic bifurcation, if causing compression, or to perform direct venous disobliteration or venoplasty are still under trial.

The Treatment of Lymphoedema.—1. *Palliative.*—For the attacks of inflammation, prolonged bed-rest, elevation, and the appropriate antibiotic are important. Even in between attacks, the patient should sleep with the foot of the bed raised and may require to use efficient elastic stocking pressure (*e.g.* Sigvaris®). Intermittent diuresis, induced by modern diuretic drugs, also is helpful. An intermittent limb compression pump can also be applied when available.

2. *Surgery* is reserved for those with severe disability. One of many surgical procedures is the removal of all the abnormal subcutaneous tissues and the covering of the exposed deeper tissues with a split skin graft (flaying operation). Another method is to bury the dermal part of the excess skin like a 'swiss-roll cake' along the whole length of the leg, so that the subdermal lymphatics may orientate themselves lengthwise and thereby assist drainage (fig. 79). Other operations seeking to divert the lymph flow through the deep fascia by removing strips of it (Kondoleon's operation) or across the obstructed zone by a skin pedicle bridge, have failed, though a bridge of mesentry and ileum, bereft of mucosa, is being tried (Kinmonth) in early cases, otherwise it is difficult to reduce the great mass of subcutaneous tissue.

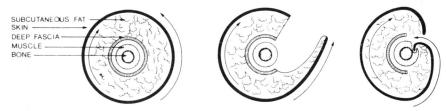

FIG. 79.—Swiss Roll operation (buried dermis) see text. (*N. Thompson, F.R.C.S., London*).

3. *Microsurgery.*—It is possible in many sites to anastomose dilated lymphatics to veins (lymphovenous anastomosis), for example in the antecubital fossa in cases of oedema of the arm (O'Brien).

Chylous Reflux.—When lymphangiography reveals a backflow of milky chyle from the cisterna chyli, with dilated lymphatics, resulting in cutaneous chylous vesicles and fistulae on the limbs, ligation and excision of the lymphatics on the posterior abdominal wall may cure the reflux, though lymphoedema persists.

LYMPHANGIOMA

Capillary Lymphangioma.—Localised congenital anomalies may be composed of capillary-like lesions in the skin. They are brownish papules or wart-like excrescences. On examination with a lens, small vesicles can be seen, which are lymphatic naevi.

Cavernous lymphangioma is often associated with the preceding variety, and consists of masses of lymphatic cysts, particularly in the neck or axilla, the condition being termed a *cystic hygroma* (Chapter 36). A similar lymphangiectatic condition may affect the lips (macrocheilia) or the tongue (macroglosia) producing sometimes gross soft tissue enlargement.

Frank Bernard Cockett, Contemporary. Surgeon, St. Thomas's Hospital, London.
Emmanuel Kondoleon, 1879–1936. Surgeon in Athens.
John Bernard Kinmonth, 1916–1982. Professor of Surgery, St. Thomas's Hospital, London.
B. McC. O'Brien, Contemporary. Director, Microsurgery Research Unit, and Assistant Surgeon, St. Vincent's Hospital, Melbourne, Australia.

LYMPH NODES

Acute Inflammation.—Lymph nodes, draining any area where there is acute infection, will also become inflamed (p. 118).

Chronic inflammation is either simple (pyogenic) or specific.

1. *Chronic Simple Lymphadenitis* is due to persistence of infection, such as occurs in recurrent tonsillitis or pediculosis capitis, and the cause should be treated.

2. *Chronic Specific Lymphadenitis*

(*a*) **Tuberculous lymphadenitis** is common in children and young adults, particularly those who have been in contact with open human tuberculosis or who drink infected milk. It also occurs in the aged. The cervical lymph nodes are most often seen to be enlarged, but the remnants of disease may be observed in the mediastinal and mesenteric lymph nodes as speckled calcification on routine x-rays. Axillary lymph nodes may be involved by spread from the mediastinum.

Tubercle bacilli most commonly reach a lymph node by lymphatics, when tubercles first form in the cortex. Microscopically, endothelial cells and lymphocytes are in evidence. Giant cells are seen with many nuclei arranged round the periphery like a horseshoe.

The stages of infection show most clearly in the neck. From the tonsillar portal of entry the infection spreads by the lymphatics to the nearest lymph node. If the disease spreads, several lymph nodes are involved. They coalesce and break down to form caseous tuberculous pus, which may perforate the deep fascia and present as a fluctuant swelling on the surface (collar-stud abscess) (fig. 80). This skin gradually becomes indurated, breaks down, and forms a sinus which if ignored will remain unhealed for years. From each of these stages resolution may take place with calcification (if caseation has occurred), and with much scarring (if sinuses have formed).

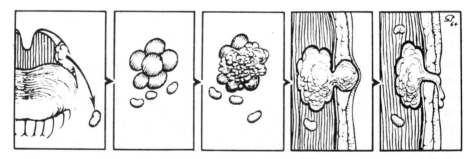

FIG. 80.—A summary of the natural history of tuberculous lymphadenitis.

Treatment.—(i) Attention to nutrition and general health.

(ii) Tuberculous material is aspirated for culture and drug sensitivity tests. A specimen must be obtained before the anti-tuberculous drugs are started.

(iii) Anti-tuberculous drugs are given immediately after the aspiration (Chapter 4).

(vi) When the patient's condition begins to improve, breaking-down tuberculous lymph nodes must be removed, because the drugs will not reach the organisms in the avascular caseous material.

(b) **Syphilitic adenitis.**—'Shotty' lymph nodes in the groin associated with a genital chancre are characteristic. Those in the submandibular region draining a chancre of the lip are softer. During the secondary stage a generalised enlargement of lymph nodes occurs. Especially noticeable are those above the internal epicondyles and along the posterior border of the sternomastoid.

3. Other Infections

Glandular Fever (syn. infective mononucleosis) is an acute virus infection. After an incubation period of five to fourteen days, enlarged, elastic and slightly tender lymph nodes appear, associated with an irregular fever and often a sore throat, a rash, and splenic enlargement. The blood examination is diagnostic, revealing an absolute and relative lymphocytosis, and an unusual concentration of sheep-cell agglutinins (the heterophile antibody of the Paul-Bunnell reaction). The condition may be mistaken for acute leukaemia or lymphadenoma. Treatment is symptomatic, and recovery is the rule, although it may be some months before the lymph nodes return to normal. The patient is isolated in the early stages.

Toxoplasmosis.—T. Gondii, a small intracellular protozoan is liable to be transmitted from mammals to humans who eat raw or underdone meat which has not been previously frozen. The most tragic manifestation is neonatal jaundice and encephalomyelitis followed by hydrocephalus or microcephaly, blindness and intracerebral calcification. Occasionally the disease manifests itself in children and adults with enlarged lymph nodes and fever. A complement fixation test is necessary.

Cat-Scratch Fever is due to a virus of the lymphogranuloma-psittacosis group. Localised inflammation occurs at the site of the lesion, associated with fever, malaise, and anorexia. This subsides in a few days, but from two to several weeks later the regional lymph nodes become enlarged. Suppuration often occurs, but the pus is sterile, and after evacuation the abscess subsides. Diagnosis is usually suggested by unilateral involvement of lymph nodes and the history of cat scratches. It is confirmed by a skin test with antigen prepared from human lymph-node pus. This distinguishes the condition from chronic pyogenic or tuberculous adenitis with which it is often confused. Broad-spectrum antibiotics help only in reducing the fever.

Generalised lymphadenopathy (in homosexuals) can be due to infection with HIV (AIDS, see Chapter 4).

LYMPHOMAS

Numerous progressive diseases arise from neoplastic change in the various elements of the lymphoreticular system.[1] The lymphomas arise from the types of stem cell (B, T or histiocyte—See Immunology section, Chapter 4), and in general, the less they are histologically differentiated, the more rapidly do they grow. In addition, they may start as slowly growing well-differentiated lesions and then become rapidly growing and more primitive as time goes on ('drift-back'). There is a great deal of variation in the histological types and while no rigid classification is entirely satisfactory the lymphomas are in practice subdivided into Hodgkin's Lymphoma (HL) (Hodgkin's disease) and non-Hodgkin's lymphomas (NHL). HL has particular pleomorphic characteristics (see below) while NHL features nodular (follicular) or diffuse lymphocytic, undifferentiated and histiocytic varieties.

Hodgkin's Lymphoma (Hodgkin's Disease)

Pathology.—Hodgkin's lymphoma is the commonest type of lymphoma and can occur wherever there is lymphoid tissue. On macroscopic section the involved

---

[1] In addition to the lymphomas are included the forms of leukaemia, myeloma and polycythaemia rubra vera.

John Rodman Paul, Contemporary. Emeritus Professor of Preventive Medicine, Yale University School of Medicine, New Haven, Connecticut, U.S.A. Described this test in a joint paper with Bunnell in 1932.
Walls Willard Bunnell, 1902–1965. Physician, Hertford Hospital, Connecticut, U.S.A.
Thomas Hodgkin, 1798–1866. Curator of the museum and demonstrator of morbid anatomy, Guy's Hospital, London. In 1832, read a paper to the Medico-chirurgical Society of London entitled 'On Some Morbid Appearances of the Absorbent Glands and the Spleen,' in which he described a number of cases of lymphadenoma. In 1865, Sir Samuel Wilks (1824–1911), Physician Guy's Hospital, London, suggested that the condition he called Hodgkin's disease, now it has been changed to Hodgkin's Lymphoma.

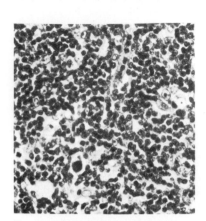

FIG. 81.—Lymphocytic predominance. (best prognosis)

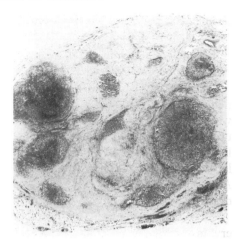

FIG. 82.—Section of whole lymph node showing nodular sclerosis (fair prognosis).

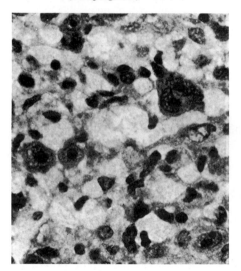

FIG. 83.—Mixed cellularity. The normal modal architecture is replaced by a cellular infiltration with lymphocytes, reticulum cells (histiocytes), eosinophils and fibrous tissue, and the characteristic Reed-Sternberg cells will be seen—a giant cell containing two large mirror image nuclei which may overlap (like pennies on a plate). This type also carries a fair prognosis, but when there is lymphocyte depletion and a preponderance of reticulum cells (histiocytes) the prognosis is poor.

nodes are pink-grey in colour and of rubbery consistency. Except in the more anaplastic forms the nodes are discrete with no periadenitis. The spleen, when involved, does not at first have the same homogeneous appearance as the lymph nodes, but as the disease advances the infiltration becomes more diffuse. Bone deposits occur in the vertebral column and pelvis. Rarely, Hodgkin's lymphoma may be confined to a single organ such as the stomach.

The histological appearance may vary with the stage of the disease but a striking feature is the cellular pleomorphism (figs 81, 82 and 83).

The nature of Hodgkin's lymphoma is still questioned. The Reed-Sternberg cell is an unusual cell in that it undergoes nuclear but not cytoplasmic division. Studies with tritiated thymidine suggest that the reticulum cell is really the basic malignant cell and that the binucleate giant cell is its product. Evidence against the malignant nature of Hodgkin's lymphoma is based upon the fact that Reed-Sternberg cells have occasionally been found in the blood of patients with other diseases—*e.g.* glandular fever. In addition the similarity between the end stage of Hodgkin's lymphoma and the graft-versus-host reaction suggests

Dorothy Reed, 1874–? Pathologist, Johns Hopkins Hospital, Baltimore, U.S.A. Described the giant cells in 1902.
Karl Sternberg, 1872–1935. Pathologist, Vienna. Described the giant cell of Hodgkin's disease in 1898.

an immunological basis. The lymphocytic and acute inflammatory cellular response seen in involved nodes are thought to represent the host's immunological reaction.

Clinical Features (fig 84 and Table).—The disease is more common in males, and usually it affects young adults (25–40 age group).

The most common presentation is painless progressive lymph node enlargement in the cervical or supraclavicular region which may or may not be associated with generalised symptoms such as malaise, fever, weight loss or pruritus. Pressure effects such as superior vena-caval obstruction from enlarged mediastinal lymph nodes may follow or even be the presenting feature. Bone pain, particularly in the back may indicate vertebral collapse secondary to bony metastases. A recognised but unexplained symptom is pain in the sites of disease induced by drinking alcohol.

On examination, the involved nodes tend to be discrete, non-tender and rubbery in consistency as opposed to tuberculosis where the nodes are matted together. In late or lymphocyte depleted cases, however, the nodes may become matted. Splenomegaly and hepatomegaly is a variable accompaniment (see below). As the disease advances irregular elevations of the temperature may occur.[1] With dissemination bony metastases, anaemia and pancytopaenia may develop. There may also be skin deposits in advanced cases. Jaundice due to excessive haemolysis of red cells or diffuse liver involvement is also seen.

The course of the disease is very variable: death may follow in weeks but long term survivals are not uncommon and with modern methods of treatment the disease may be cured.

The Clinical Staging of Hodgkin's Lymphoma (see Table).—The clinical staging of HL is necessary to determine accurately the extent of the disease, the

THE FOUR STAGES OF HODGKIN'S
LYMPHOMA

Stage 1 = Confined to one lymph node site.

Stage 2 = In more than one site either all above or all below the diaphragm.

Stage 3 = Nodes involved above and below diaphragm.

Stage 4 = Spread beyond lymphatic node system e.g. liver, bone.

(For subgroups **A** and **B** see text)

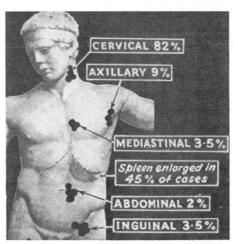

FIG. 84.—Showing the position of Hodgkin's lymphoma when the patient was seen first. In 14% of cases more than one region was involved.
(Baker and Mann's statistics.)

---

[1] The periodic Pel-Ebstein fever, originally described as a feature of Hodgkin's disease, is a mistake. This Pel-Ebstein fever was due to Brucellosis.

Pieter Klazes Pel, 1852–1919. Professor of Medicine, Amsterdam, Holland. Described a relapsing fever in Hodgkin's disease in 1885.
Wilhelm Ebstein, 1836–1912. Professor of Medicine, Göttingen, Germany. Also described the relapsing fever of Hodgkin's disease in 1887.

subsequent treatment and the prognosis. *Accurate staging may prevent unnecessary, unpleasant and dangerous treatments, e.g. cytotoxic drugs.*

The disease is subdivided into four stages (see Table). Each stage is further subdivided into groups **A** or **B** according to the absence or presence of associated generalised symptoms such as weight loss, fever, pruritus, anaemia and bone pain.

Special Investigations Leading to Clinical Staging.—The following procedures are currently in use:

A. *Node Excision Biopsy* to establish the diagnosis and accurate histological grading.

B. *Chest X-Ray* to demonstrate enlarged mediastinal nodes and tomography when indicated.

C. *Mediastinal Scanning* with Gallium 67 has been found to demonstrate involved mediastinal nodes.

D. *Intravenous Urography* may show distortion or compression of the renal calyces by retroperitoneal nodes.

E. *Lower Limb Lymphangiograms* will demonstrate both pelvic and retroperitoneal nodes. Unfortunately this investigation is associated with both false positive and false negative results.

F. *Ultrasonography* (see fig. 85).

G. *CT scan.*

H. *Laparotomy/Splenectomy/Liver and node biopsy* are used frequently to stage Hodgkin's lymphoma. This is because:

Clinical splenomegaly is unreliable in assessing splenic involvement. In one series 50% of patients with splenomegaly were found not to have splenic Hodgkin's at laparotomy. Moreover 25% of those cases without clinical splenomegaly were found to have deposits in the spleen at laparotomy. In addition this procedure may aid in decreasing the problem of hypersplenism and obviate splenic irradiation and its complications. Enlarged aortic, iliac and mesenteric nodes are sought and biopsied. While the value of this procedure must be weighed against its morbidity and mortality, its value is obvious in staging the treatment.

The Relationship between Histological Grade, Clinical Stage and Survival.—There are two clinical varieties of HL, a localised predominantly non-aggressive form, and an aggressive, progressive and fatal variety. Between these two extremes there are intermediate or changing types of disease.

Histologically inactive disease is lymphocyte predominant, clinically stage I and potentially curable. Progressive disease is characterised histologically by diffuse fibrosis, lymphocyte depletion and domination by histiocytes (reticulum cells). Clinically it is seen in stage IIIB and IV and is associated with systemic symptoms. Changing disease is characterised by mixed cellularity or nodular sclerosis in stage II or III disease. Nodular sclerosis in stage I disease however may be associated with a good prognosis.

Treatment Policy for Hodgkin's Lymphoma.—There are two forms of treatment available according to the accurate staging of the disease, namely radiotherapy (RT) and combination chemotherapy (CT). Both treatments are associated with bone marrow depression and toxic side-effects and must be carefully planned and controlled with regular blood counts. Radiotherapy is the

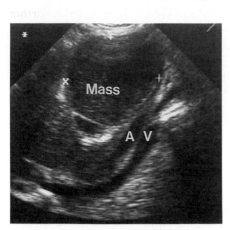

FIG. 85.—Ultrasonogram (longitudinal scan at RIF) showing large mass (NHL) lying on the external iliac vessels (A) and (V).

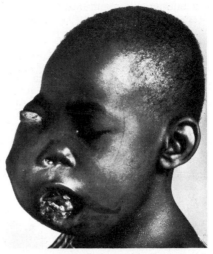

FIG. 86.—Burkitt tumour (*Dr. Denis Burkitt, London*). This rapidly growing tumour is the commonest malignant disease of children living in the equatorial regions of Africa. The age distribution is characteristic with over 80% of cases occurring between the ages of 3 and 12 years inclusive.

treatment of choice in stage I, II and IIIA disease, whilst combination chemotherapy is used in stage IIIB and IV. Megavoltage RT allows wide areas to be treated. Supradiaphramatic disease is treated by radiotherapy to cervical, axillary and mediastinal nodes. Normal tissue is protected by lead shields. RT is given in divided doses over several weeks. Infradiaphragmatic disease is treated by fields covering the para-aortic and iliac nodes (inverted Y fields). CT involves repeated courses of cytotoxic drugs and steroids as it has been shown that the drugs produce better remission when used in combination. An example of the combination commonly used is Nitrogen mustard (Mustine), Vinblastine (Oncovin), Procarbazine and Prednisone (known as MOPP). Other combinations are under trial

Results. A 5 year survival rate of 80% of cases can be achieved in the favourable cases (see above) treated by RT, and one of up to 50% of cases requiring the addition of CT.

Non-Hodgkin's Lymphoma

Non-Hodgkin's lymphoma (NHL) can in cellular and structural variety be lymphocytic, histiocytic (or mixed), well or poorly differentiated, and nodular (follicular) or diffuse. Small lymphocytes and a nodular (follicular) structure suggests a better prognosis than large lymphocytes, histiocytic dominance and a diffuse structure. While in some cases the disease can remain symptomless and apparently static for years, a drift back to more primitive cell appearance and activity is likely, with systemic as well as nodal spread. The nodes in the nodular (follicular) style are like HL, but they tend to be larger and softer in more diffusce, undifferentiated and histiocytic types (fig. 85). The blood may contain large numbers of lymphocytes making the differential diagnosis between NHL and chronic lymphatic leukaemia necessary.

The investigation and the management of the patient is broadly the same as for HL, the favourable histological types, stages and groups being likely to respond to RT but the unfavourable requiring CT as well. Cyclophosphamide is used instead of Mustine, Doxorubicin (Adriamycin®) and bleomycin also are used in the courses of treatment.

Results.—These are not as good as in HL but a 60% case remission is possible, and some cures are effected.

Mycosis Fungoides.—This red or purplish nodular skin condition which breaks down into ulcers is a T cell lymphoma with a poor prognosis.

Malignant Lymphoma of Africa (Burkitt Tumour) (fig. 86). Although this tumour is now known to occur occasionally anywhere in the world, it has only been reported in endemic proportions in tropical Africa and New Guinea. The observation that endemic distribution is limited to warm, moist climates strongly suggests the implication of some biological agent. A vectored virus was consequently considered the most likely aetiological factor. The realisation that many regions are apparently tumour-free, whereas the distribution coincides with that of hyperendemic and holoendemic malaria, suggests that variations in incidence may be dependent on malarial changes in the reticulo-endothelial system, with an added virus infection inducing malignant change. Evidence of E.B. virus infection which is now believed to be the cause of infectious mononucleosis has been almost invariably found in Burkitt's lymphoma and the two conditions may be associated.

Clinical and Pathological Features.—The tumour is multifocal, grows rapidly and is soft and relatively painless. In Africa, approximately 50% of patients present with jaw tumours which may affect one or more of the jaw quadrants. Maxillary lesions may present as oral or orbital tumours. The second commonest clinical presentation is an abdominal tumour. Renal involvement, usually bilateral, is present in 75% of all patients. In girls, ovarian involvement is particularly characteristic and paraplegia without vertebral collapse is also common. Peripheral or mediastinal lymphadenopathy or lung involvement is exceptional, but tumours are frequently observed in the thyroid, testicles, skeleton and breasts. Radiologically the tumours first appear as multiple, small osteolytic deposits which coalesce to form larger areas of bone destruction. On microscopic section dense masses of darkly staining primitive lymphoid cells interspersed with large clear histiocytes give an appearance under low power magnification of a 'starry night'.

Treatment.—The tumour is unusually sensitive to both radiotherapy and a wide range of cytotoxic drugs such as cyclophosphamide, methotrexate and orthomelphalan. A much higher proportion of long-term survivors have been reported than in any other form of childhood cancer. Several of these have followed single doses of therapy suggesting a strong host defence mechanism, possibly immunological. Surgery is not indicated with the possible exception of removing large ovarian tumours. A number of spontaneous remissions have been recorded.

Kaposi's Angiosarcoma occurs as multiple bluish or brownish nodules, especially on the limbs. In due course the nodules ulcerate and the disease disseminates widely. It may be confused with malignant melanoma. These tumours are sensitive to radiotherapy and chemotherapy. Previously considered a rarity and occurring in middle-aged male Eastern European Jews, the condition has been found to be prevalent not only in the natives of equatorial Africa, but it is occurring in young Western males. It seems to be related to Acquired Immune Deficiency Syndrome (AIDS) (Chapter 4).

Boeck's Sarcoidosis is a multisystem granulomatous disorder of unknown aetiology most commonly affecting young adults and presenting most frequently with bilateral hilar lymphadenopathy, pulmonary infiltration, skin or eye lesions. The diagnosis is established most securely when clinicoradiographic findings are supported by histological evidence of widespread non-caseating epithelioid cell granulomas in more than one organ or a positive Kveim-Siltzbach skin test. Immunological features are depression of delayed-type hypersensitivity suggesting impaired cell-mediated immunity and raised or abnormal immunoglobulins. There may also be hypercalciuria with or without hypercalcaemia. The course and prognosis may correlate with the mode of onset: an acute onset with erythema nodosum heralds a self-limiting course and spontaneous resolution while an insidious onset may be followed by relentless progressive fibrosis.

Clinical Manifestations.—It affects lungs, eyes, skin, spleen, lymph nodes, lacrimal and parotid glands, central nervous system so it presents to surgeons of different disciplines. Examination of a patient with suspected sarcoidosis comprises full physical examination, slit lamp examination of the eyes and chest radiography.

Diagnosis is based on the twin criteria of a compatible clinical picture and histological evidence of sarcoid tissue; the latter is obtained by biopsy of skin, lymph node or liver or by scalene node biopsy, mediastinoscopy or fibreoptic bronchoscopy. The Kveim-Siltzbach skin test is a simple specific outpatient technique which is positive in 80% of patients

Denis Parsons Burkitt, F.R.S., Contemporary. Medical Research Council Scientific Staff. Described this type of sarcoma in 1958.
Moritz Kaposi, 1837–1902. Professor of Dermatology, Vienna. Described pigmented sarcoma of the skin in 1872.
Caesar Peter Moeller Boeck, 1845–1917. Professor of Dermatology, Oslo, Norway. Described sarcoidosis in 1899.
Morten Ansgar Kveim, 1892–1967. Dermatologist, Oslo, Norway.
Louis Elliot Siltzbach, 1906–1980. Clinical Professor of Medicine, Mount Sinai Hospital, New York, U.S.A.

with sarcoidosis. It is an index of activity of the disease. The sarcoid granuloma in the pulmonary capillary bed produces angiotensin-converting enzyme, which can be measured in the serum (SACE). Elevated SACE levels are noted in about one-half of patients with sarcoidosis. Like the Kveim-Siltzbach test, it reflects activity of the disease. Its production is suppressed by corticosteroid therapy, so SACE is a useful monitor of response to treatment and of relapse when treatment has been discontinued.

Differential Diagnosis.—Sarcoidosis must be distinguished from a non-specific sarcoid-tissue reaction and from Hodgkin's lymphoma.

Treatment.—Corticosteroids relieve symptoms, suppress inflammation and granuloma formation, and are used for uveitis, pulmonary infiltration, hypercalciuria and renal calculi, disfiguring skin lesions, neurosarcoidosis, myocardial sarcoidosis, and involvement of spleen, lymph nodes, parotid and lacrimal glands. Alternative treatments comprise oxyphenbutazone for acute exudative disease and chloroquine or potassium-p-amino-benzoate (Potaba®) for chronic fibrotic sarcoidosis.

COMPARISON BETWEEN SARCOIDOSIS AND HODGKIN'S DISEASE

Feature	Sarcoidosis	Hodgkin's lymphoma
Age	20–50	Any
Fever	Rare	Common
Weight loss	Infrequent	Frequent
Splenomegaly	In 12%	Very common
Submental lymph nodes	No	Yes
Erythema nodosum	Common	Very rare
Pruritus	Absent	Present
Bone lesions	'Punched out' phalangeal cysts	Sclerotic lesions of spine and pelvis
Leukocytosis; lymphopenia; eosinophilia	Absent	Present (sometimes)
Hilar lymphadenopathy	Bilateral	Bilateral or unilateral
Pulmonary infiltration	Common	Uncommon
Pulmonary infiltration followed by hilar adenopathy	Never	Frequent
Secondary infections	Rare	Common
Pleural effusion	No	Yes
Radiotherapy	Unhelpful	Helpful
Corticosteroids	Therapy of choice	Helpful
Immunosuppressive regimes	Not indicated	Indicated
Prognosis	Good	Less good

CHAPTER 10

SKIN. BURNS

INFECTIONS

Boil (*syn*. Furuncle).— A boil is an acute staphylococcal infection of a hair follicle, with perifolliculitis, which usually proceeds to suppuration and central necrosis. A painful and indurated swelling appears which gradually extends. After two or three days, the centre softens and a small slough is discharged with a bead of pus, and in the large majority of cases the condition then subsides. A 'blind boil' is one which subsides without suppuration. Boils are common on the back of the neck.

Infection of the perianal hair follicle (perianal abscess), with suppuration, is likely to result in a sinus or fistula. Furunculosis of the external auditory meatus is extremely painful, as the skin is attached to the underlying cartilage, and swelling is accompanied by considerable tension.

Complications of Boils.—(i) Cellulitis, especially in debilitated subjects. (ii) Infection of the lymph nodes draining the affected part. (iii) Secondary boils due to infection of neighbouring hair follicles (*e.g.* in hydradenitis, fig. 87).

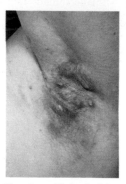

FIG. 87.—Hydradenitis-infection of axillary sweat glands and hair follicles.

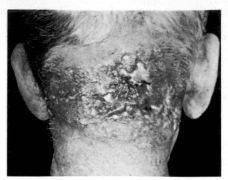

FIG. 88.—Carbuncle of the neck. (Infective gangrene of the subcutaneous tissues.)
(*Herbert Bourns, FRCS, Bristol.*)

Stye (*syn*. hordeolum).—A *stye* is due to infection of an eyelash follicle.

Treatment consists of improving the general health of the patient, since boils are frequently associated with overwork, worry, debility, examinations, or other undermining influences. Incision is unnecessary, as a touch of iodine on a skin pustule will hasten necrosis of the overlying skin so that pus can then escape. Should softening occur around a hair follicle, particularly an eyelash (stye), removal of the appropriate hair allows the ready escape of pus. The sensitivity of the organisms is determined in case the appropriate antibiotic may be needed. Washing the surrounding skin twice a day with suitable disinfectant, *e.g.* hexachlorophene, discourages the development of secondary boils. A paste, composed of anhydrous magnesium sulphate (24 parts) and glycerin (11 parts) exercises a valuable osmotic effect.

Cellulitis and Erysipelas (Chapters 3 and 4).

Carbuncle.—This is an infective gangrene of the subcutaneous tissues, due to staphylococcal infection. It is uncommon before the age of forty, and males are the usual sufferers. *Diabetes* may be present.

A carbuncle often occurs in the nape of the neck. The subcutaneous tissues become painful and indurated, and the overlying skin is red (fig. 88). Unless the condition is aborted by prompt treatment, extension will occur, and after a few days areas of softening appear, the skin gives way and thick pus and sloughs discharge. Usually there is one central large slough, surrounded by a 'rosette' of smaller areas of necrosis. Infection may extend widely and fresh openings appear on the surface and coalesce with those previously formed.

Treatment.—The general treatment and organism identification is similar to that described for boils. Many carbuncles are aborted if penicillin is used adequately in the early stages. Local treatment by osmotic pastes is often supplemented by infra-red or short-wave diathermy.

Lupus vulgaris (tuberculosis of the skin) usually occurs between the ages of ten and twenty-five, the face being the site of election. One or more cutaneous nodules appear, with congestion of the surrounding skin. On applying pressure with a glass slide the nodules are seen to be the colour of apple jelly. Extension occurs very slowly, but ulceration is likely to follow sooner or later. The resulting ulcer tends to heal in one situation as it extends to another. The mucous membranes of the mouth and nose are sometimes attacked, either primarily or by extension from the face. Oedema occurs if the fibrosis caused by the lupus obstructs the normal lymphatic drainage. Infection in the nasal cavity may be followed by necrosis of underlying cartilage. Epithelioma is prone to occur in a lupus scar (fig. 89).

Treatment is by chemotherapy (Chapter 4). If healing is slow, the lesion should be excised.

Impetigo is an intradermal infection. When caused by the streptococcus the primary lesion is bullous, which soon ruptures to form an erosion and then a crust. In the staphylococcal type, the primary lesion is also bullous, but the bullae are more durable (*e.g.* in neonatal pemphigus). The infection is contagious, and in rugby football one player so infected can spread the disease amongst his team mates and the opposing side (the condition being known as 'scrum-pox'). *Treatment* includes the careful washing of the face to remove crusts, using hexachlorophene soap and lotion (1%). Systemic antibiotics, according to the sensitivity tests, are only used in those cases which are resistant to local treatment.

Herpes Simplex can spread in a similar fashion.

CYSTS

A sebaceous cyst (*syn.* a wen) follows obstruction to the mouth of a sebaceous duct, and is therefore a retention cyst. Pathologically, it is classed as an epidermoid cyst (Chapter 8). It commonly occurs on the face or scalp (Chapter 26), but can occur anywhere except on the palms and soles, which are devoid of sebaceous glands. A typical cyst appears as a hemispherical swelling, firm or elastic in consistency, and with no definite edge. It is more or less adherent to the skin, especially if it has been previously inflamed. The punctum of the obstructed duct can sometimes be seen on the summit of the cyst, and sebaceous material expressed. An uncomplicated cyst contains yellowish-white material composed of fat and epithelial cells, of a putty-like consistency, so it can often be indented by a finger-tip. Rarely, a minute worm, *Demodex folliculorum*, which harbours in sebaceous glands, may be seen on microscopy of the cyst wall.

Complications.—(i) *Infection.*—The cyst becomes enlarged and painful, and the overlying skin is red. Recurrent attacks cause the cyst wall to become adherent

---

Carbunculus in Latin, Anthrax in Greek, is the word for Charcoal. The ancients saw in these conditions burning sores upon the skin—hence they likened them to glowing coal.
Sir Astley Paston Cooper, 1768–1841. Surgeon, Guy's Hospital, London (1800–1825). In 1821 he received a Baronetcy and one thousand guineas for successfully removing an infected sebaceous cyst from the head of King George IV.

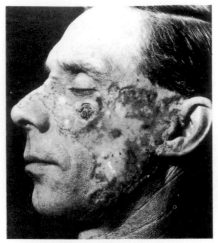

FIG. 89.—Advanced lupus vulgaris. Carcinoma has developed on the cheek.

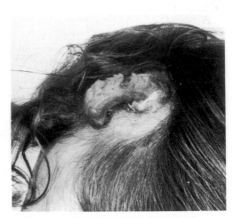

FIG. 91.—Sebaceous horn of the scalp.

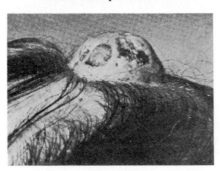

FIG. 90.—Cock's 'peculiar tumour, (infected, ulcerated sebaceous cyst).

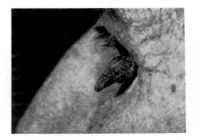

FIG. 92.—Keratin horn beside the eye, a variety of papilloma.

to surrounding subcutaneous tissue, and consequently more difficult to remove. The contents of an infected cyst become semi-liquid and usually very foetid.

(ii) *Ulceration.*—An infected cyst may discharge its contents. If an ulcerated surface remains, it can resemble an epithelioma, and to which the term Cock's 'peculiar tumour' may be applied (fig. 90).

(iii) *Sebaceous Horn.*—The contents of a cyst sometimes escape slowly from the duct orifice and dry in successive layers on the skin, forming a sebaceous horn (fig. 91 and see frontispiece).

Treatment.—(*a*) Incision-Avulsion.—Under local anaesthesia an incision is made through the skin, into the cyst. The contents are squeezed out and the cyst wall is seized with artery forceps and carefully avulsed.

(*b*) Dissection is necessary for cysts which have been previously inflamed. An incision is made over the cyst, the wall is defined, and the cyst is dissected from adjacent tissue and removed intact. Unless the wall is completely removed recurrence is probable. Incomplete removal is common if removal is attempted in the presence of recent infection.

Sequestration and **Implantation Dermoid Cysts** are described in Chapter 8.

Edward Cock, 1805–1892. Surgeon, Guy's Hospital, London.

CALLOSITIES, CORNS, AND WARTS

A **callosity** (*French: callosité*) is a localised thickened or hardened part of skin caused by friction. It is commonly occupational, *e.g.* on a gardener's hand.

A **corn** (*Old French: corn = grain*) is a horny induration of the cuticle with a hard centre, caused by undue pressure, chiefly affecting toes and feet. Most corns yield to the chiropodist, provided that footwear is suitable. Skilled treatment is important in patients with diabetes or a poor peripheral circulation, as secondary infection may precipitate gangrene. Salicylic acid in collodion (20%) applied for a few nights, followed by soaking in hot water, is often effective in removing a corn.

A **wart** (*Old English: wearte*) is a dry rough excrescence on the skin (fig. 93).

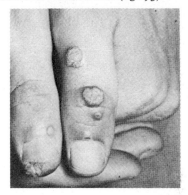

FIG. 93.—*The common wart* usually occurs on the hands, particularly in children. It is due to a virus and is infectious. As warts often disappear spontaneously, any treatment which is in use at the time will gain an undeserved reputation as a wart 'cure'. Curetting and cauterisation of the centre is the radical treatment, but further crops may appear.

Plantar warts occur in the sole, and are usually multiple. They may be so tender as to render standing or walking exceedingly uncomfortable. The nightly application of 3% formaldehyde lotion for eight weeks is effective in 60% of cases. Curettage is more certain. Under a local or general anaesthetic, a scalpel, held vertically to the skin, incises the hard skin at the boundary of the lesion. A sharp curette can be inserted beneath the wart to remove it. The footwear must be treated if re-infection by the virus is to be avoided. Cotton socks should be worn, as these can be boiled. Shoes can be disinfected by formalin vapour.

Seborrhoeic (*syn.* '*Senile*') warts, see below.

Venereal warts and moist warts (papillomata acuminata), see Chapter 60.

PAPILLOMAS AND MISCELLANEOUS SKIN LESIONS

Papilloma

A papilloma of the skin may be derived from either the squamous or the basal cell layers. The *squamous cell papillomas* include the following types: (1) *Congenital* (*syn. Naevus*[1] *Verrucosus*), which may be single or multiple, and it appears either at birth or in early life. It is a warty growth of brownish colour, but large horny excrescences may be present. (2) *Infective Wart* (*verruca vulgaris*)—the common wart—described above. (3) *Soft Papilloma*, which often occurs on the eyelids of elderly people. (4) *Keratin Horn* (fig. 92).—This is also seen in old people and is a papilloma with excess keratin formation.

Basal Cell (*Seborrhoeic, or Senile, Wart*).—Often develops in large numbers on the trunk, face, and arms of persons in or past middle life. Circular, slightly raised, warty, often brownish, they look as if they are stuck on the skin.

Molluscum[2] **Fibrosum**, are polypoid or filiform soft fleshy skin tags which occur on the neck, trunk, and face.

---

[1] Naevus (*Latin = Naevus*) = A birth mark, but often used to mean simply a mark or blemish on the skin (see Haemangioma and Melanoma).

[2] Mollusc (*Latin: Molluscus = soft*) = A soft protuberance on the skin.

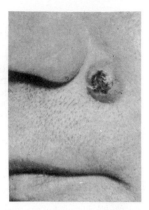

FIG. 94.—Molluscum sebaceum.

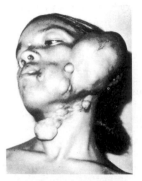

FIG. 95.—Dermatofibroma
protuberans.
(*R. Naik, MS, Durg., India.*)

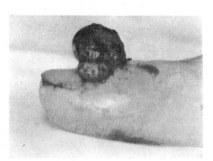

FIG. 96.—Granuloma pyogenicum. The
surface shows atrophic epidermis, but
often has crusts.

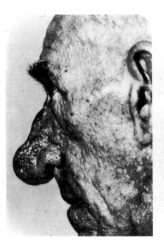

FIG. 97.—Rhinophyma.

Molluscum Sebaceum (*syn*. Keratoacanthoma).—Occurs on the face or hand
as a firm hemispherical nodule, which may reach a size of up to 2 cm in diameter
in six weeks (fig. 94). The summit of the tumour ulcerates and forms a crust
beneath which is a crater. After a time, the crust is shed and spontaneous healing
occurs with a scar. The tumour may be curetted and a caustic (*e.g.* silver nitrate)
applied to the crater. A quicker cure is obtained by excision, which permits
adequate microscopy. Undoubtedly in the past many cases were regarded as
epitheliomas and helped to swell the number of 'cures' for this condition.

Sclerosing Angioma (*Syn*. Dermatofibroma; Subepidermal Nodular Fibrosis).—This
occurs in skin as firm, indolent, single, or multiple nodules. The nodules, in adults, are
situated most commonly on the extremities. As a rule they are only a few millimetres in
diameter. Most are reddish, others are yellowish-brown (due to lipid) or blue-black (due
to haemosiderin). The latter may resemble melanoma. *Dermatofibroma protuberans* grows
persistently outwards to attain considerable size (fig. 95). It may be a low-grade fibrosarcoma.

Granuloma Pyogenicum (fig. 96).—This is a traditional but misleading name. The
lesion looks like a haemangioma but has a typical natural history. Usually single, it consists
of a red, soft or moderately firm, more or less pedunculated nodule which grows rapidly

to a size varying from 0·5 to 2 cm in diameter. Most commonly it is seen on the face, the fingers and toes. Treatment is excision.

Benign Calcifying Epithelioma (Malherbe's epithelioma).—These are solitary, hard, tumours that appear to be growing from the deep surface of the skin. They occur mostly on the face, neck and arms. The size usually varies between 0·5 to 3 cm in diameter. The tumour may arise at any age but is common in childhood. Clinically it resembles a rather hard sebaceous cyst.

Tumours of Accessory Skin Structures.—These are rare. (1) *Sebaceous naevus:* A congenital condition presenting as a pinkish-yellow plaque in the scalp. (2) *Sebaceous adenoma:* Isolated lesions are very rare. Multiple sebaceous adenomas occur in association with epilepsy and mental deterioration. (3) *Tumours of sweat glands:* Are closely related to basal cell carcinoma but present deep to the skin and are often cystic (Papilliferous cystadenoma).

Sarcoid (Boecks) Chapter 9).—This is a generalised disease which may affect skin. In the skin it occurs as reddish-brown nodules which are soft, and rarely ulcerate. Giant cells are found, but tubercle bacilli can never be isolated.

Rhinophyma (*syn.* Potato nose) (fig. 97).—This is a glandular form of Acne Rosacea. The skin of the nose, particularly the distal part, becomes immensely thickened and the openings of the sebaceous follicles are easily seen. The capillaries become dilated and the nose assumes a bluish-red colour. Surgical treatment, by paring away the excess tissue, gives a great improvement.

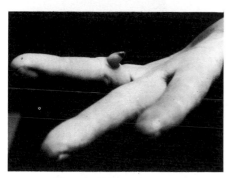

FIG. 98.—Horn of a corn.
(Dr. Sheetal Singh, Srinagar, Kashmir, India.)

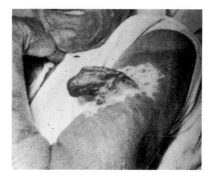

FIG. 99.—A cicatrix horn in a burn scar.
(R. R. Deskmukh, MS, Dhautoli, Nagpur, India.)

Cutaneous Horns.[1]—May be (i) Sebaceous horns, (ii) wart or corn horns, (iii) cicatrix horns, and (iv) nail horns (frontispiece, figs. 91, 92, 98, 99).

HAEMANGIOMA

A haemangioma is a developmental malformation of blood-vessels rather than a true tumour, and is therefore an example of a hamartoma (Chapter 8). It may occur in any tissue of the body, but is most common in the skin and subcutaneous tissues. A haemangioma is either capillary, venous (cavernous), or arterial in type.

Capillary Haemangioma

(1) **Salmon Patch.**[2]—This is present at birth over the forehead in the midline, and over the occiput. It disappears by the age of one year.

(2) **Port Wine Stain** (Naevus flammeus) (fig. 100).—Present at birth, it

---

[1] Sir John Bland-Sutton, 1855–1936. Surgeon, The Middlesex Hospital, London, and President of the Royal College of Surgeons, classified horns in 1911.
[2] Also called 'stork bites'! Not to be confused with the patch in syphilis.

Albert Malherbe, 1845–1915. Professor of Pathological Anatomy and Histology, Nantes, France.

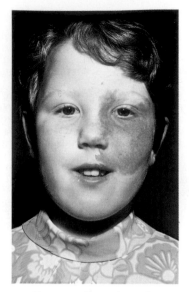
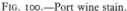
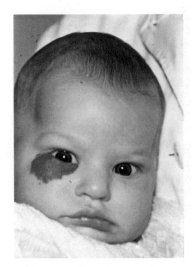

FIG. 100.—Port wine stain.   FIG. 101.—Strawberry angioma.

changes very little throughout life, although the colour may alter a little and it
may become nodular in some areas. *Treatment* is for reason of appearance. The
texture of the skin is quite normal and in a girl the blemish can be disguised by
the skilful use of cosmetics. In a boy, treatment by excision and grafting may be
considered. Radiation and other destructive treatment is disappointing. Treatment by laser destruction is being evaluated in some centres.

   (3) **Strawberry Angioma** (fig. 101).—This common condition has a typical
history. The baby is normal at birth and at the age of one to three weeks is noted
to have a red mark. This increases rapidly for some weeks or even up to three
months, until the typical strawberry or raspberry-like swelling is present. Clinically, the sign of emptying may be demonstrable. The lesion is composed of
immature vaso-formative tissue. The subcutaneous tissue as well as the skin is
often involved, and in severe cases the muscles may be affected. Sub-mucous
naevi are prone to haemorrhage, which is sometimes alarming.

   From the age of three months to one year the naevus grows with the child.
Then it ceases to grow. Eventually the colour fades and flattening occurs so that
at the age of seven or eight years involution is complete. *Treatment.*—The final
result (fig. 102) is better if natural involution is allowed to occur rather than if
regression is hastened (as it can be) by any operative or physical methods (*e.g.*
carbon dioxide snow, injection of hot water or sclerosant fluid or hypertonic
saline, *etc.*). X-ray therapy carries a high risk of disturbance of growth and is
dangerous.

   Venous Angioma (**cavernous**) is relatively uncommon. It is present at birth
and consists of a multiplicity of venous channels of varying calibre. Usually it
shows no tendency to involution and may become larger and more troublesome
later. Sometimes the whole of one limb and the adjacent part of the trunk is
affected. Occasionally the naevus is associated with a lipoma (naevo-lipoma). In

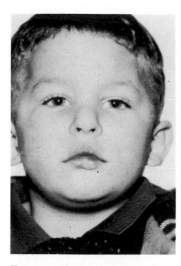

FIG. 102.—Strawberry angioma. Same case as fig. 101 with conservative treatment, about 7 years.

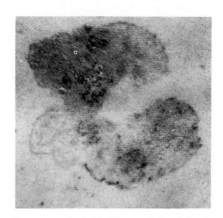

FIG. 103.—Bowen's disease of the abdominal wall.

some cases arteriovenous communications are present (Chapter 14). The skin overlying the naevus may be atrophic, and besides being in danger of severe haemorrhage from trauma, the patient may suffer from septicaemia if organisms gain entry, in which case the energetic use of antibiotics is an urgent matter. *Treatment.*—In general this is conservative. Injection of sclerosing agents (as for varicose veins) is followed by variable results, but the use of a carefully applied laser may be considered. If arteriography reveals a feeding artery, therapeutic embolisation (Chapter 14) may be possible.

Arterial (plexiform) Angioma is a type of congenital arteriovenous fistula (Chapter 14). The pulsating swelling of arteries and arterialised veins is often called a *cirsoid aneurysm* (Chapter 26).

Spider Naevus.—This may be associated with liver disease (Chapter 45) if present in the skin over the manubrium sterni, but it may occur quite innocently. It shows the characteristic sign of emptying.

Naevus tardes are small angiomas occurring *in adults*, often around the mouth. They may be associated with vasospastic conditions and scleroderma (Chapter 14).

Lymphangiomas are described in Chapter 9. Sometimes they are associated with a haemangioma (haemo-lymphangioma).

PREMALIGNANT CONDITIONS OF THE SKIN[1]

(1) **Bowen's disease** is an intradermal precancerous condition. A brownish induration with a well-defined edge appears in the skin (fig. 103). Microscopically large clear cells similar to those found in Paget's disease of the nipple (Chapter 39) are in evidence. Sooner or later carcinoma develops, and wide excision is then necessary.

(3) **Paget's Disease of the Nipple** (Chapter 39).

(3) **Leukoplakia** (Chapter 39).

(4) **Senile (or Solar) Keratosis.**—Occurs occasionally as multiple lesions on the face and backs of hands in persons past middle life. Exposure to sun is the important predispos-

---

[1] *Acanthosis Nigricans*, a pigmented hypertrophic condition of the skin folds usually in the axillae is *not* in itself premalignant, but is associated with cancer of the gastro-intestinal tract and the breast.

John Templeton Bowen, 1857–1940. Professor of Dermatology, Harvard Medical School, Boston, Massachusetts, U.S.A. Described Precancerous Dermatosis in 1912.

ing factor. Usually the lesions are less than 1 cm and have a dry, hard scale with little or no infiltration. Squamous cell carcinoma may develop.

(5) **Radiodermatitis.**—(*a*) *Early:* Erythema occurs which goes on to desquamation and pigmentation. If the dose is very great, ulceration may occur. (*b*) *Late:* Atrophy, irregular hyper-pigmentation and telangiectasis and hair loss occur. Eventually squamous cell carcinoma may develop.

(6) **Chronic Scars.**—A carcinoma which develops in a scar (Marjolin's Ulcer) presents the following characteristics.

(i) It grows slowly, as the scar is relatively avascular.

(ii) It is painless, as scar tissue contains no nerves.

(iii) Secondary deposits do not occur in the regional lymph nodes as lymphatic vessels have been destroyed. If the ulcer invades normal tissue surrounding the scar, it extends at a normal rate, and lymph nodes are then liable to be involved.

MALIGNANT DISEASE OF THE SKIN

Basal Cell Carcinoma (Rodent Ulcer).—A common tumour of low-grade malignancy which occurs in white-skinned people. Exposure to sunlight is a predisposing factor and it is therefore common in Australia. It occurs in the middle or late age and 90% of lesions are found on the face, usually above a line from the lobe of the ear to the corner of the mouth, the commonest site being around the inner canthus of the eye. Although often called a rodent 'ulcer' many of the lesions are non-ulcerated, and have a nodular appearance with a pearly or darkly translucent colour as if containing water, and with a network of fiery red blood-vessels on the surface. Thus the common types are: nodular, cystic, and ulcerated (figs. 104 and 105). An unusual type is the 'field fire' rodent (circinate spreading edge leaving central scarring).

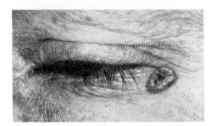

FIG. 104.—Rodent ulcer.

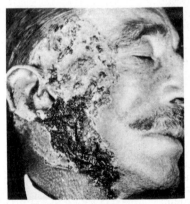

FIG. 105.—Disfigurement caused by rodent ulcer.

The ulcerated type has a typical appearance—a raised rolled edge, like a motor car tyre, with central ulceration (fig. 104). Temporary healing often takes place, to be followed by further ulceration with serous discharge and bleeding. The patient gives a history of a 'spot' which never really heals: 'it keeps scabbing over and breaking down'.

Though the tumours are slow-growing, if ulcerated they will, as the name implies, gradually erode deeper tissues, such as muscles, cartilage, and bone, producing severe disfigurement (fig. 105). Dissemination by lymphatics or the

Jean Nicolas Marjolin, 1780–1850. Surgeon, Paris. Described the development of Carcinomatous Ulcers in Scars in 1828.

blood-stream does not occur. Rarely the ulcer takes on a squamous-cell carcinomatous change.

Microscopic examination shows masses of darkly staining cells with a characteristic arrangement—an outer palisade layer of columnar cells surrounding a central mass of polyhedral cells. Cystic spaces may be seen.

Treatment.—Surgery or radiotherapy are equally highly likely to cure most lesions. The choice will depend sometimes upon the anatomical site, *e.g.* tumours invading the cartilage of the nose or pinna are best treated by excision. The surgeon (as also the radiotherapist) must include an adequate margin of healthy tissue in the treatment field; basal cell carcinoma can infiltrate more widely than is clinically suspected and histological confirmation of clearance, preferably by frozen section, is essential. For small lesions on the face the surgical defects may be closed by primary suture but, especially round the eye, a full thickness Wolfe graft (see p. 154) is often indicated to avoid distortion of the lids. Larger lesions may require pedicle flap cover. Extensive tumours invading the skull bones are often incurable but radiotherapy may provide good long-term palliation.

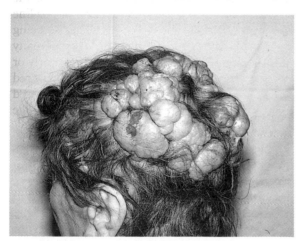

FIG. 106.—Cylindroma (turban tumour).

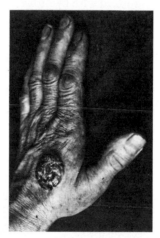

FIG. 107. — Squamous-celled carcinoma. The patient was a chemical worker.

Cylindroma (*syn.* 'turban' tumour) is so called from the arrangement of the stroma in peculiar transparent cylinders. It is considered by some to be a basal-celled carcinoma, while others classify the tumour as endothelioma (Chapter 8). The tumour gradually forms an extensive turban-like swelling extending over the scalp (fig. 106). Ulceration is uncommon, and the tumour is relatively benign.

Squamous Cell Carcinoma (Squamous Cell Epithelioma, Epithelioma) (fig. 107).—This is less common, but it is more malignant and more rapidly growing than rodent ulcer. A squamous cell epithelioma can occur *de novo* in the skin of the face of elderly people, but more often it occurs in a pre-existing skin lesion, or as a result of past irradiation. The pre-malignant conditions are listed above, and other conditions include long-standing venous ulcers, chronic lupus vulgaris lesions, and the prolonged irritation of the skin by various chemicals, *e.g.* dyes, tar or soot (Chapter 8).

A typical carcinomatous ulcer is irregular in outline, and the edges are raised and everted. The base is indurated and sooner or later becomes attached to the deeper structures. A blood-stained discharge occurs, which is increased in amount with the advent of secondary infection. The regional lymph nodes become involved, and the deposits are liable to undergo mucoid degeneration, to which secondary infection is sometimes added.

Treatment.—Treatment must be adequate. Immediately after biopsy confirmation of the diagnosis, the surgical treatment is wide excision, which may require some form of skin graft to the defect. Whether radiotherapy should be employed instead of surgery depends upon the condition of the patient, the size and attachments of the tumour, and the radiotherapy facilities.

The presence, or subsequent appearance, of enlarged mobile lymph nodes is an indication for block-dissection, unless it is considered that secondary infection is responsible, in which case the decision to operate will await the effect of the appropriate antibiotic. Fixed enlarged lymph nodes are not removable; some regression may be obtained by radiotherapy, which in special situations may be combined with cytotoxic drugs. In the anal area, combination treatments by R.T. and drugs are replacing surgery for advanced tumours (see Chapter 54).

MELANOCYTIC TUMOURS AND MALIGNANT MELANOMA

Simple Melanocytic Tumours

The melanocyte is generally believed to be derived from the neural crest. In normal skin, melanocytes appear as clear cells in the basal layer of the epidermis. They may become increased in number in the layers of the skin to form benign pigmented naevi (moles) as follows: 1. within the basal layer of the epidermis (*Lentigo*), 2. as localised aggregations projecting into the dermis (*Junctional naevus*), 3. entirely within the dermis (*Dermal naevus*) and 4. when 2 and 3 are combined (*Compound naevus*). These simple melanocytic tumours may arise anywhere in the skin including the nail bed. They are seen occasionally in the conjunctiva of the eye but are rare in other mucous membranes.

The *blue naevus* (fig. 108) is a tumour of dermal melanocytes and occurs most commonly on the face, on the dorsum of the hands and feet, and over the sacrum in certain races (Mongolian blue spot). It is very darkly pigmented and because of its overlying layer of normal, though sometimes thinned epidermis, looks shiny and blue or slate grey in colour. Malignant change is exceptionally rare.

Clinical Features.—Pigmented naevi may occur at any age but commonly appear in childhood and adolescence as small, brown, flat or slightly raised lesions in the skin. These are usually of junctional or compound type but with increasing age they either atrophy or mature into dermal naevi.

Another clinical type is seen in middle-aged patients, particularly in the face. These appear as small, rounded swellings, often non-pigmented and sometimes bear bristly hairs. They are dermal naevi.

Congenital naevi are rare. They are often darkly pigmented and may be hairy and papillary in appearance. Occasionally they cover extensive areas of skin, up to 25% or more of the body surface. They may undergo malignant change even

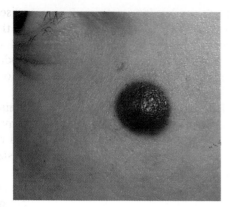

FIG. 108.—Blue naevus of face.

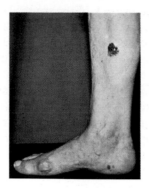

FIG. 109.—Malignant melanoma of the leg, showing pigmented and amelanotic areas.

during childhood. With this exception malignant melanoma is very rare before puberty.

Moles on the palms, soles or external genitalia were thought at one time to be especially prone to become malignant but, in fact, site is not a risk factor.

Treatment may be indicated (i) for cosmetic reasons, (ii) if by reason of its position the lesion is subject to the nuisance of repeated trauma, *e.g.* cut when shaving or rubbed by the brassiere strap, though there is no evidence that trauma causes malignant change, (iii) if the history suggests that malignant change has occurred (see below).

Surgical excision is the only acceptable treatment, and all lesions should be sent for histological examination.

MALIGNANT MELANOMA

It is now generally agreed that malignant melanoma of the skin should be regarded as a carcinoma—melanocarcinoma. A malignant melanoma may arise (i) in a pre-existing pigmented naevus or (ii) *de novo* in apparently normal skin. Pathological studies suggest that malignant change in a benign naevus occurs only in the junctional or compound varieties; the pure dermal naevus is safe. Little is known of the causation but it is commonest in fair-skinned individuals who live in hot climates and prolonged exposure to ultra violet light has been incriminated. The disease is becoming increasingly common in all Western countries.

Clinical Recognition.—Malignant melanoma is almost unknown before puberty. It should be suspected after puberty when:

1. A previously existing mole begins to enlarge, itches, weeps, scabs or bleeds, becomes ulcerated or more deeply pigmented, or produces a halo of pigment in the surrounding skin.

2. A pigmented lesion appears in an adult and grows progressively.

3. A rapidly growing, fleshy, ulcerated skin tumour appears which looks as though it may be malignant; some malignant melanomas are amelanotic, and are called amelanotic melanomas.

The commonest site in females is the lower leg (fig. 109), and in males the front or back of the trunk. In the African Negro the sole of the foot is the most frequent site; malignant melanoma does not arise from the blacker skin of the remainder of the body for reasons which are not understood. Rarely malignant melanoma arises in the eye, in the meninges or at the muco-cutaneous junction zones, e.g. anus.

Differential diagnosis is from (i) histiocytoma (sclerosing angioma), (ii) pigmented basal cell carcinoma, (iii) basal cell papilloma (seborrhoeic wart), (iv) cavernous haemangioma, blue naevus.

Spread.—Malignant melanoma may spread by local extension, by the lymphatics or by the blood-stream. Tumour cells may reach the regional lymph nodes by embolism but spread by lymphatic permeation is also seen producing local satellite nodules (fig. 110(*a*)) and/or 'in transit' deposits between the primary growth and the regional nodes (fig. 110(*b*)). Secondary lymphoedema may occur (Chapter 9). Blood borne metastases are seen in the lungs, liver, brain, bones and skin. They may also involve unusual sites, *e.g.* the breasts, small intestine and heart. Secondary deposits are typically black but sometimes contain little or no melanin, even when the primary tumour is heavily pigmented. Extensive visceral involvement may cause melanuria.

Staging and Prognosis.—A simple clinical staging system is as follows:

Stage I—primary tumour only
Stage II—enlargement of regional lymph nodes and/or satellite deposits or in transit nodules
Stage III—widely disseminated disease.

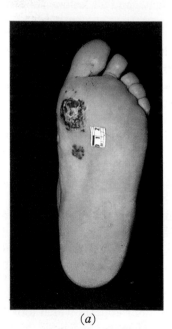

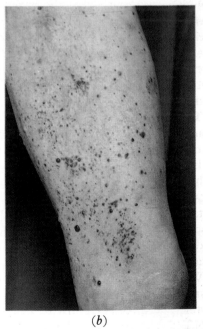

(*a*) (*b*)

FIG. 110.—(*a*) Melanoma malignum of the foot, with local satellite deposits. (*b*) 'In transit' deposits between the primary growth and the regional nodes.

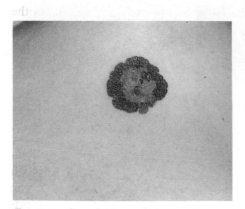

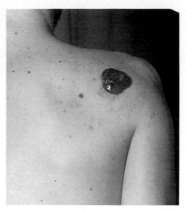

FIG. 111.—Superficial spreading melanoma. Note irregular advancing edge and central atrophy with loss of pigment.

FIG. 112.—Nodular melanoma. A thick, ulcerated lesion of poor prognosis.

Approximately 70% of patients in clinical Stage I will survive 5 years and 25% in Stage II. Most Stage III patients are dead within one year. Pathological staging of the primary melanoma can be assessed by the level of its invasion into the layers of the skin, or more simply and accurately by measuring the thickness of the tumour using an optical micrometer. Melanomas less than 1 mm in thickness seldom metastasise to lymph nodes or via the blood stream. The risk of lymph node spread increases and the prognosis worsens with increasing thickness and is grave when this exceeds 4 mm. These features correlate approximately with the clinical appearance of the lesion. The thin, superficial spreading type of melanoma (fig. 111) generally carries a favourable prognosis. The thick, nodular melanoma (fig. 112), especially when ulcerated is associated with a poor outlook. Malignant melanomas of the hands and feet are more dangerous than at other sites. The outlook is better in the female than in the male though the disease is not influenced by hormone therapy. Pregnancy makes pigmented moles darker and sometimes larger but probably does not affect their course.

Treatment.—The primary lesion is treated by surgical excision since melanoma is relatively radio-resistant. The width of excision depends on the tumour thickness. If this is less than 1 mm (tumour clinically impalpable) a 1 cm margin of healthy skin and sub-cutaneous fat is sufficient. For the tumour which is just palpable, the margin is increased to 2 cm. The frankly nodular melanoma requires wider excision, certainly no less than 3 cm all round and the sub-cutaneous fat should be removed down to but not as a rule including the deep fascia. The surgical defect is closed by primary suture where the extent of excision and laxity of the tissues permits. If not, a free skin graft or pedicled flap are used as appropriate to the local anatomy.

When the clinical diagnosis is in doubt, local excision biopsy with a narrow margin of clearance is done. It is quite safe to wait for the result of paraffin section histology provided definitive operation is not delayed for more than a few days.

N.B. Moles must never be cauterised or curetted because the vital evidence is destroyed and if the lesion is malignant the disease may be disseminated.

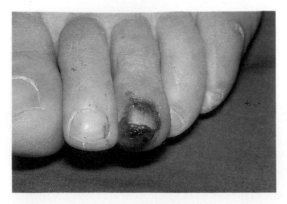

FIG. 113.—Subungual malignant melanoma.

A proven subungual malignant melanoma (fig. 113) requires amputation of the affected digit. The prognosis is poor.

Malignant melanoma may develop in the conjunctiva but unlike that of the skin can sometimes be successfully treated by careful radiotherapy.

Malignant melanomas arising in other mucous membranes, *e.g.* mouth and tongue (Chapter 32) or anal canal are by contrast highly dangerous and seldom curable.

Management of Lymph Nodes.—When the regional nodes are clinically involved they must be radically excised *e.g.* complete and meticulous block dissection of the axilla and, for the groin, dissection not only of the inguinal nodes but also those in relation to the three iliac vessels. When a primary melanoma lies adjacent to an involved lymph node field, *e.g.* on the face or neck, or near the axilla or groin, it is excised in-continuity with the nodes as a mono-block procedure. When it is situated remote from the lymph node area, *e.g.* ankle, the primary tumour and the nodes are dissected as two separate specimens.

When the regional nodes are not clinically involved, a decision must be made whether to dissect them prophylactically or to watch and wait until, in some of the patients, they become enlarged. For the thin primary, the risk of node spread is so slight that a watching policy is justified. For thicker lesions, prophylactic dissection is indicated in patients who cannot be regularly followed up. When, on the other hand, follow-up is reliable it is reasonable to reserve block dissection for those patients whose nodes do subsequently enlarge. With this policy some patients are spared the risk of an unnecessary block dissection (with the risk of post-operative lymphoedema especially for the lower limb) and there is no proof that survival is prejudiced for the remainder.

Other Methods of Treatment.—Cytotoxic agents are only of limited value when the disease is disseminated. They do however help in control of locally advanced disease in the limbs if administered by the specialised technique of isolated perfusion, where high local concentrations of the drug can be produced without generalised side effects. In this way major amputations are often avoided. Immunotherapy has been tried but its value is not yet established.

Hutchinson's melanotic freckle is an irregularly shaped flat pigmented lesion found most commonly in sun damaged skin of the cheek or temple in elderly people. Very occasionally it can appear in other exposed areas *e.g.* the dorsum of the hand. It enlarges slowly over the years and may show spontaneous regression in some areas while extending

Sir Jonathan Hutchinson, 1828–1913. Surgeon. The London Hospital. He described the melanotic freckle in 1892.

in others. Malignant change can occur after periods of the order of ten years or more, and is recognised by the formation of a nodule or nodules. This form of malignant melanoma (lentigo-maligna melanoma) is relatively less aggressive than the others and less frequently metastasises to the regional lymph nodes or systemically. It is treated by excision which does not require such a wide margin of healthy tissue as in the more usual types of the disease.

Malignant melanoma of the choroid usually presents with blurring of vision. It is treated by enucleation of the eye. As this organ has no lymphatic drainage, choroidal melanoma spreads by the blood stream frequently giving rise to visceral deposits which can be enormous especially in the liver. These metastases may not appear clinically for many years after removal of the primary tumour (Chapter 29, fig. 476).

BURNS AND SCALDS

The majority of burns are caused by heat. A scald is a burn, caused by moist heat. Other causes include actinic rays (sunburn), irradiation, chemicals, electricity and friction. A burn is a wound in which there is coagulative necrosis of the tissue. In this respect it will be appreciated that cold (*e.g.*, frostbite) also causes coagulative necrosis and that the word 'coldburn' is not really a contradiction in terms.

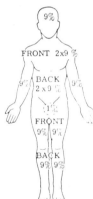

FIG. 114.—The 'Rule of Nines' may be used to estimate the body surface area of adults. By adding together the affected areas the percentage of the total body surface which is burnt can be calculated quickly. This rule does not apply strictly to infants and children. In a child aged 1 the head and neck area is 18% and in a child aged 5 it is 13% of the total body area. A useful *aide memoire* is that the patient's hand size area (one side) is 1%.
(After Wallace.)

Burn shock is contributed to by 1. the overwhelming sudden intensity of pain, but is mostly caused by 2. the loss of circulating blood volume (= hypovolaemia) in the first 24 hours through water, electrolyte and plasma protein loss in blister fluid, exudate, oedema and by evaporation. This is due to vasodilatation and increased capillary permeability of the wound, probably mediated by the liberation of histamine, kinins, prostaglandins and fibrin degradation products. Heat loss from a burned area may be considerable (see Shock, Chapter 5).

THE MANAGEMENT OF A PATIENT WITH BURNS.
A PROGRAMME

Immediate Care and Resuscitation

First Aid Directions.—*Burns and Scalds.*—Remove patient from source of heat and extinguish flames. Apply cold clean water soaks to affected areas and renew these every 3 minutes. *Electrical Burns.*—Switch off electrical supply. If the victim is unconscious exclude the presence of cardiac arrest and if necessary apply cardio-pulmonary resuscitation (Chapter 41). *Chemical Burns.*—Irrigate affected areas with copious amounts of clean water (*except* Phenol burns, where water will accelerate absorption, so polyethylene glycol should be used). With

Alexander Burns Wallace, 1906–1974. Formerly Reader in Plastic Surgery, University of Edinburgh.

acids or alkalis irrigate with water until litmus paper placed on the skin no longer reacts (irrigation may be required for several hours in severe cases).

Transport.—Burn patients must be transported with great care. A secure intravenous line is required for major cases, the burns should be covered with clean sheets and the patient wrapped in warm blankets or foil.

Severity of Injury

The factors that determine the severity of the injury include:

1. **Extent of Body Surface Burnt.**—Burn patients require intravenous resuscitation if their injury exceeds 10% body surface area in children or 15% in adults. Patients with smaller area burns may require intravenous fluid. The 'Rule of Nines' of Wallace (fig. 114) may be used to assess burn area for adults, but it should be noted that the head and neck in a small child is nearly 20% of the body surface area. The patient's own hand area is a useful guide as it equals 1%.

2. **Depth of Burn and Causative Agent.**—Burns are either '*partial*' or '*full thickness*' depending on the depth of skin destruction. Partial thickness burns heal because remnants of epidermis in hair follicles and sweat glands spread over the wound surface. Wounds caused by burning clothing, electricity or molten metal are usually full thickness, whereas flash explosions or scalds in adults are usually partial thickness (fig. 115). Children have delicate skin and minor scalds may be full thickness depending on the agent's temperature and time of contact. Partial thickness injury will usually appear moist, red and blistered, whereas a full thickness burn is usually white or brown, dry and firm to the touch. *The pin prick test* may be used to define full thickness loss (in which the nerve endings are destroyed) though partial thickness burns may also be anaesthetic.

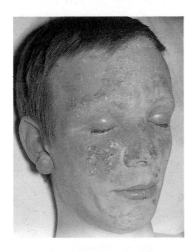

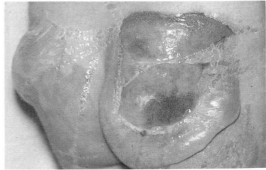

FIG. 116.—Burnt (scald) buttocks in a child, said to have sat down in a bucket of hot water.

FIG. 115.—Flash burn, a firework injury.

3. **Age of the Patient.**—Burns are tolerated poorly by individuals at the extremes of life. Note:—Children's burns may be non-accidental and the clinician must always be satisfied that the explanation of the injury is tenable (fig. 116) (see Battered Child Chapter 15).

4. **Associated Injuries or Illnesses.**—Concurrent illness increases mortality

and the presence of pre-existing renal, cardiovascular or metabolic disorders must be established. Associated fractures should be treated by closed, conservative methods and will increase the fluid requirements.

Respiratory Tract Burns

All patients with suspected respiratory tract burns or smoke inhalation should receive humidified oxygen by mask and regular pulmonary physiotherapy. Crystalloid fluid administration should be restricted to that necessary to maintain hydration and renal function. Patients with oral or nasal burns who develop stridor and respiratory distress may have laryngeal oedema and endotracheal intubation is indicated before total obstruction occurs. Tracheostomy should only be carried out if intubation is impossible or prolonged.

Lower respiratory tract burns cause oedema with bronchospasm. Treatment may include the administration of aminophylline and if bronchospasm is not relieved by bronchodilators alone, steroids are indicated. Severe cases may develop respiratory failure manifest as increasing difficulty in breathing and deteriorating arterial blood gases, in which event mechanical ventilation is indicated.

Immediate General Evaluation and Treatment

Patients should be assessed in a closed warm room and treated as follows:

Emergency Sedation. Patients must be reassured and treated in a quiet confident manner. Full thickness burns are relatively painless due to the destruction of nerve endings. The pain of partial thickness burns may be relieved by cold water compresses and dressings. Opiates may cause vomiting or respiratory depression and therefore should be used with caution in small intravenous doses. Trimeprazine tartrate (Vallergan®) is the sedative of choice for children.

Fluid Replacement Therapy.—Untreated patients can develop hypovolaemic shock because of losses from the burn wound and the formation of inflammatory oedema (Chapter 5). *The volume lost* is proportional to the area of the wound and the *rate of loss* is maximal immediately after burning, diminishing during the first 36 hours. The fluid lost resembles plasma and should be replaced with colloid solutions such as human plasma protein fraction, human albumin 4·5% or a synthetic plasma expander such as Dextran 110 (Chapter 5). A number of formulae exist to calculate the rate of administration, but the requirements must be adjusted according to the particular needs of each patient:

A Practical Guide for Fluid Replacement

Adults.—During the first 24 hours, between 1 and 1·5 litres of colloid will be required for every 10% of body surface burnt. Half of this volume is given in the first 8 hours from the time of burning (not time of admission) and the other half in the next 16 hours. On the second day about half these amounts will be required.

Children.—During the first 24 hours one plasma volume equivalent (40 ml/kg) will be required for every 15% of the body surface burnt. Half of this volume is given in the first 8 hours and the other half in the next 16 hours. On the second day about half these amounts will be required.

Clinical assessment of Progress.—Progress is assessed by examination of the patient's general clinical state with measurement of haematocrit (Chapter 5) and urine output. The clinical examination includes pulse rate, blood pressure, temperature, jugular and peripheral vein filling; and skin perfusion colour and temperature. The haematocrit should approximate to the normal expected value for that patient and the urine output should be 0·5–1ml/kg per hour at any age.

For severe cases it may be necessary to measure the central venous pressure (CVP) (Chapter 5) and continue fluid replacement for longer than 36 hours. Normal metabolic crystalloid requirements should be administered orally or intravenously in addition to the colloid burn fluid replacement.

Early Complications of severe burns include (i) *Acute Renal Failure* (Chapter 57) prevented by early and proper restoration of blood volume and maintenance of fluid balance, (ii) *Gastroduodenal erosion and ulceration* (Curling's ulcers) due to stress (Chapter 44) which can be prevented by prescribing H_2 receptor antagonists (cimetidine, ranitidine).

Initial Burn Wound Care.—The majority of burn wounds require no cleansing but adherent clothing, dirt or foreign material should be removed by gentle rinsing with warm, sterile water. It is not necessary to rupture clean blisters. If a full thickness burn encircles the trunk or limbs escharotomies are required: the dead (anaesthetic) skin should be incised along axial lines to prevent the trapped oedema producing a tourniquet effect and eventual ischaemic contracture or gangrene. This procedure may cause haemorrhage, necessitating blood transfusion.

Tetanus Prophylaxis and the Principles of Antibiotic Therapy.—Tetanus toxoid booster should be given in all cases. Patients with extensive burns should receive a 5-day course of penicillin or erythromycin. Broad spectrum antibiotics should not be given unless there is evidence of systemic infection (Chapter 3). Barrier nursing and laminar flow air help prevent secondary infection.

Nutritional Requirements.—Patients with severe burns occasionally develop paralytic ileus so for the first 12 hours the oral intake should be restricted to 50 ml of water per hour, thereafter the volume may be increased with half strength milk followed by a liquid diet. A nasogastric tube should be passed in severely burnt patients to test initially for gastric ileus, by hourly aspirations, and then to provide a route for additional calories and protein (Chapter 7).

Burn Dressings.—Burn dressings may either be oily based 'tulles', or water-based creams. Tulles may contain agents such as nitrofurazone or chlorhexidine and promote drying of the wound, but tend to adhere and cause pain at dressing changes. Water-based creams are comfortable for the patient but need to contain antibacterial agents such as silver sulphadiazine to reduce the emergence of Gram negative organisms in the wet wound environment. 0·5% silver nitrate compresses, applied once or twice daily, may be used for infected wounds. Synthetic membranes, human amnion, homograft and xenograft may be used on clean superficial wounds but these temporary skins should not be used on deep burns because they may encourage bacterial growth in necrotic tissue (see footnote on p. 151).

Hand Burns.—Burnt hands should be enclosed in polythene bags, elevated and actively exercised to reduce oedema and restore a full range of movement before digital joint capsule contracture has occurred.

Burns of the Face and Scalp.—The majority of facial burns heal spontaneously and should be treated by exposure with daily applications of 1% Povidone Iodine lotion.

Burns of the Eyes and Eyelids.—The eyes should be examined with flourescein for corneal damage as soon as possible (before oedema of the eyelids makes examination difficult); and burnt eyelids skin grafted before significant ectropion has developed.

Cold Injury.—Frost-bite may be associated with hypothermia. If the body core temperature falls below 32°C, the patient should be rewarmed slowly over a period of several hours and cardiac arrythmias controlled with intravenous lignocaine. Oxygen should be administered together with intravenous 5% dextrose prewarmed to 38°C. Areas of frost bite should be thawed with tepid water (at 40°C) and then treated as thermal burns.

Radiation Burns.—Acute radiation injury produces damage to the skin and local tissues resembling thermal burns but differs in that necrosis evolves more slowly and deeply than the initial erythema suggested. Surgery is not indicated until the wound has passed into the subacute stage characterised by the disappearance of the erythema and oedema. Subacute and chronic radiation injury should be treated as the wound appearances indicate with healing by skin grafting or flap cover.

Subsequent Care of the Burn Patient to Achieve Wound Healing

Burn Wound Care and Surgery.—*Dressings.* The majority of burns should be dressed on alternate days for three weeks to allow natural healing of the partial thickness areas. The dressings of superficial wounds may be left undisturbed for several days. *Ketamine anaesthesia* is useful for major burns dressing changes.

Skin grafting.—Full thickness burns heal slowly from the wound edges and significant areas require skin grafting. Excision and grafting may be carried out at an early stage if the patient's general condition is satisfactory, but may be associated with significant haemorrhage. Careful bacteriological monitoring of the wound is carried out prior to grafting to exclude the presence of *Streptococcus pyogenes*, which will destroy skin grafts and should be treated with flucloxacillin or erythromycin.

Skin grafts are taken from areas of normal skin with a freehand knife or mechanical dermatome (fig. 117). The graft thickness should be 15 thousands of an inch in adults and 10 in children. Areas to be grafted are cleaned with saline or aqueous chlorhexidine and residual slough excised with scissors. The grafts should be fenestrated with a scalpel blade or the mesh dermatome (fig. 118) to prevent loss from haematoma. Skin grafts may be laid in place or anchored with sutures or skin staples. The grafts should be dressed with tulle, covered by gauze, wool and elasticated bandages.

The first graft dressing should be carried out on the third post-operative day and then at two or three day intervals until healing is complete. Exposed bone, joints or tendons may require cover with full thickness flaps.

Patients with extensive burns have a limited area for skin graft donor sites. Keratinocytes can be cultured *in-vitro* to provide sheets of epidermis to assist wound healing. Cadaver or donor skin and a variety of synthetic membranes may be used as temporary skin cover. [1]

Nutritional Support.—Patients with burns exceeding 30% require a high protein and calorie diet which is usually administered by a fine bore nasogastric tube

---

[1] Cadaver or donor skin or amnion must not be used without confirmation that the source is HIV (AIDS) negative.

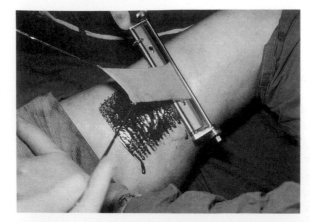

Fig. 117.—Cutting a split skin graft (*P. L. Levick, MS, FRCS, Birmingham*). The graft is taken from normal thigh skin held tense by an assistant (left). (This graft is elevated with skin hooks for demonstration purposes).

Fig. 118.—Full thickness burn wounds covered by mesh grafts (*J. P. Gowar FRCS, Birmingham*). Meshing increases the area of the skin grafts and allows blood and exudate to escape, thus minimising loss from haematoma.

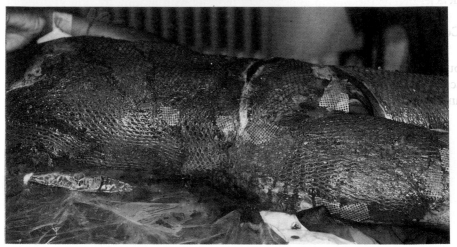

in addition to a normal diet. Milk, sugar and milk based products should be given to the formula of Sutherland:

For adults: Protein: 1 g × kg body weight + 3 g × % burn. Calories: 20 K cal × kg body weight + 70 K cal × % burn; per 24 hours.

For children the calorie and protein intake should equal that which the child normally receives at his age and weight, remembering to make good any deficiencies caused by starvation for anaesthesia.

These additional nutritional requirements are reduced as healing proceeds.

Immunology and Antibiotic Therapy.—Septic complications are the major cause of death in burn patients who are immunodepressed by the effects of the injury. The patient's immune reserves should be reinforced by the intermittent administration of fresh frozen plasma to provide antibodies and opsonins. The patient's haemoglobin level should be maintained by fresh blood transfusions. Small children have immature and inadequate immunity and may develop neutrophil polymorphonuclear leucopenia. This serious complication should be treated by fresh frozen plasma or blood together with an antibiotic if a pathogenic organism is present on the burn wound. Antibiotics should, in general, be used

Paul Lee Levick, Contemporary. Plastic Surgeon, Birmingham Accident Hospital, West Midlands, England.
John Penrose Gowar, Contemporary, Plastic Surgeon, Birmingham Accident Hospital, West Midlands, England.
Anne Sutherland, Contemporary, Plastic Surgeon, Bangour General Hospital, West Lothian, Scotland.

with caution because they may give rise to the emergence of resistant and patho-genic organisms. Burn patients are also susceptible to viral and fungal infections. Isolation and barrier nursing are essential for the most severely burnt cases.

Physiotherapy.—Regular pulmonary physiotherapy is essential for all patients with significant burns who should also be encouraged to exercise their main muscle groups and joints.

Psychological Support.—Burn patients may become severely depressed and require constant encouragement and positive reassurance to prevent them becoming lethargic and anorexic.

Late Complications include (1) *Acute Duodenal Ulcer*, which can become chronic (Chapter 44) (ii) *Protein Losing Enteropathy* causing hypoproteinaemia (oedema and delayed wound healing). (iii) *Chronic Renal Failure*. (iv) *Immune Deficiency* (see above). (v) *Consequences of Chronic Scarring*, e.g. Marjolin's ulcer, deficient temperature regulation.

Continued (Follow-up) Management and Reconstructive Surgery

Patients must be carefully encouraged to return to normal life. Deep areas of burn, whether grafted or not will invariably give rise to severe and permanent scars. These scars termed 'hypertrophic' are particularly troublesome in children and are hard, red, raised, irregular and pruritic (fig. 119 *a*, and see Chapter 1).

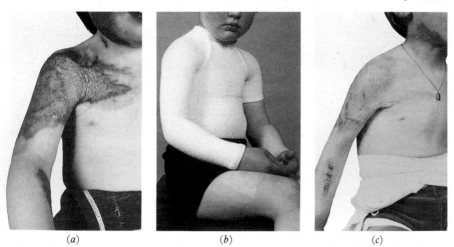

(a)   (b)   (c)

FIG. 119.—The treatment of hypertrophic scars with pressure garments. A typical example of active hypertrophic scarring (*a*) following a full thickness scald from a spilt cup of tea. Pressure garments were worn (*b*) continuously for 14 months and the scar matured with reduced contracture formation (*c*).

The process of maturation, that is, softening, flattening and the return of normal skin colour takes many months or years to completion (Chapter 1). During this period contraction of the scar tissue occurs, particularly over flexion creases. The fitting of pressure garments decreases the time of scar maturation and reduces the extent of contracture formation (fig. 119). These garments are constructed from tight fitting elasticated material and should be worn day and night, with the exception of removal for bathing and anointing of the scarred areas with moisturising cream.

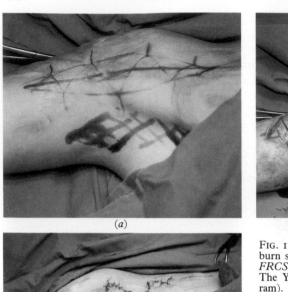

(a)

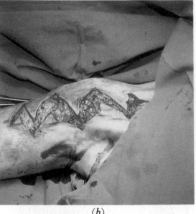

(b)

FIG. 120 (a, b, c).—Methods of releasing burn scar contractures (*P. L. Levick MS FRCS, Birmingham*) Auxillary scarring. The Y-V Plasty (Y → V → V: see diagram). The skin flaps are not undermined (unlike those of the Z plasty) and note that the axillary hair bearing skin remains undisturbed.

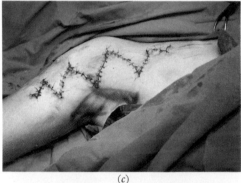

(c)

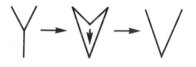

Operations for contractures.—Narrow bands of contracture should be released by the Y-V plasty technique (fig. 120) whereas broad bands are treated by incision and skin grafting (fig. 121). Areas of scar may be removed by the transposition of local or microvascular free flaps. The range of local transposition flaps is increased by 'tissue expanders', consisting of inflatable silastic balloons which are inserted under the normal skin adjacent to the area to be excised. The tissue expander is inflated over a period of several weeks by injections of saline and then removed to allow the expanded skin to be transposed.

SKIN TRANSPLANTATION
(and see Chapter 36)

Partial Thickness (Thiersch) Grafts.—Partial thickness or split skin grafts (fig. 117) contain epidermis and upper capillary dermis and are revascularised by the ingrowth of capillary buds from the underlying tissues. The graft donor areas heal within 10 days as the exposed reticular dermis is covered with new epidermis arising from the linings of the hair follicles, sweat and sebaceous glands.

Full Thickness (Wolfe) Grafts.—Full thickness grafts contain complete dermis and epidermis and have the advantage of natural skin colour in addition to reduced tendency to contraction. Revascularisation by the ingrowth of capillary buds is, however, not always reliable and may take several days, during which period the grafts require careful immobilsation. The donor defect is closed by sutures or a split skin graft.

Karl Thiersch, 1822–1895, Professor of Surgery, Erlangen (1854–1867), Leipzig, Germany. Described his method of skin grafting in 1874.
John Reissberg Wolfe, 1824–1904, Ophthalmic Surgeon. Glasgow, Scotland. Described full-thickness grafts in 1885.

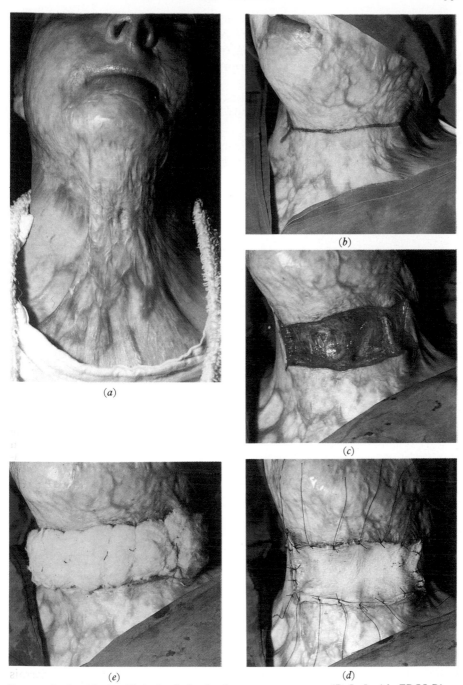

(a)

(b)

(c)

(e)

(d)

FIG. 121 (a, b, c, d, e).—Methods of releasing burn scar contractures (*P. L. Levick, FRCS Birmingham*). The 'fish tail' incision and graft method of releasing broad contractures.

Skin and Muscle Flaps.—Cutaneous flaps may be of random or axial pattern, the latter containing a recognised arteriovenous system. Inclusion of deep fascia into a cutaneous flap (the fascio-cutaneous flap) allows greater extension and mobility because the blood vessels perforating the subcutaneous adipose tissue are not disrupted.

Muscle and Myocutaneous Flaps.—Muscle or muscle including over-lying skin may be transposed as an axial pattern flap and is of particular value in covering bare bone.

Microvascular Free Flaps.—The neurovascular bundle of an axial pattern flap may be anastomosed by microvascular surgery to a donor pedicle in another area of the body.

CHAPTER 11

THE HAND

INFECTIONS OF THE HAND

Infections of the hand are encountered most commonly in manual workers and housewives who frequently suffer small abrasions or pricks in the course of their work. The infective organism is the *Staph. aureus* in 80% of cases, *Strep. pyogenes* and gram-negative bacilli. Unless the infection can be aborted suppuration will follow. The early detection of pus and its accurate localisation are of cardinal importance. Oedema is a common feature (fig. 122). Hand infections are a prime cause of loss of work, and if they are not handled properly are often followed by serious disability.

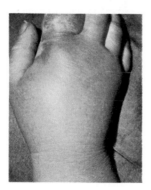

FIG. 122.—Oedema is a common feature in hand infections, being most evident on the dorsum of the hand irrespective of the site of the lesion, and is a potent cause of subsequent stiffness of the digits.
(T. J. McNair, FRCS, Edinburgh.)

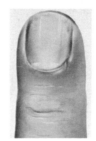

FIG. 123.—Paronychia, due to a 'hangnail'.

Acute Paronychia

Acute paronychia is the most common infection of the hand. The infection, which is subcuticular and under the eponychium, arises from a hangnail (fig. 123), careless nail paring, or an unsterile manicure instrument. Suppuration usually follows, and confined by the adherence of the eponychium to the base of the nail, the pus tends to track around[1] the cutaneous margin and, in 40% of cases, under the nail.

Treatment.—Flucloxacillin given early may abort the infection. If pus has formed it must be let out (see principles of treatment p. 164). *At operation* only the eponychium is stripped gently and completely away from the base of the nail. All pus is wiped away; loose cuticle is cut away, and should there be a pocket under the corner of the nail fold, a wedge of overlying skin is removed to ensure healing from the bottom. The loose and ragged eponychium is then excised with delicate, sharp-pointed scissors. When pus has extended beneath the nail, the undermined portion must be excised with fine-pointed, but strong, scissors. 'Floating' nail is dead nail; consequently all unattached nail must be excised. Only when pus has extended beneath half or more of the width of the nail is excision of the proximal third of the nail required.

---

[1] The colloquial American term for paronychia is 'run around'.

Chronic Paronychia[1].—The history is measured by months, rather than days, and the onset is insidious[2]; seldom does it follow acute paronychia. Today the housewife who does not wear rubber gloves when 'washing-up' is the usual sufferer. Antibiotic therapy has little or no effect, but operative treatment following the lines detailed above is often successful if the infection is a bacterial one. In many cases, however, the infection is due to a monilia or yeast. (Chapter 4). This can be settled by microscopical examination of scrapings and/or special cultures for fungi.

A useful method of treating these indolent infections is by 1:500 Bradosol (domiphen bromide) in spirit, or Penotrane® tincture (hydrargaphen) dropped into the nail-fold twice daily. Nystatin ointment can also be tried. When the pockets become filled with granulations the treatment is discontinued, and the hands must be kept as dry as possible until epithelialisation occurs.

Infection of the terminal pulp space (*syn.* Felon[3])

Pulp space infection is the second most frequent infection of the hand (about 25% of all cases). The index finger and the thumb are affected most often. The origin of the infection is usually a prick.

Surgical Anatomy.—The deep fascia, which is attached to the thin skin of the distal flexion crease, fuses with the periosteum just distal to the insertion of the deep flexor tendon, thereby closing the terminal pulp compartment at its proximal end. Through the space, which is filled with compact fat, feebly partitioned by fibrous septa, run the terminal branches of the digital artery. Thrombo-arteritis of these vessels accounts for the frequency with which osteomyelitis complicates infection of this closed space. The basal plate of the epiphysis is rarely involved (fig. 124).

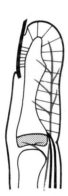

FIG. 124.—Distal pulp space to show how its proximal end is closed by attachment of the deep fascia and by the fibrous septa. The blood supply to the epiphysis does not traverse this area.

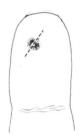

FIG. 125.—Incision for draining a pulp abscess. It is essential to drain the deep loculus of a collar-stud abscess, if such is present.

Clinical Features.—Dull pain, worse when the hand is dependent, and swelling are the first symptoms. Forty-eight hours later there are severe nocturnal exacerbations of throbbing pain, interfering with sleep. Light pressure over the affected pulp increases the pain. Frequently the corresponding regional lymph node is enlarged and tender. If the pulp is indurated and has lost its normal resilience, pus is present. Untreated, the abscess tends to point towards the centre of the pulp beneath a patch of devitalised skin. A collar-stud abscess then occurs; if still untreated, the abscess bursts. Neglected cases suffer serious loss of pulp tissue leading to a desensitised, withered finger tip.

---

[1] Called by some dermatologists (quite descriptively) chronic *perionychia*.
[2] A constant lookout must be kept for the occasional case resulting from neuropathy, *e.g.* syringomyelia.
[3] Felon (Latin, *fel* = gall). An abscess near the nail; also, one who has committed a felony.

Treatment.—In the early stages when there is no localisation large doses of flucloxacillin may bring about resolution. *Once pus is present operation without delay is the rule* (see General Principles, p. 164). A short incision as indicated in fig. 125 is made through the skin at the point of greatest tenderness. The beginner is warned not to be beguiled by entering only the superficial loculus of a collar-stud abscess. Removal of slough, which is frequently present, is most desirable, but great care must be taken not to traumatise the periosteum.

Osteomyelitis of the terminal phalanx may be a sequel of terminal pulp-space infection. That part of the bone bereft of its blood-supply will become a sequestrum and separates some weeks after the abscess has been opened, in which event the wound continues to discharge. Repeated radiographs and probing (revealing rough bone) will indicate when the sequestrum has separated. Only then must it be removed, after which healing will proceed apace. In case of a child, regeneration of the diaphysis is possible, provided the periosteum is relatively undamaged. In the adult no regeneration occurs, and the patient is left with a shortened terminal phalanx covered by an ugly curved nail.

Apical subungual infection arises from a prick (including a splinter) beneath the nail, causing infection of the space between the subungual epithelium and the periosteum (fig. 126(*a*). The lesion (fig. 126(*b*)), which is exquisitely painful, gives rise to comparatively little swelling. Tenderness is greatest just beneath the free edge of the nail, and pus comes to the surface here or beneath the nail.

Operation.—A small V is removed from the centre of the free edge of the nail, and a little wedge of the full thickness of the skin overlying the abscess is excised (fig. 126(*c*)). The amount of pus and debris evacuated is surprisingly small; commonly the abscess cavity extends down to the bone, but osteitis is unusual. Following the operation, relief of symptoms is immediate and the wound heals in about a week.

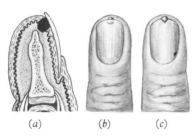

(*a*)   (*b*)   (*c*)

FIG. 126.—(*a*) Showing the anatomical relations of an apical abscess. (*b*) Apical abscess; clinical presentation. (*c*) V-exposure for evacuating the contents of the abscess.

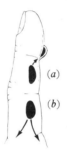

FIG. 127.—Abscess of (*a*) the middle and (*b*) the proximal volar spaces. Showing direction of spread.

Frequently a purulent blister appears in the distal flexion crease (fig. 127). In early cases it is difficult to distinguish infection of the middle volar space from infection of the underlying flexor tendon sheath; however, in the former, extreme tenderness over the proximal end of the tendon sheath is completely lacking, and movement is painful *after* (not *at*) the beginning of flexion movement.

Subcutaneous infections and abscesses can occur on the dorsal and volar surfaces at various levels (fig. 128). The volar surface of the hands of manual

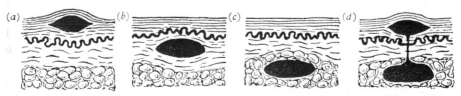

FIG. 128.—Superficial abscesses at various levels. (*a*) Intraepidermal (purulent blister), (*b*) Intradermal, (*c*) Subcutaneous, (*d*) The superficial loculus of a collar-stud abscess.
(After R. S. Pilcher, FRCS, London.)

Robin Sturtevant Pilcher, Contemporary. Emeritus Professor of Surgery, University College Hospital, London.

workers is often covered with greatly thickened epithelium. Especially in such individuals, a subcutaneous abscess may burst through the dermis and extend in the layers of the epidermis (fig. 128 (d)), in which event it is impossible to differentiate it from a purulent blister until the deeper loculus has been discovered at operation.

Treatment.—The abscess is opened. The resulting undermined flaps are cut away with scissors. The unroofed cavity is swabbed free from pus which is examined by culture for the identification of the bacteria and for tests of their sensitivity to various antibiotics. Then it is explored for a sinus leading to a deeper loculus. If such is found, the communicating channel is stretched by inserting and opening the jaws of a small haemostat.

Infections of the Volar and Web Spaces

Infection of the Middle Volar Space of a Digit (fig. 127a).—The fibro-fatty tissue occupying this space is more loosely packed than that of the terminal pulp space. The middle volar space is separated above and below by fibrous partitions while, like the proximal space, it is shut off from the dorsal cellular tissue by fibrous septa extending from the skin to the periosteum.

Clinical Features.—Infection of this space is much less common than that of the terminal pulp space. The finger is held in semi-flexion. In about one-third of cases attempts to straighten it are painful. There is tender induration over the space, while the soft tissues of the terminal and proximal segments, although swollen, are neither tender nor indurated.

Infection of the Proximal Volar Space.—This space is well partitioned from the middle volar space but it communicates freely with the corresponding web spaces (fig. 127b). Once localisation has occurred infection of the proximal volar space is comparatively easy to diagnose, and frequently the swelling is asymmetrical because of concomitant involvement of a web space (see below).

Operation.—After pus has become localised in either of the above spaces, it should be evacuated through a transverse incision made at the site of greatest tenderness. When the diagnosis is uncertain (localised tenosynovitis cannot be excluded) the space should be explored through a lateral longitudinal incision.

Infection of a Web Space.—*Surgical Anatomy.* The web spaces are the three triangular regions between the dorsal and volar skin filled with loose fat that bulges between the divisions of the palmar fascia. The spaces, when filled with pus, straddle the deep transverse ligament; consequently, although most of the pus is volar, the abscess points dorsally.

Aetiology.—The infection arises (1) from a skin crack, (2) from a purulent blister or from beneath a callosity on the forepart of the hand, or (3) via a lumbrical canal from an abscess in a proximal volar space.

Clinical Features.—As the constitutional symptoms are severe, patients with this condition are often seen before localisation of the infection has occurred. At this stage there is oedema of the back of the hand. Although the condition is strongly suspected from the location of the tenderness, a precise diagnosis cannot yet be made. The patient should be in bed with the arm splinted and elevated by suspension. Cloxacillin or tetracycline are given. Once localisation has occurred, the signs of infection of a web space become manifest.

Localising Signs.—The base of one finger is swollen, and in severe cases the fingers immediately adjacent to the space are separated. Often there is a fan-shaped blush extending from the web on to the dorsum and a small area of purplish discoloration of the skin over the affected space. The maximum tenderness is found in the web and on the anterior surface of the base of one of the fingers extending a short way into the palm. Untreated, pus can track across the base of the finger into an adjacent web space, and also along the sides of the proximal segments of the digits related to the infected web.

Operation.—A transverse incision is made on the palmar surface over the affected web space. The incision must be deepened very cautiously until the subcutaneous fat is reached. Only a few strands of palmar fascia need to be divided, and if pus does not flow it is sought with a probe or director. If the diagnosis is correct, probing is soon rewarded by a gush of pus. The opening is enlarged to reveal an abscess cavity, often the size of a thimble. The edges of the wound are cut away, so as to leave a diamond-shaped opening (fig. 129). When the abscess communicates with a dorsal pocket, a counter-incision is advisable. If, as sometimes happens, there is a twin web abscess (one on each side of the digit), each space must be opened, but there is no need to slit the communicating channel.

Deep Palmar Abscess

An abscess beneath the palmar fascia is a serious, but rare (about 1%), infection of the hand.

Aetiology.—The infection can arise as (1) a penetrating wound; (2) infection via the blood-stream of a haematoma in this situation; (3) as a complication of suppurative tenosynovitis.

Clinical Features.—As a rule the patient is a manual worker. At an early stage there is intense throbbing pain in, and deep tenderness of, the palm of the hand. Almost from the commencement this is accompanied by obvious oedematous swelling of the dorsum of the hand, which increases rapidly to become greater than that seen in any other infected lesion of the hand—so great as to give rise to what is known as 'the frog hand' (fig. 122). The fingers are held in a flexed position because the palmar fascia is more relaxed in this posture. Extension of the metacarpophalangeal joints is very painful, but extension of the interphalangeal joints is both painless and free. This is a most valuable observation in distinguishing the condition from suppurative tenosynovitis. The overlying skin temperature is raised, and regional lymphadenitis is commonly present.

As tension mounts, the normal concavity of the palm becomes flattened; a time is reached when the imprisoned pus erodes and bursts through the palmar fascia, then suddenly the intense pain passes off, but the palm becomes slightly convex. If the patient is seen for the first time after this happening, there is no means of distinguishing a deep palmar abscess with a collar-stud extension from an abscess of a subaponeurotic space, except by operation.

Operation.—Under a general anaesthesia (or regional block of the median and ulnar nerves at the wrist), a central transverse incision is made in the line of the flexion crease passing across the middle of the palm. Should pus be encountered beneath the aponeurosis, the floor of the abscess (the palmar fascia) must be probed systematically for a sinus leading to the deeper plane. In other circumstances the palmar fascia is divided *in a longitudinal direction* (to avoid digital nerves and blood-vessels). Pus is mopped up. Continued free drainage is ensured by trimming, with scissors, the skin edges as well as those of the incision in the palmar fascia. This obviates premature healing, which otherwise is prone to occur.

Lymphangitis in Hand Infections.—Organisms, nearly always streptococci, gain entrance through an abrasion that may be microscopic. Within a few hours

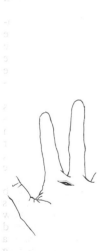

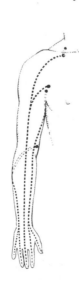

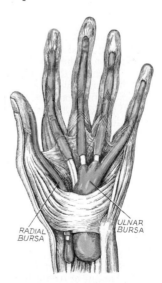

FIG. 129. — Incision for draining a web-space abscess.

FIG. 130.—The main lymphatic trunks of the forearm and arm.
(After Kanavel and Mason.)

FIG. 131.—The flexor tendon sheaths. This typical arrangement is present in 75% of cases.

RADIAL BURSA

ULNAR BURSA

Allen Bucknell Kanavel, 1874–1938. Professor of Surgery, North Western University, Chicago, Illinois, U.S.A. The fascial spaces were described in his book 'Infections of the Hand' published in 1933.

the adjacent portion of the hand becomes swollen and painful, and there is often considerable elevation of the temperature. Because superficial lymphatic vessels pursue the shortest course to the dorsum, oedema appears early and on the back of the hand (fig. 122). Red streaks, so characteristic of lymphangitis (fig. 67), are seen coursing up the arm. In lesions of the ulnar half of the hand, the first lymph node to become enlarged and tender is the epitrochlear. Where infection enters the middle finger, the first lymph node to become swollen may be *above* the clavicle (fig. 130), in which case infection is liable to enter the general circulation and give rise to septicaemia. The lymphatics of the thumb and index finger pass straight to the axillary nodes. Lymphangitis can also occur (*a*) without any other demonstrable manifestation of inflammation, or (*b*) as an accompaniment of terminal pulp-space infection and fulminating tenosynovitis. Lymphangitis responds well to the measures described in Chapter 9.

Acute Suppurative Tenosynovitis

Infection of the sheath of a flexor tendon is due to bacteria introduced by the point of a needle or other sharp object penetrating the tendon sheath. Exceptionally the sheath is infected by extension from its terminal pulp space, in some cases from the scalpel transgressing the hallowed ground of the septum that closes the proximal end of the space (fig. 124).

Acute fulminating tenosynovitis involves the whole sheath rapidly, and nearly always the infecting organism is the *staphylococcus aureus* or the *streptococcus pyogenes*. The classical local signs are:

　　1. Symmetrical swelling of the entire finger.

　　2. Flexion of the finger (the 'hook' sign) with exquisite pain on extension.

　　3. Tenderness over the sheath, especially over its proximal *cul-de-sac* (fig. 131).

Localised suppurative tenosynovitis.—Swelling and tenderness are limited to one portion of the digit, rendering confident diagnosis prior to exploration difficult.

Infection of the ulnar bursa (fig. 131) is characterised by:
　　1. Oedema of the whole hand, especially the dorsum, due to lymphatic spread.
　　2. Moderate swelling of the palm.
　　3. Sometimes a fullness immediately above the flexor retinaculum.
　　4. The flexed fingers resist extension, the maxmimum difficulty being experienced in the little, and the least in the index finger.
　　5. Especially valuable is Kanavel's sign: the area of greatest tenderness is over that part of the ulnar bursa lying between the transverse palmar creases (fig. 132).

It should be noted that the ulnar and radial bursae intercommunicate in 80% of cases, and often when an untreated infection of one has persisted for more than forty-eight hours, the other becomes involved also. In no less than 25% of cases the tendon sheath of the index, or the middle, or the ring finger communicates with the ulnar bursa, which is a fact of great surgical importance.

Infection of the radial bursa (fig. 131) is distinguished by:
　　1. The distal phalanx of the thumb is held in flexion, with rigidity and inextensibility of the interphalangeal joint. The other digits can be extended fully.
　　2. Tenderness over the sheath of the flexor pollicis longus.
　　3. Sometimes swelling just above the flexor retinaculum.

Treatment of Acute Infected Tenosynovitis.—Full doses of flucloxacillin are given. The forearm and hand, the latter being placed in the position of rest, are splinted and elevated. Clinical re-examination is made every six hours. Non-operative treatment is continued only so long as there is a good local and general response. Delay in decompressing an unresponding infection may result in sloughing of the tendon.

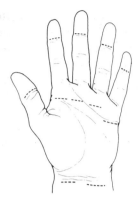

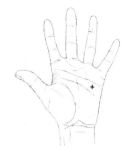

FIG. 132.—Kanavel's sign.

FIG. 133.—Sites of incision
for treating acute suppurative   tenosynovitis.   The
sheath is also exposed at the
site of the initial trauma
when such is discernible.

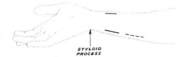

FIG. 134.—Incisions for draining the
space of Parona.

Operation.—When the site of puncture of the integument is visible, or has been indicated without hesitation by the patient, the first incision is made in a transverse direction
directly over the tendon sheath. When there is no certain information as to where the
sheath was punctured, the more distal of the two relevant incisions shown in fig. 133 is
made and deepened until the fibrous portion of the sheath is displayed. This is divided
and the thin, bulging theca comes into view. Some of the fluid within it is aspirated and
sent for bacteriological examination; the theca is then incised in a transverse direction and
its edges are pared so as to form a diamond-shaped opening. Pressure is now exerted over
that portion of the sheath proximal to the incision, and if this results in a gush of hazy
exudate, a second relevant incision (over the cul-de-sac) is made and similar steps to
prevent premature closure of the wound are taken. Employing a fine catheter, the length
of the sheath is irrigated with a solution of antibiotic, which must be water-soluble and
non-irritant.

Complications of Suppurative Tenosynovitis

Involvement of the Forearm from the Hand.—When a radial or ulnar bursa distended
with pus bursts, pus travels up the forearm between the flexor profundus ventrally and
the pronator quadratus and interosseous membrane dorsally. It is here, in the space of
Parona, that a quantity of pus can collect without giving rise to much swelling. There is,
however, brawny induration above the wrist, unless the original lesion has been incised
and continues to discharge pus. Therefore, in cases of infection of the radial or ulnar
bursa, if pus can be expressed by pressure over the wrist at the time of operation or
subsequently, it is essential that the forearm be drained by making the incisions shown
in fig. 134 and deepening them until the periosteum is reached. A haemostat is then thrust
beneath the flexor tendons, and the jaws of the forceps are opened, as a result of which
the proximal extremity of the infected bursa (or bursae) is ruptured thoroughly into the
space beneath the flexor tendons, which is then drained by a small corrugated drain.

Continuation of Suppuration.—Provided the principles set out above concerning early
decompression of infected tendon sheaths have been followed, continued suppuration is
rare. If it occurs, the first point to consider in most situations is the possibility of extension
of the infection to a fascial space or another tendon sheath. Should suppuration continue
for fourteen days, the hand should be radiographed for evidence of bone necrosis. In
relevant cases, the possibility of a non-opaque retained foreign body should also be borne
in mind. Sloughing tendon is a potent source of prolonged suppuration and much time
will be saved by excising the diseased portion, care being taken to anchor its proximal end
by sutures to prevent the cut end being carried into the forearm by muscular contraction,
and thereby spreading infection.

Francesco Parona, 1861–1910. Surgeon, Ospedàle Maggiore Novara and at Milan, Italy.

Suppurative arthritis in a related joint occurs occasionally as a complication of suppurative tenosynovitis. In these circumstances timely amputation of any digit except the thumb will reduce the period of disability (S. Bunnell).

A Stiff Digit Results.—In the case of a finger, it should be remembered that in many walks of life total amputation of a digit is less of a handicap than a stiff finger, but amputation should seldom be undertaken until the infection has subsided completely. In the case of a thumb, the surgeon's watchword for infection as well as trauma is always 'Save all possible'.

Paralysis of the Median Nerve.—When signs of median nerve palsy develop in a case of infection of the hand, early decompression of the carpal tunnel by severing the flexor retinaculum is recommended (D. Bailey). In these circumstances, involvement of the median nerve is due to compression of the nerve by the distended radial or the ulnar bursa, or (more frequently) by both bursae, which of course must be drained thoroughly at the same time.

GENERAL PRINCIPLES OF TREATMENT IN ALL CASES OF INFECTIONS OF THE HAND

The five principles in the treatment of infections of the hand can be summarised as follows:

    (i) Antibiotic therapy (Chapter 3).
    (ii) Provision of rest and elevation to the affected limb.
    (iii) Early recognition of the presence of pus and its accurate localisation.
    (iv) Evacuation of pus and, in the case of fascial spaces, debridement of the walls of the abscess cavity.
    (v) Adequate after-treatment.

To consider these principles in more detail:

Antibiotic Therapy.—Antibiotic therapy is given without delay. Because in over 90% of cases of infections of the hand the original infection is caused by staphylococci, streptococci and gram-negative organisms, flucloxacillin and tetracyline are the antibiotics of choice but the final choice of antibiotic depends upon the sensitivity tests. It is futile, damaging, and often disastrous to rely on antibiotics when suppuration has occurred. *If there is pus in any part of the hand it must be evacuated.*

Rest and Elevation of the Hand.—If it is considered possible that resolution will occur, and also following operation, the hand must be placed in the position of rest (fig. 135). When it is anticipated that in all probability some portion of the hand will become stiff, as soon as the ultra-acute stage has passed the digits should be arranged in the position of function (fig. 136). For ambulatory patients a light plaster-of-Paris slab, moulded to fit the volar surface of the hand and forearm, cannot be bettered. In addition, the forearm is supported in a sling as high as possible towards the opposite shoulder, in order to lessen oedema. For in-patients a Cramer wire splint, which is readily suspended, is both efficient and comfortable. Full elevation decreases oedema and lessens the throbbing pain.

These remarks concerning elevation do not apply to cases of uncomplicated paronychia and minor superficial abscesses; for these an ordinary sling is all that is required.

In all cases rest for an inflamed hand should be insisted upon. When the acute phase has abated, gentle voluntary movements are encouraged.

Anaesthesia.—For the distal part of the finger regional anaesthesia is employed, using 2% procaine or xylocaine (*without adrenaline*, as vaso-constriction and gangrene can occur (fig. 137)). After raising a weal, the hypodermic needle is introduced at the relevant dual

Sterling Bunnell, 1882–1957. Consultant in Hand Surgery to the Surgeon-General of the United States Army and to the United States, Navy.
David Alan Bailey, Contemporary. Surgeon, University College Hospital, London.
Friedrich Cramer, 1847–1903. Surgeon, St. Joseph's Hospital, Würzburg, Germany.

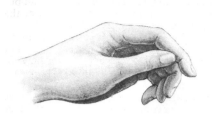

FIG. 135.—The position of rest taken up by an acutely inflamed hand. The index finger is not flexed as much as the others.

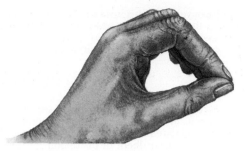

FIG. 136.—The position of function.

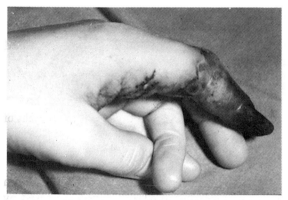

FIG. 137.—Gangrene of index finger after use of adrenaline in the injection of local anaesthetic.

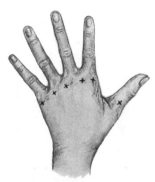

FIG. 138.—Points of puncture for anaesthetising a digit.

points shown in fig. 138. While injecting the anaesthetic solution the needle is advanced distally and forward until it is judged that the digital nerve has been reached; 0·75 ml of the anaesthetic solution is deposited here. The procedure is repeated on the contralateral aspect of the affected finger. In the case of an abscess of the hand itself, a general anaesthetic is administered, or a regional block of the median and ulnar nerves at the wrist is undertaken. On no account should a short general anaesthetic, e.g. nitrous oxide gas, be employed. Complete muscular relaxation and ample time are most desirable when operating in this area.

A bloodless field is essential. Only in the absence of bleeding can the exact site and extent of the lesion be determined and damage to tendon sheaths and nerves be avoided. The cuff of a sphygmomanometer is applied to the upper arm. The limb is then elevated for two minutes, after which the bag is inflated to a pressure of 40 mm Hg (5·3 kPa) above the systolic blood-pressure.

Operation is undertaken at a time when there is a high antibiotic level in the blood. With the exception of tendon-sheath infection, it is insufficient merely to evacuate the pus. The operation must be meticulous. Slough is removed unless it is densely adherent and, what is extremely important, granulations are abraded by gauze or scooped away with a curette, avoiding the latter in situations where it might damage the periosteum or a tendon sheath. Only after granulation tissue has been removed, leaving the walls clean and oozing blood, will the injected antibiotic from the blood enter the cavity freely. Provided every nook and cranny has been attended to in this manner, no drainage material is employed, for no further pus is expected to form; merely a little serum, at first containing blood and dead bacteria is all that oozes from a cavity thus treated. This lessens in amount about the third day, when quick healing is to be expected.

After-treatment of Serious Infections of the Hand.—In all cases dry dressings are employed. The dressings are changed at the end of twenty-four hours after operation. Thereafter often an interval of two days can elapse between re-dressings. The patient must be instructed not to get the dressings wet. These instructions differ only in the case of paronychia; in this instance the patient is instructed to wash the hands frequently, dry them thoroughly on a towel kept for the purpose, and reapply the dressing himself. Physiotherapy and exercises form an important part of the late after-treatment. In rare cases with persisting deformity, rehabilitation for a new job may be necessary.

OTHER INFECTIONS

Human Bites.—Because the wound becomes contaminated with so many types of bacteria (including Vincent's organisms from the mouth), a human bite can prove very dangerous to life or limb. Although not strictly a bite, a common type of injury of this kind is an incised wound over the knuckles resulting from a clenched fist of one combatant striking the front teeth of his opponent. The joint is usually penetrated, but the track closes when the fingers are extended. In such a case the wound must be excised and, if the capsule has been penetrated, a portion of the capsule must be included in the debridement. Because of heavy contamination, primary closure of the wound resulting from excision of a human bite is inadvisable (see Chapter 1).

Madura Mycosis (fig. 139) due to infection with Nocardia Madura is similar to Madura foot (see Chapter 12 for an account of this condition).

Orf (Contagious Pustular Dermatitis) is a parapox virus infection of the hands, transmitted in the saliva of sheep, running a self-limited course (3–6 weeks), the red papules becoming nodules of reddish blue turning grey. *Milker's nodes* is a similar condition transmitted by handling cow's udders. Treatment is conservative, but lymphangitis (pp. 118, 161) can occur.

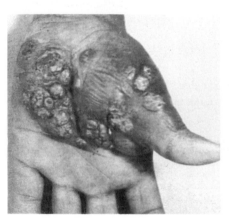

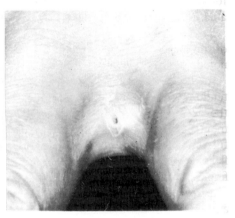

FIG. 139.—Madura Mycosis (Mycetoma) affecting the palm.
(*Prof. Dr C. Kalidas, MS, FICS, Madura Medical College, India.*)

FIG. 140.—Interdigital pilonidal sinus in a barber.

Barber's Pilonidal Sinus.—Hair clippings have a bevelled extremity like the point of a hypodermic needle. Barber's pilonidal sinus is due to the customers' clippings penetrating the skin, most frequently the web between digits 3 and 4 of the left hand. In the uninflamed state the lesion is marked by a small black dot with a collarette of epithelial scales around it; a cyst-like nodule can be palpated beneath the visible lesion. Recurrent attacks of subacute or acute inflammation (fig. 140) in the sinus cause the patient to seek relief by excision. (For the common variety of pilonidal sinus see Chapter 54).

HAND INJURIES

Classification (Based on Rank and Wakefield)

1. *Tidy Injuries.*—These are due to sharp agents, *e.g.* glass, knives, *etc.* The cuts are clean and incised. Tendons, nerves and blood-vessels (bone seldom) may be involved. These injuries must receive the correct primary treatment.

Sir Benjamin Keith Rank, Contemporary. Plastic Surgeon, Royal Melbourne Hospital, Melbourne, Australia.
Allan Ross Wakefield, Contemporary. Plastic Surgeon, Royal Children's Hospital, Melbourne, Australia.

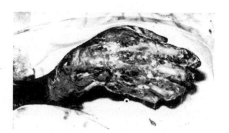

FIG. 141.—Indeterminable injury of the hand. It is impossible to know early on the full extent of the injury. One must wait to see what remains viable. During the observation stage, elevation of the arm and antibiotic cover are vital. It may be necessary to wait up to 3 weeks before proceeding with excision of dead tissue and repair.
(*E. Melmed, FRCS, Dallas.*)

2. *Untidy Injuries.*—The skin is often ragged and there may be multiple fractures. It is essential to get correct skin closure after excision of all the devitalised tissues, by suture, grafting or a flap. Primary repair of nerves and tendons in these injuries is *not* advisable.

3. *Indeterminable Injuries*, for example the severe crush or burn (fig. 141).

Evaluation of the Injury.—Careful examination of the injured hand is essential in order to ascertain the extent of injury of the following:

1. *Nerves.*—The patient may be in too much pain and may be too apprehensive for accurate sensory testing. Motor testing may be impossible because of associated injuries to tendons or bones.

2. *Arteries.*—Arterial damage is suspected by profuse haemorrhage. The state of the blood-supply to a finger distal to a laceration should always be carefully noted.

3. *Tendons and their Sheaths.*—Tendon sheaths may be lacerated without the tendon that they contain being involved. This injury can only be detected when the laceration is explored. Division of a tendon will result in lack of active movement whilst the appropriate passive movement remains possible although painful. The tendon may be visible in the wound. Isolated division of the superficial flexor tendons may be difficult to detect clinically, since flexion of the involved fingers will appear to be normal on casual examination.

4. *Bones.*—The presence of a bony injury can usually be detected clinically and can always be detected radiologically.

5. *Joints.*—Injuries to joints may be clinically obvious, or may only be detected when the wound is explored.

Treatment, in order of importance at this time, is as follows:

1. *Repair of skin.*—Skin cover is *vital* as raw areas predispose to infection and fibrosis. Fibrosis is the big enemy of hand surgery. 2. *Treatment of bone and joint injuries.* 3. *Repair of nerves.* 4. *Repair of tendons.*

Principles of Technique.—*Tourniquet.*—The use of a tourniquet in hand surgery is essential.[1] The maximum safe time for a tourniquet is 1·5 hours. Strict recording of the time of application, plus constant reminders to the surgeon of the progress of time (15 min intervals) will avoid the risk of too long application. In finger surgery, rubber tubing can be tied around the base of the finger to give an adequate bloodless field (and see Chapter 5).

Anaesthetic.—The type of anaesthesia varies with the type of injury and the general condition of the patient. If a tourniquet is used, it is often more comfortable for the patient to be under a general anaesthetic. Adequate sedation is usually necessary for a good brachial plexus or local block. Local blocks, or intravenous anaesthesia, with a tourniquet

---

[1] Bunnell said, 'Can a jeweller repair a watch in a pool of ink?'

are very useful. Adrenaline in a local anaesthetic in finger surgery is strictly contraindicated (fig. 137).

Careful Wound Toilet.—The skin, the fingernails and the wound must be thoroughly
cleansed. Any of the accepted antiseptics is adequate, *e.g.* Hibitane®. It is very important
to get rid of all the debris.

Excision (Chapter 1).—All devitalised tissue must be excised in untidy injuries.

Haemostasis is essential. In an emergency, direct pressure applied over the bleeding area
will stop haemorrhage (Chapter 5). *Not* in any circumstances should the operator grab at
bleeding points with artery forceps. After release of the tourniquet, all bleeding points
are ligated.

Antibiotics and Antitetanus Toxoid are administered routinely (Chapter 1 and 3).

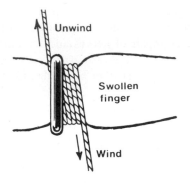

FIG. 142.—Stuck finger. The string method
for removing a ring.
(F. Exner and the 'Medical Tribune'.)

Stuck Finger. This emergency is common in children who poke fingers into small holes,
but it is also encountered when wedding and other rings require to be removed (*e.g.* for
operations). Soap or some fat may ease the ring. The string method is nearly always
successful and should be tried before resorting to saws (Exner).

REPARATIVE SURGERY

Skin Loss

Finger-tip Injuries.—On the thumb and index finger, a tender scar is a nuisance and
good sensation is essential for fine movements. In judging what operation is best suited
to his finger-tip loss, much will depend on the use to which a patient will put his hands,
e.g. a miner whose bread winning depends on early return to work which does not require
exquisite finger-tip sensation, will not appreciate the most successful delicate grafting
which may take him off work for several weeks.

(1) If skin only is lost, then a free split-thickness graft is all that is needed. With time
this may contract and hardly be noticeable.

(2) When the pulp is lost, as well as the skin, then a Wolfe graft may be needed. The
donor site is usually skin from the forearm.

(3) In 'Guillotine' injuries, with loss of pulp and bone, one must take into account the
type of work of the patient:

(*a*) Free grafting will preserve length, but the graft may adhere to bone and may remain
tender. In children the graft may contract with time and not need any further treatment
though a flap graft can always be applied at a later date.

(*b*) Repair by flap gives the best results especially for clean cut thumb and index losses.
It cannot be used in older people due to stiffness, and in children it may result in an
unsightly donor area. The Kutler repair involves the advancement over the cut end of
two lateral triangles (bases distal) of skin and subcutaneous tissues retaining an intact
neurovascular connection, a **V—Y** plasty.

(*c*) The principle of sacrificing length for primary closure, by cutting back until the
flaps will close, is only employed when it is imperative to get the patient back to work
early.

Skin Loss without Involvement or Exposure of the Deeper Structures.—On the
dorsum of the hand a split thickness (Thiersch) graft is the method of choice, due to the
simplicity and speed. These grafts are unlikely to contract as the pull of the strong flexors

William Kutler, 1903–1968. Surgeon, Polyclinic, Cleveland, Ohio, U.S.A. Described this method of repairing amputated fingers in 1944.
Frederick Blythe Exner, Contemporary. Radiologist, Seattle, Washington, U.S.A.

of the fingers overcomes this tendency. On the *palm*, a split thickness graft will contract, and thus it is necessary to use a thicker skin, *viz.* a full thickness (Wolfe) graft (Chapter 10), remembering that its viability is precarious, and thus haemostasis is essential, and adequate fixation and immobilisation vital to success.

Skin Loss with Exposure of Deeper Tissues.—Split thickness grafts will not take on the following—bare bone (devoid of periosteum), bare cartilage, or bare tendon (devoid of paratenon), and necessitates the choice between the following: (*a*) *Local Flaps: e.g.* cross finger flaps. These are extremely valuable in covering bare flexor tendon in the finger. Flaps of the dorsum and the palm are very difficult as the blood supply can easily be misjudged and necrosis will follow.

(*b*) *Distant Pedicle Flaps and transplanted flaps.* These are reserved for severe injuries.

Tendon Injuries

Timing of Tendon Surgery.—Tidy injuries may be dealt with immediately. In untidy and indeterminable injuries repair is delayed until the wound has healed.

Extensor Tendons.—Primary suture usually gives good results as these tendons are highly elastic and vascular and have a good paratenon. Moreover, the tendons act on the metacarpo-phalangeal joint and have a short movement. (The interphalangeal joints are extended by the interossei and lumbricals.)

Flexor Tendons.—(*a*) *Palm and Wrist:* Simple suture of lacerated tendons give good results as there is abundant areolar tissue which prevents adhesions. When multiple tendons are severed, it is advisable to suture only the profundus tendons.

(*b*) *Divided profundus distal to the proximal interphalangeal joint;* Simple suture is the method of choice.

(*c*) *Tendon injury between the distal palmar crease and the proximal interphalangeal joint* (the 'danger area' for tendon division): The correct procedure to be adopted is the subject of diverse surgical opinion and only an outline is given here.

(i) When both tendons are divided, most surgeons advocate excision of the sublimis tendon. Simple suture of the profundus is not favoured due to adhesion formation at the injury site with poor functional results. Most authorities advocate tendon grafting as a primary procedure.

(ii) When profundus only is divided, it may be advisable to do nothing (depending on the demand on the digit). Excision of the sublimis and primary grafting has been disappointing and it does not appear to warrant sacrifice of sublimis action. However, excision of half of the sublimis tunnel allowing primary grafting through the other half of the tunnel (Harrison) may prove to be the procedure of choice.

Thumb.—The tendon can either be sutured or grafted (if primary suture is not possible). Either way, the results are found to be adequate by most patients.

Nerve Injuries (Chapter 28).—In tidy injuries primary suture is preferable. Digital nerves, easily identified at the initial operation, may be impossible to find at a secondary procedure.

Microsurgery in Hand, and Foot, Injuries.—The value of the operating microscope and microsurgical technique in the restoration of severed digits, hands and feet speaks for itself in fig. 143.

Post-operative Care

Elevation and Prevention of Stiffness.—Oedema occurs immediately following injury (and operation). Elevation is thus essential. During the phase of elevation, immobilisation is important as movement may lead to further hyperaemia, *etc.*, with further oedema. This phase lasts 2–4 days. Immobilisation should continue until the wound is healed, *i.e.* up to 21 days with untidy or indeterminable injuries. *The aim is for early healing, not for early movement.* When bandages are removed some residual swelling is usually present which causes pain on movement. Active movement must be encouraged, however. After severe injuries the hand will need additional intensive physiotherapy, *i.e.* active exercises, combined with warmth and elevation.

Stewart Hamilton Harrison, Contemporary. Plastic Surgeon, Mount Vernon Hospital, Northwood, Middlesex, England.

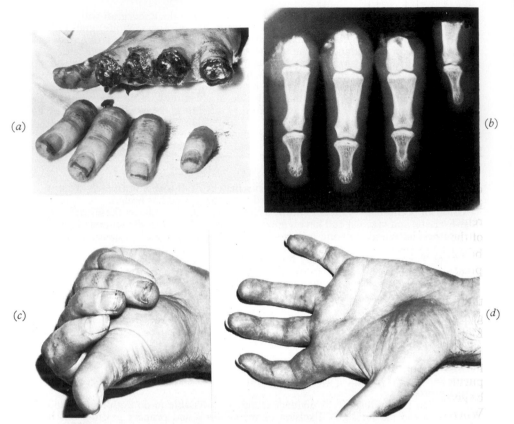

FIG. 143.—**Microsurgery** (*a*) Saw-cut amputations of 4 fingers in a young man. (*b*) x-ray of digits amputated through proximal phalanges. (*c*) Successful replantation of fingers with primary reconstruction after 1 year. (*d*) Flexion of replanted fingers of same patient at 3 years.

The severed fingers require continued cooling—*not freezing*—until vascular continuity is restored. Two operating teams are employed.

(*B. McC. O'Brien, FRCS, Melbourne, Australia.*)

Position of Splinting.—This is very important. The hand must be splinted with the metacarpo-phalangeal joints in 80° flexion, and the interphalangeal joints fully extended. This is the position in which the collateral ligaments are fully stretched and thus, should fibrosis and stiffness occur, it will be maximum in that position and on restarting active movement, it should then be possible to regain a range of full movement.

CHAPTER 12

THE FOOT

Infections of the Foot

Especially in countries where some of the inhabitants go barefooted, infections of the foot are commonplace; they also occur in the shod. In each and all of the infections of the foot about to be described it will be assumed that the reader, remembering the lymphatic drainage of the foot, will examine the lymph nodes of the groin and, in relevant cases, those of the popliteal space. The urine must be examined for sugar. It must also be remembered that arterial disease may present as an infection of the foot.

The prelude to the treatment of any of these infections is thorough washing of the foot with soap and water or, preferably, a detergent, applied with sterile gauze or cottonwool. Except in trivial infections, bed-rest with elevation of the foot must be insisted upon until the inflammation has subsided.

Infected blister is one of the most common infections of the foot. When the patient's temperature is normal and the content of the blister appears doubtfully purulent, the blister can be aspirated. If the fluid is opalescent, the patient should be given flucloxacillin and the aspirated fluid sent for bacteriological examination. When a blister is frankly purulent it should be incised.

Ingrowing Toe-Nail.—Ingrowing toe-nail (*syn.* embedded toe-nail) of the big toe, usually results from encasing sweaty feet in tight shoes, and is encouraged by cutting the nail short and convexly. The side of the nail curls inwards and grows to form a lateral spike, which causes a painful infection of the overhanging nail fold (fig. 144).

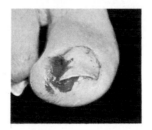

FIG. 144.—Typical ingrowing toe-nail. Conservative measures *can* be successful, depending upon the patient's willingness to help himself. The overhanging nail fold is pushed away by daily packing of the groove with a wisp of gauze soaked in mild antiseptic. The centre plate of the nail is thinned slightly by filing; this encourages the nail to become flat. The end of the nail is cut straight across or concavely. The corners must not be cut back; it is necessary for them to extend over the pulp.

Operation.[1]—The nail is like a letter protruding from a shallow envelope. The envelope is the germinal matrix and this must be included in radical removal of the affected side or the whole of the nail. Failure to remove the corners of the germinal envelope will result in the recurrence of a nail spike. The technique (Fowler) is portrayed in fig. 145. A tourniquet is essential in order that the

---

[1] Described originally by Quenu in 1887, and again by Zadik in 1950.

Alan William Fowler, Contemporary. Consultant Orthopaedic Surgeon, Mid-Glamorgan Area, Wales.
Edouard Quenu, 1852–1933. Surgeon, Paris.
Frank Raphael Zadik, Contemporary. Orthopaedic Surgeon, Sheffield.

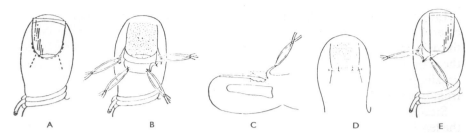

FIG. 145.—Technique of total excision of the germinal matrix. A, Skin incisions. B, Skin-flaps dissected and retracted. The epithelial layer on the deep surface of the flaps is left attached to the matrix. C, Longitudinal section showing the block of tissue to be removed. D, Skin-flaps sutured to cover the raw area. E, Segmental excision of the germinal matrix. The skin-flaps have been raised preparatory to excision of a segment of the germinal matrix.

(Courtesy British Journal of Surgery.)

germinal matrix may be seen and dissected out in its entirety. Minor degrees without chronic infection can be handled conservatively

Onychogryphosis is a thickened and crooked overgrowth of a toe-nail, usually that of the big toe. Trauma and fungus infection are implicated as causes. It occurs in elderly people, especially if bed-ridden, and it may become so curled as to resemble a ram's horn. A Gigli saw will cut through the base and the remainder can be controlled by filing. If necessary the nailbed and nail are removed as above.

Paronychia of the great toe is also common. It often occurs as a complication of an ingrowing toe-nail. An abrasion of the eponychium with contaminated scissors is also a frequent cause. The clinical features and treatment do not differ from those of a paronychia in a finger or thumb, except that when an ingrowing toe-nail is present it is necessary to deal with it radically. Washing, as described above, is carried out each time the wound is dressed.

Infected adventitious bursa (*a*) *beneath a corn* is usually the result of improper chiropody. There are signs of inflammation around the corn, the slightest pressure on which evokes excruciating pain. Drainage is accomplished by paring the corn with a sterile scalpel until pus exudes: (*b*) *over a hallux valgus* (p. 177).

Terminal pulp space infection is rare as compared with that of the hand (Chapter 11). When it occurs in the foot, usually it is the great toe that is affected.

Infection of a Web Space.—The web spaces of the foot are four in number, the space between the great toe and the second toe being the largest. The clinical features of infection of this space are similar to those of the hand, but extension from the plantar to the dorsal aspect of the web occurs earlier, and with great regularity. The treatment also is similar. In a diabetic, orthodox drainage is so disappointing that disarticulation of the relative toe, leaving the flaps unsutured, is recommended (Chapter 14).

Infection of a Plantar Interdigital Subcutaneous Space.—There are four interdigital subcutaneous spaces that lie between the five digital slips of the central aponeurosis. Infection of one of these spaces is very common among coolies who work barefooted, especially in urban areas. As a rule the patient states that a sharp stone, a nail, or a thorn penetrated the sole. The patient complains of increasing pain between the shafts of the two metatarsals that bound the infected space. Soon he is unable to walk, and the constitutional symptoms are moderately severe. Exquisite tenderness located over the infected space proclaims the diagnosis. When pus decompresses itself between the two bones into the dorsal subcutaneous space, localisation is more difficult. Drainage must be placed well away from the weight-bearing area, and consequently an incision similar to that used for drainage of a web space is advised, after which a haemostat is directed into the cavity filled with pus, and its jaws are opened. If the dorsal subcutaneous space is involved, a counter-incision should be made.

Infection of the Heel Space.—The infection is intradermal in one-third of cases, a few of these being a collar-stud extension from a deeper plane. Two-thirds of cases are due to infection of the fat-pad of the heel, which is situated in the subcutaneous portion of the posterior third of the sole. The portal of entry usually is a crack in the overlying calloused skin, and seldom, as one would think, from treading on a thorn or similar object.

Steadily increasing throbbing pain, severe enough to interfere with sleep, is the leading symptom. The patient dare not put his heel to the ground. Swelling of the soft tissues that cover one or both sides of the calcaneus is present, and in severe cases oedema of the ankle becomes manifest. Tenderness over the space leaves no doubt as to the diagnosis. As a rule, by the time the patient presents, the abscess is ready for incision, which is made through the medial or lateral side of the heel, so that the scar does not come to lie on a weight-bearing area. Fibrous septa within the abscess of the fat-pad need division with a scalpel. The lips of the cutaneous incision should be trimmed elliptically to prevent premature closing of the skin.

Deep Plantar Abscess.—The central plantar space situated deep to the plantar fascia is arranged like an apartment house of four stories, each of which is occupied by the muscles that constitute the flexors of the toes. Infection of the various floors becomes increasingly less common as one proceeds from the ground floor, upwards. For drainage of the central plantar space an incision is made parallel to, and just above, the medial border of the foot in the neighbourhood of the instep.

Infections of the Dorsum of the Foot

The dorsal subcutaneous space usually is infected by extension from a subcutaneous interdigital space or a web space, while the *dorsal subaponeurotic space* is infected either from a direct puncture or from involvement by extension from the deep plantar space. To drain the former space the incision should be placed distal to the dorsal venous arch, but in the line of the digital vessels and nerves, in order to avoid them. To drain the latter space it is best to confirm the presence of pus by attempting aspiration, and if diagnostic aspiration is positive, to make a longitudinal incision alongside the needle.

Leprosy not infrequently attacks the toes, and the initial manifestation may simulate a chronically infected corn. Leprosy is discussed in Chapter 4.

Madura foot (*syn.* mycetoma pedis) is a chronic granulomatous disease encountered especially in tropical countries, notably in certain parts of India or Africa, but with increasing frequency in territories where hitherto it has been unrecognised, such as the Southern United States, South America, and Cuba. Most cases are caused by a filamentous organism (*Nocardia madurae*) resembling actinomyces and abounding in road dust. In nine out of ten cases the organism gains entrance through a prick in those who go about barefooted. The first manifestation is a firm, painless, rather pale nodule. Soon other nodules appear. Later, the nodules become surmounted by vesicles which burst to form discharging sinuses. In the watery discharge granules can be discovered, sometimes only with perseverance. The granules may be yellow, red, or black. In 'black' madura foot, as it is called, spread is mainly in the subcutaneous plane; in the yellow and red varieties the infection burrows deeply, and bone necrosis ensues. As in actinomycosis, there is no lymphadenitis, but unlike actinomycosis, dissemination to other parts of the body does not occur. Gross swelling of the foot with flattening or convexity of the instep is characteristic. Sooner or later secondary infection supervenes, with rapid deterioration of the local condition. A similar infection can recur in the hand (fig. 139)

Treatment.—A wide-spectrum antibiotic to deal with secondary infection, followed by a prolonged course of dapsone (100 mg b.d.) improves many patients, and may obviate or postpone the necessity for amputation (Cockshott).

Guinea Worm.—This infestation is described in Chapter 8.

William Peter Cockshott, Contemporary. Professor of Radiology, McMaster University, Hamilton, Ontario, Canada.

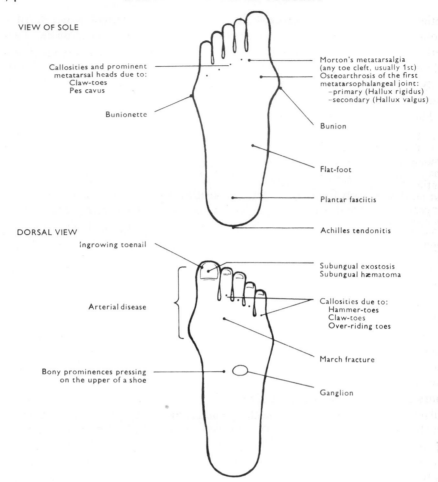

VIEW OF SOLE

Callosities and prominent
metatarsal heads due to:
　Claw-toes
　Pes cavus

Bunionette

Morton's metatarsalgia
(any toe cleft, usually 1st)
Osteoarthrosis of the first
metatarsophalangeal joint:
　–primary (Hallux rigidus)
　–secondary (Hallux valgus)

Bunion

Flat-foot

Plantar fasciitis

DORSAL VIEW

Achilles tendonitis

Ingrowing toenail

Subungual exostosis
Subungual hæmatoma

Arterial disease

Callosities due to:
　Hammer-toes
　Claw-toes
　Over-riding toes

March fracture

Bony prominences pressing
on the upper of a shoe

Ganglion

Fig. 146.—The common causes of pain in the adult foot, excluding infections (above), RA, and OA secondary to injury.

Flat Foot (*syn.* Pes Planus)

At birth the foot is flat, and the normal arch is only acquired when the infant stands. The arch is maintained in adult life by the shape of the bones of the foot, by their connecting ligaments and by the action of the muscles of the calf and sole. Flat-foot in adult life (fig. 147) may be due either to the collapse of once normal arches, or to the persistence of the infant shape.

It is often difficult confidently to attribute a complaint of pain in the foot to anatomical pes planus. Under conditions of active service in first-class infantry regiments, for example, great variations in the shape of the foot, including flat-foot, are observed in unselected groups of men not complaining of painful feet. On the other hand patients will be found complaining of significant pain in the foot who have well-formed arches.

The presence of anatomical 'flatness' is not the most important aspect of pes planus, and two other physical signs should be sought in order to decide whether a patient's symptoms can be attributed to pes planus as such. These are: (1) limited mobility of the tarsal joints and (2) localised tenderness. In general, only patients with painful limitation of movement at the sub-talar, mid-tarsal, or tarso-metatarsal joints are likely to have a mechanical disorder in the foot. Similarly, consistently localised tenderness in one part of the foot is strong evidence of a local source of organic pain.

There are 4 varieties of flat-foot:

1. **Infantile.**—This is physiological.

2. **Peroneal Spastic Flat Foot.**—An uncommon, painful condition which presents insidiously in adolescence. The foot is everted and hence the medial arch appears flat. The tendons of the peronei and long toe extensors can be seen standing out apparently in continuous contraction. Attempts passively to invert the foot are resisted by these muscles and are painful. In about 50% of cases special radiological views of the foot reveal a congenital bar of bone between the talus and the navicular, but in the remainder no abnormality is to be found. In these, the aetiology is unknown.

Treatment is unsatisfactory. Under general anaesthesia a below-knee plaster cast is applied with the foot plantigrade (muscle relaxation may be required to allow the foot to be placed in this position). The cast is worn for 2 to 3 months. Persistent recurrence, especially if a talo-navicular bar is present, may require subtalar fusion or excision of the bar.

3. **Idiopathic Adult Flat-foot.**—This is the commonest form of symptomatic flat-foot in the adult. It may be the end result of repeated episodes of 'foot-strain': an ill-defined, uncommon condition in which the foot becomes acutely painful following excessive use. More commonly, the condition is gradually progressive and presents with aching pain in the foot after long-continued standing. It is seen most commonly in people such as waitresses and hairdressers who spend long hours standing (rather than walking). The medial longitudinal arch gradually collapses causing pain centred in the medial part of the sole. Local tenderness may be found in the sole under the apex of the arch, probably because the plantar ligaments are over-stretched. Pain is provoked if these ligaments are stressed by dorsiflexing the forefoot. In later stages the foot becomes painless and the gait shuffling and inelastic. In its final stages this type of foot can be painless, though rigid and flat.

Treatment.—Treatment is only indicated if the flat-foot is symptomatic: 'prophylactic treatment' is often prescribed (mistakenly) in schoolchildren. The pain of 'foot-strain' is relieved by rest. Its prevention may require arch supports or a change of occupation. Chronic flat-foot can only be treated during the years when the foot is progressively breaking down. At this stage, arch supports moulded to the corrected shape of the foot may bring symptomatic relief but imply an acceptance of the disability. Exercises to improve the function of the intrinsic muscles of the sole and of the toe flexors may prevent further deterioration if the patient co-operates.

When the foot has finally collapsed, little can be done to improve its appearance or function and the patient should, therefore, be advised to accommodate his life to his feet by taking a sedentary job.

4. **Traumatic Flat-foot.**—This is caused by fractures which abolish the longitudinal arch. Fractures of the os calcis may produce a severe flat-foot with a rigid sub-talar joint. Fractures involving the sub-tarsal and mid-tarsal joints may lead to degenerative changes in these joints and hence to pain, the severity of which is out of proportion to the flatness of the foot.

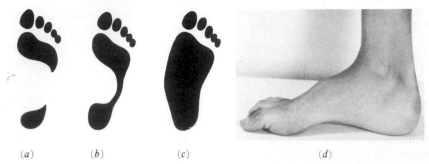

FIG. 147.—Imprints of the foot in: (*a*) Pes cavus. (*b*) Normal foot. (*c*) Pes planus. (*d*) The appearance of pes cavus.

Pes Cavus (*syn.* Claw-Foot)

Pes cavus is an uncommon condition in which there is an increased concavity of the arch of the foot, so that the instep is unduly high (fig. 147). It is typically accompanied by clawing of the toes.

Pes cavus is sometimes caused by neurological disease, for example poliomyelitis or Friedreich's ataxia, but in most cases it is idiopathic. The condition can perhaps be explained on the basis of weakness of the intrinsic muscles of the foot. These muscles flex the metatarsophalangeal joints and extend the interphalangeal joints. Without this mechanism the pull of the long flexors of the toes may cause the toes to assume the claw position and the foot to 'bunch'. Another factor which perhaps causes the deformity of pes cavus is shortening of the plantar fascia, which can be felt as a tight band stretched across the arch.

Treatment.—The treatment of pes cavus is unrewarding.

In childhood the foot is very rarely symptomatic so that the child is often not taken to a doctor or else is taken only because the parents have difficulty obtaining shoes. In such feet intrinsic exercises may be tried and, if unsuccessful, the relatively minor procedure of subcutaneous plantar fasciotomy carried out. It is difficult to justify more major procedures in a foot which is symptomless and may always remain so.

Fortunately many adult patients with pes cavus are able to play games and walk long distances. Such symptoms as are present are usually due to painful callosities under the metatarsal heads due to the 'high loading' to which a small area of skin is subjected by this shape of foot and to the difficulty of getting a shoe which fits. Therefore before considering surgical treatment of the anatomical deformity, the surgeon must satisfy himself that the patient has sufficient disability to warrant surgery and that such disability as he has cannot be corrected by making his life more sedentary and by moulding insoles to support his high arch, thus relieving weight from his metatarsal heads. In practice surgical treatment is rarely required. If it is, in adolescents or young adults with a supple foot it may take the form of an attempt to abolish the 'tie-bar' of the plantar fascia by Steindler's operation in which the plantar fascia and all the muscle attachments are erased from the lower surface of the os calcis by an open operation. The long extensor of the great toe may be transplanted to the neck of the first metatarsal to elevate this bone and so reduce the arch. In older adults with more rigid feet

Nikolaus Friedreich, 1825–1882. Chief of the Medical Clinic, Heidelberg, Germany. Described this form of ataxia in 1863.
Arthur Steindler, 1878–1959 (see footnote, p. 426).

the metatarsals may be shortened and elevated by osteotomies through their shafts.

The treatment of claw toes in the absence of pes cavus is considered below.

Hallux Valgus

Hallux valgus means lateral deviation (valgus) of the big toe (figs. 148 and 152). It is initiated by wearing footwear which is too narrow for the forefoot and which, therefore, tends to force the great toe laterally. Because women's shoes normally have a narrower forefoot than do men's, hallux valgus is much more common in women, especially the middle-aged. An abnormally broad forefoot predisposes to the condition and may be caused by a congenitally varus position of the first metatarsal (metatarsus primus varus) (fig. 148(b)). Once the valgus position of the great toe has developed, it tends to be progressive, because the direction of pull of the extensor and flexor hallucis longus tendons further increases the deformity by a 'bowstring' mechanism.

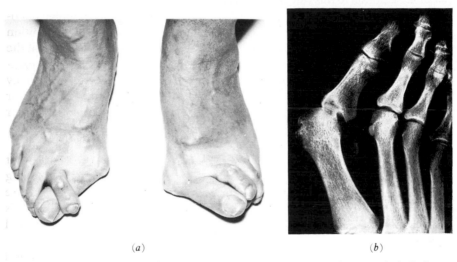

(a)   (b)

FIG. 148.—(a) The appearance of the feet with hallux valgus. A bunion is present in both feet, a bunionette only in the right. Note the variation in over-riding of the second toes: in both there is a callosity on the dorsum of the proximal interphalangeal (pip) joint. (b) X-ray of the foot with hallux valgus and metatarsus primus varus.

The following conditions are often associated with hallux valgus:

1. An exostosis on the medial side of the head of the first metatarsal, probably caused by pressure on the periosteum.

2. A *bunion*, which is an inflamed adventitious bursa, is produced over the prominent head of the first metatarsal by pressure and friction. Infection of the bursa (to produce suppurative bursitis) is common and the metatarsophalangeal joint of the big toe may be secondarily infected. A similar lesion, called a '*bunionette*', may develop over the lateral aspect of the head of the fifth metatarsal (fig. 148(a)). The skin over a bunion may ulcerate if neglected.

3. Osteoarthritis of the first metatarsophalangeal joint secondary to the malalignment of the proximal phalanx.

4. *Over-riding* or *under-riding* of the second toe by the first. In the latter condition (fig. 148(*a*)) a painful callosity may develop on the dorsum of the second toe. The second toe may be displaced laterally by the hallux to under-ride or over-ride the third (fig. 148(*a*)).

The patient may complain of an unsightly deformity, but more commonly the presenting symptom is pain caused either by pressure, infection or osteoarthritis.

Treatment.—The conservative treatment of hallux valgus is unsatisfactory. As the patient is almost invariably a woman, it is usually useless to advise the wearing of shoes with low heels, wide fronts and straight inner borders since no such shoe is available in ordinary shoe shops, and since such shoes are unsightly. A small rubber pad can be worn in the cleft between the first and second toes, but this also demands the use of a wide-fronted shoe.

Most young adults with hallux valgus will eventually require operative treatment no matter what conservative techniques are tried, but it is important not to operate merely for cosmetic purposes if the foot is reasonably comfortable. A possible exception to this rule is hallux valgus associated with significant metatarsus primus varus and without degenerative changes in the metatarsophalangeal joint: in such a foot a 'prophylactic' osteotomy of the first metatarsal so as to reduce the varus is worthwhile. The most satisfied patients after operation for the correction of hallux valgus are those in whom severe pain (as well as gross deformity) were present preoperatively: the indication for surgery in hallux valgus is pain.

Operation.—Local removal of the bunion together with the underlying osteophytes, without interference with the metatarsophalangeal joint, is not a satisfactory operation because symptoms almost always recur, and a more radical operation is later required. Exceptionally this operation may be performed in young people if the valgus deformity is slight, but the exostosis prominent.

The standard operation for hallux valgus is excision arthroplasty of the base of the proximal phalanx (Keller's operation) or of the head of the first metatarsal (Mayo's operation). The Keller procedure in younger patients can be augmented by osteotomy of the base of the first metatarsal to abduct the first metatarsal and close the enlarged gap between it and the second metatarsal. The corrected position is maintained by inserting excised bone to hold the osteotomy open on the medial aspect.

After the operation, at least 3 months will elapse before the foot will tolerate an ordinary shoe, and the patient may not feel the full benefit of the operation for as long as 6 months.

Hallux Rigidus

This condition occurs as two distinct varieties, both more common in men. In both the metatarsophalangeal joint of the great toe is stiff and painful.

(1) The adolescent type is due to synovitis of the metatarsophalangeal joint following injury, and is associated with muscular spasm. The condition is often secondary to minor trauma, for example stubbing the toe or repeatedly kicking a football with the point of the toe instead of the dorsum of the foot. There are no radiological changes. It is relieved by wearing a metatarsal bar 2 cm wide and 1·25 cm thick (fig. 150). Conservative treatment may fail to arrest the condition which then progresses gradually to present as the adult type.

(2) The adult type is nothing more than monarticular osteoarthritis (fig. 149), sometimes precipitated by injury. The limitation of movement is due to capsular

William Lordan Keller, 1874–1959. U.S. Army Surgeon, who became Head of Department of Surgery at the Walter Reed General Hospital, Washington, D.C., U.S.A. Described this operation for hallux valgus in 1904.
Charles Horace Mayo, 1865–1939. Surgeon, The Mayo Clinic, Rochester, Minnesota, U.S.A. Described this operation for bunion in 1908.

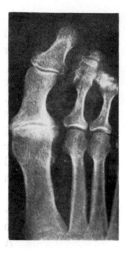

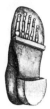

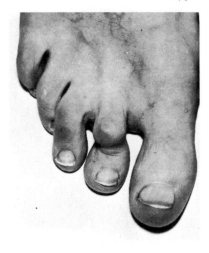

FIG. 149.—Hallux rigidus.

FIG. 150.—Metatarsal bar on shoe.

FIG. 151.—Second hammer-toe.

fibrosis, deformation of the articular surfaces, and the interlocking of osteophytes.

Treatment.—The condition may be treated by fitting a metatarsal bar or by operation. The Keller procedure is the most widely employed operation, although arthrodesis is perfectly satisfactory in men, especially if hyperdorsiflexion has developed at the interphalangeal joint of the great toe.

Hammer-toes

This condition, which may affect the second, third and fourth toes, consists of hyperextension of the metatarsophalangeal and distal interphalangeal joints, and flexion of the proximal interphalangeal joint (fig. 151). Callosities form over the bony prominence on the dorsum of the proximal interphalangeal joint, and in long-standing cases adventitious bursae develop. The tendons and ligaments become secondarily contracted.

Hammer-toes sometimes develop from overcrowding, either by small or pointed shoes, or as a result of hallux valgus. Often there is no obvious cause.

Treatment consists of correcting any predisposing cause and wearing a corrective splint or a corn plaster. If the deformity is established, arthrodesis of the proximal interphalangeal joint by the 'spike' method (Higgs) combined with extensor tenotomy and dorsal capsulotomy of the metatarsophalangeal joint is the treatment of choice. The spike operation consists of drilling the base of the middle phalanx and impaling it on the shaft of the proximal phalanx after shaping the condyles into a spike. Alternatively, the proximal phalanx may be excised.

Claw-toes

This condition differs from hammer-toes only in that (1) the toe pads do not contact the ground when the patient stands and (2), probably as a consequence of the loss of contact, the distal interphalangeal joint is flexed, not extended (fig. 152(*a*)). Because the toe pads are not weight-bearing, an increased proportion of the body-weight is borne by the corresponding metatarsal head. Because the metatarsophalangeal joint is hyperextended, often to the point of

Sydney Limbrey Higgs, 1892–1977. Orthopaedic Surgeon, St. Bartholomew's Hospital, London.

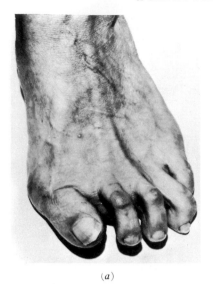 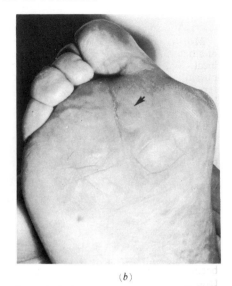

(a)   (b)

FIG. 152.—(a) Second and third claw-toes. Note that the toe pads do not touch the ground. (b) Plantar callosity (arrowed) under the second metatarsal head. Note that the pad of the second toe does not touch the ground.

dorsal dislocation, the toes are prominent dorsally and press on the upper of the shoe causing painful callosities on the dorsum of the toe and downward pressure on the metatarsal head. These two factors tend to compress the skin and soft tissues between the ground and the metatarsal heads and so cause pain and callosity formation in the skin of the sole. Eventually the fibro-fatty tissue under the metatarsal head atrophies or is displaced distally so that the metatarsal head becomes subcutaneous and easily palpable in the sole. A callosity then develops in the skin under the metatarsal head which is painful to stand on and tender when pressed (fig. 152(b)).

The condition is often associated with hallux valgus and pes cavus but may occur as an isolated entity. Its aetiology is unknown, but it is probably related to the wearing of high heels and to poor function in the intrinsic muscles of the foot. Severe claw-toes may be caused by rheumatoid arthritis affecting the metatarsophalangeal joints.

Treatment consists of exercises for the intrinsic muscles of the foot if the metatarsophalangeal joints are fully mobile. If they are not, the foot can be made comfortable by the provision of well-fitting footwear, an insole to relieve weight from the metatarsal heads, and a corn plaster on the callosity.

If conservative measures fail, the deformity can be corrected by arthrodesis of the interphalangeal joint (see hammer-toes) combined with dorsal capsulotomy and extensor tenotomy of the metatarsophalangeal joint and transfer of the flexor digitorum profundus tendon into the dorsum of the proximal phalanx. Alternatively, the affected toes may be amputated through the metatarsophalangeal joints. If pain under the metatarsal heads is the main complaint, the head of the metatarsal may be elevated by osteotomy of the shaft of one or all the metatarsal heads may be excised. The latter operation is particularly useful in rheumatoid arthritis.

OTHER CAUSES OF PAIN IN THE FOOT

Morton's Metatarsalgia.—This syndrome was thought to be due to the development of a neuroma on the interdigital nerve between the metatarsal heads, possibly caused by local compression of the nerve. It is now known that the true cause is intermetatarsal bursitis which does compress the nerve but does not cause a neuroma. The condition is rare and presents clinically with well-localised pain and tenderness between the metatarsal heads, together with paraesthesiae and hypoaesthesia in the related interdigital cleft.

Treatment is by excision of the bursa.

Plantar Fasciitis.—The aetiology is uncertain. Pain and localised tenderness occur under the heel. The pain is often severe, is felt especially at heel-strike, and interferes with walking. It is probably caused by a tear in the attachment of the plantar fascia to the os calcis, but seems sometimes to be associated with gonoccocal and non-specific urethritis. The pain is not caused, as was once supposed, by bony spurs on the plantar surface of the os calcis.

Treatment consists of advising the patient to avoid walking and standing as much as possible for 6 weeks, fitting rubber heels, and supplying insoles to weight-relieve the tender area and to take tension off the plantar fascia by supporting the medial arch. If these measures are ineffective, local injections of 25 mg of hydrocortisone and 1 ml of 1% procaine may bring relief.

Achilles' Tendonitis.—The loose connective tissue in which the Achilles' tendon slides becomes inflamed, thickened and painful. Pain may also originate, as in other forms of tendonitis, from the attachment of the tendon to the bone. The condition is often caused by a period of greatly increased walking or by the wearing of shoes with an ill-fitting heel. Occasionally it appears to be spontaneous.

Treatment consists of rest, if necessary in a below-knee plaster cast, for up to 6 weeks.

Subungual Exostosis.—Occurs on any toe but is most common on the great toe. The toe-nail is lifted from its bed and becomes painful and often infected.

Treatment is by removal of the nail and exostosis.

Congenital abnormalities of foot and toes (*e.g.* **Club-foot**) are described in Chapter 21.

Thomas George Morton, 1835–1903. Surgeon, The Pennsylvania Hospital, Philadelphia, Pennsylvania, U.S.A. Described this condition in 1876.

Achilles, the Greek hero, was the son of Peleus and Thetis. When he was a child, his mother dipped him in the Styx, one of the rivers of the Underworld, so that he should be invulnerable in battle. The heel by which she held him did not get wet and was therefore not protected. Achilles died from a wound in the heel, which he received at the Siege of Troy.

CHAPTER 13

VASCULAR DISEASE—VEINS

VENOUS THROMBOSIS

Thrombosis of veins is predisposed to by Virchow's triad:

(1) *Change in the vessel wall* with damage of the endothelium, *e.g.* inflammation or injury.

(2) *Diminished rate of blood flow*, as occurs during and after operations, and in debilitating conditions, such as typhoid fever.

(3) *Increased coagulability of the blood*, such as occurs in infections, after haemorrhage and with visceral carcinoma (Trousseau's sign) ('thrombophlebitis migrans').

The results of thrombosis are as follows:

(1) *Locally*.—The clot may organise into fibrous tissue, or the vein can become recanalised. Calcification in the form of a phlebolith is seen in pelvic veins. Infection can lead to abscess formation or pyaemia.

(2) *Distally*.—After a varying degree of oedema a venous collateral circulation soon opens up, as shown by the appearance of tortuous superficial veins.

(3) *Proximally*.—Extension into larger veins where portions of clot may become detached and, as emboli, cause pulmonary infarction (Chapter 40). Infected clot in the portal vein will cause liver abscesses (pylephlebitis).

Superficial Vein Thrombosis (Thrombophlebitis) occurs in varicose veins or in a vein which is cannulated for an infusion (Chapter 6). It occurs spontaneously in otherwise normal veins in association with conditions such as polycythaemia, polyarteritis and Buerger's disease (fig. 153). It can herald the presence of visceral cancer (thrombophlebitis migrans). The thrombosis can appear simultaneously

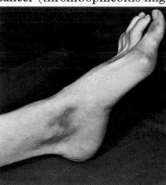

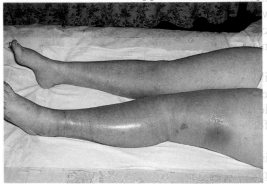

FIG. 153.—Thrombophlebitis in Buerger's disease (Chapter 14). Here the long saphenous vein is affected in front of the medial malleolus.

FIG. 154.—Phlegmasia caerulea dolens (blue leg). The leg is engorged, not as 'blue' as in venous gangrene (see fig. 156). The deep venous thrombosis is extensive in the pelvic and deep femoral veins (cf. Phlegmasia alba dolens, white leg—see text).

Rudolph Virchow, 1821–1902, Pathologist, Germany.
Armand Trousseau, 1801–1867. Physician, Hôtel-Dieu, and Professor of Medicine, Paris. Noted this sign as his own death warrant, as his own thrombosis confirmed his suspicion that he had carcinoma of the stomach.

or subsequently in other veins. A painful and cord-like inflamed area is diagnostic. The treatment includes gentle support by means of a crepe bandage (p. 188). An anti-inflammatory drug (*e.g.*, aspirin) may be helpful. A good response can follow a short course of penicillin or cotrimoxazole. As the thrombus is adherent to the intima of the vein an embolus is unusual. If an acute infection supervenes it can spread rapidly up the vein, a clinical situation in which emergency proximal ligation may be indicated.

Deep Vein Thrombosis (Phlebothrombosis[1]) follows childbirth, operations, muscular violence, local trauma of any kind, immobility, and any debilitating illness. Spontaneous thrombosis may also be indicative of the presence of a visceral neoplasm. Post-operative thrombosis is rare before the age of 40 and is particularly associated with obesity, operations for cancer and those on the prostate and the hip joint. Other epidemiological associations include the fact that it is virtually unknown in equatorial regions like Singapore, while in northern climes it appears to increase with the arrival of autumn and the winter snow. If its presence is judged in a clinical study by a radioactive ^{125}I fibrinogen uptake test the incidence is found to be as much as 30% following operations on those over 40, and of these both legs are affected in 30% (*i.e.* in around 10% of patients over 40). The incidence can be as much as 50% following major hip surgery.

The thrombus may commence in a venous tributary of a main vein, where there are eddying currents around a valve. It extends in a serpentine fashion into the main deep vein where the relatively faster stream may cause a portion to break off and so cause a pulmonary embolus (Chapter 40). The pelvic and calf veins are more commonly implicated than others. Occlusion of a length of the deep femoral vein will cause painful congestion and oedema of the leg. If in addition there is an associated lymphangitis, the swelling will increase and is likely to be protracted (*e.g.* 'white leg'—phlegmasia alba dolens). Extensive deep vein thrombosis of the iliac and pelvic veins may cause a 'blue leg' (phlegmasia caerulea dolens (fig. 154)) in which either venous gangrene or areas of infarction may threaten part of or the whole of the limb (see below and fig. 156).

Prevention of Thrombosis.—(a) *Before operation*. Stop the 'pill'.[2] When possible, grossly over-weight patients should reduce weight. Those over forty, rendered immobile during a period of in-patient investigation or other treatment, are less at risk if they have a spell of 2–3 weeks activity at home before readmission for operation. Low dose heparin may be started (see below).

(b) *During operation* it is essential that the venous return from the lower limbs is not impeded in any way. Pressure of the calf on the operating table *must* be prevented by elevating the heel on a sandbag or sorbo-rubber pad. At the end of an operation it is a good plan to elevate and massage the legs.

(c) *After operation*, conditions which predispose to a sluggish circulation such as immobility of the lower limbs, dehydration, and delayed venous return should be avoided by massage, leg movements, continued use of graduated compression stockings (TED stockings) or low dose heparin, adequate hydration, and early

---

[1] As there is likely to be as much inflammation around a deep vein as a superficial vein, the distinction given by the terms thrombophlebitis and phlebothrombosis is really inappropriate.

[2] When there is no urgency, all female patients on the 'pill' should stop this method of contraception for one month before surgery.

ambulation. Patients should not be allowed to sit out of bed with their legs dependent. In fact, patients are often more mobile in bed than in a chair.

Methods of Prevention, the efficacy of which have been confirmed by controlled trials, include:

1. *Mechanical* prevention of venous stagnation by assisting venous return on the principle of the venous pump (p. 186), by means of: (i) *Graduated static compression elastic stockings* (Kendall's Thrombo Embolic Deterrent—TED). These, by exerting pressure from below upwards, can reduce the incidence of thrombosis to below 10% (down to 20% in hip surgery). They are relatively easy to use and are 'non-invasive'. (ii) *Electrical stimulation* of the calf muscles. (iii) *Pneumatic compression.*

2. *Low Dose Heparin.* 5000 units are given subcutaneously 2 hours before operation and continued twice daily until the patient is fully ambulant. Alternatively, micro-dose heparin (Negus) can be given i.v. at a rate of one international unit/kg/h. Both low and micro-dose methods can reduce the incidence to well below 10%, but it must be remembered that they are 'invasive' techniques requiring careful procedure and should be avoided where an operation is likely to leave raw bleeding areas, or where a post-operative haemorrhage in a restricted area would be disastrous.

3. *Dextran '70'.* One regimen is to give 500 ml i.v. during the operation and 500 ml in the following 24 hours. By virtue of its property of inhibiting platelet adhesion it is, as an artificial infusate, less thrombogenic than isotonic saline (Janvrin). (See Chapter 5 for limitations.)

4. *Combination of methods* has been shown to confer additional benefit, for example heparin and stockings reduces the incidence to below 7%, and stockings with intermittent pneumatic compression to below 5%.

Detection of Thrombosis.—Phlebothrombosis is often symptomless,[1] but there may be a complaint of pain in the affected calf. Any unexplained elevation of temperature or pulse-rate should arouse suspicion of thrombosis, especially when occuring towards the end of the first post-operative week. In all cases the calves should be examined daily for tender areas of induration and alteration of the contour of the calf muscles, when compared with the other leg, due to swelling and change in tone of the muscles. Tenderness may be elicited along the course of the posterior tibial and peroneal veins. Homans' sign—pain in the calf or dorsiflexion of the foot may be present but it is rather unreliable, and may cause a thrombus to float off when the test is applied.

The Doppler principle (Chapter 14) is a useful and simple aid in the diagnosis of deep vein thrombosis. The sensing probe, placed over the femoral vein in the groin, normally transmits a venous hum (like wind in telegraph wires) and pressure on the calf, or calf muscle contractions, changes the hum into a roar, due to increased blood flow. If there is a thrombosis of the deep vein (popliteal and femoral) between calf and groin the roar does not occur. A deep venogram can show the site and extent of the obstructing thrombus (see below) in order to assist in the formulation of the correct treatment policy. However, caution should be exercised in patients who are recent or inveterate clotters, as venous gangrene has been known to occur after this investigation.

Treatment of Deep Vein Thrombosis.—(*a*) *Anticoagulants, Bandage and Rest.*—A suitable regimen includes (1) Giving anticoagulants, combining heparin and phenindione or Warfarin, and continuing the latter for three to six weeks taking care to tail-off slowly to prevent a 'rebound' of thrombosis. (2) Bandaging the whole limb with crepe or using a graduated compression stocking to increase

---

[1] Studies, using isotope-labelled fibrinogen, have indicated that symptomless thrombosis is relatively common (p. 183).

Kendall Company, Chicago, Illinois, U.S.A.
David Negus, Contemporary. Surgeon, Lewisham Hospital, London.
Simon Benest Janvrin, Contemporary. Surgeon, Crawley and Horsham Hospitals, Sussex, England.
John Homans, 1877–1955. Professor of Clinical Surgery, Harvard Medical School, Boston, Massachusetts, U.S.A. Described this sign in 1941.

the deep venous flow. (3) Resting the patient until the elevated temperature and the local signs abate, before beginning mobilisation.

(b) *Treatment based on venography.*—(i) *Fixed thrombus.*—If the thrombus is fixed to the vein wall, anticoagulants are given, heparin 40,000 units per day for 7 days, if possible, by continuous infusion (fig.48). Warfarin is begun and continued for 6 months. (ii) *Free thrombus.*—If the thrombus is loose at the top it can either be removed or be 'fixed'. Removal by thrombectomy, using a Fogarty balloon venous catheter, is not the easy procedure it might seem to be. Streptokinase or urokinase to dissolve the thrombus can be tried providing there is no further bleeding and no heparin is given but it is not often successful. Fixation of a free thrombus is achieved by blocking the vein. A ligature suffices for the superficial (not main) femoral vein, but for the vena cava a ligation, or the introduction of a filter, may be carried out. One such filter is the Kimray-Greenfield, introduced in a capsule, under x-ray control, via the neck and internal jugular vein into the inferior vena cava.

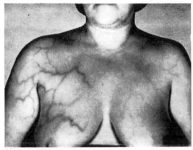

FIG. 155.—Collateral venous circulation following thrombosis of the axillary vein. Infra-red photograph.
(*Max Pemberton, F.R.C.S.*)

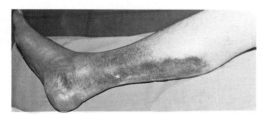

FIG. 156.—Venous gangrene due to polycythaemia vera.

Axillary Vein Thrombosis.—Thrombosis of the axillary vein is not uncommon, and can occur after unaccustomed use of the corresponding arm (*e.g.* painting a ceiling). The vein is damaged by the excessive movement that occurs between the clavicle and the first rib.[1] 'Spontaneous' thrombosis may be due to a pyjama sleeve becoming twisted around the axilla during heavy slumber, with consequent compression of the vein. The thrombosis results in painful congestion and oedema of the arm (fig. 155). As a collateral venous circulation develops, the symptoms subside; this takes about three months. The extent of the thrombosis can be limited if anticoagulant therapy is given in the early stages. Fibrinolytic therapy (*e.g.* streptokinase, urokinase) may restore the circulation if given in the first 24 hours (Chapter 14). Axillary vein thrombosis can occur after axillary dissections (e.g. during mastectomy) or radiotherapy, and occasionally complicates venous cannulation.

VENOUS GANGRENE

A rare condition, due to extensive thrombosis in peripheral veins, there being normal arterial pulsations. It may occur in the toes and forefoot without any apparent cause, though it may be a manifestation of visceral neoplasm (Trousseau's sign). It also occurs in peripheral thrombosis due to polycythaemia vera (fig. 156).

---

[1] Henry of Navarre, 1553–1610 (King Henry IV of France, 1589–1610), led his army into the battle of Ivry (1590), shouting 'Rally round the white plume of Navarre'. He used his sword to such good effect that he could not use his arm for six weeks, and probably had an axillary vein thrombosis.

Kimray Medical Associates, Oklahoma City, U.S.A.
Laser J. Greenfield, Contemporary. Surgeon, Oklahoma, U.S.A.

Treatment.—The limb is elevated and anticoagulant therapy commenced. Low molecular weight Dextran i.v. to reduce the viscosity of the blood may be helpful. Conservative surgery is performed when the final line of separation appears. It may be found that the gangrenous tissue is relatively superficial and that the deeper layers are pink and viable. Skin grafting may be helpful in this conservative approach to treatment.

VENOUS HAEMORRHAGE

Venous haemorrhage can be torrential, difficult to control, exsanguinating and fatal (Chapter 4).

Ruptured Varicose Veins.—Blood escapes from these veins under considerable pressure whether from veins in the legs (see below) or from the oesophago-gastric junction (see portal hypertension). Simple but sustained direct pressure is needed to control the bleeding prior to the institution of other effective procedures (see p. 59 and Chapter 45).

Major Veins.—Wounds in the groin and the neck, and within the chest, abdomen and pelvis whether caused by accident, assault or operation, are likely to lead to exsanguination. The first error in emergency treatment of, say, a stab wound in the groin or neck, when the wound has been tightly packed in the streets, is to assume that if there is no bleeding on removal of the pack in the A & E department the wound is of a trivial nature. It is an error realised when a sudden movement or coughing or vomiting by the patient causes resumption of an exsanguination which can be fatal. The second error at operation is to continue hopefully to mop, dab and then to jab with a haemostat forcep while blood continues to well-up and the patient continues to deteriorate. According to circumstances the surgeon has recourse to (a) extensive tight packing, say, in pelvic cancer surgery or in liver trauma—packing with rolls of gauze tied together for subsequent slow removal 24–28 hours later from a resuscitated patient or (b) precise control—ligation or repair. While direct pressure is used to control blood loss, the anaesthetist attends to adequate blood volume replacement (Chapter 5) including facilities for autotransfusion. With pressure sustained by the assistant the surgeon exposes the uninjured venous anatomy below, above and behind in order to apply soft occlusive vascular clamps. Even then other intraluminal devices (balloons, sounds and spigots) may be required to allow the surgeon to see exactly how to complete the control of the wound by ligature or suture.

VARICOSE VEINS

A vein is stated to be varicose when it is dilated, lengthened and tortuous. The condition is seen mainly in the leg (fig. 157), but spermatic, oesophageal, and haemorrhoidal veins may be affected (see appropriate chapters). Varicose veins of the legs are part of the penalty we pay for the adoption of the erect posture. Animals do not suffer from this condition.

The Venous Pump.—In the human, the return of venous blood from the lower limb to the heart requires a pump equipped with non-return valves. The pumping action is provided by the muscles. Their tone and contractions, acting within the strict confines of the encircling deep fascia, squeeze or milk the blood in the direction insisted upon by the valves, *i.e.* towards the heart. Therefore a *primary* cause of varicose veins is congenital paucity of valves, weakness or wasting of muscles, or stretching of the deep fascia—all of which impair the function of the pump. On standing, the whole weight of the column of blood from the legs to the right atrium is exerted on the valves (up to pressures of 90 mmHg (12.0 kPa), particularly on those guarding the communications between the superficial and deep venous systems of the leg (blood in the superficial system normally flows into the deep veins). The main valves affected are those at (1) the saphenofemoral lying at the junction of the long saphenous and common femoral veins, (2) the mid-thigh (mid Hunter) communication, (3) the sapheno-popliteal junction and (4) either side of the tibia and fibula (fig. 158) where there are

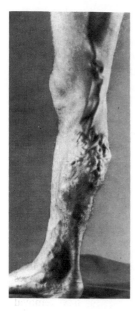

FIG. 157.—Varicose veins.

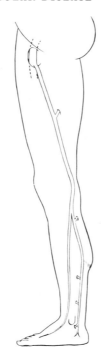

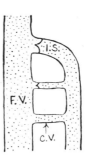

FIG. 159.—An incompetent communicating vein (C.V.), femoral vein (F.V.), long (internal) saphenous vein (I.S.).

FIG. 158.—The sites of communicating (perforating) veins between the deep and superficial (long saphenous) veins (see text). The short saphenous vein has similar communications on the lateral side of the Achilles tendon.

communications (perforators) passing through openings in the deep fascia above the ankle.

If the valves are absent or become incompetent there is not only a high back pressure on standing, but an even higher back pressure on walking and running (about 150 mmHg) as the blood is squeezed out of the veins in the deep compartment into the superficial veins (fig. 159). To some extent the long saphenous and short saphenous veins are protected by their relatively muscular walls and the brunt is borne by others in the intercommunicating network within the superficial fascia (fig. 157).

Secondary varicose veins. Varicosity is also predisposed to by any obstruction which hampers venous return, *e.g.* tumours and pregnancy, and by thrombosis of the deep veins, The predilection for females suggests a hormonal (? progesterone) factor.

Fistula varicosities. Varicose veins occuring below the age of twenty may be due to congenital arteriovenous fistula, or an extensive cavernous (venous) haemangioma. Veins leading away from an acquired arteriovenous fistula (due to trauma or deliberate shunting for dialysis purposes) also become varicose (arterialised, Chapter 14).

In severe cases of varicose veins the blood volume is increased. It is reduced by operation.

Symptoms depend on the extent of the high back pressure. The commonest is a tired and aching sensation, felt in the whole of the lower leg, and especially in the calf, towards the end of the day. Sharp pains may be felt in grossly dilated thigh veins. The ankle may swell towards evening, or the skin of the leg over the varicosities may itch. Some patients suffer from cramp in the calf shortly after retiring to bed.[1]

Examination.—The condition may either be widespread in both legs, or restricted to a single varix. Should this be at the saphenous opening, it is called a 'saphena-varix',[2] and it is readily distinguished from a femoral hernia on account of the characteristic palpable thrill when the patient coughs or the vein below is tapped with a finger.

The precise location of the incompetent or absent valves in primary varicose veins is most important, for upon it depends the success, or failure, of treatment. If an incompetent valve is present the venous flow is retrograde, so that veins when emptied fill from above; normally they should fill from below. The examination, based upon the test described by Brodie (1846) and Trendelenburg (1890), involves what has aptly been described as 'the intelligent use of the tourniquet'.

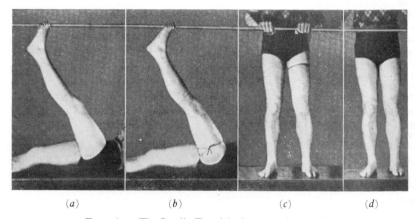

(a)   (b)   (c)   (d)

FIG. 160.—The Brodie-Trendelenburg test (see text).
(Dr S. M. Rivlin, London.)

Brodie-Trendelenburg Test.—Briefly, the patient lies upon his back and raises his leg to empty the veins (fig. 160(a)). A venous tourniquet is applied just below the saphenous opening (fig. 160(b)), and he stands up (160(c)). The constriction is then released (160(d)). If the sapheno-femoral valve is incompetent, the veins fill immediately from above; if not, the veins fill slowly from below. If the veins fill rapidly from above, with the tourniquet in place, it means that the varices are in communication with a perforating vein (one is commonly present in the lower third of the thigh), or the sapheno-popliteal junction is incompetent. In this case, the tourniquet test must be repeated, with application at successively lower sites on the thigh and leg, until the point of origin is shown by prevention of the abnormal direction of flow. Similar, and sometimes more convincing demonstration of incompetent 'perforators' is achieved by working upwards from the ankle with the tourniquet.

Treatment.—(i) **Palliative treatment** is required for varicose veins in those who are pregnant, and for those who do not wish for, who are unfit for, or who are waiting for, operation. The veins are supported by elastic stockings or crepe or elastic bandages.

---

[1] Quinine dihydrochloride (200 mg), taken on retiring, is often efficacious in relieving night cramps. Hexopal® 500 mg has also helped some patients.
[2] The word 'saphenous' is of Arabic derivation and means 'seen easily'.

Sir Benjamin Collins Brodie, 1783–1862. Surgeon, St. George's Hospital, London.
Frederick Trendelenburg, 1844–1924 (see p. 60).

(ii) **Injection-Compression (Sclerotherapy)**[1].—Sclerosants, like ethanolamine oleate[2] 5% (Ethanolamine BPC), or sodium tetradecyl sulphate 3% (Sotradecol or Thrombovar) cause a thrombosis, and later sclerosis. Satisfactory occlusion will take place only whilst the sclerosant is able to act in sufficient concentration within the superficial and communicating vein. At the same time it has to be remembered that if an excess of the sclerosant is injected at one site it may reach the deep veins in sufficient concentration to initiate a deep vein thrombosis before it becomes sufficiently diluted to render it harmless. *The minimum fully effective dose* for a sclerosant should always be known, and should not be exceeded at any one site. Injection-Compression treatment is the treatment of choice for varicose veins confined to below the knee and for recurrent varicosities after operation. It is not the ideal cosmetic treatment because of the unpredictable staining which may occur.

Technique.—In order to make the venous occlusion permanent, injections must be given into an empty vein, so that wall adheres to wall with no intervening blood clot and thrombosis which will certainly recanalise. The needle is inserted into the vein with the patient sitting down, with the leg horizontal. A latex foam pad may be put over the site of the injection (not on to the skin directly), and along the length of vein, and it is maintained by pressure bandage and a stocking overall for six weeks from the last injection or until the pain has gone from the site (Fegan). Injections are also given at the site of the perforating veins as delineated by the Brodie-Trendelenburg test (above) and at the maximum site of tenderness.

The maximum dose at any one time and any one point is 1 ml. It is usual to commence treatment with a test dose of 0.5–1 ml so that the extent of the local reaction may be gauged and the dose modified as necessary. Also it should be noted that injection or extravasation of a sclerosant into the surrounding tissue can cause necrosis.

(iii) Operations for Varicose Veins

Ligation Procedures.—The basic principle of the operative treatment of varicose veins is the ligation and division of those veins into which the high-pressure leak from the deep venous system has primarily occurred. Almost always this means ligation of the long saphenous vein where it enters the femoral vein (sapheno-femoral flush ligation). A flush ligation proximal to any tributaries is essential, otherwise a recurrence is inevitable (fig. 161). Should the short saphenous vein be the site of a high-pressure leak, it must be exposed in the

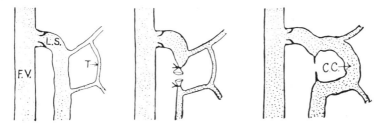

Fig. 161.—Tributaries (T.) must be ligated as well as the long saphenous vein (L.S.) flush with the femoral vein, otherwise a collateral circulation (C.C.) develops.

---

[1] A word of warning is necessary in this era of the contraceptive pill. Caution should be exercised before giving sclerosant injections to a woman practising this form of family planning. Deep-vein thrombosis and fatal thrombo-embolism have been reported.

[2] Strange to relate, Mother Nature has, from the days of the primeval swamp, provided this substance from ? platelets in the actual chemistry of natural thrombosis.

William George Fegan, Contemporary. Professor of Surgery, Trinity College, Dublin.

popliteal fossa and ligated, proximal to any superficial tributaries, close to or flush with the popliteal vein.

In other instances of incompetent valves (or 'blow outs') of the communicating veins (fig. 158), they must be ligated under the deep fascia (p. 192).

Technique of Sapheno-Femoral Ligation.—An oblique incision is made just below the groin, commencing over the pulsation of the femoral artery and extending some 6 to 7 cm medially. The proximal portion of the long saphenous vein is exposed and traced to the femoral junction, which may lie 1·25 cm deep to the fossa ovalis, *dividing and ligating all tributaries* encountered on the way. It is then tied flush with the femoral vein. The presence of an accessory saphenous vein should be excluded. It may enter the femoral vein directly and escape the necessary attention.

Dealing with the varicosities below the groin includes additional ligatures as required for 'blow outs' (see above). Other means of obliterating varicosities include multiple ligatures, injections, and minor and major avulsions (stripping).

Note: If a long saphenous vein is relatively normal (as opposed to its tributaries) it must be left alone since, in later years, it may well be needed for arterial bypass surgery.

Contraindications to Injection and Operative Treatment

(a) *Acute Infective Thrombophlebitis.*—At least three months should be allowed to pass, after this has completely subsided, before injecting.

(b) *Deep Thrombosis.*—Due to any cause or revealed by a history of prolonged confinement to bed with a painful swollen leg. Perthes' test is informative if doubt exists regarding the patency of the femoral vein:—The saphenous vein is occluded by a tourniquet applied immediately below the saphenous opening, and the patient walks 15 to 20 yards (13·5 to 18 metres). Normally, the veins below the constriction become less obvious, but if the communicating veins or the femoral vein are obliterated, these subcutaneous veins become engorged and the patient complains of 'bursting' pain.

(c) *Pregnancy, Pelvic tumours and the 'Pill'*. See footnotes pp. 183 and 189.

COMPLICATIONS OF VARICOSE VEINS

Thrombophlebitis of superficial veins reveals itself as a reddened, tender cord in the subcutaneous tissues. Ambulatory treatment is safe and convenient. Strips of foam rubber or P.V.C., the edges of which are bevelled, are laid over the inflamed vein (over a layer of bandage), and 2·5 cm above it a double thickness is placed transversely. The leg is then bandaged with an elastic bandage. The strapping is removed after a fortnight. This procedure gives immediate relief, and it need be renewed only if tenderness persists.

Eczema (chronic dermatitis) may follow minor trauma or because the patient scratches skin which itches due to extravasation and break-down of red-cells in the affected area. Alternatively, it may be an allergic manifestation resulting from ointment or strapping applied for treatment. The condition is treated by the application, twice daily, of an ointment containing zinc oxide and coal tar or, subject to careful control, one containing 1% hydrocortisone or 0·1% betamethasone.

Venous ulcers[1] (fig. 162) occur either in connection with varicose veins or follow deep-vein thrombosis in which recanalisation of the deep vein has occurred but the valves are either destroyed or incompetent due to damage. Venous stasis, favouring local anoxia and oedema, is the underlying cause of both types but lipolysis of the subcutaneous fat is an important accessory factor. It is important to be sure that the ulcer is not due to ischaemia from atherosclerotic arterial obstruction, arteritis (Chapter 14), or from syphilis (Chapter 4). A varicose ulcer responds promptly to ambulatory treatment or ligation operations, but post-thrombotic ulcers tend to be refractory to treatment, and may require bed-rest,

---

[1] John Gay, 1812–1885. Surgeon, Great (now Royal) Northern Hospital, London. Was the first to use the term Venous Ulcer.

Georg Clemens Perthes, 1869–1927. Professor of Surgery, Tübingen, Germany. Described this test in 1895.

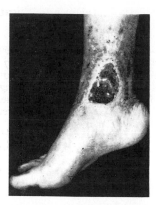

FIG. 162.—Venous ulcers with pigmentation of skin and talipes equinus deformity.

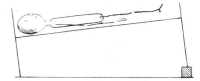

FIG. 163.—Sleeping with the foot of the bed raised.

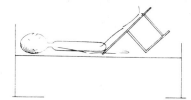

FIG. 164.—High elevation of the leg, using a chair.
(After Dickson Wright, FRCS, London.)

curettage and skin grafting. Amnion (HIV negative), applied fresh, has its advocates. Carcinomatous changes may occur in a chronic ulcer (fig. 52) (cf. Marjolin's ulcer).

A deep venogram can be particularly useful in helping the clinician to formulate treatment in difficult cases, as it will show the patency and the size of the lumen of the deep veins, the presence of valves, and the existence of high-pressure leaks in the calf:

Technique.—A fine rubber tourniquet is applied just above the malleoli to occlude the superficial veins. An injection of 20 to 30 ml of 45 to 65% Hypaque (sodium diatrizoate) is given into a superficial vein of the foot, via a fine polythene cannula. (A test injection is, of course, given first, Chapter 14.) The contrast medium is thus forced into the deep veins, and serial x-ray exposures are made of the whole leg. High-pressure conditions are simulated by tilting the patient into the semi-vertical position, or by his pinching the nostrils and endeavouring to expire forcibly (Valsalva).

Functional Venography.—With x-ray image intensification and T.V. display the function of veins, valves, communicating veins and the venous pump can be studied by injecting contrast into a superficial vein and observing flow on activating the venous pump (standing on the toes). The contrast entering the deep veins can be observed on stopping the pump. Refilling of the superficial veins via any incompetent perforator veins can be marked. This is to some extent a variation of the old Perthes' test (see above). Doppler apparatus (see next chapter) can also be adapted to indicate the direction of flow in veins (Directional Doppler).

Treatment

(*a*) **Bisgaard method.** Almost any venous ulcer can be healed by elevation, bandaging, exercises, and massage. A physiotherapy department can be most helpful in applying rigorously the Bisgaard method of treatment, which consists of:

(1) Massage in elevation to the whole leg and particularly to soften the indurated area around the ulcer.

(2) Passive movements to maintain the mobility of the foot and ankle.

(3) Active movements to the calf muscles in elevation, and in standing (with bandages on).

(4) Teaching correct walking, placing heel down first and using the calf muscles to lift the heel of the back foot, giving 'spring' to the walk and therefore improving the venous pump (p. 186).

Holger Bisgaard, 1881–1943. General Practitioner, Copenhagen. Published his method of treating varicose ulcers in 1939.

(5) A *firm* elastic (*e.g.* 'blue line') bandage is applied spirally from the base of the toes to the knee, so that movements in walking alternately stretch and relax the bandage and produce an added venous pumping effect.

(*b*) **Bandage and elevation.** Without patient compliance or facilities for properly executed Bisgaard treatment, reliance is placed upon the use of compression bandaging (*e.g.* wet Eusol and paraffin dressings or 'Viscopaste' type, under a firm spiral of elastic bandage). Proper bandaging reduces the local oedema and aids the muscular component of the venous pump. The patient should sleep with the foot of the bed raised (fig. 163) and periods of high elevation of the leg are to be strongly encouraged (fig. 164). A 'wet' bandage cannot be wound spirally round the leg without the bias of the weave cutting into the skin. It must be applied in many encircling and overlapping strips. Often a piece of felt, with bevelled edges and cut to a size larger than the ulcer, is interposed in the bandage, over the ulcer, to reduce the local oedema which so often retards healing. A crepe bandage is put on over the 'wet' bandage on top of which can be worn an elasticated TED stocking (p. 183). The patient is instructed to continue his usual work, and to wash off any discharge which may percolate through the bandage. Injection-Compression therapy may also be used as an ancillary treatment.

The first application is removed after one week, and thereafter the bandage is renewed at fortnightly intervals until the ulcer is healed. The area of the ulcer should be measured accurately at regular intervals in order to monitor the effect of a particular mode of treatment, *e.g.* by computerised stereo-photogrammetry (Bulstrode).

Additional treatment includes bacteriological control by means of culture and the use of appropriate effective antibiotics (Chapter 3), and also the control of pain by analgesics. It should be remembered that infection with Pseudomonas pyocyaneus (staining the dressings blue/green) is a cause of pain which can be alleviated by the correct antimicrobial treatment. Also in about one third of the patients suffering from severe pain there is an ischaemic element due to associated arterial disease which in turn requires proper assessment and treatment (Chapter 14).

(*c*) **Subfascial Ligation** (Cockett & Dodd Operation).—Most venous ulcers are due to incompetence of perforating veins on the inner side of the ankle (fig. 158). Therefore, when the ulcer has healed, the perforating veins should be identified and divided through an incision in the lower half of the leg 2·5 cm behind the posterior border of the tibia. The veins, which may be enormously dilated, are best secured by exposing them beneath the deep fascia. If necessary the saphenous veins are also dealt with, as already described. Occasionally a refractory indolent ulcer will respond favourably when direct incision through the hard fibrous base gives access to the normal soft tissues beneath and the large communicating veins with incompetent valves, so that ligation can be performed.

Haemorrhage from a ruptured varicose vein is usually profuse. Elevation of the leg and the application of a firm pad and bandage easily control the bleeding. *On no account* should a tourniquet be used (Chapter 5).

Calcification occasionally occurs in veins which have been varicose for many years.

Periostitis occurs in long-standing cases if the ulcer is situated over the tibia.

Equinus deformity may result from a long-standing ulcer. The patient finds that walking on the toes relieves the pain, and after some years the Achilles tendon becomes contracted (fig. 162). Cases usually respond to remedial exercises. The Bisgaard treatment (above) should prevent this complication.

C. J. K. Bulstrode, Contemporary. Reader in Orthopaedic Surgery, Oxford.
Frank Cockett, Contemporary. Surgeon, St. Thomas's Hospital, London.
Harold Dodd, 1899–1987. Emeritus Surgeon, Royal London Homeopathic Hospital, London.

CHAPTER 14

VASCULAR DISEASE—ARTERIES

Conditions encountered in arteries include: Stenosis or Occlusion, Dilatations (Aneurysms), Arteritis and small vessel abnormalities.

ARTERIAL STENOSIS OR OCCLUSION

Cause and Effect.—Arterial stenosis or occlusion is commonly caused by *atherosclerosis* but can occur acutely as a result of *emboli* (p. 207) or *trauma* (p. 212). Stenosis or occlusion produce symptoms related to the organ which is supplied by the artery: *e.g.* Lower Limb = claudication, rest pain and gangrene; Brain = transient ischaemic[1] attacks and hemiplegia; Myocardium = angina and myocardial infarction; Kidney = hypertension or infarction (fig. 165); Intestine = abdominal pain and infarction. The severity of the symptoms is related to the size of the vessel occluded, and the alternative routes (collaterals)[2] available (fig. 166).

Symptoms and signs of lower limb arterial stenosis or occlusion

Intermittent claudication[3] is a cramp-like pain felt in the muscles that: 1. Is brought on by walking, 2. Is *not* present on taking the first step (contrast osteoarthrosis—Chapter 19), 3. Is relieved by standing still (contrast lumbar intervertebral disc nerve compression Chapter 27).

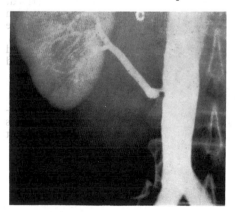 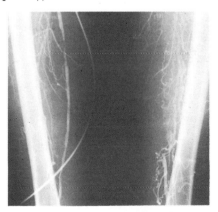

FIG. 165.—Renal artery stenosis. Arteriogram by retrograde femoral catheterisation. Note the post-stenotic dilatation.

FIG. 166.—Right superficial femoral stenosis. Left superficial femoral occlusion with collateral vessels present, causing claudication.

---

[1] Ischaemia = lacking in blood flow.

[2] Collateral circulation was demonstrated first by John Hunter 1728–1793. Surgeon, St. George's Hospital, London. He tied the external carotid artery of a stag from Richmond Park. The stag's antler fell off, but later another one grew. On re-opening the original wound, Hunter found the ligature intact, but a collateral circulation had been established.

[3] Claudication, from the Latin, claudicatio = to limp. The Roman emperor Claudius 10 B.C.–A.D. 54 walked with a limp (?due to poliomyelitis).

The distance walked is called the *claudication distance*. It is a very subjective distance which can vary from day to day in the same patient. It is altered by walking up hill or against a wind, the speed of walking, or by changes in general health such as anaemia or heart failure.

The pain of claudication is most commonly felt in the calf, but can affect the thigh or buttock.[1] Claudication less commonly occurs in the upper limb in subclavian, axillary or brachial artery obstruction, the pain being brought on by such activities as writing or manual labour.

Rest pain is severe pain felt in the foot at rest, made worse by lying down, or elevation of the foot. Characteristically the pain is worse at night, and may be somewhat relieved by hanging the foot out of bed, or by sleeping in a chair. Night cramps which are short severe muscle cramps of unknown origin should not be confused with rest pain.

Coldness, numbness and paraesthesia are common in moderate as well as severe ischaemia, but in the absence of colour changes it is essential to exclude a neurological cause.

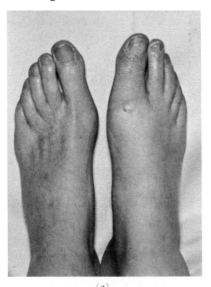 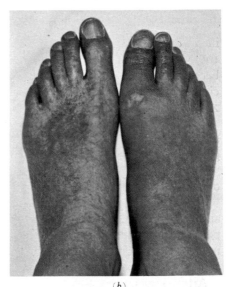

(*a*)   (*b*)

FIG. 167.—Colour changes with (*a*) elevation and (*b*) dependency (see text).

Colour changes (fig. 167).—Moderate or severely ischaemic limbs become blanched on elevation and develop a bluish-purple discoloration on dependency. Any bright red speckling is due to the extravasation of red cells through capillary walls. The angle of elevation at which blanching first occurs gives a good rough guide to the degree of ischaemia.

Ulceration and gangrene.—Ulceration occurs with severe arterial insufficiency and often presents as a painful superficial erosion between toes. Alternatively small, shallow, indolent non-healing ulcers may occur on the dorsum of the feet, on the shins, and especially around the malleoli. The blackened mumm-

---

[1] Pain in the buttock occurring on exercise (walking) and associated sexual impotence, which result from arterial ischaemia, are given the eponymous title 'Leriche syndrome' (p. 196).

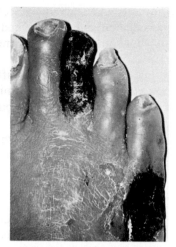

FIG. 168.—Severe chronic ischaemia.

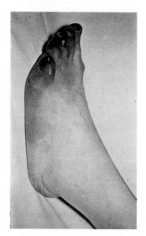

FIG. 169.—Severe acute ischaemia (embolism—too late for embolectomy!).

ified skin and tissues of frank gangrene are unmistakeable to the observer (fig. 168), but it must be remembered that in acute ischaemia a dead white limb which becomes mottled means impending gangrene and not an improvement in the circulation. Fig. 169 shows a typical case. An account of gangrene is found on p. 213.

Pregangrene.—The combination of rest pain, colour changes, oedema, hyper-aesthesia, with or without ischaemic ulceration, is frequently referred to as 'pre-gangrene'.

Temperature.—Severely ischaemic feet are usually cold but sometimes para-doxically may feel warmer than the non-involved foot.[1]

Sensation and movement.—Acutely ischaemic limbs are frequently paralytic and without sensation. These are ominous physical signs and such a limb has a poor prognosis in the absence of active treatment. Severe chronic ischaemia does not produce paralysis, but hyperaesthesia is common, especially in those areas of skin on the borderline of gangrene. Gentle handling of such limbs is essential.

Arterial pulsations.—Arterial pulsations below an occlusion in a main artery are usually absent or, in the presence of good collaterals, diminished.

In patients with vascular symptoms it is standard practice in each case to feel the pulsations in the radial arteries, the carotid arteries, the abdominal aorta, the femoral arteries in the groin, the popliteal arteries behind the knee, the posterior tibial arteries behind the medial malleoli and the dorsalis pedis artery on the dorsum of the foot. Diminution of a pulse can best be appreciated by comparing it with the pulse in the other limb, provided that this pulse is normal.[2]

---

[1] The acutely ischaemic limb tends to take on the temperature of the surroundings and may feel quite warm under the bedclothes.

[2] *Aide Memoire in eliciting physical signs (Ed. A.J.H.R.)*: Palpate abdomen for masses, especially pulsatile (aneurysm), and move downwards for palpable pulsation in common femoral, popliteal, posterior tibial and dorsalis pedis arteries. Don stethoscope and work upwards listening for bruits in midthigh, groin, iliac fossa and abdomen. Listen to heart sounds, then for bruits in neck (subclavian, carotid). Then take B.P. in both arms.

Expansile arterial pulsation with a mass may indicate an aneurysm.

In arterial occlusion with a highly developed collateral circulation, or main artery stenosis, the distal pulses may be normal to palpation. The following physical sign is then useful:

The 'disappearing pulse'.—Where peripheral pulses are apparently normal, exercising the patient to the point of claudication may unmask the effect of an arterial obstruction, by causing the previously palpable pulse to disappear. After a minute or two of rest the disappearing pulse reappears. The explanation is that exercise produces vasodilation below the obstructing lesion, and the arterial inflow, reduced by the lesion, cannot keep pace with the increasing vascular space; arterial pressure falls, and the pulse disappears.

Arterial bruits.—A vascular examination should include auscultation of the subclavian arteries in the supraclavicular fossae, the carotid arteries behind the angle of the mandible, the abdominal aorta and the femoral arteries in the groin and over the adductor (subsartorial) canal. A systolic bruit over an artery is due to turbulence, and indicates a stenosis of the artery.

Systolic bruits are conducted distally. Thus a bruit in the neck at the level of the angle of the mandible without any supraclavicular bruit frequently means a carotid artery stenosis. Where, however, a bruit is heard at both sites, its origin may be more proximal, e.g. aortic valve, aortic arch, brachiocephalic or subclavian arteries. Under these circumstances the carotid artery may prove quite normal. The patient with renal artery stenosis shown in fig. 165 had a bruit over the renal artery.

A Continuous 'Machinery' Murmur over an artery usually indicates the presence of an arteriovenous fistula.

Venous Refilling.—The limb should be elevated for thirty seconds and then laid flat on the bed. Normal refilling occurs within seconds. Reduced venous filling is often present in the severer forms of arterial insufficiency but is also common in vasospastic disease and in cold weather.

Harvey's Sign[1].—If the two index fingers are placed firmly side by side on a vein, and the finger nearer the heart is moved so as to empty a short length of vein, the release of the distal finger will allow the speed of venous refilling to be observed.

Increased venous return and varicosities of veins are associated with arteriovenous fistulas.

Impotence from failure to achieve an erection is often a feature in male patients with an occlusion in the region of the bifurcation of the aorta and the internal iliac arteries (Leriche's syndrome).[2]

The Relationship of Clinical Findings to the Site of Disease

By associating the symptoms and signs found in a case of arterial disease the site of the major arterial obstruction can be determined.

Double Blocks.—The presence of another (secondary) obstruction can usually be inferred. For example, a patient with signs of iliac artery obstruction, but with rest pain and pre-gangrene of the foot, must have a secondary obstruction since collateral circulation around an isolated iliac artery obstruction is usually excellent. The severe symptoms would indicate a secondary obstruction probably in the femoral or popliteal arteries.

---

[1] William Harvey (1578–1657), Physician, St. Bartholomew's Hospital, London. First described circulation of the blood in his course of lectures at the Royal College of Physicians of London in 1616. Harvey's book *Exercitatio Anatomica de Motu Cordis et Sanguinis in Animalibus* was not however published until 1628. The sign of venous refilling should be eponymous, as it was this observation on the direction of blood flow in the veins that confirmed Harvey's views that the blood moved in a circle.

[2] Leriche's syndrome. René Leriche (1879–1955) described Leriche Syndrome in 1940.

Relationship of Clinical Findings to Site of Disease

AORTO ILIAC OBSTRUCTION	Claudication in both buttocks, thighs and calves
	Femoral and distal pulses absent in both limbs. Bruit over aorto-iliac region
	Impotence common (Leriche)
ILIAC OBSTRUCTION	Unilateral claudication in thigh and calf and sometimes buttock. Bruit over iliac region.
	Unilateral absence of femoral and distal pulses
FEMORO-POPLITEAL OBSTRUCTION	Unilateral claudication in calf
	Femoral pulse palpable with absent unilateral distal pulses
DISTAL OBSTRUCTION	Femoral and popliteal pulses palpable
	Ankle pulses absent
	Claudication in calf and foot

The best results from surgery are obtained in patients with an *absent* femoral pulse and only claudication (without gangrene) *i.e.*, aorto-iliac disease with good distal vessels.

Investigation of Arterial stenosis or Occlusion

Many patients with symptoms due to arterial disease stenosis or occlusion do not need surgical treatment. This decision can often be made without submitting the patient to a series of special investigations (see Indications for surgery).

General.—Patients with arterial disease tend to be elderly, and atherosclerosis is a generalised disease. If surgery is indicated a full assessment is essential.

Investigations relevant to *diabetes, abnormalities of lipid metabolism, anaemia,* conditions causing *high blood viscosity* (*e.g.* polycythaemia) and *thrombocythaemia* (in small vessel disease) include a full blood count (including ESR and platelets), plasma fibrinogen, protein electrophoresis, blood and urine glucose and blood lipid profile. *A plain x-ray* of the abdomen will show the presence of arterial calcification and flecks of calcium may outline an aneurysm (fig. 170). Heart failure, myocardial ischaemia, hypertension and age related diseases such as bronchial problems and neoplasia should also be excluded.

E.C.G.—Although a normal E.C.G. does not exclude severe coronary artery disease, a grossly abnormal E.C.G. may influence the decision for surgery in patients with lower limb disease.

Blood Sugar estimation is particularly important in patients with peripheral ischaemia or those considered for surgery.

'Doppler' ultrasound blood flow detection (figs. *171 & 172*).—A continuous wave ultrasound signal is beamed at an artery and the reflected beam picked up by a receiver. The changes of frequency in the reflected beam, as compared with the transmitted beam, are due to the 'Doppler Shift', resulting from the passage of the beam through moving blood. These frequency changes are converted to audio signals. Using this principle, in conjunction with a sphygmomanometer, the systolic pressure can be measured by noting the disappearance of the signal when the cuff is inflated. This is often possible even at sites where the arterial pulse cannot be palpated.

The 'pressure index' (PI) is the ratio of the pressure measured in the posterior tibial artery at the ankle, with the cuff positioned just above the ankle, to the pressure in the brachial artery. The resting PI is normally greater than unity, values below 0·9 indicate some degree of arterial obstruction and those between 0·9 and 1·0 are equivocal. Re-testing after a standard exercise is valuable, particularly in the investigation of intermittent claudication, for differentiating vascular from neuro-orthopaedic conditions and in the

Christian Johann Doppler, 1803–1853. Austrian Physicist.

FIG. 171.—Doppler apparatus—probe, receiver and headphones.

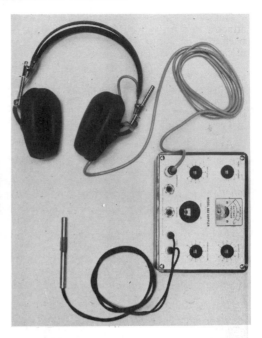

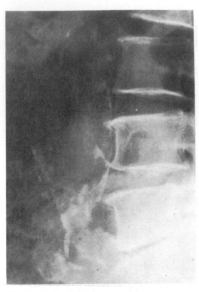

FIG. 170.—Plain lateral x-ray abdomen reveals abdominal aortic aneurysm outlined by calcium flecks.

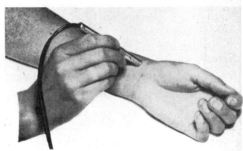

FIG. 172.—Doppler probe.

early detection of graft failure. In the absence of arterial stenosis the PI will rise after exercise.

Differences in arterial blood pressure between segments of a limb can be detected to give some indication of the sites of stenoses. In the leg the cuff is commonly placed above the ankle, at mid-calf and at mid-thigh to provide 'segmental pressures'.

Artefacts can be encountered when performing these apparently simple tests, due particularly to rigid, calcified arteries and mismatching between the size of the cuff and the diameter of the limb, particularly when mid-thigh occlusion is being attempted.

Ultrasound equipment is available which is capable of detecting the direction of flow, *e.g.* in the supraorbital artery as an adjunct to investigation of the internal carotid arteries.

Ultrasound imaging.—Ultrasound is used to image arteries and to give information on their diameters and cross-sectional areas, blood flow rates and velocities and to analyse the pulse wave. This has been achieved by the use of pulsed or continuous wave doppler and the two-dimensional images produced by the B-scan made either singly or in combination.

Plethysmography is a method of assessing changes in volume and has been applied to the investigation of arterial disease because the volume of a limb or organ exhibits transient changes over the cardiac cycle. Plethysmography in limb or digit can be performed using air-filled cuffs or mercury in rubber strain-gauges. As the pressure pulse passes through the limb segment a wave form is recorded which relates closely to that obtained by intra-arterial cannulation.

Oculoplethysmography (O.P.G.) in various forms (using fluid or air-filled cups attached to the eye by suction), particularly in combination with phonoangiography has been used extensively in North America but infrequently elsewhere for the investigation of carotid artery disease.

Phonangiography.—Low frequency vibrations of the arterial wall, caused by disturbances in blood flow can be detected as a noise (bruit) using a stethoscope or via a suitable microphone. Analysis of this sound, its location, duration relative to the cardiac cycle, and frequency distribution, can give information on arterial haemodynamics resulting from atherosclerosis and stenosis.

Treadmill.—Measurement of walking (claudication) distance.

Arteriography.—In lower limb arterial stenosis or occlusion, because it is the symptoms and their severity that decide whether surgery is indicated, *an arteriogram is undertaken only after this decision has been taken in order to find out whether or not the obstruction is anatomically suitable for a surgical procedure to be*

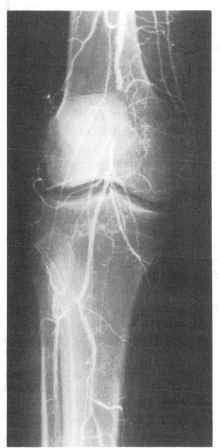

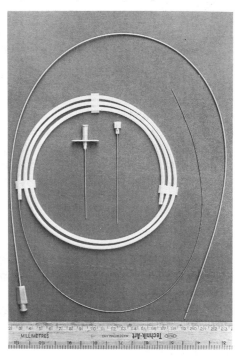

Fig. 174.—Seldinger needle and guide wire for introducing an arterial catheter.

Fig. 173.—Arterial occlusion just above the knee causing claudication of the calf; good collateral circulation.

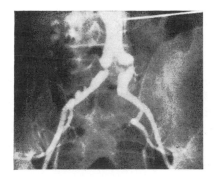

Fig. 175.—Translumbar aortography. Atherosclerotic stenosis of both common iliac arteries prevented proper visualisation by retrograde catherisation.

carried out. But, in carotid, intestinal and renal artery stenosis, an arteriogram is indicated to confirm the diagnosis and is an essential part of the assessment of the patient before the decision about operative treatment can be made.

Arteriography involves the injection of a radio-opaque solution into an artery either by a retrograde percutaneous method (usually via the femoral or occasionally the brachial artery), using the Seldinger technique (fig. 173, 174) or by direct percutaneous arterial puncture (*e.g.* translumbar fig. 175). The hazards include thrombosis, arterial dissection, haematoma, and, rarely arterial rupture. As paraplegia and anaphylaxis can occur following the injection of contrast it is necessary to confirm accurate placement of the catheter and acceptability of the material by a small trial injection.

Intravenous computerised angiography with subtraction is being developed to produce arteriograms without having to perform invasive arterial puncture.

The Management of Arterial Stenosis or Occlusion

Up to two thirds of the patients first presenting at a vascular clinic with intermittent claudication can be treated initially by *conservative methods.*

Explanation and advice.—Many patients are worried by the presence of pain on walking. Once told that walking is not doing harm, their walking distance often improves. Spontaneous improvement occurs in many patients over the first three months after an occlusive episode as collateral vessels are developed.

Adjustment of life-style.—Adjustments to everyday habits of transport can increase mobility within the claudication distance, *e.g.*, the use of a bicycle or a car.

Stopping Smoking, particularly patients with Buerger's disease (p. 231). Progression of the disease and post-surgery graft failure are more common in patients who continue to smoke.

Taking Regular Exercise, within the limits of the pain.

Diet, to reduce weight in the obese, and more specifically in the treatment of *hyperlipidaemia.*

Oral vasodilator drugs may be included in the first line of treatment immediately after an acute arterial obstruction, but it should be remembered that at this time the claudication is at its most severe and spontaneous improvement may be expected as collateral circulation improves.[1]

Lipid Abnormalities.—Serum lipoproteins contain cholesterol and triglyceride. β-lipoproteins are cholesterol-rich and pre-β lipoproteins are triglyceride-rich. The commonest abnormalities in peripheral vascular disease are Frederickson Type II hyperlipoproteinaemia (raised β lipoproteins) and Type IV hyperlipoproteinaemia (raised pre-β lipoproteins). A low cholesterol diet, or drugs such as cholestyramine are useful for Type II, and weight reduction for Type IV, abnormalities.

Diabetes and Hypertension should be treated by standard methods. In the latter case the over-zealous reduction of blood pressure by the use of beta-adrenoceptor blocking drugs can worsen claudication.

---

[1] The improvement may be attributed entirely to the vasodilator drug which thereby acquires an undeserved reputation.

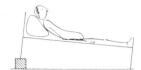

FIG. 176.—Buerger's position.

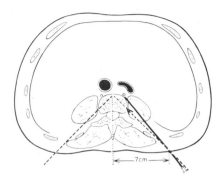

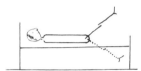

FIG. 177.—Buerger's exercises.   FIG. 178.—Lumbar paravertebral injection.

Care of the feet, avoiding socks with holes and amateur chiropody, which can spark off gangrene in the toes and heels, particularly in diabetic patients.

Heel Raise.—Claudication distance may be increased by raising the heels of shoes by 1 cm. The work of the calf muscles is reduced thereby.

Analgesics and Position.—Rest pain can be relieved to some extent in some patients by the use of analgesics, elevation of the head of the bed (Buerger's position fig. 176) and Buerger's exercises (fig. 177, repeated 2 minute elevation and dependency of the limb).

Aspirin in dispersible form may be prescribed for its anti-adhesive effect on platelets. A very small dose, one tablet (300 mg) once a week is more beneficial than, say, once a day.

Sympathectomy is not very effective in claudication but can relieve rest-pain and ulceration because the effect is mainly on skin and subcutaneous blood vessels. However, rest pain and ulceration are severe symptoms requiring surgery to improve the arterial supply whenever feasible.

Chemical sympathectomy is an alternative to surgical sympathectomy (fig. 215) but is contraindicated in the presence of anticoagulant therapy.

Technique.—Fig. 178 shows how a long (15 cm) needle is inserted, with 1% lignocaine infiltration, firstly to seek the side of the vertebral body and secondly to pass alongside it to reach the lumbar sympathetic chain. If lignocaine alone is injected the effect (warmer feet and improved venous filling) is only temporary and a more lasting result is achieved by injecting about 5 ml phenol solution in water beside the bodies of the second, third and fourth lumbar vertebrae. Care is needed to avoid penetrating the aorta or the vena cava (the plunger of the syringe must always be drawn back to exclude the presence of blood before an injection is given). The procedure is advisedly carried out under x-ray control (T.V. screening) and the likely positioning of the dilute phenol bolus can be forecast by a small injection of a contrast (*e.g.* Hypaque) solution.

Operations for Arterial Stenosis or Occlusion (Lower Limb)

Indications for Surgery.—*Claudication* is a relative indication for surgery—relative, that is, to the patient's need. A claudication distance of 30 yards may be acceptable for an elderly patient with easy access to transport to the shops, whereas a 55 year old surveyor may lose his job if he cannot walk 200 yards and so surgery may be indicated.

Rest pain is an absolute indication for surgery because of the severity of the

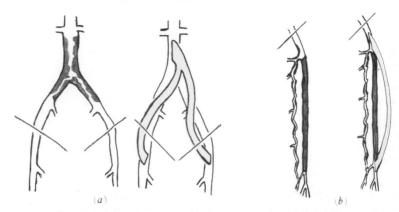

FIG. 179.—(*a*) Atherosclerotic narrowing of the aortic bifurcation. Aorto-bifemoral graft to bypass stenosis.(*b*) Superficial Femoral artery occlusion with Profunda Femoris stenosis providing poor collateral circulation. Femoro-popliteal graft used to bypass the occluded area into good 'runoff' below.

pain, provided the patient is fit to stand the operation (see general investigation), and the arteriogram shows the obstruction to be amenable to correction by surgery.

Ischaemic Ulceration that does not respond to conservative methods. Urgent surgery may be indicated in rapid deterioration of an already ischaemic limb to prevent limb amputation (often referred to as limb salvage). *Acute Occlusion due to emboli* is discussed on page 207.

Arteriography and Decision.—Once it is clear on the above clinical grounds that surgery is indicated, arteriography is performed. The site of the stenosis or occlusion is demonstrated, and then a decision is made as to whether an operation that will relieve the block is technically possible.

Site of disease and type of operation.—*Aorto-iliac artery stenosis* with good calibre vessels below this level (fig. 175) responds well to an aortofemoral bypass procedure (fig. 179*a*) or iliac endarterectomy (p. 204) which are major abdominal operations.In patients who are judged unfit for this major surgery balloon transluminal angioplasty (see fig. 181). or femoro-femoral cross-over grafts (p. 204) may be feasible.

Superficial femoral and profunda artery stenosis, often produces unilateral symptoms and these patients respond well to surgery provided the vessels below the popliteal trifurcation (posterior-tibial, tibial, peroneal) are of good calibre, and the aorta-iliac segment above does not limit flow to the common femoral artery.A femoro-popliteal bypass graft (fig. 179*b*) is used in most cases to overcome the stenosed segment. Long-term graft patency is related to the number of patent vessels supplying the pedal arch arteries and the material used as a prosthesis. The patient's own saphenous vein, if suitable, gives the best results and so assessment of the saphenous vein prior to surgery is essential. In a few patients the superficial femoral artery is occluded and the profunda femoris artery has a localised stenosis at its origin, with good collateral and distal vessels. In these patients profundaplasty (p. 204) can produce good relief of symptoms and it has the advantage of being a relatively minor procedure.

Stenosis below the popliteal artery. Direct arterial procedures are unrewarding because the small diameter of the vessels and subsequent poor flow results in early graft failure. Sympathectomy is restricted in its use, mainly for those patients with Buerger's disease and diabetes.

Prosthetic materials.—*For by-pass of the aorto-iliac segment* the favoured material is woven dacron, which unlike knitted material does not need preclotting to make it impervious to blood. *For bypass in the femoro-popliteal region* three prostheses are commonly used; *reversed autogenous saphenous vein, PTFE[1], or specially prepared umbilical vein.* The patient's own long saphenous vein has the best long-term patency and is inexpensive, but it may be found to have too small a diameter (less than 4 mm is associated with a high early graft failure), be varicose or thrombosed. In patients without a suitable vein, umbilical vein grafts have a slightly better long term patency than PTFE grafts, but umbilical vein is considerably more expensive.

In procedures such as *profundaplasty*, the incision in the artery is closed with a patch to prevent narrowing at the suture line; a vein patch being preferable to one made of, say, Dacron® velour. If possible the vein selected should be other than the long saphenous itself which may be needed for bypass surgery at a later date (including coronary artery bypass).

Suture Material.—Continuous Merselene and Prolene sutures on an atraumatic needle are used for anastomosis between aorta and graft material. Between graft and femoral artery continuous 0000 Prolene, for the distal anastomoses, for patching and closure of an arteriotomy 00000, or 000000 Prolene on an atraumatic needle is commonly used.

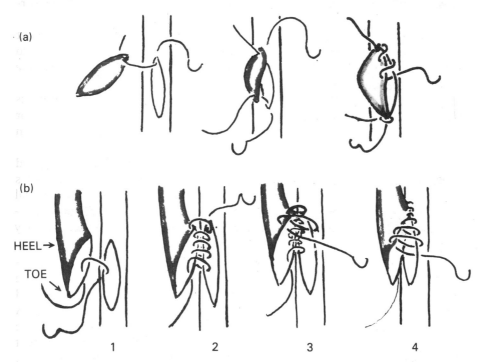

FIG. 180.—(*a*) Vein Patch and end-to-side anastomosis. The ends are fixed before working along each side. Simple *end to side anastomosis* can be performed in an identical manner to the vein patch, the obliquely cut tube taking the place of the patch. (*b*) An alternative technique makes the suturing of the difficult 'heel' area easier to visualise. (1) Suture started 1 cm from the heel of the graft. (2) Working up loosely to the angle of arteriotomy. (3) Continued for a few stitches round the heel, and then pulled tight. (4) Toe suture placed and tied. A stay stitch at the toe is useful to keep the graft stretched to length. The suture is then completed and tied to the stitch near the heel.

[1] PTFE = PolyTetraFluoroEthylene (Teflon®).

Arterial suture technique (see also Chapter 42, Anastomotic Techniques)—Vein patching prevents narrowing of an artery on closing an arteriotomy (*e.g.* profundaplasty). As already stated the piece of vein should come from, say, a branch of the saphenous vein. The vein is opened longitudinally and the adventitia cleared from the outer surface as much as possible. The patch is cut to the length of the arteriotomy and the corners trimmed before suturing (fig. 180).

Operative Details

Aortofemoral bypass graft (fig. 179*a*).—The aorta is approached through a midline or transverse abdominal incision and the common femoral arteries by vertical groin incisions. Small bowel is retracted to the right to allow the posterior peritoneum to be incised and the aorta exposed. Retroperitoneal tunnels are made from the aorta to the common femoral site. Heparin is given i.v. (*e.g.* 2,500 units) and clamps applied to the aorta, iliac and femoral vessels after dissection and the passage of supporting slings. A vertical incision is made in the aorta (often trimmed to fashion a hole) and in the common femoral arteries. Endarterectomy is performed if indicated. The graft is cut obliquely, the length being adjusted so that the level of the bifurcation lies at the level of the aortic bifurcation. The graft is then sutured to the opening in the aorta and the limbs of the graft are brought through the retroperitoneal tunnels so that the end to side anastomoses can be made with the common femoral arteries. The peritoneum is sutured over the graft in the abdomen and the wounds are closed with suction drainage to the groin wounds.

Aorto-iliac endarterectomy.—Exposure of the aorta is as above, the plaques and layers of atheroma are carefully prised away. It is possible to use a retroperitoneal approach, but proximal control is more limited.

Femoropopliteal bypass graft.—If the long saphenous vein is to be used, it will have been marked out preoperatively. The approach to the artery is along the line of the vein. After the saphenous vein is dissected and branches ligated, it is cannulated and inflated with heparinised Hartmann's solution. Once both arteries are exposed and a tunnel formed for the graft by blunt dissection, heparin is given intravenously and clamps applied. The arteries are opened and the graft is sutured end-to-side to the proximal arteriotomy. The vein must be reversed before suturing into place so that the valves do not prevent flow. The proximal clamps are released, the graft is brought through the tunnel, and the lower anastomosis is made, checking that all air and clot in the vein and popliteal artery is expelled before completing the continuous suture. The wounds are closed with suction drains to prevent haematoma formation. Antibiotic cover is advisable if artificial material is used for grafting.

Profundaplasty.—Through a vertical incision the common femoral artery and its branches are meticulously displayed, and after the usual i.v. heparin and clamping, the incision in the femoral artery is extended along the profunda branch (or branches) until relatively normal artery is found. Atheroma is gently prised away (endarterectomy) and the opening closed with a vein patch (see above).

Balloon transluminal angioplasty.—Arterial stenosis, particularly if it affects the iliac, superficial femoral (fig. 181) or renal artery (fig. 182), may be treated by passing a balloon angioplasty catheter through the stenosis and inflating the balloon with dilute contrast medium to pressures of 5–10 atmospheres for periods of 15–30 seconds. The balloons come in different sizes and when deflated the catheter has the same outside diameter as an ordinary arterial catheter and can be passed into the arterial tree using the Seldinger technique. Expansion of the balloon produces fissures in atheromatous plaques which develop an endothelial lining over the following months, and usually ruptures muscle fibres within the media.

The procedure is carried out under local anaesthesia and seems to be particularly effective if the stenosis is due to fibromuscular hyperplasia. It is sometimes possible to treat an occluded artery by advancing a guide wire through the occluded segment and then passing the balloon catheter over the guide wire.

The long-term patency is variable and is probably not as good as reconstructive surgery but the procedure can be repeated if stenosis recurs.

Other Arterial Operations and Salvage Procedures

(i) **Femoro-femoral crossover graft** is useful for relieving an iliac artery occlusion when the other iliac artery is patent with a strong femoral pulse. An 8 mm Dacron graft is tunnelled subcutaneously above the pubis and anastomosed end-to-side to the common

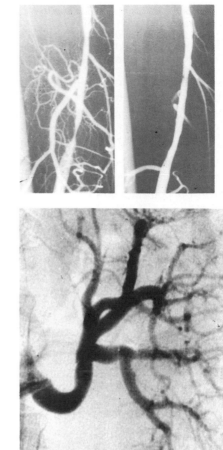

FIG. 181.—Narrowed superficial femoral artery before and after transluminal angioplasty. (J. McIvor, FRCR, London.) The advantage of this technique is that it can be done under local anaesthesia using the Seldinger technique (fig. 174) of percutaneous arterial puncture, and therefore useful in the treatment of those patients who are medically unfit for major surgery.

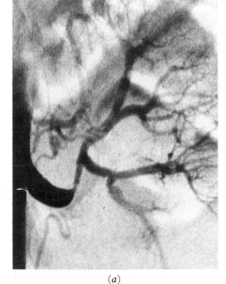

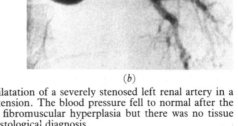

(a)   (b)

FIG. 182.—(a) Before and (b) after balloon dilatation of a severely stenosed left renal artery in a 20-year-old woman with uncontrollable hypertension. The blood pressure fell to normal after the procedure. The stenosis was probably due to fibromuscular hyperplasia but there was no tissue available for histological diagnosis.

femoral arteries on each side. Blood from the patent iliac system is then carried through this graft to vascularise the ischaemic limb.

(ii) **Axillo-femoral graft**—useful for salvaging a pre-gangrenous limb in a poor risk patient with bilateral iliac obstruction. A long 8 mm Dacron graft is tunnelled subcutaneously, from an end-to-side anastomosis with the axillary artery proximally, to reach the femoral artery of the involved limb in the groin where the distal anastomosis is made. The axillary artery will carry a sufficient volume of blood to maintain the circulation in the arm and re-vascularise the lower limb. The short-term results are usually good and in these patients with their poor general condition, the poorer long-term result is usually less important.

(iii) **Hitch-hike femoro-popliteal-tibial graft.**—A Dacron graft connects the common femoral artery to a rebored section of the upper popliteal artery. A vein graft connects the rebored section to arteries below the knee.

Salvage operations *should not* be performed for intermittent claudication alone. Gangrene and loss of limb may result if the operation should fail.

Adjuncts to Direct Arterial Surgery—(i) Lumbar sympathectomy in conjunction with direct arterial surgery, especially if the 'run-off' is poor. The other indications for sympathectomy are considered on p. 201. (ii) Blood-flow estimations (by flowmeter), or on-table arteriography at the completion of the operation are useful techniques for ensuring that there have been no errors of surgical technique before the wound is closed.

Results of Operation.—The long-term results of aorto-iliac reconstructive surgery are excellent. They are usually only marred by progressive disease producing femoro-popliteal occlusions at a later date. Femoro-popliteal surgery is less successful. The immediate post-operative success rate for vein bypass approaches 90%. Many cases fail in the first eighteen months after operation and at the end of five years the success rate is usually only 50–60%. The results of endarterectomy are less good in both short and long term and Dacron by-pass gives the poorest result with five year success rates of only 20–30%. The rather poor long-term results of femoro-popliteal surgery emphasise that these operations should only be used for clear indications.

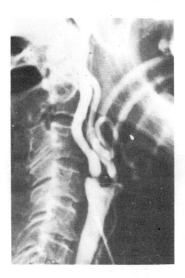

FIG. 183.—Carotid stenosis. A unilateral localised stenosis suitable for operation (see text). Also some narrowing of the external carotid. *N.B.* A rather similar double narrowing is seen in some carotid body tumours (Chapter 36).

Other Sites of Atherosclerotic Obstruction

The principles of arterial surgery as stated above can be applied to other arteries which are stenosed by the disease.

Carotid stenosis causes transient, recurrent, and progressive 'strokes' (hemiplegia). On the contralateral side to the stroke, a carotid arteriogram will show either a local stenosis at the origin of the internal carotid artery, or a complete obstruction of that artery up into the skull, to where the ophthalmic artery enters as a collateral. Only a local stenosis is suitable for the disobliteration and vein-patch operation (fig. 183). Special measures may be necessary to prevent cerebral damage occurring while the clamps are in place; postural hypertension (operating with the patient tilted head down) can be used, but a temporary silicone or polythene by-pass is more usual.

Extra/Intracranial Bypass operations using microsurgical techniques to anastomose the superficial temporal to a superficial cerebral artery are now being used in selected cases. Neurological, psychological (psychometry), arteriographic, and flow studies are included in the location of the cerebral area most under threat of ischaemia.

Subclavian artery stenosis causes ischaemic pain and a feeling of coldness in the arm and hand. Small patches of thrombus and atheroma break off as emboli, and occlude the arteries of the forearm, hand, and fingers. Endarterectomy of the second or third part of the artery may be performed.

Subclavian Steal Syndrome.—If the first part of the subclavian artery is obstructed, the vertebral artery provides collateral circulation to the arm, and its flow is reversed, as is demonstrated by arteriography. The cerebral circulation is diminished, hence the term 'steal'. Clinical features include syncopal attacks, visual disturbances, and diminished pulse and blood pressure on the affected side. A Dacron by-pass of the affected part of the subclavian artery, or thrombo-endarterectomy (rebore), relieves the symptoms. To avoid opening the chest the graft is usually taken from the common carotid artery of the affected side and anastomosed to the easily accessible third part of the subclavian artery.

Mesenteric Artery Stenosis.—Post-cibal central abdominal pain in a patient with atherosclerosis elsewhere may be shown by an arteriogram (lateral view) to be due to stenosis of the origin of the superior mesenteric artery. Usually the collateral circulation via the inferior mesenteric artery or coeliac artery has already been obstructed. The pain occurs so soon after food that the patient is afraid to eat. This classical syndrome is however a very rare cause of post-cibal pain. A by-pass graft is led from the aorta to the superior mesenteric artery, distal to the stenosis.

Renal artery stenosis may be responsible for some cases of hypertension (fig. 165). If the function of the kidney is satisfactory, the stenosis may either be by-passed or subject to balloon transluminal angioplasty (see above).

Coronary artery disease.—See Chapter 41.

Acute Arterial Occlusion

Sudden occlusion of an artery is commonly due to (A) emboli or (B) trauma.

(A) Embolic Occlusion

An embolus is a body which is foreign to the blood-stream and which may become lodged in a vessel and causes obstruction.

Simple emboli are due to blood clot. The sources of blood clot are most commonly mural thrombus following a myocardial infarct (one third of cases), mitral stenosis, cardiac arrhythmias, particularly atrial fibrillation, and aneurysms.

Emboli can lodge in any organ with resultant ischaemia and symptoms:

Lower limb—pain, pallor, paresis, pulselessness and paraesthesia (fig. 187).

Brain—the middle cerebral artery is most commonly affected, resulting in hemiplegia, permanent or temporary (transient ischaemic attacks).

Retina—Amaurosis fugax is fleeting blindness caused by the passage into the central retinal artery of a minute thrombus emanating from an atheromatous plaque in the carotid artery. Complete obstruction causes total and permanent blindness.

Mesenteric vessels—causing engorgement and possible gangrene of the corresponding loop of intestine (fig. 188).

Spleen—commonly affected with local pain and enlargement.

Kidneys—resulting in loin pain and haematuria.

Lungs—pulmonary embolism (Chapter 40) is a catastrophe which may fatally interrupt convalescence after operation.

Lower Limbs—acute arterial occlusion due to an embolus differs from atherosclerotic occlusion in that the occlusion is sudden. Indeed the clinical differences between these two causes of occlusion in the lower limb are as set out in figs. 184 and 185. It is essential to differentiate between these two causes of occlusion, because removal of an embolus within a few hours of onset of symptoms can result in a return to normal life, and prevention of amputation, whereas such dramatic results are not achieved in atherosclerotic thrombotic occlusion.

In embolic arterial occlusion

There is no preceding history of claudication.

A source for emboli can usually be found (*e.g.* recent M.I., cardiac arrhythmias, mitral stenosis, aortic aneurysm, artificial valve).

Loss of function occurs within 4–6 hours after the onset of pain (*e.g.* patient unable to move toes).

In atherosclerotic narrowing with thrombosis

There is a preceding history of claudication.

A source for emboli cannot be found.

Loss of function not present within hours (because collaterals have had time to be established).

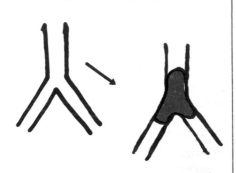

FIG. 184.—Aortic Bifurcation Embolus. Source for embolus—Recent M.I., A.F. = Severe dramatic symptoms.

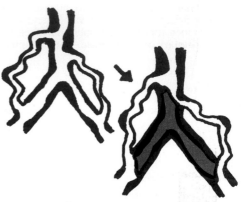

FIG. 185.—Aortic Bifurcation. Thrombosis. No source of embolus but previous claudication. Claudication worse but no dramatic event.

Embolic arterial occlusion is therefore an emergency, requiring treatment immediately the diagnosis is made (not for reassessment the next morning).

Clinical Features.—In the legs, the dramatic symptoms which occur when major vessels are occluded deserve re-emphasis—Pain, Pallor, Paresis, Loss of Pulsation and Anaesthesia (fig. 186). The limb is cold and almost immediately the toes cannot be moved (contrast venous occlusion when muscle function is not affected).

The diagnosis can be made clinically in the majority of cases. The patient, who has no previous symptoms of claudication or limb pain, and has a source of emboli, suddenly develops severe pain or numbness of the limb which becomes cold with mottled blue and white discoloration. Movement of the toes becomes progressively more difficult and sensation to touch is lost. Pulses are absent distally but the femoral pulse may be palpable (even thrusting) if the clot is lodged in a low bifurcation of the femoral artery. This is because distal occlusion results in forceful expansion of the artery with each pressure wave, despite the lack of flow.

Treatment. Because of the ensuing stasis the thrombus can extend distally and proximally. The early administration of heparin (5000–10,000 units) by continuous infusion can reduce this extension and maintain patency of the distal vessels until the embolus can be treated.

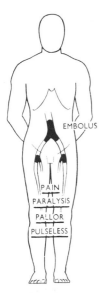

FIG. 186.—The symptoms and signs of embolism (Four P's). The fifth feature, anaesthesia, is often stated to be paraesthesia (the fifth P), but, in truth, complete loss of sensation in the toes and feet is characteristic.

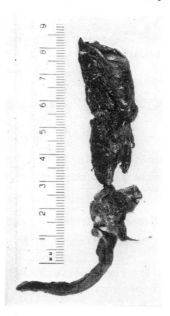

FIG. 187.—Aortic embolectomy. The extension-thrombosis extended proximally up to the renal, and distally into the iliac arteries.

The relief of pain is essential because it is severe and constant. Embolectomy is the treatment of choice in most patients with limb emboli.

Embolectomy and Thrombectomy.—Local or general anaesthesia is used, dependent upon the patient's general condition and the scope of the proposed operation. The artery, bulging with clot, is exposed and held up by slings or fine rubber tubing. Through a longitudinal or transverse incision the clot begins to extrude and is removed, together with the embolus (fig. 187). Arterial clamps are applied as bleeding occurs, special note being made of the degree of retrograde bleeding (back bleeding). *Fogarty Catheterisation.* This is the most effective method of removing proximal and distal extension thrombus and also allows an embolus or thrombus to be removed from a vessel remote from the arteriotomy. The Fogarty catheter is like a ureteric catheter, with a balloon tip, and is introduced until it is deemed to have passed the limit of the thrombus. The balloon is inflated and the catheter withdrawn slowly, together with the clot. The procedure is repeated until bleeding occurs. The method is valuable in patients with an aortic bifurcation embolus, since the clot and embolus can be extracted by insertion of balloon catheters via the common femoral arteries in the groin and the patient is saved from a laparotomy. Post-operatively, anticoagulant therapy is commenced. *Other special measures* may sometimes be required to extract extension thrombus: (*a*) application of a spiral rubber bandage from below upwards, (*b*) retrograde flushing with heparinised Hartman's solution (1000 units in 150 ml).

In *axillary artery thrombosis*, it is often necessary to expose and even open the brachial artery at the elbow to be sure that it is free of clot or another embolus.

Papaverine sulphate (1% solution) painted on to the arteries may help to relieve post-operative spasm (Kinmonth).

Prevention of further emboli is achieved by treatment of the cause whenever possible, and by reducing the chance of further thrombus formation by using long term anticoagulation with Warfarin.

Fibrinolysins.—Fibrinolytic agents (*e.g.* streptokinase, urokinase) are used to lyse an acute thrombus or embolus without resorting to surgery. They are more effective in acute thrombosis than in embolism and are usually given in an intravenous infusion. Infusion intra-arterially through a catheter whose tip is close to the obstruction is more effective but carries a higher complication rate from haemorrhage and infection. Infusion of fibrinolysins through a catheter in the right ventricle or pulmonary artery may be very effective in certain cases of severe pulmonary embolism. Certain forms of venous thrombosis (*e.g.* ilio-femoral) may also be treated. Heparin should not be used concomitantly with fibrino-

Thomas J. Fogarty, Contemporary. Surgeon, University of Oregon Medical School, Portland, U.S.A.
John Bernard Kinmonth, 1916–1982. Professor of Surgery, St. Thomas's Hospital and University of London.

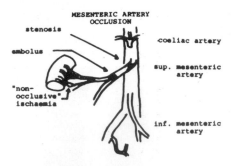

FIG. 188.—Mesenteric artery occlusion, thrombotic, embolic and non organic (non-occlusive) ischaemia (see text).

lysins. The patient should also be carefully observed for the appearance of anaphylactic reactions.

Mesenteric artery occlusion (fig. 188)

Acute mesenteric occlusion can be (1) thrombotic (following atherosclerotic narrowing), (2) embolic, or (3) non-organic in aetiology.

(1) *Thrombotic* occlusion follows progressive narrowing, and so the symptoms are progressive with *weight loss, abdominal pain* (usually postprandial) and *leucocytosis*. Once the abdominal pain becomes severe then diarrhoea, systemic hypovolaemia and haemoconcentration occur. By this stage the patient is ill out of proportion to the physical signs.

(2) *Embolic* occlusion results in sudden severe abdominal pain, with bowel emptying (vomiting and diarrhoea), with a source of emboli present (usually cardiac). Arteriography and embolectomy or bypass surgery can reduce the otherwise high mortality in these patients.

(3) *Non-organic obstruction* is due to severe constriction of the mesenteric capillary bed. It follows severe illness such as cardiac failure, systemic shock, hypotension or severe dehydration. The patients present with abdominal pain, few physical signs, but 75% have positive occult blood in the faeces. The symptoms then progress to back pain, vomiting, diarrhoea, marked leucocytosis and unexplained metabolic acidosis. Angiography and then intra-arterial injection of vasodilators via the catheter accompanied by systemic antibotics and protein infusion can reverse the otherwise high mortality (and see Chapter 51).

Other causes of Embolism

Air Embolism.—Air may be accidentally injected into the venous circulation (*e.g.* artificial pneumothorax), or sucked into an open vein. Thus venous air embolism occasionally complicates operations on the neck or axilla if a large vein is inadvertently opened, or it may be an accessory cause of death following a cut throat. The risks associated with intravenous infusion are reduced by the use of a drip chamber containing a spherical plastic float which plugs the exit when the fluid falls to a dangerous level.

When air enters the right atrium it is churned up, and the foam enters the right ventricle and causes an air-lock in the pulmonary artery, which may end in right-sided heart failure.

Treatment.—Trendelenburg's position encourages air to pass into the veins of the lower half of the body, and the patient is placed on the left side so that air will float into the apex of the ventricle, away from the pulmonary artery. Oxygen is administered to counteract anoxaemia, and to assist in the excretion of nitrogen. In serious cases the right ventricle should be aspirated by a needle passed upwards and backwards from below the left costal margin. If this fails, the heart is rapidly exposed for aspiration under direct vision.

Air may occasionally enter the left side of the heart, *e.g.* at open heart surgery, following puncture of a pulmonary vein during artificial pneumothorax or through a patent foramen ovale (paradoxical embolism). It may from there embolise coronary or cerebral arteries. Treatment is along similar lines to venous air embolism.[1]

Fat Embolism.—This condition, which is more common than generally supposed, usually follows severe injuries with multiple or major fractures. Cases have also been recorded following convulsive therapy. The fat may be derived from bone marrow or adipose tissue but recent work suggests that it is metabolic in origin, perhaps by aggregation of chylomicrons. Symptoms are evident a day or so after injury, and two more or less distinct types, cerebral and pulmonary, are recognised. In the cerebral type, the patient becomes drowsy, restless, and disorientated (delirium tremens may be suspected). Subsequently he is comatose, the pupils become small and pyrexia ensues. The pulmonary type is ushered in with cyanosis, which increases in intensity, and signs of right heart failure. White froth may occur at the mouth and nostrils. It may be mistaken for bronchopneumonia or left ventricular failure.

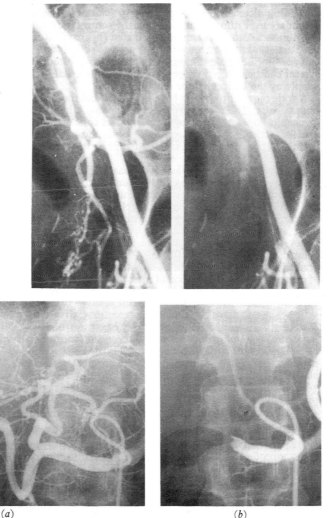

FIG. 189.—Before and after therapeutic embolisation of the internal iliac artery in a patient with gross haematuria from an ulcerating bladder carcinoma.
(*F. McIvor FRCR, London.*)

(*a*) (*b*)

FIG. 190.—(*a*) Before and (*b*) after embolisation of common hepatic artery bifurcation in a patient with the carcinoid syndrome.

---

[1]Air embolism is also a risk following Fallopian tube insufflation, and following illegal abortion. The air may travel to the brain via the paravertebral veins.

Gabriele Fallopio, 1523–1562. Professor of Anatomy, Surgery and Botany, Padua, Italy.

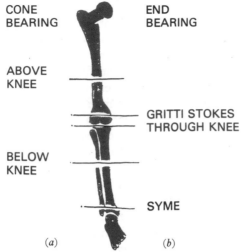

CONE BEARING

END BEARING

ABOVE KNEE

GRITTI STOKES THROUGH KNEE

BELOW KNEE

SYME

(a)   (b)

FIG. 201.—Choice of site (a) Cone bearing and (b) End bearing amputations.

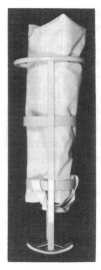

FIG. 203.—Inflatable artificial limb.

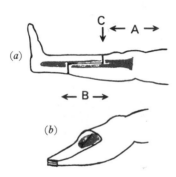

C ↓ ← A →

(a)

← B →

(b)

FIG. 202.—Below knee amputation (long posterior flap) (a) measurements. Anterior flap A = 15 cm from knee joint. Posterior flap B = 15 cm long. Anterior incision C = $^2/_5$ diameter of calf at this point. (b) Tibial stump with oblique anterior surface, and long posterior muscle/skin flap tapered distally.

than 7·5 cm) can make the end result unsatisfactory. In the severely ischaemic atherosclerotic limb, the risk of failure of stump healing with subsequent demoralising further amputation, influences many surgeons to elect in the first instance for amputation at a higher level.

Below Knee amputations

Two types of skin flap are commonly used, equal anterior and posterior flaps, and the long posterior skin flap. Whatever method is chosen it is wise to remember the old rule that the total length of flap or flaps will need to be at least one and a half times the diameter of the leg at the point of bone section. One can always trim (subtract) but not add!

Long posterior flap below knee amputation.—In cases of trauma a tourniquet is applied at the thigh, but *not* in cases of ischaemia due to atherosclerosis or embolus. Fig. 202 depicts the marking of skin flaps. Anteriorly the incision is deepened to bone, and the lateral and posterior incisions are fashioned to leave the bulk of the gastrocnemius muscle attached to the flap, muscle and flap being transected together at the same level. If bleeding is inadequate the amputation is refashioned at a higher level (a 7·5 cm bone stump being the barest acceptable minimum (see preoperative consent above)).

Blood vessels are identified and ligated. Nerves are not clamped but pulled down gently and transected as high as possible. Vessels in nerves are ligated. The fibula is divided obliquely as high as possible, using a Gigli wire saw, the skin and muscle being retracted to avoid damage. The tibia is cleared and transected at the desired level, the anterior end

Leonardo Gigli, 1863–1908. Obstetrician. Director, Santa Maria Nuova Hospital, Florence, Italy.

of the bone at section being sawn obliquely before the cross-cut is made. This, with filing gives a shape which anteriorly prevents pressure necrosis of the flap. The long muscle/skin flap is tapered (fig. 202), the area is washed with saline to remove bone fragments and the muscle and fascia sutured with catgut or O Dexon to bring the flap over the bone ends. Drains are placed deep to the muscle and brought out through a stab incision in the skin. The skin flap should lie in place with all tension taken by the deep sutures. Interrupted skin sutures are inserted. Redivac drains can be attached to the skin by adhesive tape (*e.g.* Elastoplast®) instead of sutures, thus allowing removal of the drain without taking down the stump dressing. Gauze, wool and crepe bandages make up the stump dressing.

Above knee amputation. The site is chosen as indicated above, but may need to be higher if bleeding is poor on incision of the skin. Equal anterior and posterior skin flaps are made curved to join each other laterally and of sufficient total length (one and a half times the anterior/posterior diameter of the thigh). Skin, deep fascia, muscle are transected in the same line. Vessels are ligated. The sciatic nerve is pulled down and transected cleanly as high as possible and the accompanying artery ligated. Muscle and skin are retracted, the bone cleared and sawn at the point chosen. Haemostasis is achieved. The muscle ends are grouped together over the bone by means of strong catgut mattress or purse-string sutures incorporating the fascia. Two suction drains deep to the muscle are brought out through the skin clear of the wound and affixed with Elastoplast® so that removal can take place without disturbing the stump dressing. The fascia and subcutanous tissues are further brought together so that the skin can be apposed by interrupted sutures without tension. Gauze, wool and crepe bandages form the stump dressing.

In Gritti-Stokes and Through Knee amputations, a long posterior flap is now preferred. In the Gritti-Stokes type, the section is transcondylar.

In Syme's amputation it is essential to preserve the blood supply to the heel flap by meticulous clean dissection of the calcaneum. The tibia and fibula are sectioned as low as possible to the top of the mortice joint.

Postoperative Care of an Amputation

Pain relief.—Amputation is a morally and physically degrading procedure and to add unnecessary pain is inexcusable. Diamorphine or other opiates should be given regularly, and the reader should refer to the special section concerning pain relief in Chapter 5.

Care of the good limb. Attention is focused on the amputation, but a pressure ulcer on the good foot will delay mobilisation, despite satisfactory healing of the stump. The use of a cradle to keep the weight of bed clothes off the foot, and a 'sheep skin' (p. 216) are adjuncts to good nursing care.

Exercises and Mobilisation. Immediately, the prevention of flexion deformity can be achieved by the use of a cloth placed over the stump with sand bags on each side to weight it down. Once the drains have been removed exercises are started to build up muscle power and coordination. The initial stump dressing can usually be left in place until the skin sutures are removed. The stump bandage is then applied each day to mould the shape of the stump. Mobility is progressively increased with walking between bars and the use in some centres of an inflatable artificial limb which allows weight-bearing to be started before a pylon or temporary artificial limb is ready (fig. 203). It is emphasised that the whole episode in the patient's life should be conducted in an attitude of promotion through the stages towards full independence. Early assessment of the home (part of the whole programme) allows time for minor alterations, such as the addition of stair rails, movement of furniture to give support near doors, and clearance in confined passages.

Complications.—*Early*, include the following: reactionary haemorrhage, which requires return to the theatre for operative haemostasis; a haematoma, which requires

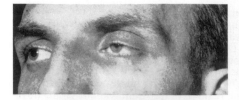

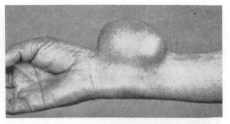

FIG. 205.—Saccular aneurysm of the radial artery.
(*Professor A. K. Toufeeq, FRCS,Lahore, Pakistan.*)

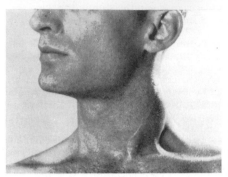

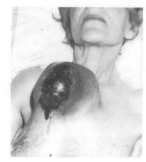

FIG. 204.—A false, and rapidly extending aneurysm of the common carotid caused by a stab wound. Note (above) the ptosis, myosis, and enophthalmos of a Horner's syndrome, due to concomitant severance of the cervical sympathetic nerve.

FIG. 206.—An aortic aneurysm has eroded the sternum and is about to rupture.
(*The late Raymond Helsby, FRCS, Liverpool.*)

evacuation; infection, usually from a haematoma. Any abscess must be drained. Depending upon the sensitivity reactions of the organisms cultured, the appropriate antibiotics are given. Gas gangrene can occur in a mid-thigh stump—the organisms coming from contamination by the patient's faeces.

Wound dehiscence and gangrene of the flaps are due to ischaemia, and a higher amputation may well be necessary. Fat embolism is another but uncommon sequel, occurring within the first two days.

Late.—Pain is usually the presenting symptom, due to: unresolved infection, *e.g.* a sinus, osteitis, sequestrum (even a complete 'ring' sequestrum); a bone spur; a scar adherent to bone; an amputation neuroma from the outgrowth of nerve fibrils which become attached to skin, muscle or fibrous tissue; a phantom limb.

Phantom Pain.—Patients frequently remark that they can feel the amputated limb and sometimes that it is painful. The surgeon's attitude should be one of reassurance that these feelings will disappear. He should on no account foster the subject and talk about phantom-limb pain in front of the patient, as it is very refractory to treatment once it is established.

Other late complications include ulceration of the stump (pressure effects of the prosthesis or increased ischaemia). Rarely, an ulcer is artefacta (fig. 64). Some patients are troubled by cold and discoloured stumps, especially during the winter.

ARTERIAL DILATATION (ANEURYSMS)

Dilatations of localised segments of the arterial system are called aneurysms. They can either be *true aneurysms*, containing the three layers of the arterial wall in the aneurysm sac, or *false aneurysms*, having a single layer of fibrous tissue as the wall of the sac (*e.g.* aneurysm following trauma fig. 204, and as a mycotic aneurysm[1]). Aneurysms can be grouped according to their *shape* (fusiform, saccu-

---

[1] 'Mycotic' is a misnomer, as the cause is not due to a fungus but to bacterial infection.

Johann Freidrich Horner, 1831–1886. Professor of Ophthalmology, Zürich, Switzerland. Described the syndrome which bears his name in 1869. The effects produced by section of the cervical sympathetic chain had been noted previously by François Pourfour Du Petit (1664–1741) in 1710.

lar (fig 205), dissecting), or to their aetiology (atherosclerosis, traumatic, mycotic, syphilitic, collagen disease (Marfan's syndrome)).

Aneurysms can occur all over the body in major vessels such as the aorta, femoral, popliteal, subclavian and carotid arteries, or in smaller vessels, such as the cerebral, mesenteric, splenic and renal arteries. The majority are true fusiform atherosclerotic aneurysms.

Symptoms.—All aneurysms can cause symptoms due to EXPANSION, THROMBOSIS, RUPTURE, or the release of EMBOLI. The symptoms relate to the vessel affected, the site supplied, or the tissues compressed by the aneurysm. Emboli from an aortic aneurysm can cause ischaemia of the toes, and thrombotic occlusion of a popliteal aneurysm can cause gangrene of the foot.

Clinical Features of an Aneurysm.—(*a*) *Intrinsic.*—A swelling exhibiting expansile pulsation is present in the course of an artery. The pulsation diminishes if proximal pressure can be applied, and the sac itself is compressible,[1] filling again in two or three beats if proximal pressure is released. A thrill may be palpable, and auscultation sometimes reveals a bruit.

(*b*) *Extrinsic.*—Neighbouring or distal structures are affected. Thus pressure on veins or nerves causes distal oedema or altered sensation. In the popliteal fossa pressure eventually will cause gangrene. Bones, joints, or tubes (such as the trachea or oesophagus), are sometimes affected, but structures which are resilient, such as the intervertebral discs, often withstand prolonged pressure.

Differential Diagnosis.—1. *Swelling Under an Artery.*—An artery may be pushed forwards, *e.g.* the subclavian by a cervical rib, and thus rendered prominent. Careful palpation distinguishes this condition.

2. *Swelling Over an Artery.*—Transmitted pulsation is liable to be mistaken for that caused by expansion. However, posture may diminish pulsation; thus a pancreatic cyst examined in the genupectoral position falls away from the aorta, and consequently pulsation is less definite.

3. *Pulsating tumours*, such as bone sarcoma, osteoclastoma, and a metastasis, especially from a hypernephroma.

4. *An Abscess.*—Before making an incision into a swelling believed to be an abscess, *e.g.* of the chest wall (fig. 206), in the groin, in the axilla, or in the popliteal fossa, it is essential to make sure that it does not pulsate! This mistake has been made many times.

5. *A serpentine artery.* (*e.g.* innominate, carotid).

ABDOMINAL AORTIC ANEURYSMS

Abdominal aortic aneurysms, the commonest type of aortic aneurysms, are found in 2% of the population at autopsy: 95% are due to atherosclerosis, and 95% occur below the renal arteries.

Symptomatic Aneurysms cause either minor symptoms such as back pain and abdominal pain, or sudden severe symptoms when they expand and RUPTURE.

Asymptomatic Aneurysms are found incidentally on physical examination, x-ray or ultra-sound investigation.

---

[1] Large aneurysms are frequently full of mural thrombus and may not be compressible.

Antonin Bernard Jean Marfan, 1858–1942. Professor of Paediatrics, Hôpital des Enfants-Malades, Paris. Described this syndrome in 1896.

Ruptured abdominal aneurysms: abdominal aortic aneurysms can rupture anteriorly into the peritoneal cavity (20%) or posteriorly into the retroperitoneal space (80%). *Anterior rupture* results in free bleeding into the peritoneal cavity. Few of these patients get to hospital, and those that do have had a prolonged period of hypotension and shock; consequently the results of surgery are poor. *Posterior rupture* produces a retroperitoneal haematoma (fig. 207). There is a brief period in many of these patients when a combination of moderate hypotension and the resistance of the retroperitoneal tissues stops the haemorrhage. The patient remains conscious, but in severe pain. If no operation is performed, the mortality is 100%. Operation results in a better than 50% survival.

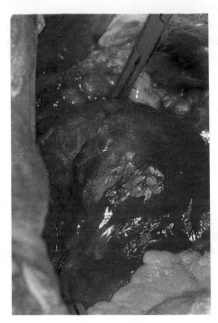

FIG. 207.—Operation for retroperitoneal hae-matoma of a ruptured aortic aneurysm. The patient is anaesthetised (on the operation table after towels have been placed—if in severe shock). Through a full length midline incision the small bowel is lifted to the patient's right side to expose the aorta and the haematoma lying behind the posterior peritoneum. The aortic pulsation is palpated through the haema-toma at its upper limit and fingers are insinu-ated each side of the aorta. With finger and thumb control the upper clamp is placed along-side and closed on the aorta. The procedure is then as for a planned case. In this illustration the clamp is at the proximal end of aneurysm, the haematoma has spread from the left para-colic gutter, to encircle the aneurysm and the aortic bifurcation.

To achieve these better results, the diagnosis must be made early. The clinical features include sudden severe back pain, accompanied in some cases by a brief loss of consciousness. The femoral pulses in one or both groins may be diminished or absent. A pulsatile mass is palpable in the abdomen, and there are signs of shock. The procedure is as follows: Two good infusion lines and a central venous pressure line must be inserted as soon as the patient arrives in hospital or the diagnosis made once admitted. Blood is sent for immediate cross-match of 15 units blood (7 litres). Infusion of saline or volume expanding fluids (Chapter 5) are given to raise the systolic blood pressure to approx 100 mmHg. Antibiotics and mannitol (p. 69) are given i.v. and a urinary catheter passed. If the patient appears to be stable, although in pain, operation may be delayed until crossmat-ched blood is ready.

Abdominal Aneurysms Without Rupture

Patients most commonly present with *pain*, usually felt in the back in the lumbar region, and upper abdomen. In addition pain can occur in the thigh and groin due to nerve compression. Gastrointestinal, urinary and venous symptoms can also be caused by abdominal aneurysm. 20% present complaining only of a *pulsatile mass*. As a general rule in the presence of a pulsatile mass, if the symptoms cannot be reasonably explained by another lesion, they must be assumed to be due to the aneurysm until proved otherwise, and the aneurysm placed in the symptomatic group.

Indication for Surgery.—1. *Symptomatic aneurysm*: without surgery, 80% with symptomatic aneurysms will be dead in one year. With surgery, 80% will be alive in one year. Surgery is indicated therefore (in patients who are otherwise medically fit). The risk of operation is increased particularly in the presence of hypertension, chronic airway disease, recent myocardial infarction and impaired renal function. Chronological age is not a bar to surgery, but few patients are fit enough for this type of procedure once over the age of 80.

2. *Asymptomatic aneurysms*: aneurysms found incidentally on examination, x-ray or ultrasound in an otherwise fit patient, need repair if they are over 7 cm in diameter on clinical examination, or over 6 cm in diameter on ultrasound. The incidence of rupture rises from 5% in aneurysms that are 5 cm in diameter to 75% in those that are 7 cm in diameter. As surgery carries a 2–10% mortality, the balance is in favour of surgery once the diameter is above 6 cm, provided there are no medical contraindications to surgery (see symptomatic aneurysms above).

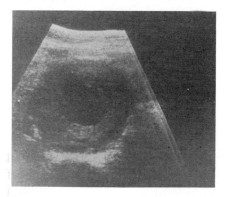 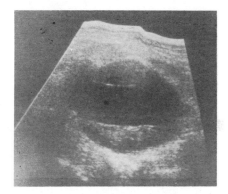

FIG. 208.—Ultrasound of an aortic aneurysm showing the large clot filled sac with a small central lumen (transverse and longitudinal scan).

Investigation: after taking a careful history and examining the patient, the following investigations are performed. Urine analysis to exclude diabetes in particular. Haemoglobin estimation, full blood count, ESR, blood group and cross match if surgery is contemplated within a few days, ECG, liver function tests, blood lipids, electrolytes and urea, chest x-ray, x-ray of abdomen, with a lateral view to show calcification in the aneurysm if present, and ultrasound of the abdomen (fig. 208).

An aortogram is *not indicated* in most cases because the cavity of the aneurysm is often filled with clot, and so the aneurysm is not demonstrated. Ultrasound gives better definition of the extent of the aneurysm, and is non-invasive. An aortogram is only indicated if it is suspected clinically that the renal arteries are

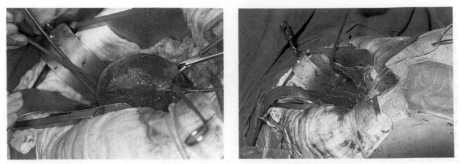

FIG. 209.—Aortic aneurysm at operation. (1) The aneurysm exposed. (2) A straight woven Dacron graft sutured within the aneurysm sac.

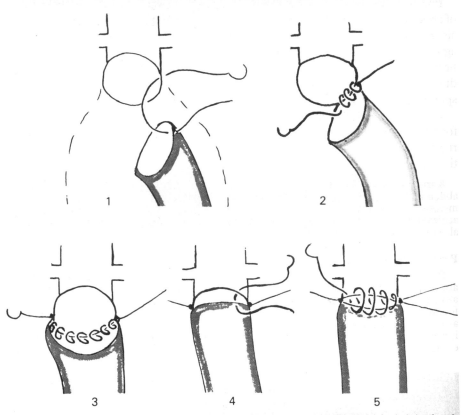

FIG. 210.—Aortic aneurysm repair (end to end within aneurysmal sac). The initial stitch is placed at '2 o'clock', leaving two-thirds of the diameter posteriorly (1). The posterior continuous sutures are placed (2) and completed (3). The anterior suture line started at the initial stitch (4) and the anterior suture line completed (5).

involved in the aneurysm (or if claudication is present). Involvement of the renal arteries by the abdominal aneurysm should be suspected if it is not possible to palpate the upper limit of the aneurysm below the xiphysternum with the patient lying flat (only 5% of cases).

Surgical procedure: (figs. 209 and 210). Under general anaesthesia, with the patient lying supine with a urinary catheter and central venous line *in situ*, a full length midline or upper transverse incision is made. The small bowel is lifted to the patient's right, and the aorta identified. The posterior peritoneum overlying the aorta is opened, and the upper limit is identified. A plane is sought between the aorta and vena cava below the left renal vein. The iliac arteries are then dissected free from surrounding structures, Heparin given, and clamps applied above and below the aneurysm. The aneurysm is opened longitudinally to the right of the inferior mesenteric artery, and back bleeding from lumbar and mesenteric vessels controlled by sutures placed from within the aneurysm sac. The graft is then sutured end to end inside the aneurysm sac (OO Prolene). The upper clamp is released and haemostasis achieved. The lower end is then sutured to the iliac bifurcation in a similar manner. Clamps are released carefully, to one leg at a time, because hypotension and arrhythmias can occur if release is too rapid. The aneurysm sac is then closed round the graft (fig. 211) and the posterior peritoneum closed to exclude the graft and suture lines from the intestine (to reduce the risk of fistula formation). The abdomen is then closed in layers.

Postoperative complications: the commonest complications following repair of abdominal aortic aneurysms are respiratory (lower lobe consolidation, atelectasis and 'shock lung'). Haemorrhage occurs in relatively few cases provided anticoagulation is not continued beyond the immediate operative period, and haemostasis is satisfactory at the end of the procedure. Ischaemia of the colon, due to lack of collateral supply occurs in 10% of all cases. It fails to resolve spontaneously in only 0.2% of cases.

Renal failure, infection of the graft and wound dehiscence are rarely seen following non-urgent procedures, but can complicate procedures for repair of ruptured aneurysms. Other complications are sexual dysfunction, fistula formation and spinal cord ischaemia.

Aorto-duodenal fistula is an uncommon but eminently treatable complication of abdominal aortic replacement surgery. It should be suspected whenever haematemesis or melaena occurs in the months or years after operation. A successful outcome is only achieved by prompt operation, separating aorta from duodenum, closing the holes, and also interposing some omentum.

Peripheral Aneurysms

Popliteal aneurysms: account for 70% of all peripheral aneurysms. Two thirds of them are bilateral. Three quarters develop complications within five years if treated conservatively. Careful examination of the abdominal aorta is indicated if a popliteal aneurysm is found because a third are accompanied by aortic aneurysms. Popliteal aneurysms present as a swelling behind the knee, or with symptoms due to complications such as severe ischaemia of sudden onset following thrombosis, ischaemic ulceration of the toes due to emboli, or pain and haematoma formation due to rupture. Surgery is indicated urgently

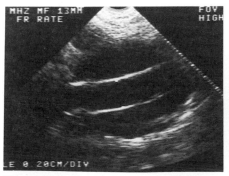

FIG. 211.—Aortic graft. Transverse scan showing the graft in the dilated aortic bed.

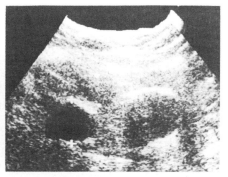

FIG. 212.—Ultrasound revealing bilateral iliac aneurysms.

in the presence of complications to prevent amputation, and in asymptomatic cases, to prevent complications. Diagnosis can be difficult, and relies on palpation of a pulsatile mass behind the knee. As a general guide, if the popliteal pulse is easily felt in a patient who is not thin, the presence of an aneurysm should be considered. Ultrasound and CT scan can be helpful in confirming the diagnosis.

Treatment: either a bypass graft with ligation of the aneurysm, or an inlay graft can be used, a local repair which is the modern application of Matas' reconstructive aneurysmorrhaphy.

Such a method is often applicable in the treatment of false aneurysms due to trauma where the opening is small and there is no infection (fig. 204).

Femoral Aneurysms.—*True* aneurysms of the femoral artery are uncommon. Complications occur in less than 3% and so conservative treatment is indicated initially. Look for aneurysms elsewhere, more than half are associated with abdominal or popliteal aneurysms.

False aneurysms of the femoral artery occur in 2% of patients after arterial surgery at this site. Mostly infective in origin, rupture is common, and so surgical treatment is indicated. Local repair with re-anastomosis at the groin under suitable antibiotic cover may be successful, but bypass, clear of the infected area, with subsequent excision of the infected part of the graft and coverage with a flap containing sartorius muscle is often the only way to prevent further problems.

Iliac aneurysms: usually occur in conjunction with aortic aneurysms and rarely occur on their own (1 in 12,000). When on their own, they are difficult to diagnose clinically and so 50% present already ruptured. Surgical treatment is indicated, with bypass, and exclusion of the aneurysm by ligation above and below the dilatation.

Aneurysms of the ascending aorta and arch require cardiopulmonary bypass for reconstruction to be undertaken. These, together with dissecting aneurysms of the thoracic aorta, and traumatic false aneurysms in that situation are considered in Chapter 41.

Arteriovenous Fistula (AVF) (**Arteriovenous Anastomosis** (AVA))—Communication between an artery and a vein (or veins) may be either a congenital malformation, or acquired by the trauma of a penetrating wound or a sharp blow. Arteriovenous fistulas are also created surgically in the forearms or legs of patients undergoing renal dialysis. All arteriovenous communications have a structural and a physiological effect.

The *structural effect* of the arterial blood flow on the veins is characteristic, as they become dilated, tortuous, and thick walled (arterialised) (fig. 213), and they also make the lesions diffuse and so render surgical procedures difficult.

Physiological Effect.—The combination of a leak from the high pressure arterial system and an enhanced venous return and venous pressure result in an increase in pulse rate and cardiac output. The pulse pressure is high if there is a large and persistent shunt. Left ventricular enlargement and, later, cardiac failure will occur. A congenital fistula in the young may cause overgrowth of a limb. In the leg, indolent ulcers may result from relative ischaemia below the short circuit.

Clinically, a pulsatile swelling may be present if the lesion is relatively superficial. On palpation, a thrill is detected and auscultation reveals a buzzing continuous bruit. Dilated veins may be seen, in which there is a rapid blood flow. Pressure on the artery proximal to the fistula causes the swelling to diminish in size, the thrill and bruit to cease, the pulse-rate to fall[1] and the pulse pressure to return to normal.

Arteriography confirms the lesion, which is noteworthy for the speed with which venous filling occurs. It is often difficult to pinpoint the actual site of the fistula.

Treatment.—*Congenital* lesions are usually stationary. Excision is advocated

---

[1] Known variously as Nicoladoni's (1875) or Branham's sign (1890).

Rudolph Matas, 1860–1957. New Orleans, U.S.A. Introduced aneurysmorrhaphy in 1902.
Carl Nicoladoni. 19th century Surgeon, Vienna.
H. H. Branham. 19th century Surgeon, U.S.A.

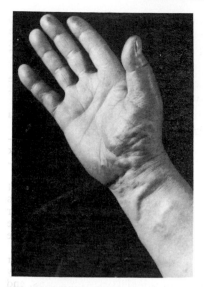

FIG. 213.—Post-traumatic arteriovenous aneurysm at the wrist. Note the prominent (varicose) arterialised veins.

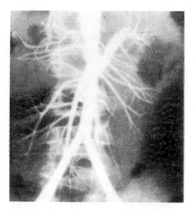

FIG. 214.—A by-pass vein graft from the aorta to the left renal artery in a little girl with bilateral renal artery stenosis, causing hypertension. The subclavian and other arteries were also occluded by Takayasu's arteriopathy (see text).

only for severe deformity or recurrent haemorrhage. It is often wise to enlist the aid of a plastic surgeon in order that proper ablation and reconstruction can be effected. Ligation of a 'feeding' artery is of no lasting value.

The *acquired* lesions tend to be progressive, and operation is indicated. The vessels are separated, and, if possible, repaired by suturing, any intervening sac being excised. Failing this, ligation of the involved artery and vein is required both above and below the lesion (quadruple ligation). Vein or Dacron grafts may be required.

ARTERITIS

Thrombo-angiitis Obliterans (Buerger's disease)

This is a condition characterised by occlusive disease of the small and medium size arteries (plantars, tibials, radial, *etc.*), thrombophlebitis (fig. 153) of superficial or deep veins, and Raynaud's phenomena occurring in male patients in a young age group (usually under the age of 30 years). Usually one or two of the three manifestations are present and occasionally all three. The condition does not occur in women or non-smokers. It is not, as used to be stated, more common in Russian Jews. Cases are seen in different races all over the world. Histologically, localised inflammatory changes occur in the walls of arteries and veins leading to thrombosis.

The usual symptoms and signs of arterial occlusive disease will be present. Gangrene of toes and fingers is common and progressive.

Arteriography sometimes shows a characteristic 'corrugation' of the femoral arteries as well as the distal arterial occlusions and helps to distinguish the condition from pre-senile atherosclerosis.

Other forms of arteritis (*e.g.* polyarteritis nodosa) must be excluded.

M. Takayasu, 1871– . A Japanese Ophthalmologist who studied in Tokyo, St. Thomas's Hospital, London and Breslau. (Conjoint MRCS, LRCP, 1896). Published paper on Takayasu's Disease in 1908.
Leo Buerger, 1879–1943. Professor of Urologic Surgery, New York Polyclinic Medical School, New York, U.S.A. Described Thrombo-Angiitis Obliterans in 1908
Maurice Raynaud, 1834–1881. Physician, Hôpital Lariboisière, and Professor Agrégé, Paris. Published his thesis 'De L'Asphyie Locale et La Gangrène Symetrique des Extrémités' in 1862.

Treatment.—The treatment is total abstinence of smoking, *i.e.* 'You can have your cigarettes or your legs, but you can't have both'! This will arrest the disease but not, of course, reverse established arterial occlusions. A mere reduction in smoking is not sufficient to prevent the relentless progression of this disease. Established arterial occlusions must be treated along the usual lines. Direct arterial surgery is not usually applicable and sympathectomy is the most useful surgical procedure. It often results in the healing of ischaemic ulcers and improvement in skin nutrition, with relief of pain. Amputations, conservative if possible, may be required.

Other types of arteritis are encountered in rheumatoid arthritis, diffuse lupus erythematosus, and polyarteritis. Treatment is similar. *Diabetes* is discussed on p. 216.

Temporal, Occipital and Ophthalmic Arteritis.—Localised infiltration with inflammatory and giant cells leads to arterial occlusion and features ischaemic headache and tender, palpable, pulseless (thrombosed) arteries in the scalp, and the major catastrophe of irreversible blindness when the ophthalmic artery is occluded.

A raised ESR and a positive scalp artery biopsy calls for immediate prednisolone therapy (20 mg tds) to arrest and reverse the process before the ophthalmic artery is involved. The dose must be reduced as soon as possible, in line with clinical improvement and a fall of the ESR, to a maintenance dose which is controlled under long term surveillance.

Takayasu's arteriopathy (obliterative arteritis of females, pulseless disease) causes narrowing and obstruction of major arteries and usually pursues a relentless course (fig. 214).

Cystic Myxomatous Degeneration.—Instances of an accumulation of clear jelly (like a synovial ganglion) in the outer layers of a main artery have been reported, *e.g.* the popliteal artery. The lesion so stiffens the artery that pulsation disappears, and claudication occurs when the limb is flexed (as on walking up stairs). Arteriography shows a smooth narrowing of an otherwise normal artery, and a sharp kink, or buckling, when the knee is flexed. Decompression, by removal of the myxomatous material, is all that is required, but the 'ganglion' may recur and require excision of part of the arterial wall and a vein-patch repair.

VASOSPASTIC CONDITIONS

Raynaud's disease usually occurs in young women, and affects the upper extremities more than the lower. The peripheral pulses are normal. The condition is attributable to abnormal sensitivity in the direct response of the arterioles to cold. When cooled, these vessels go into spasm, and as a result the part becomes blanched and incapable of finer movements. The decreased blood flow causes an accumulation of metabolites in the capillary circulation. The capillaries dilate and become filled with slowly flowing de-oxygenated blood, the part therefore becomes swollen and dusky. As the attack passes off, the arterioles relax, oxygenated blood returns into the dilated capillaries, the hands become red and a burning sensation or pain is produced by increase in tissue tension. Thus the condition is recognised by the characteristic sequence of blanching, dusky cyanosis and red engorgement. Eventually, in a minority of patients, obliterative changes may occur in the peripheral vessels, superficial necrosis occurs, the tops of the fingers undergo dry gangrene, and the distal parts of the terminal phalanges are absorbed. Early cases of Raynaud's disease must be distinguished from chilblains and vascular disturbances which are sometimes associated with the costoclavicular syndrome (Chapter 36).

Treatment.—*Conservative.*—Protection from cold, avoidance of pulp and nail-bed infections, and the use of vasodilator drugs are part of the conservative regimen that is advised for mild cases.

Sympathectomy.—The immediate results of sympathectomy are good, but after a few months the susceptibility to cold returns, although cyanosis is not so severe as before the operation, and subjective symptoms are less marked. This partial relapse is an indication that the underlying cause of Raynaud's disease is not in the sympathetic system, but is due to some abnormality in the smaller arteries and arterioles; sympathectomy apparently raises the threshold at which spasm occurs. From the practical point of view preganglionic section of the thoracic sympathetic chain can be recommended as a palliative procedure in Raynaud's disease, especially if performed before the onset of ulceration and absorption of the terminal phalanges.

Raynaud's Phenomenon.—Peripheral vasospasm also occurs secondarily to other organic diseases such as atherosclerosis, collagen diseases—especially scleroderma, Buerger's disease, cervical rib, *etc.* It also follows the use of industrial tools, *e.g.* pneumatic road drills and chain saws, which vibrate at certain frequencies. Also, in the arm, atherosclerotic stenosis of the subclavian artery, scleroderma, Buerger's disease, or cervical rib and the scalene syndrome (Chapter 36) may be responsible. Treatment is directed primarily to these causal lesions, though the conservative measures outlined above are often helpful. Sympathectomy may occasionally be required but it is not very helpful in scleroderma.

Raynaud's phenomena may also occur secondarily to atrophic changes in a limb, *e.g. after poliomyelitis, following trauma, e.g.* arthrodesis of a peripheral joint, crushing injuries, *etc.,* in cases of *severe chilblains* (perniosis) and *following frostbite.* The mechanism of the cold sensitivity in these cases is obscure but in most instances good results follow sympathectomy.

Acrocyanosis—*crurum puellarum frigidum*[1] may be confused with Raynaud's disease, but it is painless and is not paroxysmal. Affecting young females, the cyanosis of the fingers, and especially the legs may be accompanied with paraesthesia and chilblains. In severe cases sympathectomy may be necessary, and gives good results. If merely affecting the calves, a differential diagnosis is Bazin's disease.

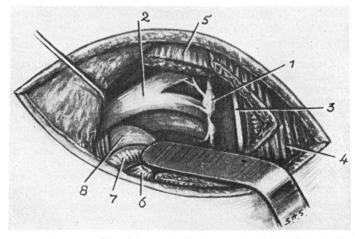

FIG. 215.—Exposure of the right cervicodorsal sympathetic chain from the front.

1. Stellate ganglion.	5. Divided scalenus anticus muscle.
2. Lower trunk of brachial plexus.	6. Divided posterior belly of the omo-hyoid.
3. Phrenic nerve displaced inwards.	7. Subclavian artery displaced downwards.
4. Partially divided sternomastoid muscle.	8. Dome of the pleura.

[1] Puellarum = of girls, frigidum = ? frigid or just cold.

Peirre Antione Ernest Bazin, 1807–1878. Dermatologist, Hôpital St. Louis, Paris.

Sympathectomy

Preganglionic Cervico-dorsal Sympathectomy.—(*a*) *Supraclavicular Method*.— Through a supraclavicular incision, the clavicular part of the sternomastoid, the posterior belly of the omo-hyoid, and the scalenus anterior muscles are divided, the phrenic nerve being displaced inwards. The subclavian artery is exposed, and the thyro-cervical trunk is divided. The subclavian artery is depressed and the suprapleural fascia is divided, so that the dome of the pleura can be displaced downwards. The stellate ganglion is identified as it lies on the neck of the first rib (fig. 215). The sympathetic trunk is traced downwards and divided below the third thoracic ganglion. All rami communicantes associated with the second and third ganglia and the nerve of Kuntz, a grey ramus running upwards from the second thoracic ganglion to the first thoracic nerve, are meticulously divided. Occasionally the approach is *under* a high arching subclavian artery.

(*b*) *Transthoracic Method*.—This gives a greater exposure and facilitates the removal of the sympathetic chain from the fifth ganglion up to the lower fringe of the stellate ganglion. It tends to give better results than (*a*), and can be employed when (*a*) has failed. In women where cosmetic effects are a consideration, the approach can be made via an axillary incision through the third space (Hedley Atkins). The sympathetic chain is easily seen and after dividing the pleura, it is dissected out, care being taken to avoid damage to the intercostal vessels, which may cause tedious haemorrhage. Care should also be taken, when making and suturing the approach wound, to avoid damage to the nerve to serratus anterior, giving rise to 'winging' of the scapula.

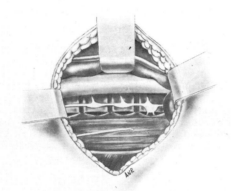

Fig. 216.—Left lumbar sympathectomy. The central retractor is holding back the peritoneum and ureter to expose the aorta and the psoas muscle, between which lies the sympathetic chain. Note that the second lumbar ganglion, adjacent to the lower pole of the kidney, has connecting rami to the spinal cord. The genitofemoral nerve is seen emerging through the fibres of the psoas.

Lumbar Sympathectomy.—Using a transverse loin incision, an extra-peritoneal approach is used in which the colon and peritoneum, to which the ureter clings, are stripped inwards so as to expose the inner border of the psoas muscle (fig. 216).

The sympathetic trunk lies on the sides of the bodies of the lumbar vertebrae, and on the right side is overlapped by the vena cava. Lumbar veins are apt to cross the trunk superficially. The sympathetic trunk is divided on the side of the body of the fourth lumbar vertebra, and is traced upwards to be divided above the large second lumbar ganglion, which is easily recognised by the number of white rami which join it. Care should be taken not to mistake small lymph nodes, lymphatics, the genito-femoral nerve or the occasional tendinous strip of the psoas minor for the sympathetic chain.

Usually both sides are done at one session.

Albert Kuntz, 1879–1957. Professor of Anatomy, St. Louis, Missouri, U.S.A.
Sir Hedley John Barnard Atkins, 1905–1983. Past President, The Royal College of Surgeons of England. Emeritus Professor of Surgery, Guy's Hospital, London.

CHAPTER 15

FRACTURES AND DISLOCATIONS—GENERAL PRINCIPLES

(INCLUDING OTHER MUSCULO-SKELETAL INJURIES)

Definitions

Fracture.–A fracture is a structural break in the normal continuity of bone. This structural break, and hence fracture, may also occur through cartilage, epiphysis and epiphyseal plate.

Dislocation.—A dislocation is a total disruption of a joint with no remaining contact between the articular surfaces.

Subluxation.—A subluxation is a partial disruption of a joint with partial remaining, but abnormal, contact between the articulating surfaces.

Mechanism of Injury

Tubular bone.—A tubular bone may be broken either by direct or indirect violence. For example the tibia may be fractured by direct violence if the bumper of a motor car strikes the bone or by indirect violence if a skier twists his body whilst the ski is held fixed. A bone fractured by direct violence is likely to be broken into several small pieces. Such a fracture is described as 'comminuted'. Indirect violence may be applied to a bone as a twisting force, in which case a spiral fracture results, or as a bending force, in which case a transverse or oblique fracture is produced. Double oblique fractures may occur so as to leave a 'butterfly' fragment separated from the two main pieces of bone (fig. 217).

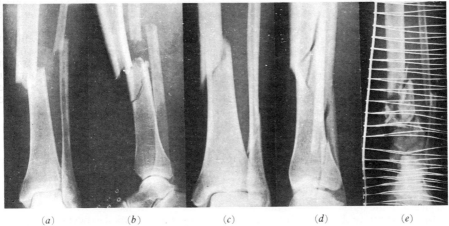

(a)	(b)	(c)	(d)	(e)

FIG. 217.—Fractures. (a) A transverse fracture. (b) A transverse fracture with an undisplaced butterfly fragment. (c) An oblique fracture. (d) A spiral fracture. (e) A comminuted fracture.

Cancellous bone.—Cancellous bone may be fractured either by compression or by tension.

Compression fractures may occur for example if a patient falls from a height and lands on his heels: the compressive force travelling up the leg and through the trunk may produce a crush fracture of a vertebral body, of the tibial or femoral condyles, or of the os calcis (Chapter 17). Such fractures are often impacted.

Traction injuries only occur in cancellous bone to which a ligament or tendon is attached, for example the medial malleolus. The bone is stressed by traction on the ligament. The fracture represents an avulsion of the bony attachment of the ligament and as such it is functionally equivalent to a rupture of the ligament. Such fractures are never impacted. Alternatively a tendon may avulse a significant fragment of bone as a result of vigorous contraction of its attached muscle, resulting in, for example, transverse fractures of the olecranon (triceps) (Chapter 16) or patella (quadriceps).

PATHOLOGY OF FRACTURE HEALING

Tubular bone.—A fracture of the shaft of a long bone disrupts the bone matrix, the periosteum and endosteum, the blood vessels in the medullary canal, in the cortex and in the periosteum, and the neighbouring soft tissues. The matrix, being inert, does not contribute to subsequent bone healing, but the blood vessels, periosteum and endosteum, and possibly the osteocytes in the involved bone do so.

The formation of callus (fig. 219).—The sequence of events in fracture healing is still subject to some dispute. *According to one hypothesis* ('haematoma' or 'induction') a haematoma is formed in the soft tissue spaces around the fracture site, the space between the fractured bone ends as well as in the medullary canal as a consequence of the disruption of blood vessels. This haematoma is invaded by granulation tissue as elsewhere in the body. Macrophages remove the haematoma at the apices of the capillary loops of which the granulation tissue is composed. At about two weeks, pluripotent mesenchymal cells derived from the surrounding soft tissues and from the endothelium of the capillaries lay down a loose connective tissue. This connective tissue which is composed of collagen fibres embedded in a dilute gel of proteoglycan subsequently becomes calcified and ossified over a period of weeks.

As the fracture haematoma becomes progressively organised and replaced by loose connective tissue, the bone ends become joined together. The repair tissue has very little rigidity or strength at this stage but from about three weeks a fibrocartilaginous tissue is formed. The matrix becomes increasingly calcified and later ossified so that the repair tissue between the fractured bone ends gradually becomes osseous. This repair tissue, known as *callus*, confers increasing rigidity and strength on the fracture and is now visible radiologically. Histologically, the repair tissue (callus) is composed of a randomly distributed mass of fibrous tissue, cartilage and woven bone. Thus, the fracture callus will be distributed throughout the area originally occupied by the fracture haematoma.

The second hypothesis of fracture healing denies the existence or participation of a fracture haematoma in the sense of a circumscribed tumorous mass. According to this hypothesis ('periosteal' or 'proliferative') the osteoprogenitor or 'bone-forming stem' cells of the periosteum and endosteum are stimulated to proliferate within hours of a fracture occurring. Over the next few days these membranes become several layers thick and in time a distinct collar of cells is formed around each fragment some distance away from the fracture site. The two *callus collars* grow progressively towards each other eventually to meet and fuse some two weeks after injury. This cellular response to injury is apparently intrinsic to the osseous tissues and has been referred to as '*primary callus response*'. It is a purposeful response to the disruption of the bone's mechanical integrity so that it is abolished by skeletal fixation (osteosynthesis) and enhanced by movement at the fracture site. The callus is not indiscriminately shed in all directions but advances from one fracture fragment to the other. It is not influenced by general systemic factors.

In addition to proliferating, the osteogenic (bone-forming) cells also begin to manifest signs of differentiation. As the cells proliferate, so do the capillaries amongst them but these do not grow as quickly as the osteogenic cells. The osteogenic cells closest to the shaft differentiate in the presence of abundant blood supply and become osteoblasts. In contrast, the cells farther away being in a relatively non-vascular environment differentiate into chondrocytes. Histologically, the fracture callus exhibits three layers merging into one another: bony trabeculae cemented to the shaft, an intermediate cartilage layer and an outer layer of proliferating osteogenic cells. In addition, the cartilaginous part of the callus is characteristically V-shaped since the wave of ossification begins from the shaft. The cartilage developing in a callus has a temporary existence only, however, and is eventually converted to bone by the process of endochondral ossification.

Whatever the mode of formation of the callus it is cemented to the original cortex. The anatomical dividing line between callus and cortical bone becomes increasingly blurred. Eventually the mass composed of callus and cortical bone is replaced by fully differentiated Haversian bone bridging the fracture site. At this point the bone returns to its original strength and rigidity but its anatomy and radiological appearance are still abnormal. Over the ensuing years, the mass of bone in the medullary canal and surrounding the fracture site is remodelled so that the anatomy of the bone gradually returns towards normal. This process involves osteoclastic resorption of redundant or poorly placed bone trabeculae and new bone formation as required.

Healing under conditions of rigid immobilisation.—When a fracture is accurately reduced and rigidly fixed with a plate and screws, the healing process is modified accordingly. An external callus is not formed, instead the fracture line gradually disappears. This has been referred to as 'primary bone healing' since it is believed that the union of the fracture fragments occurs without the participation of an intermediate tissue.

After fracture, the disruption of blood vessels and the arrest of bleeding within them leads to necrosis of bone in the areas immediately adjacent to the line of fracture. This dead bone is revitalised by the extension of the Haversian systems in the living portions. As time goes on the Haversian systems cross directly from one fracture fragment to the other. This involves osteoclasis and new bone formation so that the fracture gap is eventually sealed off. The process amounts to no more than the normal remodelling that takes place in a bone. It is slow and the patient may be dependent on his implant for several months.

Healing under conditions of non-rigid immobilisation.—Most traditional devices of internal fixation allow some movement at the fracture site. They can be regarded as bone sutures whose primary purpose is to maintain the position of the fracture fragments. Under these conditions, the external callus is still the medium by which the fracture fragments are bridged. Non-rigid immobilisation like less than perfect reduction is associated with more abundant callus formation. However, there is a limit to the amount of callus that can be formed so that ever increasing motion at the fracture site does not lead to an ever increasing amount of callus.

Cancellous bone

The pathological events following a fracture of cancellous bone are similar to those following a fracture of a tubular bone save that now the healing process occurs around a multitude of small fractures—one in each trabecula of the involved bone—rather than between the two large fracture fragments of the tubular cortex. Thus, although the histological events are similar, the *clinical and radiological appearances* are somewhat different because the fracture callus is spread evenly throughout a honeycomb of cancellous bone. Clinically, the principal difference is that abnormal motion and crepitus may never be present if the honeycomb structure is interlocked by the chance arrangement of the trabeculae at the fracture site. Such a fracture is said to be 'impacted'. Radiologically, the callus no longer appears as a bony mass surrounding the fracture site but instead may only be seen as a zone of increased radio-density (known as sclerosis) at the fracture site.

CLINICAL FEATURES AND DIAGNOSIS

There is usually a history of injury except in cases of stress fracture and some cases of pathological fracture. Immediately after the fracture has occurred the patient suffers local pain which ranges from mild to severe. The site of the fracture is tender, and within a few hours swelling and bruising appear. There is also some loss of function of the injured part which varies from minimal to complete.

If the bone ends have been displaced in relation to each other, deformity may be visible. It is often possible to elicit abnormal movement at the fracture site which is also associated with crepitus (a sensation of grating when the bone ends are moved against each other). The latter two signs should never be sought deliberately since their demonstration adds nothing to the diagnosis and merely causes pain and may result in further soft tissue damage and blood loss.

Radiography.—When a fracture is suspected on clinical grounds the diagnosis is confirmed by radiography. The bone can be seen to be fractured and the details of the fracture anatomy can be discerned. The minimum radiographic examination is only complete when radiographs of the whole bone have been obtained, including the joints in which it participates. Radiographs must also be obtained in two planes at right angles to each other (customarily antero-posterior and lateral). In certain circumstances oblique views may also be required to detect fractures, e.g. the elbow joint, the mandible.

FRACTURE DESCRIPTION

When a diagnosis of a fracture has been made, it is necessary to describe certain aspects of it fully in preparation for selecting appropriate treatment. The aspects needing description are summarised in Table 1.

TABLE 1. FRACTURE DESCRIPTION.

(1) Compound (open) or closed

(2) Site—which bone?
 —which part of bone?
- Intra-articular
- Epiphysis
- Diaphysis
- Metaphysis

(3) Fracture line
- Transverse
- Spiral
- Short oblique ± butterfly
- Comminuted

(4) Displacement
(5) Immediate complications

(1) **Compound (open) Fractures.**—A compound fracture is one in which a laceration in the skin (or mucous membrane) communicates with the fracture haematoma. Bacteria can therefore reach the fracture site. It may not always be possible to tell preoperatively whether a laceration adjacent to a fracture actually communicates with the fracture haematoma or not, but a combination of a laceration and a fracture should always be regarded as a compound fracture until surgical exploration proves otherwise. If the laceration proves not to communicate with the fracture, the latter may be termed 'technically compound'.

Lacerations associated with fractures may be caused either by a fracture fragment penetrating the skin from its deep surface (in which case the fracture is said to be compound 'from within'), or by the object causing the fracture, *e.g.* the bumper of a car, breaking the skin as well (in which case the fracture is said to be compound 'from without'). The chances of significant bacterial contamination of the fracture are greater in the latter and hence fractures which are 'compound from without' have a poorer prognosis.

However, it cannot be emphasised too strongly that the distinction between 'compound from within' and 'compound from without' is somewhat arbitrary and should not be allowed to alter the treatment recommended which is thorough exploration of the wound down to the fracture surfaces in all cases. Once there is any break in the skin surface it is possible for bone to exit and once this has occurred significant contamination of its surface can occur.

A break in the skin surface may be due to skin death from ischaemia rather than to a laceration. Fractures of subcutaneous bones with displacement may lead to pressure on the deep surface of the skin by a bony fragment and thus endanger the circulation to the skin. The reduction of such a fracture is urgent in order to preserve the skin. Injuries causing fractures by direct violence may crush the blood vessels in the skin but this may not be obvious at the time of the first examination. During the following 2 to 3 weeks the skin may slough and if this possibility is not borne in mind, a fracture may be encased in a plaster-of-Paris splint in which the skin may slough unnoticed.

There may of course be actual skin loss at the time of injury. Therefore, it must be assumed that any fracture in which the overlying skin is broken is contaminated with bacteria, either from the skin itself or from the surrounding environment. Such bacteria remain dormant in the fracture haematoma for a few hours following injury but soon thereafter start to multiply so that their number rises rapidly as time goes by. An inflammatory response develops locally and the fracture, from being contaminated, becomes infected. The chances of sterilising the fracture haematoma become increasingly remote as the number of bacteria at the fracture site rises. *Therefore the treatment of a compound fracture is a matter of urgency and should include antimicrobial precautions* (p. 245).

(2) **Site.**—In addition to recording the actual bone which is fractured it is necessary to describe the situation within the bone, especially in the case of long bones. The fracture may be at an end of the long bone in which case it will involve the joint in which the bone articulates; these are known as intra-articular fractures. Such fractures in children are known as epiphyseal fractures. The fracture may be in the diaphysis (shaft) of the bone or involve the metaphysis which is the flared region which joins the diaphysis to the articular portion of the bone.

(3) **Fracture Line.**—Reference has already been made to the various fracture lines which may result from injury, namely transverse, spiral, short oblique (with or without butterfly fragment) and comminuted. Transverse fractures are stable to compression if end to end contact is present. Spiral and short oblique fractures are unstable to compression.

(4) **Displacement.**—Displacement refers to the deformity which may be present following a fracture or dislocation and describes the position of the distal component relevant to the proximal component. For example, in the case of a posterior dislocation of the elbow the proximal forearm bones are displaced posterior to the distal humerus.

The causes of deformity are the initial force, gravity and, most importantly, the effect of contraction of muscles which are attached to the fractured fragments. Movement of the patient during administration of first aid, transport to hospital and during the course of initial assessment is also an important cause of deformity.

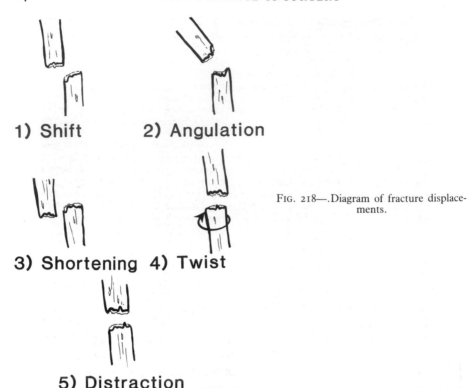

1) Shift   2) Angulation

3) Shortening 4) Twist

FIG. 218—.Diagram of fracture displacements.

5) Distraction

This can be diminished by the early application of temporary splintage.

In the case of a fracture of the shaft of a long bone there are five possible types of displacement (fig. 218):

(1) *Shift*.—This refers to loss of alignment of the cortices of the shaft.

(2) *Angulation*.—This refers to loss of the normal longitudinal axis of the shaft. Each of the above may occur in one of four directions; anterior, posterior, medial and lateral.

(3) *Shortening*.—This usually occurs due to overlap of the bone fragments but may result from impaction of one fragment into the other.

(4) *Twist (Rotation)*.—This refers to rotation of the distal fragment around the long axis of the bone, either external or internal.

(5) *Distraction*.—This rarely results from the injury but may be produced by over vigorous traction during treatment. This must be avoided because it is said to lead to delayed union of the fracture.

(5) **Immediate Complications**.—The initial assessment of a fracture is not complete without examination for immediate local complications, especially nerve and vascular status distal to the fracture and these must be recorded. Complications will be discussed later in this chapter.

Clinical Aspects of Fracture Healing

Union = the healing of a fracture by bone.—As the fracture haematoma becomes

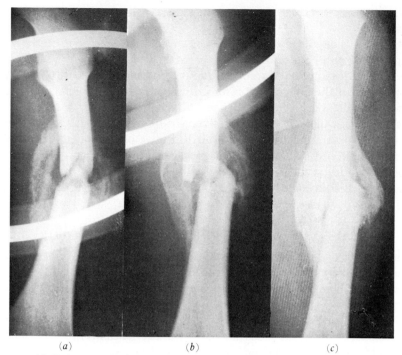

(a) (b) (c)

FIG. 219—. (*a*) Early callus formation. The calcified material does not have a bony texture and bridges the fracture site only as a vague 'cloud'. (*b*) Union. The callus now has a bony texture and bridges the fracture site but the fractured bone is easily visible, distinct from the callus. (*c*) Consolidation. The callus has a bony texture and is no longer clearly distinguishable from the femoral shaft.

TABLE 2

In general:
  (1) Lower limb fractures take twice as long to unite as upper limb fractures.
  (2) Fractures in adults take twice as long to unite as fractures in children.
  (3) Transverse fractures take longer to unite than oblique or spiral fractures.
  (4) Compound and comminuted fractures are particularly slow to unite.
  (5) No fracture unites in less than 3 weeks.

Thus, for example:
  (1) An oblique fracture of the humerus in a child takes 3 weeks to unite.
  (2) The same fracture in an adult takes 6 weeks.
  (3) A transverse fracture of the tibia in an adult takes 12 weeks, and
  (4) A comminuted fracture of the tibia in an adult may take 12–24 weeks.

organised to form fibrous tissue and subsequently woven bone, the abnormal movement originally demonstrable diminishes. Slight movement can, however, still be elicited, stressing the fracture site is painful, and local tenderness persists. At this stage the fracture is described as being 'sticky'. Between the third and sixth week following injury, the calcification and subsequent ossification occurring in the callus become visible radiologically (fig. 219(*a*)) and as this process progresses the fracture site becomes decreasingly tender and increasingly rigid and strong.

By approximately 6 weeks (the exact time varies with the age of the patient and the nature of the fracture—see Table 2) healing has progressed so that (1) no abnormal movement can be detected when the fracture is stressed, (2) stressing the fracture site is scarcely painful, and (3) local palpation provokes little or no tenderness.

This stage is described as '*clinical union*'. Radiologically, bone can be seen to bridge the fracture, but since the bone is partly woven rather than Haversian in structure, it does not have a normal radiological texture (fig. 219(*b*)). At this stage motion of the limb can be resumed without external splintage but totally unprotected stress is potentially unsafe and may lead to re-fracture.

As the woven bone of the callus is replaced by normal Haversian bone the fracture site becomes entirely painless irrespective of the patient's activity and the radiological texture of the bony mass surrounding the fracture site gradually becomes identical with that of the rest of the bone (fig. 219(*c*)). Such a fracture is described as *consolidated* and at this point the healing process can be regarded as having come to an end.

DELAYED UNION AND NON-UNION OF FRACTURES

The times by which fractured bones have usually united have been listed in Table 2, but these times are often exceeded.

Delayed Union.—When a bone still displays abnormal movement, pain when the fracture site is stressed, and tenderness over the fracture site at a time when union should have occurred, the fracture is said to display 'delayed union'. Because ossification of the callus has been delayed, the callus in such a bone may be invisible or poorly visible on an x-ray and, if visible, it may not bridge the fracture site.

Such a delayed union is known as 'atrophic' (fig. 220). A fracture displaying delayed union may continue slowly to heal until finally it unites. On the other hand there may be ample callus formation at the ends of each fracture fragment but the two fail to 'join together'. Such a non-union is known as 'hypertrophic' (fig. 221).

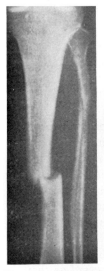 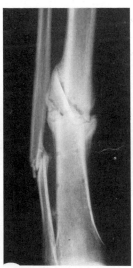 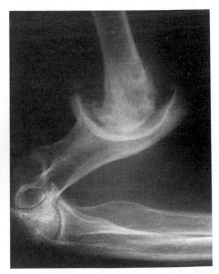

FIG. 220.—'Atrophic'   FIG. 221.—'Hypertrophic'   FIG. 222.—Pseudarthrosis.
      union.   non-union.

Pseudarthrosis.—However, the scar may be a long one and may even contain within it a cavity occasionally displaying all the tissue elements of a synovial joint. Such an abnormal joint is known as a 'pseudarthrosis' (fig. 222).

Persistent abnormal movement at a fracture site interferes with the function of a limb and the fibrous tissue in an un-united fracture is usually painful when stressed. Non-union is therefore usually unacceptable to the patient. Occasionally, however, a very firm fibrous scar forms so that, if the bone is not heavily loaded, as in the upper limb, the result is indistinguishable clinically from bony union.

The factors which influence the time for fracture healing are shown in Table 3.

TABLE 3. FACTORS INFLUENCING TIME FOR FRACTURE HEALING

Age
Constitution
Blood supply

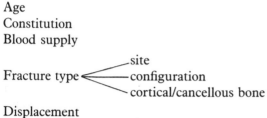

Fracture type < site
configuration
cortical/cancellous bone

Displacement
Soft tissue damage
Apposition of fragments
Immobilisation

The Causes of Delayed Union of Fracture

The causes of delayed union of fractures are shown in Table 4. Some of the more important ones are:

1. **Initial injury.**—Even in the absence of subsequent infection, compound fractures are more likely to develop delayed union. A severe initial injury, which can often be inferred by the presence of gross displacement and bone comminution, often produces delayed healing. This is most likely due to associated soft tissue damage which allows diffusion of haematoma and its contained cells into the soft tissues and somehow impairs subsequent mesenchymal cell proliferation. Extensive soft tissue damage also produces further impairment of the blood supply of the bone fragments.

2. **Infection** of the fracture haematoma usually leads to non-union and, if it occurs, is a disaster. Healing fails because the cellular elements which are required for the production of bone at the fracture site are diverted to the production of pus.

3. **Interposition of soft tissues** between the fracture fragments may so separate them that it is physically impossible for them to unite. For example, at the medial malleolus the tendon of tibialis posterior may come to lie between the medial malleolus itself and the rest of the tibia, or in spiral fractures of the femur a spike formed by one of the fracture fragments may become impaled in the muscles of the thigh. Such a fracture cannot be reduced (*i.e.* the bones ends cannot be accurately apposed) and healing by bone is obviously impossible.

4. **A poor blood supply at the fracture site** interferes with healing since the invasion of the haematoma by blood vessels is slow or absent. Cells with osteogenic potential are therefore slow to appear in the fracture haematoma. Furthermore there is some evidence that a low oxygen tension produced by a poor blood supply interferes with the production of bone by undifferentiated mesenchyme cells so that even such osteogenic cells as are present may fail to produce bone, and instead produce cartilage or fibrous tissue.

The anatomy of the fractured bone may result in a complete loss of the blood supply to one of the fracture fragments. For example in fractures of the neck of the femur, the vessels ascending in the neck of the femur to the femoral head may be ruptured by the fracture. The femoral head may then be completely infarcted, so that the healing process does not consist of the union of two vascularised bone fragments but, instead, involves the bridging of the fracture site from one side only, followed by revascularisation of the whole of the infarcted fragment. As might be expected, such injuries are either slow to unite or fail to unite altogether. Fractures of the waist of the scaphoid and neck of the talus may also be associated with similar problems.

5. **Inadequate immobilisation** leading to excessive movement at the fracture site during the healing phase may produce delayed union because the callus bridging the fracture site is constantly 're-fractured' by the movement occurring in the healing tissue. It may be speculated that shear, for example produced by torsion, is more harmful in this respect than is bending at the fracture site. Certainly minimal bending movements, such as occur in a fractured rib, are perfectly compatible with normal healing and may even promote it.

6. **Systemic disease,** for example uraemia developing as a consequence of renal failure secondary to blood loss following injury, may interfere with healing generally.

7. **Pathological fractures** due to malignant disease are often slow to unite and usually will not do so unless the local malignant disease is brought under control, for example by radiotherapy. The eventual outcome simply depends on the net result of two processes; new bone formation in an attempt to repair the fracture on the one hand and the destruction of the latter by the malignant process on the other.

8. **Distraction of the fracture fragments,** which is usually produced by the application of too much traction to the lower limb, often, but not always, leads to a delay in union. This is an iatrogenic cause of delayed union and should be avoided!

TABLE 4. THE CAUSES OF DELAYED UNION OF FRACTURES

Compound fracture	Inadequate immobilisation
Severe initial injury	Systemic disorder, e.g. uraemia
Infection	Pathological fracture
Soft tissue interposition	Distraction
Poor blood supply	

THE TREATMENT OF FRACTURES

The management of a fracture can be considered under two headings: (1) the management of the patient as a whole, and (2) the local management of the fracture itself.

General Management of the Patient

(1) **Pain.**—All fractures are painful and it should never be forgotten that the immediate responsibility of the physician is to relieve pain. This can be done by local splintage and by analgesics.

(2) **Blood Loss.**—All fractures are associated with some blood loss. This may be negligible, but in fractures of the major long bones, the spine, and the pelvis it can be considerable. Its loss, however, may not be immediately obvious. For example a patient suffering a fracture of the pelvis or of the shaft of the femur can lose 2 litres of blood into the surrounding tissues without any obvious swelling or bruising. Such blood loss must be replaced (Chapter 5).

(3) **Associated Injuries.**—Fractures are commonly associated with other injuries, for example fractures of the pelvis may be associated with injuries to the bladder, or fractures of a long bone shaft with injuries to the blood vessels or nerves in the limb. *The possibility of such injuries must always be borne in mind since they may be missed unless they are deliberately sought at the time of the first examination.*

(4) **Tetanus toxoid and antibiotics.**—In the case of compound fractures tetanus toxoid may have to be administered if the patient is not already fully protected. A broad-spectrum antibiotic which is effective against staphyloccus aureus should also be administered intravenously as soon as possible and continued for at least five days.

Local management of the fracture

General principles.—As in all branches of medicine and surgery, treatment must be based on an accurate diagnosis (fracture description) and accurate prognosis, for example if the patient is suffering from malignant disease a long period of conservative (non-operative) management is not indicated. Treatment should be selected with specific aims in mind:

(1) Pain relief.
(2) Obtain and maintain reduction of fracture.
(3) Allow and encourage union of fracture.
(4) Restore optimum function to injured limb and patient.

Treatment should be selected for the patient as an individual. Appropriate treatment for one patient may not be appropriate for another. *Treat the patient NOT the radiograph!*

A basic scheme for local management of the fracture is shown in Table 5. It is important not to forget the soft tissues which are just as important as the fractured bone.

For the soft tissues the objectives are: (1) to maintain muscle power and (2) to promote joint mobility. To some extent there is a conflict between these objectives and that of immobilising the fracture.

Severed blood vessels and nerves, and lacerations of the skin, require specific treatment.

TABLE 5. SCHEME FOR FRACTURE MANAGEMENT

Treat the patient NOT the radiograph.

1. Define fracture.
2. Detect complications.
3. Does the fracture need reduction?
4. Is the fracture unstable or stable?
5. How can the fracture be stabilised?
6. Does the fracture need immobilisation and for how long
7. How can the patient be best rehabilitated?

Reduction.—Reduction of the fracture (strictly, reduction of the deformity at the fracture site) implies restoration of normal, or perhaps more correctly, acceptable anatomy because, of course, absolutely normal anatomy is not always achieved, especially when treating fractures by closed means. If the original injury did not produce significant displacement, as for example in the fracture of the metacarpal displayed in fig. 223, no reduction is required. Should reduction be required it may be accomplished in one of several ways listed in Table 6.

TABLE 6. METHODS OF FRACTURE REDUCTION

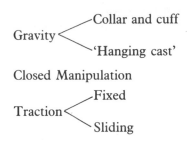

Closed Manipulation

Operation

Gravity.—Gravity can be used to reduce fractures in the upper limb, for example fractures of the surgical neck of the humerus or of the shaft of the humerus. This is achieved by placing the injured limb in a collar and cuff. The effect of gravity can be increased by adding a plaster of Paris cast which increases the weight of the limb and also provides some side-to-side stability for the fracture (fig. 224).

Closed manipulation.—Closed manipulation has the great advantage that the skin remains intact so that there is no possibility of the fracture site becoming infected. Therefore if closed reduction is possible, it is, in general, the treatment to be preferred. The patient is either given a general anaesthetic or the fracture site is rendered analgesic by local infiltration or by i.v. local anaesthesia distal to a tourniquet. Anaesthesia has the double effect of producing muscle relaxation so that the manipulation becomes easier, and of making the manipulation painless

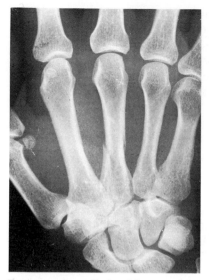

FIG. 223.—An undisplaced fracture of the shaft of 3rd metacarpal. The fracture is splinted by the neighbouring soft tissues and bones: neither reduction nor external splintage is required.

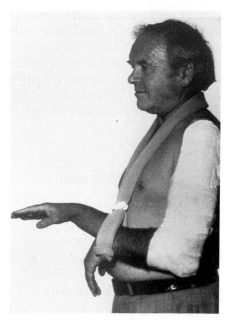

FIG. 224.—U-slab with collar and cuff sling.

for the patient. The bone ends are then manipulated in an attempt to restore the normal anatomy. The specific manipulations which are required for the reduction of common fractures are described in the following chapters, but the same general principle underlies the closed manipulation of all fractures: the surgeon seeks to reverse the mechanical events which led to the production of the original fracture. Thus an understanding of the mechanism of the injury is essential if closed manipulation is to be used intelligently.

For the reduction of some fractures, *e.g.* fractures of the shaft of the humerus or the femur, a formal manipulation is unnecessary and traction (see p. 251) alone suffices.

Traction.—Traction can also be used to reduce fractures, especially long bone fractures in the lower limb. Often it is combined with a preliminary manipulation, for example in the setting up of Thomas splint traction for a fracture of the femoral shaft. Traction is also used as a method of immobilisation and will be discussed further under that heading.

Operation.—Open reduction of a fracture may be required in the following circumstances:

(*a*) *Closed reduction may be impossible if soft tissues are interposed* between the fracture fragments. The fracture must then be exposed at operation to allow the soft tissue to be extracted and the bone ends brought into apposition.

(*b*) *Alternatively* it may be impossible to reduce a fracture by closed means because the surgeon cannot obtain any purchase on one of the two fracture fragments. For example in fractures through the anatomical neck of the humerus associated with anterior dislocation of the head of the humerus, closed manipulation is impossible since the head of the humerus is inaccessible save by operation.

(*c*) *A third situation* in which adequate reduction cannot be achieved by closed manipulation is that represented by fractures around joints in which there may be several small fracture fragments whose accurate replacement is essential if normal joint function is to be restored. Examples of such injuries are certain fracture-dislocations around the ankle and depressed fractures of the tibial condyles. Often the fragments cannot be manipulated at all, and certainly they cannot be manipulated accurately, through the skin.

Stability

A *stable fracture* is one in which the fragments do not have the potential to displace before or after reduction.

An *unstable fracture* is one in which the fragments readily displace before or after reduction.

For practical purposes, all fractures requiring reduction should be regarded as potentially unstable, because recurrence of the deformity is possible unless the fracture is stabilised (immobilised).

Stabilisation (Immobilisation)

Fractures require stabilisation to prevent mal-union and non-union. The methods available for stabilisation are summarised in Table 7.

TABLE 7. METHODS OF STABILISATION OF FRACTURES

External splint (plaster-of-Paris cast)
                External fixator

Internal splint (screws, plate, nail)

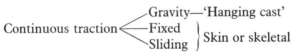

External Splint.—The strength and rigidity required in a splint are proportional to the forces applied to the fracture. Thus immobilisation is usually achieved partly by the use of splintage and partly by deliberately reducing the loads on the fracture site, for example by resting an injured arm in a sling or by walking only on the uninjured leg and crutches.

The most commonly used material for external splintage is plaster-of-Paris applied by wrapping the limb in a wet plaster-impregnated bandage. The plaster is allowed to set so as to hold the fracture in the desired position. Because it is almost impossible to obtain sufficient 'grip' on a single bone to withstand the forces imposed on the bone by contraction of the muscles attached to it, a plaster splint must always extend proximally and distally to include the joints adjacent to the fracture site. This constitutes a significant disadvantage to the use of plaster-of-Paris since it often means that when the plaster is removed the adjacent joints are stiff, the muscles weak, and the blood flow diminished. Other disadvantages include the facts that wounds cannot easily be treated in plaster, that adjustments in the reduction may be difficult to achieve, that the material is relatively heavy and radio-opaque and that it is not always easy to maintain a reduction whilst the plaster bandage is being applied. Having said this, plaster remains overall the safest, cheapest and most convenient form of splintage available. It has however one serious hazard attached to its use:

The Hazard of Plaster-of-Paris Splinting.—Plaster-of-Paris is inelastic. When a plaster is applied soon after injury it is to be anticipated that swelling will occur at the fracture site. Such swelling cannot distend the plaster and it will, therefore, result in a gradual rise in pressure in the soft tissues at the fracture site. This rise in pressure may occlude the venous return from the limb producing venous engorgement distally, and, shortly thereafter, an interruption in the arterial flow to the limb as a whole, or more commonly to a muscle compartment.

If the arterial inflow to a limb is obstructed for an hour or more, the muscles and nerves become infarcted and subsequently replaced by fibrous tissue. This sequence of events represents a significant hazard to the use of plaster-of-Paris and if it is allowed to occur, it constitutes a disaster the consequences of which are very much more grave than any which could possibly follow total failure to treat the fracture. *Thus if plaster-of-Paris is to be applied to a fresh fracture, it is essential that the plaster should not completely surround the limb.* This may be achieved either by applying a slab of plaster to the limb leaving a wide gap on one side of the limb, or by splitting a completely encircling plaster (fig. 225). Any such plaster should be well padded with wool so that swelling may occur without compressing the soft tissues and the limb should be elevated after its application.

The clinical features of an impaired blood flow are progressive in nature. The circulation in the exposed skin distal to the fracture should be examined carefully in the hours following the application of the plaster and any sign of an interruption of the blood supply (*i.e.* pallor or poor capillary filling in the limb) should be regarded as an indication that the blood supply is possibly impaired. In this event the whole plaster should be opened and all padding should be separated so that the skin is visible throughout the length of the split in the plaster. Should significant swelling occur, the patient will notice increasing discomfort and pain both at the fracture site and distal to it. These symptoms should also be regarded as an indication for easing a plaster encircling a limb. If the arterial inflow actually becomes interrupted so that the blood supply to the muscles is impaired, active movement of the muscles will become impossible (*e.g.* the fingers will be stiff) and attempts to stretch the involved muscles by passive movement will be painful. *The pulse is weak or absent. The detection of these signs is an urgent indication for the removal of plaster* and, *if this does not improve the circulation, for exploration for the appropriate main artery.* It should be emphasised however that the distal pulses may be normal in the presence of significant ischaemia to muscle compartments (see 'compartment syndrome' later in this Chapter).

If infarction is allowed to occur so that fibrosis of the muscles and nerves ensues, the resulting fibrous tissue contracts to produce deformity, stiffness, and weakness at the involved joints. This syndrome is known as *Volkmann's Ischaemic Contracture* (fig. 226).

External Skeletal Fixation.—As an alternative form of splintage to plaster-of-Paris, Steinmann or other pins may be passed through the bone proximal and

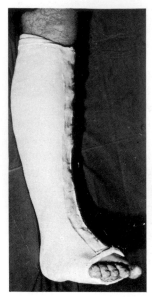

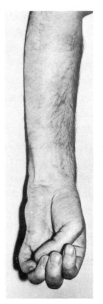

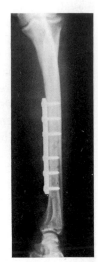

FIG. 225.—A split plaster-of-
Paris cast.

FIG. 226. — Volk-
mann's ischaemic
contracture following
a supracondylar frac-
ture of the humerus
in childhood.

FIG. 227.—Intern-
al fixation: the
onlay plate is firmly
held to the bone by
well-placed screws.

distal to a fracture and the pins then connected to a special metal frame. This method of fixation is particularly useful if the fracture is compound so that access is required to a wound. It provides very rigid fixation, is easily adjustable and is light. The disadvantage is the necessity of using pins to transfix the bone: these expose the bone to the risk of infection and are difficult to pass in other than subcutaneous bones such as the tibia. In practice therefore the method is used for compound fractures of the tibia (fig. 228).

Internal Splints.—*Methods of Internal Fixation by Operation.*—A variety of devices is available to splint fractures internally. The fracture fragments may be wired or screwed together or united by one, or rarely two, onlay plates screwed to the bone (fig. 227) or by a nail passed down the medullary canal (Chapter 17). Special devices are available for certain fractures, such as the pin and plate used for fractures of the proximal femur.

If it is felt that a fracture fragment cannot survive usefully—a decision which is sometimes made, for example, in connection with the head of the femur after fractures of the femoral neck—the bone may be removed and replaced with a prosthesis (Chapter 17).

It is argued that, if internal fixation is to be used at all, it should be as strong and as rigid as possible since this allows the joints of the limb to be mobilised early, free of external splints.

Strong, rigid implants have been designed for this purpose and techniques have been developed for enhancing the quality of fixation by applying the implant in such a way as to compress the fracture site (fig. 227). In long bone shaft

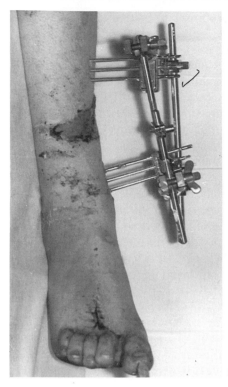

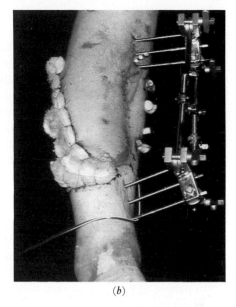

(b)

FIG. 228.—External skeletal fixators (a) Hoffmann type, (b) Thackray type. Both allow inspection and dressing of wounds (p. 249).

(a)

fractures this is done with an onlay plate, a technique known as 'compression plating'.

Internal fixation is technically difficult in comminuted fractures and in fractures through cancellous bone.

Traction.—Fractures may be immobilised by exerting traction on the involved limb. The way in which traction immobilises a fracture may be understood by likening the fracture and the adjacent joints to a bicycle chain. Each link of a bicycle chain is mobile and can be displaced on its neighbour if the chain is not under tension. If tension is applied in the long axis of the chain, the chain will straighten and movement of one link on another becomes difficult or impossible. Exactly the same principle applies to a fracture when traction is applied in the long axis of the limb.

Traction may be exerted on a limb by either (1) attaching an inelastic bandage (special materials are available) to the skin, and then a weight to the bandage (*skin traction*) or, (2) passing a metal wire or pin through the bone and attaching weights directly to the bony skeleton in this way (*skeletal traction*). The former technique has the advantage that there is no possibility of infecting the bone but it has the disadvantage that only a small weight (about 2.25 kg) can safely be attached to the skin. The weight used must be sufficient to overcome the shortening and deforming force of the muscles acting across the fracture site and thus skin traction is almost only of use in infants and children where the strength of the muscles can be matched by a pull of 2.25 kg. In adults, skin traction is only

Charles Thackray Ltd, Leeds, England.
Raoul Hoffmann, a Swiss general surgeon, described the system in 1938.

used as a temporary measure and if a fracture is to be treated definitively by traction, skeletal traction is required.

Plaster-of-Paris or the weight of the limb itself may be used to provide traction in the upper limb. For example, a fracture of the shaft of the humerus may be treated in a collar-and-cuff sling which simultaneously rests the limb and, by taking advantage of gravity acting on the elbow and forearm, exerts traction on the fracture site (fig. 224). The traction force may be increased by bandaging a slab of plaster-of-Paris to the arm. Such a slab not only provides more effective traction but also provides splintage at the fracture site ('hanging-cast'). Traction may be 'fixed', as in the use of a Thomas splint for treatment of fractures of the femoral shaft (see p. 314) or 'sliding' (see p. 314).

The Adjacent Soft Tissues.—Certain bones, for example, a single metacarpal shaft (fig. 223), are satisfactorily splinted by adjacent soft tissues, provided the violence of the injury has not displaced the bones and in so doing torn their soft tissue attachments. No additional splintage is required.

Duration of Immobilisation.—Immobilisation by external methods must be continued until the fracture has clinically united, and this obviously varies widely from patient to patient and with different fractures (Table 1).

Summary—with examples. In general, therefore, there are five possible methods of fracture treatment and these are summarised in Table 8. For example, an undisplaced fracture of the shaft of a single metacarpal (fig. 223) requires neither reduction nor stabilisation and can be treated simply by elevation of the hand and provision of an elastic bandage to decrease swelling, followed by early mobilisation of fingers. An undisplaced or minimally displaced fracture of the distal metaphysis of the radius in a child (fig. 229) does not require reduction but requires stabilisation by a plaster of Paris cast to prevent potential deformity, due to muscle pull, developing. On the other hand, a displaced fracture of the

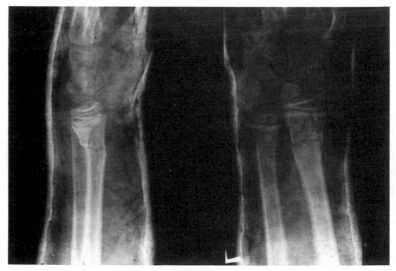

FIG. 229.—Minimally displaced fracture of distal metaphysis of the radius in a child not requiring reduction.

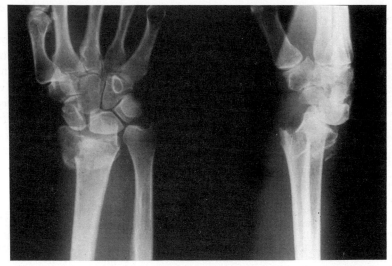

FIG. 230.—Displaced fracture of distal metaphysis of the radius requiring reduction.

distal metaphysis of the radius (fig. 230) will require closed manipulation prior to application of a full-arm plaster of Paris cast. Open reduction, which is usually always accompanied by internal fixation, may be required for a variety of reasons which are discussed later in this chapter. Finally, certain fractures, for example, displaced intracapsular fractures of the neck of the femur in elderly patients are best treated by excision of the femoral head and prosthetic replacement.

TABLE 8. POSSIBLE METHODS OF FRACTURE TREATMENT

1. Protection alone.
2. Immobilise with external splint without reduction.

3. Closed reduction ⟨ Manipulation / Traction

Followed by immobilisation with external splint or traction.

4. Open reduction and internal fixation.
5. Excision of fracture fragment and prosthetic replacement.

Indications for Operative Treatment of Fractures

The indications for operative treatment of fractures are summarised in Table 9.

1. **Compound fracture.—** A compound fracture is a surgical emergency: it must be treated urgently and with skill. Treatment aims at sterilising the fracture site, and consists of (1) wound toilet, (2) the reconstitution of skin cover, and (3) the use of antibiotics.

Wound Toilet and Closure.—It is imperative that this operation be carried out carefully, in optimal operating conditions, with a good light. If possible, a tourniquet should be applied to the limb following exsanguination so that the fracture site can be examined thoroughly. The wound in the skin is extended if necessary and the damaged soft tissues inspected. All the guidelines for wound operative surgery and closure set out in Chapters 1 and 2 should be revised here, and followed rigorously. At the end of the procedure all remaining bone and soft tissues should be surgically clean, and demonstrated to be viable by releasing the tourniquet to see that the tissues bleed.

A swab should be sent for culture and sensitivity. A sutured wound of any size should be drained by closed suction.

Once the skin wound has healed satisfactorily without infection of the fracture site, the fracture itself may be treated as if it were simple. While the skin is healing the fracture should be reduced and splinted, but splintage should never (save in experienced hands or in the presence of severe associated soft tissue injuries) take the form of internal fixation since the foreign material which must necessarily be used to produce internal fixation hinders sterilisation of the fracture site by the local inflammatory response and by antibiotics. So far as possible, external splintage should allow for inspection of the wound: external skeletal fixation is ideal in this context (see External Skeletal Fixation and fig. 288).

Antibiotics and prophylaxis against tetanus and gas gangrene are discussed in Chapter 4. In general a broad-spectrum bactericidal antibiotic should be used which is effective against Staphylococcus aureus. It should be administered in adequate dosage intravenously. The ideal duration of antibiotic therapy is not known for certain and there is considerable variation from one surgeon to another. The author prefers a five day course (unless there are indications to extend this), three days intravenously and two days orally.

TABLE 9. INDICATIONS FOR OPERATIVE TREATMENT OF FRACTURES

1. Compound fracture.
2. Reduction of fracture.
3. Stabilisation of fracture.
4. Time factor—metastatic disease.
5. Soft tissue management.
6. Management of complications—vascular injury
                                    —head injury

For each of the above, closed treatment may be impossible, inadequate or futile.

2. **Reduction and stabilisation of fracture.**–Open reduction of a fracture will be required if closed treatment is impossible, for example; a small deeply placed fragment; a fragment trapped within a joint; or soft-tissue interposition between the fracture fragments. Closed treatment may be too inaccurate for intra-articular fractures or fractures of forearm bones and only open reduction will achieve perfect anatomy. Open reduction will also be indicated if it is not possible to hold a reduction by external splintage because no satisfactory splint is available to immobilise a small fragment or to overcome muscle pull. Small fragments requiring immobilisation are commonly adjacent to joints (as, for example, the head of the femur, fragments around the ankle, or the tibial condyles). Although it may be possible to immobilise the fragments by external splintage, this will involve immobilisation of the whole joint. Unfortunately a combination of severe injury and prolonged immobilisation may produce serious joint stiffness and, therefore, in skilled hands, better results may be obtained by internal fixation of the fracture so as to allow early mobilisation of the joint. The opportunity provided by the internal fixation of any fracture to mobilise muscles and joints early after injury, consitutes an argument for operating even when closed means of management

are available, such as for example in fractures of the shafts of the femur or tibia. This advantage has to be balanced carefully against the disadvantages, of which the most serious is the risk of sepsis. Unless the surgeon is experienced, closed means are preferable.

The inability of external splintage to overcome muscle pull is illustrated by transverse fractures of the patella, after which the quadriceps muscle may pull the proximal fragment of the patella upwards into the thigh. The two fragments can be pressed together through the skin under anaesthesia, but even if the knee is then splinted in full extension, the gap between the fracture fragments opens again as soon as the quadriceps muscle contracts. Thus the restoration of normal anatomy is impossible unless the two fragments of the patella are fixed together at operation.

The maintenance of reduction may be possible by closed means but may be hazardous to the general health of the patient. Thus in fractures through the intertrochanteric region of the femur it is possible to immobilise the fracture either by applying a plaster-of-Paris spica or by the use of traction, and both of these techniques are employed in the young. In the elderly, the prolonged immobilisation in bed which either form of treatment requires is hazardous to the patient's general health since pressure sores, deep vein thrombosis, pulmonary embolism, and hypostatic pneumonia are all common complications of bed rest in this age group. Thus for this fracture in the elderly, operation is required to produce internal fixation of the fracture so as to allow the patient to be mobilised out of bed.

3. **Time factor.**—In the case of pathological fractures resulting from metastatic disease the patient may not have long to live and it is, therefore, appropriate to carry out internal fixation of the fracture, if possible and especially in the lower limb, so as to allow an early return to the home environment.

4. **Soft tissue management.**—*Fractures associated with damage to vital soft tissue* may be best treated by internal fixation of the fracture so as, for example, to allow a ruptured artery to be repaired.

Operation may also be required to apply an external skeletal fixator so as to allow access to the limb for the management of skin loss (fig. 228).

5. **Management of complications.**—In addition to internal fixation in association with vascular repair, patients suffering from head injury may be unconscious or confused and restless, making management in plaster casts or traction impossible. In these circumstances it is often appropriate to carry out an internal fixation, for example intra-medullary nailing of a humeral shaft fracture.

MANAGEMENT OF THE SOFT TISSUES

Muscles may be injured at the time of the fracture or they may be affected indirectly by adhesion formation between themselves and the fracture site. Their function must be preserved as far as possible by encouraging the patient to contract all the muscles in the injured limb statically, and regularly to move through a full range of all those joints which have not been immobilised. If the muscles are not exercised, they waste and adhere to the bone and other soft tissues, and the venous return from the limb is impaired. Muscular exercise is obviously much easier if the fracture has been neutralised by internal fixation to leave the joints free.

Immobilisation of *joints* produces gradual obliteration of the synovial space with fibrous tissue, and damages articular cartilage. This results in stiffness of the involved joint.

Immobilisation of a joint may be an inevitable consequence of immobilising a fracture, but wherever possible it should be avoided. Thus plaster-of-Paris splints should not include joints if their immobilisation is not essential to the mobilisation of the fracture, and any joint which is not immobilised in plaster should be actively exercised.

Fracture of a limb also results in loss of circulatory control which results in oedema formation which further leads to the development of adhesions around joints and subsequent stiffness. It is important to prevent this series of events by elevation of the injured limb, active movement of unsplinted joints, isometric muscle exercises and the provision of an elastic support bandage after removal of plaster casts.

COMPLICATIONS OF FRACTURES

Complications of fractures may be local and general (remote) and occur (1) immediately, (2) early and (3) late.

TABLE 10. IMMEDIATE COMPLICATIONS OF FRACTURES

Local
Skin
Vascular
Neurological ⟨ Nerve / Spinal cord and roots
Muscular
Viscera ⟨ Abdominal / Thoracic

General (Remote)
Multiple injuries
Haemorrhage → shock
Crush syndrome

1. Immediate Complications

These are summarised in Table 10. Skin damage (compound fracture) has already been considered earlier in the Chapter. The major artery of a limb may be damaged by external compression by haematoma and displaced fracture fragments, 'spasm', contusion with secondary thrombosis or actual division. The symptoms and signs of vascular impairment in a limb are the five P's and are listed in Table 11 (see Chapter 14 and note on Paraesthesia).

Recognition of damage to the major artery to a limb is of paramount importance in order to allow repair and restoration of circulation in order to prevent the onset of gangrene and muscle necrosis and subsequent fibrosis. The injuries which are particularly liable to be associated with vascular damage are supracondylar fracture of the elbow, elbow dislocation, fracture of lower third of femoral shaft, knee dislocation and fractures of the proximal tibial shaft. The management of vascular injuries is considered in Chapter 14.

Acute compartment syndrome.—This syndrome may occur after any injury to a limb, even in the absence of a fracture. In the forearm and lower leg there are 'closed compartments' consisting of unyielding bone, interosseous membrane and the investing layer of deep fascia, in which are the muscles, nerves and vessels. If swelling occurs within the 'closed compartment' there is obstruction of venous outflow which leads to further swelling and later leading to muscle ischaemia which, if not relieved, leads to necrosis and subsequent fibrosis.

The importance of this condition is that the distal circulation to the skin *and* the pulses may be completely normal and mislead one into a false sense of security. Patients suffering from an acute compartment syndrome do suffer severe pain, which is much greater than expected for the type of injury sustained, as a result of muscle ischaemia, and in addition have marked muscle tenderness and may have distal sensory disturbance such as loss of sensation in the first dorsal cleft of the foot with anterior compartment syndrome of the lower leg. There is also muscle weakness and passive stretching of the involved muscles is especially painful, for example the 'finger extension test' produces severe pain in patients suffering acute compartment syndrome of the flexor compartment of the forearm. If this diagnosis is suspected, all encircling bandages and plaster casts must be immediately split from top to bottom and if this does not immediately relieve the symptoms then a fasciotomy must be undertaken immediately.

TABLE 11. VASCULAR IMPAIRMENT IN A LIMB

Pain
Paraesthesiae
Pallor   } 5 P's (see note and fig. 186 Chapter 14)
Paralysis
Pulseless

Neurological.–Peripheral nerves may be damaged as a result of closed and compound fractures of the limb and the spinal cord or its emerging nerve roots may be damaged in association with injuries of the spinal column. These are considered in more detail in Chapters 27 and 28 respectively.

TABLE 12. EARLY COMPLICATIONS OF FRACTURES

Local
1. Sequelae of immediate local complications:—
   (a) Skin necrosis and gangrene.
   (b) Volkmann's ischaemia.
   (c) Gas gangrene.
   (d) Venous thrombosis.
   (e) Visceral complications.
2. Joint—infection.
3. Bone—infection
        —avascular necrosis.
4. Fracture blisters.

Remote
1. Fat embolism.
2. Pulmonary embolism.
3. Pneumonia.
4. Tetanus.
5. Delirium tremens.

2. Early Complications of Fractures

The early complications of fractures are summarised in Table 12. Some of these are further discussed in other chapters: gas gangrene, Chapter 4; venous thrombosis, Chapter 11; fat embolism, Chapter 10; pulmonary embolism, Chapter 40; tetanus, Chapter 4:

Bone and joint infection may follow compound injuries of bone and joint despite adequate initial management and must be treated by administration of appropriate antibiotics in large doses by an intravenous route during the early stages. Adequate drainage must also be provided surgically and dead bone and soft tissue excised.

Fracture blisters often occur in the skin overlying fractures, especially around the ankle (fig. 231) and may pose problems for placement and healing of skin incisions required for open reduction and internal fixation of the fracture. If surgical treatment of a fracture is clearly indicated it is best to carry this out at the earliest possible opportunity after injury.

Avascular necrosis.—Certain fractures may damage the blood supply to significant parts of bone and result in avascular necrosis of that part of the bone. The commonest fracture associated with this is the intracapsular fracture of the proximal femur which often results in avascular necrosis of the femoral head. Other sites are the proximal scaphoid, humeral head, and body of the talus after

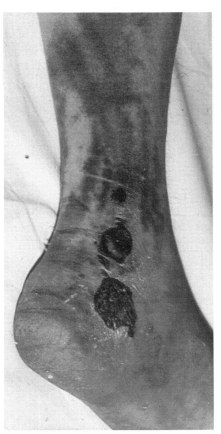

FIG. 231.—Fracture Blisters.

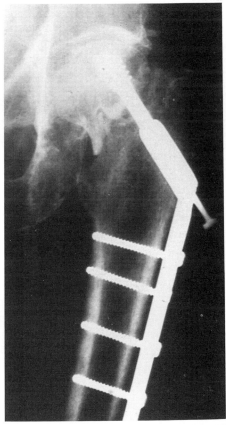

FIG. 232.—Avascular necrosis of the head of the femur following intracapsular fracture. Note bone density and non-union.

fractures of the waist of the scaphoid, proximal humerus and neck of the talus respectively.

Avascular necrosis of bone may lead to changes in density of the affected part on a radiograph. Usually the density increases (fig. 232) but not always. Avascular necrosis is also associated with delayed and non-union of the fracture and, at a later stage, when the fracture has united there may be fracture of sub-chondral bone which results in collapse of the articular surface and secondary degenerative osteoarthritis.

Delirium tremens.—Alcoholic patients who sustain fractures and are admitted to hospital find themselves suddenly separated from a source of alcohol. It is not uncommon for them to suffer from delirium tremens and this must also be remembered as a possible cause of confusion and restlessness in these patients.

3. Late Complications of Fracture

The late complications of fracture are summarised in Table 13. Joint stiffness is common after prolonged immobilisation and after intra-articular fractures, especially if these are treated by immobilisation. Certain joints, for example the elbow and shoulder, are particularly prone to stiffen even after short periods of immobilisation. Knee stiffness is also not uncommon in association with femoral shaft fractures when treated by prolonged immobilisation in a Thomas splint. In part this is due to adhesions developing between the quadriceps muscle and the fracture. Secondary osteoarthritis may develop as a result of intra-articular fractures which result in articular cartilage damage. Avascular necrosis of bone may also lead to secondary osteoarthritis of the hip, for example, after intracapsular fracture of the proximal femur.

TABLE 13. LATE COMPLICATIONS OF FRACTURES

Local
1. Joint—stiffness
        —secondary osteoarthritis
2. Bone—mal-union
        —delayed and non-union
        —growth disturbance
        —chronic infection
        —disuse osteoporosis
        —Sudeck's atrophy
        —re-fracture
3. Muscle—myositis ossificans
        —late tendon rupture
        —tissue atrophy
        —tendonitis
4. Nerve—tardy[1] nerve palsy

Remote
1. Renal calculi
2. Accident neurosis

---

[1] Tardy = slow to come on.

Mal-union of fractures.—A fracture which unites in a position of deformity is said to be mal-united. For example, a long bone shaft fracture may unite with significant angulation at the fracture site. This complication of normal healing may result from imperfect reduction or failure to stabilise a previously satisfactory reduction. Mal-union usually, but not always, results in impaired function and cosmetic loss.

Non-union of fractures.—As already described, delayed or non-union may be 'atrophic' (fig. 220) or 'hypertrophic' (fig. 221). If an obvious cause of non-union such as infection is evident, the underlying pathology should be treated. Commonly there is no obvious cause of non-union, and in this event treatment relies upon two factors: (1) absolute fixation and (2) the use of a bone graft.

Absolute fixation cannot be produced by external splintage alone, but may be achieved by internal fixation either with an intramedullary nail or with sufficiently rigid on-lay plates combined if necessary with external splintage. The periosteum adjacent to the fracture is elevated and a bone graft is applied subperiosteally around the fracture site without disturbing the fibrous non-union itself. A bone graft, combined only with external splintage, is adequate if only a very little movement is permitted at the fracture site by the fibrous tissue crossing the fracture. The bone graft ideally should consist of the patient's own bone since the cells of the graft then contribute to new bone formation. Cortical bone is relatively ineffective in this context since per unit of mass it contains relatively few cells with osteogenic potential. Autogenous cancellous bone is, therefore, the material of choice and a convenient site for this is the patient's iliac crest. The matrix of the graft acts as a scaffold upon which new bone is formed and may also induce new

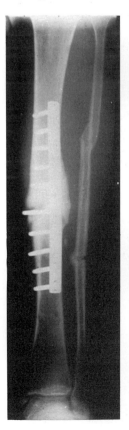
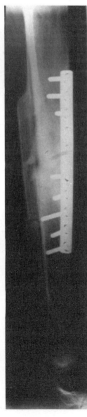

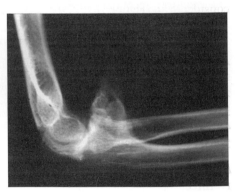

FIG. 234.—Myositis ossificans following a supracondylar fracture.

FIG. 233.—Rigid immobilisation of a hypertrophic non-union of tibia with an A-O plate.
(A-O = Association for Osteosynthesis, begun in Switzerland by Allgower and Müller).

bone formation. Subperiosteal new bone formation is probably induced by the surgical elevation of the periosteum and the rawing of the subjacent cortical bone as well as by the graft itself.

Atrophic non-unions must always be treated by internal stabilisation and application of a bone graft but hypertrophic non-union can be treated by rigid internal fixation alone (fig. 233). In practice the fracture non-union is usually 'taken apart' and anatomical alignment obtained prior to application of internal fixation.

Following a fracture, there is normally an increase in the blood flow through the injured area associated with a loss of bone matrix (*i.e.* osteoporosis, Chapter 23) in the skeleton adjacent to the fracture. Immobilisation also causes these changes so that if an injured limb has to be immobilised, they may be severe. Occasionally very marked osteoporosis, associated with thickening of the soft tissues, vascular stasis, pain and joint stiffness complicates a fracture irrespective of its severity. This syndrome is known as *Sudeck's Atrophy*. Its aetiology is unknown but it is thought to have either a reflex vascular basis or possibly to be due to the extreme reluctance of some patients to use the limb after the removal of splintage, a reluctance which accentuates the changes normally produced by immobilisation. The patient should be encouraged, with supervision in a physiotherapy department, to use the limb. No other specific treatment is available, although a local intravenous infusion of guanethidine below a proximal arm tourniquet may be of benefit in some cases. Myositis ossificans is a complication of certain fractures and dislocations, for example supracondylar fracture of the elbow and elbow dislocation in children, where deposition of bone occurs in an area of injured muscle (fig. 234). It frequently leads to increasing stiffness of the elbow.

Complications of Dislocations

The complications of dislocations are summarised in Table 14. These will be considered in relation to specific dislocations in the subsequent chapters.

TABLE 14. COMPLICATIONS OF DISLOCATIONS

Immediate local
1. Skin (compound dislocation)
2. Vascular
3. Neurological
4. Ligamentous
5. Associated fracture

Early local
1. Infection
2. Avascular necrosis

Late local
1. Joint stiffness
2. Instability
3. Recurrent dislocation
4. Secondary osteoarthritis
5. Sudeck's atrophy
6. Myositis ossificans

SPECIAL TYPES OF FRACTURE

In addition to the usual traumatic fracture there are the following special types of fracture:

1. Fractures in childhood
   - Birth fracture
   - Incomplete fracture
   - Epiphyseal fracture
   - Battered child syndrome
2. Stress (fatigue) fracture
3. Pathological fracture

Fractures of Childhood

Fractures occurring in children differ from those in adults in 6 important

Paul Hermann, Martin Sudeck, 1866–1938. Professor of Surgery, Hamburg, Germany. Described this type of osteoporosis in 1900.

respects: (1) the fractures unite more readily, (2) mal-union can to some extent be corrected by growth, (3) joint stiffness is rare after immobilisation, (4) the fractures may involve the epiphyseal plate and hence interfere with growth, (5) the bone may fracture incompletely, and (6) the patient is often unable to protect himself and to give a history, a combination which gives rise to the Battered Baby Syndrome (see below). The first 3 differences make fractures in children much easier to treat than in adults, and make immobilisation by external splintage almost invariably the method of choice.

Union is almost invariable following all fractures in childhood: a fracture of the neck of the femur is an occasional exception. Not only is union invariable, but it occurs in about half the time required for an adult.

The correction of mal-union by growth seems to occur most readily when the residual angulation occurs about an axis parallel with that of the movement permitted at the adjacent joint. Thus, for example, in supracondylar fractures of the humerus backward angulation of the distal fragment (*i.e.* extension) can be corrected by growth but a varus deformity (*i.e.* adduction) cannot. Torsional deformities correct less well than angular.

Joint stiffness is rarely caused by immobilisation in a child. Following the removal of splintage, children quickly use the injured limb and usually regain a full range of movement rapidly and without physiotherapy.

Occasionally fractures occur during birth. Although this usually implies that the fracture is pathological, for example in cases of osteogenesis imperfecta, occasionally fracture occurs through normal bone as a result of trauma sustained during the delivery (fig. 235).

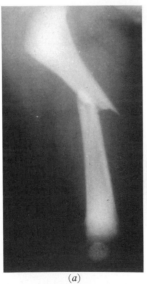

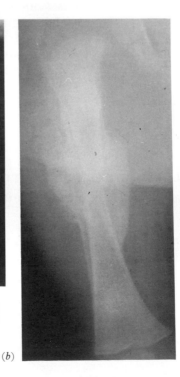

(a)

FIG. 235.—Birth fracture (a) at birth, (b) massive callus at 7 days.

(b)

FIG. 236.—A buckle, or incomplete, fracture of one cortex of the radius. Note the bending of the cortex ('greenstick').

Incomplete fractures are of three types. Simple buckling of one or both cortices, usually in the metaphyseal region of a long bone, results from compression failure after axial loading from, for example, a fall on the outstretched hand (fig. 236). Traumatic bowing may occur without any evidence of acute angular deformity, especially in the ulna and fibula.

A *greenstick fracture* results from angulation beyond the limits of bending; there is failure on the tension side of the bone and the compression side bends (fig. 236). The resultant angulation may be hard to correct without completing the fracture.

Fractures of the epiphysis usually involve the growth plate but occasionally occur in isolation; for example, avulsion at a site of ligament attachment or an osteochondral fracture of the patella. Injuries to the growth plate and epiphysis are very common and form approximately one third of skeletal trauma in children. The fracture line usually runs through that part of the growth plate lying between the calcified and uncalcified cartilage. Several patterns of separation may be produced as described and classified by Salter and Harris (see below).

EPIPHYSEAL (GROWTH PLATE) INJURIES
(classification after Salter and Harris)

I = Separation of the epiphysis from the metaphysis, but without fracture.

II = Separation, but with fracture of a small triangular piece of metaphysis.

III = Intra-articular fracture extending from the joint surface through the plate with separation of the portion.

IV = Intra-articular fracture, the line going through the plate *and* through part of the metaphysis.

V = Severe 'end-on' crush.

Although epiphyseal injuries may lead to a disturbance of growth they do so surprisingly rarely. When growth disturbance does occur it is usually due to one of the following:

Avascular necrosis of the plate.
Crushing or infection of the plate.
Formation of a callus bridge between the bony epiphysis and the metaphysis.
Non-union.
Hyperaemia producing local overgrowth.

Most growth-plate fractures can be treated by closed manipulative reduction, if displaced, and immobilisation in a plaster of Paris cast. Salter Type III and IV fractures often require open reduction and internal fixation to restore joint surface anatomy and prevent growth disturbance resulting from callus bridge formation (Type IV).

The Battered Child—.The term 'battered child' is used to describe a child who has received serious, deliberately inflicted injuries at the hands of his parents or some other adult. The true incidence of this type of injury is not known, but it is undoubtedly common. For every case diagnosed there must be dozens which are unrecognised. The injuries occur because the child is unable to protect himself, and are unsuspected because he is unable to give a history.

Robert Salter, Contemporary. Professor of Surgery, Children's Hospital, Toronto.
W. R. Harris, Contemporary. Orthopaedic Surgeon, Toronto, Canada.

The injured children are usually under the age of 2 years. They are taken to the general practitioner or to hospital, often after a suspicious delay, and the parents are either unable to explain the injuries or suggest some minor accident, such as falling off a sofa, which is quite inappropriate to the severity of the injuries. In more than half the cases there is a history of radiological evidence of previous injury. The commonest injuries are soft tissue bruises and abrasions, burns (Chapter 10), fractures of the ribs and long bones, epiphyseal injuries, and sub-dural haematoma with or without a fractured skull.

Since this type of child-abuse is repetitive, it is vital, for the safety of the child, to make the diagnosis and take appropriate action as soon as possible. The doctor who first sees the child should be aware of the condition and ready to suspect it. Suspected cases must be admitted to hospital immediately in order to protect the child while the paediatrician and the medical social worker undertake the investigation necessary to establish the diagnosis.

'Stress' Fractures

High, oft-repeated loads applied to the skeleton may produce lesions known as 'stress' fractures (but for which a better term would be 'fatigue' fractures).

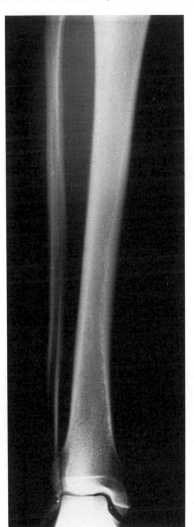

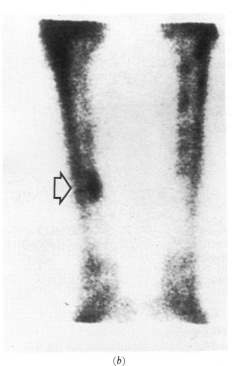

(b)

FIG. 237.—Stress fracture in a marathon runner. (a) Radiograph of tibia which is normal. (b) Bone scan (Technetium 99m) showing hot spot at site of stress fracture (arrow).

(a)

Typical examples occur in the tibiae of runners training on town pavements, in the femoral necks of newly-induced infantrymen carrying out fully-laden route marches (see Intra-Capsular Fractures of the Neck of the Femur, Chapter 17), and in the metatarsals (see march fractures, Chapter 17). The bone in question becomes painful and is tender. Radiologically, the fracture, which is nearly always incomplete, is invisible at first but later is revealed by a zone of increased radiodensity due to callus formation.

In the early stages when the radiograph is normal, a bone scan, using Technetium 99m labelled diphosphonate, will reveal an area of increased uptake of the tracer ('hot spot') at the fracture site (fig. 237). The only treatment necessary for most stress fractures is rest.

Pathological fractures

The foregoing discussion has been concerned entirely with injuries to normal bones. Bone may be the seat of a number of pathological processes, for example neoplasm or osteoporosis, which significantly weaken it either generally or locally, and hence make it liable to fracture in the face of trivial forces. Such fractures are known as pathological fractures.

Pathological fractures due to secondary neoplasm should be treated by internal fixation, if the local state of the fracture and the general state of the patient allow, in order to make the patient more comfortable. Following internal fixation, radiotherapy may arrest the growth of the tumour and allow union to occur.

INJURIES TO ARTICULAR CARTILAGE
(see also Transchondral Fractures, Chapter 22)

Pathology.–Mitosis of human adult chondrocytes does not occur following injury and therefore true healing is impossible. In this sense the chondrocyte is similar to the neurone. Experimental defects involving only the cartilage do not heal; the corresponding lesion in man is only detected as an incidental finding during the exploration of a joint and its fate is presumed to be the same as that in experimental animals. An osseo-cartilaginous defect, produced by a fracture extending through the articular surface, results in bleeding from the bony surface into the joint. The defect fills with granulation tissue arising from the bone and this is eventually converted into fibro-cartilage. Such a fracture is known as an osteochondral fracture (fig. 238).

Clinical Features.—There are no specific clinical features of a cartilage injury, but because an injury producing cartilage damage usually produces an effusion or bleeding into the involved joint (haemarthrosis), swelling and fluctuation in the involved joint usually accompany cartilage damage. In the absence of treatment, some wasting always occurs in the muscles acting on the joint during the weeks after the injury. A loose fragment may fail to gain attachment to the synovial membrane and may then mechanically block movement in the joint, a symptom known as 'locking' of the joint.

Blood in a joint tends to remain liquid because of the presence of haemolysins in the synovial fluid, but it eventually clots and subsequently becomes organised into fibrous tissue. This organised haematoma adheres to the cartilage surfaces and to the synovial membrane, so that movement in the damaged joint is mechanically limited. Immobilisation—imposed either by pain or in the course of treatment—can be shown, experimentally, to damage cartilage and to lead to the

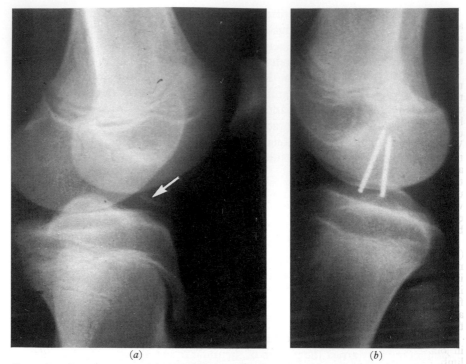

(a)   (b)

FIG. 238.—Osteochondral fracture. (a) Thin radiodense line within the joint cavity. (b) Replacement
and fixation with fine pins.

proliferation of fibrous tissue in the synovial cavity. Immobilisation and injury
also result in adhesion formation between peri-articular soft tissues such as tendons, ligaments and muscles. Thus articular injuries commonly lead to stiffness
in the injured joint.

Because it is rare for defects in the articular surface to be perfectly reconstituted, irregularities persist after these injuries which may eventually result in
osteoarthrosis.

Osteochondral fracture fragments frequently contain enough subchondral
bone for them to be seen on the radiograph as a thin radio-dense line lying within
the joint cavity (fig. 238a). Arthroscopy should be performed in order to assess
the exact size and site of the defect. If the fragment is sizeable and from a weight-
bearing portion of the joint it should be replaced surgically with fine pins
(fig. 238b). Smaller fragments can be removed and discarded.

INJURIES TO LIGAMENTS AND TENDONS

Pathology.—Ligament injuries may be either simple sprains or ruptures. In a simple
sprain some of the collagen fibres of which the ligament is composed are torn but the
ligament as a whole is mechanically intact. Blood vessels in the ligament are ruptured so
that local swelling and bruising occur. Nerve fibres running in the ligament may suffer a
traction injury. In a rupture, the same pathological events occur but to a greater extent,
so that the ligament is broken into two and all the blood vessels, collagen fibres and nerve
fibres in the involved ligament are divided. Following a rupture, the joint is mechanically
unstable.

Tendons rarely rupture, save in pathological circumstances, for example if they become avascular or have been subject to persistent attrition over a roughened bony edge. Traction injuries to a healthy bone/tendon/muscle unit usually produce a rupture at the tendon muscle junction or an avulsion of the tendon from the bone. Tendons, especially those in the hand, may be involved in lacerations anywhere in their length.

Clinical Features.—Injuries to ligaments and tendons heal by the formation of a haematoma around the injured structure which subsequently becomes organised to form fibrous tissue. At this stage the divided ends of the ligament are connected by a scar in which the collagen fibres run at random and in which the ends of the original structure can be seen histologically. Such a scar gradually becomes replaced by well-orientated collagen fibres until eventually the histological appearances of the structure have been reconstituted. Whether or not the mechanical properties of the ligament return to normal, depends upon the length of the resulting scar, upon its strength, and upon the extent to which the scar adheres to the surrounding tissues. A tendon, when divided, usually retracts because of the contraction of its parent muscle. Such retraction may produce a gap so wide as to be unbridgeable and as a consequence healing does not occur. If the tendon does not retract, vessels invade the tendon from the surrounding tissues so that the scar tissue which eventually forms, involves both these tissues and the tendon itself. Thus the tendon becomes adherent, its excursion is limited and its function impaired.

Clinically, simple sprains result in two specific physical signs—localised tenderness (usually over the bone/ligament junction) and pain when the ligament is stressed. Ligament ruptures result in three physical signs—localised tenderness, pain when the ligament is stressed and in addition, mechanical instability. The demonstration of mechanical instability is diagnostic of a ligament rupture and in particular distinguishes a rupture from a simple sprain. These physical signs are well illustrated by ligament injuries at the ankle and knee (Chapter 17). Bruising, local swelling, an effusion into the joint and, with time, muscle wasting are usual, but non-specific, concomitants of these injuries.

Damage to the nerve fibres and mechanoreceptor endings in ligaments, and especially in joint capsules, breaks the postural reflex arcs of which these fibres form the afferent limb. As a consequence the muscles acting across the joint lose their normal postural co-ordination so that in the lower limb, the joint tends to be unstable: for example at the ankle the patient complains that the foot 'gives way'.

If a tendon has been divided, the active movement for which it is responsible is lost. Passive movement remains but may be painful. Loss of active movement may not be obvious clinically if other muscles are available to take over the function of the severed tendon, e.g. the profundus flexor tendons can flex the proximal interphalangeal joints and hence replace sublimis, and all the muscles passing behind the ankle can plantarflex the foot, so masking a rupture of the Achilles' tendon.

Disturbances of Normal Healing.—Failure to heal, the analogue of non-union in bone, may occur in tendons and ligaments if the ends of the divided structure are too widely separated. With lesser degrees of separation, an elongated scar may be produced allowing abnormal movement in the involved joint (in the case of a ligament) or a loss of part of the active range of movement (in the case of a tendon). The collagen fibres in the scar may fail to become well orientated so that the scar is persistently painful when stressed.

Failure to co-apt the ends of the ruptured structure will certainly result in imperfect healing. Absence of tension in the healing tissue may also play a part in poor collagen orientation since it has been shown in tissue culture that collagen fibres tend to array themselves parallel to lines of tension.

Treatment.—If tendons have been lacerated and their ends separated, they will not heal unless they are sutured together. Suture should be carried out as soon as possible provided the sterility of the wound can be ensured. Following suture, the tendon should be immobilised by external splintage of the joints across which it acts for 3 to 6 weeks. The detailed management of tendon injuries in the hand is discussed in Chapter 11.

Ruptured ligaments may be treated either by immobilisation of the involved joint or by suture. Immobilisation is satisfactory provided that the ends of the ruptured ligaments are lying in contact with each other. Unfortunately in a number of ligaments (for example the medial collateral and cruciate ligaments of the knee) the ends of the ligament may retract: it is then preferable to explore the ligament and suture the ends together.

The joint should be immobilised until it is felt that the ruptured ligament will withstand the loads applied to it by protected movements—usually a period of 3 to 6 weeks. Ideally a sutured ligament should be sufficiently secure to allow such movement to occur immediately post-operatively, but in practice the sutures are usually not secure enough to permit this.

In some ligaments, for example the lateral collateral ligament of the ankle, significant separation of the ends of the ligament rarely if ever occurs, and normal movements cause no significant separation of the two halves of the ligament. Such ruptures can be treated by early non-weight-bearing mobilisation without causing material elongation of the ligament as it heals.

Following a ligament injury, the muscles acting across the joint become weak and unco-ordinated and the joint stiff, sequels which are treated by appropriate active exercises.

CHAPTER 16

FRACTURES AND DISLOCATIONS. UPPER LIMB

INJURIES OF THE SHOULDER GIRDLE

Classification

The injuries to be described may be classified as follows:

Fractures of the shoulder girdle:

Fractures of the clavicle.

Fractures of the scapula.

Injuries of the shoulder and related joints:

Dislocation of the sternoclavicular joint.

Subluxation and dislocation of the acromio-clavicular joint.

Dislocation of the shoulder.

Fractures of the Clavicle

Fractures of the clavicle are common and usually result from a blow to the shoulder, producing a shearing effect in the middle third of the S-shaped bone. The potential deforming forces are the weight of the arm which depresses the distal fragment and the pull of the sterno-mastoid muscle which elevates the proximal fragment (fig. 239). Most fractures occur in the middle third (shaft) (80%) but fractures can occur in the outer third (15%) and inner third (5%).

Fractures of the outer third may be minimally displaced (because both fragments are attached to the scapula by ligaments) or displaced (coraco-clavicular ligament ruptured). Fractures of the outer third may also involve the articular surface of the acromio-clavicular joint.

In the absence of displacement no specific treatment is required. If displacement occurs (rupture of the coraco-clavicular ligament) the injury should then be treated in an exactly similar way to an acromio-clavicular dislocation.

Fractures of the middle third (shaft) of the clavicle medial to the point of attachment of the coraco-clavicular ligament are common, especially in children and young adults. The injury is caused by direct violence and in children the fracture is often of the greenstick variety. In adults there is usually more angulation and displacement than in children. Significant displacement so that the bone ends are not in contact is rare, because the soft tissues attached to the clavicle tend to hold the bone ends together.

On *clinical examination* there is tenderness and often obvious angulation of the clavicle at the fracture site. The diagnosis is usually obvious radiologically.

Treatment.—No attempt should be made to reduce the fracture, since it is impossible to hold the reduction even if it is achieved. Most surgeons rely only

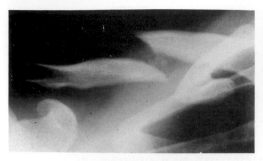

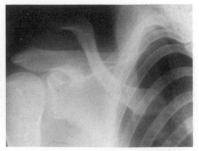

Fig. 239.—Fracture of the clavicle.   Fig. 240.—Acromio-clavicular dislo-
                                                           cation.

on a broad arm sling for the injured limb, combined with analgesics. The sling
should be worn for approximately three weeks.

The fracture almost always unites. Mal-union is common but is of no functional
significance and is rarely a significant cosmetic problem. Non-union may occur
when there is substantial displacement at the fracture site. Established non-union
can be treated by plating and bone grafting if the non-union gives rise to pain.
Fortunately, most ununited fractures of the clavicle are painless. Since it is difficult to achieve union even with a bone graft, non-union should not be treated
unless it gives rise to symptoms.

Fractures of the scapula.—The commonest fractures of the scapula involve the body
or neck of the bone. Comminuted, stellate fractures occur in the body of the scapula
following direct violence. They should be treated symptomatically by resting the arm in
a sling until the pain has diminished enough to allow mobilisation of the shoulder. It is
important to look for and exclude an associated chest injury.

Fractures of the neck of the scapula also result from direct violence; the fracture line
usually runs from the suprascapular notch to below the coracoid process. Treatment is by
application of a broad arm sling and early active shoulder movement as pain subsides.

Dislocation of the sterno-clavicular joint.—This is a rare injury which usually results
from a blow to the front of the shoulder which results in an anterior dislocation of the
sterno-clavicular joint. Occasionally, a direct blow to the medial end of the clavicle results
in a posterior dislocation which may result in tracheal obstruction by the clavicle. The
former type of injury is treated by accepting the deformity and encouraging early shoulder
movement. In cases of tracheal obstruction urgent reduction will be required. This is
usually possibly by closed means and is stable after reduction.

Acromio-Clavicular Dislocation

This injury is due to traction on the arm or to a violent downward blow on the
point of the shoulder. Dislocation of the acromio-clavicular joint can only occur
if the capsular ligament of the joint, and also the coraco-clavicular ligament,
ruptures. If both these structures are torn, the scapula falls under the weight of
the arm whilst the clavicle is drawn upwards by the pull of the sternomastoid
muscle (fig. 240).

Clinical Features.—An obvious prominence is present at the outer end of the
clavicle where this bone is displaced upwards relative to the acromion. The
acromio-clavicular joint is tender.

An antero-posterior x-ray should be taken of both acromio-clavicular joints so
as to compare one with the other. The presence of a 'step' is diagnostic of an
acromio-clavicular dislocation.

Treatment.—Primary treatment of the dislocation is difficult. Strapping can be applied so as to lift the point of the elbow relative to the clavicle, but this is very uncomfortable, hard to maintain, and if really effective may cause pressure sores. It is preferable to reduce the dislocation by passing a screw through the clavicle to engage in the coracoid and thus draw the coracoid up to the clavicle. The screw should be removed about 3 months following the injury since it will inevitably work loose as the scapula moves on the clavicle. Alternatively wires can be passed from the tip of the acromion process across the joint and into the clavicle. These should also be removed after about six weeks and before vigorous movement of the shoulder is started.

Since (1) the disability from this injury even if untreated is slight (although in women the prominence of the clavicle may be thought to be unsightly), (2) strapping is usually ineffective and (3) operative treatment leaves a scar, many surgeons prefer only to rest the arm in a sling and then mobilise the shoulder when pain has settled. Osteo-arthrosis in the acromio-clavicular joint is an occasional late sequel which can be treated by excision of the outer end of the clavicle.

Acromio-clavicular subluxation.—If only the acromio-clavicular ligaments are ruptured and the coraco-clavicular ligaments remain intact then the condition is known as acromio-clavicular subluxation. The deformity is much less obvious and the treatment is by sling immobilisation and early active shoulder movement when pain subsides.

Dislocation of the Shoulder

This is a common injury. The head of the humerus usually dislocates forwards from the shoulder joint so as to lie beneath the coracoid process, to produce a sub-coracoid anterior dislocation of the shoulder.

The injury is produced by forced extension and external rotation of the abducted arm. The head of the humerus is forced against the anterior capsule of the shoulder and either ruptures the capsule or avulses the labrum from the glenoid. The latter injury, since the glenoidal labrum is avascular, rarely heals. Having torn the anterior soft tissues of the shoulder, the humerus passes over the anterior margin of the glenoid and in so doing the posterior part of the articular surface of the head may suffer a compression fracture. Once dislocated from the shoulder joint so as to lie beneath the coracoid, the humerus is locked in this position by muscle spasm.

Rarely the humerus may dislocate posteriorly, and very occasionally, particularly in women with poor musculature, may subluxate vertically downwards. Rarely the head dislocates downwards with the arm in full abduction (Luxatio in Erecta).

The clinical features of anterior sub-coracoid dislocation are classical. The outer aspect of the shoulder is flattened and the arm appears to take origin from a point under the junction of the middle and outer thirds of the clavicle. The shoulder cannot be moved and the arm is held in a position of slight abduction (fig. 241). The patient often appears supporting the elbow of the injured arm by the other hand. The distance between the point of the elbow and the axillary skin is reduced, and the axillary concavity is obliterated.

Posterior dislocation of the shoulder may be difficult to diagnose clinically, since the appearance of the shoulder is essentially normal.

X-ray.—Radiologically an anterior dislocation of the shoulder may be diagnosed on an antero-posterior view because the head of the humerus can be seen to be lying beneath the coracoid (fig. 242). A posterior dislocation is less easily diagnosed since the head of the humerus does not move appreciably in a medial direction. Thus in an antero-posterior projection the appearances of the shoulder

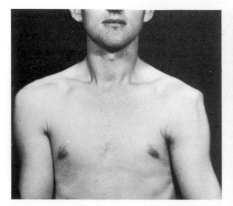

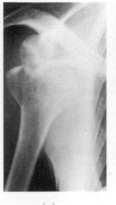

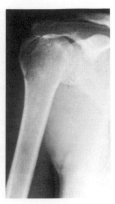

FIG. 241.—Sub-coracoid dislocation of the left shoulder.

(a)   (b)

FIG. 242.—(a) Sub-coracoid dislocation of the shoulder with fracture of the greater tuberosity of the humerus. (b) Satisfactory reduction.

are not grossly abormal. An axillary view, however, will display the head of the humerus lying either anterior or posterior to the glenoid.

Treatment.—Reduction of a dislocated shoulder is easy if the patient is given a general anaesthetic producing muscle relaxation. If the surgeon is skilled, it is possible to reduce a dislocated shoulder without anaesthesia and even without analgesia, but if the surgeon is unskilled this will simply frighten and hurt the patient and possibly damage the shoulder joint. Thus in general it is desirable to anaesthetise the patient with muscle relaxation. When this is done reduction of a dislocated shoulder can be accomplished simply by pressure in an appropriate direction over the head of the humerus. There are however two classical methods by which an anterior dislocation can be reduced and it is occasionally necessary to resort to one of these manoeuvres even in a patient whose muscles are relaxed. The more satisfactory of the two is the method described by Kocher. The alternative method (of Hippocrates) is not now regarded as safe. It entailed traction on the arm with counter-pressure by the unshod foot of the operator in the axilla.

Technique of Reduction of an Anterior Dislocation of the Shoulder (Kocher's Method).—The patient lies on his back. If the left arm is injured, the surgeon stands on the patient's left side and grasps the injured elbow with his left hand. Traction is exerted in the long axis of the humerus for approximately 2 minutes and then, using his right hand, the surgeon gradually externally rotates the patient's humerus by flexing the elbow and using the forearm as a lever. When full external rotation has been obtained, traction is maintained and the elbow is brought across the patient's body so as fully to adduct the shoulder. The patient's hand is then brought across to his opposite shoulder so as fully to rotate the shoulder internally (fig. 243). At some point during this manoeuvre an obvious reduction is felt and the contour of the shoulder returns to normal. Reduction is confirmed by putting the shoulder through a full range of movement under anaesthesia.

The arm is then immobilised in a sling and bandaged to the side so as to maintain full adduction and internal rotation of the shoulder for a period of 3 weeks. At the end of 3 weeks the sling is removed and progressive mobilisation of the shoulder commenced, avoiding only external rotation in abduction. (The position in which the shoulder dislocates.)

Whether or not prolonged immobilisation decreases the risk of subsequent recurrence is not known for certain. The risk of recurrence in older patients

Emil Theodor Kocher, 1841–1917. Professor of Surgery, Berne. Described this method of reducing a dislocated shoulder in 1870

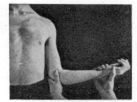 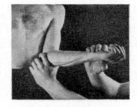 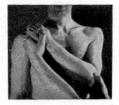

(a)

FIG. 243 (a).—Kocher's method for the reduction of a dislocated shoulder.

FIG. 243 (b).—Kocher's method is 3000 years old. Detail sketch from wall painting in the Metropolitan Museum, New York, from Ramesside Tomb.
(M. K. Hussein, FRCS, Cairo from Jnl. of Bone & Joint Surgery. By permission of E. & S. Livingstone.)

(b)

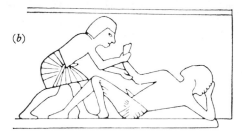

sustaining the injury for the first time is small and they should be treated by early mobilisation after reduction in order to prevent troublesome shoulder stiffness.

Complications of anterior dislocation of the shoulder are commonly associated fracture (neck of humerus, greater tuberosity), axillary nerve damage and, later, recurrence of the dislocation. An associated fracture should be treated on its own merits. Patients with axillary nerve damage should be treated expectantly as most cases recover spontaneously.

Recurrent Dislocation of the Shoulder.—If correctly treated, the majority of dislocations of the shoulder heal to give no further disability. Occasionally the shoulder becomes unstable and recurrently dislocates after trivial violence. Finally the patient may acquire the knack of actively dislocating and reducing the shoulder for himself. If the patient cannot reduce the dislocation for himself, and indeed even if he can, this instability may cause significant disability and require treatment.

Treatment.—Recurrent dislocation of the shoulder is treated by operation. An anterior approach is made to the shoulder. The original lesion in the capsule or glenoidal labrum is displayed and may be repaired by re-attaching the labrum by suturing it to the bony rim of the glenoid (Bankart procedure).

The subscapularis muscle and anterior capsule are then overlapped in front of the joint so as to reinforce the anterior aspect of the joint and thereafter to limit external rotation (Putti Platt procedure).

Alternatively the coracoid process, with the coraco-brachialis and biceps muscles attached to it, is transposed to the anterior lip of the glenoid so as to form a bone block which prevents further anterior dislocation of the shoulder.

Recurrent posterior and downward dislocation of the shoulder occurs occasionally, and is treated (but with difficulty) by operation.

FRACTURES OF THE HUMERUS
Classification

Proximal⟨ surgical neck
anatomical neck
greater tuberosity

Shaft
Distal

A. S. Blundell Bankart, 1879–1951. Consulting Surgeon, Royal National Orthopaedic Hospital, London.
Sir Harry Platt, 1886–1986. Emeritus Professor of Orthopaedics, Manchester.
Vittoria Putti, 1880–1940. Institute Rizzoli, Bologna, Italy.

Fractures of the Proximal Humerus

The humerus may fracture through the surgical neck following a fall on to the outstretched hand which drives the humerus upwards against the acromion and glenoid. The anatomical neck may fracture following a fall on to the point of the shoulder which drives the humerus directly against the glenoid. Fractures of the greater tuberosity also usually result from falls on the shoulder.

Fractures through the surgical neck are common in the elderly and are usually associated with osteoporosis. These fractures are best classified according to the 4-segment classification proposed by Neer. The four segments are: articular segment, greater tuberosity, lesser tuberosity and shaft. If any segment is displaced greater than one centimetre or greater than 45° the fracture is classified as displaced. If the segment is displaced less than one centimetre and less than 45° it is minimally displaced.

1-Part fracture—minimal displacement (any number of segments)
2-Part fracture—one segment displaced
3-Part fracture—two segments displaced
4-Part fracture—four segments displaced

Clinical Features.—The patient complains of pain in the shoulder and usually cannot move the joint. Occasionally, however, in minor impacted fractures through the surgical neck, limited movement is possible. The diagnosis is made radiologically.

Approximately 80% of fractures of the proximal humerus are undisplaced because the fragments are held to each other by the soft tissues enclosing the proximal end of the humerus and are impacted into each other. Treatment of these fractures is simple. The arm is rested in a sling until pain has subsided sufficiently to allow early active mobilisation of the shoulder to be commenced in order to prevent shoulder stiffness. In approximately 20% of cases one or more fragments are displaced. The fragments often cannot be reduced by closed means and are unstable after reduction. There may also be associated rotator cuff damage and avascular necrosis of the humeral head, especially in 4-part fractures.

Treatment.—*In young patients* if the greater tuberosity is fractured and has retracted greater than one centimetre from the rest of the humerus under the pull of the short rotators, the fragment should be surgically replaced and held with a screw or wires. Post-operatively the patient's arm should be rested in a sling and active abduction deferred for at least three weeks. *2-part fractures* with displacement between the articular segment and shaft can usually be treated by closed manipulation or by simple application of a collar and cuff to allow gravity to reduce the fragments. This should be followed by early passive mobilisation to prevent shoulder stiffness. *3-part fractures* are best treated by open reduction and wire loop fixation and associated rotator cuff repair. *4-part fractures* have a high incidence of avascular necrosis of the humeral head and are probably best treated by prosthetic replacement of the head, cuff repair and wire loop fixation of the tuberosities.

The complications of proximal humeral fractures are:
   1. Shoulder stiffness—this is common, especially *in the elderly* who may never

Charles Sumner Neer, Contemporary. (See footnote p. 369.)

regain a full range of movement. *The fracture is usually, therefore, disregarded in this group of patients and treatment directed towards early passive followed by active mobilisation.*

2. Nerve injury—occasionally injury to the axillary nerve will occur. This is manifested by the patient's inability to contract the deltoid muscle during attempted abduction of the shoulder, and by numbness over a small area of skin at the outer side of the upper arm. Treatment is expectant and gradual recovery usually occurs.

3. Mal-union is not uncommon but compatible with excellent function in many cases.

4. Avascular necrosis of the head of the humerus is common in 4-part fractures.

5. Non-union is not common but may occur.

6. Dislocation of the shoulder—rarely the fracture is associated with a dislocation of the shoulder. In these cases the dislocation should be reduced first, by operation if necessary, and then the fracture should be treated along the usual lines.

Most patients have for at least six months after injury, shoulder stiffness, pain at extremes of motion and 'weather ache'.

Fractures of the Proximal Humeral Epiphysis in Children.—This is a not uncommon injury in childhood. The injury is usually a Salter Type II separation of the proximal humeral epiphysis (fig. 244) which may be minimally displaced (usual) or totally displaced (unusual). In most cases the deformity can be accepted as extensive re-modelling usually occurs. Treatment is by application of a collar and cuff for approximately three weeks followed by active mobilisation of the shoulder.

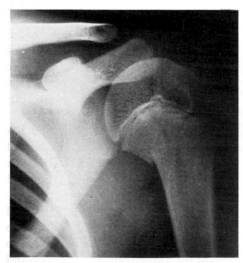

FIG. 244.—Fracture of the proximal humerus in a child.

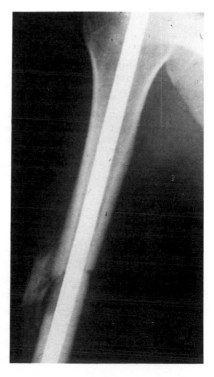

FIG. 245.—Fracture mid-shaft of humerus fixed by intramedullary nail.

Fracture of the Shaft of the Humerus

Mechanism.—These injuries are due either to a twisting injury to the arm or to a direct blow over the shaft of the humerus. The former injury produces a spiral fracture which may include a 'butterfly' fragment, the latter produces a transverse fracture which may also have a 'butterfly' fragment, but usually a smaller one. These injuries may also result from a fall on the hand.

Clinical Features.—The physical signs of tenderness, swelling, deformity and abnormal movement usually make the presence of a fracture obvious and this is confirmed radiologically.

Displacement.—Fractures occurring above the insertion of the Pectoralis major muscle usually result in abduction and internal rotation of the proximal fragment. Fractures occurring between the insertions of Pectoralis major and deltoid usually result in adduction of the proximal fragment (Pect. major) and abduction of the distal fragment (Deltoid). Fractures occurring below the deltoid muscle insertion result in abduction of the proximal fragment with or without overriding.

Treatment.—Acceptable reduction of these fractures can usually be obtained by gravity acting on the arm which exerts steady traction which tends to correct any angulation and overriding that may occur.

Because the shoulder is a multi-axial joint, any angulation which may persist at the fracture site does not interfere materially with function and, surprisingly, up to 20° of angulation at the united fracture produces no clinically obvious deformity (Klenerman). It is necessary only to rest the arm in a collar-and-cuff (not a sling since a sling supports the weight of the arm and hence removes the traction force on the fracture site) and, for pain relief, to bandage the arm to a slab of plaster running from the top of the acromion, down the lateral side of the arm, under the elbow and up the medial side of the arm for 5 cm (fig. 224).

For further security the arm, splinted by the U-slab, may be bandaged to the chest wall. Immobilisation should be maintained for 3 weeks during which the hand and, as far as possible, the elbow are kept mobile. From 3 to 6 weeks the arm is removed daily from the collar-and-cuff to mobilise the shoulder.

Alternatively a '*hanging cast*' can be applied which consists of a complete plaster-of-Paris cast extending from axilla to wrist. Because this is heavier the action of gravity becomes more effective, however, the disadvantage is that the elbow cannot be mobilised during treatment. Most fractures unite in approximately eight weeks.

Occasionally it is not possible to obtain a satisfactory position using the above methods and then it is preferable to proceed to an open reduction and internal fixation using a plate, or if the fracture is transverse and near the middle of the shaft, an intra-medullary nail (fig. 245). It is preferable to insert this nail from below, entering just above the olecranon fossa, in order to prevent damage to the rotator cuff which often occurs with insertion through the greater tuberosity.

Complications.—(1) Radial nerve damage occurs in approximately 5–10% of fractures. It is commonest in spiral fractures of the distal third. The treatment is expectant because the nerve is usually in continuity and there is full recovery in most cases. It is important to prevent the development of fixed flexion of the wrist and fingers by a combination of splintage and passive mobilisation whilst recovery is awaited. If reinnervation of the most proximal muscle has not occurred in the expected time, as calculated from the distance between the site of injury and the neuro-muscular junction, the nerve should be explored. It is

Leslie Klenerman, Contemporary. Orthopaedic Surgeon, Northwick Park Hospital, Harrow, Middlesex, England.

not usually possible to carry out an end-to-end suture at this stage and therefore the repair must be effected by a nerve graft. Because the results of this form of treatment are unpredictable, many surgeons prefer to tackle the problem by tendon transfer. A satisfactory procedure is as follows: the pronator teres is transferred to the extensor carpi radialis brevis to extend the wrist; flexor carpi ulnaris or flexor carpi radialis is transferred to the extensor digitorum and extensor pollicis longus to extend the fingers and thumb; and palmaris longus is transferred to the abductor pollicis longus to provide abduction of the thumb away from the palm.

(2) Non-union may occur in transverse fractures as a result of soft tissue interposition or distraction produced by over-enthusiastic use of the 'hanging cast'. Treatment is by open reduction, rigid internal fixation and cancellous bone grafting.

Fractures of the Distal Humerus

Classification

Supracondylar
Transcondylar
Intercondylar (T or Y)
Condyle—Lateral
        —Medial
Articular surface—Capitulum
                —Trochlea
Epicondyle—Medial
        —Lateral

Supracondylar Fracture of the Humerus in Adults.—Unlike the fracture in children this is an uncommon injury in adults. The flexion type of fracture results from a direct force applied to the posterior aspect of the elbow and the extension type of fracture results from a fall on the outstretched hand. Undisplaced fractures should be treated in a full-arm plaster cast for six weeks and displaced fractures by closed manipulation or open reduction and rigid internal fixation to allow early active elbow movement in the hope of reducing later elbow stiffness.

Supracondylar Fracture of the Humerus in Children

This injury is one of the most serious fractures in childhood and poses considerable therapeutic problems.

Mechanism and Morbid Anatomy.—The injury is most commonly caused by a fall on to the outstretched hand with the elbow slightly flexed to produce the so-called 'extension type' (99%). The fracture line runs transversely through the distal metaphysis of the humerus (fig. 246). The fracture is greenstick in 50% of cases and complete in 50% of cases. A 'flexion type' occurs in 1% of cases as a result of a fall on a flexed elbow.

The displacement of the distal fragment may be minimal, but more commonly there is substantial, complex displacement. This consists of the following elements: 1. backward shift of the distal fragment, 2. backward angulation of the distal fragment, and 3. pronation of the distal fragment (because the hand is usually pronated at the time of the injury). Pronation produces internal rotation of the distal fragment (the two movements are really the same). As a consequence,

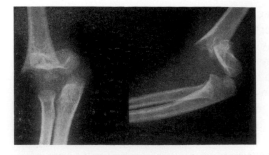

FIG. 246.—Supracondylar fracture of the humerus; there is danger to the neuro-vascular structures between the fragments in this very displaced fracture. (See fig. 226)

the medial cortex of the distal fragment moves posteriorly relative to the medial cortex of the shaft of the humerus, whilst on the lateral side of the fracture the fragments often remain 'hitched' to each other. The pull of the arm muscles then draws the medial side of the distal fragment proximally, posterior to the shaft of the humerus, whilst leaving the lateral side roughly in its original anatomical position. The effect of this displacement is to adduct the distal fragment relative to the shaft of the humerus. Thus pronation results in internal rotation and adduction of the distal fragment. There is also usually either medial or lateral shift of the distal fragment.

Clinical Features.—The elbow swells rapidly following this injury so that gross swelling may obscure the other physical signs within 3 or 4 hours. During this time bruising is not obvious. The child is unable to move the elbow. If significant swelling has not occurred, the posterior prominence of the point of the elbow is obvious and it is possible to palpate the medial and lateral epicondyles and the point of the olecranon so as to establish that they are normally related to each other (fig. 251). This finding distinguishes the injury clinically from a posterior dislocation of the elbow.

The possibility of an interruption of the blood supply to the forearm following this injury must be paramount in the mind of the surgeon from the moment that he first sees the child. This complication may occur at the time of the injury if the brachial artery is contused or lacerated by the anterior aspect of the proximal fragment of the humerus. In this event the radial pulse will not be palpable. More commonly the radial pulse is present at the time of the injury but is obliterated by swelling and flexion of the elbow following reduction. It is therefore imperative to examine carefully the blood supply to the hand on the injured side at repeated intervals over the first 2 or 3 days following injury.

The details of the injury may be difficult to make out radiologically, since ossification of the distal end of the humerus is complex and presents a confusing radiological picture. Further difficulty is created by the fact that the elbow cannot be extended to take an x-ray. These difficulties can to some extent be overcome by x-raying the other elbow in the same position of flexion for comparison.

Treatment.—Undisplaced fractures are treated by application of a posterior plaster slab and collar and cuff with the elbow flexed for three weeks. Greenstick fractures with angulation >20° are treated by manipulation (elbow flexion only) under anaesthetic followed by immobilisation for three weeks. Reduction of displaced fractures is difficult, and if the surgeon has not already had the opportunity of reducing the fracture himself he should if possible consult an experienced surgeon urgently so that the latter has the opportunity of assisting the manipulation before gross swelling has made palpation of the normal anatomy impossible.

Technique of Manipulation of a Supracondylar Fracture

The assistant grasps the upper arm whilst the surgeon holds the injured hand as if he were 'shaking hands'. The surgeon then exerts firm steady traction for a period of 2 minutes or more in the *long axis of the forearm*: that is to say he does not attempt to extend the elbow until traction has drawn the distal fragment beyond the proximal fragment. This reduces the chance of damaging the brachial artery with the distal end of the proximal fragment when the elbow is extended in the next stage of the manipulation, or of entrapping it in the fracture site when the elbow is subsequently flexed. Following traction in the flexed position, the surgeon extends the elbow, feeling the radial pulse as he does so. When full extension has been obtained, the forearm is fully supinated to correct the pronation described above. The fact that the hand and distal fragment are fully supinated is confirmed by fully supinating the uninjured hand and externally rotating the shoulder: the two hands should now have assumed the same attitude. Next, the carrying angle at the elbow is corrected by eye. The surgeon then grasps the upper arm with his second hand placing his fingers over the biceps muscle so that his thumb rests on the olecranon. He then changes the position of the hand exerting traction, placing it so that he grasps the distal forearm with his index on the radial pulse. He then slowly flexes the elbow using the hand with which he is exerting traction to produce a combination of flexion and continuous traction in the long axis of the forearm. The thumb over the olecranon presses the olecranon (and with it the distal fragment) forwards into flexion; the fingers of this hand exert counter-traction against the hand pulling in the long axis of the forearm. Flexion is continued until a point just beyond 90° is reached. Throughout this manoeuvre the radial pulse is felt and if it is obliterated by flexion (which may be due either to impingement of the brachial artery on the distal end of the proximal fragment of the humerus or to compression of the brachial artery as the swollen forearm 'folds' into it) the elbow is extended until the pulse returns. When the maximum degree of flexion has been obtained compatible with the presence of a radial pulse, a light back slab is applied over padding to hold this position and the reduction is checked radiologically.

If reduction is satisfactory a collar and cuff is added and **the child must be admitted to hospital for observation of the circulation to the forearm and hand.** The upper limb is elevated by resting the elbow on pillows to reduce swelling of the fingers. Throughout the following 48 hours the state of the circulation in the hand is examined regularly and any suggestion that the circulation is impaired is treated instantly by removal of the plaster and increased extension of the elbow. If extension of the elbow does not return the circulation to normal, the brachial artery must be explored to ensure its patency.

The triceps muscle wrapped around the back of the fracture holds the fragments in a position of reduction provided adequate flexion has been obtained. X-rays are taken at 48 hours and again 1 week after injury to check that reduction has been maintained, but it is difficult to obtain a view in which the fracture fragment can be adequately displayed. The best view is one taken 'shooting through the elbow' at right angles to the distal end of the humerus.

The fracture unites in 3 or 4 weeks. The sling is then removed and the child's arm gently mobilised.

If a satisfactory reduction cannot be obtained by manipulation or, having obtained a satisfactory reduction, it is not possible to flex the elbow enough to stabilise it (on account of swelling) then the fracture should be treated by skin traction with elbow in extension or by open reduction and fixation with two wires passed across the fracture site from the medial and lateral epicondyles respectively.

Complications.—(1) Nerve palsy—damage to the median, ulnar and radial nerves may occur and should be looked for. Treatment is expectant as almost all recover.

(2) Vascular—this has already been discussed. It should be emphasised again

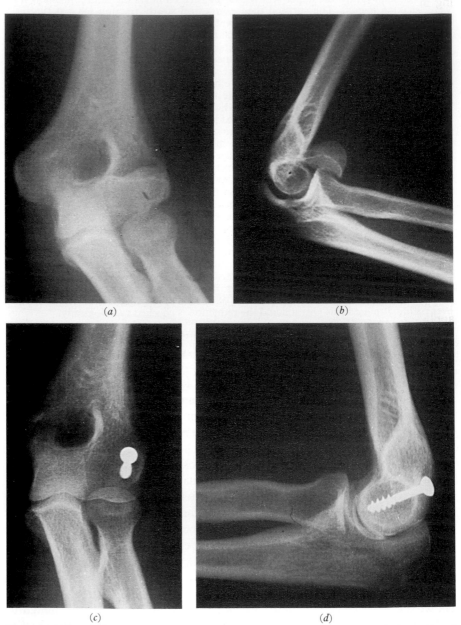

(a)

(b)

(c)

(d)

FIG. 247.—Fractured capitulum, lower end of humerus (a) and (b) AP and lateral views. (c) and (d) AP and lateral views after open reduction with fixation by a screw.

that an acute compartment syndrome may also occur with this fracture in the presence of an adequate distal pulse (p. 256). The treatment is fasciotomy.

(3) Elbow stiffness is common after this injury and it usually takes at least three months for full return of movement. Full extension may take even longer to return.

(4) Mal-union may occur due to failure to reduce the fracture properly, resulting in the so-called 'gunstock' deformity which consists of a combination of residual varus, internal rotation and extension. The latter two will usually correct by re-modelling but residual varus angulation will not.

(5) Myositis ossificans.

Intercondylar Fracture of the Humerus in Adults.—These injuries are rare but difficult to treat. They usually result from a fall onto the point of the elbow which results in the olecranon being driven upwards against the articular surface of the distal humerus. The fracture line runs vertically upwards from the centre of the distal articular surface of the humerus and then diverges in T or Y fashion to reach the medial and lateral cortices in the supracondylar region. There may be comminution of the fragments.

The diagnosis is made upon the clinical evidence of injury to the elbow combined with the obvious x-ray appearances.

Treatment.—In young adults attempts must be made to reduce this fracture accurately but this is difficult. The best method of achieving accurate reduction is by open operation followed by rigid internal fixation which will allow early active movement of the elbow to prevent stiffness. It is the achievement of rigid fixation which is difficult in the presence of comminution.

In the elderly the fracture should be ignored, the elbow rested in a plaster cylinder for 2 weeks, and then gradually mobilised regardless of displacement at the fracture site. A surprisingly good range of movement is often obtained in this way.

Fractures of Condyles and Articular Surfaces

These are rare injuries in adults. Undisplaced fractures can be managed by application of a full arm plaster cast for six weeks. Displaced fractures should be treated by accurate open reduction and internal fixation followed by early movement of the elbow (fig. 247). The commonest complication of these fractures is elbow stiffness.

Fracture of the Lateral Condyle in Children.—This injury is due to a varus angulation of the elbow resulting from a fall on the outstretched hand. The lateral condyle is avulsed by the lateral ligament of the elbow. The injury is a Salter Type IV epiphyseal separation (fig. 248). Clinically there is usually marked swelling, bruising and tenderness over the lateral aspect of the elbow. The diagnosis is confirmed by radiography. The fracture may be undisplaced or grossly displaced, being angulated through approximately 90° in two planes by the extensor muscles of the forearm.

Treatment.—Undisplaced fractures are treated in a full arm plaster cast with the elbow flexed to 90% and the wrist extended and supinated. Check radiographs are required every four days for two weeks. The plaster is removed after three weeks. Displaced fractures must be treated by accurate open reduction, through a lateral approach, and internal fixation with one or two wires. Following operation a full arm plaster cast is applied for three weeks and the wire(s) removed at six weeks.

Complications.—(1) Mal-union may result from failure to reduce the fracture accurately which results in a callus bridge developing between bone of the epiphy-

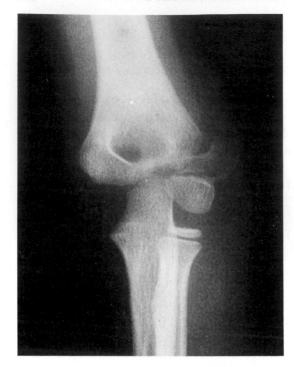
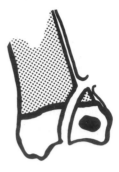

Fig. 248.—Fracture of the lateral epicondyle in a child and diagram of lateral condyle fracture (Salter IV, p. 263).

sis and bone of the metaphysis. Growth is therefore arrested on the lateral side of the elbow and continued growth on the medial side leads to a valgus deformity of the elbow.

(2) Non-union may occur if the fracture is not accurately reduced.

(3) Tardy[1] ulnar palsy may occur due to stretching of the ulnar nerve in association with a valgus deformity of the elbow.

Fracture of the Medial Epicondyle.—This is a fairly common injury in children. It represents an avulsion injury of either the humeral attachment of the wrist and finger flexors, or of the medial collateral ligament of the elbow, following a valgus strain to the elbow.

Treatment.—If the fragment is only slightly displaced (fig. 249) the elbow should be rested for three weeks in a plaster-of-Paris backslab and then gently mobilised. Even if fibrous union occurs it is of no consequence. If the fragment is displaced significantly there is debate about the best method of treatment. Some advocate reduction, which can only usually be achieved by open reduction and wire fixation, while others accept any displacement. Certainly if medial instability of the elbow joint can be demonstrated by applying a valgus strain then open reduction and internal fixation should be performed.

Occasionally the fragment becomes trapped within the joint and then open reduction will always be required to extricate it. The ulnar nerve may be damaged in association with a medial epicondyle fracture and its function should always be tested. Occasionally late ulnar nerve symptoms develop due to irritation from

---

[1] Tardy = slow to come on.

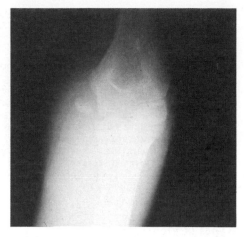

FIG. 249.—Displaced medial epicondyle fracture.

associated bony irregularity; the treatment for these cases is anterior transposition of the ulnar nerve.

THE ELBOW

The elbow is very liable to become stiff following an injury, regardless of its exact nature. It is uncertain why this is so: commonly no specific explanation for the stiffness can be found and it is presumed that adhesions have formed within and around the capsule of the joint. It seems likely that too vigorous an attempt to move the joint in the first few weeks after an injury may promote stiffness of this kind and therefore in general it is wise to rest the elbow for a short period following injury (immobilisation may, of course, be inevitable as a consequence of the nature of the injury). Movement is then gently encouraged under close supervision in a physiotherapy department, making repeated measurements of the precise range of flexion and extension that has been obtained.

Myositis Ossificans.—This is a condition, midleadingly named, which may occur following musculo-skeletal injury anywhere in the body but which is particularly common following injuries at the elbow. Why it should be common at the elbow is unknown.

Pathologically, the condition consists of ossification in a haematoma. This may occur following a fracture, or may follow a purely soft tissue injury in which periosteum has been avulsed. It is believed that the periosteal cells proliferate within the haematoma and ossify it. Since the new bone replaces the haematoma, the bone tends to lie between the muscles rather than to involve the muscles themselves. Thus myositis ossificans is not, as its name implies, an ossifying inflammatory disease of muscle.

Clinically, at the elbow the development of the condition may first be suggested by a failure of the range of movement gradually to increase following gentle mobilisation. *If exercises are then pressed strenuously, the range of movement actually decreases rather than increases and pain in the elbow becomes worse.* At this stage (about 3 or 4 weeks after injury) there are no abnormal radiological signs. By 4 to 6 weeks after injury a faint cloud of new bone formation with indistinct edges can be seen in the area destined to become ossified. The new bone gradually becomes more dense and more organised until finally it takes on the radiological appearance of mature bone (fig. 233).

Treatment is difficult. When the condition is first suspected the elbow should be rested absolutely in a plaster cylinder until pain and tenderness have settled. Remobilisation should then be started extremely gently taking care to measure the range of movement at least twice a week in order to detect the earliest sign of any reduced mobility since this implies that the attempt to mobilise the joint is increasing the amount of new bone formation and thus making the condition worse, not better. Attempts have been made to remove the new bone surgically. This should never be attempted until the bone has a radiologically mature appearance, since if it is, the haematoma produced by the operation is liable to ossify in its turn. The removal of a block of mature new bone is often surgically difficult and may give a disappointing increase in the range of movement since by the time that the operation is possible, fibrous adhesions have formed between all the soft tissues around the elbow. However the condition is treated, some permanent limitation of movement is the usual outcome.

Types of Elbow Injury

The important injuries are:

Elbow dislocation

Fractures of radial head

Fractures of the proximal ulna ⟨ olecranon / coronoid process

Fractures of the distal humerus, which have already been described, can also be considered under the heading of elbow injuries.

Dislocation of the Elbow

This usually occurs in a posterior direction, following a fall on the outstretched hand with the elbow slightly flexed. The coronoid process of the ulna passes posteriorly below the distal end of the humerus. Spasm of the triceps muscle then locks the elbow in a position of posterior dislocation (fig. 250).

The forearm is usually also displaced laterally so that the commonest (80%) type of elbow dislocation is postero-lateral. The dislocation can occur in other directions, anterior, medial or lateral. On occasions the radius or ulna may dislocate in isolation or the radius and ulna dislocate in opposite directions (*divergent dislocation*).

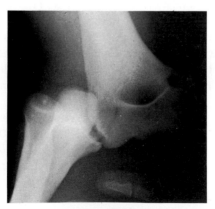 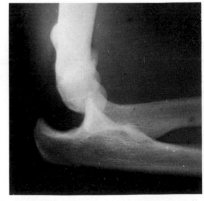

FIG. 250.—Posterior dislocation of the elbow.

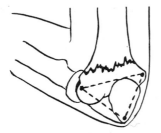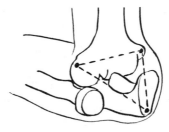

FIG. 251.—Bony points in the elbow. 1. In the normal elbow and in the elbow after a supracondylar fracture, the triangle formed by the tip of the olecranon and the two epicondyles is roughly equilateral. 2. When the elbow is dislocated the tip of the olecranon is displaced and the triangle is no longer equilateral.

Clinical Features.—The patient is unable to move the elbow from a position of slight flexion. The point of the olecranon can be felt to be abnormally posterior to the humeral epicondyles: a clinical feature which distinguishes this injury from supracondylar fracture of the humerus (fig. 251). Radiological examination reveals the dislocation and may show associated fractures either of the coronoid process, of the head of the radius, or of the distal articular surface of the humerus. The fractures are often best, or only, seen in a post-reduction radiograph, an investigation which should never be omitted.

Treatment consists of giving the patient a general anaesthetic to produce muscle relaxation. It is then easy to reduce the dislocation by applying traction in the long axis of the (slightly flexed) ulna. The sensation of reduction is usually obvious and, once achieved, the elbow can be put through a full range of movement. The reduction is stable because of the bony configuration of the elbow, but it must be remembered that this injury can only occur if the capsule and ligaments of the elbow have been ruptured. The elbow should therefore be immobilised in a plaster back slab and a sling for 3 weeks and thereafter *gently* mobilised. Check radiographs should be obtained after one week because re-dislocation may occur occasionally despite the plaster back slab.

Complications: (1) Associated fracture—radial head or coronoid process.

(2) Irreducible dislocations occasionally occur but are rare. Treatment is by open reduction.

(3) Median or ulnar nerve damage may occur but is uncommon. The function of these nerves should always be tested before and after reduction.

(4) Vascular injury may also occur but is also unusual except in cases of open dislocations with wide displacement of the arm and forearm bones.

(5) Myositis ossificans (see above).

Children.—Dislocation of the elbow in children is rare without an associated fracture. The usual combination is a postero-lateral dislocation in association with a fracture of the medial epicondyle which may become trapped in the joint after reduction. *Treatment* is by closed reduction following which the fracture is treated on its own merits. Remember that if the medial epicondyle appears to be 'missing' on the post-reduction film it may be in the elbow joint; treatment is by surgical removal followed by replacement in its correct position and internal fixation.

In the child aged 1–4 a condition known as '*pulled elbow*' may occur. This usually results from a sudden pull on the extended elbow. The child will not move the elbow which is held flexed and pronated. The radiographs are normal. This condition is due to a tear in the distal attachment of the annular ligament allowing subluxation of the proximal radial epiphysis (radial head) through the tear and the proximal part of the annular ligament is then able to slip into the radio-humeral joint where it is 'pinched' when the radial head slips back. *Treatment* is simply by full supination to the slightly flexed elbow followed by application of a sling for two weeks.

Rupture of the Collateral Ligaments of the Elbow

Forced abduction of the forearm bones on the humerus may rupture the medial collateral ligament or avulse its bony attachment to the medial epicondyle. Adduction may produce a similar injury to the lateral collateral ligament.

Clinical Signs.—There is marked tenderness, bruising, and swelling in the region of the injured ligament. Mechanical instability of the joint may be suspected clinically, and can be proven by examining the elbow under an anaesthetic, if necessary taking a stress radiograph.

In the absence of a fracture, the arm is treated in the same way as following the reduction of a dislocation of the elbow. The treatment of an associated fracture of the medial epicondyle (an injury equivalent to a rupture of the medial collateral ligament) is discussed on p. 282.

Fractures of the Proximal Ulna

Two fractures of the proximal ulna may involve the elbow: fracture of the olecranon and fracture of the coronoid process.

Fracture of the olecranon is usually caused by a fall on to the point of the elbow, the olecranon being broken by the distal end of the humerus. The fracture line is transverse and runs through the narrowest point of the olecranon. The pathological and clinical features of the injury and its treatment are closely paralleled by transverse fractures of the patella.

Clinical Features.—It is essential to decide clinically whether or not the triceps expansion is intact over the fracture site. If it is, there will be local bruising, swelling and tenderness, but active extension of the elbow against gravity will be possible. There will be no clinically detectable gap at the fracture site, and radiologically there will be no separation of the fracture fragments. If the triceps expansion is ruptured, active extension against gravity is impossible and the proximal fragment is drawn up into the arm by the triceps muscle creating a palpable gap at the fracture site and an obvious separation of the fragments radiologically.

Treatment.—If there is no significant separation of the fracture fragments and active extension is possible, the elbow may be treated by 6 weeks' immobilisation in a padded plaster cylinder followed by gentle mobilisation or by internal fixation. If the fracture fragments are separated, the fracture must be reduced and immobilised by internal fixation since the fracture cannot be completely reduced even by full extension of the elbow, and immobilisation of the fully extended elbow may result in disastrous stiffness of the joint. The fracture should therefore be treated by open reduction and internal fixation, using the tension band principle, carried out with two parallel wires and a figure-of-eight wire (fig. 252). Following sound internal fixation early movement of the elbow should be commenced. In cases where the proximal fragment is very small, or where gross comminution is present, the fragments can be excised and the triceps tendon re-attached to the proximal ulna.

Complications.—(1) Loss of some movement, especially full extension is not uncommon after this fracture.

(2) Ulnar nerve damage may occur but is rare.

(3) Secondary osteoarthrosis may develop in cases where irregularity of the joint surface remains after inadequate treatment.

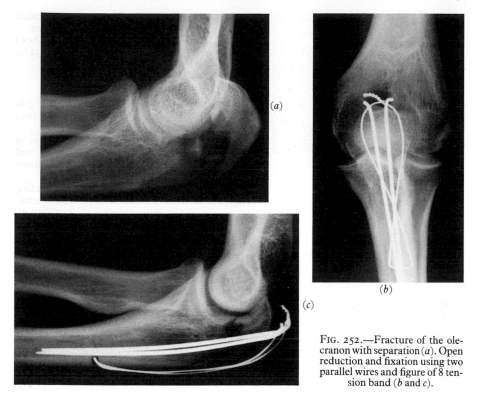

Fig. 252.—Fracture of the olecranon with separation (a). Open reduction and fixation using two parallel wires and figure of 8 tension band (b and c).

Fracture of the coronoid process is uncommon and usually accompanies dislocation of the elbow. The coronoid process is usually approximated to the ulna by reducing the dislocation. If it is not, open reduction is required.

Fractures of the Proximal Radius

These fractures occur as a consequence of a fall on the outstretched hand. If the thrust goes directly up the long axis of the radius, the neck of the bone may be fractured and is often impacted: a mechanism similar to that which produces fractures of the neck of the humerus. More commonly the fracture line runs vertically to split off a fragment of the head (fig. 253). The fracture may be undisplaced, marginal with displacement (impaction, angulation or depression) or comminuted. The fracture may also occur in association with dislocation of the elbow.

The clinical signs are often trivial and do not suggest that a fracture has occurred. There is commonly very little bruising and minimal swelling. The only significant physical signs are painful limitation of movement combined with tenderness over the head of the radius. The injury is revealed radiologically.

Treatment of undisplaced fractures is by encouragement of early movement as soon as pain begins to decrease at 48 hours. Some also advocate aspiration of the elbow to reduce pain and increase range of movement. *Treatment of displaced marginal fractures* is controversial and ranges from immediate excision of the radial head, to internal fixation, to conservative treatment as in undisplaced

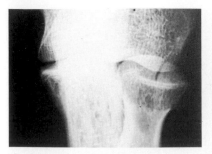

FIG. 253.—Vertical fracture of the head of
the radius.

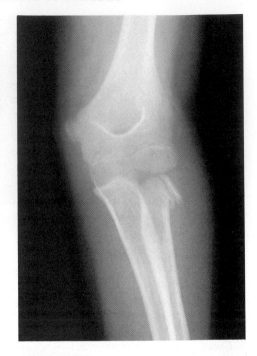

FIG. 254.—Fracture dislocation of the
proximal radial epiphysis (Salter II type).

fractures. Comminuted fractures should be treated by early excision of the whole head. Complete excision should be confirmed at the time of surgery by intra-operative radiography.

Fracture of the radial head in association with elbow dislocation should be treated on its own merits after reduction of the dislocation.

Children.—Fractures of the proximal radius also occur in children following falls on the outstretched hand. The fracture is usually situated in the proximal metaphysis (neck) and only occasionally is there a true separation of the proximal radial epiphysis of the Salter II type or very rarely Salter I type. Treatment is by closed reduction if angulated >30°; if this fails then open reduction should be performed (fig. 254).

FRACTURES OF THE FOREARM

Classification

Fractures of olecranon ⎫
Fractures of radial head ⎭ discussed under elbow injuries.
Fractures of shafts of radius and ulna.
Monteggia fracture.
Galeazzi fracture.

Fractures of the Shaft of the Radius and Ulna

Fractures of One Forearm Bone without Angulation.—A fracture of the radius or ulna, without angulation, may occur as a consequence of a blow applied directly to the forearm. The fracture requires immobilisation in an above-elbow plaster for 6 weeks in an adult, 3 weeks in a child. (See also: Monteggia and Galeazzi Fracture-dislocations, p. 290.)

Fractures of Both Forearm Bones.—These fractures usually occur at approximately the same level and are caused by a direct blow, which in effect bends the bones at the point where the blow is received. Occasionally the bones may be fractured by torsion of the forearm: in this case the fractures are oblique and are disposed at different levels in the two bones.

Treatment.—In the adult it is imperative that an absolutely perfect reduction be achieved since otherwise a loss, often substantial, of pronation and supination will occur. In the child residual angulation of about 5° can be accepted as it will be corrected by remodelling. Residual rotation (pronation or supination) at the fracture site cannot be corrected by remodelling.

Perfect reduction is usually impossible by closed manipulation. Therefore in the adult the fractures should be treated by open reduction and compression plating.

Following mechanically adequate internal fixation no plaster is required provided the patient undertakes only gentle activities with his arm. If plates have been applied which maintain reduction but which are not mechanically sound, they will need the support of an above-elbow plaster for at least 6 weeks. In a child, an acceptable reduction can usually be obtained conservatively but if it cannot the fractures should be treated by internal fixation using oblique wires across the fracture site or small onlay plates supplemented by a full arm plaster-of-Paris cast.

Complications.—1. Non-union may result from inadequate fixation or in the presence of infection. With good fixation non-union of the radius and ulna occur in less than 5% of cases.

2. Mal-union results from poor reduction and is preventable with adequate treatment.

3. Nerve injury is uncommon after this injury.

4. Acute compartment syndrome may occur and the symptoms and signs of this condition should be constantly sought so that the appropriate treatment can be instituted (Chapter 15).

5. Synostosis (cross-union) between radius and ulna occasionally occurs.

In cases where more than one third of the circumference of the shaft of the radius or ulna are comminuted, plating should be accompanied by cancellous bone grafting.

The Technique of Closed Manipulation.—The elbow is flexed to 90° and the surgeon applies traction to the hand against counter-traction applied by an assistant grasping the upper arm. Traction corrects angulation and disimpacts the fractures so that the bones in the distal part of the forearm can be pronated or supinated to align them with those in the proximal part. If the radial fracture is distal to the insertion of pronator teres, the proximal radius will lie in mid pronation, but if the fracture is proximal to the insertion of pronator teres, the proximal radius lies in full supination and this is therefore the position in which the surgeon places the hand. When the fracture has been reduced, an assistant applies an above-elbow plaster whilst the surgeon maintains traction. The fracture is x-rayed immediately the plaster has been applied, at 48 hours and then weekly for 3 weeks. The plaster is maintained for 6 weeks. If at any time the position of the bones is seen to be unsatisfactory, the fracture is treated by open reduction.

Undisplaced fractures should be treated by application of a full arm plaster cast with 90° elbow flexion and neutral rotation, for approximately 6–9 weeks. Regular check radiographs should be obtained during the first three weeks.

Monteggia and Galeazzi Fracture-dislocations

Monteggia fracture-dislocation consists of a fracture of the ulna and dislocation of the superior radio-ulnar joint.

The Galeazzi fracture-dislocation consists of a fracture of the radius and dislocation of the inferior radio-ulnar joint.

The presence of a fracture of one forearm bone should always raise the suspicion that the inferior or superior radio-ulnar joint has been dislocated as well. This suspicion is confirmed if angulation occurs at the fracture site, for this is only possible in a fracture of a single forearm bone if the ligaments connecting the angulated bone to its opposite number have been torn. *Thus the general rule that a fracture somewhere in the shaft of a long bone demands an x-ray, not only of the bone itself but of the proximal and distal joint, is particularly well exemplified by this fracture.*

The commonest type (60%) of Monteggia fracture is the 'extension type' which consists of anterior angulation (apex anterior) of the ulna and anterior dislocation of the radial head. 'Flexion' and 'Lateral' types also occur but less commonly. *Treatment* is by open reduction and compression plating of the ulna and closed reduction of the radial head followed by the application of a full arm plaster cast for six weeks. Open reduction of the radial head and repair of the annular ligament is only undertaken if closed reduction fails.

Complications.—(1) The full extent of the injury is often missed, especially in children! (This error can be avoided—see below.) (2) Posterior interosseous nerve injury occasionally occurs.

In Children a Monteggia fracture is frequently missed. The reason for this is probably that the ulna may not actually fracture but simply bend enough to allow dislocation of the radial head. It should be remembered that a line passing along the longitudinal axis of the radius should pass through the capitulum in all radiographic views. If it does not, a dislocation of the proximal radius is present unless proved otherwise. *Treatment* is usually possible by closed manipulation followed by immobilisation in a full arm plaster cast for six weeks.

The Galeazzi fracture usually consists of a transverse or short oblique fracture at the junction of the middle and lower thirds of the radial shaft with dorsal angulation and dislocation of the inferior radio-ulnar joint (fig. 255). *Treatment*, in the adult, is by open reduction and compression plating of the radius.

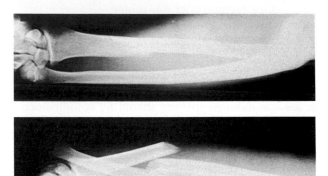

FIG. 255.—Galeazzi fracture (see text).

In Children a Galeazzi fracture is much less common. *Treatment* is usually possible by closed reduction of the radius which usually produces automatic relocation of the inferior radio-ulnar joint; the upper limb is immobilised in a full arm plaster cast for six weeks.

FRACTURES OF THE DISTAL RADIUS AND ULNA

Classification

Adult	*Children*
Colles' Fracture	Fracture distal radial epiphysis
Smith's fracture	
Barton's fracture	Fracture distal radial metaphysis
Radial styloid fracture	

Colles' Fracture

This is a fracture of the distal end of the radius produced by a fall on to the palm of the outstretched hand. The injury is uncommon below the age of 50. After this age, it becomes increasingly common so that overall it is one of the commonest fractures. It is particularly common in women, as are fractures of the proximal femur, and, like fractures of the proximal femur, its increasing frequency with age has been attributed to the development of osteoporosis in post-menopausal women. The association of the fracture with increasing age is probably also due to the fact that the elderly are more liable to fall than are the young.

Morbid Anatomy.—The fracture line lies approximately 2 cm proximal to the distal articular surface of the radius. The fracture is often comminuted, especially

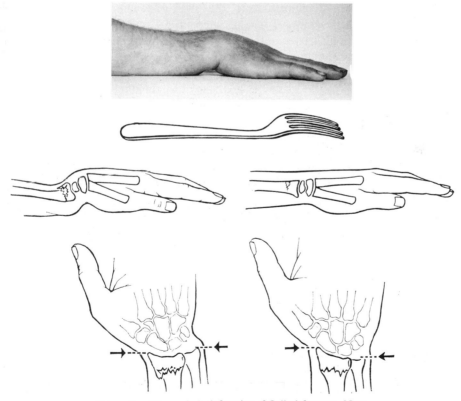

FIG. 256.—Dinner-fork deformity of Colles' fracture. Note the levels of the radial and ulnar styloid processes before and after reduction.

Abraham Colles, 1773–1843. Professor of Surgery, Royal College of Surgeons in Ireland (1804–1836) and Surgeon Dr. Steven's Hospital, Dublin. Described this fracture in 1814.

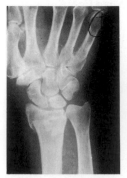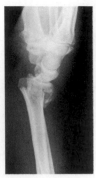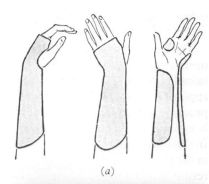

FIG. 257.—Colles' fracture.

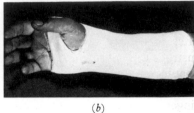

FIG. 258.—Colles' plaster. (*a*) Plaster slab in ulnar deviation and slight palmar-flexion applied immediately after the reduction of a Colles' fracture. (*b*) The completed plaster.

(*a*)

(*b*)

on the dorsal surface. The distal fragment is: (1) shifted dorsally, (2) angulated dorsally, (3) driven proximally into the shaft, (4) angulated radially and (5) supinated. There is always an associated injury to the inferior radio-ulnar joint: the articulating surfaces of these bones are displaced relative to each other and their connecting ligaments (including the triangular cartilage) are torn or the ulnar styloid is avulsed. It is uncertain whether the latter injury is due to avulsion of the ulnar styloid by the triangular cartilage or by the ulnar-collateral ligament of the wrist. The fracture lines may extend into the radio-carpal and radio-ulnar joints.

Clinical Features.—The appearance of the wrist is typical and is described as a 'dinner-fork' deformity (fig. 256). Viewed from the side the dorsal aspect of the wrist is unduly prominent; viewed from the dorsum the lateral aspect of the wrist is slightly prominent and the hand is radially deviated. The fracture site is tender. The radial styloid is no longer distal to the ulnar styloid; instead the two styloid processes are approximately at the same level, a reflection of shortening in the radius (fig. 256). Radiologically the fracture, the extent of the displacement, and the degree of comminution will be obvious (fig. 257).

Treatment.—The fracture is reduced by manipulation and immobilised with a plaster back-slab which is completed to form a Colles' plaster (fig. 258) 24 hours after the injury.

Manipulation of a Colles' Fracture.—The patient is given a general anaesthetic or a regional block using either intravenous anaesthesia distal to a tourniquet or a brachial plexus block. An assistant grasps the upper arm whilst the surgeon grasps the injured hand as if he were 'shaking hands'. He then exerts firm traction in the long axis of the limb in order to disimpact the fragments of the radius. When this has been accomplished, he presses the distal fragment into palmar-flexion and ulnar-deviation using the thumb of his other hand. At the same time, he draws the patient's hand into pronation, ulnar-deviation and palmar-flexion. A plaster slab is then applied to the lateral, dorsal and medial aspects of the forearm, wrist and hand from the elbow to the metacarpal heads holding the wrist in palmar-flexion and ulnar-deviation (fig. 258 (*a*)). Satisfactory reduction is confirmed by x-ray. The slab is converted to an encircling Colles' plaster if the circulation to the fingers is satisfactory 24 hours later.

The plaster is maintained for 6 weeks. If extreme palmar-flexion and ulnar-deviation is required to maintain the reduction, this position should be maintained only for 3 weeks, at the end of which time the plaster is removed and re-applied with the wrist more nearly neutral. It should be noted that although pronation is required to correct the supination element of the deformity, a plaster is applied which does not control the movements of pronation and supination. In this sense a Colles' plaster is inadequate for this injury: it is used only because, in the age group involved (the elderly), the injury to the inferior radio-ulnar joint results in a greater limitation of pronation and supination if these movements are restricted than if they are permitted. Loss of forearm rotation is a more serious disability than mal-union. The fingers should be actively mobilised immediately after the injury since otherwise they may become stiff. Patients should be instructed to elevate the arm above the head several times per day to prevent shoulder stiffness. These latter two aspects are probably more important than treatment of the fracture itself in terms of functional outcome. If progressive finger swelling occurs, the patient must return to hospital. The patient may need to be admitted for a period of in-patient elevation of the upper limb and mobilization of the fingers under physiotherapy supervision.

Complications.—(1) Mal-union.—While union is almost invariable, there is often some residual deformity because (*a*) even if the initial reduction is perfect, recurrent backward angulation of the distal fragment is common if the dorsal cortex of the radius is comminuted and, (*b*) a Colles' plaster does not control the supination element of the deformity.

(2) Stiffness of wrist, shoulder and fingers.—When the plaster is removed, the wrist is often stiff and may require remobilisation in a physiotherapy department. The inferior radio-ulnar joint is also commonly stiff and may be very difficult to remobilise. Occasionally persistent limitation of pronation and supination combined with significant displacement of the distal radius relative to the distal ulna may, in younger patients, require excision of the distal ulna (a procedure which can be regarded as an excision arthroplasty of the inferior radio-ulnar joint).

(3) Carpal tunnel syndrome is not uncommon as a late complication of a Colles' fracture. Treatment is by surgical division of the flexor retinaculum after confirmation of the diagnosis by nerve conduction studies.

(4) Rupture of the extensor pollicis longus tendon over the dorsal aspect of the wrist may also occur as a late complication. Surprisingly this is commoner in undisplaced fractures. Treatment is by tendon transfer if the resultant disability is troublesome to the patient (which it is not always!).

(5) Sudeck's atrophy – see Chapter 15.

Smith's Fracture.—This is the reverse of Colles' fracture, the distal fragment being palmar-flexed rather than dorsiflexed. It is uncommon. The injury is conventionally attributed to a backward fall on the outstretched hand but it seems more likely that it is in fact due to a fall on the dorsum of the palmar-flexed wrist, not to a fall on the palm of the outstretched hand at all. Reduction is by reversal of the original mechanism and immobilisation in an above-elbow plaster for 6 weeks or, better, by internal fixation using an Ellis plate.

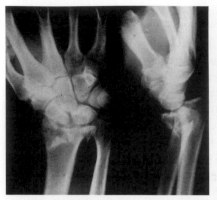 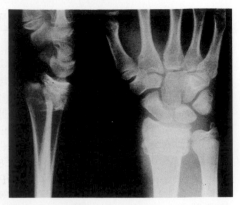

FIG. 259.—Barton's fracture—intra-articular (see text).

FIG. 261.—Child's Colles' fracture; fracture separation of the distal radial epiphysis.

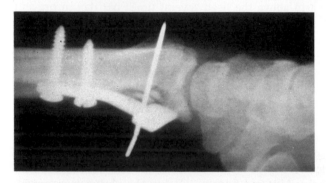

FIG. 260.—Barton's fracture. Open reduction and fixation by an Ellis T-plate.

Barton's Fracture.—This is an intra-articular fracture of the distal radius with volar displacement of a small triangular fragment along with the whole of the carpus (fig. 259). Although the injury can be managed by closed reduction and application of a full-arm plaster cast in supination, redisplacement is very common and the fracture is best managed by open reduction and application of an Ellis T-plate (fig. 260).

Fracture of the Radial Styloid.—This injury occurs following a direct blow on the wrist (the injury used to be called 'chauffeur's fracture', when cars were started with a starting handle, since if this kicked back it often struck the wrist on its lateral aspect) or occasionally following a fall on the wrist. The fracture line runs proximally and laterally through the radial styloid roughly from a point opposite the articulation between the scaphoid and the lunate. Displacement is uncommon and the only treatment required is the application of a Colles' plaster for 6 weeks.

Fractures of Distal Radial Epiphysis.—*This is the child's Colles' fracture.* The injury is usually a Salter type II fracture separation of the distal radial epiphysis resulting in a displacement similar to the Colles' displacement (fig. 261). Reduction, if displaced significantly, should be carried out under general anaesthesia followed by application of a Colles' plaster cast for four weeks. The fracture may be surprisingly difficult to reduce. Growth disturbance is rare.

Fracture through the Distal Metaphysis of the Radius in Children.—This may occur at any level proximal to the epiphyseal plate. The fracture may be of the greenstick variety or may be complete. The former is often almost undisplaced and only requires support in a Colles' plaster for 3 to 4 weeks. The fracture may however be complete, with marked angulation (concave dorsally) at the fracture site. This is a deceptive injury for it is often regarded by the inexperienced as the equivalent of a Colles' fracture and treated in the same way. If it is, so that pronation and supination are not controlled by the plaster which is applied, significant re-angulation commonly occurs at the fracture site leading to malunion and marked limitation of pronation and supination. Following reduction, the fracture should be held by a well-moulded plaster which extends above the elbow with the hand palmar-flexed, ulnar-deviated and in neutral rotation, the elbow itself being at right angles so that pronation and supination are controlled. Both undisplaced and displaced fractures should be x-rayed one week after reduction to ensure that angulation of the fracture has not occurred in plaster. If it has, re-manipulation is required.

INJURIES OF THE CARPUS

Any of the bones of the carpus may be fractured and some may also be dislocated. However, the common and important injuries are:

Scaphoid fracture
Lunate dislocation
Peri-lunate dislocation
Dorsal chip fracture

Fractures of the Scaphoid

By far the commonest injury of the carpus is fracture of the scaphoid (60–70%). The injury occurs following a fall on the outstretched hand, typically in young adults. It is uncertain precisely how this causes fracture of the scaphoid, but it seems possible that the bone is 'bent' at its waist over the radial styloid.

The patient presents with a complaint of pain in the wrist, but function of the wrist may not be grossly impaired. On examination there is tenderness over the scaphoid in the anatomical snuff-box, a little swelling and no bruising. These physical signs often appear trivial and suggest a 'sprained wrist' rather than a fracture. Radiological examination (which should include not only an antero-

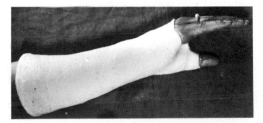

FIG. 262.—A scaphoid plaster.

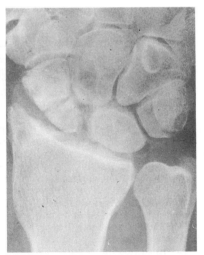

FIG. 264.—Non-union of a fracture of the waist of the scaphoid with secondary osteoarthrosis of the wrist.

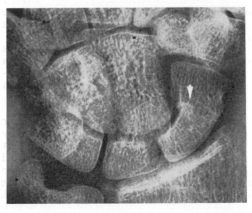

FIG. 263.—Fracture through the waist of the scaphoid.

posterior and lateral view of the wrist, but also two oblique views) may not display the fracture immediately after injury since no displacement occurs at the fracture site.

Because this fracture does not produce substantial clinical and radiological signs it is often missed and wrongly diagnosed as a 'sprained wrist'. The wrist is then treated with strapping and as a consequence the fracture may not unite. Therefore any 'sprained wrist' in which a fracture of the scaphoid cannot be excluded should be treated for 2 weeks in a scaphoid plaster (fig. 262). Two weeks after the injury, the plaster should be removed and the wrist re-x-rayed. By this time bone resorption will have occurred at the site of a scaphoid fracture so that the injury will be radiologically obvious (fig. 263). The fracture may be in the proximal pole, waist, or distal pole of the bone and may be displaced or undisplaced. The fracture may involve the tubercle of the scaphoid only.

Treatment.—If the fracture is diagnosed at the time of the injury or at re-x-ray 2 weeks later, a scaphoid plaster should be applied for 8 weeks. This treatment will result in bony union in 90% of uncomplicated cases. Some surgeons advocate primary internal fixation for this fracture, expecially if there are strong social, athletic or personal reasons for not using a plaster cast. Certainly, if there is non-compliance on the part of the patient it is probably advisable to procede to internal fixation as this will probably reduce the overall non-union rate. If internal fixation is carried out, the fracture should be fixed with a small compression screw. Some surgeons also advocate primary internal fixation of displaced fractures but whether or not this is necessary in all cases remains to be substantiated.

Complications.—(1) Non-union occurs in approximately 10% of cases and can even occur after adequate immobilisation of the fracture although most cases seen in practice are young men in whom the diagnosis was made late or not at all or did not comply with plaster immobilisation. The treatment is by bone-grafting with or without internal fixation.

(2) Avascular necrosis of the proximal fragment may occur because the blood supply to the proximal part of the bone often enters entirely through the distal pole. Thus when the waist of the scaphoid is fractured the proximal pole is infarcted. The fracture then fails to unite and avascular changes, similar to those seen in the femoral head (Chapter 17), may develop in the proximal half of the bone. These changes may lead to osteoarthrosis of the wrist (fig. 264).

Fracture of the tubercle of the scaphoid occurs occasionally and is an insignificant injury. It is functionally immaterial whether the fracture unites or not, and the wrist need only be treated by such immobilisation as is necessary to relieve pain. The essential difference between this injury and fractures of the waist of the scaphoid is that in this injury no articular surface is involved, whereas after fractures through the waist of the scaphoid the mechanism of the wrist may be prejudiced by an unsound fibrous non-union.

Lunate and Perilunate Dislocation of the Wrist.—A fall on the palm of the out-stretched, dorsiflexed hand may dislocate the whole of the carpus backwards in relation to the radius and lunate. This is a perilunate dislocation of the wrist. The dislocation may persist, spontaneously reduce, or reduce but in so doing displace the lunate forwards. This third possibility produces a dislocation of the lunate. These dislocations may be complicated by a fracture of the waist of the scaphoid. If they are, the proximal pole of the scaphoid remains with the lunate, and the distal pole with the rest of the carpus.

Surprisingly, it is not uncommon for these injuries to be missed clinically and radiolog-ically. Clinically the wrist and fingers are stiff and the wrist swollen and tender. If the lunate has dislocated, it may compress the median nerve to cause median nerve signs. A well-centred lateral x-ray clearly reveals the dislocated lunate in front of the carpus or the posterior displacement of the carpus, but a poor, slightly rotated lateral view may conceal the dislocation. The antero-posterior view at first sight may be passed as normal, but close inspection will show that the bones of the proximal row of the carpus (scaphoid, lunate and triquetral) are not disposed round the head of the capitate with the intervention of a regular joint space as in the normal wrist, and, if the lunate has dislocated, the lunate appears tri-angular rather than quadrangular in outline because it is rotated as it is dislocated forwards.

Treatment.—Isolated dislocation of the lunate can usually be treated by closed reduction. If this fails then open reduction is mandatory. Avascular necrosis of the lunate may occur after this injury. Trans-scaphoid perilunate dislocation should be treated by open reduction and internal fixation of the fractured scaphoid and repair of the disrupted volar carpal ligaments.

Dorsal chip fracture.—This consists of a ligamentous or capsular avulsion of a flake of bone from the dorsal aspect of the carpus. It is a not uncommon injury resulting from forced palmar flexion of the wrist. Treatment is symptomatic with early mobilisation of the fingers and wrist.

INJURIES OF THE HAND

Fracture of the Terminal Phalanx.—This bone is commonly fractured by crushing injuries. The skin and pulp are also crushed so that the skin is often lacerated and the fracture is compound. Perhaps because these injuries involve a small bone, they are often regarded as trivial. This is a mistake, for if the injury to the terminal phalanx and to the overlying soft tissues does not heal satisfactorily, the finger tip becomes permanently tender to touch and often painful in cold weather. Permanent tenderness of a finger tip is a severe disability: the patient tends to use the other fingers and to guard the affected finger so that it gradually becomes stiff. If the digit involved is the thumb, the situation is even more serious for loss of the thumb is functionally almost equivalent to loss of the arm.

Treatment, if the fracture is compound, consists of careful wound toilet and loose suturing of the skin followed by the application of a pressure dressing. The dressing should be changed at 48 hours and thereafter at regular intervals in order to inspect the skin. A broad spectrum antibiotic and tetanus toxoid are administered. If the skin dies or is lost, it may require replacement with full thickness skin on the pulp or split skin elsewhere on the digit (Chapter 11). If the fracture is simple, a pressure dressing should be applied until the pain has subsided.

Mallet Finger.—This injury consists of a rupture, or avulsion-fracture, of the terminal slip of the extensor tendon to the distal phalanx. If the tendon is avulsed, the bony insertion of the tendon can be seen as a small fracture fragment on the dorsal aspect of the terminal interphalangeal joint (fig. 265). The injury is caused by forced flexion of the terminal phalanx whilst the extensors of the finger are contracting. It may occur, for example, during bed-making when the hand is thrust under the mattress to tuck in the sheets: the finger tip catches in the mattress and is forcibly flexed at a time when the patient is holding the interphalangeal joints actively extended. It is a well known cricket injury (catching the ball) especially in wicket keepers.

The patient complains of localised pain and swelling and an inability actively to extend the terminal phalanx. Passive extension is possible but when the finger is released the terminal phalanx falls back into a position of 30° of flexion under the influence of the long flexor tendons (fig. 266).

Treatment.—If a fracture fragment has been avulsed and can be seen radiologically to be rotated from its bed, the fragment should be sutured back into place. If no fragment has been avulsed, or if an avulsed fragment is not significantly displaced, the injury should

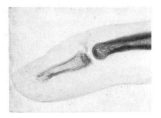

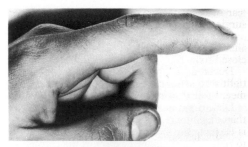

FIG. 266.—Mallet finger.

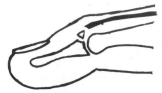

FIG. 265.—Mallet finger. Avulsion of a flake of bone to which the long extensor tendon is attached.

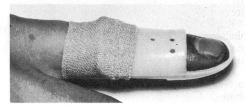

FIG. 267.—A Stack mallet finger splint.

be treated in a splint holding the terminal phalanx in full extension for 6 weeks (fig. 267). On this regime most tendons unite so that the patient regains active extension, but occasionally the deformity persists. The patient should be advised to accept this deformity since firstly, it often improves gradually over the year following the injury; secondly, the disability it causes is very slight, save in certain occupations such as playing the guitar; and thirdly, late treatment (by suture of the tendon) tends to stiffen the distal interphalangeal joint.

Fractures of the Middle and Proximal Phalanx.—These fractures may be caused by a direct blow (when the fracture is often comminuted) or by bending or twisting the finger (when the fracture is transverse or spiral). The fracture is usually unstable, and if it is, is angulated forwards. The tendons adjacent to the fracture may adhere to the fracture as it heals and hence limit movement in the finger.

Treatment is difficult since it is not easy to maintain reduction and to immobilise the fracture without stiffening the joints of the finger. If the fracture appears to be stable and there is little displacement, the fracture can be splinted satisfactorily whilst *allowing movement* at the joints of the finger by strapping the finger to its neighbour for 4 weeks. Care must be taken when this is done to ensure that there is no rotational deformity at the fracture site, for if there is, the finger will deviate as it flexes so as to inferfere with its neighbour. If the fracture is displaced, it is reduced by traction followed by immobilisation on an aluminium splint applied to the flexion aspect of the finger and palm. The interphalangeal joints should be immobilised in extension and the metacarpo-phalangeal joint in flexion in order to minimise subsequent stiffness.

If the fracture is not soundly united when the splint is removed after 4 weeks, the fracture may require a further period of splintage provided by strapping the finger to its neighbour. If accurate reduction cannot be obtained by manipulation and splintage, the fracture should be reduced at operation and the reduction held by crossed Kirschner wires.

Following this the finger should be strapped to its neighbour, leaving the inter-phalangeal joint free, and early active mobilisation encouraged.

Dislocation of the interphalangeal and metacarpo-phalangeal joints.—Dislocations of the proximal interphalangeal joints are the commonest. The displacement is usually dorsal but may be lateral and much less commonly anterior. Dorsal dislocations result from forceful hyperextension which also results in rupture of the volar plate. Closed reduction is usually easily carried out by traction and flexion of the finger. After reduction the integrity of the collateral ligaments must be checked. The finger is strapped to its neighbour for three weeks and actively mobilised. Lateral dislocations result in a complete

Martin Kirschner, 1879–1942. Professor of Surgery, Heidelberg, Germany. Described the use of traction wires in 1909.
Hugh Graham Stack, Contemporary. Orthopaedic Surgeon, Harold Wood Hospital, Essex, England.

tear of one collateral ligament and are probably best treated by closed reduction and surgical repair of the torn ligament.

Occasionally the head of the proximal phalanx 'button holes' through the capsule or alternatively the long flexor tendon may become interposed in the joint. In these cases closed reduction is impossible and open reduction should be performed.

Dorsal dislocations of the distal interphalangeal joint are often compound due to the tight soft tissue envelope surrounding the joint. Reduction is usually possible by closed means followed by a short period of volar splintage.

Dislocations of the metacarpo-phalangeal joints of the fingers are much less common than dislocations of the metacarpo-phalangeal joint of the thumb. When they do occur it is usually the two border fingers which are affected. These dislocations may be difficult to reduce by closed means because of interposition of soft tissues, for example the volar plate or the head of the metacarpal may be locked between the long flexor tendons and the lumbrical muscle in the case of the fingers, and between the two slips of flexor pollicis brevis in the case of the thumb. In these cases open reduction must be carried out.

Ruptures of the Collateral Ligaments.—Forced adduction or abduction at the inter-phalangeal or metacarpo-phalangeal joints may rupture the collateral ligament on the tension side of the joint. The joint momentarily subluxates but reduces spontaneously unless the ruptured collateral ligament becomes interposed between the joint surfaces.

Clinically, the joint is tender on the side of the ruptured ligament and mechanical instability can be appreciated. Instability can be confirmed by a stress x-ray. There is no abnormality in ordinary radiographs unless the bony attachment of the involved ligament has been avulsed and is radiologically visible, or the ligament is interposed in the joint space in which case persistent malalignment of the finger will be noticed.

Treatment.—The finger should be immobilised on an aluminium splint. If the collateral ligament is interposed in the joint surface or an avulsed bony fragment is displaced, the joint should be opened and the collateral ligament or fracture fragment sutured in its anatomical position.

Fractures of the Metacarpals.—Fractures of the shaft or neck of one or more of the medial four metacarpals are produced by the knuckles striking objects (*i.e.* by punching), or by blows on the dorsum of the hand. Fractures of a single shaft are splinted by the adjacent metacarpals and suffer little displacement. Fractures through the neck are usually associated with some forward angulation of the head of the bone but this deformity, even if gross, results only in recession of the knuckle and a minimal loss of extension at the metacarpo-phalangeal joint. This is of no significance if full movement at other joints and a good grip is achieved by early mobilisation. Transverse fractures of the metacarpals are sometimes slow to unite, but all other fractures unite well.

Treatment.—The associated finger should be strapped to its neighbour and a plaster back slab added for further protection. Early active mobilisation should be encouraged.

It should be explained to patients with angulated fractures of the neck of the metacarpal that, if no specific treatment other than early mobilisation is undertaken, their hand will return to normal save for a 'dropped knuckle' and perhaps a small extensor lag. If they prefer not to accept this disability, an attempt should be made to reduce the fracture by flexing the metacarpo-phalangeal joint to 90° and then pressing the proximal phalanx, and with it the distal fragment, dorsally in relation to the shaft of the metacarpal. The reduction is held by placing the finger on a volar splint with the interphalangeal joints extended and the metacarpophalangeal flexed to 90°. Union usually takes place in three weeks.

If the fracture is very unstable it can be held reduced by one or two percutaneous wires inserted through the neck of the metacarpal into the neck of the neighbouring metacarpal.

Fractures of 3 or more metacarpal shafts require reduction and splintage since the metacarpus as a whole is unstable. This is probably best achieved by open reduction and insertion of oblique longitudinal wires. These injuries may be associated with gross swelling in which case the patient should be admitted to hospital for elevation of the hand and early active mobilisation of the fingers under physiotherapy supervision.

Fracture-Dislocation of the Base of the First Metacarpal (Bennett's Fracture).— This injury is caused by a blow to the point of the thumb. An oblique fracture of the base of the metacarpal occurs extending proximally to involve the articular surface. The shaft of the bone is drawn proximally by the pull of the long muscles of the thumb, so that it subluxates from the carpo-metacarpal joint (fig. 268).

Treatment.—The fracture-dislocation is easily reduced by traction, extension of the thumb, and pressure over the dorsal aspect of the base of the first metacarpal (fig. 268). The difficulty is to maintain reduction. This can be done if the 1st metacarpal is immobi-

Edward Hallaran Bennett, 1837–1907. Professor of Surgery, Trinity College, Dublin. Described this fracture in 1882.

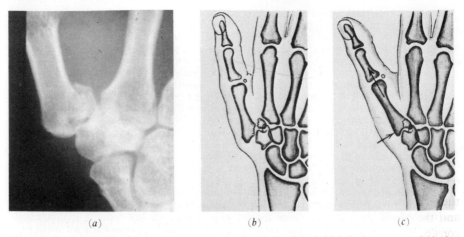

(a)   (b)   (c)

FIG. 268.—(<i>a</i>) Bennett's fracture dislocation, (<i>b</i>) the nature of the initial displacement and (<i>c</i>) the principles of reduction.

lised in plaster in almost full extension at the carpo-metacarpal joint whilst direct pressure is applied over the dorsum of the base of the bone as the plaster sets, so as to press the shaft medially against the palmar fragment. Unfortunately a reduction held in this way often slips. Therefore some surgeons apply continuous traction to the thumb by means of a plaster cast applied to the forearm, in which is incorporated a loop of thick wire to take adhesive traction applied to the end of the thumb. Alternatively the fracture may be fixed internally with a wire.

Lacerations of the Hand. (These are discussed in Chapter 11.)

CHAPTER 17

FRACTURES AND DISLOCATIONS. LOWER LIMB AND PELVIS

FRACTURES OF THE PELVIS

The pelvis is a bony ring consisting of the two iliac bones and sacrum linked by the very strong sacro-iliac, sacro-tuberous and sacrospinous ligaments posteriorly and the symphysis pubis and related ligaments anteriorly. This bony ring has considerable inherent stability. The posterior two thirds of this ring transmit weight from the spine to the hip during walking and standing. The anterior third of the ring transmits weight to the ischial tuberosities during sitting.

Fractures of the pelvis usually result from road traffic accidents in patients under 60 years of age and falls in the home in patients over the age of 60. They are associated with a considerable mortality (5-20%).

The diagnosis of a fractured pelvis is suspected on the history, and the findings of localised tenderness and pain on stressing the pelvis. It is proved radiologically.

TABLE. 1 CLASSIFICATION OF PELVIC FRACTURES

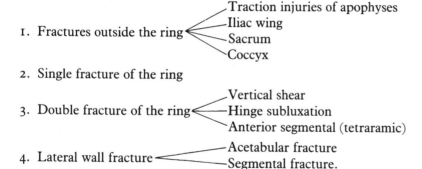

1. Fractures outside the ring
   - Traction injuries of apophyses
   - Iliac wing
   - Sacrum
   - Coccyx

2. Single fracture of the ring

3. Double fracture of the ring
   - Vertical shear
   - Hinge subluxation
   - Anterior segmental (tetraramic)

4. Lateral wall fracture
   - Acetabular fracture
   - Segmental fracture.

Fractures outside the ring.—Traction injuries of the apophyses may result from muscular violence in teenage athletes. Most commonly the anterior inferior iliac spine is avulsed by the rectus femoris tendon (fig. 269) or the ischial tuberosity by the hamstring tendons. Occasionally the anterior superior iliac spine is avulsed by sartorius. There are usually no complications and no specific treatment is required, other than rest until pain settles, unless the fragment is widely displaced.

Comminuted fractures of the iliac wings usually result from direct violence and there is usually little displacement because the iliacus muscle on the inner side, and the gluteal muscles on the outer side, support the bone. The patient should be treated by bed rest until symptoms settle, which usually takes two to

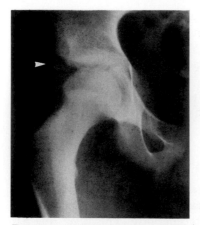

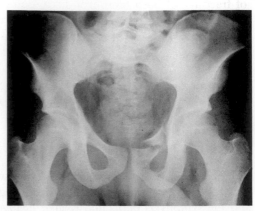

FIG. 269.—Avulsion of the anterior inferior iliac spine.

FIG. 270.—Fracture of pubic ramus (single fracture of the ring).

three weeks. Occasionally a paralytic ileus may develop as a result of the retro-peritoneal haematoma.

Fractures of the sacrum are usually transverse at the lower border of the sacro-iliac joint and result from a direct blow from behind. These fractures are often difficult to visualise on radiographs. They may be associated wtih sacral nerve damage and this should be looked for. Treatment is by bed rest until pain settles.

The Coccyx.—The coccyx may be fractured as a result of kicks or falls. Pain, which is often severe, occurs on walking, sitting or with actions which involve contraction of the levator ani, such as defaecation or coughing. Rectal examination reveals local tenderness and occasionally deformity. No specific treatment is needed and the symptoms settle spontaneously in about 6 weeks.

If symptoms persist for months, in spite of adequate rest and symptomatic treatment by sitting on soft cushions or anaesthetic injections, excision of the coccyx may have to be considered. There should be no haste in making this decision as persistent symptoms are often psychological in origin. In some cases these symptoms occur without fracture or even injury. This condition, known as *coccydynia*, is of unknown aetiology. The treatment of the pain is the same as that for pain occurring after fracture.

Excision of the coccyx does not usually relieve the symptoms completely, if at all, and the patient should be warned of this before going ahead with surgery.

Single fracture of the ring.—These injuries are very common and result from compression either from a crush injury or a force transmitted through the femur to the pelvis, for example, after a fall. The compressed pelvic ring usually gives way at the weakest point, the anterior rami, resulting in a fracture of one or more usually two pubic rami on the same side with minimal displacement (fig. 270).

The pelvis is a rigid osseo-ligamentous ring. If it is broken in only one place, no significant displacement can occur at the fracture site and the only treatment which is needed is for the patient to rest until the pain has settled. The fracture usually unites in about six weeks. A rare complication is bladder perforation by a spike of bone.

Double fracture of the ring.—Fractures through two places in the ring consti-tute a far more serious injury since (1) the pelvis is no longer a stable weight-bearing structure, (2) the separated fragment may be displaced and (3) the frac-ture may be difficult or impossible to reduce. A vertical shear fracture consists of fractures of both rami or a disruption of the symphysis pubis at the front, coupled with a fracture of the ilium or sacrum or a disruption of the sacro-iliac joint posteriorly (fig. 271) The mobile hemi-pelvis tends to be pulled upwards by the anterior and posterior trunk muscles and rotated outward by the weight of the leg.

This type of pelvic fracture is associated with the highest mortality and morbidity. The injury usually results from either direct antero-posterior or lateral compression from a crushing injury or indirect lateral compression through the lower limb. The aims of treatment are to reduce the displacement by applying skeletal traction to the leg to correct leg length and application of a pelvic sling to reduce outward rotation of the hemi-pelvis. The patient should remain on traction for 6–8 weeks following which mobilisation can begin but no weight-bearing on the injured side should be allowed until 12 weeks after injury.

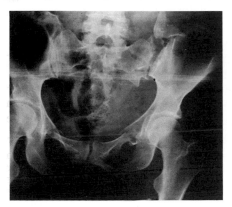

FIG. 271.—Double fracture of the pelvic ring with disruption of left sacro-iliac joint.

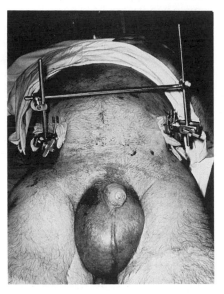

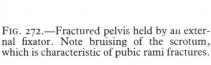

FIG. 272.—Fractured pelvis held by an external fixator. Note bruising of the scrotum, which is characteristic of pubic rami fractures.

The most important immediate complication is the liability to severe, internal and therefore concealed haemorrhage, and to injury of the viscera—the male urethra commonly, the bladder in both sexes occasionally, and the rectum and vagina rarely. Systemic signs of blood loss should be sought and blood transfused if necessary. Blood escaping from the external urinary meatus in the male immediately suggests rupture of the urethra.

The management of bladder and urethral injuries are discussed in Chapters 58 and 60 respectively. Other complications include injury to nerve roots, arteries and occasionally entrapment of bowel or lumbo-sacral trunk.

Hinge subluxation occurs when there is a disruption of the symphysis pubis with wide separation in addition to disruption of one sacro-iliac joint with little separation. Stability of this injury is variable and a common complication is urethral injury.

Treatment is by reduction using a pelvic sling or alternatively an open reduction can be carried out and a plate applied to the posterior aspect of the symphysis. An external fixator can also be applied to each hemi-pelvis as a means of reducing and holding this type of fracture (fig. 272) Weight-bearing on the affected side should not be allowed for 12 weeks.

An anterior segmental (tetraramic) fracture usually results from direct violence to the symphysial region. Fractures of all four rami occur with displacement of a segment and attached uro-genital diaphragm. The urethra is often sheared off at the apex of the prostate in a male. Uncomplicated fractures require bed-rest for approximately 4–6 weeks.

Lateral wall fractures.—Fractures of the acetabulum may be linear in which case they may be undisplaced or displaced. Undisplaced fractures require treatment in bed with traction applied to the leg in order to prevent subsequent displacement. Traction can be removed after six weeks but the patient must remain non-weight bearing on the affected limb for a further six weeks. Displaced fractures require open reduction and internal fixation in order to restore normal acetabular anatomy, although occasionally this can be obtained by a combination of longitudinal and lateral skeletal traction applied to the lower limb.

Sometimes the acetabular fracture will be comminuted resulting in irreparable shattering of the acetabulum including the weight-bearing area of the roof. The femoral head may be subluxated or dislocated centrally or upwards. Treatment is by a combination of longitudinal and lateral traction to the lower limb for 4–6 weeks followed by a further six weeks longitudinal traction during which time the hip can be actively mobilised.

A segmental fracture occurs when a segment of the lateral wall of the pelvis, containing the intact acetabulum, is displaced inward. The fractures occur through both pubic rami and the wing of the ilium. Treatment is by lateral traction for 8–12 weeks.

Complications of pelvic fractures.—1. *Blood loss.*—40% of all patients with pelvic fractures require blood transfusion. As already mentioned, blood loss is a major problem in those with double fractures of the pelvic ring. Blood loss from torn iliac vessels is the usual cause of death resulting from a fracture of the pelvis.

2. *Injury to bladder and urethra.*—This is discussed in chapters 58 and 60 respectively.

3. *Deep vein thrombosis* is not uncommon in patients treated on bed rest following a pelvic fracture.

4. *Mal-union* is common but does not usually present significant problems except in females of child-bearing age. Caesarean section may be required for delivery.

5. *Secondary osteoarthritis* is common after disruptions of the sacro-iliac joints and acetabular fractures.

THE HIP—DISLOCATION

This injury is relatively uncommon because of the depth of the acetabular cavity and the strong support afforded to the joint by its ligaments and muscles.

The injury usually occurs when the hip is flexed, especially if it is also adducted, because in this position the head of the femur is covered posteriorly by capsule

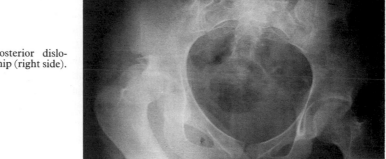

FIG. 273.—Posterior dislocation of the hip (right side).

rather than bone. Thus a force applied in the long axis of the femoral shaft may dislocate the head over the posterior lip of the acetabulum. Such a force is commonly provided either by a weight falling on the back of a person in a stooping position, as may happen if a coal-miner is struck by a 'fall of roof', or, more commonly, in car and motor cycle accidents in which, for example, a front seat passenger in a car is thrown forwards so that the knee strikes the dashboard. The dislocation may be *posterior (fig. 273) (by far the commonest), anterior or central.*

Posterior Dislocation of the Hip

In the usual posterior dislocation, the head of the femur escapes into the sciatic notch (where rarely the sciatic nerve may be damaged), and then passes up on to the dorsum of the ilium. The leg is flexed, adducted, and internally rotated, so that the sole of the foot rests upon the opposite instep. Pain is sometimes referred along the sciatic nerve, which may be involved by direct injury. X-rays should always be taken to confirm the dislocation and to detect any associated fracture.

The commonest associated fracture is a posterior acetabular rim fracture which may be small or large and displaced or undisplaced. Other fractures may be present and should be looked for; these are fractures of the femoral head and neck, shaft, knee and acetabulum. Sciatic nerve function should be tested and documented prior to reduction if possible.

Reduction is usually easy provided that the injury is recent, and the anaesthetist obtains full muscle relaxation. The patient is placed on a mattress on the floor, and the iliac crests are steadied by an assistant. The surgeon stands over the limb and flexes the knee and thigh, bringing the head of the bone beneath (*i.e.* posterior to) the acetabulum. The femur is then adducted and pulled vertically upwards so as to draw the head forward from its posterior position. The essence of the reduction lies in the vertical lifting of the femur. Usually reduction will occur with this vertical traction alone but sometimes the hip must be internally rotated while upward traction is being exerted before the head of the femur suddenly snaps into its socket.

Usually the reduction is quite obvious when it occurs, and if the acetabulum is intact the reduction is stable—especially so when the hip is extended, abducted and externally rotated. Reduction is usually adequately maintained by skin traction applied to the lower limb and this should be continued for three to six weeks, during which time the hip is mobilised.

Complications.—1. *Sciatic nerve injury* occurs in approximately 10% of cases. The whole nerve may be affected or, as is more usual, the lateral popliteal component. Treatment is expectant and the patient should be provided with a cosmetic drop foot splint on toe spring.

2. *Avascular necrosis* of the femoral head (p. 310) occurs in approximately 15% of cases if reduction is carried out soon (less than 8 hours after injury) but in as many as 50% of cases if there is delay in obtaining reduction of the dislocation. The abnormal radiological features associated with this complication may not appear until 2–3 years after the injury. Because there is no evidence to suggest that revascularisation occurs more quickly or completely if the patient remains non-weight bearing for a prolonged period after the injury and because there is no way of knowing if and when revascularisation is complete, this old practice has nothing to commend it and should be abolished! The important message is to reduce the dislocation as soon as possible after the injury.

3. *Associated fractures* may occur as already described. These should be treated on their own merits after reduction of the dislocation. Fracture of the femoral neck must be treated by operation since in no other way can the fracture and the dislocation be reduced. Avascular necrosis is almost invariable. Posterior rim fractures of significant size should be treated by open reduction and internal fixation, especially if they are associated with post-reduction instability.

4. *Secondary osteoarthritis* may occur following dislocation of the hip even in the absence of an associated fracture and avascular necrosis.

Anterior Dislocation of the Hip.—This is rare. The femoral head may lie either in the obturator or pubic position: in both cases the limb is in a position of flexion, abduction, and external rotation.

Central Dislocation of the Hip.—This may be caused by a blow in the greater trochanter, driving the head of the femur through the floor of the acetabulum. This injury amounts to a comminuted fracture of the acetabulum and may be accompanied by other fractures of the pelvis.

Treatment is difficult and unsatisfactory. The femoral head can often be pulled out to its anatomical position by traction on the leg (sometimes combined with a side pull applied via a wire or nail in the greater trochanter). Unfortunately the weight-bearing part of the acetabulum rarely reduces with the head of the femur and, even if it does, the floor of the acetabulum does not accompany the reduction. The fracture can be reduced by operation but this is difficult. Therefore probably the best form of management is to accept the displacement and mobilise the hip with tibial skeletal traction as soon as pain allows. Osteo-arthrosis usually develops eventually, regardless of treatment.

FRACTURES OF THE FEMUR

Fractures of the femur are common and can be classified as follows:

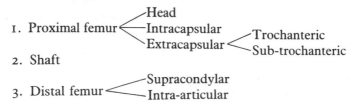

1. Proximal femur — Head
                   — Intracapsular
                   — Extracapsular — Trochanteric
                                   — Sub-trochanteric
2. Shaft

3. Distal femur — Supracondylar
                — Intra-articular

Fractures of the Proximal Femur

Since the days of Sir Astley Cooper these fractures have been divided into *intra-capsular* and *extra-capsular*. Intra-capsular fractures occur in that portion of the neck of the femur which lies within the capsule of the hip. Extra-capsular fractures occur in the remainder of the neck down to approximatley three inches below the lesser trochanter and are divided into trochanteric (occurring through the trochanteric mass) and sub-trochanteric (occurring through or just below the lesser trochanter). Rarely, fractures of the femoral head itself may occur in association with dislocation of the hip.

Intra-capsular Fractures of the Neck of the Femur: Pathology.—These fractures are anatomically sub-divided into subcapital and (more distally) transcervical. It is possible however that they all consist of a fracture starting superiorly at the junction of the head and neck (*i.e.* 'subcapital'), which propagates downwards through the head-neck junction until it encounters the medial trabecular system, and which may then be deflected distally by this column of strong bone so that it emerges inferiorly somewhere in the neck (*i.e.* to be 'transcervical'). Two features of this fracture make treatment difficult: (1) the blood supply to the proximal fragment is often impaired and (2) the proximal fragment can be neither manipulated nor immobilised by conservative means.

The blood supply of the head of the adult femur can best be summarised as follows:

(1) An extracapsular arterial ring located at the base of the neck and formed from branches of the medial and lateral femoral circumflex arteries.

(2) Ascending cervical branches of the extracapsular arterial ring which lie sub-synovially on the surface of the neck. These are known as retinacular arteries and enter the head by piercing the bone at the junction of head and neck.

(3) Arteries of the ligamentum teres which, in the adult, are not always patent and, if they are, probably only supply a small area of bone around the fovea capitis.

In addition terminal branches of the ascending nutrient arteries are present within the neck of the femur which also received branches from the retinacular arteries. It is the intra-osseous and retinacular vessels, the major source of blood supply to the head, which are frequently damaged in association with an intracapsular fracture. The greater the displacement of the fracture the greater is the risk of vascular damage.

Damage to the blood supply frequently occurs and leads to avascular necrosis of part or the whole of the femoral head.

Classification.—There are several classifications which have been proposed for intra-capsular fractures of the neck of the femur but, for practical purposes, they are only useful from a clinical point of view and the following is, therefore, suggested:

(1) Stress fractures
(2) Undisplaced/impacted fracture
(3) Displaced fracture ± comminution

Displacement is usual at the fracture site and takes the form of external rotation and adduction of the distal on the proximal fragment. Occasionally subcapital fractures are impacted: no rotation then occurs and the fracture appears to be abducted, rather than adducted.

Rarely and in young adults stress fractures may occur in the femoral neck of those exposed to unusual and unaccustomed physical activities such as route marches with a full military pack. Treatment is by relief of weight bearing until healing occurs.

Clinical features.—These fractures are very much more common in elderly women in whom they are associated with seemingly trivial domestic stumbles. The fact that these fractures seem to be produced by very slight violence is perhaps due to the fact that osteoporosis has weakened the femoral neck. There is now however evidence that the fracture is due to fatigue in these patients, not to a fall; *i.e.* that the patient falls because the bone fractures, not that the bone fractures because the patient falls.

In unimpacted fractures the leg is short and lies in external rotation; there is tenderness over the fracture site in the groin; attempted movement of the hip is painful; and the patient is unable to lift the leg off the examination couch. *In impacted subcapital* fractures there is tenderness over the fracture site but otherwise there may be no abnormal physical signs. These fractures are therefore easily missed clinically.

An exact diagnosis requires x-ray examination. Even on x-ray, impacted fractures with minimal displacement may be missed.

In young adults the fracture may occur following severe violence applied in the long axis of the femur so as to shear the femoral neck. Such fractures may be associated with dislocation of the hip.

Treatment.—To some extent this remains the 'unsolved fracture' and the best method of treatment remains controversial and will vary from one hospital to another. Treatment is invariably operative because the proximal fragment cannot be controlled conservatively. Undisplaced and impacted fractures (fig. 274) in patients of all ages should be treated by internal fixation, preferably with a sliding compression screw attached to a single-piece two-hole plate. *For displaced fractures, if the patient is under 65* closed reduction followed by internal fixation as above should be carried out. If a satisfactory closed reduction cannot be obtained an attempt at open reduction should be performed. The reason for using a sliding screw is that, if collapse occurs at the fracture site as it unites, the screw can back out without fixation being lost or the femoral head being penetrated.

If the patient is over 65 the treatment of choice is replacement of the head and neck of the femur with a prosthesis (hemi-arthroplasty), for example a Thompson prosthesis (fig. 275 (*a*) & (*b*)). The reason for this is that the chance of non-union or of avascular necrosis is substantial and the ability of the patient to withstand a second operation (see 'Complications') is slight. If the patient is suffering from rheumatoid arthritis or on steroid medication the treatment of choice is primary total hip replacement.

After operation the patient can be allowed out of bed as soon as the general condition allows and encouraged to mobilise fully weight-bearing if an adequate fixation has been achieved or a prosthesis is *in situ.*

The Technique of Internal Fixation.—The patient is placed on a special operating table incorporating traction to the feet and counter-traction via a post in the perineum.

Frederick Roeck Thompson, Contemporary. Professor of Orthopaedic Surgery, New York Polyclinic Medical School, New York, U.S.A.

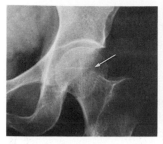

FIG. 274.—Impacted undis-placed intracapsular fracture of neck of femur.

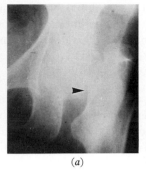

(a)

(b)

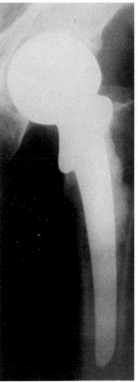

FIG. 275.—Displaced fracture neck of femur (a). Replace-ment of head and neck of femur (hemi-arthroplasty) with a Thompson prosthesis (b).

The table also allows for the use of an image intensifier in two planes (antero-posterior and lateral). The fracture is reduced by manipulating the leg in flexion, internal rotation and occasionally by additional lateral traction to disimpact the fragments. The leg is then brought into extension and the foot secured to the foot plate of the table to maintain reduction by traction in extension and internal rotation. The reduction is checked using the image intensifier. A lateral incision is made over the greater trochanter and extended down the lateral aspect of the thigh. A guide wire is inserted into the femoral neck and head of the femur using an angled guide which matches the angle of the plate. Using the image intensifier the wire is placed so that it lies in the middle of the neck and head in both the antero-posterior and lateral planes. A hole is then reamed in the neck and head using a cannulated reamer which is inserted over the guide wire. The large cancellous bone screw is then inserted along this tract after tapping its distal extent. The barrel of the fixed angle plate is then attached to the shank of the screw and the plate screwed to the lateral aspect of the femur with cortical bone screws. Compression can be applied to the shank of the cancellous screw in order to compress the fracture fragments together. The wound is closed and the patient returned to bed without external splintage.

Complications

1. **Non-union** occurs in approximately 30 to 40% of all intra-capsular frac-tures, partly because adequate immobilisation is difficult to achieve even by internal fixation and partly because fragment frequently has a poor blood supply. In addition healing is impeded because there is little or no periosteum or sur-rounding soft tissues around the neck of the femur and synovial fluid may lyse the blood clot which acts as a scaffold for callus formation. Non-union can be treated by:

(i) *In the elderly*, total hip replacement.

(ii) In young patients, if the head is viable with an intact blood supply (a bone scan may be useful here) the internal fixation should be repeated and a fibular bone graft inserted. This operation may also be combined with a valgus sub-trochanteric osteotomy to reduce the shearing stress on the fracture produced by weight-bearing.

2. **Avascular necrosis.**—As a result of this fracture a part or the whole of the femoral head may be rendered avascular in 15–35% of cases. This is the commonest cause of avascular necrosis of the femoral head which may also occur in alcoholics, patients receiving steroid therapy, after irradiation, and spontaneously for no apparent reason. Avascular necrosis is also seen in men who breathe compressed air, for example, deep sea divers; this condition is known as Caisson disease of bone. Due to loss of blood supply an infarct of the femoral head occurs which itself is symptomless. At a later stage there develops a fracture through the necrotic bone or through the revascularised and repaired bone as a result of which collapse of the articular surface occurs leading to secondary osteoarthritis; at this stage pain becomes a dominant symptom. Treatment is that of osteoarthritis of the hip. These secondary changes of femoral head collapse may take several years to develop. The characteristic change seen on the x-ray is usually an increase in bone density of the femoral head. In the early stages following fracture this is a relative increase in density due to disuse osteoporosis occurring in the surrounding vascularised bone which cannot occur in the avascular femoral head. Later there may be an absolute increase in density due to new bone formation on the surface of the original dead trabeculae which leads to an overall increase in the amount of bone present within the femoral head. These latter changes may also take several years to develop.

3. **Thrombo-embolism** occurs in 25% of the elderly patients with intracapsular fracture of the neck of the femur.

4. **Mortality** is approximately 20% during the first three months after fracture in the elderly subjects and is closely related to the pre-fracture level of activity and mental test score.

Extra-capsular Fractures of the Proximal Femur.—Fractures distal to the base of the neck of the femur are known as extra-capsular fractures of the proximal femur and are sub-divided into two groups; trochanteric fractures down to the level of the lesser trochanter and sub-trochanteric from the lesser trochanter to 2–3 inches below. Trochanteric fractures may be undisplaced or displaced.

In contrast to intra-capsular fractures, all the bone involved in extra-capsular fractures—especially in those fractures involving the cancellous bone of the trochanters—has a good blood supply so that non-union and avascular necrosis of the femoral head are almost unknown. The proximal fragment can be controlled conservatively and hence operative treatment, although frequently used, is not mandatory.

Trochanteric fractures in the elderly are probably due to a sideways fall producing a blow over the greater trochanter. In the young they occur following violent trauma—for example in road traffic accidents.

Clinically the diagnosis is made, as in the case of the intra-capsular fracture, by the combination of external rotation and shortening of the leg, tenderness over the fracture, and the patient's inability to raise the leg from the examination couch. In pertrochanteric fractures the leg tends to be more externally rotated than in fractures through the neck.

Treatment.—It is a relatively simple matter to treat a pertrochanteric fracture without operation, merely by applying traction to the limb and confining the patient to bed for 3 months until the fracture is clinically united. The traction will restore length, and the deformities of adduction and external rotation are corrected by abducting and internally rotating the leg. This method of treatment is perfectly acceptable for young adults. Most of these fractures, however, occur in the elderly and in this age group 3 months of bed rest would frequently result in *bed sores, pneumonia, venous thrombosis, pulmonary embolism and death*. Hence in this age group the fracture is invariably fixed internally so that the patient need not stay in bed.

The fracture can be internally fixed in a similar manner to that described for intracapsular fractures except that a six-hole plate is used to secure the compression screw within the proximal fragment to the shaft of the femur (fig. 276). Providing good bone to bone contact is restored in the medial cortex of the trochanteric region, the fracture is considered to be 'stable' and the patient is allowed out of bed as soon as the general condition allows and is permitted to walk weight-bearing on crutches or with a walking frame.

Complications.—Mortality and thrombo-embolism occur in similar frequency to that occurring after intracapsular fractures. Avascular necrosis and non-union are rare. Mal-union is not uncommon, especially in fractures treated by conservative means. The usual deformity is one of shortening, adduction (varus) and external rotation.

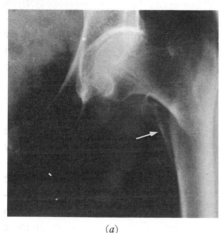

(a)

(b)

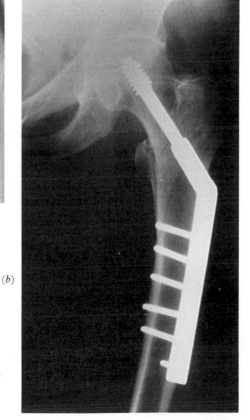

Fig. 276.—Extracapsular fracture of neck of femur (a) fixed by closed reduction and internal fixation with a sliding compression screw and six-hole plate (b).

Subtrochanteric fractures are much less common in the elderly but may occur in young patients as a result of major trauma. Treatment is by open reduction and internal fixation with a compression blade-plate. In young patients, especially in the presence of comminution of the medial cortex, cancellous bone grafting should also be performed.

Avulsion of the Lesser Trochanter.—This injury is sometimes caused by sudden contraction of the ilio-psoas muscle, and is common at about puberty. The condition is unlikely to be diagnosed without the assistance of x-rays. Treatment consists in immobilising the limb for 4 weeks in slight flexion.

Fractures of the proximal femur in children.—Fractures of the proximal femur do occur in children but are rare, especially an intracapsular fracture. The latter type of fracture results from severe violence and may be a Saiter Type I epiphyseal separation or, more usually, fracture through the neck itself. Undisplaced fractures are treated by traction or a plaster hip spica and displaced fractures by closed or open reduction followed by internal fixation with pins supplemented by traction or a hip spica. The risk of complications such as avascular necrosis, non-union and mal-union is high. Extracapsular fractures can usually be treated satisfactorily by skin traction for 3–4 weeks followed by application of a plaster hip spica.

Fractures of the Shaft of the Femur

Fractures of the shaft of the femur occur in children of all ages and adults, especially in young adults. In the latter group, the injury is usually due to severe violence so that associated injuries are common. The fracture may be a simple crack or spiral with minimal displacement but more often is transverse with comminution and gross displacement of fragments. On occasions the fracture may be segmental which results from two transverse fractures which isolate a separate segment of diaphysis between the two fracture sites. There may be significant loss of blood supply to this segment with serious implications for healing. Fractures of the shaft of the femur are not infrequently compound in young adults involved in road traffic accidents.

Displacement depends upon the direction of violence, muscular contraction and gravity. In the upper third of the shaft, the proximal fragment is flexed by the iliopsoas muscle, abducted by the gluteal muscles, and everted by the external rotators. The lower fragment is adducted by the adductor muscles, drawn proximally by the hamstrings and quadriceps, and everted by the weight of the limb.

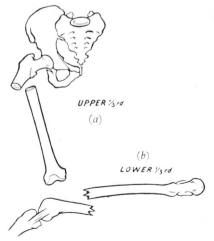

Fig. 277.—Characteristic deformities following fractures in the upper and lower thirds of the shaft of the femur.

UPPER ⅓rd
(a)

(b)
LOWER ⅓rd

In middle-third and lower-third fractures, the deformity is one of backward angulation of the distal fragment and shortening (fig. 277).

The diagnosis is usually obvious and is confirmed radiologically.

There is no obvious bleeding in a simple fracture of the shaft of the femur, but bleeding into the thigh—*often in excess of a litre*—is invariable in adults and such blood loss must be replaced (Chapter 5).

X-rays of the pelvis *must* be obtained in all cases of femoral shaft fracture to rule out the possibility of an associated dislocation of the hip or fracture of the proximal femur. The knee must also be examined clinically and radiographically for evidence of an associated ligamentous injury or fracture. Finally the vascular status of the limb distal to the fracture must be assessed.

Treatment.—As in any other fracture, the aims of treatment are: (1) reduction (*i.e.* restoration of alignment and of length), (2) immobilisation of the fracture and (3) the prevention of knee stiffness.

1. *Restoration of alignment* is essential in the femur because mal-alignment throws an abnormal strain upon the knee joint, so that osteo-arthrosis is prone to develop in later life. Residual posterior angulation results in an extensor lag and hence in instability of the knee.

2. *Restoration of adequate length* is essential unless the patient is to wear an ugly raised shoe. Severe shortening tends to occur at the fracture site because (1) it is often produced by the initial injury, (2) the powerful thigh muscles pull the distal fragment proximally and (3) substantial bleeding at the fracture site is invariable and tends to 'balloon' the thigh to produce an increase in girth and decrease in length. Full restoration of length is not necessary: up to 2 cm of shortening is acceptable as this amount is easily concealed by pelvic tilt.

3. *Immobilisation of the fracture site* can be achieved by traction and counter-traction, by internal fixation, or by plaster-of-Paris fixation (but in the adult this involves a very heavy, extensive plaster and is ineffective in overcoming muscle pull).

4. *Severe knee stiffness* is a common complication of fractures of the shaft of the femur, especially in the distal half, as a result of scarring in the thigh muscles and adhesion formation in the joint. Delayed union is especially prone to result in permanent knee stiffness. Distraction seems to cause non-union and it is preferable to have a femur which is a little short but united with a fully mobile knee, than a femur which is of full length but in which union is delayed and knee movement is limited.

Conservative Treatment (Traction and Counter-traction).—Because of the muscular contraction by the powerful muscles of the thigh, an untreated fracture of the femur may easily develop 10 cm of shortening ('over-riding'). The maintenance of length against this constant tendency to shorten is the special problem presented in this fracture. It is, therefore, essential to have a clear understanding of the principles of traction and counter-traction.

In most fractures, other than in those of the shaft of the femur, it is common practice to overcome shortening by a manipulation under anaesthesia and, if the bone ends can be successfully 'hitched' against each other, to maintain this length merely by encasing the limb in plaster. This is quite impossible in the femur because, even if the fragments could be 'hitched', the soft bulk of the thigh would allow them to slip again soon after the plaster was applied. If the fracture is oblique or comminuted, it is impossible to obtain stable end-to-end contact in the first place because the thigh muscles are so powerful. Thus the reduction has to be maintained by the continuous application of traction.

In applying traction to the distal fragment so as to hold the thigh to an acceptable length, it is always necessary to use counter-traction to the proximal fragment to prevent the trunk and pelvis following the traction force and again allowing the thigh to shorten.

There are two entirely different methods of applying traction and counter-traction: (1) Sliding traction and (2) Fixed traction.

1. **Sliding Traction** (*syn*. Weight Traction, Balanced Traction).—There are many modifications of detail in applying sliding traction, but the essential principles are:

(*a*) Traction is applied to the distal fragment by weights and pulleys attached to the limb either by skin strapping or by skeletal traction. Skeletal traction is to be preferred in the adult as it is more comfortable and can be more powerful. It is secured by driving a 4 mm stainless steel Steinmann or, better, Denham pin through the upper end of the tibia. Skin traction is perfectly adequate in children.

(*b*) Counter-traction is provided by using the weight of the body. This is brought into action by elevating the foot of the bed so that the patient's trunk and pelvis tend to slide away from the source of traction. With a traction force of 9 kg the foot of the bed is raised about 22 cm (fig. 278).

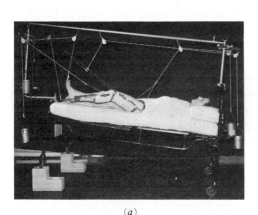 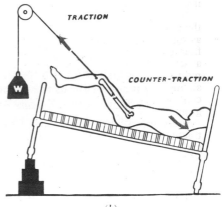

(*a*)   (*b*)

FIG. 278.—The principal elements in sliding traction: traction and counter-traction.

(*c*) The normal forward bowing of the shaft of the femur is maintained by support for the back of the thigh. Because of the tendency for the thigh to sag under the influence of gravity, the original deformity of backward angulation tends to persist, and must be controlled by slings or supports under the thigh.

Further apparatus permits knee movement, holds the foot in dorsiflexion (to prevent equinus deformity), and counterpoises the whole apparatus so that it 'floats' with the patient as he moves in bed.

Sliding traction is attractive because it is comfortable, and does not expose the patient to the risk of an infected fracture which may occur following open reduction and internal fixation. The main danger of the method is that bone contact may be lost ('distraction') due to excessive traction. As muscle spasm passes off then any given weight in the traction system becomes more effective. The weights may have to be reduced if check radiographs show evidence of distraction developing. A modification of sliding traction is the so-called 'split bed technique' in which the bottom half of the bed is removable to allow early knee flexion in an attempt to prevent knee stiffness.

2. **Fixed Traction** depends entirely on the use of the Thomas splint. Cords are attached to the distal fragment, either by skin extensions or by a skeletal pin, and after passing the

Robin Arthur Denham, Contemporary, Orthopaedic Surgeon, Royal Portsmouth Hospital, Portsmouth, Hants, England. The Denham pin is similar to the Steinmann save that it is threaded to obtain a better grip on the bone.
Hugh Owen Thomas, 1834–1891. Surgeon, Liverpool, England. Though he never held a hospital appointment, preferring to attend patients in their homes, he is regarded as the founder of orthopaedic surgery. He introduced his splint in 1875.
Fritz Steinmann, 1872–1932. Surgeon, Berne, Switzerland. Described a pin for skeletal traction in 1907.

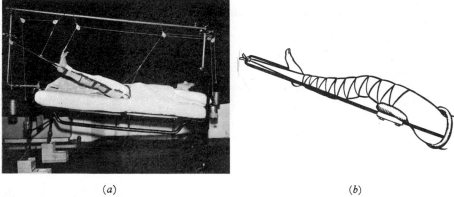

(a)   (b)

FIG. 279.—Fixed traction applied with a Thomas splint and adhesive strapping to the skin.

Thomas splint over the limb so that the padded leather ring takes a purchase against the ischial tuberosity, traction is applied by tying the cords to the foot of the splint. Counter-traction is thus exerted by pressure of the ring against the soft tissues and the ischial tuberosity (fig. 279).

Backward angulation of the shaft of the femur is controlled by slings passed between the side-bars of the splint behind the thigh. Fixation of the fracture is obtained by enclosing the limb and the splint in a bandage.

It is evident that this method can exert only a relatively slight traction force, because the skin of the perineum would not be able to withstand a counter-traction force as great as that used in sliding traction. The great art of the method is therefore to hold the fracture with minimum force. To do this, the fracture must be capable of reduction under anaesthesia and the Thomas splint with fixed traction is then used merely to retain a reduction already achieved. This method has been modified by Bonnin, who adds skeletal sliding traction to fixed traction in order, not so much to treat the fracture (which is controlled by the fixed traction), but to draw the ring of the Thomas splint away from the groin.

Fixed traction provides more effective immobilisation of the fracture than does sliding traction and hence is said to result in a higher incidence of union. On the other hand, early knee stiffness is more marked after treatment by this method, although at the end of one year there is little difference in the range of knee movement obtained by either method.

After a period of approximately six weeks on traction and if early callus formation is observed on the x-ray and the fracture is in the middle third of the shaft some surgeons prefer to apply a cast brace and allow the patient to mobilise on crutches taking partial weight through the injured limb. A cast brace consists of a thigh plaster cast which incorporates a special quadrilateral socket proximally for ischial weight-bearing. Distally the leg is encased in a below knee walking or non-walking plaster cast. The thigh and leg casts are joined by a flexible hinge which allows knee movement. Although this method of treatment shortens the period of traction and therefore hospitalisation there is no doubt that there is some risk of the development of late deformity and the treatment process must be monitored by regular check radiographs. There is no place for this treatment in non-compliant patients.

Union.—A transverse or comminuted fracture of the shaft takes at least 12 weeks to unite in an adult if treated by traction. During this time the muscles of the leg must be exercised, at first statically but later with knee movement. Lateral mobility of the patella must be maintained manually from the moment of injury.

Josiah Grant Bonnin, Contemporary. Formerly Orthopaedic Surgeon, Central Middlesex Hospital, London.

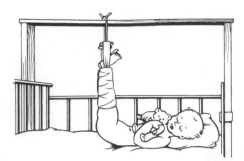

FIG. 280.—a 'Gallows' splint. Traction is applied by means of strapping, and the legs are slung up to the crosspiece, so that the pelvis is just lifted from the mattress (a position which is very convenient for nursing purposes). The child's weight acts as counter-traction. Alternatively, children of this age can be treated in a plaster spica.

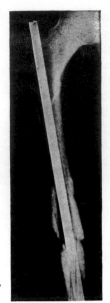

FIG. 281.—Küntscher intramedullary nail in the femur.

When the fracture is judged to be united, the traction is removed and the patient allowed to mobilise the leg in bed. If the fracture site remains comfortable, the patient is allowed up on crutches and gradually returns to full weight bearing.

Fractures of the femoral shaft in children can usually be managed satisfactorily by skin traction in a Thomas splint. For children less than 2 years old and *weighing less than 25 pounds* a gallows splint can be used (fig. 280).

Operative Treatment: Internal Fixation.—Conservative treatment has the following disadvantages: (1) it involves prolonged treatment in hospital, (2) knee stiffness is common, (3) reduction may be impossible if muscle is interposed between the fracture fragments and (4) it requires constant intelligent attention to detail in order to ensure that the reduction is not lost and that pressure sores do not develop, *e.g.* over the Achilles' tendon and in the groin, or over the lateral popliteal nerve in the region of the neck of the fibula resulting in a lateral popliteal nerve palsy. These disadvantages can be circumvented by open reduction and internal fixation using a blade-plate in the sub-trochanteric region of the shaft or an intramedullary nail in the second and third quarters of the shaft (fig. 281). The nail can be inserted either by exposing the fracture site, or a 'closed nailing' can be carried out using x-ray control with an image intensifier.

Provided the fracture is not too comminuted, no external splintage is required post-operatively and the patient can get up on crutches, progress to weight-bearing and start knee flexion within a few days of operation. These advantages have to be set against the occasional disaster of a surgically induced infection.

On balance, there is little to choose between conservative and operative treatment unless reduction cannot be achieved conservatively in a mid-shaft fracture, or the fracture is in the proximal shaft of an adult, for then the abduction and flexion of the proximal fragment is sometimes impossible to control conservatively. Operative treatment is never necessary in children.

Gerhard B. G. Küntscher, 1900–1972. Medical Director, Hafen Hospital, Hamburg, Germany.

Complications.—(1) Vascular injury may occur especially with displaced fractures at the junction of the middle and lower thirds of the femoral shaft. Treatment is by immediate repair of the femoral artery and stabilisation of the fracture by internal fixation.

(2) Nerve injury is unusual as a result of fracture but may occur during treatment from pressure on the lateral popliteal nerve by the outer bar of a Thomas splint.

(3) Non-union is not common but does occur and is treated by internal fixation and cancellous bone grafting. The possible causes include distraction, infection (following a compound fracture or operation), insufficient mobilisation and soft tissue interposition.

(4) Mal-union may occur with inadequate treatment. Shortening, varus and external rotation are the usual deformities.

(5) Knee stiffness is common after this fracture as already described. If less than 90° flexion is present then consideration should be given to improving this by quadricepsplasty.

(6) Re-fracture should be prevented by a gradual return to activity. If it occurs then treatment is by a short period of traction followed by application of a cast brace.

Fractures of the distal femur

Supracondylar fractures of the femur present a special problem, since the gastrocnemius muscle tends to flex the distal fragment, producing posterior angulation at the fracture site. This is very difficult to control conservatively, although it is possible to do so, using two Steinmann pins, one through the tibial tubercle to provide traction in the long axis of the femur and one through the distal fracture fragment to provide forward traction at right angles to the long axis of the femur. Preferably the fracture should be treated by internal fixation of the fragments using a blade-plate, followed by early mobilisation of the knee. Complications are similar to those occuring after femoral shaft fracture except that delayed and non-union is not as common.

Intra-articular fractures of the distal femur.—These may take the form of T or Y fractures, which are similar to those occurring in the distal humerus, or involve one condyle only (fig. 282). They may be due to indirect violence (by a mechanism similar to that which produces ruptures of the collateral ligaments). Alternatively they result from direct violence: a direct blow applied to the anterior aspect of the flexed knee (*i.e.* to the patella) may drive the patella backwards into the femur, splitting the two femoral condyles from the femoral shaft so as to produce a '*Y' shaped fracture of the femoral condyles*. This fracture may also be produced by falls from a height on to the heels.

The diagnosis is suspected clinically by obvious deformity, bruising and swelling of the knee. The details of the injury are made out radiologically.

The treatment of fractures of the condyles is difficult. In young adults an attempt should be made to reconstruct the joint surfaces, but if comminution is extreme, this is often impossible. If reconstruction seems possible, it should be attempted by open operation with internal fixation of the fracture fragments. In more elderly

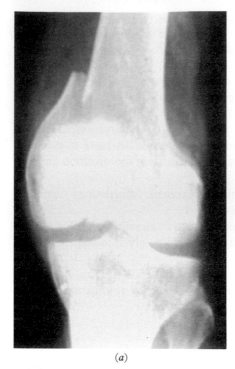

(a)

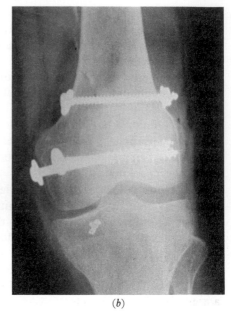

(b)

FIG. 282.—Displaced fracture of medial condyle, an intra-articular fracture (a). Reduced by open operation and internal fixation (b).

patients or in young adults with minimally depressed fractures good results can be obtained conservatively either by treating the knee with early mobilisation on skeletal traction, or alternatively by immobilising the knee for 3 to 6 weeks in a plaster cylinder followed by active mobilisation in a physiotherapy department. Whatever form of treatment is employed, weight-bearing should be avoided for 3 months. Osteo-arthrosis is a common late complication.

Injuries of the distal femur in children usually result in Salter Type II separations of the distal femoral epiphysis. The injury is usually one of hyper-extension which results in anterior displacement of the epiphysis, or valgus angulation which results in lateral displacement of the epiphysis. If the epiphysis is significantly displaced, a closed reduction is carried out by manipulation and the leg placed in a full length plaster cast for six weeks with the knee flexed 60°.

FRACTURES OF THE PATELLA

Fractures of the patella may be due to indirect violence, *i.e.* to forced flexion of the knee when the quadriceps are contracting (in which case the fracture runs transversely across the patella) or to direct violence, for example a blow on the anterior aspect of the flexed knee (in which case the fracture is usually comminuted, although sometimes only one or two fragments are broken from the main body of the bone). The latter fractures are described as 'stellate' and are sometimes compound.

Fractures of the patella can be classified as follows: Undisplaced transverse; Displaced transverse; Upper or lower pole; Comminuted (stellate); Vertical (marginal); Osteochondral.

Transverse fractures of the patella may be isolated injuries: the two fragments of the patella do not then become displaced since they are held in their normal position by the pre-patella expansion of the quadriceps tendon and the patella retinaculae. Should force continue to be exerted on the extensor apparatus after the patella has fractured, the fracture may extend as a tear into these soft tissues. The quadriceps muscle then draws the proximal fragment of the patella proximally so that a substantial gap opens at the fracture site (compare Fractured Olecranon, Chapter 16).

Undisplaced fractures may be suspected by the demonstration of local tenderness and with care can be visualised radiologically (their demonstration is not easy since in an antero-posterior view the shadow of the patella is obscured by that of the distal end of the femur). Active extension of the knee is possible (but painful) without an extensor lag. Treatment is by immobilisation of the knee in a plaster cylinder for 6 weeks combined with quadriceps exercises, followed by mobilisation in a physiotherapy department.

Fractures with separation are obvious clinically because the gap is palpable. They are also obvious radiologically. Active extension of the knee is impossible. Treatment is by open reduction and internal fixation using two parallel wires and a 'tension-band system' (fig. 283). It is important to accurately reduce the fracture to restore the articular surface. Following open reduction and internal fixation by this method the knee can be actively mobilised soon after operation in order to prevent knee stiffness.

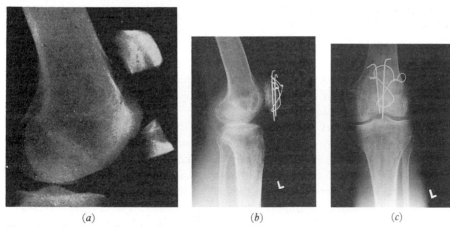

(a)   (b)   (c)

FIG. 283.—Transverse fracture of the patella (a), fixed internally by means of two wires and a figure of 8 tension band (b & c).

Should the fracture line traverse the patella so as to produce one large and one very small fragment it is often best to excise the small fragment rather than to attempt reconstruction. Following this the quadriceps tendon or the infra-patellar tendon is sutured into drill holes in the proximal or distal aspect of the patella respectively.

Comminuted fractures of the patella cannot be accurately reduced and they therefore invariably result in significant irregularity of the posterior, articular surface of the bone. Such irregularity predisposes to osteoarthrosis of the patello-femoral joint. These fractures should therefore be treated by removal of all the fragments of the patella (*i.e.* by patellectomy) followed by reconstruction of the soft tissue components of the extensor apparatus. Following this operation, powerful, active extension of the knee is possible but there may be some loss of flexion. Surprisingly, the appearance of the knee is nearly normal. Alternatively some surgeons prefer to leave the patella *in situ* and treat the fracture by immobilisation in a cylinder for six weeks. If the patient subsequently develops troublesome symptoms related to patello-femoral osteoarthritis patellectomy can be performed. Vertical fractures separating one or two small fragments from the lateral or medial border of the patella can be treated symptomatically if the extensor mechanism is intact. (Radiologically, these fractures may be confused with congenitally bi-partite patellae.)

An osteochondral fracture of the patella usually occurs as a complication of a dislocation of the patella. An area of articular cartilage attached to a piece of subchondral bone is sheared off the posterior aspect of the patella. The fragment is usually removed surgically and discarded. Complications of fractures of the patella are secondary osteoarthritis and chondromalacia patellae (Chapter 19).

Dislocation of the patella over the lateral femoral condyle may occur following a direct blow on the medial side of the patella or without significant violence if some predisposing anatomical abnormality exists in the knee. Following direct violence, the medial patella retinaculum is ruptured and the patella passes over the lateral femoral condyle to lie on its lateral aspect. Once in this position, the patella remains there unless replaced by the patient himself or by a physician, and thus the knee is locked. The anatomical abnormalities which predispose to this condition are a small patella, a high patella, an unusually low lateral femoral condyle, marked knocked knee (so that the extensor mechanism tends to bowstring across the lateral aspect of the knee), or marked internal rotation of the legs (producing 'kissing patellae'). Minor degrees of misalignment in which the patella does not actually dislocate may be responsible for some cases of Chondromalacia Patellae (Chapter 19).

Once the patella has dislocated it is prone to do so repeatedly, and spontaneously. This condition is known as '*Recurrent Dislocation of the Patella*' and results in repeated locking or giving way of the knee. It is attributable to chronic elongation or rupture of the medial patella retinaculum so that the transverse, distal fibres of the vastus medialis muscle no longer stabilise the patella in a medial direction when the quadriceps muscle contracts. The clinical features of the initial dislocation are obvious. Recurrent dislocation is also usually obvious, but occasionally if the dislocations reduce spontaneously the patient is not aware that the patella is dislocating and merely complains that his knee repeatedly locks or gives way.

The treatment of an initial dislocation is reduction of the patella, followed by immobilisation of the knee in a plaster-of-Paris cylinder for 6 weeks to give the medial patella retinaculum a chance to heal. Following removal of the plaster the knee is mobilised and particular attention is given to developing the quadriceps muscle.

Recurrent dislocation of the patella requires operative treatment. Numerous procedures have been described, but the most commonly employed is medial transposition of the tibial tubercle combined with release of the lateral patellar retinaculum and 'double-breasting' of the medial retinaculum.

In patients who have not yet reached skeletal maturity the reconstruction should be confined to soft tissue procedures only.

SOFT TISSUE INJURIES OF THE KNEE

No joint sustains so wide a range of injuries as does the knee. This is because it is a commonly injured, major weight-bearing joint whose stability depends almost entirely upon soft tissues (ligaments and muscles). Its ligaments are both extra- and intra-articular and alone amongst the major joints it contains menisci. Injuries to the knee may be divided into those which affect the ligaments, the menisci, the extensor apparatus, and the tibial and femoral condyles. (Fractures of the tibial and femoral condyles are described under fractures of the tibia and femur respectively.)

The Ligaments

Mechanism of Injury.—A blow on the lateral side of the knee when the patient is bearing weight on the leg abducts the tibia on the femur and stresses the *medial collateral ligament*. If the violence is relatively minor, some of the fibres of the ligament give way, but the ligament as a whole remains intact. Such an injury is a simple sprain. Should the violence be more severe, the ligament may be ruptured, usually at its femoral attachment. Because the medial meniscus is attached to the medial collateral ligament, peripheral detachment of the medial meniscus is commonly associated with this injury. Further forced abduction of the tibia stresses the cruciate ligaments, one or both of which may be sprained or ruptured, and extends the rupture of the medial collateral ligament anteriorly and posteriorly through the capsule. If the medial collateral and cruciate ligaments are ruptured, the tibia becomes grossly unstable on the femur in abduction so that the knee can be subluxated.

The reverse mechanism (*i.e.* adduction of the tibia on the femur) is far less common (because the knee is more commonly struck on its lateral than on its medial aspect) and the results in an injury first to the *lateral collateral* and then to the *cruciate ligaments*. As a result of this latter type of injury the lateral popliteal nerve may sustain a traction injury.

The *posterior cruciate ligament* may be injured if the anterior aspect of the tibia is struck when the knee is flexed, an injury which not uncommonly occurs to the front-seat passenger in a motor car if he is thrown violently forward against the dashboard.

Isolated *anterior cruciate ruptures* may occur if the knee is forcibly hyperextended.

Clincial Features.—It is important to obtain an exact description of the injury and of the ensuing events, since this often helps to distinguish one soft tissue lesion from another. A description of the injury itself will suggest the mechanism and hence, as indicated above, the pathology. If bleeding has occurred into the joint (a haemarthrosis), the knee swells within 1 or 2 hours and this suggests the presence of serious intra-articular damage. Should the knee swell, but only over the course of 12 or 24 hours, the swelling is likely to be due to an effusion. This implies the existence of a less severe injury. As fluid collects in the joint, the knee becomes increasingly painful and movement becomes more difficult. When a moderately large effusion has developed, only a few degrees of movement are possible and the knee is held in about 10° of flexion (a situation which must be distinguished clinically from locking of the knee (p. 324)).

It is important to remember that with a complete rupture of a collateral ligament it is possible for the haemarthrosis to escape from the joint and it will not therefore always be obvious clinically. Also, major ligament injuries are sometimes surprisingly painless in the early stages following injury and these latter two factors may lead the examining clinician into a false sense of security.

Physical Signs.—It is vital that the student should have an accurate understanding of the surface anatomy of the knee, since the diagnosis of soft tissue injuries and the distinction of meniscus injuries from ligament injuries depends upon the accurate localisation of tenderness in relation to the underlying structures (fig. 284). Soon after the injury an effusion or haemarthrosis can be demonstrated but not always as indicated above. Localised tenderness can be elicited over the collateral ligaments if these are injured. No clearly localised tenderness is demonstrable if a cruciate ligament is injured.

If a ligament has been sprained rather than ruptured, stressing the ligament will not demonstrate abnormal movement but will provoke pain in the injured ligament. Thus, for example, if the tibia is abducted on the femur, pain will be elicited from a simple sprain of the medial collateral ligament. If the ligament has ruptured, the knee as a whole may be too painful to allow the ligament to be stressed. The knee should then be examined under anaesthesia.

With the knee in full extension the tibia is abducted and then adducted on the femur and any abnormal movement which occurs is compared with that in the uninjured knee. Excessive movement suggests the presence of a rupture of the appropriate collateral ligament *and* the posterior capsule. The absence of abnormal movement when testing in full extension does not rule out the possibility of a collateral ligament tear because an intact posterior capsule will stabilise the knee in full extension. In order to overcome this the test is repeated with the knee in about 30° of flexion to relax the posterior capsule. Any excessive movement which is detected can be recorded by taking a stress x-ray of the knee.

If the tibia is flexed to 90° on the femur, the anterior cruciate ligament resists forward glide of the tibia on the femur: excessive forward glide therefore indicates a rupture of the anterior cruciate ligament. Excessive posterior glide indicates a rupture of the posterior cruciate ligament.

If a ligament injury, especially a rupture, is missed soon after injury and hence goes untreated, the pain will settle, but the knee will not become sign- and symptom-free. The patient complains that the knee feels insecure and it may be recurrently painful and swollen. If the joint is examined some months after injury, mechanical instability and often an effusion may be demonstrated and marked quadriceps wasting will be seen.

Radiological Appearances.—At the time of injury, there are usually no abnormal radiological features. The cruciate ligaments, when stressed, may sometimes avulse their tibial attachment rather than rupture in their length and the lateral collateral ligament may avulse its fibular attachment: the resultant fractures can be seen radiologically, especially if the bone fragment is significantly displaced. Rarely, there may be slight persistent separation of the medial femoral and tibial condyles if the medial collateral ligament has

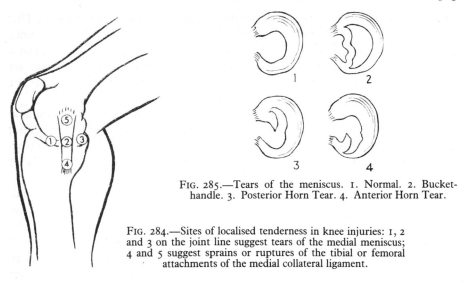

FIG. 285.—Tears of the meniscus. 1. Normal. 2. Bucket-handle. 3. Posterior Horn Tear. 4. Anterior Horn Tear.

FIG. 284.—Sites of localised tenderness in knee injuries: 1, 2 and 3 on the joint line suggest tears of the medial meniscus; 4 and 5 suggest sprains or ruptures of the tibial or femoral attachments of the medial collateral ligament.

ruptured and become interposed in the joint space. Some weeks following injury, new bone formation may be seen at the femoral attachment of a collateral ligament if the periosteum has been avulsed at the time of injury (a condition known as Pellegrini-Stieda's disease).

Treatment.—Simple sprains of the collateral ligaments require only limitation of normal activities combined with mobilisation and quadriceps exercises for 3 to 6 weeks.

The treatment of ruptures of these ligaments is controversial, both immediately after injury and later should instability persist.

The cruciate ligaments when ruptured never lie with their ends in apposition. The collateral ligaments also commonly recoil. Therefore if simple immobilisation is employed, the ligaments may not heal because their ends are not apposed. For this reason many surgeons explore a rupture of any ligament of the knee immediately after injury so that the ends of the ligaments can be sutured together. This operation is technically difficult in the case of cruciate ligaments and most surgeons do not attempt primary repair of these except in the case of avulsion of the posterior cruciate ligament from its tibial attachment, with a significant fragment of bone. In these cases the fragment and attached ligament should be replaced and fixed with a small screw. In the case of the collateral ligaments most surgeons perform, what is a relatively simple, primary repair. Whether or not the overall long term results are better than with conservative treatment is still debatable.

Following operation the knee is immobilised in a few degrees of flexion in a plaster cast extending from the groin to the metatarsal heads for six weeks.

Alternatively the knee may be immobilised, without operation, in the hope that the ruptured ligaments will then unite spontaneously. Whilst in plaster, quadriceps exercises are begun and as soon as the plaster is removed the knee is actively mobilised and the thigh muscles exercised. Weight-bearing should be deferred for three weeks from the time of injury.

Chronic Ligament Injuries.—If a rupture of a ligament of the knee fails to heal normally, the knee may no longer be mechanically stable. It is then liable to 'give way', especially when stressed in sport, to swell and to be intermittently painful. The instability often results in repeated injuries so that the condition tends to become worse as time goes by. This is a very serious state of affairs for professional sportsmen.[1]

---

[1] As a result the subject of knee injuries and their sequelae in sportsmen has almost become a subspeciality in orthopaedics and represents a large part of sports medicine.

Augusto Pellegrini, Contemporary. Surgeon, Ospedale Mellini, Chiari, Italy.
Alfred Stieda, 1869–1945. Professor of Surgery, Konigsberg, which was in Germany until 1945 but is now Kaliningrad in the U.S.S.R.
Pellegrini described traumatic calcification of the collateral tibial ligament in 1905; Stieda published his account of the condition in 1908.

Because of the complexity of the ligaments stabilising the tibio-femoral and patello-femoral joints, because the same symptoms (*i.e.* 'giving way', swelling and pain) can be caused by meniscal injuries or loose bodies, because more than one lesion may coexist in the knee, and because the exact nature of the instability which occurs when the patient runs (for example abnormal, uncontrolled rotation of the femur on the tibia in flexion) may be difficult to demonstrate on the examination couch, these lesions are hard to diagnose and even harder to treat. Experts in the field are not in full agreement but, in general, clinical and radiological examination is used to define the nature of the lesion and the resultant instability. This is then controlled, if possible, by a brace or by surgery. The latter may involve an attempt to re-suture ruptured ligaments but since this is often difficult or impossible, surgery usually takes the form of the transfer of tendons in the hope of restoring the function of the ligaments by substitution. The use of prosthetic ligaments has been tried but so far without great success.

The Menisci[1] (The Semi-Lunar Cartilages)

Mechanism of Injury.—The menisci are commonly torn in sports injuries or when rising from a kneeling position. Tears of degenerate menisci occur in the osteoarthrosic knee. The mechanism is rotation of the tibia on the femur in the flexed, weight-bearing knee, for example, if a games player stands on one leg with the knee slightly bent and then twists his body. The medial meniscus tends to be damaged if the femur is internally rotated on the tibia, the lateral meniscus if the femur is externally rotated. Medial meniscus injuries are more common than lateral meniscus injuries in a ratio of about 20 to 1 and both are less common in women.

Morbid Anatomy.—Tears may occur in the anterior horn, the posterior horn or as bucket-handle tears in the body of the meniscus (fig. 285). Following an initial tear, progressive damage to the meniscus is common, so that eventually the original anatomy of the tear may not be discernible. The menisci are avascular and once torn do not heal.

The lateral, and commonly the medial, meniscus may occasionally be congenitally discoid in shape rather than semi-lunar. Discoid menisci are more prone to tear than the normal meniscus and, even if untorn, occasionally give rise to very loud 'clunks' in the knee.

Clinical Features.—Patients suffering meniscus injuries may not necessarily attend a doctor at the time of the original injury. Physical examination of the knee is often not diagnostic and the diagnosis rests largely upon the history. In the history the important features are an accurate description of the original injury, a complaint of locking or unlocking, and the lateralisation of any pain or clicks.

The mechanism of the injury has already been described. Following injury, the knee swells overnight as an effusion collects, and usually comes to be held in about 10° of flexion, from which position movement is painful. As the effusion settles, the range of movement gradually increases until after about 6 weeks it is nearly full. However, at the time of the injury the torn portion of the meniscus may become interposed between the femoral and tibial condyles so as mechanically to prevent either full extension or (much more rarely) full flexion of the knee. (Such a mechanical block to flexion or extension is known as 'locking'.) The patient may notice this at the time of the injury but more commonly it is

---

[1] Meniscus (Greek) = a crescent.

masked by the more obvious events of pain, swelling and the consequent limitation of movement. The displaced meniscus sometimes returns to its original position (so as to unlock the joint) as the effusion settles and thus the original episode of locking may never be noticed by the patient. Usually, however, it becomes obvious that the knee is locked as the effusion subsides.

Subsequent events.—Following a return to apparent normality, the knee may still be prone to two sequelae: recurrent episodes of locking and 'giving way'. These events are attributable to displacement of the torn segment of the meniscus between the articulating femoral and tibial condyles. Such displacements may suddenly prevent either full extension or full flexion of the knee ('locking'). A sudden inability fully to extend the joint is always obvious to the patient and is accompanied by pain in the appropriate compartment of the joint. The patient may not notice the contrast in the loss of the last few degrees of flexion. Sometimes the knee unlocks spontaneously or it may have to be manipulated by a physician or by the patient himself in order to regain a full range of movement. The history of sudden unlocking with a click located in one or other joint compartment is almost diagnostic of a torn meniscus (but it may be due to the presence of a loose body in the knee).

'Giving way' denotes a condition in which the knee suddenly flexes under the patient so that he falls to the ground, or, more commonly, the knee may feel as if it is about to give way (*i.e.* may feel unstable) without actually collapsing. This symptom may be caused by a torn meniscus or may be due to damage to the mechano-receptors in the capsule of the knee upon whose normal activity the co-ordination of the thigh muscles depends. Quadriceps weakness may produce the same symptom. (Since the stability of the knee is dependent upon the accurate, co-ordinated contraction of the thigh muscles, any injury producing muscular weakness and inco-ordination may cause a feeling of instability in the joint.)

Physical Signs.—Soon after injury the meniscus is tender. As with ligament injuries, the demonstration of such tenderness depends upon an accurate knowledge of the surface anatomy of the knee. Tenderness over the anterior or posterior horns of either meniscus cannot easily be confused with tenderness over any other structure, but tenderness over the central part of the meniscus cannot be distinguished from tenderness over a collateral ligament (fig. 284). Wasting of the quadriceps muscle is invariable within 2 weeks of injury. If the knee is locked, a full range of movement cannot be obtained and gentle attempts to force a full range will produce a sensation of elastic resistance and pain localised to the appropriate compartment of the joint. If a meniscus is torn, there will usually be an effusion (albeit sometimes a small one) but not always.

On the other hand effusions occur in other conditions so that their presence is not diagnostic of a meniscus injury. McMurray's sign (the demonstration of a painful click if the flexed tibia is rotated upon the femur) is sometimes positive. The distinction between a medial and a lateral meniscus injury depends entirely upon the localisation of tenderness and lateralising features in the history but this is *not* always reliable.

In summary.—It is often difficult to make a confident clinical diagnosis of a torn meniscus unless the knee is locked. The significant features in the history are recurrent locking, effusions and medial or lateral pain. On examination the diagnosis is suggested by an effusion, appropriately localised tenderness (and a block to full movement if the knee is locked).

Investigation.—There are no abnormal radiological features in routine x-rays but meniscal tears can be demonstrated by arthrography or by arthroscopy. However plain x-rays must never be omitted because they may reveal other

Thomas Porter McMurray, 1887–1949. Professor of Orthopaedic Surgery, Liverpool, England.

pathology which is the cause of pain, for example a loose body, osteochondritis dissecans and, on rare occasions, a bone tumour.

Treatment.—If a definite diagnosis of a torn meniscus is made, the meniscus or the torn part of it should be removed if the patient is sufficiently troubled by the condition, which is not always the case. Because the meniscus is avascular, except at its peripheral attachment, a tear will not heal spontaneously.

Commonly, the diagnosis cannot be made with certainty and surgery should then be deferred. The patient is treated with quadriceps exercises so as to build up his thigh muscles and the knee is watched. Should symptoms suggestive of a meniscus injury persist, it may be inferred that the meniscus is torn, and the knee is investigated by arthrography or arthroscopy in an attempt to make a precise diagnosis before exploring the joint and to localise which meniscus is torn.

If the knee is locked at the time when it is first examined, the patient may rapidly be made more comfortable by admission to hospital followed by a diagnostic arthroscopy, and if this confirms the diagnosis, in most patients proceed to a menisectomy (partial or total depending on the findings).

Menisectomy

The leg is exsanguinated using an Esmarch's bandage (Chapter 4) and an inflatable tourniquet. The cartilage is exposed by an oblique incision running from the appropriate femoral condyle downwards towards the tibial tubercle. The torn cartilage is steadied by a blunt hook and its anterior attachment to the tibia is divided. The cartilage is then grasped by forceps and pulled forwards, dividing its attachment to the coronary ligament. When the cartilage has been freed as far posteriorly as it can be displaced, it is dislocated into the inter-condylar notch and the posterior horn divided. The synovial membrane and capsule are sutured with plain catgut and the skin sutured with interrupted nylon sutures. A well padded bandage consisting of alternating layers of wool and dommette[1] is applied before the tourniquet is removed so as to limit bleeding into the joint. Post-operatively quadriceps exercises are started immediately.

Alternatively, some surgeons now practice arthroscopic menisectomy by which it is possible, using an arthroscope and special fine cutting and grasping instruments, to remove the whole or part of a meniscus without a formal arthrotomy. The advantage of this method of treatment is that it probably results in a more rapid return to full activity. This technique should not be used by those who have not had special training in the method.

Cysts of the Menisci.—A cyst of a meniscus is due to myxomatous degeneration occurring in the substance of the cartilage itself. The lateral cartilage is affected perhaps 20 times more commonly than the medial.

Clinically a tense swelling, often more obvious when the knee is flexed, appears over the joint line. The cyst sometimes appears suddenly. Pain follows exertion but may occur at rest. It is commonly described as being like toothache.

Treatment.—The cartilage together with the cyst should be removed if symptoms are persistent, but like a ganglion in any other site it can be ignored and often disappears spontaneously after a number of years. Local removal is unsatisfactory as recurrence is inevitable.

The Extensor Apparatus

The extensor apparatus of the knee comprises the quadriceps muscle, the

---

[1] This type of bandage was introduced by Robert Jones.

Johann Friedrich August von Esmarch, 1823–1908. Professor of Surgery, Kiel, Germany. Introduced this bandage in 1869 for use on the battlefield.
Sir Robert Jones, 1858–1933. Orthopaedic Surgeon, Royal Southern Hospital, Liverpool, England. He was the nephew of Hugh Owen Thomas (see footnote p. 314) and did much to spread the knowledge of his uncle's work.

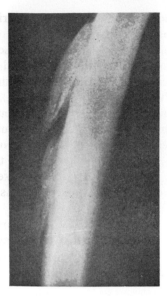

FIG. 286.—An ossifying haematoma overlying the femur.

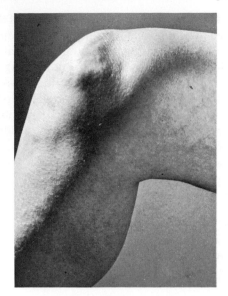

FIG. 287.—Rupture of the insertion of the quadriceps muscle into the patella.

tendinous insertion of the quadriceps muscle into the patella, the patella retinaculae, the patella itself, the ligamentum patellae and the insertion of the ligamentum patellae into the tibial tubercle. This apparatus constitutes a single functional unit and provides the active extension of the knee which is vital to normal gait. The apparatus may be injured anywhere in its length either by direct or by indirect violence (*i.e.* by a direct blow or by forced flexion of the knee when the quadriceps muscle is contracting).

Contusion of the quadriceps muscle results from direct violence. Localised pain follows attempts at contraction of the muscle and an extravasation of blood occurs within the muscle sheath. The extravasated blood may appear subcutaneously some distance from the site of the contusion, for example near the patella. Rest and pressure dressings are required for the first few days and thereafter the knee is progressively mobilised.

Contusion of the deep fibres of the quadriceps muscle may be associated with avulsion of the periosteum from the femur. The resulting haematoma may ossify to produce a radiologically demonstrable and occasionally palpable bony swelling on the anterior aspect of the femur (fig. 286). (This pathological process is sometimes referred to, wrongly, as myositis ossificans (Chapter 16).

Rupture of the muscle belly of the rectus femoris occurs at about mid-thigh level in young athletes as a consequence of very forceful, but resisted active extension of the knee. Extension of the knee is still possible after the pain of the rupture has subsided. When all local oedema has disappeared, the proximal end of the muscle stands out as a visible lump when the patient contracts the thigh. Distal to this lump there is a palpable gap in the muscle. No surgical treatment is possible (since the muscle will not hold sutures), nor is surgical treatment necessary because the injury causes no permanent disability.

Rupture of the tendinous insertion of the quadriceps muscle into the patella is an uncommon injury which usually occurs in middle-aged and elderly patients, often after a trivial indirect injury such as stumbling. It may, however, occur in athletes. It is probable that the underlying pathology in the middle-aged is similar to that in ruptures of the Achilles' tendon, namely ischaemic necrosis of the tendon. The gap is easily visible and palpable a few weeks after injury (fig. 287) but is less obvious immediately after injury when the space is filled with haematoma, the tissues are swollen and the quadriceps inhibited. Soon after the episode the diagnosis may therefore be missed. The tendon should be repaired with mattress sutures.

Ruptures of the ligamentum patellae occur, although rarely, in young athletes following extreme violence. The diagnosis is obvious, since the patella is drawn upwards to create a considerable, palpable gap. The knee is bruised, swollen and tender. Active extension is impossible. Treatment is by suture of the ruptured ligament followed by immobilisation of the leg in a plaster cylinder for 6 weeks.

Avulsion of the tibial tubercle occurs very rarely in adults. Minor avulsion injuries are not uncommon in adolescents, a condition known as Osgood-Schlatter's Disease (see Chapter 22). A similar condition occurs, more rarely, at the distal pole of the patella and is known as Sinding-Larsen's disease (Chapter 22).

FRACTURES OF THE TIBIA

Fractures of the tibia are considered in three groups:
(1) Fractures of the proximal tibia.
(2) Fractures of the shaft.
(3) Fractures of the distal tibia (ankle fractures).

Fractures of the Proximal Tibia

Fractures of the proximal tibia are classified as articular or non-articular. The commonest type of articular fracture is a fracture of the lateral tibial plateau (fig. 288a). This usually results from a direct blow to the lateral aspect of the knee (as for example when a car bumper strikes the knee) which causes the tibia to be abducted on the femur and the lateral femoral condyle is driven downward into the tibial plateau thus fracturing it. There may also be damage to the medial collateral ligament. Falls from a height may result in a fracture of one or both tibial condyles; in these cases the fracture line passes outwards from the intercondylar eminence, thus sparing the actual articular surface of the plateau. Sometimes the two types of fracture are combined. Undisplaced and minimally displaced fractures can be treated by early active mobilisation of the knee provided that the patient remains non-weight bearing for at least six weeks and regular check x-rays show that no displacement is occurring. Displaced fractures should be treated by accurate open reduction, including elevation of depressed fragments, and internal fixation (fig. 288b). Following this the knee is mobilised early to prevent knee stiffness. The commoner complications of these fractures are, knee stiffness and secondary osteoarthritis. Non-articular fractures include fractures of the intercondylar eminence and tibial tuberosity. If the former fracture is displaced it is usually possible to reduce this by placing the knee in full extension in a plaster cylinder for six weeks. If a satisfactory reduction cannot be

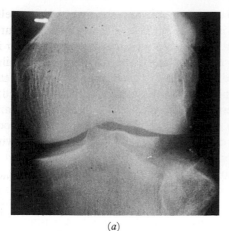

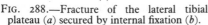
(a)

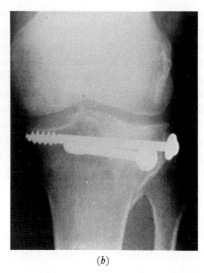

FIG. 288.—Fracture of the lateral tibial plateau (a) secured by internal fixation (b).

(b)

achieved then open reduction and internal fixation should be performed. Isolated fractures of the tibial tuberosity are rare; if displaced the treatment is by open reduction and screw fixation to restore the extensor mechanism of the knee.

Fractures of the Shaft of the Tibia and Fibula

Fracture of the Shaft of the Tibia Alone.—This fracture is usually due to torsion causing a spiral fracture which may appear to be oblique on x-ray. Diagnosis is easy, as the bone is subcutaneous so that deformity and localised tenderness are readily detected.

Treatment.—When the fibula remains intact, the displacement of a fractured tibia is relatively slight, and as angulation is rarely more than 5°, it is usually sufficient to apply an above-knee plaster cast without any attempt at reduction. Though it might appear that fractures of the tibia when the fibula is intact would be unlikely to give rise to difficulty in treatment, in fact delayed union is not uncommon. It is probable that this is because the intact fibula acts as a 'strut' to prevent the fragments of the tibia coming into close contact.

Fracture of the Shaft of the Fibula Alone.—This fracture results from direct violence to the fibula or occurs in association with external rotation and abduction injuries of the ankle joint (p. 335). It is, therefore, important to exclude an associated ankle fracture or ligament injury when a diagnosis of a fibular fracture has been made. *Treatment* of a fracture of the fibula alone need be nothing more rigorous than the application of an adhesive elastic strapping. The common peroneal nerve may be damaged in association with fractures of the proximal end of the fibula.

Fractures of the Tibia and Fibula

These fractures occur as a result of either direct or of indirect violence. Road traffic accidents are the commonest cause of fractures due to direct violence. For example, the bumper of a car strikes the leg and fractures the tibia and fibula by a mixture of impact and bending. Similar mechanisms operate as a result of motor cycle accidents. The fractures occur at about the same level in the two bones, are transverse or oblique and are frequently associated with a butterfly fragment or more extensive comminution. These fractures are frequently compound as a result of the impact tearing the skin and there is usually significant displacement. Direct violence to the tibia can also result from kicks during football which result in minimally displaced transverse fractures which may also be compound.

Indirect violence may be applied to the tibia and fibula either in the form of torsion (the body turning during a fall on the fixed foot), or by bending (the foot and lower tibia being fixed while the body falls sideways, bending the tibia as it does so). The former injury is common in ski-ing, the latter in football. Both injuries may be compound, often trivially so, from within.

Fractures of the tibia are more commonly compound than those of any other bone and skin closure is particularly difficult because the bone is subcutaneous. When the skin has healed, compound fractures may be treated as if they had been simple in the first place. The treatment of compound fractures is discussed in Chapter 15.

It is also necessary to consider the *exact location of the fracture* (proximal, middle or distal third), fracture pattern, displacement, presence or absence of comminution and whether the fracture is compound or not. The prognosis for healing of these fractures is closely related to the *degree of initial displacement, the degree of comminution and the severity of the associated soft tissue wound.*

Treatment.—Fractures of the bones of the leg can be treated in 3 ways:

(1) By plaster after manipulative reduction. This form of treatment is used for fractures in patients under the age of 16, and for fractures in older patients, in whom a stable reduction can be obtained, for example after obtaining end-to-end opposition of the fragments of a transverse fracture. It is the most widely used and the safest form of treatment. If a stable reduction cannot be obtained, an alternative method is to insert a transverse skeletal pin above and below the fracture and then incorporate these two pins in a full leg plaster cast in order to hold the bones out to length and prevent shortening. One disadvantage of this technique is the possibility of distracting the fragments during the formal manipulation following which the fragments will be held apart by this method, leading to delayed union.

The Technique of Closed Reduction of a Fractured Tibia and Fibula.—Several methods are available, of which the following is the simplest if the surgeon is single-handed. The patient is anaesthetised to produce muscle relaxation and is placed supine with his knees flexed over the end of the operating table. The surgeon is seated facing the injured leg and the height of the table is adjusted until the foot just clears the surgeon's knee. An inelastic bandage is tied over plaster wool as a 'halter' round the ankle and looped under the surgeon's foot.

Following closed reduction and application of a full leg plaster cast, extending from groin to metatarsal heads with the knee in 20° flexion and the foot plantargrade, regular x-rays are required during the first four weeks after injury to check that the position is not lost.

Up to 10° of angulation at the fracture site can be corrected at any time in the next few days by cutting the plaster circumferentially at the level of the fracture, wedging it open on the concave side of the angulation, and then completing the plaster.

(2) By skeletal traction through the lower end of the tibia or the os calcis

with the leg in a special frame or a plaster cast. Traction may render formal manipulation unnecessary. This form of treatment is used if a stable reduction cannot be maintained by plaster alone. A variant of this method, in which pins are passed into the tibia both above and below the fracture and are then fixed to an external metal frame can be used to immobilise the fracture rather than to apply traction (Chapter 15). This latter method is particularly useful in the treatment of compound fractures because the fragments can be accurately reduced during wound debridement and exploration and following this held reduced by the external fixator. Because no plaster cast is then necessary, excellent access to the wound is allowed for the purposes of dressings, skin grafts or flaps *etc*.

(3) By internal fixation with a compression plate or an intramedullary nail. This form of treatment should only be used in expert hands. It is particularly indicated in multiple fractures and in closed fractures in non-elderly patients where an acceptable reduction cannot be obtained by closed means. It is contra-indicated in compound fractures. It has the advantage that the joints can be mobilised early, but the disadvantage that the fracture may be infected at operation.

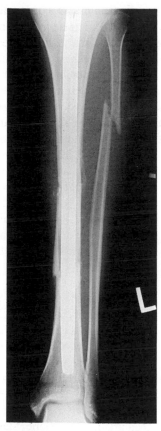

FIG. 289.—Segmental fracture of the tibia treated by A—O intra-medullary nail.

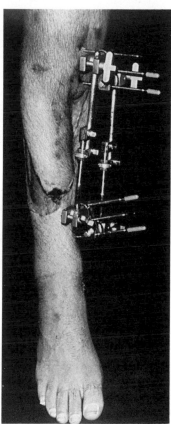

FIG. 290.—Compound fracture of the tibia with skin loss. External fixator facilitates skin flap or grafting methods.

Where possible an intramedullary nail should be used for fixation because it is a much stronger method of fixation than a plate, and allows the patient to fully weight bear soon after operation. However, it can only be used in non-comminuted transverse fractures of the middle third of the diaphysis (fig. 289).

The tibia usually takes about 12 weeks to unite. It is rarely fit to take weight without support under 16 weeks but if the fracture is stable, weight bearing may be allowed shortly after injury in a plaster cast, with the aid of internal fixation, or in an appliance (a 'cast-brace') composed of a cast around the skin to which is attached a brace which transmits some weight from the shoe directly to the proximal fragment.

Should the fracture be ununited at 3 months, further immobilisation in an above-knee plaster cast, preferably with weight-bearing, is required. If union has still not occurred after a further 6 weeks, immobilisation can be continued, but many surgeons prefer to reduce the duration of treatment by bone-grafting the tibia, with or without the addition of internal fixation (Chapter 15).

Complications.—(1) *Skin damage*—these fractures are frequently compound, often with extensive skin damage and loss. Treatment is by stabilisation using an external fixator with early skin cover provided by split skin grafting or local skin flaps (fig. 290).

(2)*Vascular injury*—displaced fractures of the proximal shaft may damage the trifurcation of the popliteal artery.

(3) *Delayed and non-union* of fractures of the tibial shaft is common, probably occurring in as many as 20% of all cases. If union is not present 16–20 weeks after fracture most surgeons will proceed to internal fixation and cancellous bone grafting for atrophic non-union and rigid internal fixation alone for hypertrophic non-union (Chapter 15). The following factors predispose to delayed and non-union:

a. Significant initial displacement.
b. Soft tissue damage.
c. Comminution.
d. Infection.
e. Distraction (pins 'above and below', traction)
f. Inadequate immobilisation.
g. Location of fracture (mid-shaft).
h. Intact fibula.

(4) *Mal-union* is not uncommon after poor closed treatment, especially shortening, mal-rotation and varus and valgus deformities. Residual varus and valgus deformities >10° may lead to later secondary degenerative osteoarthritis of the ankle joint.

(5) *Infection* may occur after compound fractures even with adequate treatment. It is frequently associated with delayed and non-union and presents significant problems of management. The treatment programme will often be lengthy and consist of the following: excision of dead and infected bone, stabilisation of the fracture (usually by an external fixator), administration of appropriate intravenous antibiotics in high dosage, cancellous bone grafting and early provision of full thickness skin cover if a skin defect is present.

(6) *Ankle and sub-talar joint stiffness.*

(7) *Compartment syndrome* (see Chapter 15).

Fractures of the tibia in children.—Fractures of the tibial plateau are rare in children. Salter Type II separations of the proximal tibial epiphysis do occur but are much less common than those of the distal femur; treatment is along the same lines. Fractures of the shafts of the tibia and fibula are common and are usually relatively undisplaced. Most can be managed by closed manipulative reduction, if necessary, followed by application of a full leg plaster cast for 6–12 weeks, depending on the age of the child.

ANKLE FRACTURES

Mechanism and Morbid Anatomy.—The ankle is usually injured by indirect violence: the foot being externally rotated, inverted (adducted), everted (abducted) or, more rarely, internally rotated on the tibia. Rarely the ankle may be injured by a force which shears the talus transversely relative to the tibia, or which drives it vertically up into the tibia. Each of these mechanisms of injury produces a characteristic fracture pattern, so that these injuries can be classified, although with some over-simplification, on the basis of the mechanism.

Although the mechanism is described as if the foot moved (*e.g.* into inversion) on a fixed tibia, in practice these injuries nearly always occur with the foot fixed, for example by a hole in the ground or in a ski, whilst the tibia continues to move, driven by the momentum of the body weight. The foot is inherently more stable in eversion than in inversion and hence injuries due to inversion are more common than those due to eversion. Because during normal walking the feet are placed in a little external rotation relative to the line of travel, a sudden arrest of the weight-bearing foot whilst the tibia continues to move forward has the effect of externally rotating the foot on the tibia. (The student can demonstrate this for himself by walking, stopping his foot dead as it is placed on the ground, and noting the direction in which his tibia moves as he tends to fall forward.) Thus inversion and external rotation are the two most common mechanisms of injury.

The important factor in ankle injuries is the stability of the tibio-fibular mortice. If the mortice is stable, that is to say if no abnormal motion is possible between the tibia and the talus, the injury is relatively trivial. If abnormal motion is possible, the injury is potentially serious since persistent instability at an anatomically abnormal mortice causes pain and ultimately osteo-arthrosis of the ankle. Thus if the mortice is stable, the aim of treatment is to protect the ankle until healing has occurred; but if the mortice has been disrupted it must be reconstructed (reduced) and held (immobilised) until bone and soft tissue healing is complete.

External Rotation Injuries[1].—The fracture pattern which results from an external rotation injury depends upon whether the foot is supinated or pronated at the time of injury.

Supinated foot.—If the foot is supinated (inverted) at the time of sustaining an external rotation injury then the medial soft tissue structures are relaxed and do not fail first. The talus is not free to rotate fowards on the medial side but rotates backwards pivoting on the intact medial structures. The talus pushes the lateral malleolus posteriorly producing a rupture of the anterior tibio-fibular ligament

---

[1] External rotation fractures are traditionally known as Pott's fractures.

Percival Pott, 1714–1788. Surgeon, St. Bartholomew's Hospital, London. Described this fracture–dislocation of the ankle in 1765.

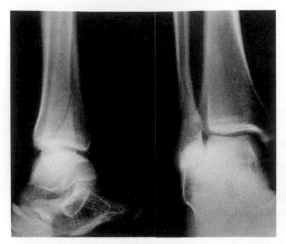

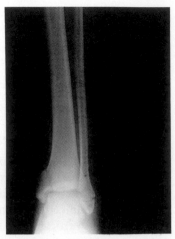

FIG. 291.—Ankle fracture first degree. The characteristic line of the fracture of the fibula is seen on the lateral view (see text).

FIG. 292.—Ankle fracture. Medial compression failure results in a near vertical fracture line because it is 'pushed off'.

followed by an oblique fracture of the distal fibula with a characteristic fracture line which runs downwards and forwards to the level of the ankle joint (*first degree injury*). The fracture fragment, which includes the malleolus, has a spike which lies posterior to a second spike projecting from the fibular shaft. The malleolar spike is attached to the tibia by the posterior inferior tibio-fibular ligament. Thus the lateral malleolus is attached to the tibia and the mortice is stable. Furthermore there is no damage to the medial structures of the ankle and therefore lateral talar shift cannot occur. This type of fracture is probably the commonest type of ankle fracture.

The fracture is often not obvious on an antero-posterior radiograph but can be seen on a lateral view (fig. 291). If the force continues to act then the medial structures fail either by rupture of the deltoid ligament or an avulsion fracture of the medial malleolus (*second degree injury*). The mortice is now unstable. There is no diastasis because the inter-osseous and posterior tibio-fibular ligaments remain intact. In addition to the above fractures the rotating talus may 'push-off' a small posterior malleolar fragment (so-called 'third malleolus') from the posterior aspect of the distal articular surface of the tibia (*third degree injury*).

Pronated foot.—If the foot is pronated (everted) then the deltoid (medial) ligament is taut and, as the talus externally rotates, the deltoid ligament itself ruptures or avulses a fragment of bone from the tip of the medial malleolus. The talus is then free to rotate on a lateral axis producing torsion of the fibula which results in a rupture of the anterior tibio-fibular ligament and inter-osseous tibio-fibular ligament followed by a spiral fracture of the fibula which may be situated at any level from the upper border of the syndesmosis to the neck of the fibula. This also results in a *partial diastasis* (movement of the fibula away from the tibia) of the inferior tibio-fibular joint. Sometimes during this sequence of events the tibia may move medially off the talus under the influence of body weight resulting in the fibula being carried away from the tibia producing an oblique bending fracture of the fibula with rupture of the posterior tibio-fibular ligament also and a *complete diastasis*.

Inversion (Adduction) Injuries.—*Inversion (adduction) injuries produce a lateral traction force and medial compression force.*

Failure of the lateral structures due to traction usually precedes failure of the medial structures due to compression. Lateral traction failure results in a rupture of the lateral ligament (partial or complete) or an avulsion fracture of the lateral malleolus at its tip or transverse at the level of the ankle joint. Medial compression failure results in a fracture of the medial malleolus with a near vertical fracture line because it is 'pushed off' (fig. 292). The first stage of this injury results therefore in a sprain or rupture of the lateral ligament (fig. 293).

A rupture starts at the anterior fasciculus and extends backwards through the lateral ligament and medially through the anterior capsule, allowing the talus to tilt more and more in the mortice as it does so. Sprains and ruptures of the lateral

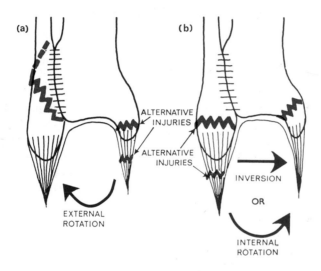

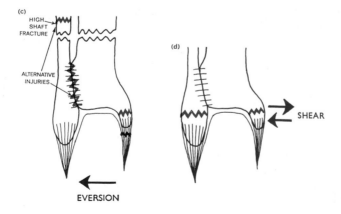

FIG. 293.—Varieties of ankle fracture.

ligament are the commonest ankle injuries and are usually loosely diagnosed as a 'sprained ankle'. Ruptures cannot be differentiated from sprains clinically but the distinction can be made by stress radiography (fig. 294).

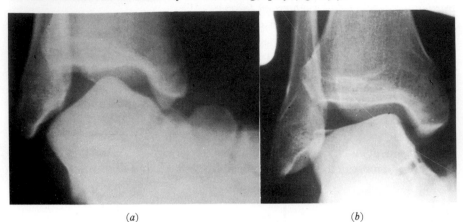

(a)   (b)

FIG. 294.—Inversion stress x-rays of two ankles with ruptures of the lateral ligament. (a) An AP view showing gross talar tilt indicating a complete rupture of the lateral ligament. (b) Less marked talar tilt, but note the transchondral fracture of the dome of the talus where the talus strikes the fibula. A routine AP x-ray of both these ankles revealed no abnormality.

Eversion (Abduction) Injuries.—*Eversion (abduction) injuries of the ankle produce a medial traction force and a lateral compression force.* The former results in a rupture of the deltoid ligament or a 'pull-off' fracture of the medial malleolus. The latter produces an oblique fracture of the lower fibula extending upwards and outwards from the level of the ankle joint with comminution of the lateral cortex. Because the anterior and posterior tibio-fibular and the interosseous ligaments are all under tension simultaneously, the fibula is held to the tibia and no diastasis occurs. The damage to the medial structures usually precedes damage to the lateral structures. The first stage of the injury is therefore an isolated fracture of the medial malleolus (fig. 295) or a rupture of the deltoid ligament and the second stage of the injury, if the force continues to operate, is a fracture of the lower fibula as described.

Internal Rotation.—This mechanism is rare and produces injuries similar to those produced by inversion.

Vertical compression injuries.—These result from falls on to a dorsi-flexed or plantar-flexed ankle. The former injury results in an anterior compression fracture of the distal tibial articular surface and the latter injury in a posterior compression fracture. Occasionally combinations occur, resulting in comminution of the whole of the distal articular surface of the tibia.

Classification.—It is much simpler to classify ankle fractures according to the actual injuries sustained rather than by how they were sustained and the method outlined in Table 2 is suggested. It is important to emphasise that the differentiation between a stable first degree injury and an unstable second degree injury resulting from a combination of malleolar fracture and tear of opposite collateral ligament may be difficult. It can only be done by a combination of inspection of radiographs *and clincial examination of the patient* to detect signs of soft tissue damage (bruising, tenderness and swelling) over ligament sites.

TABLE 2 CLASSIFICATION OF ANKLE FRACTURES

First degree	—fracture one malleolus —no talar shift —stable
Second degree	—fracture 2 malleoli *or* fracture 1 malleolus + ligament tear —unstable
Third degree	—fracture 3 malleoli —unstable in medio-lateral *and* antero-posterior directions
Fourth degree	—high fibular fracture —tear of inferior tibio-fibular ligaments —diastasis; unstable in all directions
Fifth degree	—vertical impaction of distal tibial articular surface.

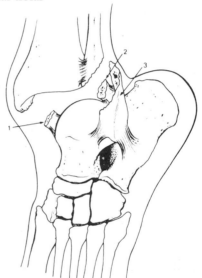

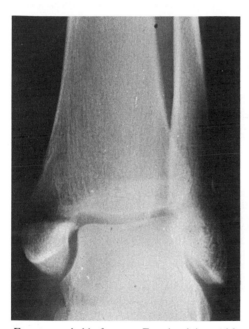

FIG. 295.—Ankle fracture. Eversion injury with isolated fracture of medial malleolus.

FIG. 296.—The morbid anatomy of a third degree external rotation injury of the ankle. Note that the medial malleolus (1), the third malleolus (2) and the lateral malleolus (3) are all attached directly or indirectly by ligaments to the talus or os calcis and hence that they move with the foot. (For clarity, the talus is shown in this figure as lying distal to the tibia. In fact, it lies behind the lower end of the tibia.)

One should also beware of the combination of a deltoid ligament tear and a high fibular fracture. This is an unstable injury but the ankle radiograph may be normal if displacement has not already occurred!

Treatment of Ankle Fractures.—The objective is to restore:

1. The anatomical position of the talus in the ankle mortice.
2. The joint line parallel to the ground.
3. The smooth articular surface, and to
4. Stabilise until the fracture(s) unite by plaster cast or internal fixation.

In general, unstable displaced fractures in 'young' patients should be treated by accurate open reduction and internal fixation and in 'older' patients by closed reduction and application of a plaster cast, see Techniques (below). Unstable undisplaced fractures in patients of all ages should be treated by application of non-weight bearing plaster casts and careful follow up with regular check-x-rays. A stable fracture should be treated by application of a weight bearing below knee plaster cast for six weeks.

Ligament Injuries.—1. *The Lateral Ligament.*—Sprains of the lateral ligament should be treated by compression bandaging, early mobilisation within the limits of pain and swelling, and co-ordination exercises. Ruptures (which in everyday clinical practice are as common as simple sprains but are often not diagnosed as such since the diagnosis requires stress radiography) should be treated by the same regime save that for the first 3 weeks the patient should not bear weight on the injured foot.

2. *The Inferior Tibio-Fibular Ligaments (Inferior Tibio-Fibular Diastasis).*—Rupture of these ligaments is best treated by internal fixation using a screw passed through the fibula into the tibia. Plaster-of-Paris is applied for 6 weeks postoperatively.

Complications.—1. Mal-union results from failure to reduce and stabilise unstable fractures.

2. Non-union occasionally occurs in fractures of the medial malleolus, probably as a result of infolding of periosteum producing soft-tissue interposition. For this reason this fracture is always best treated by internal fixation.

3. Secondary degenerative osteoarthritis often results if there is residual joint surface incongruity.

4. Ankle stiffness.

The Technique of Closed Reduction of a Fracture-Dislocation of the Ankle

As judged from the pre-reduction x-rays of a severely displaced fracture, it may appear unlikely that a satisfactory reduction could ever be obtained without operation. This impression is often misleading, reduction being possible because all the fragments are attached to the bones of the foot (fig. 296). The essential feature of the reduction is to concentrate on restoring the alignment of the foot to the tibia, rather than on reducing the separate fragments by local manipulation of the individual fractures. The manipulation consists of reversing the direction of the forces which caused the original injury (a general principle in the reduction of all fractures).

The direction of forces which caused the injury can often be deduced by studying the fracture pattern as already described in the previous section on Mechanism and Morbid Anatomy. Thus abduction injuries are reduced by adduction, and adduction injuries are reduced by abduction, of the foot on the tibia. In the case of external rotation injuries with a posterior malleolar fracture and backward displacement of the foot the reduction is carried out as follows. Traction in the long axis of the limb is applied so as to draw the talus clear of the distal end of the tibia, followed by forward displacement of the talus on the tibia, and then internal rotation and medial displacement of the foot. The talus cannot be 'over-reduced' anteriorly because the tissues posterior to the ankle will not permit it, nor into excessive internal rotation because the fibular 'spikes' interlock, nor medially because the dome of the talus strikes the root of the medial malleolus.

Having appreciated the sensation of reduction (see legend fig. 297), a well-padded below-knee plaster is applied whilst an approximate reduction is maintained. The surgeon then grasps the foot and tibia as before, but now through the plaster, and repeats the manoeuvre leading to reduction, taking care to hold the foot plantigrade as the plaster sets. If the ankle is very unstable, external rotation should be controlled by extending the plaster to the thigh with the knee flexed to 90° for 3 weeks. *The plaster should be split and*

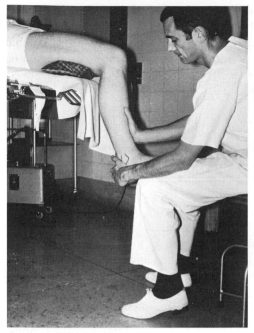

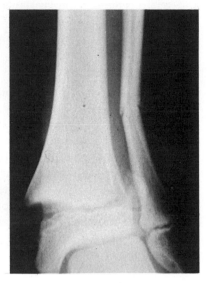

FIG. 297.—The technique of reduction of a third degree external rotation injury. The anaesthetised patient lies supine with the knees flexed over the end of the operating table. The surgeon sits at the foot of the table and grasps the injured heel with his left hand (if the right ankle is injured) placing his thenar eminence behind the lateral malleolus. Steadying the tibia with the right hand, the surgeon then exerts traction on the injured foot and draws it forwards so as to bring the talus beneath the articular surface of the tibia. He then internally rotates the foot and displaces it medially until firm resistance is encountered.

FIG. 298.—Ankle fracture in a child. Salter type II separation of distal tibial epiphysis with accompanying greenstick fracture of the fibula.

the patient admitted to hospital for 24 hours so that the circulation to the toes can be observed.

The Technique of Internal Fixation of Fractures of the Ankle.—A number of implants are available for the treatment of these fractures the details of which are beyond the scope of this text. The essentials, however, are: (1) to operate either before swelling has developed or after it has subsided, *i.e.* after 10 days of elevation and immobilisation; (2) to employ a scrupulously aseptic technique; (3) to concentrate particularly upon secure fixation and accurate reduction of the medial malleolus since the medial side is the key to the long term health of the ankle; and (4) to reduce the 'third malleolus' if this is displaced and constitutes more than one-third of the articular surface of the tibia as seen in a lateral x-ray. After internal fixation the ankle may or may not require external splintage in plaster but weight-bearing should certainly be avoided for 9 weeks.

Fractures of the ankle in children.—Ankle fractures do occur in children and the following are the commoner ones encountered:

1. Salter Type I separation of the distal fibular epiphysis results from an inversion (adduction) injury. There is usually little or no displacement and treatment is by application of a below knee walking plaster cast for three weeks.

2. Salter Type II separation of the distal tibial epiphysis occasionally occurs as a result of a plantar flexion and inversion injury; there is often an accompanying greenstick fracture of the fibula (fig. 298). Treatment is by closed manipulation if significant displacement is present followed by application of a full leg plaster cast for six weeks.

3. Tillaux fracture.—this is a Salter Type III fracture of the lateral part of the distal tibial epiphysis, usually occurring at the age of 13–14 after the medial half of the distal tibial

Paul Jules Tillaux, 1834–1904. French surgeon.

growth plate has closed. The injury represents avulsion of the lateral half of the epiphysis by the attached anterior tibio-fibular ligament following an external rotation injury. Treatment is by application of a below knee walking plaster cast for six weeks if undisplaced or by open reduction and internal fixation if significantly displaced.

4. Fractures of the medial malleolus may be Salter Type III or IV injuries. If displacement is present then treatment should be by accurate open reduction and internal fixation to restore a perfect articular surface and prevent growth disturbance from fusion of the growth plate in the Type IV injury (and see p. 263).

Rupture of the Achilles' Tendon

The Achilles' tendon is the commonest tendon to rupture, and since the injury is frequently diagnosed incorrectly, special note should be made of its clinical features. It is an injury most common in middle-aged men and, though it can occur during games and severe exertion, it often happens as a result of a trivial stumble, the sensation of rupture being mistaken for a blow on the back of the leg. Such ruptures apparently occur because the tendon is ischaemic and weaker than normal. The rupture usually takes place about 3 cm above the insertion of the tendon into the os calcis. A gap is easily palpable, and sometimes visible, at the site of the rupture. The foot can be dorsiflexed to a greater extent than the normal foot. The power of plantar-flexion is reduced so that the patient cannot stand on tiptoe on the injured foot, but it is to be noted that it is never completely absent. This is the most important point, because the surgeon can be led to imagine that the tear must be incomplete by the fact that some power of plantar-flexion exists. This power is, of course, exerted by the long flexors of the toes, the tibialis posterior, and the peronei. Very few cases of suspected 'partial' rupture of the Achilles' tendon are in fact incomplete and it is dangerous to make this diagnosis because suture of the tendon is much more difficult if the operation is delayed.

The diagnosis of 'rupture of the plantaris tendon' is occasionally made in patients younger than those typically sustaining the classical Achilles' tendon rupture. It is probable that 'plantaris rupture' is an imaginary condition, and that the clinical picture is that of a partial tear of the calf muscle fibres at a much higher level than the true Achilles' rupture.

Treatment.—Early suture of the Achilles' tendon followed by immobilisation of the ankle in a plaster cast for 6 weeks gives excellent results, but late suture is usually disappointing because the proximal end has retracted and lost its elasticity, so that the gap sometimes cannot be closed even by plantar-flexion of the foot and flexion of the knee (in which position the gastrocnemius and soleus muscles are relaxed).

THE FOOT

Fractures of the talus are uncommon but may occur as a result of a fall from a height or forced dorsiflexion of the ankle. The neck of the talus is the usual site of fracture, being shorn through by the sharp anterior articular surface of the tibia. The fracture may be undisplaced or displaced and may also be associated with dislocation of the body of the talus from the ankle mortice or a sub-talar dislocation. More rarely fractures may occur in the body or head of the talus. In both the latter sites the fractures may be of the osteochondral type.

As in the case of the os calcis, considerable swelling rapidly develops and obscures the diagnosis, which is often established only after radiography. Infarction of the bone within

Achilles (see footnote p. 181).

the body of the talus is not uncommon because the blood vessels supplying the region are torn as a result of the neck fracture. Avascular necrosis of the body of the talus results which may be associated with non-union and later secondary osteoarthritis of the ankle (compare fractures of the neck of the femur (p. 307) and of the scaphoid (Chapter 16).

Treatment.—If the body of the talus is dislocated, closed reduction, using skeletal traction through the os calcis, is sometimes successful, but usually operative reduction is necessary followed by internal fixation of the fracture of the neck using one or two lag screws. Reduction is required urgently because of the risk of pressure necrosis of the overlying skin produced by the displaced body of the talus, and occasionally pressure occlusion of blood vessels supplying the foot. Displaced fractures without an associated dislocation are treated by open reduction and internal fixation. Post-operatively and for undisplaced fractures of the body or neck of the talus the ankle is rested in a below knee plaster cast for eight weeks.

Fracture of the Os Calcis.—Is caused by falls from a height. The bone is shattered like an eggshell and the fracture usually involves the sub-talar joint (fig. 299). The degree of displacement varies according to the violence. In some cases there is little or no displacement; in others the whole os calcis is flattened and widened. The Achilles' tendon tends to pull the posterior part of the bone upwards and the heel is always everted.

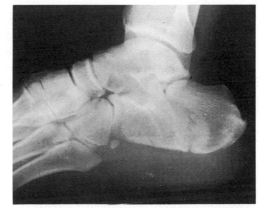

FIG. 299.—Fracture of the os calcis involving the sub-talar joint.

This injury, especially if it involves the sub-talar joint, is likely to leave the foot stiff regardless of treatment. As a consequence, walking on sloping or uneven surfaces is difficult and often painful. Though the foot is often painful for months, pain nearly always subsides eventually. Stiffness on the other hand is usually permanent, but tolerable to the patient.

There may be associated injuries to the spine, for example a fracture of a lumbar vertebral body, and the patient should be questioned about pain in the lumbar region.

Treatment.—This is controversial; most surgeons accept the deformity and concentrate on early non-weight bearing mobilisation combined with elevation and compression by wool and crepe to control swelling. Weight bearing is started after eight weeks. Some surgeons prefer to carry out an open reduction and internal fixation of the displaced fracture of the important weight bearing posterior articular facet of the os calcis (fig. 300). Fractures which do not involve the sub-talar joint are treated by early non-weight bearing mobilisation.

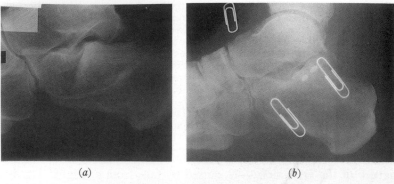

(a)   (b)

FIG. 300.—Fracture of the os calcis with displacement of the posterior facet (a) pre-operation (b) following elevation and internal wire fixation (seen between two 'marker' paper clips).

Complications.—The two commonest complications are persistent stiffness of the sub-talar joint which produces difficulty in walking over uneven surfaces, and later secondary osteoarthritis of the sub-talar joint. The latter complication is treated by sub-talar arthrodesis.

Fractures of the shafts of the metatarsals are caused by crushing injuries, for example by weights falling on the feet or the wheels of vehicles running over them. When these fractures accompany severe crushing of the foot, the broken bone may be the least significant part of the injury: the soft tissues are also crushed so that a not-infrequent end result is a foot which is thickened, stiff and painful, even though the fractures have united.

Treatment.—If only one or two metatarsals have fractured, reduction is not required unless some part of the shaft, in a grossly displaced fracture, is projecting into the sole of the foot. Splintage is also unnecessary and early mobilisation with non-weight-bearing exercises is to be encouraged. Return to activity is achieved by taking weight on the heel as soon as the patient feels he can, which may be in 2 to 3 weeks. Full function is possible in 8 to 12 weeks.

If more than two bones are broken, the fractures are usually unstable and the foot must be immobilised in a plaster boot for 4 to 6 weeks. Active mobilisation of the foot is required thereafter.

Tarso-metatarsal dislocation (Lisfranc dislocation).—An uncommon but important injury of the foot, because it is often missed, results from a twisting injury resulting in dislocation of some or all of the metatarsals from the tarsal bones, usually in a lateral direction. There are often associated fractures of the metatarsal bones, especially the second. This injury is also usually accompanied by massive swelling of the foot and may be complicated by damage to the dorsalis pedis artery and toe ischaemia. *Treatment* is by open reduction and internal fixation by wires (fig. 301).

Avulsion of the styloid process of the fifth metatarsal is a common, minor injury which causes unnecessary inconvenience if treated in a walking plaster. The styloid process is avulsed by the pull of the peroneus brevis contracting during forced inversion of the foot. The fragment is frequently detached by 2 mm or more, but even if bony union does not occur, a fibrous non-union is always symptomless. The foot should not be immobilised and it is unnecessary to apply anything more than adhesive strapping to support the foot and control swelling.

Jacques Lisfranc, 1790–1847, French Surgeon. He described the joint but not the dislocation.

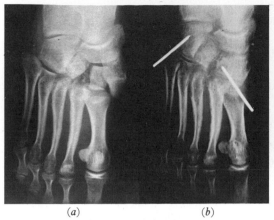

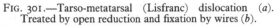

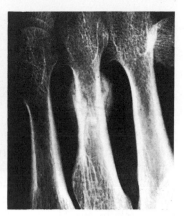

(a)   (b)

FIG. 301.—Tarso-metatarsal (Lisfranc) dislocation (a). Treated by open reduction and fixation by wires (b).

FIG. 302.—March fracture of the third metatarsal.

Fracture of the neck of the second or third metatarsal may occur not as a result of a single violent episode, but as a result of fatigue (*march fracture*). The fracture usually follows excessive walking—hence the term march fracture. It is predisposed to by a short first metatarsal which causes undue stress to fall on the necks of the second and third metatarsals during the toe-off phase of gait. Sudden pain, localised over the dorsal aspect of the bone, is characteristic. An immediate x-ray will often fail to reveal the crack, but if repeated in 3 weeks callus will be obvious (fig. 302). The only treatment needed is strapping and restricted activity.

CHAPTER 18

INFECTIONS OF BONES AND JOINTS

ACUTE OSTEOMYELITIS

Acute osteomyelitis used to be a common and serious, indeed often a fatal, disease in children. Over recent years there has been a fall in the incidence of the disease, probably due to an improvement in the general health of children. At the same time antibiotics have made the disease less serious: it need never now be fatal and should be curable.

Aetiology.—The bacteria reach the bone by the blood-stream. A primary focus may be obvious in the form of a boil or an infected graze, but not uncommonly no obvious source of infection is evident. Rarely the disease may be secondary to a frank septicaemia or pyaemia. More commonly the blood-borne infection takes the form of a bacteraemia.

It has been suggested that a lowered general resistance on the part of the patient, and local trauma, may predispose to this disease, but the evidence in support of these suggestions is unconvincing.

The usual causative organism is the *staphylococcus aureus*. Other organisms which may be responsible include the streptococcus, pneumococcus, *haemophilus influenzae*, staphylococcus albus and a number of other organisms, no one of which is present commonly.

Pathology.—The disease always, or nearly always, begins in the metaphysis. The infective process progresses through the thickness of the cortex via the Haversian canals and as it does so causes thrombosis of the vessels in the bone. As a consequence, by the time the infection reaches the sub-periosteal region of the bone a variable amount of the cortex may have been infarcted. In the first 24 or 48 hours after the onset of the infection, an inflammatory exudate forms deep to the periosteum, elevating the membrane from the bone. Periosteal elevation is painful and, since the periosteum is inelastic, the inflammatory exudate deep to it is under tension. As a consequence the patient rapidly develops marked toxic signs. Approximately 48 hours after the first symptom, frank pus develops sub-periosteally. Partly as a consequence of the resistance of cartilage to invasion by the septic process, and partly because of the very firm attachment of the periosteum (more accurately the perichondrium) to the epiphyseal plate, transgression of the plate itself and consequent interference with growth is rare. The inflammatory process progresses along the length of the medulla causing venous and arterial thrombosis as it does so. Sub-periosteally, pus tracks both longitudinally and circumferentially around the bone, stripping the periosteum and interrupting the periosteal vessels. Thus progressively larger areas of the cortex become infarcted and involved in the inflammatory process.

In the absence of treatment pus finally bursts through the periosteum and tracks through the muscles to present subcutaneously. Eventually the skin breaks down and pus discharges from a sinus which connects the bone with the skin surface.

The bone infarct in acute osteomyelitis is known as a *Sequestrum*. Surrounding the sequestrum, the elevated periosteum lays down new bone which entombs the dead bone within. This ensheathing mass of new bone is known as the *Involucrum*. In the places where pus has broken through the periosteum to form a defect in it, sinuses develop which are represented in the involucrum by holes known as *Cloacae*[1] (fig. 303). The development

---

[1] Cloaca (Latin) = A drain.

of such advanced pathology is now rarely seen since modern treatment if adequate, aborts the disease before pus has formed, and certainly before a significant amount of bone has died.

Two factors are responsible for the chronicity of this disease: the presence of dead, infected bone which cannot be resorbed; and the fact that the intraosseous abscess cavity cannot be obliterated because it has rigid bony walls. As a consequence of these factors the body's normal defence mechanisms (leucocytes and antibodies) together with any antibiotics that may be given therapeutically are unable to reach all the bacteria in the bone. Accordingly, although the disease process may be sterilised in the living bone, recurrence is always likely.

Clinical Features.—Pain is the presenting symptom.

It is essential that an accurate history is taken so that the onset of the first complaint of local pain can be timed exactly. The significance of this feature of the history is discussed further under *Treatment*. The pain gradually increases in severity, and the child becomes increasingly febrile and toxic, at a rate dependent upon the toxicity and virulence of the infective organism. It is usual for the mother to seek medical advice within 48 hours of the onset of the first symptom.

Physical Signs.—The essential physical sign is localised tenderness. When the doctor first examines the child, the child is likely to be irritable and to resent examination. It is imperative that the physician should be patient, and gently palpate the child's limbs until the exact area of maximum tenderness has been identified. If this tenderness lies over the metaphysis of a long bone, the diagnosis of acute osteomyelitis should be presumed until it can be proved otherwise. The adjacent joint may contain an effusion, raising the differential diagnosis of suppurative arthritis. The joint itself however is not tender and although the child resists movement of the limb, with patience it is possible to demonstrate that some movement of the joint is allowed. This contrasts with acute suppurative arthritis in which absolutely no movement is permitted. The temperature is raised, often markedly so, and an associated increase in the pulse rate occurs. Some days after the onset of the first symptom noticeable swelling and heat may be detected in addition to tenderness. Finally the area of the abscess (for such it is by this time) is fluctuant.

It is absolutely essential that blood cultures should be undertaken before antibiotic treatment is commenced. In order to provide the maximum possible chance of a positive culture, three separate venipunctures should be made and from each venipuncture three aliquots[1] should be cultured separately. The child's body surface should be searched minutely for possible primary foci of infection and if these are found they should be cultured.

Special Investigations.—Other investigations are of no diagnostic value early in the disease. The E.S.R. and white cell count are usually raised but this is entirely non-specific.

X-ray.—There are no abnormal radiological features in the first few days of the infection. As time goes by, new bone can be seen deposited by the elevated periosteum, but this sign does not appear until more than 10 days after the onset of the disease and will then be demonstrable whether or not the disease has been sterilised: it depends entirely upon the presence or absence of periosteal elevation. Some rarefaction in the bone due to local hyperaemia will also occur after 2 or 3 weeks but again does not distinguish continuing osteomyelitis from the sterilised disease. The radiological appearances of chronic osteomyelitis are dealt with elsewhere (p. 348).

---

[1] Aliquot (L.) Alius = Other. Quot = How many. In this case 3 other samples.

Treatment.—The child is admitted to hospital and the limb is splinted, but in such a way that easy access to the tender area is retained. The outline of the tender area is marked on the skin.

If the patient is first seen within 48 hours of the appearance of the first symptoms, antibiotic treatment is begun immediately after appropriate samples have been taken for blood culture. Acute osteomyelitis is one of the few diseases in which it is justifiable to begin antibiotic treatment without waiting for bacterial sensitivity, a peculiarity which stems from the fact that if the disease can be sterilised within the first 48 hours, complete resolution can be guaranteed. If sterilisation fails or is not attempted in this time, the disease may become chronic, so generating life-long disability and a possible cause of death. The great majority (about 80%) of the isolates from osteomyelitis are *Staphylococcus aureus* and cloxacillin should be administered at a dosage of 100–200 mg/kg body weight in divided doses intravenously until the child is clinically well, has no fever and the local signs have decreased. Oral therapy, with flucloxacillin can then be given. In addition, benzyl penicillin should be given intravenously (0.25–1.0 million units every six hours). For penicillin-hypersensitive patients a cephalosporin may be given intravenously. In children under three *Haemophilus influenzae* may be a responsible organism and especially affects the small bones of the hands and feet. At the present time ampicillin 250 mg q.d.s. intravenously is recommended. Unfortunately antibiotic resistance amongst organisms causing osteomyelitis creates problems. The staphylococci are usually resistant to benzyl penicillin and ampicillin and therefore require a penicillinase-stable penicillin. Most strains of *Haemophilus influenzae* are currently susceptible to ampicillin but if failure to respond is thought to be due to a resistant organism, chloramphenicol should be substituted (but see p. 32). Other antibiotics may be substituted if they are dictated by the sensitivity tests.

If the patient is first seen 48 hours or more after the onset of the first symptom, the possibility arises that pus is present. If pus is present, it may be sterilised by antibiotics, but the general surgical principle applies to bone as to other tissues that *an abscess requires surgical evacuation.* The presence of pus may be difficult or impossible to detect with certainty since fluctuation is late to develop. Fluctuation cannot be demonstrated in the early stages of abscess formation because the periosteal membrane is tense, the involved bone is often deep to muscle, and the area is too tender to palpate firmly. Therefore the surgeon has to rely upon his general impression as to the severity of the disease and his knowledge of its duration in deciding either to treat the patient initially with antibiotics, or to combine this therapy with incision of the tender area.

If it is decided to rely on antibiotic therapy alone in the belief that no pus is present, antibiotics should be given and the effect of this treatment upon the toxic signs and upon local tenderness should be watched very closely. If the antibiotic is controlling the disease, and if no pus is present, the temperature will subside to become normal within 2 or 3 days and tenderness will progressively disappear. If, on the other hand, the antibiotics are inappropriate to the sensitivities of the organism or pus is present, the temperature is likely to settle but not to normality: spikes up to 38°C will continue. If this occurs, the tender area must

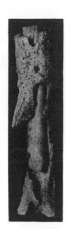

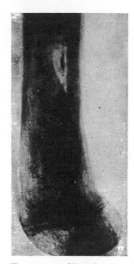

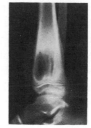

FIG. 303.—Sequestrum enveloped by an involucrum which is pierced by cloacae.

FIG. 304.—Chronic osteomyelitis of the femur with a cavity containing a sequestrum.

FIG. 305.—Brodie's abscess of the lower end of the tibia, revealing a band of sclerosis surrounding a central lucent area.

be explored surgically with a view to evacuating pus if any is present and to obtaining the organism for culture and sensitivity.

Operation.—Operation is carried out under general anaesthesia and is preceded by exsanguination of the limb by elevation and the use of an inflatable tourniquet. An incision is made over the tender area and carried down to the bone where pus is usually found deep to the periosteum. The abscess cavity is fully opened and the pus evacuated. A swab is taken for culture and sensitivity at this stage. There is controversy as to whether or not this procedure should be followed by drilling the cortex in order to enable any pus that may be present in the medullary cavity to drain to the surface. The wound is then closed with interrupted sutures over a closed sterile suction drain. Antibiotics and local splintage are continued post-operatively.

Complications.—These may be divided into two types, general and local. The general complications are septicaemia and pyaemia which may give rise to metastatic abscesses. Either complication, if uncontrolled, may prove fatal. Amyloid disease may develop as a complication of chronic osteomyelitis (below).

The local complications include: (1) secondary involvement of the joint if the epiphyseal line is intra-articular, e.g. the hip joint in association with osteomyelitis of the proximal femur; (2) spontaneous fracture which is rare provided the limb is splinted and the disease adequately treated, (3) deformity which, surprisingly, is rare, and (4) chronic osteomyelitis.

Differential Diagnosis

Acute Suppurative Arthritis.—Here the sepsis is intra-articular, and therefore the patient allows no movement of the joint. In the 'sympathetic' effusion associated with acute osteomyelitis, a certain range of painless movement can usually be obtained if the patient is examined gently. The maximum tenderness is near the end of the bone in osteomyelitis rather than over the joint in suppurative arthritis.

Acute Rheumatic Arthritis is usually polyarticular and fleeting in any one joint. There is a history of a sore throat and cardiovascular signs are often present.

Haemarthrosis may occur in haemophilia. The patient is usually a known haemophiliac and aspiration, if necessary, reveals blood.

Scurvy.—Sub-periosteal haematomata are sometimes very tender, and if near an epiphysis may be confused with acute osteomyelitis.

Acute Exanthemas and Typhoid Fever.—These conditions may be suspected on account of the profoundly toxic and even comatose condition of the patient. If careful palpation over a localised area of the end of a long bone induces resentful movements or moaning, the possibility of osteomyelitis should be considered.

Ewing's Tumour.—See Chapter 20.

Acute Traumatic Osteomyelitis

This condition arises as a result of infected wounds, for example compound fractures, and operations on bones. The constitutional disturbances are less severe than in acute (infective) osteomyelitis, as the causative wound provides some measure of drainage. Treatment consists of more extensive opening of the wound, removal of dead bone, and antibiotics. The prevention of this condition depends upon the adequate initial treatment of compound fractures (Chapter 15) and upon sterile operating conditions.

CHRONIC OSTEOMYELITIS

Pathology.—Acute haematogenous osteomyelitis may pass into chronic osteomyelitis if early treatment is not available, or is inadequate so that infected bone dies to form a sequestrum. The disease may take two forms. The pathology of the more common variety in which a large volume of bone is involved has been described under acute osteomyelitis (p. 344). The incidence of this condition has been greatly reduced by the modern treatment of the acute infection, but some cases remain as a legacy of the pre-antibiotic era, and more will probably occur in the future if the acute infection is inadequately treated. The second variety is known as *Brodie's abscess*. The infection in this form of the disease is closely contained so as to create a chronic abscess within the bone composed of pus or jelly-like granulation tissue surrounded by sclerotic bone. The lesion may be the sequel to a pyogenic septicaemia from which the patient has recovered, leaving a bone abscess which may remain dormant for years. On the other hand, it may be found in a patient who is known to have had osteomyelitis (but not septicaemia) affecting a bone other than the one in which the Brodie's abscess is discovered.

Clinical Features.—Chronic osteomyelitis may remain quiescent for months or years, but from time to time acute or sub-acute exacerbations occur. An exacerbation is ushered in with constitutional upset and local evidence of inflammation, which may culminate in a discharge of pus, often from a pre-existing sinus. An x-ray sometimes reveals a sequestrum which has separated from the surface of the bone or which lies in a cavity (fig. 304). Tomographs may help to demonstrate a sequestrum and a sinogram may delineate an abscess cavity in the bone.

A Brodie's abscess causes intermittent local pain and occasionally transitory effusions in the adjacent joint during an exacerbation. Examination may reveal tenderness and thickening of the bone. A radiograph is diagnostic (fig. 305). The amount of bony sclerosis is variable, ranging from dense sclerosis extending a considerable distance round the cavity to, more commonly, a faint line of sclerosis at the junction of the abscess with the cancellous bone.

The chronicity of a Brodie's abscess is the result of the physical characteristics of bone, because the abscess can never close by collapse of the walls as happens in soft tissues. Moreover, the infection kills the hard, bony walls of the abscess and provokes new bone deposition, thus preventing leucocytes, antibodies and antibiotics from reaching the contents of the cavity.

Treatment of exacerbations in chronic osteomyelitis consists of immobilisation

Sir Benjamin Brodie, 1783–1862. Surgeon, St. George's Hospital, London.

of the limb and the administration of antibiotics. On this regime the exacerbation often subsides, but only to recur again later in life.

Surgical intervention in chronic osteomyelitis has as its objective the removal of dead bone and the elimination of dead space. Dead bone in the form of a sequestrum may be detected by probing a sinus or by x-ray. Seams of dead bone dispersed within living bone cannot be detected with certainty but may be suspected if an x-ray shows an area of sclerosis. An appropriate antibiotic (which is chosen in the light of the sensitivity of the causative organism) is administered for some days prior to operation. Access to the bone is usually gained through a previous scar. The soft tissues are stripped from the bone, and the involucrum is removed to reach the sequestrum. If a cavity is present, the over-hanging walls are removed with an osteotome, until it is 'saucerised'. Sclerotic bone is removed *en bloc* if this is practicable. The wound is drained and closed in such a way as to eliminate dead space as far as possible. Modern approaches to this problem include insertion of gentamycin-impregnated beads following debridement of the affected area. These are removed 14 days later and the dead space obliterated by packing the cavity with cancellous bone chips, or filling it with a local muscle flap.

So difficult is it to guarantee that an operation will cure chronic osteomyelitis affecting a large volume of bone, that operative intervention is not be be considered lightly unless a sequestrum is known to be present. If, however, a sequestrum is present and is removed, sinuses will often close and the disease may be cured. If only a cavity or sclerosis is present in the bone without a sequestrum, the attempt to 'saucerise' may fail and still leave a sinus. There are many patients for whom, if the discharge is slight and easily controlled by a dressing, it is preferable to retain the sinus and dressings permanently. Amyloid disease need be feared only when a copious discharge of pus has persisted for some years.

Amputation may be advisable if exacerbations are frequent or prolonged, in order to rid the patient of recurring periods of painful disability, and to forestall the onset of amyloid disease.

A Brodie's abscess should be treated by surgical evacuation and curettage of the cavity under antibiotic cover followed, if the cavity is of moderate size, by packing with cancellous bone chips.

ACUTE SUPPURATIVE ARTHRITIS

Like acute osteomyelitis, this used to be a common disease especially in children, but is now rare. Acute infection of a joint occurs as a result of:

1. Direct infection, as by a penetrating wound or a compound fracture which involves the joint.

2. Local extension, from some neighbouring focus, such as acute arthritis of the hip joint from osteomyelitis of the femoral neck.

3. Blood-borne infection, the usual organisms being the streptococcus, staphylococcus, and pneumococcus, and less commonly the gonococcus and *B. typhosus*.

The knee joint, owing to its large size and exposed position, is the commonest joint to be involved by penetrating wounds, while suppurative arthritis from blood-borne infections is the more common cause in other joints.

Clinical Features.—The patient complains of steadily increasing pain, inability to move the joint and malaise. On examination the patient is often severely toxic with a raised temperature and pulse rate. The joint is held in the position of its greatest capacity (the 'position of ease') and, if subcutaneous, it can be seen to be swollen (see Table below). Palpation reveals increased heat, tenderness and an effusion. Movements are prevented absolutely by muscular spasm, and attempts at either active or passive movement cause severe pain.

Treatment.—*1. Immobilisation.*—The joint must be immobilised until the infection has been cured. As any case of suppurative arthritis may be followed by ankylosis, it is the duty of the surgeon to anticipate this possibility by immobilising the joint in the best position for ankylosis (*i.e.* the position of optimum function), as indicated in the table below. The limb is supported and fixed by a suitable splint or appliance in the correct position, an anaesthetic being administered if necessary. Traction is used in cases of septic arthritis of the hip to prevent dislocation.

2. Antibiotics are administered systemically as in acute osteomyelitis.

3. Aspiration is useful for both diagnostic and therapeutic reasons. The nature of the fluid can be ascertained, and the organism cultured to obtain its antibiotic sensitivity.

Joint	Position of ease	Site of maximum swelling	Position for ankylosis
Shoulder	Adducted	Under the deltoid along the tendon of the biceps and in the axilla.	40° to 50° of abduction, with elbow joint just anterior to the coronal plane and hand in front of the mouth.
Elbow	Flexed at a right angle and pronated	On either side of the triceps tendon	Flexed at a right angle semi-pronated. If both sides, one elbow at 75° of extension, the other at 135°. These positions enable the patient to reach the external orifices.
Wrist	Slight flexion	Under extensor and flexor tendons	Slightly dorsi-flexed to allow a firm grasp.
Hip	Flexed, adducted, and externally rotated	Upper part of Scarpa's triangle	20° to 30° of flexion to allow sitting, and in neutral position as regards abduction and rotation.
Knee	Flexed	Suprapatellar bursa, and either side of patellar tendon	5° to 10° of flexion to allow foot to clear ground in walking.
Ankle	Slightly plantar-flexed (and inverted at the subtalar joint)	Anteriorly and on either side of the Achilles tendon	At a right angle.

Aspiration reduces the tension within the joint, thereby relieving pain, and limiting the stretching of ligaments and capsule. It has the disadvantage that a previously uninfected 'sympathetic' effusion may be infected if the needle traverses a septic focus on its way into the joint. On balance, the advantages outweigh this disadvantage. If frank pus is aspirated, the joint is opened (see below).

4. Aspiration and Injection.—After fluid has been aspirated, antibiotics may be injected into the joint. Repeated injections of antibiotic into a joint are unnecessary, since systemic administration is adequate.

5. Arthrotomy and Drainage is only done if the joint is found on aspiration to contain frank pus, or if bone destruction has involved the articular surfaces so that some degree of ankylosis is all that can be expected when healing has occurred. The joint is opened, washed out, and closed suction drains are placed down to the synovial cavity. This technique is nowadays less often needed, because the disease, if diagnosed early, can be treated by antibiotics and aspiration.

Extra-articular abscesses sometimes require to be opened and drained. In the case of the knee joint, pus is particularly liable to track upwards beneath the quadriceps, where its presence may be overlooked.

6. Excision.—Nowadays this too is rarely required, but if the condition of the patient deteriorates in spite of treatment, or if suppuration is prolonged, drastic surgical ablation of the diseased bone is necessary.

Complications.—*Early complications* include destruction of articular cartilage, pathological dislocation, and necrosis of the epiphysis resulting from damage to the blood supply (especially in the case of the proximal femoral epiphysis). *Late complications* include secondary degenerative osteoarthritis, joint stiffness and fibrous or, particularly, bony ankylosis.

TUBERCULOUS ARTHRITIS AND OSTEOMYELITIS

Pathology.—Bone and joint tuberculosis is haematogenous in origin. The primary focus is related either to the gastro-intestinal tract if the disease has been acquired by the ingestion of bovine tubercle, or to the lungs if the disease has been by the inhalation of the human strain. With the eradication of bovine tuberculosis in diary herds and of human pulmonary tuberculosis, bone and joint tuberculosis has become rarer in the United Kingdom except in certain cities, e.g. Leicester, with a large immigrant population. However, in countries where bone and joint tuberculosis is still common it is usually due to the human strain of the organism since little milk is drunk.

The disease starts either in the *synovial membrane* or in *intra-articular bone*. The disease may develop in any synovial joint (especially those with extensive synovial membranes such as the hip and knee), in tendon synovial sheaths (especially those of the finger flexors), or in bursae (such as that over-lying the greater trochanter). The spine is also commonly involved and tuberculosis here carries the eponymous description of 'Pott's Disease'. The vertebral bodies—almost always those of two neighbouring vertebrae—are involved first.

Typical tubercles develop in the synovial membrane which becomes bulky and inflamed, and an infected effusion collects in the synovial cavity. If the infection can be diagnosed and cured at this stage, full function may be restored to the joint. If, on the other hand, the pathological process progresses, articular cartilage is destroyed and the

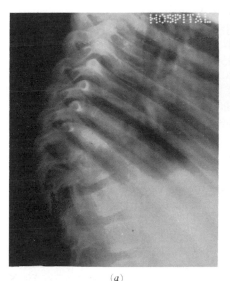
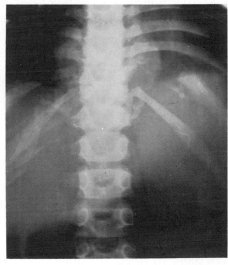

(*a*)   (*b*)

FIG. 306.—Tuberculosis of the 11th and 12th dorsal vertebrae. (*a*) Collapse of two vertebral bodies into a wedge. (*b*) Perispinal abscess shadow.

Percival Pott, 1714–1788. Surgeon, St. Bartholomew's Hospital, London.

adjacent bone is involved. At this stage some loss of function is certain since healing leaves a fibrous ankylosis, not two healthy surfaces of articular cartilage separated by the synovial cavity. If the disease starts in intra-articular bone, the synovial membrane rapidly becomes involved. For practical purposes involvement of both the synovial membrane and of the bone must be assumed when a diagnosis is made of tuberculous arthritis.

In the spine, the diagnosis is rarely made until the bodies of two neighbouring vertebrae are significantly involved so that the end result, at best, is the replacement of an intervertebral disc and of the diseased bone by fibrous tissue. Should treatment for spinal disease be delayed, abscess formation occurs and the vertebral bodies collapse (fig. 306). The pus tracks along tissue planes to present superficially in places often distant from the involved vertebrae; for example, pus arising from D12/L1 may track along the psoas muscle to present in the groin. Vertebral collapse produces forward angulation of the spine (a 'Kyphus': fig. 307) and the combination of pus formation and spinal angulation compresses and may damage the spinal cord. The cord may also be prejudiced by interference with its blood supply from the anterior spinal arteries. As a consequence paraplegia (Pott's paraplegia) may develop.

Tuberculosis of the shaft of a long bone occurs in miliary tuberculosis, but is rare.

Clinical Features

Symptoms.—These may arise from the diseased joint, from the primary focus, and from the systemic effects of the disease.

Locally the patient complains of an ache in the joint, at first mild in nature, which is worse on exertion or at night. If the joint is subcutaneous, it may be noticed to be swollen, a feature made more obvious by the wasting of the associated muscles. As the disease progresses the joint becomes increasingly stiff, partly because movement is painful and partly because movement is limited by adhesion formation, muscle spasm and bone destruction. As the bone is destroyed, the joint may dislocate until local deformity is obvious. In the spine swelling is not visible until a considerable quantity of tuberculous pus has collected and stiffness may be too slight to be noticed by the patient: thus a mild ache may be the only symptom of a potentially crippling disease. A kyphus appears late in the disease.

Systemically the patient feels unwell in himself, listless and febrile—the latter especially at night when he may have 'night sweats'.

Physical Signs.—If the joint is superficial, the synovial thickening and effusion may be visible. The muscles acting on the joint are markedly wasted. The joint is held in its position of ease (Table, p. 350).

On palpation, the synovial thickening and effusion can again be made out and the joint will be found to be moderately tender. The skin overlying the joint, even if abscess formation has occurred, is not red and is only slightly warm: a feature which is characteristic of tuberculous inflammation and abscess formation, so that such abscesses are known as 'cold abscesses'. Active and passive movement of the joint will be limited and painful.

In the spine the only physical signs of the disease in its early stages are tenderness on percussion of the spinous processes of the involved vertebrae and minimal limitation of movement. Later, a kyphus may be seen (fig. 307 (b)) and abscesses may be visible in the groin or posteriorly in the triangle of Petit. A kyphus in the lumbar spine may be masked by the normal lumbar lordosis.

Special Investigations.—*Haematology and Immunology.*—The ESR and white cell count are raised, the latter with a lymphocytosis. The Mantoux test is positive—sometimes violently so. The haemoglobin concentration should be measured since anaemia is common and requires correction.

Jean Louis Petit, 1674–1750. French Surgeon.
Charles Petit Mantoux, 1877–1947. Physician. Le Cannet, France.

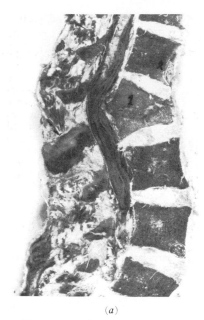 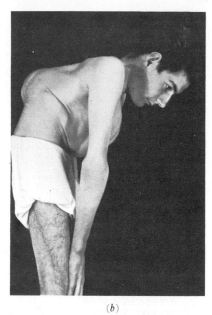

(a)   (b)

FIG. 307.—(a) Tuberculosis of the spine. L1 and L2 (1) have collapsed to produce wedging (and hence kyphus). A further tuberculosis lesion is present in D12 (2). (b) The clinical appearance of kyphosis due to tuberculosis of the spine.
(From London Hospital Museum.)

Radiology.—The early radiological signs are not dramatic: the bone adjacent to the joint is a little less dense than normal and it may be possible to make out a soft tissue swelling. As the disease advances, the joint space or disc space narrows and bone destruction becomes visible as an area of osteolysis. Thus in the spine a characteristic appearance now develops: the disc space narrows, and lytic lesions, typically anterior, appear in the bone of the adjacent vertebral bodies. Further bony destruction is accompanied by abscess formation so that diseased bone is seen to lie in and around a soft tissue shadow containing loose fragments of bone and calcified soft tissue (figs. 306 (b) and 308). At this stage deformity can be radiologically obvious (fig. 306 (a)).

A chest x-ray should always be taken and may reveal active tuberculosis.

Histology.—Early accurate diagnosis is imperative, since tuberculous arthritis can be cured (to leave the patient with no loss of function) provided it is adequately treated before bone and cartilage are destroyed. Since early in the disease the clinical, haematological, immune and radiological features are not diagnostic, histological examination of biopsy material (revealing acid-fast bacilli and typical tubercles) is essential.

1. *Removal of Lymph Nodes.*—An involved node draining the diseased joint may be removed. The disadvantage of this method is that a negative result does not exclude the presence of the disease.

2. *Arthrotomy and Biopsy of the Synovial Membrane.*—This method allows the appearance of the joint to be noted and provides certain histological diagnosis. The disadvantage is the risk of sinus formation through the operative wound. Provided the operation is carried out under antibiotic cover (see below) this risk is negligible. This is therefore the method of choice.

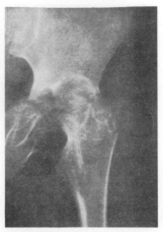

FIG. 308.—X-ray appearances in active tuberculosis of the hip joint in a child.

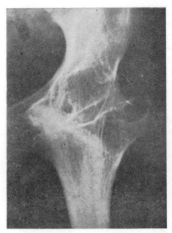

FIG. 309.—Brittain's ischio-femoral, extra-articular arthrodesis of the hip (see text).

3. *Needle biopsy* of radiologically involved tissue. This is the method of choice in the spine because direct surgical access may be difficult.

Bacteriology.—Joint aspirate, biopsy material, sputum and urine should be cultured for tubercle bacilli and inoculated into the guinea-pig. A positive culture may take some weeks to obtain. A diagnosis should have been made by this time on the basis of the histology, and treatment started. Bacteriology is therefore confirmatory only.

Differential Diagnosis.—Tuberculous arthritis may be confused with rheumatoid arthritis in a single joint, infective arthritis, and haemarthroses occurring in haemophilia. In the spine the differential diagnosis is from osteomyelitis due to other organisms (especially staphylococcus, typhoid bacillus), ankylosing spondylitis, back pain due to disc prolapse and degeneration, and neoplasm.

Treatment.—1. Antibiotics.—Immediately the diagnosis is made, the guidelines advocated on page 36 should be followed for at least 12 months (isoniazid plus rifampicin and/or ethambutol/streptomycin). If the diagnosis depends upon synovial biopsy, antibiotics are started immediately post-operatively, without awaiting the histological result.

2. Immobilisation.—The diseased joint is immobilised in the position of function (see Table, p. 350) until local symptoms have settled. In the case of the spine, immobilisation requires the use of a collar for the cervical spine lesion, or bed rest until local symptoms have subsided. In countries where hospitalisation may be difficult, tuberculosis of the lumbar spine has recently been treated by antibiotics alone, the patient remaining ambulant throughout the period of treatment.

3. General Management.—The general health of the patient should of course be improved as far as possible by providing an adequate normal diet and by giving an iron supplement or even blood transfusion if there is significant anaemia. Should there be coincidental pulmonary tuberculosis with tubercle bacilli in the sputum, it will of course be necessary to isolate the patient until this aspect of the disease is brought under control. Sanatoria, sunshine and special diets are not necessary.

H. A. Brittain, 1904–1954. Orthopaedic Surgeon, Norfolk and Norwich Hospital, England.

4. Surgery.—Surgery is not required at the synovial stage of the disease since the disease can then be arrested by antibiotics alone. If, however, the synovial membrane is very markedly inflamed and thickened, synovectomy and joint toilet may be helpful.

If abscess formation has occurred, the abscess is incised and evacuated 3 or 4 weeks after the commencement of antibiotic treatment. When the abscess has been evacuated, the originally articulating bones terminate in the abscess cavity. The joint will never regain its normal function: it is stiff, movement is painful, and weight bearing in the spine and legs is particularly painful or impossible. Some form of arthrodesis is required in order to provide the patient with a painless stable, although stiff, joint. Before antibiotics became available, arthrodesis of a tuberculous joint was carried out avoiding, if possible, the infected tissue (fig. 309). Such operations ('extra-articular arthrodeses') were technically difficult. Since the advent of antibiotics, the bone ends can be brought into apposition across the evacuated abscess cavity and sound bony fusion can commonly be obtained in this way.

In the spine, exactly the same surgical principles apply. The disease, however, is rarely diagnosed before bone involvement has taken place so that some form of arthrodesis is nearly always required. If no significant pus formation has occurred when antibiotics are given, it is usually possible to sterilise the lesion in the vertebral bodies with little or no vertebral collapse. The lesion itself can then be ignored surgically and the spine stabilised by a posterior fusion. Should pus formation have occurred, the abscess requires evacuation through an antero-lateral approach. At the same time as the abscess is evacuated bone grafts are packed between the involved vertebral bodies so that healing results in an anterior body-to-body fusion.

Occasionally the disease leaves a joint which is replaced by short firm fibrous tissue (a 'sound fibrous ankylosis'). Tissue of this kind may be sufficiently stable to allow the joint to function as if it were arthrodesed, especially in the non-weightbearing upper limb, so that no surgical arthrodesis may be necessary.

Prognosis.—The prognosis for this disease is now excellent. Death either from the tuberculous process itself or from secondary amyloidosis is now rare. Disability of any kind can often be prevented by early, adequate antibiotic treatment combined with appropriate immobilisation. At the worst the patient may spend 3 to 6 months in hospital and although finally cured of the tuberculous process, have a permanently stiffened joint.

Tuberculous Tenosynovitis.—This may take two forms:

(*a*) The endothelial lining of the sheath is replaced by oedematous granulation tissue containing miliary tubercles. Very little free fluid is present. A soft elastic swelling appears and if the disease progresses, pus may form and track into neighbouring sheaths or joints.

(*b*) An effusion occurs in the tendon sheaths and 'melon-seed' bodies are usually present in large numbers, so that a soft, coarse crepitus is detected on pressing fluid from one part of the sheath to another. Melon-seed bodies resemble grains of boiled sago. They are composed of collections of fibrin, cellular debris and occasional tubercle bacilli (fig. 310). The term 'compound palmar ganglion' is applied to this condition when it occurs in

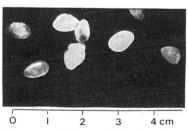

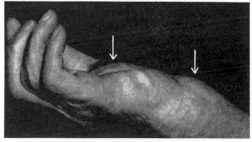

FIG. 310.—'Melon-seed' bodies from tuberculosis synovitis at the wrist.

FIG. 311.—A compound palmar ganglion (tuberculous flexor synovitis at the wrist). The swelling in the palm communicates with the swelling above the wrist.

connection with the flexor tendons of the fingers. A soft, painless swelling appears (fig. 311), and fluctuation may be transmitted above and below the anterior carpal ligament. As with all forms of tuberculous disease of bone, joint or tendon, obvious wasting of adjacent muscles is present. Treatment consists of general measures, the use of antibiotics and the application of an appropriate plaster cast to immobilise the involved tendon sheath. If the condition progresses, careful dissection and removal of the tendon sheath is indicated.

CHAPTER 19

THE RHEUMATIC DISEASES

OSTEOARTHROSIS (OSTEOARTHRITIS)(OA)[1]

Aetiology.—Normal synovial joints may be regarded as being in a state of equilibrium between the mechanical properties of the articular cartilage and the mechanical stresses imposed upon this tissue. If the loads applied to the joint rise or the same loads are applied through unusually small areas (i.e. the joint becomes abnormally incongruous), this equilibrium will be disturbed because the applied stresses rise. The equilibrium will also be disturbed if disease damages the cartilage so as to prejudice its mechanical properties. OA can perhaps be viewed as the outcome of any such dis-equilibrium and, as such, as the final common path travelled by any joint whose mechanics have been disturbed. Thus, OA is perhaps best thought of, not as a specific disease entity, but rather as a constellation of clinical and anatomical features, analogous to heart failure: indeed it might with advantage be renamed 'joint failure'.

There is some evidence that OA is not initiated by abrasive wear caused by a breakdown in lubrication. Thus, if OA be loosely regarded as 'wear' in a joint, it is probably wear in the sense that linoleum 'wears' when walked over by stiletto heels, not wear in the sense in which it occurs in a poorly lubricated bearing.

Secondary OA.—Here, predisposing causes either damage cartilage or reduce the contact area in a joint. Thus, injuries to articular cartilage, especially if they interrupt the normal contour of the subchondral bone to produce 'high points' in the articular surface, render the joint liable to develop osteoarthrosic changes over the ensuing years. Diseases which make the joint surface irregular (such as Perthes' Disease or Slipped Femoral Epiphysis (Chapter 22) predispose to OA by reducing the contact area in the joint and hence raising the contact pressure on the cartilage so as to damage the tissue mechanically.

Articular cartilage may also be damaged enzymatically in septic arthritis, tuberculous arthritis, or rheumatoid arthritis (RA), and all these conditions may cause Secondary OA. (In RA the late disability is not always strictly attributable to the rheumatoid process but rather to secondary osteoarthrosic changes superimposed upon a burnt-out rheumatoid joint.) Recurrent haemarthroses (as in haemophilia), and chemical infiltration of cartilage with pigment (*e.g.* ochronosis), or calcium pyrophosphate (chondrocalcinosis), also damage articular cartilage and may result in OA.

---

[1] The Rome Conference of the International League Against Rheumatism in 1961 proposed that this condition should be named alternatively *osteoarthritis* or *osteoarthrosis*. These alternatives were accepted by the American Rheumatology Association in 1963. The term *osteoarthrosis* is now in almost universal use amongst British rheumatologists and is to be preferred to *osteoarthritis* since the latter implied, misleadingly, that the condition is an inflammatory disease of joints.

Most cases of OA at the hip in Caucasians are idiopathic and are sometimes (misleadingly) called 'Primary'. Although the aetiology is unknown, there is mounting evidence that (1) a number of anatomical variants, not easily detectable in life, may exist at the hip and produce high local contact pressures on the cartilage and (2) that the repeated application of these pressures may cause fatigue failure in the collagen network in cartilage thus initiating the destruction of the tissue. In Caucasians radiological evidence of the disease is most frequent at the knees but disability severe enough to require surgery is most common at the hip.

Pathology.—The first visible abnormality in primary OA affects articular cartilage, the surface of which becomes roughened (a change known as 'fibrillation'). This surface roughening signifies fragmentation of the collagen network in the tissue and is accompanied by a loss of matrix proteoglycan and by softening. Fibrillation extends progressively deeper into the tissue until bone is exposed, a condition described pathologically as ulceration.

Fragments of cartilage become detached from the subchondral bone as ulceration occurs. They may form loose bodies in the joint, but most eventually become attached to the synovial membrane. Here they set up a low-grade inflammatory response which spreads to involve the capsule. The resulting gradual fibrosis of the synovial membrane and capsule shortens the capsule and thus limits joint movement. Endochondral new bone formation occurs around the periphery of the joint surface (where the articular cartilage is usually preserved because it is not exposed to significant load carriage) and leads to typical excrescences around the joint known as 'osteophytes'. In the bone adjacent to the joint there is an increase in vascularity very early in the disease, indeed it is suggested by some authorities that the alteration in bone haemodynamics represents the initial change in the disease process. Later, as the cartilage becomes destroyed, the subchondral bone and trabeculae become thickened, a change known as 'sclerosis', and areas of soft tissue ('cysts'), often liquefied in the centre, form in the cancellous bone adjacent to the joint. The bone separating such cysts from the synovial cavity may collapse into the cyst leading to progressive deformation of the bony articular surfaces and the separation of loose fragments of bone.

Clinical Features

Symptoms. The initial complaint is always of pain felt on exercise and/or at night. The pain on exercise gets gradually more severe as the joint is used, a

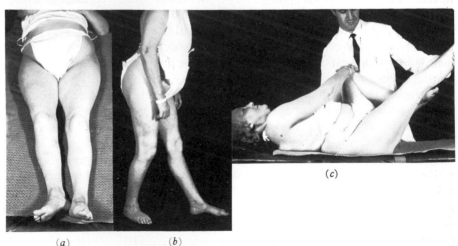

(a)　　　　　　(b)

FIG. 312.—OA right hip. (a) Note external rotation, adduction and shortening. (b) Fixed flexion causing lumbar lordosis and protruding buttocks when the patient tries to stand erect. (c) Thomas's test to reveal fixed flexion (here 45°) at the right hip. The patient flexes her left hip fully and in so doing straightens her lumbar spine until it touches the couch. The right leg rises from the couch to reveal fixed flexion at the hip. The surgeon places his right hand under the spine to ensure that the lumbar lordosis is fully flattened and with his left hand supports the right leg to prevent pain but does not attempt to flex the hip.

Hugh Owen Thomas, 1834–1891. Surgeon, Liverpool, England. See footnote Chapter 17.

symptom particularly noticeable in the weight-bearing joints such as the hip and knee. Pain is also felt when the joint is first moved after a period of immobility. Pain at night may be so troublesome as to be a predominant symptom: it is not uncommon for a patient with OA of the hip to be woken several times every night by pain. As the pain increases, the joint gradually loses movement because of muscle spasm, reluctance to move the joint, fibrosis of the capsule, and the bony changes described above. In the joints of the lower limb pain and stiffness combine to produce a limp. As the disease progresses the stiffness becomes increasingly severe until all movement at the joint is lost. By this time the joint usually lies in the position of 'ease' (Table, Chapter 18) which may well be a position which is functionally useless, for example the hip typically becomes fixed in flexion, adduction and external rotation (fig. 312). This development of complete stiffness in a functionally inappropriate position constitutes deformity. Thus the patient, especially if more than one joint is involved, may be completely crippled and either bed-ridden or forced to use a wheelchair.

Physical Signs.—On inspection the abnormal position of the joint may be evident and a swelling attributable to a small synovial effusion may be visible in subcutaneous joints such as the knee. On palpation the joint may be mildly tender and fluctuation produced by an effusion may be detectable. When the patient is asked to move his joint, the loss of movement in certain directions will be evident and in the subcutaneous joints a sensation of grating can be appreciated if the hand is placed over the joint as it moves. This sensation is known as 'crepitus'. At the hip the tendency for the joint to become stiff in adduction and flexion leads to apparent shortening of the leg (fig. 312). True shortening may also occur as the femoral head and acetabular roof collapse.

Radiological Appearances.—These are characteristic (fig. 313). In the first instance they consist merely of narrowing the joint space: a space which is of course occupied by radiolucent articular cartilage. As this cartilage thins and ulcerates the radiologically apparent joint space diminishes. Shortly thereafter bone changes become evident: sclerosis in the subchondral bone is the first abnormal feature to appear followed by cyst and osteophyte formation. Finally the bone collapses. The very marked new bone formation (manifest as sclerosis and the presence of osteophytes) distinguishes this disease radiologically from rheumatoid arthritis, in which the predominant radiological feature is one of bone loss.

Treatment.—There is no specific pharmacological treatment for OA. In the early stages the patient can be helped by advice as to how to keep his joints mobile whilst loading them as little as possible, and by simple analgesics. Physiotherapy helps to build up in strength the muscles acting across the involved joint and to regain a full range of active movement. Weight loss is desirable, and the use of a walking stick and of a raise to the heel of the shoe (if the leg is short) also assists those with OA of the joints of the leg. Operative treatment has to be considered if these measures fail (p. 362).

Chondromalacia Patellae.—A condition which has been thought to be analogous to primary OA affects the patello-femoral joint of young adults (especially women). In this disease the articular cartilage covering the patella and subsequently that covering the patellar articular surface of the femur becomes softened, fibrillated and finally ulcerated.

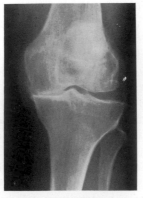

FIG. 313.—OA of the knee affecting the medial compartment to cause a varus deformity (genu varum). This is a weight-bearing x-ray: films taken with the patient supine may grossly underestimate the deformity. (See also figs. 316, 317, 318).

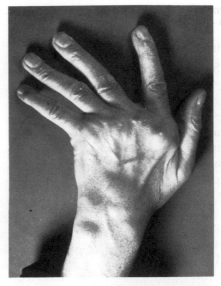

FIG. 314.—The hand in rheumatoid arthritis.

Although this sequence of events is identical with that seen in primary OA elsewhere, in this joint it occurs in early life as a normal event so that its pathological significance is hard to ascertain. The condition has been treated by various surgical procedures aimed directly at the cartilage (drilling and shaving). It is doubtful if these procedures are beneficial, although the regeneration of fibrocartilage following drilling of the patella in advanced OA of the knee has been described. Recently the view has gained ground that the condition is due to an increase in the contact pressure between the patella and the lateral femoral condyle caused by a tendency for the patella to be drawn laterally in involved knees. Treatment based on this view takes the form of division of the lateral patellar retinaculum and occasionally of transposition of the tibial tubercle. Useful pain relief has been reported after these operations. As a last resort the patella may be excised.

RHEUMATOID ARTHRITIS (RA)

Aetiology.—The aetiology of RA is unknown, but a number of theories have been advanced of which probably the most widely credited today rests upon the belief that the disease is immune in nature. Certainly, the disease is systemic in that its manifestations are not only applied to the joints.

Pathology.—In the joints, the tissue first affected in rheumatoid arthritis is the synovial membrane, which becomes inflamed and bulky. A striking histological feature in the synovial membrane is the presence of numerous lymphocytes and plasma cells which can be shown to be actively synthesizing antibodies. In addition an effusion accumulates so that the volume of material (synovial fluid and membrane) within the capsule of the joint becomes very considerably increased. As the synovial tissue enlarges, it gradually encroaches upon the articular cartilage where it is known as *pannus*[1]. Beneath the synovial pannus, the articular cartilage is destroyed and never subsequently regenerates. Intra-articular structures, such as the cruciate ligaments in the knee, may also be destroyed. The bone adjacent to the joint is eroded by the intrusion of exuberant synovial membrane. It also becomes osteoporotic, partly as a consequence of the hyperaemia associated with the disease, but sometimes partly as a consequence of its treatment with steroids. The

---

[1] Pannus (Latin) = cloth or apron.

combination of a loss of cartilage and osteoporosis may lead to rapidly progressive, severe bone collapse and hence to instability and deformity of the involved joint.

Clinical Features

Symptoms.—The disease may commence in childhood, when it is known as Juvenile Chronic Polyarthritis or Still's disease, or at any time in adult life. RA developing in the elderly seems to run a more benign course than the disease developing in the young adult. Women are more commonly affected than men. The disease is typically poly-articular and often starts in the small joints of the hands or feet. Thereafter all the synovial joints of the body may become involved simultaneously or consecutively. Each joint as it is involved is painful, stiff and swollen. The activity of the disease tends to wax and wane both in the patient as a whole and locally in the involved joint, so that a joint may be painful, stiff and swollen for a period of 2 to 3 months and then gradually settle to be followed after an interval by a similar episode in another joint. The patient often feels unwell in himself and is mildly febrile.

Physical Signs.—The involved joints, especially those of the hand, show marked synovial thickening and as the disease advances typical deformities develop (fig. 314). On palpation the synovial thickening, together with the presence of a synovial effusion, may be obvious. The joint can often be felt to be mechanically unstable and movement is painful and limited. As the disease progresses, limitation of movement, muscle wasting and deformity gradually develop at involved joints so as to cripple the patient.

Radiological Features.—The joint space is initially narrowed as in OA (fig. 315 (a)) but the intrusion of affected synovium into the bone produces typical lytic lesions in the latter. In contrast to OA, osteophytes are small or absent and the bone adjacent to the joint becomes increasingly porotic so that it collapses under the compressive loads to which it is subject (fig. 315 (b)). As the

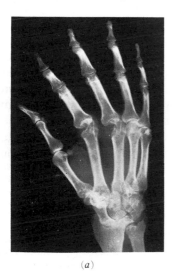 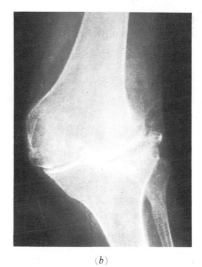

(a)   (b)

FIG. 315.—(a) The hand in rheumatoid arthritis: note loss of joint space, erosion of the metacarpal heads and disorganisation of the wrist. (b) The knee in rheumatoid arthritis. Gross collapse of the lateral tibial and femoral condyles.

Sir George Frederic Still, 1868–1941. Professor of Diseases of Children, King's College Hospital, London.

disease advances, a combination of bone destruction and capsular stretching allows the joint to subluxate and finally to dislocate.

The active rheumatoid process may remit in a particular joint, leaving its articular cartilage destroyed. Thereafter the joint may progressively develop osteoarthrosic changes so that the final x-ray appearances are to some extent those of OA.

The sequence of events by which the pathological process in RA causes the clinical features is discussed in relation to surgical treatment below and on p. 367.

Special Investigation.—The ESR is raised and an abnormal immune globulin known as the *rheumatoid factor* may be demonstrated in the blood by use of the Latex or Rose Waaler tests. The demonstration of rheumatoid factor is not, however, diagnostic of RA since it is found in healthy individuals and in those suffering from various chronic infections; neither is rheumatoid factor always present in RA. These abnormal haematological findings are in sharp contrast to OA in which the blood picture is entirely normal and in which there is no systemic disturbance of any kind.

Treatment.—The conservative treatment of RA consists of exercises and splintage to maintain joint function and to prevent deformity, combined with drug therapy. The reader is referred to specialised texts regarding the use of pharmacological substances (first-line analgesics, anti-inflammatory analgesics, local corticosteroid injections, and second-line drugs, *e.g.* corticosteroids, gold *etc.*). Surgery may be used to remove involved synovial tissue, to relieve the disability of a destroyed joint, or to treat isolated soft tissue lesions such as compression of the median nerve in the carpal tunnel (Chapter 24).

The Rationale of Surgery in Relation to Pain, Stiffness and Deformity

Operative surgical treatment of OA and RA is never curative: rarely, the pathological process may be arrested or even reversed, more commonly its existence and progression have to be accepted and surgery offered to provide palliation of the patient's disability—pain, stiffness and deformity. The exact causation of this disability is sometimes obscure, but an attempt must be made to explain it if the rationale of operative surgery is to be understood.

Pain in OA and RA appears to arise in three tissues: *the bones of the joint, its capsule and the muscles acting on it.* Cartilage is not innervated and accordingly is insensitive to pain. Synovial membrane is poorly innervated and experiments with human volunteers have shown that it is almost insensitive to pain arising from mechanical stimulation. No doubt active inflammation of the synovial membrane, as of the capsule, is painful, but active inflammation of these tissues in the rheumatic diseases is not treated surgically.

Bones.—Nerve fibres which might be pain afferents have been described in bone, but the effective stimulus for the provocation of pain in bone is unknown. Experimentally, pain may be induced when the intra-osseous venous pressure is raised and venous engorgement of juxta-articular bone has been demonstrated in OA. (Traction on the periosteum is painful but this is not relevant to pain induction in intra-articular bone where the true periosteum is replaced by cartilage or synovium.) Whatever may be the precise nature of the effective stimulus for bone pain, it may be regularly observed in clinical practice that if the arthritic bony surfaces are replaced with appropriate prostheses securely fixed to the skeleton, the patient's arthritic pain both at rest and on weight-bearing is abolished

Harry M. Rose, Contemporary. Professor of Medical and Surgical Research Chemistry, Department of Microbiology, Columbia-Presbyterian Medical Centre, New York.
Erik Waaler, Pathologist, Ullevaal Hospital, Oslo, Norway.

at once. This observation proves that the major component of the pain of arthritis originates in bone and it may be speculated that this is due to the generation of abnormally
high stresses in the bone, possibly leading to trabecular micro-fractures and hence to
vascular engorgement.

Capsules and ligaments of all joints are well innervated both with mechanoreceptor
afferents subserving perceptual and reflex proprioception and with pain afferents. The
effective mechanical stimulus for the provocation of capsular pain appears to be excessive
tension in the capsule. In the context of the rheumatic diseases excessive capsular tension
may be brought about by two pathological events: firstly, an increase in the volume of
material within the capsule, that is to say by an increase in the bulk of the synovial
membrane or by an accumulation of intra-articular fluid, and secondly, by capsular fibrosis
leading to shortening and tethering of the capsule. Joint movement and position affect
the severity of this pain in two ways. In all joints some position within the normal range
draws the capsule most tightly against the synovial contents and it is this position which
provokes pain when the bulk of the intracapsular tissues is increased. Secondly, the pain
arising from capsular fibrosis is provoked only or chiefly when the capsule has shortened
to such an extent that it limits movement: when this limited movement is attempted by
the patient with sufficient force to apply tension to the capsule pain is provoked. Thus
capsular pain interferes with movement and in an attempt to avoid it the patient tends to
hold the joint immobile in a position of capsular relaxation.

Muscular pain is probably provoked by local anoxia or by the accumulation of metabolic
end-products, arising from abnormally sustained muscular contractions. Such contractions—known clinically as muscle spasm—have not been convincingly demonstrated elec-
tromyographically but their existence may be inferred from the fact that the passive range
of movement in a diseased joint is often increased under a general anaesthetic producing
muscle relaxation. Muscle spasm of this type appears to be a reflex consequence of joint
disease and imposes immobility in the affected joint.

Joint stiffness is a loose term covering two disturbances of function—a sense
of added resistance encountered by the patient when he attempts to move the
affected joint, and a total inability to move the joint through some part of its
normal range. The first factor is perhaps in part due to a rise in intra-articular
friction caused by disruption of the normal cartilaginous bearing surface, but
seems mainly attributable to articular and extra-articular soft tissue thickening,
adhesion, and oedema, and probably to over-contraction ('spasm') of the antagonist muscles.

A reduction in the passive range of movement may be due to pain and muscle
spasm—in which case the range will return under anaesthesia—or to such mechanical factors as capsular and peri-capsular fibrosis, osteophyte formation and
collapse of the articulating bony surfaces.

Deformity in its early stages may be regarded simply as a loss of part of the
normal range of movement. For example, a patient who is unable fully to extend
his knee may be said to have a flexion deformity or contracture of that joint.
Deformity may progress to a point at which the two articulating bones start to
take up a position in relation to each other which does not occur anywhere in the
normal range of movement: in other words the joint becomes *subluxated* and
finally *dislocated*.

Dislocation implies a mechanical derangement of the tissues of the joint and
the presence of a deforming force. The factor chiefly responsible for dislocation
in the rheumatic diseases is the collapse of the bony articular surfaces. In the leg
the ligaments stretch little, if at all, but at the hand they are said to do so sufficiently to permit dislocation. The deforming forces at work consist of the body
weight and the play across the joint of muscles of normally unequal power (such
for example as the finger flexors and extensors), muscles in 'spasm', or muscles

suffering progressive fibrosis. In the leg, the position of a joint may be normal until weight-bearing is attempted. The deforming force of the body weight may then be sufficient to subluxate the diseased joint. Subluxation or dislocation of this kind affects particularly the knee and is referred to as *instability*.

SURGERY IN RELATION TO THE PATHOLOGY OF OSTEOARTHROSIS (OA)

Osteotomy. The bone adjacent to a joint is divided to allow the fragments to be displaced relative to each other in such a way as to bring residual cartilage into the area of the joint transmitting the major loads. For example: in OA of the tibio-femoral joint the cartilagenous and later, the bony defect initially affects one compartment (medial or lateral) only. Such defects produce an angular deformity in the weight-bearing knee concave towards the side of the defect. Thus for example a defect in the medial tibial condyle will produce a varus deformity. Any such deformity will displace the line of action of the resultant of the forces acting through the knee towards the concavity, that is to say towards the defect (fig. 316). Thus a vicious circle is established in which the defect results in a deformity which increases the loads acting on the defect to cause increasing deformity and pain. One way in which this vicious progress could be interrupted is to angulate the tibia, by osteotomy, so as to return the overall alignment of the leg to normal (or even a little towards over-correction), thus off-loading the defect and bringing the relatively healthy cartilage on the other side of the joint back into the line of action of the load (fig. 317).

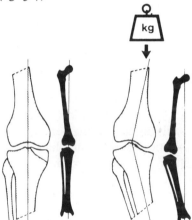

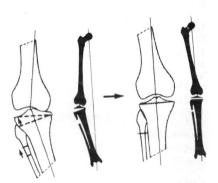

Fig. 316.—The normal non-weight-bearing knee is shown on the left. Note that the centre of the hip, knee and ankle lie in a straight line. If a bone defect (unshaded) were to be created in the medial tibial condyle, the femoral condyle would collapse into the defect on weight-bearing to produce varus malalignment as shown on the right.

Fig. 317.—On the left the varus malalignment shown in fig. 316 is present. The bone resected from the proximal tibia and from the shaft of the fibula by a closing wedge osteotomy, is marked with dotted lines. When this bone is removed and the osteotomy surfaces are approximated, the leg is restored to its normal alignment as shown on the right.

In early OA of the hip, cartilage is often lost from the superior surface of the head and preserved elsewhere. Intertrochanteric osteotomy followed by angulation of the shaft of the femur may now rotate the femoral head sufficiently to allow intact cartilage to become weight-bearing.

Osteotomy apart, nothing can be offered surgically which might, even theoretically, restore the tissues of the joint to their original, normal state. Thus if it is felt that a joint has become too destroyed for osteotomy to be useful, the joint must be stiffened (arthrodesed) or replaced.

Arthrodesis.—The bone ends are resected and then held in contact in the hope that they will fuse together. If they do, pain is relieved and deformity corrected, but at the

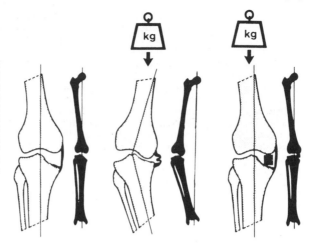

FIG. 318.—The left hand diagram shows a knee with a medial tibial defect but without a soft tissue contracture. When load is applied to this knee, the joint collapses into varus as shown in the middle diagram and in fig. 261. The knee may be restored to normal alignment by blocking open the defect with a prosthesis, shown diagramatically, on the right.

price of loss of movement. This price may be acceptable, as for example in the joints of the foot, or very undesirable as for example in the hip and knee. In the former joints, arthrodesis therefore offers the possibility of permanent pain relief at an acceptable price and for this reason it is frequently employed, for example, for osteoarthrosis of the subtalar joint or ankle. Unfortunately OA of these joints is relatively rare whereas it is very common in precisely those lower limb joints where movement is vital (the hip and knee). Thus arthrodesis has only a small part to play as a primary procedure in the surgery of OA.

Joint Replacement Surgery.—A major surgical problem therefore exists in OA of the hip and knee: the disease is common, cannot satisfactorily be treated by arthrodesis and frequently presents too late to be treated by osteotomy (which is anyway an unreliable procedure). No similar problem exists in the upper limb since here OA is rare and does not usually cause severe pain. It is therefore particularly for the hip and knee that an alternative is needed. This alternative is replacement surgery.

The rationale of joint replacement is simple: the defective bone and cartilage is removed and replaced by a prosthesis in much the same way as an area of caries is removed from a tooth and replaced by a filling. If the height of the defect is restored precisely, deformity and instability will be corrected (fig. 318) whilst movement is permitted and pain is relieved by covering the opposing, exposed bone surfaces with prostheses (of appropriate shapes and made of inert materials) attached to the skeleton in such a way that they do not move against the bone. The materials in use today are high density polyethylene for the concave component of the joint and one of the implantable metals for the convex surface, both bonded to the skeleton by a cold curing acrylic (polymethyl-methacrylate). The technicalities of these procedures are outside the scope of this text.

The immediate outcome of a successful replacement is easy to describe: pain is abolished and the joint is rendered mobile and stable. Technically however these procedures are not easy to perform and if a component becomes loose or infected, the pre-operative disability may return in full and may then be difficult or impossible to relieve. Since the chances of loosening or infection are related in part to the length of time the implant is required to function, joint replacement procedures should be used with great caution, if at all, in the young. For patients over 60 however they represent the treatment of choice for OA of the hip and knee that is causing severe disability.

Procedures for Joints affected by OA

The Hand.—The only joint in the hand commonly requiring surgical treatment for primary OA is the carpo-metacarpal joint of the thumb. Here the disease may be treated by *arthrodesis* of the diseased joint by *excision arthroplasty* of the trapezium, or by osteotomy of the base of the thumb metacarpal. At their best these operations give indistinguishable results with an excellent return of painless function. Heberden's nodes occasionally cause pain at the TIP joints.

The Wrist.—Secondary OA following injury is treated, if the pain is sufficiently severe, by arthrodesis.

William Herberden, 1710–1801. Physician, London, England.

The Radio-Ulnar Joints.—The distal radio-ulnar joint may be affected by secondary OA following fractures adjacent to the joint, such as Colles' fracture. The proximal radio-ulnar joint is similarly affected following fractures of the head of the radius. In both cases the treatment of choice is *excision arthroplasty;* in the distal joint by excision of 2·5 cm of the distal ulna, in the proximal joint by excision of the head of the radius.

The Elbow Joint.—Primary OA may affect all components of the joint. Should the joint be so painful as to require surgery, which is rare, the most commonly employed procedure is *arthrodesis* of the humero-ulnar joint in sufficient flexion to allow the patient to feed himself and wash, together with excision of the head of radius.

The Shoulder.—The shoulder is rarely affected by OA, primary or secondary, but if so, it may be treated by *arthrodesis*. Although fusion is not easy to secure, it is easier than in RA because the bone is hypertrophic rather than porotic. The functional results of a sound arthrodesis in the position of function (*i.e.* approximately the position taken up by the shoulder when the hand is brought to the mouth) are good.

The Toes.—OA and other degenerative changes affecting the toes are considered in Chapter 12 and page 369.

The Foot and Ankle.—OA, primary or secondary, occasionally affects any of the tarsal (especially the subtalar) joints or the ankle. If surgical treatment is necessary, arthrodesis is the only procedure available at joints other than the ankle. The latter however can now be replaced.

The Knee.—The knee, after the hip, is the joint most commonly affected by OA.

Arthrodesis should not now be carried out as a primary procedure. It is used as a last resort if one of the modern forms of total joint replacements fail and cannot be revised. Several methods of arthrodesis have been described but the Charnley arthrodesis is perhaps the most reliable and widely used.

Excision arthroplasty of the patella has a part to play in OA confined to the patello-femoral joints, *e.g.* after fractures of the patella.

Total replacement arthroplasty is now giving very encouraging results. At the time of writing its place in OA cannot be defined but it is being used on a steadily increasing scale and may well displace all other surgical procedures in patients over 60 years of age in the next 5 years. A variety of prostheses is available (p. 369).

Osteotomy is indicated in patients under the age of 60 with early osteoarthrosis causing disabling pain with neither significant loss of flexion nor fixed flexion deformity. The disease at this stage is unicompartmental, causing a varus deformity if it affects the medial side of the joint (fig. 313) and a valgus deformity if it affects the lateral side. If the defect in the articular surface affects the tibia, the bone is divided above the tubercle and angulated so as to correct the deformity. Defects in the femoral condyle are treated by supracondylar femoral osteotomy. By realigning the knee in this way the force acting on the diseased compartment is reduced and this in turn eases pain and retards the progression of the disease.

The Hip

Total replacement arthroplasty using a prosthesis replacing the acetabulum as well as the head of the femur was introduced by McKee and Charnley (both in England) in the late 1950s. The device now most widely used in the UK is the Charnley prosthesis in which the acetabulum is constructed of high density polyethylene, and the head of the femur of stainless steel. Both components are attached to the bone with a cold-curing acrylic 'cement'. Post-operatively, the convalescence is short, weight-bearing may be allowed within days of operation, and the prolonged, tedious and sometimes painful physiotherapy which some other procedures require is unnecessary. This operation is now the treatment of choice for most cases of OA of the hip: at the present time, because of uncertainty surrounding the long-term results, the operation is avoided if possible in patients under 60 years of age unless the prognosis for life is shortened by intercurrent disease.

Osteotomy is employed—at the intertrochanteric level using internal fixation of the osteotomy site (fig. 320)—when pain, especially night pain, demands surgical relief but the range of movement is still good: the presence of 70° of active flexion being taken as a rough dividing line between a hip suitable for osteotomy and one suitable for arthroplasty. Since total replacement arthroplasty is avoided in patients under 60 years of age, osteotomy is employed particularly in this age group: over the age of 60 it has been generally replaced by total replacement arthroplasty. In some centres the operation has been abandoned in favour of replacement in younger age groups as well.

Abraham Colles, 1773–1843. (See Footnote, p. 291.)
George Kenneth McKee, Contemporary, Norwich, England.
Sir John Charnley, 1911–1982. Professor of Orthopaedic Surgery, University of Manchester, England.

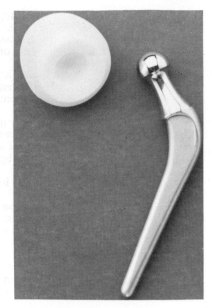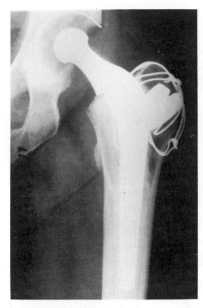

FIG. 319.—Total replacement of the hip using the Charnley prosthesis.

Osteotomy brings significant relief of pain, especially of night pain, to about 60% of patients who have the operation. Stiffness is often not relieved, however, so that in terms of the return of function osteotomy is by no means an entirely satisfactory procedure.

SURGERY IN RELATION TO THE PATHOLOGY OF RHEUMATOID ARTHRITIS (RA)

It might be thought that the likelihood of surgical procedures being useful in RA would be slight: the disease is after all said to be due to a chronic, progressive synovitis which unless arrested would be expected to destroy a joint however it might be reconstructed surgically.

Synovectomy. Based on the view of the pathology, synovectomy was widely used in joints with an accessibly synovium such as the knee and the joints of the hand. The results were disappointing: synovitis recurred in the regenerated synovium and the long-term fate of the joint was not influenced for the better. Nevertheless the procedure may still have a part to play in the hand with severe synovitis, resistant to rest and medication, involving the tendon sheaths and joints.

Osteotomy has little or no place in RA. The destruction of articular cartilage in RA affects the whole of the joint surface, so little benefit can be expected (nor is it obtained) by attempts to alter the areas of the articular surface subjected to load.

Arthrodesis should be avoided if at all possible in RA since to stiffen a joint imposes additional stresses on its neighbours, and in this disease these joints are likely to be abnormal (limited exceptions are mentioned below).

Joint Replacement.—Thus the surgery of RA is a matter of joint replacement with limited exceptions in the small joints of the feet, the hand, wrist and spine where synovectomy (perhaps in the hand) arthrodesis and excision arthroplasty have a part to play.

It might be thought that, however attractive in theory, it would be impracticable to treat established RA surgically since in principle every joint in the body is involved. Closer inspection makes the situation seem more hopeful. The disability in the upper limb although significant, is frequently tolerable since pain is not usually severe whilst the presence of other mobile joints and the astonishing versatility of the hand make it possible to offset significant handicap in one joint or even one limb: Nelson won Trafalgar with one arm. It is in the lower limb that pain may be intolerable and because the patient cannot walk he or she becomes unemployable, unable to care for herself and socially

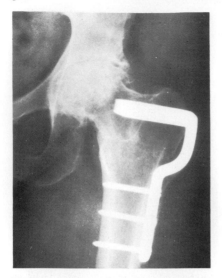

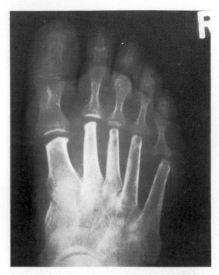

FIG. 320.—Intertrochanteric osteotomy at the hip with internal fixation using a Müller-Harris splint.

FIG. 321.—Excision of the metatarsal heads (Fowler's operation).

isolated. Fortunately one joint—the knee—is responsible for the majority of severe disability. Involvement of the hip is relatively uncommon but when it occurs (in about 3% of patients) it is crippling. The foot is almost always involved but although this involvement is painful it is often not crippling. Thus replacement of the knees—now in some centres a routine and reliable procedure—may abolish, perhaps indefinitely, the major disability in RA. Hence surgery, especially replacement surgery of the knee, has a major part to play in the treatment of RA.

Procedures for Joints affected by RA

The Hand and Wrist.—*Synovectomy* is employed at the metacarpo-phalangeal joints of the fingers, the radio-carpal and inferior radio-ulnar joints, and for the extensor (and, less commonly, flexor) tendon sheaths.

At the metacarpo-phalangeal joints of the fingers the synovial tissue erodes the cartilage and bone. As a consequence the joints subluxate and finally dislocate. Since the finger flexors are stronger than the extensors, dislocation takes the form of palmar and then proximal displacement of the phalanx on the metacarpal. A similar mechanism produces anterior dislocation of the wrist, and disruption of the inferior radio-ulnar joint. The extensor tendons may rupture as a consequence of a nutritional disturbance, combined with abrasion over the prominent dorsum of the distal radius and ulna. As the fingers deviate ulnar-wards the extensor tendons come to lie to the medial side of the metacarpal head so that their line of pull tends to exacerbate this deviation.

By removing the synovium before subluxation has taken place this evolving deformity may be arrested. At this stage, however, marked pain from capsular distension is not a feature so that the surgical decision is a difficult one: probable slowing of the progression of deformity and some pain-relief have to be set against the loss of movement which often follows this procedure.

At the time of synovectomy the capsule may be incised and reefed so as to stabilise the joints and re-align the extensor tendons. The tendons themselves may be repaired if they have ruptured and their synovial sheath may be excised if their bulk interferes with the function of the hand.

Once deformity has occurred, and especially when the metacarpo-phalangeal and wrist joints have subluxated, operations on the bones of the hand are indicated.

Arthrodesis of the radio-carpal joint is an excellent procedure and is one of the mainstays in the surgical treatment of the rheumatoid hand. The wrist can be rendered stable and pain-free so that the power of the grip is much improved. The loss of movement compared

Maurice E. Müller, Contemporary. Formerly Professor of Orthopaedic Surgery, Berne, Switzerland.
Nigel Henry Harris, Contemporary. Orthopaedic Surgeon, St. Mary's Hospital, Harrow Road, London.
Alan William Fowler. (See Chapter 12)

with that occurring in the normal wrist impairs function very little: compared with the pre-operative state of the wrist any loss is insignificant. Replacement of the wrist is starting to show encouraging results.

Excision arthroplasty of the metacarpal heads and of the bases of the phalanges from dislocated metacarpo-phalangeal joints makes it possible to realign the fingers with the metacarpus. The consequent improvement of function is limited by stiffness at the false joint due to adhesion formation. In an attempt to improve range *total replacement arthroplasty* may be employed. Excision of the dorsally dislocated distal ulna from the inferior radio-ulnar joint (a second example of *excision arthroplasty*) usually combined with fusion of the radio-carpal joint, produces a useful increase in the range of painless supination and pronation.

The Elbow.—*Synovectomy* is occasionally useful when the joint is painful, the synovial membrane thickened, but the bone intact.

Arthrodesis is occasionally indicated to confer painless stability, but the objections to this procedure in RA—that fusion is difficult to obtain and that the presence of other involved joints makes loss of movement functionally objectionable—usually outweigh the advantages.

Excision arthroplasty of the radial head may increase the range of painless motion—especially of pronation and supination. Excision of the entire joint may provide a good range of painless movement but the associated instability is such that little increased function is obtained.

Total replacement arthroplasty of the humero-ulnar joint is now giving increasingly encouraging results.

The Shoulder.—*Synovectomy* is not undertaken at this joint since the membrane is relatively inaccessible surgically and its bulk is hard to assess clinically.

Arthodesis is hard to secure in RA, but is occasionally indicated in a severely painful joint. The loss of total shoulder movement is not as severe as might be expected since scapulo-thoracis motion is unaffected and by itself provides a useful range of shoulder movement.

Excision arthroplasty of the humeral head may be undertaken as an alternative to arthrodesis: the operation and the after-care are less arduous than for arthrodesis and the pain relief is comparable. However the false joint is too unstable to allow effective abduction so that the functional result is worse than that following arthrodesis. *Partial replacement arthroplasty* using a prosthetic replacement for the humeral head (the Neer prosthesis) has proved useful in RA. *Total replacement arthroplasty* is available but the results are not encouraging.

The Toes.—The commonest consequence of RA requiring surgical relief in the feet is a claw toe deformity. As a result of this deformity—which consists of dorsal dislocation of the phalanges on the metacarpal heads and flexion contractures of the proximal inter-phalangeal joints—the dorsum of the involved toes rubs on the upper of the shoe whilst the head of the metatarsal is driven painfully downwards through the sole on weight-bearing.

Synovectomy has not been used extensively in an attempt to prevent this deformity in the foot in the way in which it has been used in the hand. However *excision arthroplasty* of the metatarsal heads, together occasionally with excision of the base of the proximal phalanx, is used commonly (fig 321). At the time of excision arthroplasty, the extensor tendons may be divided. This procedure allows the toes to be brought into line with the forefoot and very successfully relieves pain under the metatarsal heads. Post-operatively the gait lacks the 'toe-off' spring of normal gait, but such a spring has already disappeared by the time the operation becomes indicated. At the metatarso-phalangeal joint of the great toe the deformity is that of a hallux valgus rather than a claw toe, but again the operative treatment is *excision arthroplasty*.

As an alternative to excision arthroplasty, grossly deformed toes may be amputated through the metatarso-phalangeal joints.

The Midtarsal and Ankle Joints.—Pain arising from the midtarsal and ankle joints is best treated by well-fitting shoes or boots with appropriate insoles. Isolated involvement of one of these joints may merit arthrodesis, or, at the ankle, total replacement.

The Knee.—Total replacement has now supplanted all other forms of surgical treatment for the arthritic knee. As at the hip therefore the basic surgical decision is simple: if the patient's disability is tolerable it should be accepted; if it is not the knee should be replaced. A number of procedures and prostheses is available, one of which is illustrated in fig. 322.

Charles Sumner Neer II, Contemporary. Orthopaedic Surgeon, Columbia-Presbyterian Medical Center, New York.

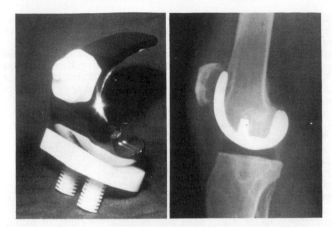

FIG. 322.—Replacement of the knee with the ICLH
(Imperial College—London Hospital) prosthesis.

The Hip.—*Total replacement arthroplasty* using the implants already described (p.366) is now the standard, indeed the only, surgical treatment for the hip in RA: at its best the operation results in almost normal hip function.

Synovectomy is not undertaken at the hip for the same reasons as those which apply to the shoulder. *Arthrodesis* is never indicated since it suffers from the same objections as those which apply to arthrodesis of the elbow and knee. Furthermore joints in addition to the involved hip have to be immobilised in plaster-of-Paris to obtain fusion, and in RA this risks disastrous stiffness affecting several joints. *Excision arthroplasty* is only used as a salvage procedure after failure of total replacement arthroplasty and takes the form of removal of the femoral head and proximal femoral neck (the Girdlestone operation). This operation relieves pain and permits a sufficient range of movement to enable the patient to lie and sit comfortably. The hip, however, is unstable so that walking is difficult and usually requires the aid of two sticks. *Interposition arthroplasty* and partial replacement has now been abandoned in favour of total replacement.

The Spine.—RA may affect all the facet joints of the spine but surgery is indicated only in the cervical spine, especially at the atlanto-axial joint, where the disease may lead to instability of the atlas on the axis with consequent danger to the spinal cord. This complication of RA is treated by *arthrodesis* (called 'fusion' when applied to the spine) of the unstable level.

ANKYLOSING SPONDYLITIS

Pathology.—This is a crippling disease which, although it has some features in common with RA, forms a distinct clinical entity and is regarded as such in the U.K. On the other hand the initial histological appearances of this disease are so similar to those of RA that in the U.S.A. ankylosing spondylitis is regarded as a variant of RA.

The disease is essentially a process of calcification and then ossification of the ligaments and capsules of joints, which results in complete bony ankylosis of the central articulations of the body. (This contrasts with rheumatoid arthritis which is not predominantly an ankylosing disease and which affects the small, distal joints of the extremities first). Whereas RA affects mainly females, ankylosing spondylitis is more common in men, starting in early adult life. Recognised associations include aortic valve disease, urethritis, amyloidosis and pulmonary fibrosis.

It has recently been shown that the tissue antigen HLA-B27 occurs in 96% of patients with ankylosing spondylitis, while present in only about 6% of general Caucasian populations. Tissue typing may thus help in diagnosing the condition, but the mechanism by which this genetic factor operates in predisposing to the disease is not yet established.

The joints most affected, in order of frequency, are the sacro-iliac joints, the joints of the spine (ascending from the lumbar level), the hips, the costal joints, and the shoulders. In addition to developing bony ankylosis, the spine becomes flexed so that eventually the patient is bent double and can no longer see forwards (fig. 323).

Garthorne Robert Girdlestone, 1881–1950. Nuffield Professor of Orthopaedic Surgery, Oxford.

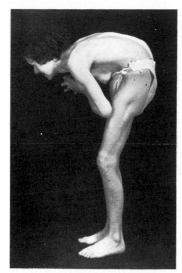

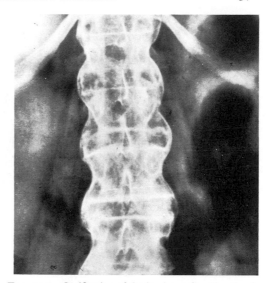

FIG. 323.—Ankylosing spondylitis.   FIG. 324.—Ossification of the lumbar spine ('bamboo' spine).

Special Investigations.—The diagnosis is confirmed by the finding of a raised ESR (an investigation which should never be omitted in the examination of young adults complaining of low back pain), by the radiological demonstration of bony obliteration of the sacro-iliac joints, and finally by the presence of ossification in the spinal ligaments ('bamboo spine') and ankylosis of other involved joints (figs. 324 and 325).

Treatment.—There is no specific treatment for this condition. Fortunately the disease sometimes arrests spontaneously before the full picture of spinal ankylosis in gross deformity is reached. Patients in whom the thoracic cage is ankylosed and the spine is flexed, may die of pulmonary infection because of the reduction in their vital capacity. Simple analgesics help to relieve pain and postural exercises may help prevent increasing deformity. Osteotomy of the spine is occasionally indicated to correct severe deformity. Pain and stiffness in the hips may be relieved by arthroplasty.

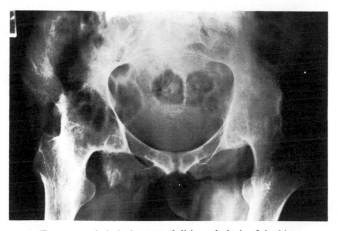

FIG. 325.—Ankylosing spondylitis: ankylosis of the hips.

CHAPTER 20

TUMOURS OF BONES AND JOINTS

All primary bone tumours are rare: the incidence of osteosarcoma, the common-est primary malignant bone neoplasm (excluding myeloma), is only 1 per 230,000 of population. From the collective standpoint of the community therefore they are unimportant, almost insignificant. From the individual standpoint of the patient and his family, however, they may represent a tragedy, for many of the malignant tumours occur in the young (at which age they constitute one of the commonest malignant tumours), they are usually fatal, and the attempt to cure them involves mutilating surgery.

Nomenclature and Classification.—These tumours are named after the pre-dominant type of tissue matrix formed by the tumour. The benign tumours take the suffix—'oma' and the maligant tumours the suffix—'sarcoma'. Thus a benign tumour forming bone and/or osteoid is named an osteoma and the corresponding malignant tumour an osteosarcoma. Tumours forming a cartilaginous matrix are named chondroma and chondrosarcoma, the fibrous series fibroma and fibrosar-coma. Tumours differentiating to a synovial pattern are named synovioma and synovial sarcoma. A number of primary bone tumours arise from the cells con-tained in the bone marrow and these are also named, so far as possible, after

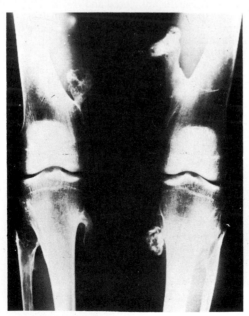

FIG. 326.—Multiple osteochondromas (exostoses) each of a typical hooked shape growing away from the epiphysis, of all the bones round the knee.

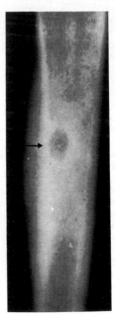

FIG. 327.—Osteoid osteoma in the tibia (see text).

the type of tissue differentiation. The matrix of some tumours is too poorly differentiated to allow specification classification.

BENIGN TUMOURS

Most of the benign tumours of bone occur in children and young adults and often stop growing with the cessation of skeletal growth. Such lesions might more properly be regarded as localised dysplasias rather than neoplasias, and indeed those which are multiple, for example multiple osteochondromas and chondromas, may well be viewed in this light.

The exceptions to the general rule that the tumour ceases to grow at skeletal maturity are giant cell tumours, probably better regarded as locally malignant, and osteoid osteomas, the precise pathological nature of which is unknown. Aneurysmal bone cysts are almost certainly not neoplastic.

Osteochrondroma is almost certainly the result of a localised disturbance of bone growth at an epiphysis. A portion of epiphyseal cartilage remains in the periosteum of the metaphyseal segment of the bone and endochondral ossification takes place in it, usually in continuity with the metaphyseal cortex. The cartilage cap proliferates, endochondral ossification continues, and thus the osteochondroma grows. With continued bone growth the osteochondroma moves away from the epiphysis and tends to become 'hooked', its tip pointing away from the epiphysis (fig. 326). Usually it ceases to grow when skeletal growth is complete. The lesion may be solitary or multiple (Chapter 21). The growth or growths may form an appreciable mass or they may interfere with the action of an adjacent soft tissue such as a tendon. The complaint of severe or persistent pain in such a tumour should raise the suspicion of malignant change. The radiological features are shown in fig. 326.

Compact Osteoma (syn. Ivory Exostosis) consists of a small knob of extremely hard, dense, but otherwise normal bone usually arising on the inner or outer table of the skull.

Osteoid Osteoma.—This 'tumour' consists of a small area of arborescent trabeculae of osteoid and bone with a vascular connective tissue ground work. The tumour itself is usually less than 1 cm in size and provokes dense new bone formation around it. Its neoplastic nature is unsure, and the lesion may possibly be a low grade osteitis. The tumour is most commonly seen in patients between 10 and 25 years old, is slightly more common in males, and usually occurs in the long bones. Any bone may be involved, the most commonly involved bones being the femur and the tibia. Lesions over 1 cm in size are sometimes designated 'Osteoblastoma', but are histologically indistinguishable from Osteoid Osteomas. Alone amongst the benign neoplasms of bone, osteoid osteoma presents with pain which is severe, unrelieved by rest, but often specifically relieved by salicylate. The only abnormal physical sign is bone tenderness, and even this is often absent so that patients with osteoid osteomas may sometimes be regarded as hysterical. Radiologically, the bone in the area of the tumour is densely sclerotic. Towards the centre of the sclerotic area and often obscured by it, there is a radio-opaque 'nidus' in a radiolucent zone which represents the tumour itself (fig. 327). If the tumour lies in cortical bone, there may be overlying subperiosteal new bone formation. Tomography may be required to demonstrate the nidus.

Chondroma.—This tumour consists of a lobulated mass of cartilage. The tumour may arise in any bone, but is most frequent in the metacarpals, phalanges or metatarsals. Occasionally the tumours arise in synovial membrane. If situated in the medulla (*enchondroma*), the bone is thinned or expanded by the tumour causing pain and deformity. Pathological fracture is common. Tumours on the surface of the bone are known as *ecchondromas*. The matrix of the tumour may calcify and sometimes ossify. Like osteochondromas, chondromas may be solitary or multiple (Chapter 21). Malignant change is rare in solitary tumours, but may occur when the tumours are multiple.

Fibroma.—These occur in bone as islands of fibrous tissue of characteristic radiographic appearance. They range from small oval cortical defects to quite large lesions. Areas of fibrous dysplasia are distinguished from fibromas by the presence within them of new bone.

Aneurysmal Bone Cysts.—These occur mainly in the ends of growing long bones. They form expanding osteolytic lesions containing bloody fluid through which pathological fractures may occur. Callus formation following such a fracture may obliterate the cyst. Care must be taken to distinguish them from osseous haemangiomas.

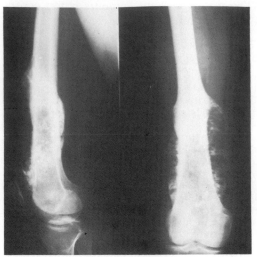

FIG. 328.—Osteosarcoma of the femur. Note Codman's triangle well seen in the proximal part of the tumour and 'sunray spicules'.

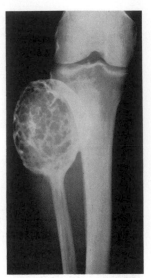

FIG. 329.—Giant cell tumour of fibula.

Biopsy.—A diagnosis of a benign tumour can usually be made on the basis of clinical and radiological appearances but, as a general rule, the lesion should always be biopsied, or when possible excised, since histological examination is advisable.

Treatment of Benign Tumours.—Osteomas can be ignored unless they give rise to symptoms which demand treatment. They should then be removed.

Lesions which significantly weaken bone such as chondromas or aneurysmal bone cysts should be treated, even if symptomless, to prevent pathological fracture. The lesion is excised by curettage and the resulting cavity in the bone is packed with autogenous bone chips. In multiple chondromatosis (Ollier's disease), it may, of course, be impractical to treat all the tumours in this way.

MALIGNANT TUMOURS

Osteosarcoma.—This is a highly malignant tumour: reported 5 year survival rates vary, but few exceed 15%. Osteosarcomas arising in hitherto normal bone, occur mainly in the second and third decades of life and tend to occur in the metaphyseal region of the long bones, especially those of the leg. Paget's disease predisposes bone to develop a sarcoma, about 60% being osteosarcomas. Such tumours develop late in life (because Paget's disease is a disease of the elderly), arise in any bone involved by Paget's disease, and are almost invariably fatal. Excessive irradiation also predisposes bone to sarcomatous change.

The tumour is composed of pleomorphic cells which invade and destroy the bone producing a radiologically osteolytic lesion with ill-defined edges. Although they destroy normal bone, the tumour cells themselves produce abnormal bone of irregular structure. If the tumour has invaded the soft tissue, neoplastic bone can be seen radiologically outside the confines of the normal bone, where it tends to be deposited as irregular spicules of bone radiating away from the shaft to give a 'sunray' appearance (fig. 328). As the tumour grows in size, the periosteum is elevated so that above and below the tumour reactive new bone may be deposited subperiosteally. Radiologically, this bone appears as a triangle of new bone (*Codman's triangle*, fig. 328)

Louis Ollier, 1830–1900. Professor of Surgery, Lyon, France.
Sir James Paget, 1814–1899. Surgeon, St. Bartholomew's Hospital, London.
Ernest Amory Codman, 1869–1940. Surgeon, Massachusetts General Hospital, Boston, Massachusetts, U.S.A.

Metastasis occurs via the blood-stream to produce pulmonary secondary deposits. Locally, pathological fracture may take place. Finally, if the tumour is untreated, it fungates to produce an infected malignant ulcer sometimes overlying a painful pathological fracture.

Chondrosarcoma.—This tumour arises usually in hitherto normal bone. It may however appear as a complication of any pre-existing cartilagenous tumour. It may arise in any bone, with a predilection for the flat bones and ribs. Unlike osteosarcoma, it occurs mainly in middle-aged persons, is very rare in children, and uncommon in teenagers.

Although malignant, the tumour may be slow-growing and mitoses so infrequent that malignancy may be impossible to decide on biopsy material. The tumour is locally invasive and, although often slow to metastasise, it may give rise to blood-borne pulmonary secondaries which are eventually fatal. The matrix of the tumour is more or less cartilagenous. It may ossify in patches but more commonly calcifies.

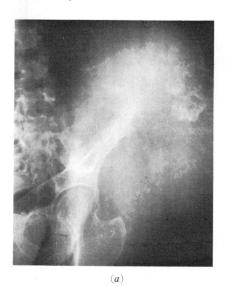
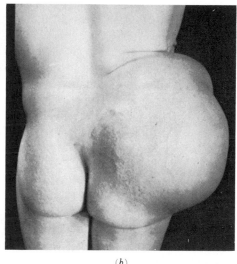

(a) (b)

FIG. 330.—(a) Chondrosarcoma of the ilium. (b) The clinical appearance of the buttock shown in (a).

The tumour invades and destroys bone, transgresses the periosteum and invades the adjacent soft tissues. In the spine, where it is rare, the tumour usually manifests itself whilst it is still small by causing collapse of a vertebra or by invading or compressing the cord or a nerve root. In the pelvis, on the other hand, the tumour may reach a considerable size before the patient notices a mass (fig. 330).

Fibrosarcoma.—These tumours are usually composed of spindle-shaped fibroblasts which produce a collagenous matrix but they may be pleomorphic. In bone, the tumour arises centrally or periosteally. (The tumour may, of course, also arise in any soft tissue.) They are of varying malignancy, produce blood-borne pulmonary secondaries, and are associated with a 5 year survival rate of about 30%.

Synovial Sarcoma. This is histologically a bi-phasic tumour composed of elements simulating synovium mingled with malignant fibroblasts. It is extremely malignant, and may appear at any age.

The tumour usually arises close to a major joint (most often the knee, ankle or wrist) but it may arise, apparently primarily, in connective tissue, in muscle or subcutaneously. Metastasis appears to occur via the blood-stream, the lymphatics and by the migration of cells through the tissue planes of the limb. Secondary involvement of regional lymph nodes is not unusual.

Giant Cell Tumour.—It is uncertain from what cell this tumour arises. It is composed of undifferentiated spindle cells and multinucleate giant cells in a vascular stroma. Microscopically it is indistinguishable from the so-called 'brown tumour' of hyperparathyroidism and this condition must be excluded by biochemical and radiological investigations (Chapter 23).

The tumour occurs most often in the third and fourth decades of life and tends to be more common in women. The epiphyseal regions of the long bones, especially around the knee, are the most common sites of origin but tumours of the humerus, radius and ulna occasionally occur.

The tumour is osteolytic and expands the bone with thinning, often perforation, of the cortex to cause a pathological fracture in some cases. The bone is destroyed irregularly so that the tumour is traversed by remnants of the original bone and comes to lie in a cavity with heavily trabeculated walls. As a consequence, it has a typical 'soap-bubble' radiological appearance (fig. 329). It rarely invades soft tissues but may do so when fracture occurs. Thus locally the tumour is only of low-grade malignancy. Metastasis is rare, but occurs via the blood-stream to the lungs. Recurrence following local removal is common, and such recurrences are more likely to be frankly malignant than the original tumour.

Secondary Tumours in Bone.—Two thirds of all secondary malignant tumours in bone arise from carcinomas of the breast or prostate. One sixth arise from a variety of other primary neoplasms (especially those of the bronchus, kidney, and thyroid). In the remaining one sixth, no primary tumour is found at the time when the secondary presents. The majority of tumours are osteolytic but a few, mostly arising from the prostate, stimulate new bone formation and are then called 'osteosclerotic'.

Clinical and Radiological Features of Malignant Bone Tumours (Table I).— Regardless of the pathology, these tumours present by causing pain, a noticeable lump or tender area, or a pathological fracture.

The diagnosis depends upon the clinical features of the tumour, its radiological appearance and its histology (biopsy). An exact diagnosis cannot be made in approximately 10% of tumours.

Clinically the important features are the mode of presentation (the more malignant the tumour the more likely it is to present with severe pain or pathological fracture rather than as a mass), the age of the patient, the fact that on physical

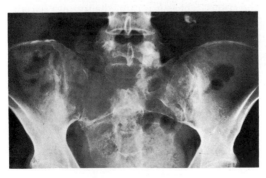

FIG. 331.—Multiple osteolytic secondaries in the pelvis.

TABLE I. *Malignant Tumours of Bones and Joints*:
Principal Clinical and Radiological Features

Tumour	Presentation	Age of Patient	Location of Tumour	Radiological Appearance
Osteo-sarcoma	Pain, swelling and/or pathological fracture	2nd and 3rd decades. Elderly in Paget's disease	Ends of shafts of long bones, esp. femur, tibia, humerus. Any Paget diseased bone	Bone destruction with ill-defined edges. Extension into soft tissues (shadow). Codman's Triangle. Sunray spicules. Pathological fracture. Secondaries in lungs
Chondro-sarcoma	Mass	4th–6th decades	Ribs, Ilium, Scapula, Proximal ends of femur and humerus	Bone destruction with ill-defined edges. Extension into soft tissues (shadow). Large tumour (in flat bones) with ossifying or calcifying matrix
Fibro-sarcoma	Mass or pathological fracture	Any age, mainly 25–60	Any bone. May occur in Paget's disease	Area of bone destruction
Synovial Sarcoma	Soft tissue mass	Any age	Usually a joint	Soft tissue swelling ± spotty calcification
Giant Cell Tumour	Pain, swelling ± fracture or joint symptoms	3rd and 4th decades	Epiphyseal region of long bones especially distal femur, proximal tibia and fibula	Expands the bone. Sharp edges unless frankly malignant. Soap bubble appearance
Secondary Neoplasm	Pain and/or pathological fracture	Middle-aged and elderly	Any bone	Bone destruction with ill-defined edges. Occasionally marked sclerosis in adjacent bone

examination the tumour is attached to bone, the location of the tumour, and the presence of any evidence of a primary neoplasm elsewhere.

Radiologically two features suggest malignancy irrespective of the exact nature of the tumour. These are:

1. The presence of an ill-defined osteolytic lesion in the bone. Although the lesion is osteolytic, tumour new bone or calcification may occur within it or reactive new bone may occur around it.

2. Evidence that the tumour has breached the periosteum and invaded soft tissues.

The distinguishing radiological features of the commoner tumours are summarised in Table I and illustrated in figs. 328–331

Biopsy.—Histological material should always be obtained by biopsy before treatment is undertaken. If possible, open biopsy is undertaken: the naked-eye appearance of the tumour is noted and material is taken from the edge of the tumour together with adjoining normal tissue. The cell morphology of the tumour, the type of matrix formed, the presence of abnormal mitoses, and the invasion of adjacent tissues permit a diagnosis of malignancy and usually serve to identify the tumour. Needle biopsy may be employed for tumours of the spine but since this technique yields only a restricted sample of tissue it is not as reliable as open biopsy.

Treatment

Osteosarcoma.—There is no general agreement as to how this tumour should be treated but the most widely followed practice today follows certain principles. Local control of the tumour must be obtained by surgery, either amputation or wide local resection with replacement of the defect by a custom-made prosthesis or allograft. In addition most surgeons advise adjuvant chemotherapy in an attempt to control or to prevent the development of metastatic disease. This may be given pre-operatively as well as post-operatively.

Amputation should be carried out at the site of election through the bone or joint immediately proximal to that involved in the tumour. Thus for example, osteosarcoma of the tibia should be treated by amputation through the femur, and at the proximal end of the femur disarticulation of the hip or hind-quarter amputation is required. Solitary pulmonary secondaries have been successfully treated by lobectomy.

Chondrosarcoma.—In spite of the difficulty that this tumour nearly always arises in the proximal limb skeleton, treatment is by amputation or wide local resection and insertion of a custom-made prothesis or allograft. The tumour is nearly always large when first diagnosed, and when large is radio resistant. Hence radiotherapy has no part to play in its treatment.

Fibrosarcoma.—This tumour is treated by early amputation or by wide block resection.

Synovial Sarcoma.—This tumour carries an extremely poor prognosis regardless of treatment: few or no survivors have been reported after 5 years. The tumour should be treated by a proximal amputation together with irradiation of the stump of the limb.

Giant Cell Tumours are treated where possible (for example in the proximal fibula or distal radius) by block resection of the tumour and adjacent bone. Unfortunately such a resection is often disabling since the tumour may be located, for example, in a tibial condyle, block resection of which would render the knee useless. An attempt should then be made to eradicate the tumour by curettage followed by packing the cavity with bone chips. Unfortunately, the incidence of recurrence following curettage is high. Recurrent tumours may be frankly malignant and require amputation or local resection and insertion of a custom-made prosthesis or allograft.

Ewing's Tumour

There is uncertainty about the pathology of this lesion. Some hold that it is a malignant endothelioma arising from the endothelial cells in the bone marrow, others that it arises from immature reticulum cells or the myeloid cell. The tumour usually occurs in the middle of a long bone in childhood or early adolescence. Radiography shows a number of layers of sub-periosteal new bone formation expanding the shaft and giving the characteristic appearance of a cut onion. Clinically a painful hot swelling is noticed and the patient may show intermittent elevations of temperature. In this way the condition may be difficult to distinguish from acute haematogenous osteomyelitis. Several lesions may be present

James Ewing, 1866–1943. Professor of Oncology (Tumours), Cornell University Medical College, U.S.A.

when the patient is first seen. Treatment is by radiotherapy to the whole of the involved bone and adjuvant multidrug chemotherapy. Several different schemes of polychemotherapy have been devised, but are beyond the scope of this chapter. The prognosis for these patients has improved dramatically over the past few years.

CHAPTER 21

CONGENITAL DISEASES OF BONES AND JOINTS

The congenital diseases of bones and joints are of two kinds: developmental anomalies and dysplasias.

The developmental anomalies are characterised by the fact that the fundamental abnormality of growth occurs *in utero* and is static at birth: the evolution of the disease thereafter is due to secondary changes.

The dysplasias are characterised by abnormal growth both *in utero* and through-out the period of post-natal skeletal development. Many dysplasias are clinically detectable at birth and hence are certainly congenital; others remain undetected until later in life. It is assumed, almost certainly correctly, that in the latter a tendency to abnormal growth was present at birth and hence that they are also congenital.

Some congenital diseases are genetic in origin, some are thought to be due to disturbances in the intra-uterine environment. For the majority, the aetiology is unknown.

CONGENITAL DISLOCATION OF THE HIP (CDH)

Overall Incidence.—Before it was realised that instability of the hip could be diagnosed at birth (fig. 332*a* & *b*) CDH was diagnosed in 1 child in 1000. The reported incidence of unstable hips (see below) is much higher, varying from 8 to 20 per 1000 live births.

Pathology.—The hip may be either dislocated or dislocatable at birth. The precise details of the morbid anatomy at birth are not certain, but the essential practical fact is that the bones of the pelvis and femur are broadly within normal limits, but the ligaments of the hip are unduly lax so that the femoral head can be dislocated from the acetabulum. The infant may lie with the hip in the dislocated position, or the hip may be in the reduced

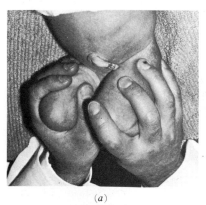 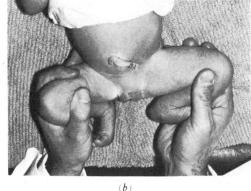

(*a*)   (*b*)

FIG. 332.—Congenital dislocation of hip. Von Rosen's or Barlow's sign. (*a*) The hip in full adduction. (*b*) The hip in full abduction: note that the knee touches the couch.

position but be easily dislocatable. Over the first few months of life the ligaments of the hip shorten so that if the femur is maintained in the acetabulum during this period, the hip becomes stable and normal development results. On the other hand, if the femoral head is allowed to remain out of the acetabulum during this period, shortening of the ligaments makes reduction of the dislocation increasingly difficult. If the hip is allowed to remain dislocated until the child crawls and then walks, the acetabulum and femur fail to develop normally. It is then difficult to return the hip to normal whatever treatment is instituted, and osteoarthrosis in the involved hip may develop early in adult life.

Aetiology.—The condition may be unilateral or bilateral, and is familial. Three factors appear to be important in its aetiology:

1. *An hereditary predisposition* to joint laxity: the patient's relatives may either have dislocated hips themselves or may have hypermobile joints so that they can perform 'party tricks' such as extending their wrists and fingers until the fingers lie parallel with their forearm or extending their thumb until the thumb touches the radius.

2. *Female sex* on the part of the infant: the condition is 3 to 5 times more common in girls. This may be due to the fact that maternal *relaxin* crosses the placental barrier to enter the foetus. If the hormonal environment of the foetus is also female, relaxin acts on the foetus' joints in the same way as it does on those of the mother to produce joint laxity in the pelvis.

3. *Breech malposition* of the foetus: for infants who are either delivered in the breech position or who spend a substantial part of the last 2 months *in utero* in this position the incidence of instability of the hip is about 10 times as great as for infants with a vertex presentation. It is possible that in the breech position the uterus presses on the foetal legs in such a way that, if the hip ligaments are already lax, dislocation may occur.

Clinical Features.—It is imperative that this condition be diagnosed in the first few days of life. This will only be done if the physician or midwife attending the delivery is aware of the existence of the condition and knows how to demonstrate its presence.

Diagnosis at Birth.—At birth the appearance of the infant is normal, and the hips can be put through a full range of movement. If the hip is dislocated, telescoping can in theory be demonstrated but in practice it is extremely difficult for the examiner to convince himself that this is occurring in a neonate. Thus, conventional clinical examination of the hip reveals no abnormality. Radiologically, the epiphysis of the femoral head does not appear until the first year of life and the acetabulum is largely cartilaginous so that, even if the hip is dislocated (rather than dislocatable), there is no obvious radiological abnormality. Thus, there is no way of detecting a dislocatable or dislocated hip at birth save by a specific examination designed to elicit instability. It is imperative that every doctor supervising a pregnancy should be familiar with this physical sign which is elicited as follows:

The Demonstration of Instability of the Hip at Birth.—The demonstration consists of eliciting a click from the hip, and is known as Barlow's or von Rosen's sign. The legs are held as shown in fig. 332. The hip is then flexed to 90° and adducted. Whilst adduction is taking place, gentle pressure is exerted by the examining hand in a proximal direction along the long axis of the femoral shaft. As the femoral head rolls over the posterior lip of the acetabulum it may, if

Thomas Geoffrey Barlow, 1915–1975. Orthopaedic Surgeon, Salford Royal Hospital, Salford, England.
Sophus von Rosen, Contemporary. Orthopaedic Surgeon, Malmö General Hospital, Malmö, Sweden.

dislocatable (but not if dislocated), slip out of the acetabulum. The sensation which the examining hand receives as the hip slips over the posterior lip of the acetabulum is difficult to describe but is composed of a mixture of the feeling of abnormal posterior movement plus a distinct 'clunk' as the femoral head leaves the acetabulum. If the hip is dislocated by this manoeuvre or if it is already dislocated prior to examination, the second half of the physical sign can now be elicited. The hip is kept 90° flexed and, starting from a position of full adduction, is gently abducted. Now instead of exerting pressure proximally in the long axis of the femoral shaft, the examiner exerts pressure distally in the long axis of the shaft via his little finger placed proximal to the greater trochanter. The femoral head can now be felt to reduce with a soft 'clunk' into the acetabulum somewhere during the course of movement from full adduction to full abduction. As abduction continues the femoral head remains in the acetabulum, demonstrating that the hip is stable in this position.

Occasionally a soft click can be felt in the hip which is noticeably different to the experienced examiner from the 'clunk' of an unstable hip. The origin of these clicks is uncertain but they presumably come from soft tissue around the hip. Should the physician attending the delivery detect either a 'click' or a 'clunk' the patient should be referred immediately for an orthopaedic opinion.

There are perhaps a few dislocated hips which cannot be reduced at birth. The diagnosis of dislocation in these hips at birth appears to be difficult or impossible.

The Treatment of CDH in the Newborn Infant. The incidence figures quoted above show that in the absence of neonatal treatment only a minority of unstable hips at birth will develop into a persistent dislocation. All that is required to ensure that no unstable hip develops in this way is to place the femoral head in the acetabulum by the method described for the elicitation of von Rosen's sign and to keep it there until the hip is clinically stable and normal development is occurring radiologically.

Various splints have been devised to do this by keeping the hip in a position of 90° flexion and abduction (a position in which the femoral head is stable in the acetabulum) for a period of three months. All are satisfactory. One such splint is the von Rosen splint which is illustrated in fig. 333.

The Diagnosis of CDH in a child of one year's age or more. It is very much to be hoped that no medical practitioner in the United Kingdom will ever in future have occasion to concern himself clinically with this problem. Unfortunately, because the method of making the diagnosis in the first week of life is not yet universally appreciated and implemented, it still happens that children present later in life with dislocated hips. This is a tragedy.

If one hip is dislocated, the skin creases in the groin and around the buttocks are asymmetrical (fig. 334). The affected hip has a full range of flexion, extension and rotation but cannot be fully abducted in 90° of flexion. In the infant, the normal hip will abduct until the knee nearly touches the examination couch. The dislocated hip will abduct only to about 45° (fig. 335). Telescoping may be demonstrated.

If the patient is old enough to stand, Trendelenburg's sign is positive. This sign is elicited by asking the patient to stand on the affected leg and noting the position taken up by the pelvis. If the sign is negative (*i.e.* the hip is normal), the pelvis

Friedrich Trendelenburg, 1844–1924 (see footnote, p. 60). Described this sign in 1895.

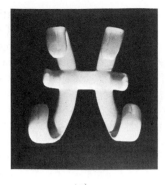

(a)

(b)

FIG. 333.—(a) and (b) The von Rosen splint made of padded malleable metal.

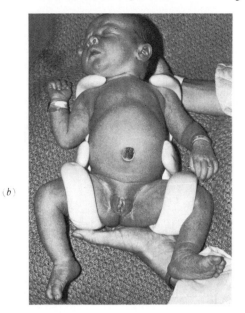

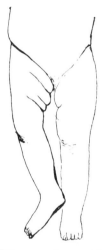

FIG. 334.—Asymmetrical skin creases.

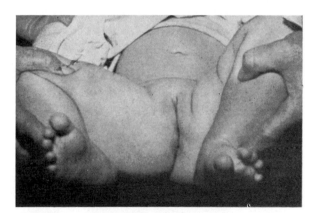

FIG. 335.—Limited abduction of the left thigh in CDH.

rises on the unsupported side (figs. 336 and 337 (b)). If the sign is positive, the pelvis drops on the unsupported side (fig. 337 (a)). A positive sign is produced by any pathology which interferes mechanically with the abductor mechanism of the hip, for example dislocation of the hip, fracture of the neck of the femur, or paralysis of the abductors. If Trendelenburg's sign is positive, the patient has a typical gait lurching downwards towards the unsupported side during the stance phase on the affected leg.

If both hips are dislocated, asymmetry of the groin creases is absent and the symmetry of the 'waddling' gait (there being a Trendelenburg limp on both sides) often misleadingly makes it appear normal. Accordingly bilateral dislocation of the hips in infancy can be missed more easily than can unilateral dislocation.

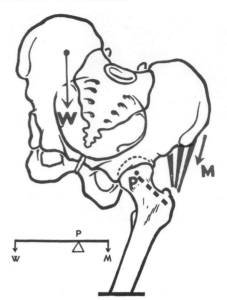

FIG. 336.—The physio-
logical basis of
Trendelenburg's sign.
Contraction of the glu-
teus medius elevates the
pelvis

W=weight of body
M=muscle pull
P=pivot (the hip)

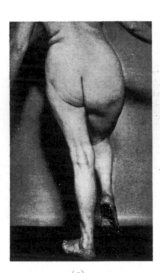

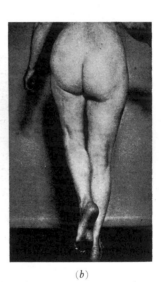

(a)   (b)

FIG. 337.—(a) Trendelenburg's sign positive—standing on the defective hip. (b) Trendelenburg's sign negative—standing on the sound hip.

X-ray Examination.—In contrast to the situation in neonates, the hip is radiologically
abnormal (fig. 338). The significant features are:

1. Lateral and upward displacement of the epiphysis of the femoral head. This displacement can be demonstrated by drawing 2 lines, one horizontally through the triradiate
cartilage and one vertically through the superior lip of the bony acetabulum: in CDH the
femoral epiphysis lies above the first line and lateral to the second.

2. A break in Shenton's line. Shenton's line is a fortuitous radiological appearance
consisting of the continuous curve produced by the inferior margin of the superior pubic
ramus and the medial cortex of the femoral neck and shaft. If the hip is dislocated, this
line will be broken by a step—because the femur moves upwards.

Edward Warren Hine Shenton, 1872–1955. Surgical Radiographer, Guy's Hospital, London.

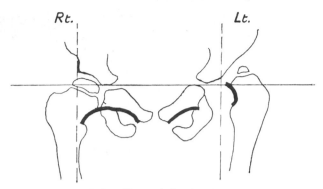

FIG. 338.(*a*).—CDH (Lt). Shenton's line (black) broken on the left side. Note the small ossific nucleus on the dislocated side above the horizontal and lateral to the vertical line, and the shallow acetabulum with its undeveloped bony roof.

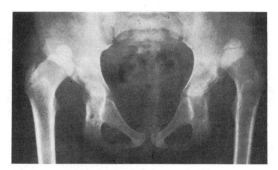

FIG. 338.(*b*).—Bilateral CDH in a six-year-old girl.

3. The capital femoral epiphysis is late to develop and when it does so is smaller than that on the unaffected side.

4. The superior lip of the bony acetabulum is also slow to develop so that it appears radiologically that the acetabulum is unduly shallow. If the hip continues to be dislocated throughout childhood, the final bony acetabulum is truly shallow. In infancy, however, the true acetabulum is often not particularly shallow since the cartilagenous development of the superior lip is not grossly abnormal.

Treatment between the ages of 6 months and 7 years (for unilateral dislocation) or 4 years (for bilateral dislocation).—Weight-bearing at the infant hip begins when the infant crawls at about 6 months. From this age until about 7 years for unilateral dislocation, and until about 4 years for bilateral dislocation, it is possible to reduce the hip and finally obtain fair function. Above these age limits, reduction is difficult and it is probably unwise to attempt it for reasons set out below; see Treatment in the Older Child (p. 387).

Treatment aims to replace the femoral head in the acetabulum and to keep it there whilst normal development occurs. Reduction is impeded by the fact that (1) the soft tissues have by this time developed in such a way as to conform with the abnormal position of the femur, and (2) the acetabulum has become filled with a mass of fibro-fatty tissue. Maintenance of reduction is difficult because: (1) the acetabulum is abnormally shallow and vertical, (2) the femoral head is smaller than normal, and (3) the femoral neck is usually retroverted on the shaft.

Closed 'Manipulation'.—It is sometimes possible under general anaesthesia to replace the femoral head in the acetabulum without any force being exerted on the leg. Should force be required the manoeuvre is unwise, since it is likely to result in damage to the blood supply of the femoral head. If closed reduction under anaesthesia is thought likely to fail, it should be preceded by a period of traction in progressively increasing abduction, and for this a variety of special splints have been devised. The femoral head may reduce spontaneously during a period of traction, or it may be reduced under anaesthesia after a period of traction. Open adductor, and sometimes psoas, tenotomy is often needed to allow the hip to be fully abducted without forcibly compressing the femoral head.

Open Reduction is indicated if closed reduction fails. It may be difficult to determine if the femoral head has been truly replaced in the acetabulum by closed manipulation, or whether on the other hand it has been brought opposite the acetabulum, but held out from a full reduction by fibro-fatty tissue in the acetabulum or by the presence of a fold of capsule and acetabular labrum (the limbus) intruding between the femoral head and the superior part of the acetabulum. The presence of such an impediment to reduction may be suspected if the femoral head persistently 'stands off' radiologically after an apparently satisfactory reduction, and may be confirmed by arthrography. The presence of a limbus, or clear-cut inability to reduce the dislocation by conservative means, are indications for open reduction. The hip is exposed and the soft tissues obstructing reduction are excised or released, so that the head can be repositioned in the acetabulum.

Maintenance of Reduction.—If the hip has been replaced either by closed or open means it must be maintained in the acetabulum for a period of months by some form of *splintage*. This may be done initially by traction on an appropriate splint or by a double hip spica applied with the hips held in the position of maximum stability. Not all hips are best immobilised in the same position, but stability is usually obtained in a position of abduction and flexion with some degree of external or internal rotation (fig. 339). Extreme internal or external rotation should be avoided since this tends to 'wring out' the vessels in the capsule of the hip and may interfere with the blood supply to the femoral head so that changes similar to those seen in Perthes' disease (Chapter 22) develop. After 3 to 6 months a hip spica may be exchanged for a Denis Browne splint if the child is under 2 years of age.

If reduction has been deferred until the bones of the hip have developed abnormally, *surgical reconstruction* of the hip may be required in addition to open reduction. The available procedures consist of:

1. *Pelvic Osteotomy* (Salter) which aims to rotate the acetabulum into a more horizontal position to cover the femoral head.

2. A *Shelf Operation* in which the superior lip of the acetabulum is reconstructed (so

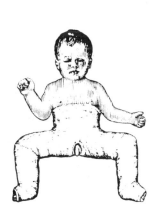

FIG. 339.—Congenital dislocation of the hip.—Plaster-of-Paris spica for the maintenance of the reduction of a bilateral CDH in neutral rotation and 90° abduction (see text).

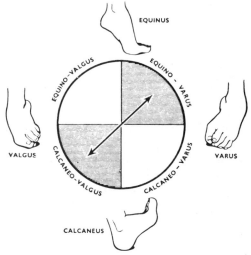

FIG. 340.—Nomenclature of talipes. Shaded quadrants indicate the common varieties.

Sir Denis John Wolko Browne, 1892–1967. Surgeon, Hospital for Sick Children, Great Ormond Street, London.
Robert B. Salter, Contemporary. Professor of Orthopaedic Surgery, University of Toronto, Ontario, Canada.

that it covers the femoral head) by a bone graft or by medial displacement of the acetabulum relative to the ilium after a pelvic osteotomy just above the hip.

3. *Intertrochanteric Rotation Osteotomy of the Femur* in which the proximal fragment is rotated, bringing the femoral head squarely into the acetabulum.

Treatment in the Older Child.—Putti suggested that the results of treatment in bilateral dislocations of the hip over the age of 4 years and in unilateral dislocations over the age of 7 years are worse than the results of the disease itself and thus that no treatment is indicated for these children in childhood. A lower age limit applies to bilateral dislocation because (1) the limp is less noticeable; (2) as a consequence these patients, although they have a slightly abnormal posture and an abnormal gait, tend to live normal lives until their 40's or 50's when secondary osteoarthrosis may develop; (3) there is a danger that treatment may be more successful in one hip than in the other so that a bilateral dislocation is converted into a unilateral dislocation and (4) treatment may stiffen the hip, a tolerable outcome in one hip but a significant disability if it affects both.

CLUB FOOT (TALIPES)

Nomenclature.—'Club Foot' is a loose term used to describe a number of different abnormalities in the shape of the foot. If the foot is fixed in a position of plantar-flexion so that it cannot be fully dorsiflexed, the deformity is described as one of 'equinus'. The opposite deformity is described as 'calcaneus'. If the foot is inverted and adducted at the mid-tarsal joint so that it cannot be fully everted the deformity is described as 'varus'. The opposite deformity is described as 'valgus'. Almost invariably two or more of the deformities are combined and by far the most common congenital combination is 'equino-varus'. The Latin synonym for club foot is 'talipes' and the descriptive nomenclature for a club foot combines this term with the Latin description of the deformity. Thus the most common variety of congenital club foot is known as 'Talipes Equino-Varus' (fig. 340).

Aetiology.—It has been suggested that raised intra-uterine pressure forces the lower limbs of the foetus against the wall of the uterus so as to mould the feet into the position of deformity. The presence of lesions in the skin over the convex aspect of the foot in talipes equinovarus which very much resemble healed pressure sores, lends support to this belief. It has alternatively been suggested that the primary disturbance is in the muscles of the calf of the soft tissues of the foot where some form of contracture, possibly ischaemic in nature, has been visualised as drawing the foot into a position of deformity. Neither of these postulated aetiological mechanisms has received widespread support and the most commonly held view is that the primary disturbance is a developmental defect of the soft tissues of the legs affecting particularly the ligaments on the concave side of the curve, or possibly, in the case of talipes equino-varus, the development of the neck of the talus.

Congenital club foot may also be paralytic, and secondary to myelodysplasia (Chapter 25). The deformities in arthrogryphosis multiplex congenita may include club feet. The club foot in this disease is gross, and nearly always associated with other deformities, in particular with clubbing of the hand (p. 392).

Morbid Anatomy.—Surprising as it may seem, there are relatively few accurate descriptions of the morbid anatomy of untreated club foot at or before birth and therefore the nature of the original morbid anatomy is uncertain. Within a few months of birth the morbid anatomical features are as follows:

1. Adduction and external rotation of the bones of the forefoot. The adduction occurs at the mid-tarsal and tarso-metatarsal joints, but also to some extent affects the bones themselves which are curved so as to be concave medially. The adduction may be so gross as to result in medial dislocation of the navicular from the talo-navicular joint. The external rotation is produced by torsion of the shafts of the metatarsals.

2. Inversion of the os calcis and of the navicular on the talus. The inverted os calcis and navicular carry the rest of the foot into inversion with them.

3. Plantar-flexion of all the bones of the foot including the talus. The talus, although

Vittorio Putti, 1880–1940. Professor of Orthopaedic Surgery, University of Bologna, Italy.

plantar-flexed, is not as plantar-flexed as the other bones so that the head of the talus tends progressively to dislocate from the mid-tarsal joint in a dorsal as well as a lateral direction.

4. There is possibly an early abnormality in the neck of the talus which, it has been suggested, is angulated so that the head of the talus is displaced downwards and medially. Secondary changes occur in the head of the talus.

5. The os calcis may be small. As a consequence the heel is small.

6. All the ligamentous structures on the medial side of the foot and to some extent in the sole are shortened, but are histologically normal.

7. The muscles of the calf are hypoplastic, but histologically normal. As a result, the flexors of the foot and toes and the invertors of the foot are short. As growth takes place, hypoplasia commonly persists in spite of effective treatment for the deformity, so that finally the whole of the foot and calf are smaller than normal.

8. The skin shows adaptive shortening on the concave side of the curve, a fact which may present difficulties in skin closure following surgical treatment. On the convex side of the curve dimples are often present which may in extreme cases resemble scars, especially over the lateral malleolus.

The extent of these deformities is variable. In the mildest cases the deformity consists only of adduction and some rotation of the forefoot. In extreme cases the foot is so deformed that the sole rests on the medial side of the tibia (figs 341(a) and (b)).

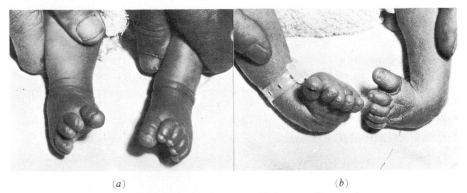

(a)   (b)

FIG. 341.—(a) Mild talipes equino-varus. (b) Severe talipes equino-varus.

Clinical Features.—The condition should be diagnosed at birth. If the deformity is severe the diagnosis is obvious, but mild deformities may be difficult to distinguish from the normal because the new-born infant tends to posture the foot in a position of equino-varus. The normal new-born foot has a greater range of dorsiflexion and eversion than the normal adult foot: it can be dorsiflexed until the dorsum touches the anterior aspect of the shin. If this is impossible, a minor degree of talipes equino-varus exists. Thus part of the examination of a new-born infant should include putting the foot through a full range of movement. If a club foot is detected, the spine and all other joints should always be examined carefully to exclude myelodysplasia and arthrogryphosis. Since the bones of the foot are at this stage largely cartilagenous, radiography is useless.

It must be appreciated that in the world as a whole most deliveries are not supervised by a physician and that therefore a club foot may not present until infancy or later life. By this time the deformity which was present at birth has become fixed and callosities will have developed on the skin of the foot where it bears weight. By adult life (fig. 342) secondary degenerative changes develop in the deformed joints.

Conservative Treatment.—If the deformity is slight, so that the foot can be

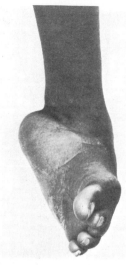

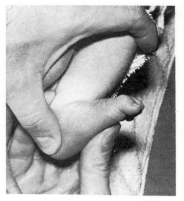

FIG. 343.—The technique of manipulation of the foot (in this case the left) in the treatment of talipes equino-varus. Note the range of dorsi-flexion at this normal infant's foot. The physician's left thumb everts the heel while his right thumb dorsiflexes and everts the foot by pressing on the base of the fifth metatarsal.

FIG. 342.—Untreated tal-ipes equino-varus in an adult.

dorsiflexed to a little beyond the plantigrade position, the mother should be taught to manipulate her child's foot after every feed. The foot is dorsiflexed and everted as shown in fig. 343. Sufficient pressure should be exerted by the mother to blanch her own fingers and this pressure should be maintained for about 2 seconds. The pressure should be released and re-applied over a period of about 5 minutes. Minor deformity can usually be corrected on this regime but the infant should be examined at monthly intervals to ensure that the deformity does in fact steadily diminish.

If initially the foot cannot easily be brought beyond the plantigrade position, the maximum correction obtained by manipulation must be maintained and gradually increased by serial splintage. The neonatal foot is too small to be treated satisfactorily in plaster-of-Paris but correction can usually be maintained by strapping. The foot may be taped to a padded aluminium splint using zinc oxide plaster by the method shown in fig. 344. The splint is removed and reapplied with a little more correction every week. By this method gradual correction of the deformity may be achieved so that, if all goes well, by 3 months the deformity can easily be corrected to beyond the plantigrade position. Splintage is then discontinued and maternal manipulation substituted. If by the age of 1 to 2 months the position of the foot is not satisfactory, plaster-of-Paris is substituted for the aluminium splint: a padded above-knee cast is applied with the knee at 90° of flexion so that the femur can be used to gain a purchase against which to abduct the foot. The cast is applied with the foot in the position of deformity and the foot is manipulated gently into a position of maximum correction as the plaster dries. The plaster is changed at 3 weekly intervals (a procedure in which in an infant may require sedation) until a satisfactory correction has been achieved.

On this regime most club feet should have been corrected by the age of about

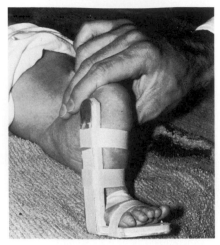

FIG. 344.—Splintage of the foot in the treatment of mild talipes equino-varus.

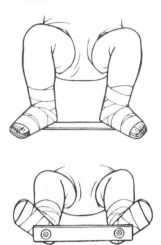

FIG. 345.—Denis Browne splint.

3 months. If they have been, splintage can be discontinued and maternal manipulation substituted.

Denis Browne splints (fig. 345) may be used throughout the day instead of maternal manipulation until the child walks and thereafter they may be used at night.

Treatment by Operation.—A minority of club feet cannot be satisfactorily corrected by manipulation and splintage by the age of 6 weeks. In this event, the soft tissues on the medial side of the foot should be released surgically, the posterior capsule of the ankle divided, and the Achilles tendon elongated sufficiently to render the foot plantigrade.

The Operation of Medial Release and Elongation of the Achilles Tendon for Talipes Equino-Varus.—Through a curved incision posterior and distal to the medial malleolus the ligaments on the medial side of the ankle, talo-navicular and navicular-cuneiform joints are divided. The tendons of tibialis anterior, tibialis posterior, flexor hallucis longus and flexor digitorum longus are divided and elongated by Z-plasty. Division of these structures should allow the forefoot to be abducted and the foot to be everted. When this is done gaps open at the ankle, talo-navicular and navicular-cuneiform joints. Post-operatively, the cartilage covering these bones proliferates rapidly so as to fill the gaps. The Achilles tendon is then elongated by Z-plasty. This may be sufficient to produce the required slight over-correction of the equinus deformity, but if it is not, the posterior capsule of the ankle joint is divided. During this operation the neurovascular bundle posterior and distal to the medial malleolus is carefully safeguarded. Closure of the skin may be difficult in the corrected position. Post-operatively the foot is splinted in a position of slight over-correction using an above-knee plaster as described above.

Treatment of 'Relapsed' Club Foot.—No matter what regime is employed for the initial treatment of club foot, there is a tendency for the condition to relapse over the early years of life and therefore children whose feet have been satisfactorily treated in infancy should be supervised until they are adult. If relapse occurs in a child less than 4 years of age, a soft tissue release as described above is usually sufficient, but in children over the age of 6 this procedure is insufficient. Children presenting with unsatisfactory feet at this age require not only medial release but also resection of bone from the lateral side of the foot. The foot may be likened for this purpose to a horse with two reins: the operation aims to pay out the medial rein (by medial release) and to pull in the lateral rein so as to turn the forefoot in a lateral direction. The lateral rein is shortened by resecting the articular surfaces of the calcaneo-cuboid joint and stapling the calcaneum to the cuboid so as to achieve calcaneo-cuboid fusion. Once calcaneo-cuboid fusion has been obtained, growth of the lateral side of the foot is slowed so that the tendency to relapse is diminished.

Achilles (see footnote Chapter 12).

In adolescent children presenting with an unsatisfactory club foot, the foot may be corrected by the resection of laterally based wedges (followed by fusion of the exposed bony surfaces) from the mid-foot (to correct forefoot adduction) and the os calcis (to correct inversion of the heel).

If the condition presents in adult life, subtalar (triple) fusion with an appropriate resection of bone so as to bring the sole into a plantigrade position is the treatment of choice. Astragalectomy is the alternative if the deformity is severe.

OTHER ANOMALIES

Absence of the Proximal Femur is rare. Radiologically the proximal third of the bone always appears to be absent, but the condition varies in severity since in some patients a cartilagenous femoral head is present although not radiologically visible. Treatment is difficult and the limb tends to become grossly short.

Absence of the Fibula is associated with forward bowing of the tibia, an equino-valgus deformity of the foot and absence of the 5th toe. The condition has some similarity to absence of the radius and its associated deformities. In both these conditions the fibrous tissue replacing the absent bone appears to grow more slowly than adjacent normal tissue so as to draw the limb into a curve concave on the side of the absent bone.

Absence of the Tibia is exceedingly rare and is inevitably followed by amputation.

Congenital Pseudarthrosis of the Tibia is probably a developmental abnormality although some are associated with neurofibromatosis and the possibility cannot be excluded that it is due to an ununited intrauterine fracture. Clinically the condition presents with marked forward angulation of the tibia at birth. Radiologically, a bony discontinuity can be seen at the junction of the middle and lower thirds of the bone and the adjacent bone is sclerotic and thinned. Treatment is difficult, and various procedures have been advocated which range from McFarland's operation in which the angulation is ignored, and a bone graft is placed posterior to the tibia extending from normal bone above to normal bone below the site of the pseudarthrosis, to multiple corrective osteotomies, and, more recently, free vascularized grafts of bone and surrounding muscle.

Congenital Vertical Talus is a rare condition producing a congenitally flat foot. The long axis of the talus is vertically disposed so that the head of the bone is dislocated ventrally from the talo-navicular joint. The os calcis is in a position of equinus. As a consequence of these deformities the sole of the foot is convex downwards and the foot is rigidly flat. The condition must be distinguished from the normal flat foot of infancy in which, although the foot has no medial arch, the sole is flat rather than convex downwards and the foot is mobile. Treatment is difficult and consists of surgical reposition of the talus.

Abnormalities of the Toes correspond to those which may occur in the fingers (see below). In addition one toe, commonly the fifth, may override its neighbour. This is a familial condition which gives rise to no disability and which does not respond to simple conservative measures in infancy. No treatment should be given in infancy but the toe may require either correction or amputation in adult life.

Phocomelia[1] is a condition in which a limb (arm or leg) may totally or partially fail to develop. Although the condition occurs spontaneously attention has been drawn to it recently by the discovery that certain drugs, for example thalidomide, may interfere with the development of the foetus *in utero* to produce phocomelia. Such drugs are known as teratogens.

Treatment.—Under no circumstances should any portion of a phocomelic limb, for example a remnant of a finger attached directly to the trunk at the shoulder, be removed even though it is apparently useless, since such vestiges may enable the child to activate a powered prosthesis if they are capable of the slightest movement.

Minor degrees of phocomelia are represented by the *absence of one or more fingers*. The least rare anomaly of this kind is 'the lobster hand' which has a thumb and only one finger. Function is surprisingly good in hands of this kind and no treatment is indicated.

Syndactyly or Webbed Fingers may be primary, secondary or acquired. Primary syndactyly is often familial and in this condition not only does the skin bridge the two fingers but the bones of the fingers are fused as well. No treatment is successful. Secondary syndactyly is possibly due to amniotic adhesions and in this condition only the skin bridges

---

[1] Phoco (L)=a seal. *i.e.* Like a seal's flipper.

Bryan Leslie McFarland, 1900–1963. Professor of Orthopaedic Surgery, University of Liverpool, England.

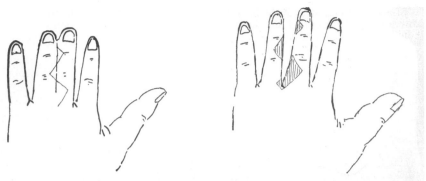

FIG. 346.—Syndactyly. The fingers are divided by means of a modified 'Z' plasty. There is insufficient skin to bridge the gap totally; the defect is therefore covered with a split thickness graft to both fingers. (Simple division with 'Z' plasty will nearly always result in scar contracture across each interphalangeal joint.)

the fingers. They can be separated by plastic surgical procedures (fig. 346). Acquired syndactyly may follow burns and can also be treated by plastic surgery.

Absence of the Radius is a rare anomaly as a consequence of which there is gross radial deviation of the carpus and hand ('club hand'). The thumb is often absent as well. Treatment consists of splintage to hold the deformity, but this is commonly unsuccessful. Fusion of the carpus to the ulna with an extensive release on the lateral side of the wrist may be required followed by pollicisation of the index finger to replace an absent thumb.

Radio-Ulnar Synostosis is an uncommon condition in which the radius and ulna are fused, usually in the proximal 2·5 cm of the bone. Pronation and supination are impossible. No treatment is advised.

Sprengel's Shoulder is a condition in which the whole shoulder girdle, including particularly the scapula, is higher on the affected side than on the opposite side. No treatment is available.

Webbing of the Neck occurs as part of the Klippel-Feil syndrome.

Congenital Pseudarthrosis of the clavicle is a condition similar to congenital pseudarthrosis of the tibia (p. 391). It is confined to females and only the right clavicle is affected.

Cervical rib is dealt with in Chapter 36.

THE SPINE

Fusion of cervical vertebrae occasionally occurs but is not noticeable clinically unless it is part of a more complex deformity such as the Klippel-Feil syndrome.

Hemivertebrae, especially in the dorsal region, may cause scoliosis (Chapter 22).

Myelodysplasia may occur in the sacral or more proximal spine.

Spondylolysis at L5 and L4 may possibly be congenital in origin although it is now widely regarded as being a fatigue fracture. The condition may progress to Spondylolisthesis (Chapter 27).

Sacralisation of the 5th Lumbar Vertebra, Lumbarisation of the 1st Sacral Vertebra and False Joints between the Transverse Processes of L5 and the Sacrum or Ilium are common congenital abnormalities. They may be revealed as a chance x-ray finding, sometimes in patients complaining of back pain. It is uncertain whether or not they themselves are actually responsible for back pain.

BONE DYSPLASIA[1]

These diseases are sometimes referred to as Dysplasias, sometimes as Dystrophies. The term 'dystrophy' strictly implies that the condition is due to faulty

---

[1] There is a regrettable tendency to expect the student to remember the names of all the many dysplasias of bone: very little useful purpose is served by doing so. Many have been given exotic names constructed from a random mixture of Latin and Greek, and in addition have been eponymously named.

Otto Gerhard Karl Sprengel, 1852–1915. Surgeon, Grossherzogliches Krankenhaus (Grand Ducal Hospital), Brunswick, Germany. Described congenital high scapula in 1891.
Maurice Klippel, 1858–1942 and André Feil, 1884–   , both of whom were neurologists in Paris. Described this disease in a joint paper in 1912.

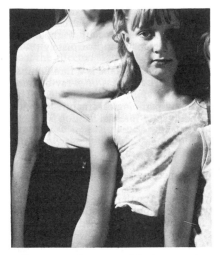

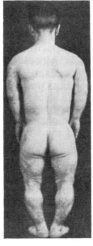

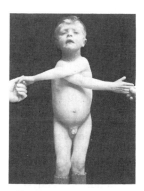

FIG. 347.—Exostoses of the humerus in three sisters.

FIG. 348.—Achondroplasia.

FIG. 349.—Cleidocranial-dysostosis.

nutrition, the term 'dysplasia', to faulty development. Since there is no evidence that any of these diseases have a nutritional basis, the term dysplasia is to be preferred. In some diseases the dysplasia appears to be genetic in origin but in many the cause is unknown. They may affect the skeleton generally, or may be localised to certain areas.

Dysplasias of Orthopaedic Significance

Brittle Bones (Osteogenesis Imperfecta).—The bones are unduly fragile (and the sclerotics of the eyes are blue). Multiple fractures occur following trivial injuries which, because of their multiplicity, result in progressive deformity. The severity of the disease varies; some patients have only one or two fractures, others have many. A child prone to a great many fractures may die before reaching adult life but if it survives, the tendency for the bones to break seems to diminish and even to disappear when skeletal growth ceases. The blood chemistry is normal. The bones are histologically normal and fractures unite uneventfully.

Radiologically the long bones are often osteoporotic, bent and slender; the bone ends may appear large and sometimes cystic.

Treatment.—Individual fractures should be treated on their merits. Should a long bone become unduly deformed it may be cut into several segments and each segment threaded on to an intramedullary nail to correct the deformity.

Multiple Exostoses (Diaphyseal Aclasis) (see also Osteochondroma Chapter 20).—This is a familial disorder more common in males (but see fig. 347). It appears to be due to a failure of bone remodelling at the metaphysis and perhaps to a failure of the control of circumferential growth at the epiphyseal plate. A variable number of exostoses develop in the metaphyseal region of the long bones. The exostoses usually stop growing at the completion of skeletal growth. They may occasion deformity and interfere with the movement of local soft tissues. Patients are otherwise unaffected by the disease, although they are often a little shorter than normal.

Five per cent of patients develop malignant changes in an exostosis. It is unfortunately impracticable to remove all a patient's exostoses in order to prevent this, but should an exostosis become painful, or should it continue to grow after the completion of skeletal growth, it should be removed *en bloc* and sent for histology.

Multiple Chondromatosis (Dyschondroplasia, Ollier's Disease) (see also Chondroma, Chapter 20).—This disease is rare and is not familial. Ossification of the cartilage at the epiphyseal plate is faulty and islands of cartilage remain unossified within the shaft and continue to grow. The disease tends to be unilateral and the affected limb is short.

Louis Xavier Édouard Léopold Ollier, 1830–1900. Professor of Surgery, Lyons, France. Described dyschondroplasia in 1899.

CHAPTER 22

DISORDERS OF THE GROWING SKELETON

Disorders of the epiphyseal plate may manifest themselves functionally, as *disturbances of growth,* or structurally because the epiphyseal plate is a point of mechanical weakness in a long bone, so that *displacement of the epiphysis* may occur. Certain other disorders of the epiphysis affect both its bony and cartilaginous portions and hence are termed '*Osteochondritis*'.

DISTURBANCES OF GROWTH

The spine and limbs normally remain straight as they grow because growth on the two sides proceeds at an equal rate. If the growth rate on one side exceeds the growth rate on the other, the structure will become curved, being convex on the side of more rapid growth. Unequal growth in the spine is the possible cause of idiopathic scoliosis; in the leg it produces bow leg or knock-knee. Torsional deformities are not so easily explicable.

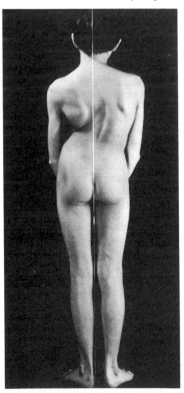

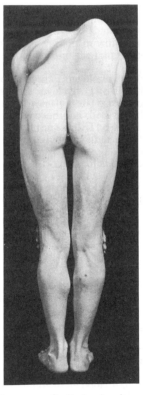

FIG. 350.—Scoliosis: the appearance of the back.

FIG. 351.—Scoliosis showing 'rib hump' revealed in flexion.

Scoliosis

Scoliosis is defined as a lateral curvature of the spine, but the lateral curvature is always complicated by a rotational deformity which, in the thoracic region, is transmitted to the ribs and produces asymmetry of the thorax (figs. 350 and 351). Scoliosis is classified according to its aetiology:—*Idiopathic, Congenital, Paralytic, Postural, Pulmonary.*

1. **Idiopathic Scoliosis.**—This is the most common form of scoliosis, and next to the paralytic form is responsible for the most severe curves, usually in the dorsal spine.

The fundamental cause of idiopathic scoliosis is, as the name implies, unknown. It has been attributed to paralysis of the intrinsic muscles of the spine caused by subclinical poliomyelitis, but its incidence appears to have been unaffected by the control of poliomyelitis, and girls are more commonly affected than boys (whereas poliomyelitis affects both sexes equally). The absence of paralysis in any other muscle group is also against the presence of a paralysing disease. It is, in fact, the complete normality of the rest of the body which distinguishes this condition from paralytic and other forms of scoliosis. A genetic element is almost certainly involved since the disease has a slightly increased familial incidence. Whatever the ultimate cause of the deformity, the proximate cause is a disturbance of vertebral growth.

Clinical Features.—In order that the patient may stand upright, the primary curve in the spine is balanced by secondary curves in the opposite direction above and below it. These compensatory curves bring the shoulders over the pelvis so that in mild primary curves, no gross abnormality may be visible when the patient is dressed. On the other hand, a severe scoliosis is very disfiguring for two reasons: firstly there is a loss of as much as 15 cm of height as the spine becomes 'concertinaed', and secondly a rib hump develops which gives the appearance of a hunchback. Thus the adult picture in a severe case is that of a hunchbacked dwarf. The curves in the spine in a child are to some extent fixed (structural) and to some extent mobile. The latter are caused by the spine collapsing like a concertina under the influence of gravity: if the child is picked up by the head or the axillae, the mobile part of the curve straightens so that only the structural component remains.

The rib hump is characteristic of idiopathic scoliosis and early in the disease is best demonstrated by standing behind the unclothed patient and asking her to touch her toes. Even in the absence of any very marked clinical deviation of the spine, this test will show the asymmetry of the chest (fig. 351). The rib hump is produced by rotation of the dorsal vertebrae (when they are involved in the curve) and, with them, of the ribs. The vertebrae rotate in such a way that the tips of the spinous processes move towards the concave side of the curve and hence, clinically, diminish its apparent severity. On the convex side of the curve, vertebral rotation displaces the ribs posteriorly to form the rib hump. Thus the appearance of the back is a poor guide to the severity of the spinal curve: rotation of the spine diminishes the appearance of the deformity in so far as it brings the spinous processes nearer the midline, but increases it in so far as it produces a rib hump. The only way that the spinal curve can be assessed accurately is by the measurement of x-rays (fig. 352).

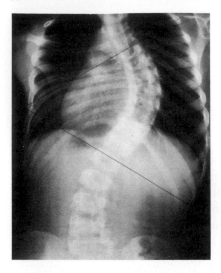

FIG. 352.—The radiological appearance of the spine in scoliosis. The curves are measured accurately on these x-rays; it is useless to depend upon clinical impressions of the appearance of the spine. The angle of the curve is measured by the angle subtended by the upper surface of the first and the lower surface of the last vertebra in the primary curve.

Because of the deformity of the ribs and dorsal spine, a dorsal scoliosis reduces the vital capacity, often seriously so. As a consequence the patient may eventually die of pulmonary infection. Alternatively, secondary pulmonary fibrosis may lead to Cor Pulmonale and right sided heart failure.

Clinical Management.—Idiopathic scoliosis may appear in infancy, in childhood, or during adolescence. In infancy it may resolve spontaneously but a few curves become progressive. All curves, once established as structural and irreversible, may deteriorate rapidly, particularly during periods of skeletal growth. After the completion of spinal growth (which coincides with the fusion of the iliac crest apophyses), deterioration may continue at a slower rate, or, more commonly, will come to a halt. Once advanced structural deformity has developed, nothing can be done to restore the spine to normal. Thus untreated, the condition may rapidly progress until the patient is an irrevocably dwarfed hunchback. Early diagnosis and, if necessary, treatment are therefore essential.

The rate of progression of deformity is hard to predict when the patient is first seen, so that the patient must be examined frequently once the deformity has been noticed. Comparable anteroposterior x-rays of the entire spine should be taken every 3 months during the first year and thereafter at longer intervals until skeletal growth is complete (fig. 352). Without careful radiological supervision a deformity may develop, within a year of the curve first being noticed, which is too severe for full correction.

Treatment.—In most patients who develop a severe curve, a rapid deterioration takes place in the 2 or 3 years prior to skeletal maturity. Mild curves under 20% may be treated *expectantly*, the spine being checked regularly by comparable anteroposterior radiographs, taken in the erect position, until growth is complete.

Conservative or non-operative treatment by the Milwaukee brace[1] and exercises may be successful in preventing deterioration or even producing improvement in curves which advance beyond 20° but do not exceed 40° to 45°. The brace may be used in more severe deformity, particularly in young children, as a holding device until the child reaches the age of ten to twelve years, when definitive surgical treatment can be carried out.

---

[1] The Milwaukee brace was introduced in 1946 by Walter Putnam Blount and his associates at Milwaukee, Wisconsin, U.S.A..

Operative treatment is reserved for those patients who deteriorate during conservative treatment or who have severe curves (over 50°) when first seen. It is preferable to defer surgery until near skeletal maturity because of the unpredictable effects of further growth after spinal fusion. Fusion of the spine is also more difficult to achieve in the young child. Nevertheless correction and fusion in a young child is sometimes carried out where deterioration cannot be controlled in any other way.

The aim of all surgery for scoliosis is correction and fusion of the primary curve. Correction may be pre-operative or it may be part of the surgical procedure.

Techniques of Pre-operative Correction

1. *Risser Turnbuckle Cast.*—This was widely used to obtain pre-operative correction. Method:—A plaster cast is applied, including the head and one thigh, with the patient's spine flexed laterally to produce the maximum correction of the mobile portion of the curve which can be tolerated. The cast is heavily padded with sorbo rubber at the points where pressure is encountered. When the cast is dry it is cut at the level of the apex of the primary curve and angulated so as to produce progressive correction. The new position is held by means of metal turnbuckles incorporated into the plaster. In this way a slow correction can be obtained from week to week and checked by x-ray. When the primary curve has been sufficiently corrected from the cosmetic and functional standpoints (which may not be the point of complete correction in an originally severe curve), a window is cut in the back of the plaster over the primary curve and through this the spine is fused posteriorly. The fusion must extend to include the vertebrae immediately above and below the primary curve. The bone used is generally taken as small chips from the patient's own spine and iliac crests, but the volume can be increased by adding banked bone. If the primary curve is very long, the operation may be performed in stages. After operation, the patient remains in a Risser jacket for 6 months whilst the fusion consolidates. The following year is spent in a carefully moulded corset or Milwaukee brace so that the soft new graft is not subjected to severe bending forces.

2. *Risser Localiser Cast.*—This is applied on a special frame. The patient lies on a narrow strip of canvas and correction is obtained by a combination of longitudinal traction and the localiser which applies pressure over the rib hump to correct the angular and rotation deformities. A well fitting plaster cast is applied in the corrected position. A series of such casts may be used to obtain gradual correction.

3. *Cotrel Dynamic Traction.*—Mobilisation of a rigid curve and some correction may be obtained by this method. The pelvis is anchored to the foot of the bed by a leather harness. A leather head halter is connected via a pulley at the head of the bed to a pair of stirrups through which the child applies longitudinal traction by extending the legs.

4. *Skeletal Traction* may be applied to the skull by means of a 'halo'. This may be combined with skeletal traction to the femora or pelvis. Great forces can be applied by this means and the method requires most careful supervision to avoid neurological and other complications.

Operative Correction

Harrington Instrumentation is the most widely used method of operative correction of scoliosis. After exposure and stripping of the posterior elements of the spine, hooks are applied to the vertebrae beyond the end vertebrae on the concave side of the primary curve. These hooks are connected by a rod which has a ratchet device so that gradual distraction can be applied to produce correction (fig. 353). A compression rod and hooks are sometimes used on the convex side of the curve.

Dwyer's Procedure.—Through an anterior approach the vertebral bodies are exposed on the convex side. A wedge of disc and body is removed at each level of the primary curve. The gaps so created are closed by means of a series of screws in the vertebral bodies. A tension cable passes through the heads of the screws. As each level is corrected the screw head is crimped on to the cable.

Technique of Fusion.—Correction, whether pre-operative or intra-operative, is always combined with spinal fusion. This may be an anterior fusion between the vertebral bodies, or a posterior fusion of the laminae and transverse processes. Or a combination of the two is sometimes used. Additional bone, preferably autogenous bone from the ilium, is commonly employed.

Joseph Charles Risser, Contemporary. Professor of Orthopaedic Surgery, Loma Linda University, Los Angeles, California, U.S.A.
Cotrel, Contemporary. French Orthopaedic Surgeon.
Paul R. Harrington, Contemporary. Associate Professor of Orthopaedic Surgery, Baylor University, Houston, Texas, U.S.A.

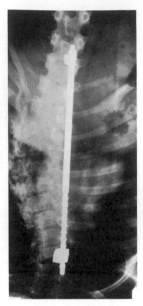

FIG. 353.—A single Harrington rod used to extend and internally fix the concave side of the curve.

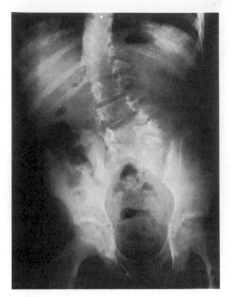

FIG. 354.—Congenital lumbar scoliosis due to a hemivertebra at L.3 fused to L.4. Note associated spina bifida, in this case occult.

Standard posterior fusion consists of meticulous stripping of the primary curve from the midline to the tips of the transverse processes. This is followed by excision of the apophyseal joints and decortication of the laminae and transverse processes. Additional bone is packed into the bed so prepared and the wound is closed.

Following spinal fusion a corrective plaster is maintained until the graft is mature and solid. This may take about a year.

2. Congenital scoliosis is associated with congenital spinal anomalies, such as hemivertebra (fig. 354), errors of segmentation, spina bifida, diastematomyelia, *etc*. Associated anomalies are common particularly of the spinal cord and kidneys. A myelogram and intravenous pyelogram are therefore indicated if surgery is contemplated.

3. Paralytic Scoliosis (Chapter 25).

4. Postural Scoliosis.—This affects children of school age and is characterised by being a simple C curve without rotation of the vertebrae. The deformity is fully mobile and correctable. Formerly quite common, the condition is now almost non-existent, possibly because of the improvement in the general health of the population, the provision of physical education in schools and the avoidance of bad posture when sitting at school desks. Treatment is by gymnastics and lessons in deportment.

5. Pulmonary Scoliosis.—Pulmonary disease may produce scoliosis if disease of one lung results in contraction of the chest wall on that side. In the past the most severe deformities followed the treatment of empyema by prolonged drainage through tubes in the chest wall, but the modern treatment of chest disease has made this one of the rarer causes of scoliosis.

Angular and Torsional Deformities of the Leg

Perfectly normal infants may be noticed by their parents to have some degree of knock-knee or bow-leg (fig. 355), in-toeing or splay-foot when they first stand and begin to walk. These 'deformities' often worry the parents, although they

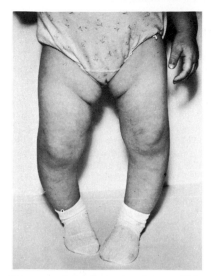

FIG. 355.—Infantile bow-leg. This appearance is within the limits of normal at this age.

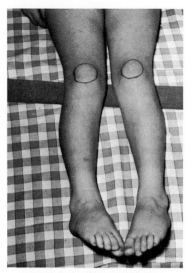

FIG. 356.—Internal tibial torsion (the patellae are ringed) causing in-toeing, and associated knock-knee.

do not upset the child. Typically, medical advice is sought when the child is 3 to 4 years of age. Of the two deformities, knock-knee is slightly the more common.

Knock-Knee and Bow-Leg.—Knock-knee and bow-leg occur as part of the normal pattern of growth, and are only viewed as deformities if they are severe and progressive. Bowing of the knees is normal in the newborn, involving the femur and tibia. This physiological bowing corrects spontaneously during the first 2-3 years of life and usually requires no treatment. Between the ages of 3-7 developmental (idiopathic) knock-knee may be present; all but 2% of these correct spontaneously without treatment.

In countries where malnutrition is common, knock-knee is a frequent complication of rickets, but in the U.K. Vitamin D deficiency rickets is almost non-existent, save in immigrants. Rickets occurs (rarely) as a consequence of a metabolic disorder or malabsorption syndrome (Chapter 50). Epiphyseal dysplasia may cause bow legs (tibia vara) or less commonly knock-knee. Blount's disease, a variety of epiphyseal dysplasia, common in the West Indies, affects only the postero-medial segment of the proximal tibial epiphysis and metaphysis causing bow legs but no other deformity.

The degree of knock-knee can be measured by noting the distance between the medial malleoli. Bow-leg can be measured by noting the distance between the medial femoral condyles. The severity of both 'deformities' is prone to increase when the child stands, so that a measurement should be made both non-weight bearing and weight bearing and should be related to the length of the leg.

In-toeing is somewhat more common than *splay-foot* and is due to torsion of the bones of the legs. If the child is placed supine on the examination couch with the patellae pointing directly forwards, the degree of tibial torsion is revealed by the position taken up by the foot (fig. 356). Most of the torsion is usually in the tibia but some may be in the femur. Here it affects particularly the angle made

Walter Putnam Blount, Contemporary. Orthopaedic Surgeon, Milwaukee, Wisconsin, U.S.A.

in the coronal plane between the femoral neck and the back of the femoral condyles (the 'angle of femoral anteversion').

Treatment.—No form of splintage, or adjustment to the footwear, has any effect upon any of these deformities. No treatment is indicated until the age of 6, since the deformity is usually self-correcting before that age. The parents should therefore be reassured and the child left to live a normal life. If significant deformity persists after the age of 7, the legs can be straightened by osteotomy or by slowing growth on the convex side of the curve. Growth can be slowed either by placing staples across the epiphyseal plates at the knee on the convex side of the limb or by excising this portion of the epiphyseal plate and fusing the epiphysis to the metaphysis with a bone block. The latter operation (epiphyse-odesis) has the advantage over stapling of being more reliable, but the disadvantage of being irreversible. These operations must be carefully timed in relation to the child's growth potential so as to avoid over-correction and under-correction.

Torsional deformities very rarely require correction, but in girls severe in-toeing, as well as being a slight functional disability, may represent a significant cosmetic defect. Should it be severe enough to merit treatment, the only treatment available is to divide the proximal shafts of the femora and de-rotate the bones at the osteotomy site. If the deformity really merits operations of this magnitude, they should be carried out when the child is about 11 years of age.

DISPLACEMENT OF EPIPHYSES

Slipped Femoral Epiphysis

Displacement of the proximal femoral epiphysis may occur in the face of the loads imposed by normal activities—possibly because the normal loads applied to this epiphysis are high, because the epiphyseal plate may not be disposed at right angles to the line of action of the resultant force applied to it, or because the epiphyseal plate is not mechanically normal. The latter possibility is entirely hypothetical. No other epiphysis is liable to displacement in this way. Rarely the normal epiphysis may be displaced by significant violence: this is really a fracture of the femoral neck which happens to involve the epiphyseal plate.

The condition affects children between the ages of 10 and 18 years. It is particu-larly common in boys in a ratio of 3:2 and in over-weight 'hypogonadal' children. It is bilateral in about 20% of patients, the two sides being affected at about the same time. Dunn has observed that, when unilateral, the side of the dominant hand is usually affected first. Relative to the neck, the epiphysis slips downwards and posteriorly. This is the equivalent of the femoral shaft and neck moving into adduction and external rotation in relation to the head.

Two varieties of slipped epiphysis are encountered: 1. acute (*i.e.* sudden) displacement and 2. chronic (*i.e.* slow) displacement.

1. Acute Slipped Epiphysis.—Careful questioning will often reveal that the acute slip is really a final episode in what has been a slow slip, but the symptoms prior to the acute slip can be so slight as to pass without notice. The acute slip often follows an injury of some magnitude, such as a fall off a bicycle or at football, after which the patient is unable to move the hip and experiences severe pain. The clinical signs are identical with those of a subcapital fracture in an adult, and indeed this condition is a subcapital 'fracture' through the epiphyseal plate. X-rays show complete displacement of the epiphysis (fig. 357).

Treatment is similar to that of a subcapital fracture of the femur in a young adult: the epiphysis should be reduced under anaesthesia without undue delay (by internal rotation and abduction) and fixed internally with 3 Moore's pins

Denis Michael Dunn, Contemporary. Orthopaedic Surgeon, Essex County Hospital, Colchester, Essex, England.
Austin Tally Moore, 1899–1963. Orthopaedic Surgeon, Columbia Hospital and the Moore Clinic (which he founded in 1939), Columbia, South Carolina, U.S.A.

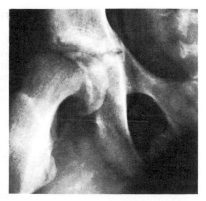

FIG. 357.—Slipped femoral epiphysis.

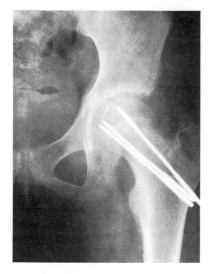

FIG. 358.—Internal fixation of a slipped femoral epiphysis with 3 Moore's pins.

(fig. 358) under x-ray control. The child should remain in bed for 3 weeks, use crutches for 6 weeks, and then walk normally. Contact sports and physical education should be avoided for 1 year. If the child is overweight, he should diet.

2. **Chronic Slipped Epiphysis.**—In this condition the child complains of pain in the hip, thigh or knee, and of a limp, but is able to walk. Pain in the knee may be the only complaint, and if the hip is neither examined nor x-rayed in two planes, the diagnosis will be, and often is, missed; *i.e.*, when the slip is in the early stages and readily treated by pinning *in situ*. On first examination muscle spasm usually causes limitation of movement in all directions, suggesting an inflammatory process in the hip (for example early tuberculosis). Rest in bed for a day or two relieves the pain and spasm: isolated limitation of internal rotation and abduction, and slight apparent shortening of the leg, are then demonstrable.

X-rays will reveal the displacement of the epiphysis (figs 357 and 359) although if only a small slip has occurred it is very difficult to detect in an antero-posterior view. In a lateral view of the hip, however, the posterior displacement of the

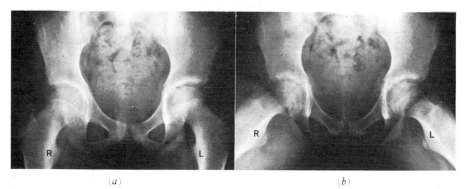

(a)   (b)

FIG. 359.—A minimal slip of the right femoral epiphysis. (a) Apparently normal antero-posterior x-ray. (b) Minimal slip revealed on a lateral x-ray of the femoral neck.

epiphysis is obvious. Therefore a *lateral view of the hip should always be obtained if a slipped femoral epiphysis is suspected clinically.*

In the absence of treatment there is a period of disability during which the slip progresses. This may be followed by spontaneous remission if healing occurs at the epiphyseal plate so that the head of the femur 'unites' with the neck in the slipped position. The patient then recovers almost full function, though with the permanent physical signs of limited abduction (due to the adduction element in the deformity) and limited, or absent, internal rotation (due to the external rotation element in the deformity). Later in life, osteoarthrosis may be expected to develop. Alternatively the period of slow, progressive slipping may culminate in an acute slip.

Treatment.—Attempts to reduce a chronic slipped epiphysis are difficult or impossible, and the attempt may damage the blood supply to the head. If the slip is slight, the position should be accepted and treatment should aim only to prevent further displacement by internal fixation of the epiphysis as for an acute slip. Because this condition is commonly bilateral, the other hip should be watched for any sign of a slip or should be pinned prophylactically.

If gross slipping has occurred by the time the patient is first seen, an osteotomy, either in the neck or trochanteric region of the femur, should be performed to correct the external rotation and adduction deformity. These operations are technically difficult and osteotomies of the neck run the risk of interfering with the blood supply to the epiphysis.

Displacement in Response to Significant Violence.—This may occur at any epiphysis: the condition is really a fracture through or adjacent to a previously normal epiphyseal plate and is described in Chapters 16 and 17.

Cartilage Necrosis (*Waldenstrom's Disease*).—Especially in Negro children, the articular cartilage in the hip may die after the epiphysis has slipped. The aetiology of this condition is unknown. The radiological joint space becomes reduced and the hip loses movement, sometimes completely. No specific treatment is available. Care should be taken to see that the hip, if it does become stiff, does so in the position of function (see Table, Chapter 18). Movement sometimes recovers to some extent spontaneously after a long period of stiffness.

Subclinical Displacement.—It has recently been suggested by Murray that children, especially athletic boys, may sustain subclinical slips which are responsible in later life for many examples of so-called primary osteoarthrosis of the hip.

OSTEOCHONDRITIS

It is a confusing misfortune for the medical student that this one term is used to describe widely differing pathological processes all of which affect epiphyses. The exact nature of the pathological process occurring in the diseases which are given the title 'Osteochondritis' is uncertain because adequate human histological material has rarely been available. It is only possible here to state that three pathological processes appear to be at work: *infarction of epiphyses, traction injuries to epiphyses,* and *transchondral fractures in epiphyses.*

Infarction of Epiphyses

This disorder affects particularly the proximal femoral epiphysis where it is known as Legg-Calvé-Perthes' desease, the distal epiphysis of the second metatarsal bone, where it is known as Freiberg's disease, the navicular where the whole

Johan Henning Waldenstrom, 1877– . Swedish Surgeon.
Ronald Ormiston Murray, Contemporary. Radiologist, Royal National Orthopaedic Hospital, London.
Arthur Thornton Legg, 1874–1939. Orthopaedic Surgeon, The Children's Hospital, Boston, Massachusetts, U.S.A.
Jacques Calvé, 1875–1954. Orthopaedic Surgeon, La Fondation Franco-Américaine, Berck-Plage, France.
Georg Clemens Perthes, 1869–1927. Professor of Surgery, Tübingen, Germany. Legg. Calvé and Perthes all described osteochondritis of the head of the femur independently in 1910.
Albert Henry Freiberg, 1868–1940 (see p. 408).

bone may be regarded as the epiphysis and where it is known as Köhler's disease, and the lunate where it is known as Kienböck's disease. The last three examples may well be due to trauma. Of these, Perthes' disease is the most common and has the most serious consequences for the patient.

Perthes' Disease

Pathology.—Since this disease is not fatal and there is no therapeutic indication for removal of the femoral head in patients suffering from the disease, there have been very few observations of the morbid anatomy of this disease in man. On the basis of the histology obtained from epiphyses infarcted experimentally in animals, the little human histological material that is available, and the radiological appearances of the epiphysis in experimental animals and in man, it may be speculated that the sequence of events in Perthes' disease is as follows:

The presence of an epiphyseal plate results in a peculiarity of the blood supply to the bone of the epiphysis, for blood vessels do not cross the epiphyseal plate. Thus the blood supply to the epiphysis is derived entirely from vessels passing around the periphery of the plate and along the ligamentum teres. (In the adult on the other hand blood not only reaches the head of the femur by the original route, but also by a route within the bone itself across the fused epiphyseal plate.) Since the epiphysis is entirely intra-articular all the epiphyseal vessels run beneath the synovial membrane before entering the epiphysis itself, and thus the epiphysis could be infarcted if, for example, fluid collected in the joint under sufficient pressure to occlude the vessels. It has been suggested that this is in fact the mechanism of infarction in Perthes' disease. (Why certain small bones such as the navicular may also infarct, is uncertain.)

That the spontaneously occurring variety of the disease is caused by infarction of the epiphysis is supported by the fact that similar changes in the femoral head may follow events which would clearly be expected to interrupt its blood supply such as traumatic dislocation of the hip and fractures of the femoral neck in children, immobilisation of the hip in positions in which the capsule is twisted around the femoral neck (as for example occurs in the treatment of congenital dislocation of the hip by immobilisation of the hip in positions of extreme internal or external rotation), and tense haemarthroses in the hip in haemophiliacs.

When the blood supply to the epiphysis has been interrupted the bone dies but the cartilage, nourished from the synovial fluid, survives and proliferates. Thus the bony epiphysis on the infarcted side appears smaller (because it fails to grow) and the radiological joint space appears larger (because the cartilage grows, and possibly because an effusion is present in the joint).

Although the cartilage survives for some weeks upon synovial nutrition, some chondrocytes eventually die, especially in the basal layers, perhaps because proliferation of the overlying cartilage makes it impossible for them to receive an adequate supply of nutrients by diffusion from the synovial surface. Dead cartilage (1) is probably softer than normal so that it may deform under normal loads, and (2) may not ossify.

Granulation tissue invades the infarcted epiphysis by overgrowing the margins of the epiphyseal plate. The dead bone is partly resorbed and partly entombed in new bone deposited on a scaffold of the old; a process known as creeping substitution. Before it is replaced, the dead bone may fail mechanically (*i.e.* may fracture) especially if the cartilage is soft, perhaps because it fatigues. Thus, the bony nucleus of the epiphysis, like the cartilaginous portion, may deform in response to normal loads.

Once the trabeculae become crushed, creeping substitution can no longer occur and the necrotic area must be removed or replaced by a fibrocartilaginous material having some of the appearances of immature cartilaginous fracture callus. This material is soft and biologically 'plastic' so that it may be moulded. As healing occurs it is replaced by woven bone by a process of membraneous ossification.

The epiphyseal plate is abnormal in all cases with loss of normal architecture and also a failure of normal ossification producing some widening of the growth plate. This will result in a growth disturbance which will further contribute to the deformity of the femoral head.

As the bone is revascularised the deeper layers of the overlying cartilage are progressively, but patchily, converted into bone by endochondral ossification. The combination of creeping substitution of the bony nucleus and patchy endochondral ossification in the

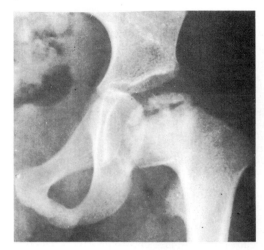

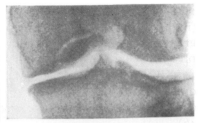

FIG. 361.—Osteochondral fracture frag-ment separating from the medial femoral condyle.
(Professor Carl Krebs, Aarhus, Denmark.)

FIG. 360.—Radiological appearance of Perthes' disease of one year's duration.

cartilage makes the epiphysis appear radiologically dense, fragmented, and deformed. Although the bony nucleus of the epiphysis always appears to be deformed radiologically, the femoral head itself may not be so: a fact which can be observed experimentally with the naked eye or clinically by arthrography.

Clinical Features.—Boys are affected more commonly than girls in the ratio of 4 to 1. The reason for this is uncertain. The condition usually presents between 3 and 10 years. 18% of cases are bilateral. The child presents with pain often felt in the anterior thigh and knee, and is noticed by the parents to limp particularly in the evening and after exercise. There may be a history of injury in the past but there is commonly a silent period between this incident and the onset of symptoms.

Clinical examination will reveal apparent shortening of the limb, wasting of the quadriceps and restriction of hip movements by muscle spasm with pain at the extremes of movement. This muscle spasm will commonly resolve in a few days of bed rest with skin traction. Routine examination should exclude the presence of inguinal hernia and genito-urinary anomalies as there is known to be an association between these conditions and Perthes' disease. All haematological investigations are normal.

Radiological Features.—This process passes through a series of stages. At first the ossific nucleus appears normal save that it is smaller than that on the other side. The radiological joint space however becomes greater than the opposite side. In part this is due to an effusion and in part to the continuing growth of the cartilaginous portion of the femoral head. In the second stage part or all of the bony epiphysis becomes crushed or fragmented producing a broad and flattened femoral head in many cases (fig. 360). In the long term the prognosis varies with the degree of this involvement (Catterall). In the third phase the crushed area is reabsorbed and finally replaced by bone. This is followed by a long phase of remodelling continuing throughout the remainder of growth.

At the stage of fragmentation it is possible to predict radiologically those cases in which severe flattening will occur. These cases may be considered to be 'At Risk' and have the following radiological signs: (i) A lytic area in the lateral part

Anthony Catterall, Contemporary. Orthopaedic Surgeon, Charing Cross and Royal National Orthopaedic Hospitals, London.

of the epiphysis and adjacent metaphysis, (ii) calcification lateral to the epiphysis, (iii) lateral subluxation, (iv) extensive metaphyseal change and (v) a horizontal growth plate. Treatment is indicated when two or more of the 'At Risk' signs are present.

It is important to differentiate the changes already described from those conditions which produce a Perthes-like change. They are multiple epiphyseal dysplasia, cretinism, infection, sickle cell disease and Gaucher's disease (Chapter 46).

Prognosis.—The long term complication of this disease is osteoarthritis of the hip. The symptoms of this may be delayed for 30–40 years. The more deformed the femoral head at the time of healing the greater the chance of early symptoms. The prognosis depends on the age of the child at the onset of the disease. This is because young children are lighter and less likely to damage the epiphysis and also have longer to remodel the femoral head after the disease has healed. Girls have a worse prognosis than boys.

Treatment.—There is no specific treatment for the underlying pathology. The object of treatment must be to prevent severe flattening of the femoral head. In the past it was the practice to confine the child to bed for 2–3 years to prevent this deformation but subsequent research has demonstrated that this will not alter the natural history.

Because the femoral head, particularly its lateral cartilaginous part, is outside the acetabulum and also because the movements of the hips are reduced, the principles of treatment have been redefined as: (1) Restoration of movement by (i) Containment of the femoral head within the acetabulum (ii) Mobilisation of the reduced hip (2) Prevention of further ischaemia by (i) Relief of further stress to the hip (ii) Prevention of injury.

Containment of the femoral head within the acetabulum may be achieved by a broomstick ('Broomstick plasters') holding the legs apart in abduction and internal rotation. Active movement is encouraged while the legs are in the plaster, to restore the normal range of movement to the hip.

Once the movement of the hip has been restored the clinician must decide how to maintain the reduction achieved. He can either do it by retaining the broomstick plaster or by realigning the leg leaving the femoral head in the reduced position. This may be achieved by femoral osteotomy of the varus (adduction) and rotation type or by the innominate osteotomy of Salter. It must be stressed that 60% of cases achieve a good result without treatment and therefore in mild forms of the disease where there is a minor involvement and a good range, simple out-patient supervision is all that is required.

Infarction of the Navicular (Köhler's disease).—This condition presents with physical signs and radiological appearances analogous to those of Perthes' disease. The affected bone becomes painful and tender and apparent radiological deformation occurs. Treatment consists of relieving weight from the affected foot until revascularisation and a normal bony radiological appearance have been achieved.

Avascular Necrosis of the Lunate (Kienböck's Disease).—This may follow serious injury, for example dislocation, in which all the soft tissue attachments of the bone are ruptured so that the bone is infarcted. It may also follow trivial injuries, sometimes after an interval of years. Sometimes there is no history of trauma at all. The wrist becomes painful and stiff. Radiologically the lunate is dense and deformed. Long-standing cases are complicated by osteo-arthrosis.

Treatment.—The patient should be advised to adjust his occupation so as to limit the demands on his wrists. If this is impossible, the lunate is excised and replaced by a silastic implant or the wrist can be arthrodesed.

Infarction of the Head of the Second Metatarsal (Frieberg's disease).—This condition is not entirely similar to the two foregoing diseases in that infarction occurs in a rather

Robert Salter, Contemporary. Professor of Orthopaedic Surgery, Hospital for Sick Children, Toronto, Ontario, Canada.
Alban Köhler, 1874–1947. Radiologist, Wiesbaden, Germany. Described this disease of the tarsal scaphoid in 1908.
Robert Kienböck, 1871–1953. Professor of Radiology, Vienna. Described this condition in 1910.
Albert Henry Freiberg, 1868–1940. Professor of Orthopaedic Surgery, Cincinatti University, Cincinatti, Ohio, U.S.A. Described infarction of the second metatarsal bone in 1914.

older age group, namely in adolescents aged between fifteen and twenty-five years. The 'disease' may in fact be due to a compression fracture of the epiphysis rather than to infarction (see Transchondral Fractures below). Treatment is difficult and consists of attempting to weight-relieve the affected bone by an appropriately placed insole. If pain persists, the head of the second metatarsal should be elevated by an osteotomy of the shaft, or by an excision arthroplasty (excising the base of the proximal phalanx).

Traction Injuries to Epiphyses

Pathology.—Because the epiphyseal plate represents a point of weakness in the long bones, mechanical failure may occur in the region of the epiphyseal plate which is imposs- ible in the adult. Slipped femoral epiphysis (p. 402) is one example of mechanical failure of this kind. Certain epiphyseal plates may be loaded in tension, a mode of loading which they do not appear to be well able to withstand, so that traction injuries form another example of such lesions. These injuries produce physical and radiological signs which in some ways resemble those associated with other disorders of the epiphysis and which for this reason have been named as 'Osteochondritis'.

These injuries occur in the knee, the heel, and the spine. In the knee the tibial tubercle, which is part of the proximal tibial epiphysis, may gradually be avulsed from the shaft, which is part of the metaphysis. This condition is known as '*Osgood-Schlatter's disease*'. A corresponding condition may occur at the distal pole of the patella where the condition is known as '*Sinding Larsen's disease*'. At the heel the posterior epiphysis of the os calcis may be partially avulsed by the Achilles' tendon. This condition is known as '*Sever's disease*'.

In the spine the disease may occur in the vertebral bodies where it is known as '*Scheuer- mann's disease*'. The disease affects particularly the 6th to the 10th thoracic vertebrae, and the lumbar spine. The vertebral bodies become narrowed anteriorly, especially in the thoracic region, to produce a smooth, rigid kyphosis. In the lumbar region slight anterior narrowing occurs but this is not clinically evident since the normal lumbar spine is lordotic. The epiphysis may fail to fuse with the rest of the vertebral body and thus appears as a separate island of bone in the adult. Probably because the disease is associated with a disturbance of the intervertebral disc, the corresponding disc spaces are narrowed. It may even be that this condition is not strictly a traction injury to the epiphysis at all, but rather represents an extrusion of nuclear material through the epiphyseal plate, separating the epiphysis from the metaphysis. Whatever their cause, these events alter the mechanics of the spine and thus may cause back pain.

Treatment consists of resting the involved epiphysis until pain and tenderness have subsided. This usually takes about 6 weeks. No persistent disability follows these con- ditions save in the spine where there may be a permanent increase in the normal dorsal kyphosis, sometimes accompanied by back pain.

Transchondral Fractures (Osteochondritis Dissecans). Loose Body (and see Chapter 15).

Pathology.—A transchondral fracture is one in which the fracture line runs entirely in articular bone, that is to say in bone covered by articular cartilage. Because articular cartilage is more elastic than bone, strains which fracture the bone may not break the cartilage. Thus the bony fragment may be held in its bed by an intact bridge of cartilage. The cartilage is nourished from the synovial fluid and hence remains healthy. In contrast the bone dies because its blood supply is completely interrupted at the fracture line. If the cartilage all round the fracture breaks at the time of injury, the fragment separates to form a *loose body* in the joint. If the cartilage remains partly or completely intact, the fracture may unite and the fragment may become revascularised. Sometimes, however, especially if the fragment is large, revascularisation fails and the dead fragment of cartilage- capped bone may then separate to form a *loose body* long after the injury. Such injuries may occur in adults as well as in children, but in the latter, if the bone has an epiphysis, it is the epiphysis which is involved.

The connection between the injury and the formation of the loose body is often unprov- able because the violence required to produce the fracture is slight and because the injury and the formation of the loose body are widely separated in time. The suspicion therefore arises that the formation of some loose bodies may not be due to injury at all. This suspicion is strengthened by the occasional spontaneous development of loose bodies in several joints of the same patient. It has been suggested that this may be due to thrombosis

Robert Bayley Osgood, 1873–1956. Professor of Orthopaedic Surgery, Harvard University, Boston, Mass., U.S.A.
Carl Schlatter, 1864–1934. Professor of Surgery, Zurich, Switzerland. Osgood and Schlatter described osteochondritis of tibial tubercle independently in 1903.
Christian Magnus Falsen Sinding Larsen. Norwegian Surgeon. Described this disease of the patella in 1921.
James Warren Sever, 1878–1964. Orthopaedic Surgeon, Children's Hospital, Boston, Mass., U.S.A. Described apophysitis of the os calcis in 1912.
Holger Werfel Scheuermann, 1877–1960. Radiologist, Municipal Hospital, Sundby, Copenhagen. Described juvenile kyphosis in 1920.

of an end-artery supplying the involved bone. In these cases of uncertain aetiology, it is reasonable to retain the term *Osteochondritis Dissecans*.

Clinical Features.—The condition may affect any convex articular surface but is particularly common in the femoral condyles, and the capitellum. Less commonly it occurs in the head of the femur and the dome of the talus (fig. 294 (*b*)). An unseparated fragment causes aching pain and an effusion in the joint. The lesion can be displayed radiologically but only if views are carefully chosen so as to place the lesion on the 'skyline' (fig. 361). Tomographs may be required. A separated fragment forms a loose body which may lock the joint. Radiologically the loose body and its parent cavity can be seen.

Treatment.—If the fragment separates totally, the loose body must be removed. The crater from which it was derived should be ignored and will gradually be filled with fibrocartilage. If the fragment is not displaced from its parent cavity when first detected, a state of affairs which applies particularly to the knee, it should be held in place by two pins. (Smillie pins) in the hope that it will eventually re-unite. If the end-result of a transchondral fracture is an irregular articular surface, osteoarthrosis is likely in later life.

Ian Scott Smillie, Contemporary. Emeritus Professor of Orthopaedic Surgery, Dundee, Scotland.

CHAPTER 23

GENERALISED DISEASES OF BONE

Paget's Disease (syn. Osteitis Deformans)

The disease, of unknown aetiology, is rare under the age of 40 but becomes progressively more common as age advances, finally reaching an incidence of about 10% in people over 90 years of age. Males are slightly more commonly affected than females. The condition can affect any bone in the body and many bones may be affected in the same patient. The spine, the skull, the pelvis, the femora and the tibiae are the most commonly involved bones.

The pathological process begins with osteoclastic resorption of existing bone. This is followed by osteoblastic regeneration of a primitive coarse-fibred bone which is highly vascular. This process affects both cortical bone, which becomes increasingly thick and less well demarcated from adjacent cancellous bone, and cancellous bone where massive ill-formed trabeculae replace the normal structure. Finally the affected bones assume the mosaic pattern of lamellar bone.

Clinical Features.—Most cases of Paget's disease are discovered incidentally. However as the disease gives rise to visible thickening of the involved bones, a

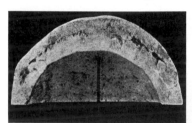

FIG. 362.—Paget's disease of the skull
(*R.C.S. Museum.*)

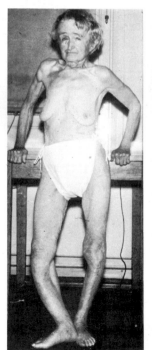

FIG. 363.—Paget's disease affecting the skull, which is large, and the legs (especially the right tibia) where the bones are thickened and bowed.

FIG. 364.—Paget's disease involving the tibia showing thickening of the bone, bowing, a pathological fracture anteriorly, and mottled sclerosis.

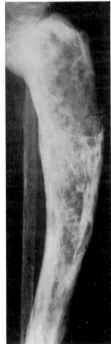

FIG. 363.

FIG. 364.

Sir James Paget, 1814–1899. Surgeon, St. Bartholomew's Hospital, London. In three classical papers (1877, 1882 and 1889) he described the advanced polyostotic form of the disease and most of the known complications.

complaint of increased thickness may be the presenting symptom. This applies particularly to the skull (fig. 362) where an inability to wear his normal size of hat may draw the patient's attention to the first changes. Also the pathological process may be painful, especially in the weight-bearing bones where deformity is taking place: the patient will then present complaining of a dull, continuous aching pain localised in the involved bone. The new bone formed is less strong than normal bone and, either because it deforms under load or because its deposition is irregular, it tends to bend producing typical bowing of the involved bones especially in the leg (fig. 363). The consequent deformity may be noticed by the patient. Attention is not infrequently drawn to the presence of the disease by the development of one of its complications (see below).

Physical Signs.—Subcutaneous bones may be obviously thickened and bowed, but otherwise there are no significant findings. Because of the massive increase in vascularity of the bones, the involved parts of the skeleton may become the functional equivalent of arterio-venous fistulae and as a consequence lead to left ventricular failure.

Radiological Appearances.—The involved bone is bigger than normal, the cortex is thickened, and the medullary cavity is patchily sclerotic. The normal clear line of demarcation between cortex and medullary canal becomes blurred. The long bones may be deformed. The final appearance of the bone is one of predominant sclerosis with a typical mottled appearance (fig. 364).

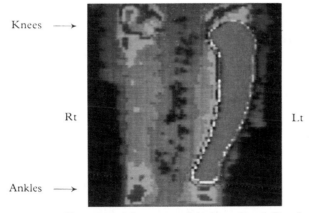

FIG. 365.—A bone scan of the lower legs in Paget's disease showing markedly increased uptake in the involved tibia on the left.

Special Investigations.—The serum calcium and serum phosphorus are usually within normal limits. The serum alkaline phosphatase is often very high, but this finding is in no way specific for it is a feature of most diseases associated with an increase in osteoblastic activity. The urinary excretion of hydroxy-proline is often elevated because of the increase in bone turnover, and can be used to monitor the effects of treatment. A bone scan, using one of the bone-seeking isotopes, shows markedly increased uptake in the involved areas of the skeleton (fig. 365).

Treatment.—The pain of Paget's disease can now be relieved by treatment with calcitonin. The extent to which this hormone also reverses the pathological process is uncertain but current evidence suggests that it does so to a significant extent. Whether or not it affects the incidence of complications, especially of malignant change, remains to be seen.

Complications

1. **Osteogenic sarcoma** develops in approximately 5% of patients with Paget's disease. The neoplasm is extremely malignant and death is almost invariable once this complication has developed. Treatment should be along the lines described for osteogenic sarcoma in general (Chapter 20).

2. **Pathological fracture** may occur through long bones involved with Paget's disease. The fractures are usually transverse and the appearance of a transverse fracture in the tibia or femur in a patient over the age of 40 whose bone looks a little thickened should raise the suspicion of Paget's disease. Union may, but not always, occur uneventfully whether treatment is by internal fixation or by external splintage. Internal fixation may be indicated because of the age of the patient, but is usually difficult since the medullary canal has been lost, the bone is extremely vascular, and can be either very hard or very soft.

3. **Osteoarthrosis** occasionally develops in joints adjacent to deformed bone, but it is by no means certain that the incidence of osteoarthrosis is in fact higher than in the uninvolved population of similar age.

4. **Paraplegia** is a rare complication of involvement of the vertebrae.

5. **Heart failure** (high output) may occur due to the arteriovenous shunts within the affected bones.

6. **Deafness** may occur due to bony involvement of the middle ear.

Osteoporosis

This condition may occur in a localised form following local inflammation or disuse (due for example to paralysis or immobilisation). A generalised form may develop either primarily, and as such represents an almost invariable concomitant of increasing age, or secondarily following endocrine disorders or certain drugs (*e.g.* steroids).

Senile osteoporosis first becomes manifest in women shortly after the menopause and in men at around the age of 65, but it is rarely a clinical problem in women before the age of 65, and in men before the age of 85. There is no precise dividing line between normality and osteoporosis and the latter can be detected radiologically only when about 40% of the skeleton has been lost. There is now evidence that the major cause of osteoporosis in ageing women is the change in their hormonal environment after the menopause. Disuse (secondary to the generally reduced level of activity in the elderly) may also play a part. It is also suggested that loss of bone in the elderly may be due in part to osteomalacia (p. 413) as well as to osteoporosis.

The condition is characterised by a reduction in the amount of bone in the skeleton, which is only radiologically manifest when approximately 40% of the skeleton has been lost. At this time the cortices of the long bones are noticeably thinner and cancellous bone less dense than normal. As a consequence of the latter change, the invertebral discs may intrude into the centres of the vertebral bodies to produce a typical 'fish head' appearance. Histologically the bone is perfectly normal and there are no demonstrable metabolic changes.

The disease itself is symptomless and only constitutes a clinical problem in so far as osteoporotic bone is more liable to fracture than normal bone. Fractures commonly associated with senile osteoporosis include Colles' fracture, fractures of the proximal humerus, crush fractures of the vertebral bodies, fractures of the femoral neck and intertrochanteric fractures of the femur. The first two and the last of these fractures are always associated with a clear-cut history of a fall and as such are perhaps as much due to the unsteadiness of the elderly as to their osteoporosis. Fractures of the vertebral bodies and of the femoral neck, on the other hand, may occur without history of injury and there is now evidence that they represent the end-result of progressive fatigue fracture of isolated trabeculae. Such fractures can be attributed to the increased stresses which osteoporotic bone must encounter because of its reduced mass.

Fractures present either obviously, in the case of the Colles' fracture or fracture of the femoral neck, or as back pain in the case of compression fractures of vertebral bodies. The fracture should be treated on its own merits, ignoring the presence of osteoporosis, which does not interfere with healing. No specific treatment is available for osteoporosis itself.

Deficiency Diseases Affecting Bone

A deficiency of certain vitamins may lead to abnormalities in the skeleton. In this section these diseases will be mentioned only in the briefest outline in so far as the bony complications demand orthopaedic treatment. The student is referred for a more detailed treatment of the diseases themselves to appropriate textbooks.

Rickets.—Rickets is due to a dietary or absorption deficiency of vitamin D. Uncalcified bone matrix is deposited normally but fails to calcify. Histologically, the bone contains large areas of uncalcified matrix which is known as osteoid. The disease affects both bones formed by endochondral ossification and bones, such as the skull, which ossify in membrane.

The disease usually presents in infants, but may develop at any time during the period of growth if the diet becomes deficient in vitamin D. Clinically, characteristic abnormalities develop in the skeleton: the costochondral junctions enlarge to cause the 'ricketed rosary', the skull develops frontal bosses, the pelvis becomes triradiate and the long bones bow under the body weight (particularly the lower third of the tibia which bows forwards and outwards with buttress formation on the concave side). In general the stature is stunted.

Treatment.—The treatment of the disease itself consists of the administration of vitamin D. Early bone deformities may respond to appropriate splinting, but if they are more than trivial they will require correction by manual breaking of the bone (osteoclasis) in the third and fourth year of life, or osteotomy thereafter. The tibia is the bone most commonly requiring orthopaedic treatment.

Osteomalacia is the analogue of rickets occurring in the adult skeleton. Once again excessive osteoid is demonstrable histologically and the bones become unduly soft so that they deform under the body weight. Treatment consists of correction of deformities by osteotomy where necessary and practicable, together with the administration of vitamin D.

Other Causes of Excessive Osteoid in Growing and Adult Bones.—In children phosphaturia (synonyms—renal tubular rickets, vitamin D resistant rickets), and Fanconi's syndrome (amino acid-uria) both produce the changes of rickets. In adults renal tubular acidosis produces the changes of osteomalacia. Renal failure occurring from whatever cause in children may produce dwarfism and occasionally the appearance of rickets, whilst in the adult it occasionally produces osteomalacia and/or osteitis fibrosa. Osteoid tissue is often present in excess in hyperparathyroidism, together with the more specific lesion of osteitis fibrosa.

Guido Fanconi, Contemporary. Emeritus Professor of Paediatrics, Zürich, Switzerland. Described this syndrome in 1936.

Scurvy.—Scurvy is a deficiency disease attributable to a lack of vitamin C. In the skeleton endochondral ossification ceases but chondrocyte proliferation continues. As a consequence a chaotic state of affairs develops in the epiphyseal line: fractures may occur following insignificant trauma and haemorrhages are common. Haemorrhages occurring either around the epiphyseal line or subperiostally in the shaft, may ossify to give rise to bony swellings.

Treatment consists of the administration of vitamin C.

Endocrine Diseases Affecting Bone

Adrenalcorticosteroids in excess produce osteoporosis. This may occur either second-arily following increased stimulation from the pituitary, or primarily as a consequence of an adrenal cortical tumour. High doses of steroids administered therapeutically have the same effect of reducing skeletal mass. This complication occasionally develops during the course of the treatment of rheumatoid arthritis and greatly increases the disability due to the disease itself.

Disorders of the pituitary may affect the skeleton not only indirectly via the adrenal cortex, but also directly. A deficiency of growth hormone developing during the growth phase produces pituitary dwarfism. Excessive growth hormone consequent upon the development of a pituitary adenoma produces pituitary gigantism if the tumour develops before the epiphyses have closed, and acromegaly if it develops after the epiphyses have closed. No orthopaedic treatment is available for any of these conditions.

Hyperparathyroidism affects the skeleton. The disease itself is dealt with in Chapter 38. The bone changes in hyperparathyroidism retain the name (osteitis fibrosa cystica[1]) which they were given when they were thought to represent a separate disease entity. Histologically, marked osteoclastic activity can be seen and the resorbed bone is replaced with fibrous tissue to produce the so-called 'brown tumours' (see Giant Cell Tumour, Chapter 20). As a consequence, patchy osteolytic lesions develop throughout the skeleton and pathological fractures may occur through them. It is of particular diagnostic import-ance that resorption affects the terminal phalanges in the hand and the alveolar margins in the jaws, so that the radiological appearances of the hands and jaws are characteristic. The blood chemistry is abnormal: the serum calcium is raised, the serum phosphorus lowered, and the alkaline phosphatase usually somewhat raised.

Orthopaedic treatment is required only for pathological fractures. These are treated on their merits. They unite satisfactorily provided the underlying endocrine disease is treated.

---

[1] Osteitis fibrosa cystica is also known as one of von Recklinghausen's disease (see p. 106).

CHAPTER 24

DISEASES OF MUSCLES, TENDONS AND FASCIAE

NON-ARTICULAR RHEUMATISM

'Non-articular Rheumatism' is a poor, but not easily abandoned, name for a group of common conditions, the pathology (or pathologies) of which are not understood. The conditions present as pain localised to the aponeurotic attachment of muscle to bone. The commonest sites for this to occur are 1. the attachment of the extensor muscles of the forearm to the lateral epicondyle of the humerus (where the condition is called 'tennis elbow'), 2. the attachment of the flexor muscles to the medial epicondyle ('golfer's elbow'), 3. the attachment of the rotator cuff of shoulder muscles, especially the portion made up by the tendon of the supraspinatus muscle, to the greater tuberosity of the humerus, 4. the attachment of the ligamentum patellae to the patella or the tibia, 5. the attachment of the Achilles' tendon to the os calcis, 6. the attachment of the plantar fascia to the os calcis. Similar symptoms commonly develop in the muscles of the back and it is possible that here they are due to the same pathological process affecting the bony attachment of one of the back muscles. In the back, however, localised pain of this kind has been attributed to reflex muscular spasm arising from some (unknown) deep-seated lesion in the spine or alternatively to 'fibrositic nodules'. (The terms 'fibrositic nodule' and 'fibrositis', like the term used here 'non-articular rheumatism', are meaningless and do not advance our understanding of the condition but at least the latter does not imply a knowledge of the pathology.)

The tender area, especially at the lateral epicondyle of the humerus and at the attachment of the rotator cuff, has been explored on various occasions but significant morbid anatomical features have not always been demonstrated. It seems that the condition may be caused by a tear in the collagen fibres attaching the muscle to the bone which, because it is repeatedly loaded does not heal satisfactorily. The tear may be caused by overt injury, by the loads imposed by excessive but normal activity (as for example, at the elbow, by typing or tennis: hence 'tennis elbow') or by weakening of tissues following an interruption of their blood supply (as for example happens in the rotator cuff and possibly the Achilles' tendon).

The specific features of these lesions are as follows:

Tennis Elbow.—The patient complains of pain in the elbow at rest and in particular when he uses the hand and hence contracts the wrist and finger extensors. The attachment of the extensor muscles of the forearm to the lateral epicondyle is tender, and active resisted contraction of the extensor muscles of the fingers or the wrist provokes pain at the elbow.

Golfer's Elbow.—This is a precisely similar condition to tennis elbow, save that it affects the attachment of the flexor muscles of the forearm to the medial epicondyle. Tenderness is often less well localised than in tennis elbow (and treatment is even less satisfactory).

Supraspinatus Tendonitis.—In this condition pain is felt in the shoulder, especially on abduction and rotation, and localised tenderness is present over the insertion of the supraspinatus tendon.

A feature of supraspinatus tendontis or of any painful pathological process around the shoulder is the rapid onset of shoulder stiffness. This is probably to be attributed to the close proximity of the humerus to the acromion so that adhesions readily form between the two bones (involving the rotator cuff and the sub-acromial bursa) which limit movement of the humerus on the scapula.

In supraspinatus tendonitis, the pathology is a little more clearly understood than in other examples of this condition. Injection studies of post-mortem material have shown that the blood supply to the supraspinatus tendon commonly becomes defective in middle and later years—probably because of compression of the tendon between the acromion and the proximal humerus. As a consequence the tendon is prone to degenerate and may even rupture spontaneously (see Tendon Ruptures, p. 417). Progressive calcification of the tendon may develop and be obvious radiologically (fig. 366).

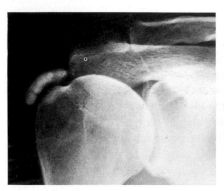 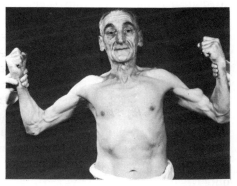

FIG. 366.—Supraspinatus calcification. Shadow of calcium seen lying above the head of the humerus lateral to the outer margin of the acromion.

FIG. 367.—Spontaneous rupture of the tendon to the long head of the left biceps muscle. Note that when the muscle contracts the long head bunches near the elbow.

Pain occurs on moving the humerus, especially as the inflamed portion of the supraspinatus tendon passes between the head of the humerus and the acromion: this occurs in the middle third of the abduction arc so as to give a typical clinical picture, described as the *painful arc syndrome* in which the patient is freely able to abduct his arm through the initial 60°, has pain raising the arm through the next 60°, but thereafter is able to abduct the arm painlessly. Pain recurs as the arm is brought down to the side through the same mid 60° of abduction. As a consequence of the pain provoked by movement, such patients naturally tend to protect the shoulder by holding it still. Adhesions now form which limit shoulder movement mechanically. Thus the patient initially complains of pain in the shoulder and soon thereafter notes stiffness. The pain and stiffness tend, in the absence of treatment, gradually to increase for 3 months but thereafter remain static—usually for a further period of 3 months. During the latter half of this second period pain gradually settles in the shoulder so that now the patient finds it is more comfortable to move it. Probably as a consequence of increasing comfort, the range of movement gradually increases until by about the end of 9 months the whole cycle is completed and the joint returns essentially to normal. This sequence of events has been given several names of which probably the best is *frozen shoulder*. It should be clearly understood that a frozen shoulder is not a specific clinical or pathological event: it is merely a response of the shoulder to any locally painful pathological process.

Patellar Tendonitis.—Occasionally the ligamentum patellae may become painful and tender in adults either at its attachment to the patella or at its distal attachment to the tibia. Pain is felt on active extension of the knee.

Plantar Fasciitis is described in Chapter 12.

Achilles' Tendonitis is described in Chapter 12.

Treatment.—No satisfactory treatment is available for these conditions. The patient should be advised that the condition is normally self-limiting and that he should, so far as possible, avoid powerful contraction of the involved muscles without keeping the joint itself still: movement in the absence of powerful muscular activity is the objective. Local injections of steroid and local anaesthetic into the tender area sometimes bring about dramatic relief. When the supraspinatus tendon is calcified it may suddenly become excruciatingly painful. Such pain can be relieved by incision and evacuation of the calcareous deposit. Surgical treatment is required, rarely, if these conditions persist and are severely painful. The procedures aim to release or decompress the involved tendon but, like conservative measures, they do not always bring symptomatic relief.

PATHOLOGICAL TENDON RUPTURES

The supraspinatus tendon may rupture spontaneously following interruptions in its blood supply in middle-aged or elderly adults. The tear may include only the supraspinatus tendon or may extend throughout the rotator cuff. The rupture often occurs following insignificant violence or even as part of normal everyday activities. The patient complains of sudden pain in the shoulder the severity of which usually masks the important physical sign: an inability to initiate abduction. For this reason and because once abduction has been started passively (for example by the patient tilting his body to the affected side so that abduction is initiated by gravity) the deltoid can continue abduction in a normal way, the diagnosis is frequently missed.

The disability, even if the lesion is left untreated, is very slight. This is fortunate since the only form of treatment available is suture of the tendon and this is frequently unsatisfactory—partly because the tendon holds sutures poorly, and partly because the operation often results in adhesion formation and hence in a stiff shoulder. Thus if the patient is prepared to accept the disability, it is probably best to leave the condition untreated.

The long head of biceps brachii may rupture in the bicipital groove. This is probably due to attrition and again occurs spontaneously. The patient complains of sudden pain in the upper arm followed occasionally by a little bruising. The diagnosis is made by asking the patient to flex the elbow against resistance where-upon the affected biceps muscle bunches distally leaving a gap proximally (fig. 367).

Once again the disability is usually trivial and if the patient is prepared to accept it no treatment should be offered. Should the patient miss the slight loss of elbow flexor power which follows this injury, it is feasible to reattach the proximal end of the biceps to the humerus itself.

The rectus femoris muscle may be ruptured by normal loads at its attachment to the patella. This condition is discussed in Chapter 17.

The Achilles' tendon may rupture after insignificant violence—probably because it is weakened by vascular insufficiency as is the supraspinatus tendon. This condition is discussed in Chapter 17.

TENDON SHEATH DISORDERS

Simple Tenosynovitis.—This condition follows excessive or unaccustomed use, and is commonly seen in connection with the extensor tendons of the hand and the Achilles' tendon. Pain and local oedema are present and a characteristic soft crepitus (like the rustling of tissue paper) is sometimes palpable when the fingers are moved. The condition is treated by resting the tendons involved, which in the case of the extensors of the hand must of course involve the fingers. A minimum of 3 weeks absolute rest in a splint is usually required, followed by a period of gentle but progressive activity.

Suppurative Tenosynovitis.—This condition affects particularly the flexor tendons of the hand since these sheaths are far more commonly injured than those elsewhere in the body. The condition is discussed in Chapter 11.

Stenosing Teno-Vaginitis.—This is a condition of unknown aetiology in which the sheath of a tendon thickens, apparently spontaneously, so as to entrap the tendon. Pain and limitation of movement result. The condition is most common at the common sheath of the abductor pollicis longus and extensor pollicis brevis tendons of the wrist (*de Quervain's disease*) and at the retinaculae of the flexor tendons of the fingers and thumb in the palm ('*trigger finger*'). In the palm, the flexor muscles are sufficiently strong to continue forcing the tendon through the diminished gap in the flexor reticulum. The flexor tendon as a consequence gradually develops a constriction under the retinaculum and a bulge distal to it. Finally, the flexor muscles may force the bulge through the retinaculum but the extensor muscles may be insufficiently powerful to extend the finger thereafter. The finger now snaps as it passes through the constriction and finally locks in a position of flexion from which attempts passively to extend the finger are painful.

Both de Quervain's disease and trigger finger can be cured by dividing the appropriate retinaculum surgically. It might be expected that following this oper-ation the involved tendon would subluxate but in practice this never occurs.

Carpal Tunnel Compression of the Median Nerve.—The carpal tunnel is formed by the flexor retinaculum anteriorly and by the distal row of the carpus posteriorly. The median nerve and the flexor tendons pass through it. Sometimes as a consequence of some clearly demonstrable pathology such as rheumatoid arthritis involving the synovial sheaths of the flexor tendons, the contents of the

Fritz de Quervain, 1868–1940. Professor of Surgery, Berne, Switzerland. Described Stenosing Teno-Vaginitis in 1895.

tunnel increase in bulk and compress the median nerve. Usually, however, signs of median nerve compression develop without any obvious increase in bulk in the contents of the tunnel. The aetiology of this condition is unknown but it may be an example of *stenosing teno-vaginitis*, in this case affecting the flexor retinaculum. The condition usually occurs in otherwise normal individuals but is associated with myxoedema (Chapter 37), pregnancy, and after a Colles' fracture.

The patient complains of pain which classically is localised to the distribution of the median nerve in the hand but which may be felt anywhere in the arm. The poor localisation of the pain may make the diagnosis difficult since it is easy to confuse the condition with other causes of pain in the arm, for example with cervical spondylosis. Commonly the pain is worse at night and the patient may notice that he is then relieved by hanging the hand over the edge of the bed, a feature of the history which is almost diagnostic of carpal tunnel compression of the median nerve. As the compression increases in severity more obvious neurological symptoms develop including paraesthesiae, numbness, inco-ordination, and finally frank weakness in the muscles of the hand innervated by the median nerve (of which the easiest to examine is abductor pollicis brevis, wasting of which is obvious). The fingers, apart from being inco-ordinated, may also feel stiff, especially first thing in the morning, a symptom which is probably attributable to compression of the flexor tendons themselves. Examination of the hand is frequently negative but may demonstrate slight tenderness over the carpal tunnel, an increase in pain if the fingers and wrist are held fully flexed for a new moments, and the presence of abnormal neurological signs in the distribution of the median nerve in the hand. Conduction studies on the median nerve demonstrate delay at the carpal tunnel.

Treatment.—Whatever may be the pathology, simple decompression of the tunnel by longitudinal incision of the flexor retinaculum cures the condition, often in a dramatic fashion. Rheumatoid tenosynovitis may in addition require synovectomy.

FASCIAE

Dupuytren's contracture is a localised thickening of the palmar, and rarely the plantar, fascia. The fascia thickens to form nodules and contracts so that eventually the affected fingers are drawn into flexion. The overlying skin of the palm adheres to the fascia. Most commonly the disease starts near the base of the little finger and soon draws that finger into the palm of the hand (fig. 368). Later it involves the ring finger and, less often, the long and then index fingers, in the same way. In long-standing cases permanent changes take place in the metacarpophalangeal and the proximal interphalangeal joints which render futile any attempt to straighten the fingers.

The pathology of the condition is unknown. In the past it was believed to be due to repeated trauma to the palm. However, it is known to be familial and is frequently seen in patients who have never experienced such trauma. That it is so often bilateral and may involve the feet is also against any traumatic origin. It is more common in men than in women and may be seen in cirrhotics and epileptics who take sodium hydantoin. It may also develop in diabetics.

Baron Guillaume Dupuytren, 1777–1835. Surgeon, Hôtel Dieu, Paris. Described Contracture of the Palmar Fascia in 1831.

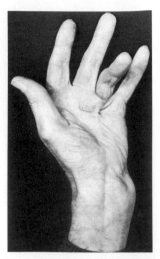

FIG. 368.—Dupuytren's contracture; note puckering of adherent skin in the palm.

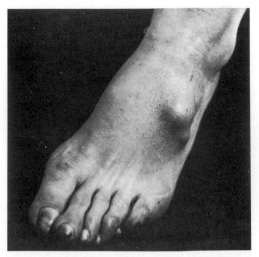

FIG. 369.—Simple ganglion on the tendon of the peroneus brevis muscle.

Treatment.—Early cases can be treated by night splintage and gentle stretching by the patient. More advanced changes require excision or (less satisfactorily) multiple division of the affected fascia. This operation can give excellent results in all but severe longstanding cases where permanent joint changes have developed. In these cases it may be advisable to amputate the affected finger.

GANGLIA

Ganglia are localised, tense (but often painless) cystic swellings containing clear gelatinous fluid. They often communicate with, and are always adjacent to, a tendon sheath or the capsule of a joint. Their origin is uncertain but they are probably caused by myxoid degeneration of fibrous tissue of capsule, ligaments and retinaculae. They are sometimes predisposed to by injury. Simple ganglia are most commonly found on the dorsum of the wrist and the foot (fig. 369). Occasionally minute ganglia develop on the flexor aspect of the fingers which although small, are exquisitely painful and tender.

Treatment.—Traditionally, ganglia were burst by striking them with the family Bible! Today, if they do not resolve spontaneously, they are excised. The patient should be warned that 'recurrences' are common, and may choose to have no treatment.

BURSAE

Simple Bursitis.—Acute traumatic bursitis follows injury or unaccustomed exercise, for example inflammation of the bursa anterior to the Achilles' tendon may follow a cross-country run.

Chronic Bursitis.—This is the result of repeated pressure or slight injuries, to anatomical bursae. Examples are involvement of the *prepatellar bursa* (housemaid's knee, fig. 370) or *olecranon bursa* (students or miner's elbow, fig. 371), and subsartorial bursitis (fig. 372).

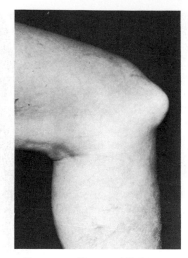

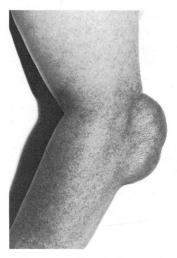

FIG. 370.—Housemaid's knee.

FIG. 371.—Chronic olecranon bursitis.

Involvement of the *semimembranosus bursa* occurs particularly in children (fig. 373). The cyst is aspirated if it causes disability, but most cysts disappear spontaneously. Semimembranosus bursae, if they communicate with the knee joint, sometimes enlarge when there is an effusion in the joint, for example as a result of osteoarthrosis, and form one variety of *Baker's cysts*. (In general, synovial cysts in the popliteal fossa, which are known as Baker's cysts, may arise as described above from the semimembranosus bursa or, in rheumatoid arthritis of the knee, from a posterior rupture of the capsule of the joint.)

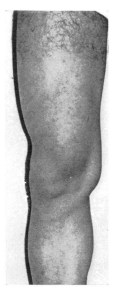

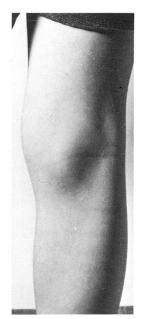

FIG. 372.—Subsartorial bursitis.

FIG. 373.—Semimembranosus bursitis.

William Morrant Baker, 1839–1896. Surgeon, St. Bartholomew's Hospital, London. Described these cysts in 1877.

Acute Suppurative Bursitis.—This is due to direct infection by penetrating wounds, or by the spread of local cellulitis. The prepatellar bursa is the most commonly involved. A 'sympathetic' effusion in the knee joint sometimes follows. Confusion with infective arthritis should be avoided, as in the latter condition any attempt to move the joint is painful, and at the knee pain is elicited by pressure in the popliteal space (see Chapter 18). The infection usually responds to chemotherapy, but if pus is already present incision and drainage will be necessary.

Excision of Bursae.—Persistent trouble with a subcutaneous bursa (*e.g.* olecranon, prepatellar) may only be resolved by complete excision of the whole of the endothelial lining and surrounding 'capsule' under a general anaesthetic.

Adventitious bursae form as a result of prolonged pressure over bony prominences. The term 'adventitious' means that no anatomical bursa was present at the site of the newly formed cyst, and that it was generated in connective tissue as a result of repeated shearing motion in the tissue. One of the commonest of such bursae is that over the medial aspect of the head of the first metatarsal in hallux valgus (Chapter 12). Like anatomical bursae, adventitious bursae can become infected.

CHAPTER 25

NEUROLOGICAL DISORDERS AFFECTING THE MUSCULO-SKELETAL SYSTEM

In spite of the wide variety of diseases which affect the nervous system the consequences for the locomotor system tend to follow a common pattern so that it is possible to lay down certain principles of management which have a general application. The loss of motor power and sensory faculty require separate consideration, although both are commonly found together.

MOTOR LOSS—PARALYSIS

The consequences of paralysis are twofold:

1. *Loss of Function.*—This results from the failure of action of the affected muscles and, while many of its consequences are self evident, the loss of joint stability is of particular importance.

2. *Liability to Deformity.*—In the adult this is seldom a serious problem for although there is a tendency for contractures to develop in the non-paralysed muscles these are relatively easily controlled by passive movements and splintage. In the growing child however the problem is much more serious for here there is a disturbance of growth. For reasons not well understood the non-paralysed muscle becomes relatively shorter than its paralysed fellow so that the joints concerned become fixed in the direction of the acting muscles. These changes may be followed by secondary bony deformity leading to even greater fixity of the joint. In addition to these particular deformities there may be an overall shortening of the limb, again for reasons which are not readily apparent.

It is important to appreciate that these forces of unbalanced growth are almost irresistible and just as a solid pavement yields before the persistence of a penetrating weed so also will splints and calipers fail if they are used alone in an attempt to correct or even to control these deformities. On the other hand it must be remembered that a totally paralysed limb has no tendency to deform since there is no imbalance to distort it, although its overall dimensions are usually reduced. In these circumstances gravitational force may have some distorting effects particularly in the production of equinus deformity of the foot, but this is easily resisted.

The Management of Paralysis.—This has 3 main objectives as follows:

1. **The Elimination of Deformity.**—In the adult the emphasis should be on prevention, with the institution of passive movements and splintage as soon as possible. If fixed deformity does develop simple tenotomy will usually be sufficient to bring it under control.

In the child splintage alone will not suffice and it will usually be necessary surgically to divide the contracted structures and in particular the tendons of the unopposed muscles acting on the joint. Once these deforming forces have been eliminated it may be possible to complete the correction by serial casts and splintage. Bony deformity may also be corrected at this stage providing that the epiphyses are not interfered with.

2. The Prevention of Recurrent Deformity.—In the child this implies the restoration of muscle balance across the joint. This can be achieved by reinforcing the paralysed group or by weakening the non-paralysed muscles, although in practice the methods are often combined.

Reinforcement of the Paralysed Group.—This may be achieved by *tendon transfer* in which the tendon of a normally acting muscle is inserted in a new site while preserving the origin of the muscle and its nerve supply thereby altering its mode of action. If this is to be undertaken there are certain principles which must be observed.

(i) The transferred tendon should itself be working to full power. Tendon transfer results in a significant loss of strength so that if the tendon of a partially paralysed muscle is transferred it may be reduced to total impotence in its new situation.

(ii) Deformity in the joint must have been previously eliminated. Tendon transfer alone cannot be relied upon to correct an established deformity.

(iii) The action which is expected of the transferred tendon should be as close as possible to its original action to facilitate re-education. This is of particular importance in the lower limb where the powers of re-education are limited.

(iv) The path of the transferred tendon should be as direct as possible.

(v) The transferred tendon should if possible be re-inserted into bone rather than into another tendon.

Weakening of the Non-paralysed Group.—This is the only method available if tendon transfer is not possible. It must always be remembered that a flail joint will not deform, so that if only one muscle is left acting across a joint muscle balancing will be impossible and it is better to eliminate all activity. Methods for weakening an active group are:

(*a*) *Tenotomy.*—Spontaneous reconstitution is possible so that if permanent loss of power is required it is better to resect a length of tendon.

(*b*) *Elongation.*—Z-elongation of a tendon results in a considerable but not total loss of power.

Both of these procedures may be indicated for correction of the deformity and it is often convenient to carry out the rebalancing procedures at the same time.

Denervation.—Division of the motor nerve to the overacting muscle is sometimes indicated (for example, the soleus and adductor group).

3. The Re-establishment of Joint Stability and the Restoration of Function.—Joint stability may already have been achieved by tendon transfer together with some restoration of function, but if not, then the choice lies between arthrodesis of the joint, which is normally possible only in the adult, or external splintage which is the solution usually adopted in children until they are old enough for bony procedures. The methods commonly employed in the lower limb are as follows:

Subtalar Instability.—Below knee iron and T strap (fig. 374). The iron is usually placed on the side of greater weakness. Thus if the foot tends to valgus

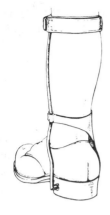

Fig. 374.—Outside iron and inside 'T' strap to control valgus deformity.

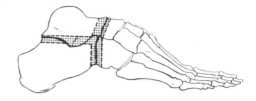

Fig. 375.—Shaded areas denote the bone to be removed in triple arthrodesis (triple fusion).

an outside iron and inside T strap is normally used. In many instances it is better to use a double iron. When skeletal maturity of the foot is attained (about 12 years) arthrodesis of the subtalar complex (triple fusion) can be undertaken (fig. 375) and the appliance discarded. Stabilisation at an earlier age can be achieved by means of an extra-articular graft between talus and calcaneum inserted across the sinus tarsi (Grice). Since this does not interfere directly with joint cartilage the disturbance to growth is minimised.

Ankle Instability.—A double leg iron is used. If there is a tendency to equinus this is restricted by a torsion bar in the heel or a toe-raising spring. An appropriate stop can be incorporated if there is calcaneus deformity. A cosmetically more attractive solution for drop foot has become available more recently with the development of new plastic materials. This consists of a flexible back splint which is worn inside a normal shoe. Ankle arthrodesis is usually inadvisable and definitive correction of equinus or calcaneus deformity of the foot is usually obtained at the subtalar level by a modification of triple fusion.

Knee Instability.—This can be controlled by a double leg iron extending up to a thigh corset and may be provided with an unlocking device to permit sitting. Again these are gradually being replaced in suitable cases by more acceptable plastic orthoses.[1] The stability of the knee is dependent on the quadriceps muscle and if this is paralysed the patient cannot normally stand without a brace. If the knee is entirely flail, however, some patients can achieve stability by a trick action in which the knee is forced into hyperextension (fig. 376). Note that in this position the ankle is in some equinus. Arthrodesis of the knee is seldom indicated for paralysis.

Hip Instability.—This is usually caused by paralysis of the glutei. Loss of the abductors results in a lurching gait which may be improved by the use of sticks but if the gluteus maximus and hamstrings are paralysed the patient is usually unable to stand upright without the trunk falling forwards. In these circumstances the bracing may need to be carried above the waist. Some patients with flail hips are able to stand by hyperextending the joints relying on the strong anterior capsule of the joint to support them. Arthrodesis is never indicated for paralysis affecting the hip.

---

[1] Orthosis = a form of splint.

David Stephen Grice, 1914–1960. Professor of Orthopaedic Surgery, University of Pennsylvania School of Medicine, Philadelphia, U.S.A.

Gluteal paralysis creates a special problem for the hip if it arises within the first few years of life. In the presence of functioning adductor and flexor groups dislocation is likely and must always be looked for when there is flexion and abduction deformity.

Tendon Transfer.—The use of tendon transfer in the prevention of deformity has already been mentioned and these procedures may also be used for the restoration of function. The very fact that a joint has been arthrodesed may liberate certain muscles for this purpose.

On the whole tendon transfers are very satisfactory in the upper limb where each muscle appears to have separate cortical representation so that rapid re-education can be expected. In the lower limb, however, there appears to be central representation of whole joint movements rather than of individual muscles so that re-education of a single muscle within a group is more difficult. The expectation of useful function from a lower limb transfer is therefore much less than in the upper limb particularly if it is expected to act in a different phase of the gait than formerly and the ability to convert shows much individual variation. The chief value of such transfers is probably the prevention of deformity although certain operations, such as the lateral repositioning of the tibialis anterior and forward transfer of tibialis posterior through the interosseous membrane can usually be relied on to produce worthwhile function for the ankle.

PROCEDURES FOR PARALYSIS FOLLOWING PERIPHERAL NERVE INJURIES
(CHAPTER 28)

Approximately 18 months after nerve division irreversible changes will have occurred in the motor endplates unless re-innervation has occurred, so that further recovery cannot be expected after this time and secondary reconstruction may be indicated. The procedures which are commonly carried out are as follows:

Circumflex Nerve.—Loss of shoulder abduction is the complaint and a useful range of this can be restored by arthrodesing the shoulder providing that the scapular rotators are intact. It must be remembered that this will entail a loss of rotation of the arm.

Musculocutaneous Nerve.—The brachioradialis may provide sufficient flexor power at the elbow to make reconstruction unnecessary but if not, additional flexor power can be obtained by advancing the origin of the forearm flexors further up the humerus (Steindler).

Radial Nerve.—Various combinations of tendon transfers are available depending on the level of the lesion but at least one wrist flexor should be preserved to prevent hyperextension. A suitable combination for a high lesion is as follows:

Pronator teres into extensor carpi radialis, longus and brevis.

Flexor carpi ulnaris into long finger extensors.

Palmaris longus into long thumb extensor.

Median Nerve.—In the more common low lesions of the nerve the main disability results from the sensory loss and weakness of opposition. The latter may be improved by tendon transfers, the simplest of which employs the flexor sublimis tendon to the ring finger. The direction of pull of the tendon is made appropriate by causing it to pass first through a pulley constructed on the ulnar side of the wrist. In high lesions the disability is much greater but some improvement in hand flexor function can be achieved by transfers using the brachioradialis and one of the wrist extensors.

Ulnar Nerve.—The disability from a lesion of this nerve is often slight and

Arthur Steindler, 1878–1959. Professor of Orthopaedic Surgery, State University, Iowa City, Iowa, U.S.A.

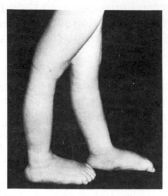

FIG. 376.—Complete quadriceps palsy in the right leg. The patient is able to stabilise the knee by bracing it back into hyperextension.

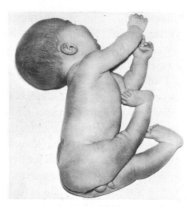

FIG. 377.—Child with meningomyelocele. There is fixed flexion and adduction of the hips, extension of the knees and calcaneus deformity of the feet. Voluntary innervation was absent below the fourth lumbar segment.

reconstruction may not be called for. However, paralysis of the adductor pollicis results in weakness of the pinch grip which may be reinforced by tendon transfer usually with one of the radial wrist extensors which has been suitably prolonged.

Brachial Plexus.—A wide variation in the pattern of residual paralysis can result from this and some of the above procedures may be appropriately combined. A total unrecovered paralysis results in a flail arm which is usually best treated by amputation through the humerus, together with arthrodesis of the shoulder. If the scapular rotators are preserved some abduction at the shoulder will then be possible and may be used to activate a prosthesis. The decision to carry out this procedure should not be too long delayed or the patient will have become permanently adapted to the one-armed way of life.

Lateral Popliteal Nerve.—Many patients are content to control their foot drop with a toe-raising spring or orthosis but some active dorsiflexion may be achieved by a transfer of the tibialis posterior through the interosseous membrane on to the dorsum of the foot. Alternatively, a triple fusion operation may be performed, removing the greater part of the under surface of the talus (Lambrinudi). As a result when the foot is in 'neutral' the ankle is in maximum plantar flexion so that further footdrop is impossible.

MENINGOMYELOCELE (SEE CHAPTER 27)

This is the commonest of the severe forms of spina bifida and is almost invariably accompanied by some paralysis in the lower limbs which is often extensive and comprises a mixture of both upper and lower motor neurone types. Deformities are often present at birth particularly flexion adduction contractures at the hips, which may be dislocated, and deformities of the foot (fig. 377). These are not to be regarded as separate associated abnormalities; they are secondary deformities and usually correspond with the distribution of the paralysis. Without treatment progressive deformity corresponding with the imbalance can be expected.

Constantine Lambrinudi, 1889–1943. Orthopaedic Surgeon, Guy's Hospital, London.

Management.—The management follows general principles with the object of providing straight limbs with plantigrade feet at the same time preserving joint mobility and the important ability to sit comfortably. Certain special features should be mentioned:

Foot Deformity.—This has the first priority in the orthopaedic management. Corrective splintage may be used as in non-paralytic talipes but caution must be used since the feet are anaesthetic. In very resistant cases it may be wise to perform early division of the deforming tendons. Once the deformity has been corrected muscle rebalancing should be carried out if possible but in many instances there will be insufficient muscles under voluntary control to do this. Spastic muscles should not be used for transfer and in these circumstances it may be better to abolish all muscle activity in the foot and to support it in a caliper until 11 or 12 years of age when it can be stabilised by triple fusion.

Hip Deformity.—Gluteal palsy is common in this condition. Where the flexor and adductor groups are strong the hips will either be dislocated at birth or will dislocate in the first few months. By the end of the first year about half of all untreated children with the condition will have dislocated hips. The deformity should be reduced as soon as possible by open tenotomy of the adductors, holding the hip reduced by some form of splintage in abduction and extension. As soon as the child is old enough (about 1 year) the muscle imbalance must be corrected. The adductors have already been weakened and the flexors must now be treated similarly by dividing the tendon of the iliopsoas which is the most important deforming force. At the same time an attempt may be made to reinforce the missing abductors and extensors by transferring the iliopsoas tendon to the back of the greater trochanter (Sharrard).

Rotation and other deformities at the hip may be corrected by femoral oste-otomy at any age since the epiphyses are not interfered with.

CEREBRAL PALSY (SPASTIC PARALYSIS)

This condition which presents in childhood is the result of intracranial damage involving the cerebral hemispheres or the basal ganglia. It sometimes results from a congenital malformation of these structures, whilst in others the damage is acquired either during birth or soon after. The result in all is a varying degree of limb paralysis of the upper motor neurone type in which spasm is prominent, together with difficulties in co-ordination (ataxia) and uncontrolled purposeless movements (athetosis).

The pattern is very varied and one or all limbs may be involved. The common-est pattern is of a symmetrical spastic paresis of the lower limbs with a tendency to flexion and adduction of the hips with flexion of the knees and equinus of the feet. In the upper limb there is typically flexion of the wrist and fingers with adduction of the thumb and pronation of the forearm but ataxia and athetoid movements are often present in addition.

The mechanism of deformity and disability is very complex and is by no means exclusively due to the overactivity of the spastic muscles. Some muscle groups may exhibit normal tone and yet be significantly weakened and, particularly in younger children, the limbs may be held in particular attitudes due to the persist-

William John Wells Sharrard, Contemporary. Orthopaedic Surgeon, Sheffield Royal Infirmary, Sheffield, England.

ence of primitive reflexes such as the tonic neck reflex. Many children have serious difficulties with balance and orientation in space and these may have an over-riding effect on their locomotor performance.

Management.—Physical therapy is important, particularly in the reinforcement of weak muscle groups by exercise. Passive stretching of muscles and splintage may help to lessen deformity but their limitations should be recognised. Severe fixed deformity can only be corrected by surgery.

When operations are planned the objectives must be clear. Deformity may require correction in order to assist with the child's general management as, for example, when tight adductors interfere with dressing and toilet care. If, on the other hand, improved function is the aim then this must be realistic, taking into account the child's I.Q., overall muscle power, co-ordination, *etc.* Failure to do this will lead to unduly ambitious and unnecessary surgery.

The objects of treatment are as before: the elimination of deformity and the restoration of muscle balance, but in the latter tendon transfer can play only a limited part because of the difficulty in finding wholly normal muscles to transfer. Rebalancing therefore has to be confined to procedures which weaken the strong groups.

Hip.—Adduction deformity and spasm is the commonest problem and if it interferes with walking or toilet care is an indication for adductor tenotomy.

Adductor Tenotomy.—A skin crease incision is made close to the inguinal ligament and the tendons of adductor longus, brevis and gracilis divided through their tendinous parts as close to the pelvis as possible. It may also be necessary to divide the pectineus and even part of adductor magnus. Both branches of the obturator nerve should be identified. If spasm is prominent it may be justifiable to divide the anterior branch but the posterior branch must be preserved. If there is also flexion deformity the tendon of the iliopsoas can be divided or elongated through the same wound. The legs are immobilised in an abduction and extension cast for 3 weeks.

Flexion and adduction predominance predisposes to hip subluxation which will proceed to full dislocation over a number of years, and strict radiological vigilance is required in its presence. Adductor/abductor imbalance may be restored by weakening the adductors by adductor tenotomy and anterior branch neurectomy and in this way the tendency to dislocate is controlled. Once dislocation has occurred restabilisation is extremely difficult. Another common problem at the hip is produced by internal torsion of the femur tending to an ungainly intoeing gait. This may require a rotation osteotomy for its correction.

Knee.—Flexion deformity is the usual problem and is best dealt with by Z elongation of the hamstring tendons behind the knee.

Foot.—Equinus of the heel is extremely common and the child walks on his toes. Sometimes the contracture involves only the gastrocnemius in which case the deformity disappears on flexing the knee. In these circumstances division of the gastrocnemius part of the Achilles' tendon is required. If the entire group of calf muscles is involved an elongation of the Achilles' tendon is indicated. This must be done cautiously as overcorrection may lead to intractable calcaneus deformity.

Upper Limb Deformities.—The results of surgery in the upper limb are often disappointing usually due to deficient sensation and proprioception. If these are intact there may be a place for a flexor slide operation to reduce finger flexion contracture and for procedures to eliminate the common 'thumb in palm' deformity.

POLIOMYELITIS (INFANTILE PARALYSIS)

This is an acute febrile disease caused by a neurotropic virus whose permanent effect is an irregularly distributed flaccid paralysis caused by injury to the anterior horn cells. New cases of the disease have been practically eliminated in the United Kingdom as a result of mass immunisation. Occasionally cases of paralysis present without a clear history of the acute infection. These are recognisable by the distribution of the flaccid paralysis and the wasting which is almost invariably asymmetrical, involving particularly the proximal part of the lower limbs and the spine and trunk musculature. Sensory disturbance is absent.

Management.—In the initial and recovery phases of the disease orthopaedic management is confined to simple splintage to minimise deformity, but after 2 years or so no further recovery can be anticipated and definitive reconstruction can begin. Although almost any pattern of paralysis is theoretically possible a number of deformities occur with some regularity.

Foot.—*Pes equinus due to paralysis of the dorsiflexors of the foot.* This can be corrected in childhood by a Z elongation of the Achilles' tendon possibly accompanied by a posterior capsulectomy of the ankle. Anterior transfer of tibialis posterior will help to control recurrence.

Pes calcaneus due to calf paralysis.—This can be treated by a transfer of the peronei and the tibialis anterior through the interosseous membrane to the heel. Triple fusion will be required eventually in most cases (fig. 375).

Knee.—The ability to stabilise a knee with a paralysed quadriceps has already been mentioned (fig. 376), and if present represents a strong contraindication to correction of equinus deformity of the foot which may result in a loss of power to hyperextend the knee. If the knee flexors are strong it will again be impossible to hyperextend the joint, when elongation of the hamstring tendons may be helpful. Alternatively they may be transferred forward into the patella to act as extensors.

Hip.—If the paralysis occurs in infancy and affects the abductors, subluxation or dislocation may occur. After dividing the adductors transfer of the iliopsoas to the great trochanter to act as an abductor (Mustard) will prevent progressive subluxation and may also improve the Trendelenburg gait. There is a tendency for the femoral neck to become valgus in these circumstances, further destabilising the hip. Varus osteotomy may therefore be indicated.

Leg Length Discrepancy.—This may amount to many centimetres so some correction is required. The normal limb may be shortened by driving staples across the growth plates of the upper tibia and lower femur so that normal growth is slowed or in an adult the bone shortened by excising its segment of diaphysis. Alternatively the short limb may be lengthened up to 6 cm by dividing the tibia or femur in a step cut fashion and producing gradual distraction with skeletal fixation and a screw apparatus. When the maximum correction has been obtained the osteotomy is secured with a plate and a bone graft applied. This procedure is more satisfactory in the tibia than in the femur where the risk of complications is significantly higher.

Scoliosis—Muscle imbalance around the vertebral column may produce severe scoliosis with rotary changes as in idiopathic scoliosis (Chapter 22). However, the curve usually remains a good deal more mobile than in the latter condition. In its most severe form there is a collapsing spine so that the patient cannot even sit up and respiration is embarrassed.

Treatment.—Treatment follows the same lines as in idiopathic scoliosis with correction usually in plaster casts followed by fusion to maintain the correction attained. It should be recognised that this represents a conflict with the basic rules of management since the muscle imbalance remains uncorrected, but there is no alternative in this situation. It is not surprising therefore that there is often recurrence of deformity.

DISSEMINATED (MULTIPLE) SCLEROSIS

This is a slowly progressive disorder resulting from patchy demyelination of the central nervous system. It results in progressive spastic paralysis, usually of

William T. Mustard, Contemporary. Orthopaedic Surgeon, Hospital for Sick Children, Toronto, Canada.

the lower limbs. There is a tendency to deform and in particular to develop flexion of the knees and flexion and adduction of the hips. Treatment should therefore be prophylactic with the use of splints and passive joint movement. Unfortunately late cases are often seen and although no growth forces are involved deformity is often severe as it may represent the end result of many years of neglect.

The knees may be treated by tenotomy of the hamstrings followed by serial plasters to increase extension. Flexion and adduction of the hips may be so extreme that surgery in the groin is physically impossible. In these circumstances division of the psoas in the pelvis through a retroperitoneal approach with an intrapelvic division of the obturator nerve will make the situation more manageable. Tendon transfer is never indicated in this condition.

HEMIPLEGIA FOLLOWING A CEREBROVASCULAR ACCIDENT

The pattern of deformity here is very similar to that in cerebral palsy but since the patients are adult it is more easily controlled particularly if physical therapy and splintage are instituted early enough. Occasionally fixed deformity of sufficient severity to require surgery is encountered. Equinovarus of the foot is the commonest problem and this can very satisfactorily be dealt with by elongation of the Achilles' tendon and a division of the tibialis posterior through the same incision. Hamstring tenotomy may sometimes be needed for knee flexion deformity. Upper limb surgery may also be occasionally indicated.

SENSORY LOSS

This has consequences for both skin and the bones and joints.

Skin.—Because of the lack of protective sensation ulceration is likely particularly in weight bearing areas of which the classical illustration is the perforating ulcer over the metatarsal heads. The latter is particularly liable to occur if there is accompanying equinus deformity from associated motor loss. In the fingers sensory loss is of particular significance for, apart from the liability to damage,

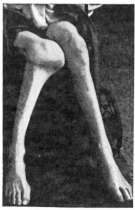

Fig. 378.—Charcot's disease
of the right knee.
(Dr. Worster-Drought, London.)

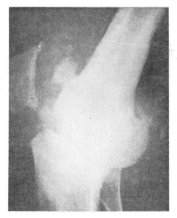

Fig. 379.—Charcot's knee joint.
Hypertrophic type.

an insensitive finger will not be used even if its motor function is perfect. All attempts at finger reconstruction therefore must make provision for restoration of some innervation. If nerve repair is impossible sensation to the pulp may be restored by a pedicle graft of innervated skin from the tip of another finger, the pedicle including an intact digital neurovascular bundle.

Neuropathic Joints.—Tertiary syphilis was formerly the commonest cause of this condition but as this disease disappears an increasing proportion have become due to other causes including syringomyelia, peripheral neuritis (*e.g.* diabetes) and the rare condition of congenital indifference to pain.

Clinical diagnosis is usually easy due to the remarkable combination of a joint showing obvious gross disorganisation with deformity, swelling and grotesque hypermobility together with remarkably little pain (fig. 378)—the so-called Charcot joint.

Function is often astonishingly well preserved. The accompanying features of the underlying disease will also be present. Radiography shows a grossly disorganised joint with destructive features and irregular areas of new bone formation (fig. 379).

Treatment.—Although arthrodesis would appear to be the logical treatment this is often difficult to achieve in this condition and it is usually sufficient to stabilise the joint with a suitable appliance—a brace in the lower limb or a moulded leather support in the upper limb.

Jean Martin Charcot, 1825–1893. Physician, La Salpêtrière, Paris. Described tabetic arthropathy in 1868.

CHAPTER 26

THE HEAD (SCALP, SKULL AND BRAIN)

THE SCALP

The **scalp** consists of four layers—skin, subcutaneous tissue, epicranial aponeur-osis or galea, into which is inserted the occipito-frontalis muscle, and the sub-aponeurotic areolar layer. The scalp is well supplied with blood-vessels, and the walls of the arteries are adherent to the fibrous tissue in the subcutaneous layer. Therefore scalp wounds bleed freely, as the muscular coat of a divided artery cannot retract readily when the vessel is severed.

Wounds of the scalp.—The great vascularity of the scalp indicates that wounds heal well, and areas which at first sight seem necrotic may in due course prove to be viable and heal. If scalp is lost due to trauma or surgery, repair of a relatively small resultant defect requires extensive flaps or free grafts. For these reasons any excision or 'debridement' of the edges of scalp wounds should be reduced to the minimum and only portions grossly contaminated or necrotic should be removed (Chapters 1 and 2). While all coverings of the brain are important (*e.g.* dura and skull), the scalp is the one layer which is essential, and must, therefore, be preserved.

Scalp wounds should be managed by shaving the hair over an area at least 3 cm clear of the wound, which is then cleaned, avoiding soapy solutions. Bleeding from the wound edges is best controlled by simple pressure, and it is rarely necessary to apply artery forceps to the galea. It is difficult and potentially dangerous to probe wounds to determine the presence of depressed fractures and foreign bodies, which can only be detected with certainty by radiography (fig. 408 and legend). Therefore, after shaving, cleansing and application of a temporary dry dressing, radiographs should be done (see p. 449 for indication for x-ray of skull) before wounds are closed in two layers, galea to galea and skin to skin, with interrupted black silk sutures. When the wound edges and layers are much disorganised it is reasonable to close the wound loosely in one layer, avoiding any tension; in these circumstances extending the incision in an S-shaped manner may ease the closure.

Haematoma of the scalp may be subcutaneous, subaponeurotic or subperi-cranial. Subaponeurotic haematomas spread extensively beneath the epicranial aponeurosis and are only limited by the attachment of the aponeurosis around the base of the calvarium. Subpericranial haematomas are limited by the suture lines which border the underlying bone, to which the pericranium is attached.

Infections of the scalp occur most commonly in association with wounds, particularly when lacerations are not dealt with for several days. However, the vascularity of the skin tends to promote healing, and infection usually remains localised. Rarely infection may spread widely in the loose avascular areolar tissue beneath the galea. Post-traumatic scalp infection requires indentification of the organism and appropriate antibiotics after wound toilet; occasionally extensive subgaleal pus will require drainage through multiple incisions. When there is much soiling of scalp wounds, tetanus and occasionally gas gangrene are potential dangers.

Subperiosteal infection, with or without osteomyelitis, is rare and is usually the result of chronic frontal sinusitis. The associated external swelling due to subperiosteal pus and scalp oedema is termed Pott's puffy tumour (p. 465). The condition has serious implications because of the association with intracranial abscess, either extradural or subdural, and therefore any patient with signs of subperiosteal infection should be referred for further investigations.

LUMPS ON THE HEAD

General principles.—Accurate clinical diagnosis, with radiography of the skull when indicated, is an essential prerequisite before any attempt at surgical removal or biopsy. In general lumps in the midline should be approached with particular caution because they are likely to be in continuity with intracranial structures such as the meninges and sagittal venous sinus; radiography is obligatory. Surgery should be undertaken only by those able to deal with associated intracranial pathology; any lump removed must be examined histologically. The usual principles of examination of any lump are relevant and particular features include:

(*a*) *Hardness and fixation to the skull.* This indicates that the lump is arising from or involving bone. Primary intracranial pathology includes meningioma (especially parasagittal), and meningeal sarcoma. Lesions arising from the skull include benign osteoma (exostosis), metastases, osteogenic sarcoma (sometimes arising in Paget's disease, Chapter 23); chronic infection with osteomyelitis may mimic a bony tumour.

(*b*) *Lumps which are firm* include sebaceous cysts, and dermoid cysts. Soft fluctuant lumps include meningoceles (especially in the midline) which may be translucent and have a cough impulse.

Sebaceous cysts (*syn.* wens) (Chapter 10) are often multiple (fig. 380). The surrounding scalp becomes bald if pressure interferes with its blood supply. Infection and ulceration are described in Chapter 10 (and see frontispiece).

Dermoid cysts are most frequent over the external angular process (fig. 469). X-ray shows bone defect with a sclerotic margin (fig. 381). Although congenital they may not appear until the patient is some years old or in adult life. Communication with an intracranial dermoid may take place by a narrow neck which passes through the inner table and which is visible on x-ray. An impulse on coughing is only detected if the communication is wide.

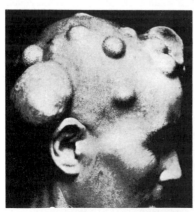

FIG. 380.—Sebaceous cysts of the scalp.

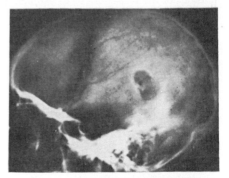

FIG. 381.—Lateral x-ray showing dermoid cyst of the diploe. The inner table has been penetrated by intracranial extension.

Treatment.—Superficial cysts are excised locally. Extensions are approached by osteoplastic craniotomy. The intracranial portion may be larger than the superficial.

Squamous and Basal-celled carcinomas (Chapter 8), which begin as a small ulcer which bleeds repeatedly when the hair is combed, are easily overlooked in their early stages. Over the course of months or even years such a tumour may spread widely in the scalp and involve all layers and erode the skull. Treatment is by early biopsy and excision, and extensive rotation flaps may be needed to close the resulting scalp defect.

Papillomas are common and cause discomfort on combing the hair. Constant irritation of this nature encourages malignant changes.

Lipomas arise from fatty tissue incorporated with the areolar layer (Chapter 8).

Melanomas may be unrecognised, owing to the small growth being hidden by hair. If malignant changes supervene, the appearance of secondary deposits should lead to the discovery of the tumour.

Fibrosarcoma has already been described (p. 109).

Cirsoid aneurysm is rare. Capillary naevi sometimes occur in the skin, beneath which abnormal arteries communicate directly with distended veins. The superficial temporal artery and branches are most commonly affected. The underlying bone becomes thinned by pressure which also causes the hair to fall out. Radiography may show perforations in the skull which indicate that part of the tumour is intracranial. These tumours tend to enlarge slowly with a risk of serious haemorrhage if ulceration occurs (fig. 382).

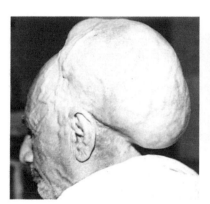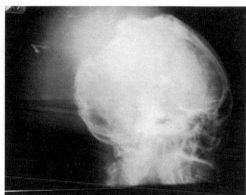

FIG. 382.—Cirsoid aneurysm. X-ray shows erosion and perforation of the skull.
Dr. Shanmugasundaram M.S., Chinglepet (Tamil Nadu), India.

Treatment consists in extirpation of the tumour in the early stages (ligation of one or both external carotid arteries is advisable as a preliminary step to local excision). If its size forbids such radical treatment, then the main vessels are ligated, but this is often unsuccessful, as a large tumour on the surface usually possesses intracranial connections which maintain the blood supply.

THE SKULL

Microcephaly may be associated with agenesis of the brain and imbecility, or result later from premature synostosis in a normal child.

Oxycephaly (*syn.* steeple-head, Gk. *oxus* = sharp) is a condition in which the skull is egg-shaped, following premature obliteration of sutures. Most cases develop increased intracranial pressure.

Synostosis, or premature fusion of sutures (coronal and/or sagittal) may produce deformities of the skull, and raised intracranial pressure. The complications include protuberance of the eyes and deterioration in visual acuity. The principle of surgical treatment is the opening of the sutures and prevention of re-fusion by interposition of material such as plastic. The surgery is specialised and results not always satisfactory.

Meningocele.—*Clinical Features.*—Protrusions of a pouch of dura mater through a congenital defect in the skull can occur at the root of the nose or over the occipital bone (fig. 383). Trans-sphenoidal projections protrude through the base of the skull into the

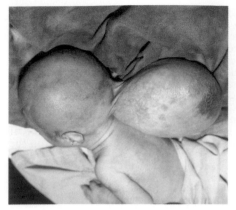
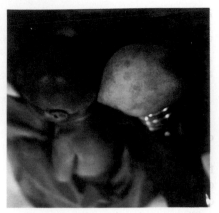

FIG. 383.—Meningocele.—A tense rounded swelling, pedunculated and translucent.
Dr. Shanmugasundaram, M.S.

naso-pharynx and have been mistaken for nasal polypi: attempted removal has resulted in meningitis. A meningocele is present at birth, and forms a tense rounded swelling which is translucent and sometimes pedunculated, and which yields an impulse when the child cries or coughs. The lower end of the spine should be examined as there is frequently a meningocele through a sacrococcygeal defect as well. Growth of the skull may occlude the neck of a small sac; in this case a cyst remains which is non-pulsatile and unaffected by coughing.

An encephalocele is a similar condition, but some portion of the brain is also extruded (fig. 384). Should this cerebral extrusion contain part of a ventricle, it is known as a *hydroencephalocele*. In these conditions vascular pulsation is present. Such children are often still-born or severely disabled.

Infections of the skull.—Osteomyelitis of the skull occurs either as a result of chronic frontal or ethmoid sinusitis, mastoid infection or following inadequate treatment of a compound depressed skull fracture. Chronic sinus or mastoid infection may be associated with intracranial abscess (p. 464), irrespective of osteomyelitis, but the presence of osteo-myelitis increases the risk of intracranial abscess, probably through emissary veins. Patients with osteomyelitis in association with ENT sepsis should be closely observed and investigated for intracranial infection.

Tuberculous disease of the skull is uncommon, but occasionally occurs in association with tuberculous lesions elsewhere. As with other bones, the infection commences either

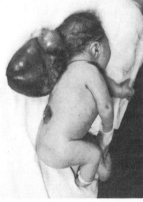

FIG. 384.—An encephalocele. A myelocele is also present.

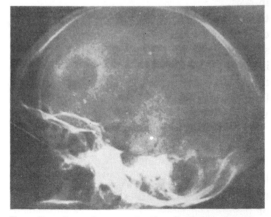

FIG. 385.—Lateral x-ray showing irregular clear area produced by a secondary deposit from carcinoma of the breast.

in the pericranium or in the medulla, *i.e.* the diploe. The diseased bone should be removed widely, otherwise abscesses are likely to form and erode the scalp. Antituberculous drugs are given (Chapter 3).

Syphilitic pericranitis is nowadays a rare affection. Localised swellings occur which are slightly tender and fixed to the bone. Under suitable treatment disappearance is usual, although a small bony swelling occasionally remains.

NEW-GROWTH OF THE SKULL

Innocent tumours are rare. An *ivory* osteoma occasionally arises in the region of an air sinus (Chapter 20).

Malignant new-growths resemble those of other bones. *Pericranial sarcoma* forms a tumour, the consistency of which depends upon its vascularity and rate of growth. Thus it may be pulsatile or of an almost bony hardness. *Osteoclastoma* occasionally develops in the diploe.

The commonest malignant tumour is secondary carcinoma, usually derived from primaries in the breast, thyroid, prostate, or suprarenal.

Hypernephromas produce rapidly growing vascular tumours, which pulsate when the outer table is eroded. Secondary deposits usually produce a single clear area on the skull x-ray with irregular margin (fig. 385). Deposits from carcinoma of the breast are often multiple.

CRANIO-CEREBRAL INJURIES

Introduction.—**In most countries the primary and continuing care of patients who have sustained a head injury is the responsibility of general and orthopaedic surgeons rather than neurosurgeons. Despite the expansion of neurosurgical services this situation is likely to continue and therefore the general surgeon requires a knowledge of principles and practice in this field. Since the majority of patients do not require any neurosurgery, the major steps in the care of such patients are medical, diagnostic and nursing and it is these steps which will determine the outcome far more frequently than any surgical manoeuvres. Indeed the avoidance of unnecessary cranial surgery is an important principle, because such surgery may be harmful. At the same time the general surgeon must be aware of the indications for specialised intracranial investigation which usually requires transferring the patient to a neurosurgical department. Finally he must be able to decide when there is a clear indication for urgent surgery without specialised investigation, either because the rate of deterioration does not allow any further delay, or because the facilities for intracranial investigation do not exist. Thus, in many parts of the world, patients must still be managed without C.T. scanning.**

INJURIES OF THE BRAIN

Mechanism and Pathology.—At the moment of impact a diffuse neuronal lesion is inflicted on the brain which is responsible for the immediate clinical picture of brain injury. Secondary changes of brain swelling or intracranial haemorrhage take time to develop. The rise in pressure resulting from these causes leads to a deterioration in the patient's level of consciousness a few hours after injury; the clinical picture in the early stages results from the neuronal lesion

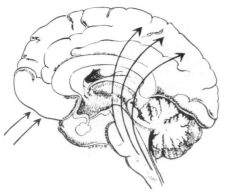 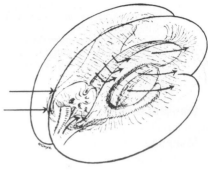

FIG. 386.—Lines of force acting on the hypo-thalamus and brain stem as the result of posterior displacement of the hemisphere.

FIG. 387.—Lines of force acting on the corpus callosum and one peduncle as the result of anterior displacement of one hemisphere.

alone. All degrees of brain injury resulting in loss of consciousness, concussion, contusion, or laceration of the brain are produced by one mechanism, namely displacement and distortion of the cerebral tissues occurring at the moment of impact.

The main factors which determine the severity of cerebral injury are:

1. *Distortion of the brain.*—The brain has 'mobility' in several respects. In life it is a soft structure which is readily distorted and therefore one part of the brain may move in relation to another. The mobility due to the consistency of cerebral tissue is accentuated by the presence of the fluid (CSF) and vascular compartments. This creates 'shearing' forces which will produce widespread damage to neurones, nerve fibres, supporting tissues (glia) and blood vessels. These effects may be diffuse and therefore far removed from the site of the blow to the head (figs. 386, 387). The clinical effect of this distortion may be the initial loss of consciousness, and, if the deterioration produces significant neuronal damage, persisting loss of consciousness and/or focal neurological deficit. Changes in level of consciousness are due to distortion and neuronal damage in the lower central structures (*e.g.* mid brain) which may be momentarily distorted in a vertical or lateral direction. Such distortion may produce transitory damage or persisting damage in the brain stem reticular formation, the groups of cells which are responsible for normal consciousness, probably through the activation of cortical mechanisms. This explains the persisting loss of consciousness in patients who have little external evidence of trauma over the skull vault.

2. *Mobility of the brain in relation to the skull and membranes.*—The dura mater is more or less firmly attached to the skull, and merges into the falx and tentorium. Between the brain and the dura is a space which varies in depth, and consists of the true subdural space and deep to that the subarachnoid space containing the CSF. The brain is not, therefore, held firmly by the skull, falx and tentorium and considerable movement between the brain and the dura may occur following 'acceleration' or 'deceleration' injuries, which increase the damage to the brain. With age the brain shrinks, and the mobility increases. A secondary effect of this movement is rupture of veins which cross the subdural space and which drain

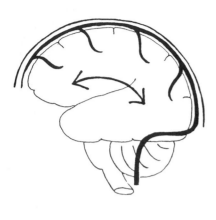

FIG. 388.—Suspension of the brain in the slings formed by the superior cerebral veins.

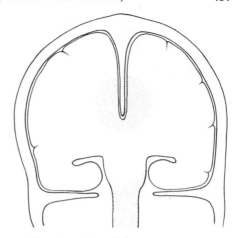

FIG. 389.—Sites of falxine and tentorial damage.

blood from the cerebral hemispheres into the dural venous sinuses, especially the superior sagittal sinus (fig. 388).

3. *The configuration of the interior of the skull.*—The degree of brain damage due to distortion and movement of the brain will be affected by the internal configuration of the skull, falx and tentorium. Where the skull is 'smooth' (convexity) brain damage is usually less severe than where it is 'rough', 'sharp' or the cavity relatively confined. Thus the temporal lobe will be damaged by the sharp sphenoid ridge and confined middle cranial fossi; the frontal pole by the rough anterior cranial fossa floor and the confined anterior corner of the anterior fossa; the occipital pole by the meeting of falx, tentorium and occipital convexity; the corpus callosum by the 'sharp' edge of the falx; the cerebral peduncles by the 'sharp' edge of the tentorium (fig. 389).

4. *Deceleration and acceleration.*—The majority of severe cranio-cerebral injuries due to traffic accidents are the result of rapid deceleration when the moving head strikes an immovable object (*e.g.* the road). This produces the features of distortion aggravated by the brain's mobility (see above). The converse is the 'acceleration' injury when the stationary skull is struck by a moving object (*e.g.* assault). The skull will rapidly accelerate and therefore distort the stationary brain. The complexity and extent of the brain damage may be increased if there is loss of consciousness, the subject falls to the ground and the brain suffers a severe 'deceleration' injury.

5. *The pre-existing state of the brain.*—The ageing brain has fewer reserves than the younger brain and therefore the lasting effects of an injury are likely to be greater in the elderly.

CEREBRAL CONCUSSION, CONTUSION AND LACERATION

The older clinico-pathological terms which were used to describe brain injury, concussion, contusion, and laceration of the brain *merely* indicate minor and major degrees of injury and *do not imply* any individual difference in mechanism.

In cerebral concussion the distortion is slight. There is a brief temporary physiological paralysis of function without organic structural damage, which results in a transient loss of consciousness, followed by complete recovery.

Cerebral contusion indicates a more severe degree of damage with pathological changes which might be diffuse or relatively localised. Changes include bruising and swelling of cortical gyri, localised or generalised 'oedema', shearing damage to nerve cells and axons either superficially or more deeply between grey matter and white matter, and haemorrhage due to tearing of small blood vessels within the brain substance. In patients who have survived for long periods after such injuries, autopsy may ultimately reveal diffuse degenerative changes in grey and white matter. So-called 'brain oedema' is one of several pathological processes which contribute to brain swelling. Oedema, that is accumulation of fluid, may be intracellular or extracellular. Congestion and dilatation of vessels with increase in the brain's blood volume also contributes to the swelling.

In cerebral laceration the internal changes are the same as those seen in contusion, but the brain surface is torn, with effusion of blood into the cerebrospinal fluid owing to laceration against bony ridges and the edges of dural septa during brain displacement.

Early Secondary Pathology. A. Intracranial Factors

Brain swelling.—The brain often reacts to any insult, be it ischaemic, neoplastic inflammatory or traumatic, by swelling due to *oedema*. The accumulation of fluid is both extracellular and intracellular. Macroscopically oedema may be localised, at least initially to the part of the brain most damaged, but it may extend rapidly throughout one or even both cerebral hemispheres, causing a severe rise in intracranial pressure and, at an earlier stage, features of a relatively localised space occupying or compressing lesion which may mimic a compressing haematoma.

Brain Necrosis.—This is seen most frequently in the so-called 'burst temporal lobe' syndrome. By a combination of swelling (oedema and venous engorgement), ischaemia leading to haemorrhagic infarction, and necrosis, there may be a relatively localised mass occupying the anterior and middle parts of one of the temporal lobe; similar changes may also occur in one or both anterior poles of the frontal lobe. This produces all the clinical features of a lateralised supratentorial mass lesion, usually presenting some hours or even a few days after injury, and may require urgent craniotomy and temporal or frontal lobectomy.

Haematoma.—The surgically remediable intracranial haematomas may be extradural (p. 442), subdural or intracerebral (p. 444/5). They may be the result of arterial or venous bleeding, and therefore vary in their time of presentation in relation to the injury. The deeper the haematoma, the more likely it is to be associated with primary brain damage, oedema, and necrosis and therefore the results of surgical evacuation are poorer. It is rare to have an intracerebral haematoma due solely to the rupture of one major vessel; usually such haematomas are due to the tearing of many small vessels, and it is often difficult to determine the relative part played by the haematoma in the clinical problem.

Vascular changes.—Consequent to rising intracranial pressure disturbance in cerebral blood flow may occur which causes further brain damage through ischaemia, and the ischaemia itself may produce an increase in brain oedema. In normal life there are auto-regulatory mechanisms which, to some extent, protect the cerebral circulation despite changes in blood pressure and intracranial pressure. When the intracranial pressure rises severely, the autoregulatory mechanism fails and irreversible ischaemic changes occur. In addition following brain injury there may be dilatation and engorgement of the venous system which will further increase the brain swelling, and therefore the intracranial pressure and increase the brain oedema by impeding the normal drainage of tissue fluid and worsen the cellular ischaemia.

Coning, or herniation of the contents of the supratentorial compartment through the tentorial hiatus, or the contents of the infratentorial compartment through the foramen magnum, may accompany a rise in pressure in the appropriate compartment (fig. 390). The pathological sequelae to the tentorial hiatus include herniation of the medial part of the temporal lobe (the uncus) on the side of the supratentorial mass which causes pressure upon the ipsilateral third cranial nerve, and upon the mid brain. The mid brain is distorted and displaced away from the side of the mass, where the free edge of the tentorium indents or 'notches' the cerebral peduncle, and interferes with the descending motor pathways from the hemisphere opposite to that which is being compressed. In addition the compression of the mid brain contributes to obstruction of the CSF flow in the aqueduct, which contributes further to the rise of intracranial pressure. These changes produce a deterioration in the level of consciousness, dilation of the pupil on the side of the compressing mass, and a hemiparesis on the *same* side as the mass. This situation is called 'Kernohan's Notch'.

Coup and Contre-Coup.—These words are used to indicate the types of cranio-cerebral damage which may occur either on the side of the blow to the head (*coup*), or opposite (and often diagonally opposite) to the position of the blow (*contre-coup*). Provided it is clear where, and where alone, the head was struck, this knowledge can provide a useful guide to pathology when used in conjunction with the lateralising signs of a compressing lesion (see Coning, above).

COUP AND CONTRE-COUP INJURIES

Coup	Contre-coup
Scalp Laceration	—
Skull Fracture	—
Extradural Haematoma	—
Subdural Haematoma	Subdural Haematoma
Cerebral Laceration and Contusion	Cerebral Laceration and Contusion
Brain Oedema	Brain Oedema
Intracerebral Haematoma	Intracerebral Haematoma

Early Secondary Pathology. B. Extracranial Factors

Respiration.—Respiratory failure or inadequacy is one of the most potent factors which can aggravate or precipitate the development of severe brain oedema and venous congestion, leading rapidly to irreversible changes. Of the two factors, the arterial pO_2 and pCO_2, a rise in pCO_2 is the more potent. It is therefore essential that pCO_2 and pO_2 are maintained at *normal* levels in any patient who has sustained a severe head injury. Although at times hyperventilation has been employed in order to reduce intracranial pressure, abnormally low pCO_2 levels may cause a reduction in cerebral blood flow and subsequent cerebral ischaemic damage, and it is therefore safer to achieve normal levels.

Systemic blood pressure and blood volume.—When the brain is at risk from

James Watson Kernohan, Contemporary. Emeritus Consultant in Pathology, Mayo Clinic, Rochester, U.S.A.

ischaemic damage following injury it is obviously essential that a normal cardiac output is maintained and that blood loss from other injuries is adequately replaced. Recent work has confirmed that, when the intracranial pressure is high, protective cerebral blood flow regulatory mechanisms are impaired and a fall in cardiac output is particularly likely to result in irreversible cerebral ischaemic damage.

Fluids.—Although the onset of brain oedema is usually the result of the primary brain injury and ischaemia, the state of the vascular compartment will influence its course. Thus, if hypotonic fluids are given intravenously, the plasma osmolality may be lowered, particularly if there is any delay or defect in renal excretion of the excess 'water', and therefore by an osmotic effect fluid may be drawn into the brain tissue and brain swelling increased. With disturbance of the normal blood-brain barrier (which is poorly understood) these effects may be increased. Therefore intravenous fluids should be isotonic, and the volumes used (apart from replacement of blood loss by blood) should be dictated by normal requirements and renal function. Problems with fluid and electrolyte balance may be exacerbated by inappropriate secretion of pituitary anti-diuretic hormone as a cerebral response to the cerebral injury. This may produce dangerously low levels of plasma sodium.

Temperature.—When the body temperature rises the metabolic demands of all tissues rise and the accumulation of catabolites increases. When cells or particular groups of cells are damaged, increased metabolic demands will aggravate the cellular failure or aggravate the manifestations of poor function. This is well seen following severe head injury when a rise in body temperature will cause a further deterioration in neurological state.

THE ACUTE COMPRESSING INTRACRANIAL HAEMATOMAS

These are 1. Acute Extradural Haematoma, 2. Acute Subdural Haematoma and 3. Acute Intracerebral Haematoma.

Acute Extradural Haematoma.—Extradural haemorrhage may arise from branches of the *internal maxillary* or *anterior meningeal* vessels torn by fractures of the anterior fossa. In such cases a deterioration in level of consciousness occurs in association with an antero-basal fracture.

The majority of cases of acute extradural haematoma are due to an injury associated with fracture of the temporal or parietal bone whose bleeding results in an extracranial extravasation producing a boggy swelling deep to the temporal muscle.

The classical syndrome of extradural haemorrhage results from injuries of the anterior or posterior branches of the *middle meningeal artery*. In such cases the injuring force, which comes from a lateral direction, is often relatively trivial, such as a blow from a golf or cricket ball which strikes the thin bone of the temporal plate, inflicting a fracture which drives the dura inwards and tears a meningeal artery or vein at a point where it leaves the bony canal in the pterion and crosses to gain attachment to the dura mater. In the elastic skull of children the injury may occur without fracture, as it may, but less commonly, in adults.

From the torn vessel blood passes in three directions:

(1) Outwards through the fracture to form a boggy swelling under the temporal muscle, the finding of which is an additional indication for the *admission for observation of a conscious patient.*

(2) Downwards into the middle fossa.

(3) Upwards over the parietal region.

The development of the extradural compressing mass depends upon the ease with which the dura can be stripped away from the inner surface of the skull. With advancing age the dura becomes more adherent to the skull and, with the 'elasticity' of the skull, is one factor in the greater incidence of extradural haematoma in children and young adults. During the 'lucid' interval (below) the haematoma gradually enlarges and it is not until it has reached a size sufficient to cause a severe rise in intracranial pressure and critical distortion of the mid brain at the tentorial hiatus, that the conscious level deteriorates, often rapidly (fig. 390).

Finally, impaction of a mid-brain cone produces decerebrate rigidity and fixed dilatation of *both* pupils, at which stage the case is probably too late to remedy by operation.

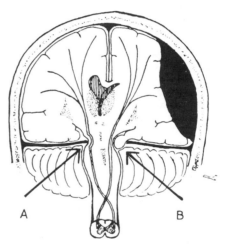

FIG. 390.—Acute extradural haematoma. (A) Impaction of the opposite crus against the opposite rim of the tentorial opening. (B) Displacement of the inner edge of the temporal lobe (uncus) descending into the tentorial opening (mid-brain cone).
(*G. B. Northcroft, FRCS, London.*)

Clinical Features.—Usually a laterally directed blow of small magnitude causes a short initial period of concussion, followed by a characteristic **lucid interval**, during which the haematoma is collecting intracranially and also forming a swelling under the temporal muscle. An example is an unconscious footballer who was carried off the field but later recovered sufficiently to finish the match; headache and drowsiness supervened so that he retired to bed early and was later found dead from middle meningeal haemorrhage.

Although the 'lucid' interval is one of the 'classical' features of an acute extradural haematoma, the 'lucidity' may be only relative compared to the subsequent deterioration. In these circumstances the clinical diagnosis is less obvious, and the consequent delay in diagnosis may reduce the prospect of a favourable outcome. The practical difficulty in such cases is to decide what degree of primary cerebral injury may be present with persisting low level of consciousness, but nevertheless an acute extradural haematoma may yet supervene. It is the awareness of this possible 'non-classical' presentation which has prompted the move towards greater use of the CT scan (see below).

The next change is in the level of consciousness. The patient becomes confused and irritable, and at this stage is in danger of being arrested if found wandering and smelling of alcohol; therefore, beware of the patient brought to Casualty in a confused state with a bruise in the temporal region. Persons alleged to be found drunk have been locked in cells only to be found dead in the morning, the unconsciousness and stertorous breathing of compression being mistaken for a drunken stupor. Confusion changes to drowsiness, and there may be evidence of hemiparesis. At the same time inward displacement of the temporal lobe causes the inner portion of the lobe to press against the third nerve above the edge of the tentorium (fig. 390(B)), causing constriction (rarely observed), rapidly followed by dilatation of the pupil on the side of the haemorrhage. If the pressure is not relieved, displacement of the brain stem at the tentorial opening forces the opposite crus against the rim of the tentorium, producing a hemiparesis, which this time occurs on the same side as the haematoma (fig. 390(A)).

Posterior branch bleeding is less than one fifth as common. Here the clot is situated at a distance from the motor cortex, the surface bruising is situated farther back, or there may be a steady arterial haemorrhage from the ear when the fracture line involves the middle ear. The level of consciousness deteriorates, and the patient passes into a stage of cerebral irritation or stupor with a dilated pupil from pressure inwards on the third nerve, but there may be no motor paralysis for several days, or the paralysis appears on the same side of the body as the haemorrhage as the result of brain shift and impaction of the contralateral crus. The site of operation is determined by the site of the fracture, surface bruising, and dilatation of the pupil.

Extradural haemorrhage of venous origin is produced by fractures which injure the major sinuses or by tearing of a meningeal vein. Injury of the superior longitudinal sinus produces a massive subgaleal haematoma, together with evidence of clot compression, causing rapid deterioration of consciousness with unilateral or bilateral leg weakness if the clot is over the upper end of one or both motor cortices.

Acute Subdural Haematoma.—Following severe head injury there is commonly a thin layer of clot over the brain in the subdural space. This does not usually constitute a significant compressing lesion which is more likely to be produced by the underlying cerebral swelling and contusion. A significant subdural haematoma is produced either by rupture of a large cortical vein as it crosses the potential subdural space to reach the fixed dural venous sinuses (fig. 391) or by laceration of the cortex and subsequent venous or arterial haemorrhage.

The *presentation* and *management* of acute subdural haematoma may be similar to that of acute *extradural* haematoma, but tend to differ in certain respects.

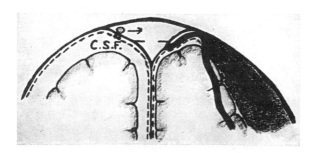

FIG. 391.—Position of a subdural haematoma produced by tearing of the superior cerebral veins at the level of the arachnoid. The diagram also shows the partial or occasionally complete septum which divides the superior sinus. Cerebrospinal fluid drains into the upper compartment through the arachnoid granulations. The superior cerebral veins drain into the lower.
(G. B. Northcroft, F.R.C.S., London.)

1. There is often severe primary brain damage (*e.g.* laceration) and therefore initial and persisting loss of consciousness. A truly lucid interval is unusual.

2. Deterioration tends to occur sooner than in extradural haematoma.

3. The haematoma may be 'coup' or 'contre-coup' (p. 441).

4. The haematoma is often extensive and may cover an entire hemisphere extending both subfrontally and subtemporally.

5. Effective surgical action is unlikely without special investigation (CT scan or arteriogram, p. 455).

6. Effective surgery involves an extensive craniotomy; even then the results are poor due to the primary and often widespread brain damage and brain oedema.

When the presentation is less dramatic and delayed by several days (so-called sub-acute subdural haematoma) it is very difficult to determine the part played by the haematoma as opposed to the underlying brain damage and especially increasing brain oedema. Without the CT scan surgical opinions are frequently without foundation, and surgery ineffective.

7. Very rarely a large acute subdural haematoma may occur in the elderly following a trivial injury or shaking of the brain with rupture of a 'bridging' vein.

Acute Intracerebral Haematoma.—This is the least common of the significant and remediable compressing intracranial haematomas. It is rare for a major intracerebral vessel to rupture as a result of trauma and produce an expanding haematoma which is the sole cause of cerebral compression. When there is a totally lucid interval before such an event it is more likely that haemorrhage has occurred from a pre-existing vascular lesion such as an aneurysm or arteriovenous malformation. If time permits arteriography before surgery is advisable.

Usually traumatic intracerebral haematomas are associated with cerebral laceration, contusion, oedema and necrosis, the compressing lesion being formed by all these elements. Therefore in these circumstances the benefit of removing the clot is unpredictable and often disappointing. Occasionally the removal of such traumatic masses in the anterior part of the temporal lobe or in the frontal pole may be effective, but pre-operative diagnosis with CT scan or arteriogram is essential.

CLINICAL DIAGNOSIS AND MANAGEMENT

Primary and later neurosurgical management must include the following, which will be considered in clinical sequence:

1. Casualty reception
2. Indications for admission
3. Radiography
4. Continuing care and observations
5. Deterioration
6. Indications for surgery without special investigation (decision making)
7. Special investigations
8. Non-surgical therapy: osmotic diuretics, steroids
9. Miscellaneous early complications

1. Casualty Reception.—The reception of the severely injured patient is a large subject which has been dealt with elsewhere (Chapter 1). In the following paragraphs the essential points relate to patients whose main reason for admission is a major head injury. There are certain *general principles*:

(*a*) Patients are more likely to die from airway obstruction than from any remediable intracranial lesions.

(*b*) Surgically remediable intra-thoracic and intra-abdominal lesions take precedence over any intracranial procedures.

(*c*) In normal civilian practice patients are brought rapidly to a casualty department; therefore compressing intracranial haematomas are unlikely to present when the patient is first seen.

(*d*) The initial clinical assessment and its recording especially of the level of consciousness is of crucial importance if any later deterioration is to be gauged accurately.

(*e*) The immediate institution of the correct care of the unconscious patient does more to lower the morbidity and mortality from major head injury than any other single measure.

In receiving and assessing a patient in casualty the essential steps in chronological order can be summarised as follows:

(i) *Protection of the airway* (see oedema).—All the usual measures for the protection of the airway in an unconscious patient should be taken immediately; removal of false teeth, positioning prone or on one side with the head low, mouth suction and insertion of a pharyngeal airway. The presence of a compound skull fracture with exuding brain tissue is not a contraindication to lowering the head. In the majority of patients these measures will suffice. However if they do not a cuffed endotracheal tube should be inserted, which is in itself a test of the need for that manoeuvre.

(ii) *General assessment.*—The general assessment is often as important as the neurological because intra-thoracic and intra-abdominal injury may require immediate action. These aspects are dealt with elsewhere (Chapter 1) but it should be stressed that the picture of 'surgical shock' should not be ascribed to the head injury unless the presence of another major injury has been excluded.

(iii) *Neurological assessment*

(*a*) Level of consciousness.—This is the single most important neurological observation, and one that causes greatest difficulty in accurate description and recording. Terms and gradings which require definition (*e.g.* 'coma', 'stupor') should be avoided. A brief description in simple words which include the degree of alertness, ability to communicate or obey commands, and type of spontaneous or reflex limb movements is often satisfactory. The Glasgow Coma Scale (fig. 392) is a valuable method of recording consecutive observations, and of observing progressive changes but without requiring previous definition of terms used.

(*b*) Pupils.—When *both* pupils are small on admission and later *one* dilates, that provides the most accurate clinical guide to the lateralisation of a supratentorial compressing lesion (see Coning, p. 441). If however one pupil was known to be dilated immediately after the injury it is usually due to direct injury related to the orbit and neither pupil can be used later as a guide to lateralisation. Therefore the first assessment and recording of pupillary size is of extreme importance; size and equality rather than reaction to light is the more important feature, and should be recorded graphically or verbally.

(*c*) Limbs.—The types of spontaneous or reflex limb movements are an essential part of the assessment of the level of consciousness (see above). Hemiplegia

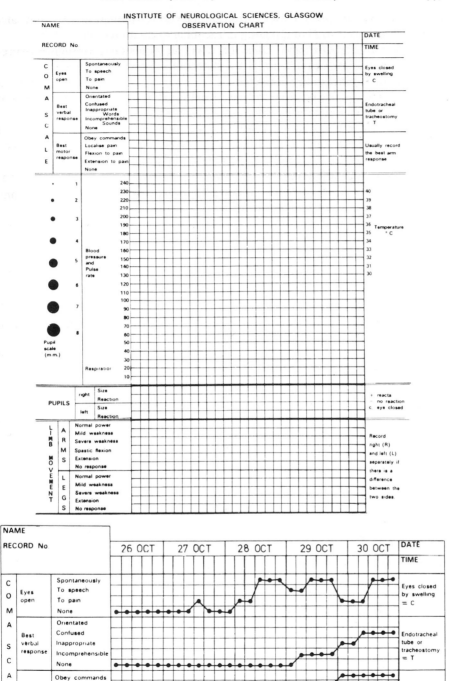

FIG. 392.—(a) The Glasgow Coma Scale; (b) details of a case.
(Institute of Neurological Sciences, Glasgow.)

is as likely to be due to a 'stroke' prior to injury as to trauma; in the acute state it is very rarely due to a compressing intracranial haematoma, but may be due to the primary cerebral damage. Alone it is never an indication for urgent surgery. Of more immediate significance is the detection of paraplegia or quadriplegia indicative of a spinal injury (Chapter 27).

(d) Cranium.—The position and nature of the external trauma should be noted accurately, the wound over an obvious fracture should be cleaned with saline and surrounding hair removed for a distance of at least 5 cm, and a head dressing applied. The presence of CSF rhinorrhoea, or otorrhoea is noted, and special note made of any mandibular or facial fracture which might lead to further difficulties with the airway.

(e) History of injury.—With the severely injured the initial assessment and resuscitation is usually done before a history of the injury can be obtained. However, that information is important, particularly if a preceding medical condition has led to the injury. Information from witnesses, ambulance attendants and relatives should be sought. *Alcohol* poses particular problems, which are often greater in those who have been less severely injured, and it makes accurate assessment of neurological lesions more difficult, and may be misleading when deterioration in conscious level due to an intracranial haematoma occurs.

2. Indications for Admission.—Following head injury patients are admitted to hospital for two main reasons: (A) For continuing hospital care, for those who have suffered serious injury and who are in obvious need of care and possibly surgery. (B) For observation in case a complication should develop, despite the patient being perfectly well at the time of admission. The first category presents little difficulty about the indication for admission, but the second presents considerable difficulty. Remediable complications (*e.g.* acute extradural haematoma) may occur following very trival injury, but there is some evidence that they are more likely to occur after transient change in consciousness, when a skull fracture is present and when the patient complains of persisting headache. However, although the incidence of haematoma is very low in the absence of these features it is currently a matter of debate whether transient clouding of consciousness alone should remain an indication for admission. Accepting that there are these grounds for debate, the following are reasonable guidelines:

(i) *Indication for skull radiographs after recent injury.*
   1. Loss of consciousness or amnesia at any time
   2. Focal neurological symptoms or abnormal signs
   3. Suspected penetrating injury
   4. Scalp bruising or swelling
   5. Alcohol intoxication
   6. Difficulty in assessing the patient

(ii) *Indications for Admission.*
   1. Any degree of depression of level of consciousness on examination
   2. Skull fracture
   3. Focal neurological signs
   4. Persistent headache or vomiting
   5. Other medical conditions such as patients on anticoagulants, haemophilia
   6. Uncertainty about the degree of alcohol intoxication

7. Circumstances of injury unknown

8. Crime

9. Absence of responsible relatives or friends.

If the absence of a skull fracture is used as one of the reasons for *not* admitting a patient, the radiographs *must* be of acceptable quality. If patients are not admitted, a responsible relative or friend should be given *written* instructions about the possible complications and appropriate action.

The duration of observation is arbitrary, but since it is exceptional for acute extradural haematoma to present more than 18 hours after injury, overnight admission is sufficient.

3. Radiography.—The purpose of *skull radiographs* includes:

(i) The demonstration of a skull fracture whose position may provide a valuable guide to the *site* of an extradural haematoma which might develop later.

(ii) The presence of a skull fracture provides some indication of the severity of the injury, and is one of the indications for admission.

(iii) The demonstration of a depressed fracture which may require surgery.

(iv) The demonstration of a calcified pineal gland and its position relative to the midline, which may change in subsequent radiographs.

(v) The presence of intracranial air.

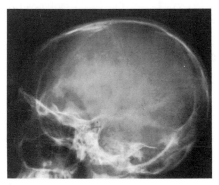 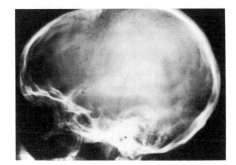

FIG. 393.—Skull radiograph of poor quality fails to show fracture.   FIG. 394.—Good quality radiograph shows fracture.

Therefore the radiograph on admission may provide an essential base line when later deterioration occurs, and in the early management it can be argued that the radiographs are more important in patients who are relatively well than in those who are deeply unconscious. Unless radiographs are of reasonable quality they are valueless and may be dangerously misleading (figs. 393, 394), and in those circumstances it is wiser to defer radiography until films of good quality can be obtained. The skull radiographs usually required are the right and/or left lateral, the half-axial (35°) and the antero-posterior (20°). However a *chest radiograph* is essential, as is a *lateral radiograph of the cervical spine* to demonstrate clinically undetectable fractures or fracture dislocation (Chapter 27). If patients are in urgent need of intensive care, time should not be wasted in trying to obtain skull radiographs.

4. Continuing Care.—The objects of further care are: (*a*) by nursing and other intensive care measures to enable the patients to survive a period of 'unconsciousness'. (*b*) By repeated observation to detect at the earliest possible moment the development of complications which may need surgical or medical action.

Care of the 'unconscious' patient.—The quality of care given, which largely depends upon the availability of experienced nursing staff will determine the outcome in the majority of patients. Attention to airways, skin, eyes, mouth, bladder and bowels, limb joints, nasogastric tube feeding and intravenous infusions are very demanding and the surgeon must take a personal interest in these matters if morale is to be maintained. *Controlled ventilation* is used widely if spontaneous respiration is inadequate to maintain normal levels of pCO_2 and pO_2. *Tracheostomy* is very rarely necessary in the first few days after injury because an endotracheal tube may be used for up to seven days; thereafter if the airway or respiration is inadequate, tracheostomy may be required. As the level of consciousness improves there may be a stage of irritability which is difficult to control; drugs are best avoided because all *sedatives* tend to depress respiration to some extent, which may lead to a gradual rise in the pCO_2 and deterioration due to brain swelling even ten days after injury. Clearly if the patient is conscious enough to experience severe pain from other injuries (*e.g.* limbs) it is inhumane to withhold *analgesics* such as codeine phosphate (100 mg), but morphia is best avoided. Because *epilepsy* is a major cause of deterioration (see below) all patients should be on prophylactic *anticonvulsants*; adult drugs and dosages are phenobarbitone 60 mg 8-hourly, or phenytoin 100 mg 8-hourly, and neither will depress the level of consciousness.

5. Deterioration.—The most important indication of deterioration following head injury is a decline in the level of consciousness. Its recognition requires accurate observation and accurate sequential recording (see Glasgow Coma Scale, fig. 392). The major causes of deterioration are:

(i) Airway obstruction/hypoventilation *causing* brain swelling *causing* rising intracranial pressure.

(ii) Brain swelling *causing* rising intracranial pressure.

(iii) Intracranial haematoma.

(iv) Epilepsy.

(v) Fluids and dehydration.

(vi) Fever—infection—meningitis.

(vii) Blood loss from other injuries.

(viii) Aerocele.

Although swelling is a more frequent cause of deterioration than compressing intracranial haematoma, it must be assumed that the deterioration is due to a haematoma until proved otherwise. The exceptions to this rule are: epilepsy, fluid imbalance, infection and fever, and blood loss. Unfortunately airway obstruction and inadequate ventilation may not only cause increased brain oedema, but also the addition of brain oedema in the presence of a haematoma and therefore it is not always safe to assume that oedema alone is the cause of the deterioration following airway obstruction.

Epilepsy may cause rapid deterioration in level of consciousness and if a convulsion is not witnessed it may be difficult to differentiate this from the occasionally rapid effects of cerebral compression. A convulsion does not necessarily indicate the presence of a compressing haematoma.

Fever from any cause will produce deterioration. *Meningitis* may follow injury especially with basal skull fractures and tends to present at the third to fifth day after injury. At that time, in the presence of fever and neck stiffness diagnostic lumbar puncture is indicated.

Fluid imbalance and particularly dehydration may produce a gradual deterioration over the course of 48 hours; clinical examination, review of fluid charts and plasma electrolytes should detect the imbalance, and the level of consciousness improves with correction.

6. Indications for Surgery without Special Investigations (Decision Making).

The SIGNS OF CEREBRAL COMPRESSION are DETERIORATION IN LEVEL OF CONSCIOUSNESS, SLOWING PULSE, RISING BLOOD PRESSURE and SLOWING RESPIRATION.

In the presence of these signs, and having reasonably excluded other causes (see above), the conclusion must be that:

This patient has a compressing haematoma until proved otherwise.

In these circumstances neurosurgical advice should be sought because either (*a*) The patient should be transferred to a neurosurgical department or (*b*) Surgical action must be taken without delay and without special investigations. The decision taken will depend upon the rate of deterioration, dilatation of one or both pupils, the travelling time to (rather than the distance from) the neurosurgical department, the experience of the surgeon and the availability of special surgical instruments.

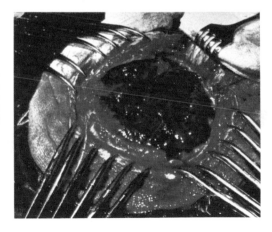

FIG. 395.—Acute extradural haematoma. (*M. B. Yorston, FFARCS, Southampton*): When the burr-hole is made, the clot has the appearance of blackcurrant jelly and obscures the dura and bleeding dural artery.

Surgery without special investigations.—The prime purpose of such surgery is to locate and evacuate, or exclude an *acute extradural haematoma* (fig. 395), an essentially remediable lesion, in a patient who is rapidly deteriorating. (The clinicopathological aspects of acute extradural haematoma are described on p. 442 and the reader may need to refer to this section before that which follows.)

The major decisons before embarking upon urgent exploratory surgery concern:

(i) *The presence or not of a haematoma* (determined by the signs of rising pressure, see above).

(ii) *The side for exploration.*—For this the essential guides are in order of reliability (*a*), the shift of a calcified pineal on x-ray and (*b*) the side of the first pupil to dilate, provided it was not dilated immediately after injury. (See casualty reception.)

(iii) *The position of exploratory burr holes* on the appropriate side. In order of importance the guides are:

(*a*), the position of a vault or squamous temporal fracture; (*b*), the site of external trauma; and (*c*), the standard temporal position (see below).

Pre-operative.—Ideally general anaesthesia with endotracheal intubation and controlled ventilation should be used. However, if that is not available, time should not be lost, an endotracheal tube should be inserted, and operation done under local anaesthesia. Having determined the likely side of the compressing lesion (see above) the patient is positioned supine with a sandbag under the appropriate shoulder and the face turned to the opposite side. It is wise to remove all the hair, or at least that of the appropriate half of the head, and that side is shaved. The sterile towels should be arranged in a way that allows access to frontal, temporal and parietal regions. Blood should be available, but surgery should not be delayed if it is not.

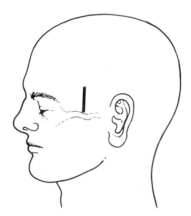

FIG. 396.—Incision for standard temporal burr hole.

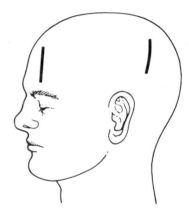

FIG. 397.—Incisions for frontal and parietal burr holes.

Operation

The exploratory burr hole (position see above).—A 3 cm vertical incision is made *down to bone*; a self-retaining mastoid-type retractor is inserted and opened forcefully thus controlling scalp and muscle bleeding. The incision for the *standard temporal burr hole* is *immediately* above the zygomatic arch mid-way between the posterior margin of the orbit and the external auditory meatus (fig. 396). At that level the squamous temporal bone lies relatively deeply, but no damage can be done in reaching it, and it is essential to use the self-retaining retractor to control the scalp and muscle bleeding. Using a brace and bit with first the sharp point, and, when the inner table of the skull is pierced, the reamer which has a protective flange, a burr hole is made. *If a significant extradural clot is present the dura will not be seen* because the dura will have been separated from the brain by the clot which has the appearance of blackcurrant jelly. For the same reason the responsible bleeding dural artery (*e.g.* middle meningeal) will not be seen.

Further action.—A. Extradural clot is not present.—Bearing in mind that the essential purpose of this exploratory surgery is the exclusion or evacuation of an *extra*dural clot it is unwise to open the dura at this stage. If the first burr hole has been placed over or next to the fracture, it is reasonable to make a second burr hole in the *standard temporal position*. If that also is negative it is reasonable to make a frontal or parietal burr hole if the original guides have not already included those positions (fig. 397). If none of these burr holes on one side have revealed an extradural clot two further questions arise:

1. *Should the dura be opened?* The assessment of the thickness and therefore significance of an acute *subdural* clot by inspection through a burr hole is extremely difficult. Only specialised radiology can assess this accurately and show the extent as well as the thickness of the lesion. Whenever there is primary brain damage (contusion, laceration) there is some clot in the subdural space but this is rarely a significant compressing lesion. Furthermore the satisfactory evacuation of a significant subdural clot requires a major and often larger craniotomy (osteoplastic flap) with a wide dural opening; these procedures require particular neurosurgical expertise and facilities, and the surgery itself may lead to further technical problems such as herniation of a swollen brain. Therefore if an extradural haematoma is not found, *the dura should not be opened*, ventilation should be continued, an osmotic diuretic given (mannitol, p. 456) and the patient transferred for special radiology.

2. *Should a burr hole be made on the other side?* If the radiologically demonstrated shift of the pineal has been used to determine the side of the compressing lesion nothing will be gained by making a burr hole on the opposite side. If the side of the first dilating pupil and the side of the fracture and/or site of external trauma coincide, a contralateral burr hole need not be made. If however the fracture or evidence of external trauma (*e.g.* bruising and swelling on the temporal region) is on the side opposite to the first dilating pupil, the compressing lesion is likely to be *contre-coup* (p. 441). However, very rarely the pupil may mislead and therefore a final burr hole should be made over the fracture and/or site of external brusing swelling.

Further action.—B. Extradural clot present.—Assessment of thickness of the clot is made by using a blunt-nosed brain cannula with centimetre marks and feeling the resistance of the dura; any clot greater than 0·5 cm thick is significant. Sometimes the burr hole will have been placed just at the edge of the haematoma which is not, therefore, immediately visible; only by gently inserting a dissector and depressing the dura will the clot be detected (fig. 398).

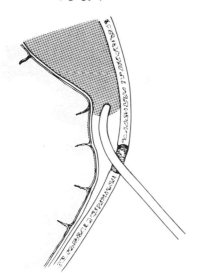
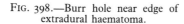
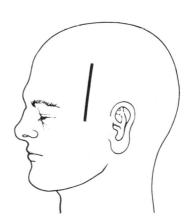

FIG. 398.—Burr hole near edge of extradural haematoma.

FIG. 399.—Extension of incision for craniectomy.

Evacuation of clot.—(*a*) *By craniectomy:* The burr hole incision is extended in a straight line to a length of about 8 cm (fig. 399), a second self-retaining retractor is inserted and with bone nibblers the burr hole is enlarged to a craniectomy of at least 7 cm diameter (fig. 400). The clot is then gently lifted off, this and the bone removal decompressing the brain. Small fragments of clot adherent to the dura are left because their removal only produces troublesome oozing from the dura to which 'Oxycel' may be applied. If a major

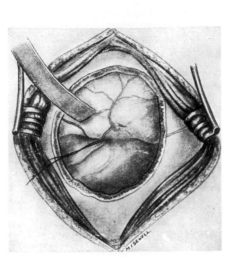

FIG. 400.—Craniectomy and control of meningeal artery by dural stitch.

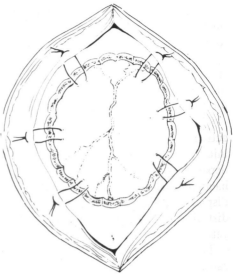

FIG. 401.—Dural 'hitching' stitches.

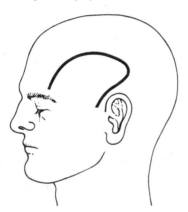

FIG. 402.—Incision for temporal craniotomy.

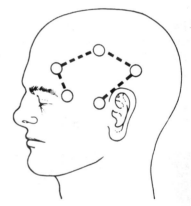

FIG. 403.—Burr holes and saw cuts for temporal craniotomy.

dural vessel is bleeding it is controlled either by diathermy or by a stitch passed under the vessel. The dura is then 'hitched' to the surrounding bone by passing sutures (*e.g.* black silk) through the superficial layer of the dura and the surrounding muscle or pericranium; this step is essential to prevent the re-accumulation of a haematoma (fig. 401). The muscles, temporal fascia, galea and skin are then closed in layers without drainage and a full head dress using gauze and a crepe bandage is applied.

(*b*) *By craniotomy and osteoplastic flap.*—In experienced hands this gives wider access without any appreciable loss of time in decompressing the brain and is generally used in neurosurgical departments, but does require familiarity and neurosurgical instruments. The stages are the turning of a scalp flap, the placing of multiple burr holes which are then joined by a Gigli saw and the raising of a quadrilateral bone flap hinged at its base upon the temporal muscles (figs. 402 and 403).

Postoperative.—As soon as the conscious level permits the patient should be mobilised; skin sutures are removed on the second or third day. Antibiotics are not used routinely. Prophylactic anticonvulsant drugs (see Continuing Care) should be continued for about six weeks in the absence of any other indications for their longer term use.

Leonardo Gigli, 1863-1908. Obstetrician. Director, Santa Maria Nuova Hospital, Florence, Italy. Introduced his saw for pubiotomy in 1894, and adapted it for craniotomy in 1898.

7. Special Investigations.—Once the decision has been taken that there is time for the deteriorating patient to be transferred to a department with access to special neuroradiological facilities, it is reasonable to give osmotic diuretics (p. 456) to gain temporary improvement during transfer. However, even in neurosurgical departments, there are occasions when, with patients who are deteriorating very rapidly and whose second pupil is dilating, there can be no further delay for radiology and exploratory burr holes are made (see '6').

Computed Axial Tomography (CT scan).—This non-invasive type of investigation provides the most accurate guide to intracranial pathology following injury, and is available in all neurosurgical departments and to many general departments. It has revolutionised the investigation of head injury, intracranial haemorrhage and infarction, and space occupying lesions. When available it displaces the use of arteriography and air study. The investigation causes no disturbance to the patient and eliminates exposure to conventional x-ray investigations.

The patient lies on a motorised couch in order that the part to be examined can be positioned within the scanning gantry. The head is scanned from above downwards in a series of transversing planes like a tomograph from vertex to base of skull by tilting the x-ray tube and detector array within the gantry at each scan.

The information is fed to a computer and produces a record in which high density objects such as bone, clot or tumour appear white, the brain substance appears grey, areas of oedema a dark mottled colour and the ventricular fluids black. Collectively the scanner produces a complete picture in which tumours, clots, infarction, ventricular displacement or hydrocephalus are readily distinguished.

Its major value is in the differentiation between brain swelling, contusion

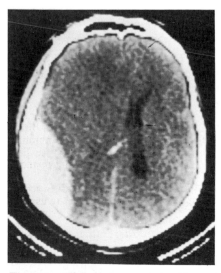

FIG. 404.—CT Scan. Acute extradural haematoma.

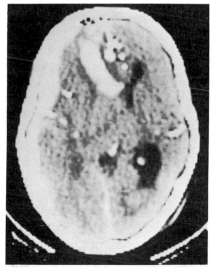

FIG. 405.—CT Scan show left hemisphere swelling, ventrical displaced to right, contusion, intracerebral blood and subdural clot.

and compressing haematoma, and the accurate demonstration of the extent and thickness of a haematoma, and therefore the need for surgical evacuation. The demonstration of oedema provides a guide to the use of osmotic diuretics (below) and of controlled respiration (figs 404, 405). So valuable is this method of investigation that there are now strong grounds for transferring all patients with severe head injuries to hospitals where CT scan is readily available. It has largely replaced other methods of investigation.

Carotid arteriography, in the absence of CT scan, remains a valuable method of investigation particularly in the demonstration of extracerebral haematomas (extradural and subdural). In those conditions there may be displacement of the middle cerebral artery, the anterior cerebral artery may be displaced from its midline position away from the side of the haematoma and the cortical vessels do not reach the inner table of the skull (fig. 406).
Ultrasound has been of value in demonstrating the position of midline structures by their characteristic echo but it does not approach the accuracy of the calcified pineal visible on plain radiographs or the information gained from CT scan.
Intracranial pressure monitoring is a very specialised method of investigation which may be of value in continuing and postoperative care but is not relevant to the acute situation on admission to hospital.

8. Non-surgical Therapy

Osmotic diuretics.—The basis for the use of these substances is that by raising the osmolarity of the plasma, fluid will be drawn from the brain extravascular compartment into the blood, thereby reducing brain oedema and swelling. Therefore solutions given intravenously for this purpose must be hyperosmolar, non-diffusible (*i.e.* they should not pass across the blood-brain barrier), non-irritant and be not excreted too rapidly by the kidney, or metabolised rapidly. In the past 5% sucrose was used but to little effect; lyophilised urea was more effective but because it was diffusible there was a considerable rebound' effect. Today *mannitol* as a 20% solution given intravenously to an adult as a volume of 250 ml (or in dire circumstances 500 ml) over the course of 20 to 30 minutes is the agent in general use. It may be used repeatedly at 6 or 8 hour intervals but the following must be noted:

(*a*), There should be satisfactory renal function; (*b*), if a diuresis has not occurred following mannitol, further administration should be delayed; (*c*), fluid and electrolyte replacement should be meticulous, particularly with the loss of electrolytes with each diuresis; (*d*), if hyper-osmolarity of the blood is to be produced, the rate of administration is critical.

There are *potential dangers* in the use of mannitol before either a diagnosis has been established or a course of action instituted. Thus although the cause of a patient's deterioration may well be brain oedema, giving mannitol may produce temporary improvement in the presence of a large haematoma, soon to be followed by profound deterioration. Therefore mannitol should not be used in the acute stage following injury unless the possibility of an intracranial haematoma has been excluded in a patient who is deteriorating, except to gain time prior to surgery. It should never be used as a diagnostic test to differentiate between oedema and haematoma.

Frusemide (40–80 mg by intramuscular injection) is an alternative agent which

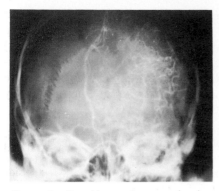

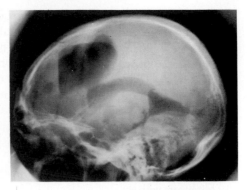

Fig. 406.—Carotid arteriogram showing mid-line shift and bare area over cortex due to clot.

Fig. 407.—Frontal aerocele and spontaneous ventriculogram fracture through frontal sinus.

produces a very rapid diuresis and thereby raises the osmolarity of the vascular compartment. It is non-irritant, but requires good renal function for its effect.

Cortico-steroids (Dexamethasone and Betamethasone).—In high doses (up to 24 mg a day) these drugs are effective symptomatically in malignant brain tumours, the main effect being upon surrounding brain oedema. In the management of severe head injuries they have been used widely for some years, often in doses of up to 60 mg a day. Unfortunately this practice is based more upon tradition than objective evidence, *because at present there is no evidence that their use improves the outcome in severe head injury.*

9. Miscellaneous Complications—Early

'Brain-stem injury.'—This term is used loosely to describe a clinical picture which is ascribed to primary damage in the brain-stem (medulla and pons). It should be stressed that the changes may follow unrelieved supratentorial compression. The patients are often children or young adults, the latter being motor cyclists who, wearing crash helmets, suffered an acute flexion/extension movement of the neck at the moment of impact on the vertex. Signs of external trauma may be absent, but the patient is 'unconscious', with spontaneous extensor spasms of all four limbs, arching of the trunk (opisthotonus), a rapid pulse, rapid and often shallow and therefore inadequate respiration, small pupils, pyrexia and sweating. Any stimuli will tend to increase the tendency to extension. If this state has been present from the time of injury the likelihood of a compressing haematoma is remote. Prognosis depends upon intensive nursing care, and control of respiration; the ultimate intellectual deficit may be considerably less severe than following major supratentorial brain damage, but there is often marked spasticity and inco-ordination.

Posterior Fossa Compression.—Compression of the cerebellum and medulla by posterior fossa haematoma is rare. However in the presence of a fracture which passes towards the foramen magnum and therefore crosses the lateral sinus an extradural haematoma may occur. These tend to present somewhat later than the supratentorial extradural haematoma, usually after 48 hours and the most important physical sign is *slowing and irregularity of respiration,* which may precede other evidence of deterioration. Special investigation by CT scan or ventriculogram is needed prior to a posterior fossa craniectomy.

CSF Rhinorrhoea.—For CSF rhinorrhoea to occur there must be a communication between the intracranial (intradural) cavity and the nose. Therefore CSF rhinorrhoea indicates a tear of the dura (usually basal) and a fracture involving the paranasal sinuses, frontal, ethmoid or sphenoid. At the moment of impact not only does the dural tear and fracture occur but also a plug of brain may be forced into the dural tear; although this may temporarily seal the defect it also prevents dural healing and therefore the CSF rhinorrhoea may persist and the patient be at risk from meningitis which is usually pneumococcal. CSF rhinorrhoea may occur in association with displaced fractures of the middle third of the face (Chapter 30).

Although there are different views on the management of CSF rhinorrhoea a reasonable course is:

1. Initially the patient is given prophylactic antibiotics (penicillin and sulphonamides).

2. Fractures of the middle third of the face are reduced; in many cases the rhinorrhoea may cease.

3. The indications for anterior fossa exploration are CSF rhinorrhoea persisting for more than ten days, the presence of a fracture involving the frontal or ethmoid sinus, an aerocele (see below), and an attack of meningitis which has been treated. Factors such as age, neurological state, and degree of disruption of the anterior fossa floor are taken into consideration.

Aerocele.—Entry of air into the cranial cavity usually occurs in association with CSF rhinorrhoea. Air may enter the subarachnoid space and ventricular system (a 'spontaneous ventriculogram') or the substance of the frontal lobe because the brain is adherent to the margin of the dural defect. This occurs particularly if the patient blows his nose. Rarely a frontal aerocele may cause compression and therefore deterioration about two or more weeks after injury (fig. 407). Surgery is similar to that for CSF rhinnorrhoea.

Meningitis.—Apart from its association with CSF rhinorrhoea and otorrhoea, meningitis may occur after any major head injury particularly if a basal skull fracture is present but often undetected (see p. 460). Bleeding into the subarachnoid space is common with head injury, and neck stiffness immediately after injury is *not* an indication for lumbar puncture. Meningitis when it occurs does so after the first 48 or 72 hours and, therefore, provided there are no signs of cerebral compression, fever and neck stiffness are, at that stage, an indication for lumbar puncture. If there are also signs of cerebral compression the patient should be transferred for urgent intracranial investigation before lumbar puncture.

Pituitary Failure.—Occasionally basal fractures may pass across the pituitary fossa causing acute pituitary damage and endocrine failure. This may lead to a profound fall in blood pressure, tachycardia, pallor and hypothermia with deterioration in level of consciousness. Once the condition is recognised high doses of steroids should be given (hydrocortisone 200 mg 6 hourly for the first 24 hours, followed by reduced and then maintenance dosage).

Fat Embolism.—Systemic fat embolism may cause diagnostic difficulties when patients with multiple injuries which include a head injury show neurological deterioration at about 48 hours after injury or surgery for limb fractures

(Chapter 14). Neurological features which suggest fat embolism rather than an intracranial haematoma are the time of deterioration, the delayed onset of features of a brain-stem injury (see above), pupils which vary in size from moment to moment but which remain equal, the presence of small retinal haemorrhages, and the absence of any firm lateralising signs. The finding of fresh petechiae over the upper part of the trunk and in the axillae is of help. However in the absence of positive signs of fat embolism, it is usually wise to check the position of the pineal if it is visible, or to obtain a CT scan.

FRACTURES OF THE SKULL

Fractures of the vault and base of the skull are produced: (1) by compression of the sphere; (2) by local indentation; (3) by tangential injury. A traditional primary classification of skull fractures is:

A. *Closed.*—The scalp is not breached, but there may be bruising or grazing of the scalp as distinct from a full thickness laceration.

B. *Open.*—There is an open laceration of the scalp with exposure of the underlying fracture.

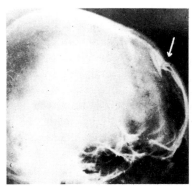

FIG. 408.—Sharp bone spicules penetrating the dura. Probing of an open wound to determine the type of fracture is potentially dangerous because a spicule of bone plugging a laceration in a large vein or dural sinus may be dislodged, and cause uncontrollable bleeding.

This simple classification, which is analgous to that of fractures elsewhere, gives some guide to the likelihood of foreign tissues being present in the wound and the relative danger of subsequent infection at any depth. However given that the primary management of the *scalp* injury is satisfactory the differentiation between closed and open fracture is of less surgical importance than the classification of the type of fracture, which can *only* be established radiologically. Unless there is a very obvious skull defect beneath an open wound in which brain tissue is visible, attempts to differentiate between simple and depressed fractures clinically are rarely accurate. Furthermore probing of such wounds to determine the type of fracture is *potentially dangerous* (see fig. 408 and legend, and see Scalp Lacerations).

1. **Simple and Comminuted Linear Fractures of the Vault.**—These are the most common types of fracture, and in themselves do not require surgery. The surgical management is simply that of the overlying laceration if present. The significance of such fractures (apart from those in special sites) is that their presence gives some indication of the severity of the injury, the degree of deceleration or acceleration primary brain injury, and the likelihood of delayed complications.

Indeed extradural haematoma is more common in the presence of a simple linear fracture than with depressed fractures. A linear fracture of the squamous temporal bone is of special significance in that respect, and should make very frequent observation of the patient, particularly a child, obligatory.

2. **Linear Fractures of the Skull Base.**—The clinical indications of the presence of such fractures include bruising within the orbital margins involving the eyelids and conjunctiva (anterior cranial fossa), and bruising in the mastoid region, Battle's sign[1] (middle cranial fossa and petrous bone). Such fractures are the result of skull distortion, and indicate that a considerable force was applied to the skull at the moment of impact. These fractures may be difficult to demonstrate radiologically, unless special skull views are taken. Since accurate diagnosis of such fractures is rarely essential for management, basal views of the skull should be done with circumspection because the position of hyper-extension of the neck is potentially dangerous in the presence of any degree of cervical instability, or in the presence of cervical spondylosis.

Skull base fractures may be associated with immediate and often irreversible damage to cranial nerves, *e.g.* olfactory, optic, oculo-motor, facial and auditory. A delayed lower motor neurone facial weakness may be due to contusion and swelling of the facial nerve in continuity within the facial canal. Anterior fossa fractures may be associated with CSF rhinorrhoea (see above). Middle fossa and petrous bone fractures increase the risk of meningitis, which may occur after an interval of several days. *CSF otorrhoea* indicates a basal fracture with disruption of the dura over the petrous bone, and rupture of the tympanic membrane. Management is by prophylactic antibiotics for Gram-negative and Gram-positive organisms until the otorrhoea stops; meningitis due to continued leakage of CSF from the middle ear through the Eustachian tube is very rare.

3. **Linear Fractures of the Posterior Fossa and Foramen Magnum.**—These are rare and can be seen clearly only on the half-axial skull radiographs. Their significance lies in the rare association with a posterior fossa extradural haematoma, of which the presenting clinical feature may be a decline in respiration which precedes deterioration in level of consciousness. If such a fracture is present, it is wise to observe the patient for at least 3 days.

4. **Linear Fractures involving the Frontal Paranasal Sinus.**—If such fractures are associated with a linear tear of the dura, CSF rhinorrhoea may occur (see above). Even if CSF rhinorrhoea is not present it is wise to check that it cannot be provoked by positioning the patient with his head low, before he is discharged from hospital. The indications for surgery in the absence of CSF rhinorrhoea are debatable.

5. **Depressed Fractures.**—Traditionally a fracture is said to be 'significantly' depressed if the degree of depression is greater than the depth of the inner table of the skull. The possible complications of depressed fractures are:

(*a*) *Dural tear.*—This is the most important indication for surgery. The greater the depression of the bone fragments, and the more the fragments are angled inwards, particularly a spicule, the more likely is the dura to be torn; even in the absence of such features it may be very difficult to exclude a dural laceration by

---

[1] Battle's sign = discoloration appearing over the mastoid process.

William Henry Battle, 1855-1936. Surgeon, St Thomas's Hospital, London.

the radiological appearances of a depressed fracture.

(*b*) *Underlying Haematoma.*—It is unusual to have a significant compressing clot beneath a depressed fracture. If there are clinical indications investigation (*e.g.* CT scan) should be done before elevating the fracture.

(*c*) *Pressure upon the Cerebral Cortex.*—In practice this very rarely contributes to the clinical effects of a depressed fracture.

(*d*) *Epilepsy.*—A depressed fracture may be one of several factors contributing to early or late post-traumatic epilepsy. Elevation of the fracture may diminish the risk of epilepsy, although in individual cases this may be debatable.

(*e*) *Cosmetic Defects.*—In the adult this is rarely a problem; but the simple depressed 'pond' fracture of infants following obstetric manoeuvres may need elevation for cosmetic reasons, although such fractures often undergo spontaneous elevation.

(*f*) *Pressure upon Dural Venous Sinuses.*—Very rarely a depressed fragment of bone may compress and obstruct the superior saggital or lateral sinus, leading to raised intracranial pressure. Of greater importance is the risk of severe haemorrhage if depressed fractures over the sinuses are elevated; therefore fractures in these sites *should not be elevated*.

SURGERY OF DEPRESSED FRACTURES

When the injury is compound prophylactic antibiotics covering Gram-positive and Gram-negative organisms should be started on admission, and continued for 10 days after surgery.

There are different views about the timing of surgery for depressed fractures. Emergency elevation is not required, but as soon as the patient's general condition is stable, especially in respect of other major injuries, operation for the compound fracture should be done. When the fracture is simple (*i.e.* closed) operation may be delayed for 2 or 3 days, particularly if there is doubt over the patient's neurological progress, and intracranial investigation may become necessary.

Important points in surgical technique are:
  (i) The hair should be shaved widely round the wound.
 (ii) Care is taken to remove all foreign material from the laceration.
(iii) A wound may be extended in a linear fashion, or be made part of a skull flap.
 (iv) Because the scalp is the most important of the tissues covering the brain, *scalp should not be excised*, and debridement should be kept to an absolute minimum.
  (v) The pericranium is detached from the bone using a rougine, and preserved for closure.
 (vi) A burr hole is made in the normal skull next to the depressed area, but away from the midline of the vault. Bone is nibbled away towards the depression, the underlying dura is gently separated from the overlying bone fragments using an Adson's elevator.
(vii) The depressed fragments are cautiously lifted out *and kept*, so that the dura beneath the depression is fully exposed and any dural tear can be seen.
(viii) If there is a dural tear, the edges of the dura are gently separated from the underlying brain using the Adson's elevator.
 (ix) Any indriven fragments of bone or foreign bodies are cautiously removed, but *only obviously necrotic and extruding brain tissue* may be sucked away.
  (x) Any bleeding from the brain can be controlled by diathermy or tantalum clips.
 (xi) The edges of the dural laceration are brought together using interrupted sutures. If there has been loss of dura, a free graft of pericranium may be inserted.
(xii) If the area of exposed dura is greater than 3 cm diameter, 'hitching' stitches should be inserted (see fig. 401).

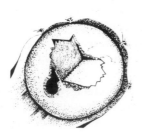

FIG. 409.—Formation of burr hole beside a fractured area to allow unlocking of the bone fragment.

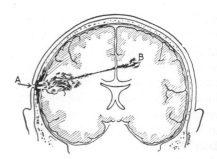

FIG. 410.—Transverse penetrating wound, entry at (A) showing: (1) Protrusion of brain through the dura at entry site forming hernia cerebri. (2) Pulped brain and bone close to entry. (3) A metal fragment at (B) has crossed the open superior fissure.

(xiii) The removed bone fragments should be cleaned and replaced in a mosaic fashion, and the pericranium and scalp closed carefully in layers without drainage.

Skull Reconstruction.—Areas of skull defect are restored at intervals of three to six months after injury, by the insertion of moulded tantalum plates or acrylic inlays. Concealed horseshoe or transverse incisions within the hair line are used for these purposes.

Head Wounds due to Missiles.—The outcome depends on the explosive impact of the missile in the cranium, which is the commonest cause of fatality, and the relation of the wound track to the great vessels and the ventricles. Through-and-through tracks, from side to side or front to back, may be survived. Survivable injuries can be transported to a suitable hospital. Projection of the swollen brain through the dura at the site of entry or exit forms a hernia cerebri, which seals off the subarachnoid space during transport (fig. 410). A pressure dressing is applied. Immediate controlled ventilation has reduced the mortality from missile injuries (Chapter 2).

Operation consists of the excision of the surface wound and suction, cleansing, and removal of foreign material from the track. The dura is closed by suture or grafting at entry and exit points.

Penetrating wounds produced by sticks are always to be regarded very seriously. Although scissors or pokers may enter the roof of the orbit when a child falls and thereafter be successfully withdrawn, a stick which goes in through the orbital roof, or backwards behind the orbit into the temporal lobe, cannot be withdrawn intact; portions which are left behind may, from previous contact with the ground, be infected with gas gangrene or tetanus, with probable fatal infection.

LATE EFFECTS OF HEAD INJURY

Chronic Subdural Haematoma

This is produced by rupture of the veins passing from the cerebral hemispheres to the venous sinuses as the result of displacement of the brain inside the skull. Usually the superior cerebral veins are ruptured, producing haemorrhage over the convexity of the hemispheres; very rarely veins passing from the temporal lobe to the sphenoid or petrosal sinuses may produce clots which collect on the under-aspect of the brain. This complication, which is potentially fatal, is produced particularly by blows of small magnitude applied to the front or back of the head which may be insufficient to produce even transient concussion, but which are sufficient to move the brain suddenly. Cerebral atrophy renders this displacement easier, and hence the condition becomes commoner with advancing age. The superior cerebral veins pass from the convexity of the hemispheres and pierce the arachnoid membrane before crossing the potential subdural space to join the inner aspect of the dura 2·5 cm or more from the middle line; they then run inwards to drain into the lower compartment of the superior longitudinal sinus. Sudden displacement may snap the vein at the level of the arachnoid, allowing blood to pass downwards into the potential subdural space between the arachnoid and dura. Frequently, corresponding veins on both sides are affected and the condition is bilateral in 50% of cases. The haematomas are often large, bilateral collections up to 60 ml a side or unilateral collections of 120 ml being quite usual. There is a progressive change in the nature of the subdural fluid which becomes thinner, lighter in colour and eventually is similar to CSF.

Clinical Features.—The symptoms may follow a preceding concussion, but owing to the slight nature of the force required to produce displacement, this complication may occur without preceding loss of consciousness and without the head being even struck. It can follow a sudden jolt, as when a driver is thrown against the steering-wheel of a car, or be produced by knocking the head against the lintel of a door, or landing heavily on the feet when jumping from a height; it has followed dental extraction and electroconvulsive therapy. The interval between 'trauma' and onset of symptoms may be of weeks or months.

The symptoms are undramatic and consist of mental apathy, slowing of cerebration, slowness of response to questions merging into stupor. When the stupor develops, it comes and goes as the brain volume varies, the patient being inaccessible at times and then rousing sufficiently to answer questions accurately, but very slowly and after a considerable pause. When the level of consciousness deteriorates further the operative mortality rises to 30%; hence the significance of the early symptoms.

Physical signs vary. In older patients, where more room is available and if the fluid collects slowly, there may be no signs, or at most a unilateral or bilateral extensor plantar response from pressure on the motor cortex or brain-stem displacement. Pupillary changes occur last when the brain stem is affected and pressure-cone formation is imminent. Lumbar puncture shows a fluid at low pressure with protein increased to 120 mg/100 ml (1·2 g/l), often stained yellow from the transudation of pigment, but no cells. Papilloedema is exceptional. Success in treatment comes from acting on suspicion and employing skull radiographs for the position of the pineal, CT scan, or exploratory burr holes. Carotid arteriography should be avoided in the elderly.

Treatment.—Bilateral posterior parietal burr holes are made under local anaesthesia to expose the dura which often has a blue-green tinge. On incising the dura there is a gush of brown fluid. This should be allowed to flow out of the burr hole spontaneously, aided by lowering the head. The brain surface will frequently remain at a considerable distance from the dura. If the CT scan has shown a large collection of fluid but only a small amount has been obtained from the posterior parietal burr hole, another burr hole should be made further forward on that side (fig. 411A and B).

Post-operatively the patient is nursed flat initially and the subdural space can be re-tapped using a blunt-nosed brain cannula through the closed burr hole wounds.

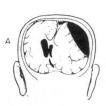

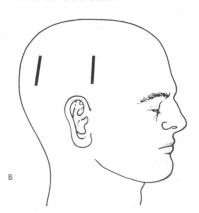

FIG. 411.—(A) Site of clot. (B) Incisions for burr holes for chronic subdural haematoma.

Post-Traumatic Epilepsy.—Epilepsy occurring soon after injury does not indicate the presence of a compressing intracranial haematoma. It reflects degrees of primary brain damage which may be trivial and from which total recovery occurs. Children are more susceptible to early epilepsy than adults, and it is probably a reflection of an inherent epileptic tendency. *Epilepsy within one week* of injury occurs in about 10% of all cases admitted to hospital with a head injury; factors which tend to increase the incidence are prolonged post-traumatic amnesia, intracranial haematoma and depressed fracture. In these circumstances prophylactic anti-convulsants should be given for about six weeks, but for up to three years in those who have suffered from any post-traumatic epilepsy.

Late Post-Traumatic epilepsy has an overall incidence of about 5% but of up to 25% in those who have suffered from early epilepsy, and therefore similar factors are involved. It probably represents cortical scarring and reactive gliosis. The epilepsy may be focal, general or essentially temporal, and although in the majority of patients its onset is within the first year, in about 20% the onset is delayed for more than four years. When the onset is very late (*e.g.* 10 years) it may be wiser to investigate the patient as a case of 'late onset epilepsy' rather than assume that the epilepsy is post-traumatic. The use of long-term prophylactic anti-convulsants, *e.g.* for 3 years, is advisable in those who have suffered early epilepsy, major compound fractures with dural and cortical laceration, and intradural compressing haematomas.

Post-Traumatic Hydrocephalus.—Late deterioration with apathy and mental retardation may rarely be caused by post-traumatic hydrocephalus requiring the insertion of a ventricular shunt (see p. 484).

Post-Traumatic Headache is not always cerebral in origin. Referred pain of spinal origin resulting from associated strains in upper cervical joints may be referred through the great occipital and posterior auricular nerves to the vertex, forehead, or temple. The post-traumatic state, with vertigo, defective memory and concentration, abnormal fatigue, irritability, and defective emotional control, may result from temporary or permanent cerebral lesions.

Patients with minor injuries recover speedily, but in serious cases prolonged convalescence is needed. Usually some symptoms of the post-contusional state consisting of headache, giddiness, defective memory, defective concentration, irritability, impaired emotional control, impaired sleep, or susceptibility to alcohol, persist for a period of eighteen months. Post-traumatic dementia constitutes a permanent handicap sometimes necessitating institutional care. Schizophrenia is a rare complication of even a minor injury.

INTRACRANIAL ABSCESS

Intracranial abscess is of three types (1) Extradural. (2) Subdural. (3) Intracerebral.

Extradural abscess is produced by osteomyelitis of the skull (p. 436 for causes), and is usually secondary to spread of infection from the middle ear or frontal sinus. In the case of the middle ear, infection most commonly reaches the

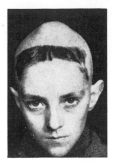

FIG. 412.—Pott's puffy tumour.
(The late Professor Lambert Rogers, FRCS, Cardiff.)

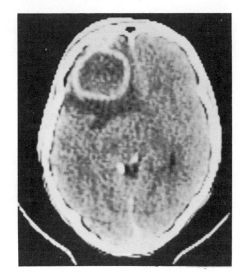

FIG. 413.—CT scan showing frontal abscess and oedema.

extradural space by extending through the tegmen tympani. Following frontal sinusitis, a large collection may form behind the frontal bone, infection having passed through the posterior wall of the sinus. Spread in the diploic veins may carry the infection to bone areas an inch or more above the ear or frontal sinus and cause local sequestration.

Acute localised headache, tenderness on local percussion of the skull, and localised pitting oedema of the scalp over the affected area, collectively form Pott's puffy tumour (fig. 412).

Subdural Abscess.—This condition, at one time invariably fatal, can now be treated. The mortality has been reduced to 10%, although much depends upon the patient's level of consciousness on admission. It is produced by septic thrombophlebitis spreading usually from infections of the frontal sinus or accessory air cells. Infection extends from the superior sinus to the cerebral veins, and thus infects the subdural space. The abscess extends in this space over the cerebral hemispheres, often bilaterally, and must be treated before it spreads to the inner or under aspects of the hemispheres.

Intracerebral Abscess.—Success in treatment is determined far more by the pathological type of the abscess than by the method of treatment adopted. Some abscesses rapidly spread to infect the ventricle; others localise readily, becoming walled off, and pass into the favourable subacute or chronic stages.

Intracerebral abscesses are produced by: (1) Local extension of adjacent infection as in sepsis in the middle ear and air sinuses. (2) Blood-borne infection as from intra-thoracic sepsis. (3) Local implantation as in head injury, which is rare.

Local extension abscesses are produced by septic thrombosis spreading from foci of infection in the ear or frontal sinuses. Usually three out of five abscesses arising from the ear are situated in the corresponding temporal lobe; the others are in the cerebellum. Frontal lobe abscesses are usually on the same side as the infected frontal sinus.

Very rarely, aberrant abscesses may occur, for example, contralateral frontal abscesses produced by infection crossing the superior sinus, or frontal or parietal abscesses from ear disease. Three stages may be recognised—acute, subacute, and chronic.

Percival Pott, 1714-1788. Surgeon, St. Bartholomew's Hospital, London. Described this condition in 1760.

In the acute stage there is septic encephalitis without pus formation. This may extend to produce ventriculitis or localise to form an abscess.

The subacute stage commences at three weeks by the formation of a glial wall, the thickness of which is determined by the local blood supply and is therefore thickest towards the cortex and thinnest towards the ventricle. A unilocular or multilocular cavity is produced, containing active organisms. The wall becomes thick within six weeks and the chronic abscess persists and may enlarge, behaving as a space occupying lesion which mimics a tumour.

Metastatic abscess is a complication of intra-thoracic sepsis, especially subacute bacterial endocarditis, lung abscess, bronchiectasis and empyema; it may occur in other infective states. Infected clot from the lung passes to the left heart, thence via the carotid, usually into the middle cerebral circulation, which forms a direct continuation of the carotid system; hence the infection is implanted deep in the white matter of the parietal or temporal lobe close to the ventricle. The blood supply of the brain is poor in the white matter, but rich in the cortex; tissue reaction is therefore feeble, and the septic encephalitis spreads rapidly and produces fatal septic ventriculitis within a matter of days or there may be multiple parietal abscesses.

Diagnosis and Management

The clinical diagnosis and management of intracranial abscess is a matter of urgency. The results of treatment are directly related to the neurological state and especially to the level of consciousness when neurological management starts. Cerebral abscess is often associated with surrounding brain oedema (fig. 413), which increases the mass effect of the abscess and causes a rapid rise in intracranial pressure. Rupture of an untreated cerebral abscess into the ventricular system may be rapidly fatal. Therefore once the suspicion of intracranial abscess arises the patient should be referred for urgent intracranial investigation.

Clinical diagnosis depends upon three aspects:

1. Evidence of past or present infection, especially in the middle ear, paranasal sinuses or thorax.

2. Focal neurological symptoms and signs.

3. Symptoms and signs of raised intracranial pressure.

1. **Evidence of infection.**—Chronic suppurative otitis media, an attic perforation and recent mastoidectomy should immediately raise the possibility of intracranial abscess which may be temporal subdural, temporal intracerebral or cerebellar. Chronic frontal sinusitis raises the possibility of frontal subdural or cerebral abscess; even an acute history of upper respiratory tract infection such as a heavy cold without positive radiological evidence of sinusitis, may be relevant.

General features of infection may be few or absent. Thus, fever is frequently absent as is tachycardia. The peripheral white blood count, especially with intracerebral abscess, is above 10,000 in only 50% of patients and above 20,000 in only 10%. The ESR (erythrocyte sedimentation rate) is raised (45-50 mm/ hour) in the majority of patients.

2. **Focal neurological symptoms and signs.**—These will depend upon the site of the lesion. *Epilepsy* is a common early symptom in subdural abscess and frontal intracerebral abscess and may be a reflection of the early cortical thrombophlebitic stage, or of an area of focal infarction in which infection develops later. *Dominant temporal lobe abscess* produces dysphasia, and a contralateral hemiparesis, and *cerebellar abscess* nystagmus and inco-ordination on the side of the lesion.

3. Symptoms and signs of raised intracranial pressure.—As with other intra-cranial space occupying lesions these are:

Symptoms	Signs
Headache	Depressed conscious level
Deterioration of level of consciousness	Papilloedema
Vomiting	Slowing pulse
Failing vision	Rising blood pressure

The particular features relevant to intracranial abscess are persisting headache, vomiting, deterioration in the level of consciousness and a slowing pulse. Because the history is often relatively short, failing visual acuity does not occur and *papilloedema is frequently absent.*

Differential diagnosis between abscess and meningitis.—Chronic suppurative otitis media may cause meningitis, or a meningeal reaction leading to headache, drowsiness and neck stiffness. However these signs may also be present with intracranial abscess. *Lumbar puncture in the presence of an abscess is dangerous* because it may precipitate coning and rupture of the abscess. At the same time the early diagnosis of meningitis is essential for satisfactory treatment. Furthermore the CSF findings in cerebral abscess are often unhelpful. In view of the dangers and diagnostic difficulties a guide is:

If meningitis is suspected *lumbar puncture should not be done* if (*a*), There is evidence of a focal neurological disturbance or (*b*), There are symptoms or signs of raised intracranial pressure.

The patient should be referred for urgent intracranial investigation to exclude an abscess.

Often the symptoms and physical signs of a chronic abscess develop immediately or within a day after operation has been performed on the ear or frontal sinus for the relief of a chronic headache—in these cases operation reveals an abscess with thick walls. Clearly a subacute or chronic abscess was present at the time that the operation was performed, and was itself the cause of the head pain for which the operation had been conducted. The local disturbance of the operation causes a reaction in the abscess cavity, and stimulates the early post-operative onset of physical signs. It is important to realise that the presence of well-marked localising signs developing within a period of days usually indicates re-activation of a chronic abscess requiring immediate treatment.

In every case of suspected cerebral abscess it is important to examine all possible sources of infection. In many cases the probable cause is evident, but discharge from an ear may cease when intracranial complications develop, for hindrance to discharge by inspissated pus predisposes to the extension of infection.

Further Management

Intracranial investigation and localisation.—In the past EEG, ventriculography and carotid arteriography have been very valuable and are still used. Isotope brain scanning provides a useful guide to the presence of supratentorial abscesses. However the investigation of choice today is the CT scan (fig. 413).

Surgery.—Surgery is both diagnostic and therapeutic. Drainage, formerly the recognised method of treatment, has been replaced by repeated aspiration of the abscess cavity or by excision. As soon as an abscess has been demonstrated radiologically, a burr hole is placed in the appropriate position, the dura opened and a blunt brain cannula inserted (fig. 414); if an abscess is entered the pus is gently aspirated, an antibiotic inserted (*e.g.* penicillin 20,000 units), and, if CT scan is not available, a radio-opaque contrast medium (*e.g.* Steripaque 1 ml) also inserted.

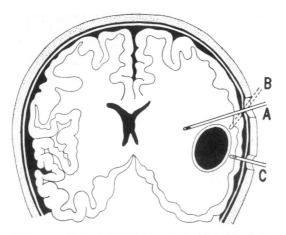

FIG. 414.—Method of localisation of abscess by burr-hole exploration. Needle at A encounters resistance at B. Puncture is performed by a second burr hole over the site of the abscess C.

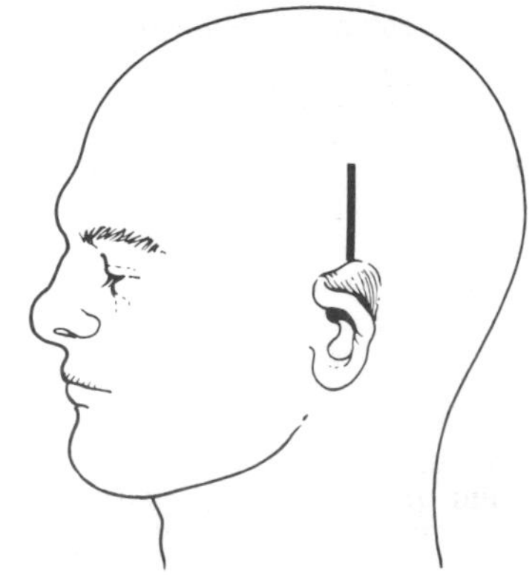

FIG. 415.—Incision for burr hole for temporal lobe abscess.

Further surgical management consists of repeated aspiration through the burr hole, the progress being assessed by the clinical state, and the shrinkage of the abscess as shown by CT scan or the injected contrast medium. Some surgeons favour early excision of the abscess; others only if the abscess fails to shrink.

There are occasions when time does not permit special investigations if the patient is deteriorating rapidly or special investigations are not available. The most critical of situations is that of a patient who has chronic suppurative otitis media, deterioration of level of consciousness and a dilated pupil. A burr hole must be made immediately above the down-turned ear and the temporal lobe needled (fig. 415).

The surgery of cerebellar abscess is more difficult and although an an emergency measure exploratory needling through a posterior fossa burr hole may be done, it is desirable to excise the abscess at a formal posterior fossa craniectomy.

Antibiotics.—The pus aspirated must be examined immediately for organisms and culture set up. Since streptococci are still the most common organisms to be found, the patient should be started on high doses of penicillin intravenously (up to 24 mega units in 24 hours). Other organisms commonly isolated include bacteroides and proteus(Chapter 3). Therefore metronidazole and chloramphenicol should be given with penicillin until the organisms have been isolated and the sensitivities are available. Even when progress is rapid it is wise to combine appropriate antibiotics in smaller doses for six weeks. Prophylactic anti-convulsants should be given for six months.

Treatment of implantation abscess.[1]—In the acute stage the track is explored from the surface, bone and foreign material are removed, and pus is evacuated by repeated aspiration or tube drainage. Antibiotic treatment is given freely. Chronic abscesses may be excised intact.

INTRACRANIAL TUMOURS

Tumours arise in connection with the meninges, nerve sheath, or cerebral substance (gliomas). Tumours of the pituitary gland, vascular malformations, gummas, tuberculomas, blood-clots, and chronic abscess contribute to the total. *Secondary carcinoma is far more common than primary intracranial tumour.* Secondary deposits are most common from the lung, but may originate from any organ in the body and from the naso-pharynx. When these have been excluded, an average surgical series will be as follows:

[1] Pietro de Marchettis, a monk in Padua, treated such cases successfuly by the insertion of lampwick drains in 1665.

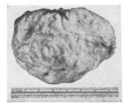

FIG. 416.—Characteristic globular
meningioma. (⅓ scale.)

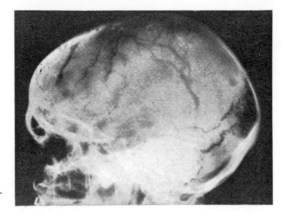

FIG. 417.—Converging vascular markings overlying a meningioma.

Meningioma, 18%.

Schwannoma, 8%.

Glioma, 43%.

Pituitary adenoma, 12%.

Craniopharyngioma, 5%.

Metastatic carcinoma, 6% (not previously excluded on clinical grounds).

Blood-vessel tumour, 2%.

Granulomas and unclassified and rare tumours make up the rest.

Meningiomas, 18%, vary in structure and vascularity and include psammomas (calcified meningioma, usually spinal), fibroblastomas, endotheliomas, and angioblastic meningioma. They are usually globular (fig. 416), but occasionally form a carpet, meningioma *en plaque*, which spreads widely in the meninges. Arising from the arachnoid, the tumour gains secondary attachment to the dura, the arteries and veins of which enlarge to provide a tumour circulation (fig. 417). Dilated emissaries between the bone and dura carry the venous return to the veins of the diploe and scalp, and along these veins tumour cells invade the bone, causing bone destruction and reactive hyperostosis (fig. 418).

Meningioma occurs in the following situations:

(1) **Parasagittal**—arising from the lateral lacunae and pressing down on to the upper aspect of the frontal parietal and occipital lobes.

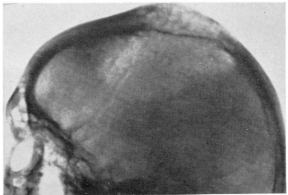

FIG. 418.—A large meningioma
hyperostosis extending from the
right to left parietal bones. Successfully removed together with
underlying tumour. This necessi-
tated a nine-hour operation.

(2) **Fronto-basal**—occurring on the cribriform plate, outer, middle, and inner third of the sphenoid wing and tuberculum sellae, pressing on the olfactory, oculomotor and optic nerves as well as the brain.

(3) **Posterior fossa**—in the region of the cerebellopontine angle, foramen magnum and under surface of the tentorium.

(4) They may also arise from the falx or from the choroid plexus within the ventricle.

Schwannoma, 8%, is usually found on the sheath of the auditory nerve (eighth nerve tumour), and may be multiple in association with von Recklinghausen's disease and sometimes occurs in association with multiple cerebral or spinal meningiomas.

Gliomas, 43%.—The malignancy of the tumour varies in proportion to the degree of reversion to the primitive type of cell:

Astrocytoma in its most adult form is composed of star-shaped cells which resemble adult neuroglial tissue. It occurs in three forms: (1) The diffuse or infiltrating, which cannot be totally removed as its margins are unrecognisable and it often affects the brain stem. (2) The solid, relatively circumscribed. (3) The cystic, in which the nodule of tumour secretes fluid from its surface, forming a cystic cleft between itself and compressed normal brain. The tumour projects into the cyst cavity, and removal of this nodule may produce a complete cure depending upon the histological grade of malignancy. Astrocytoma occurs throughout the cerebral hemispheres, cerebellum and brain stem. However, most astrocytomas contain a variety of cells, the proportion of which varies in different parts of the same tumour. Biopsy from a single favourable point may thus give a totally erroneous impression of a tumour's malignancy. In the modern classification of Kernohan, astrocytic gliomas are classified Grades 1, 2, 3, 4, according to the proportion of adult and primitive cells which they contain. Grade 1 corresponds to the pure astrocytoma. Grade 4 to glioblastoma multiforme (*Bailey* and *Cushing's* Classification).

Oligodendroglioma.—An adult cell tumour consisting of cells with short stunted processes affects the hemispheres in adults. It is often less malignant that other gliomas.

Spongioblastoma polare arises from primitive uni- or bi-polar spongioblasts and affects inaccessible regions, such as the optic chiasma, third ventricle, and hypothalamus in young subjects. It is irremovable, somewhat radio-sensitive, and rarely produces seedling metastases in the cerebrospinal fluid.

Medulloblastoma occurs usually in young children, affecting the vermis of the cerebellum. It grows rapidly and produces seedling metastases in the CSF pathways and the fourth ventricle. It is radio-sensitive.

Ependymoma may occur throughout the cerebral hemispheres and in the fourth ventricle. The cells resemble the ependymal cells lining the ventricles. In the cerebral hemispheres they vary in malignancy and tend to behave like the malignant astrocytomas. In the fourth ventricle they are less malignant.

Clinical Features.——All tumours have an initial silent period which varies in length according to position and rate of growth. If the tumour is not near any area which will produce symptoms or signs, it will take up space provided in the subarachnoid cisterns; it will flatten and displace the ventricle and brain until it can gain no more room, and it will then produce symptoms of raised intracranial pressure, such as morning headache, effortless vomiting, and papilloedema. It may be several years or more before this occurs in the case of a meningioma. If the tumour is situated in an important area, it may, by its local effect, produce

CLINICAL COURSE OF CEREBRAL TUMOUR

Stage 1	Stage 2	Stage 3	Stage 4
Initial period of silent growth.	Focal syndromes. Epilepsy.	Raised intracranial pressure.	Brain displacement. False localising signs. Cone formation.

Friedrich Daniel von Recklinghausen, 1833-1910. Professor of Pathology, Strasbourg.
Percival Bailey, 1892-1973. Professor of Neurology, Chicago, Ill., U.S.A.
Harvey Cushing, 1869-1939. Professor of Surgery at Johns Hopkins and Harvard University.

symptoms of epilepsy or progressive neurological syndromes before any evidence of intracranial pressure is produced. Hence the absence of headache, vomiting, and papilloedema does not exclude a tumour.

Epilepsy arising for the first time in adult life should always be suspected as being due to a tumour until this possibility has been disproved (fig. 419).

FIG. 419.—The principal causes of epilepsy at different ages.

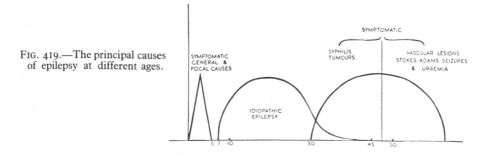

Idiopathic epilepsy does not occur before the age of six. Ninety per cent of cases of idiopathic epilepsy have their first seizure before the age of thirty. After the age of thirty, epilepsy is usually symptomatic, and in patients between the ages of thirty and fifty tumour is a common cause. However, the incidence of so-called idiopathic epilepsy depends upon the extent of investigation. With the increasing use of CT scanning and more recently magnetic resonance imaging, structural lesions such as small tumours, angiomas, infarction and even demyelination can be demonstrated in patients who would otherwise be regarded as having idiopathic epilepsy.

Progressive focal syndromes should likewise be regarded as indicating a tumour until this possibility is disproved. Degenerative conditions such as disseminated sclerosis are characterised by periods of remission and exacerbation. Vascular lesions occur instantaneously and are followed by some degree of improvement. If repeated on several occasions, as in multiple emboli, an appearance of steady progression is produced, but there is only one condition that will produce a steadily progressive syndrome, and that is a tumour.

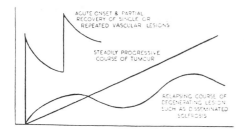

FIG. 420.—Clinical courses of vascular, neoplastic and degenerative lesions.

The stage of raised intracranial pressure can develop in association with focal symptoms or be the sole evidence of tumour formation, occurring earliest in midline and posterior fossa tumours which obstruct the flow of fluid from both ventricles, producing an internal hydrocephalus.

The Symptoms of raised intracranial pressure are:
1. Headache
2. Deterioration of level of consciousness
3. Vomiting
4. Deterioration of visual acuity

The Signs of raised intracranial pressure are:
1. Lowered level of consciousness
2. Slowing pulse
3. Rising blood pressure
4. Papilloedema

It is the presence and severity of these symptoms and signs rather than focal features which indicate the degree of urgency of treatment.

The Stage of Coning.—Certain patients do not present until cone formation is imminent. When intracranial pressure becomes high, the inner border of one hemisphere may be forced under the falx plugging the superior longitudinal fissure and blocking one pathway for the cerebrospinal fluid absorption. The temporal lobe may be forced down from above into the tentorial opening. The cerebellar vermis may be pushed up into this opening or the cerebellar tonsils may be forced down into the foramen magnum. Ominous signs of a threatened cone include violent paroxysmal headache, drowsiness, slow cerebration, slow pulse, and neck stiffness. Unilateral pupillary dilatation is an urgent sign. *Lumbar puncture must be rigidly avoided* at this and earlier stages if the diagnosis of an intracranial space-occupying lesion is probable (cf fig. 390).

Frontal lobe tumours if deeply situated produce a progressive change in personality, with lack of insight, neglect of normal pastimes, occupations, and duties, and an alteration in emotional reaction particularly noticeable to relatives, consisting usually of a simplicity and unwarrantable cheerfulness (euphoria) or irritability. Epilepsy is generalised in type, and localising signs are limited to contralateral facial weakness.

Parietal lobe tumours produce Jacksonian epilepsy and progressive hemiparesis. Examination reveals loss of touch analysis resulting in astereognosis. Deeply situated left-sided tumours may exhibit defects of spatial relationship and loss of power of calculation (acalculia).

Occipital lobe tumours.—Epilepsy is generalised in type, preceded by an aura of flashing lights in the contralateral visual field. Signs, other than homonymous hemianopia, are few.

Temporal lobe tumours on the left side may produce progressive aphasia or visual or auditory hallucination sometimes with generalised convulsions. Lesions of the uncinate region produce uncinate hallucination of smell and taste and dreamy states of unreality. Right-sided lesions may cause similar uncinate attacks of generalised epilepsy without aura. Localising signs include hemiparesis and superior quadrantic hemianopia.

Parasagittal meningioma overlying the various lobes produces similar syndromes but with characteristic skull x-ray changes (figs. 417 and 418).

Basal meningioma produces involvement of the olfactory and optic, oculomotor, and trigeminal nerves, in addition to pressure on the brain. Bone changes in the region of the orbit may cause proptosis or fullness in the temporal fossa.

Midline tumours always produce bilateral internal hydrocephalus with pressure symptoms.

Tumours of the third ventricle.—Colloid cysts at first cause a ball-valve obstruction producing intermittent blockage of the foramen of Monro. Later, persistent bilateral hydrocephalus is accompanied by severe pressure symptoms or progressive cerebral atrophy and dementia. Glioma of the floor of the ventricle causes hydrocephalus associated with endocrine disturbance, disturbances of sleep rhythm, and sexual precocity.

Pineal tumours by pressure on the quadrigeminal plate produce hydrocephalus with

Alexander Monro, 1733-1817. Professor of Anatomy, Edinburgh.

paralysis of the oculomotor nuclei with loss of upward, lateral, and downward movement of the eyes.

Subtentorial Tumours.—Tumours of the posterior fossa distort the aqueduct and fourth ventricle, and by obstructing the escape of CSF, produce raised intracranial pressure. The effect of the hydrocephalus varies with the age of the patient:

Cerebellar vermis tumours are usually medulloblastomas and occur in young children before the sutures have united. The hydrocephalus causes progressive enlargement of the head. At a later age, when the sutures have united, there are serious pressure symptoms and stiffness of the neck from herniation of both cerebellar tonsils into the foramen magnum. Since the vermis controls the co-ordination of trunk and legs, localising signs are only seen if the child is taken out of bed, it will then be seen to walk with the feet wide apart and have a tendency to fall over forwards when standing with the feet together.

Cerebellar hemisphere tumours are often astrocytomas. They produce hydrocephalus and pressure symptoms in older subjects. Since the hemisphere controls the co-ordination of the corresponding side of the body, there is deviation to the affected side on walking and unilateral inco-ordination of the arm. Nystagmus may or may not be present.

Acoustic neuroma grows from the auditory nerve at the internal auditory meatus and produces enlargement of this structure, visible on x-ray. Arising from the eighth nerve the first symptom is unilateral deafness, which is often first detected by the patient on the telephone. The tumour projects into the cerebello-pontine angle and presses upon the adjacent seventh, sixth, and fifth nerves, causing a syndrome of unilateral deafness, facial weakness, and sometimes squint. The corneal reflex is reduced from pressure on the fifth nerve. There may be trigeminal neuralgia from this cause or trigeminal anaesthesia. Later the tumour presses upon the cerebellum and brain stem, producing cerebellar signs and raised pressure. Finally it grows up into the tentorial opening from below, and here it not only blocks the up-flow of cerebrospinal fluid but assumes a position anterior to the brain stem coming into close relationship with the basilar artery and twisting the pons. Cerebrospinal fluid protein is always high, often over 200 mg/100 ml (2·0 g/l). Audiometry may detect an early symptomless acoustic neuroma.

The investigation of cerebral tumour must define the site and nature of the tumour.

History taking.—The history alone will sometimes indicate the site of the tumour and also give a hint as to its pathological type. If symptoms have been long-standing, they suggest a slowly growing and favourable tumour. A short history may, however, be due to the final breakdown of adaptation in a slowly growing tumour or indicate a rapid malignant growth.

The history may suggest a primary disease to which the cerebral condition is secondary. Since metastatic carcinoma, especially bronchial, is far more common than primary cerebral tumour, particular attention must be paid to history of loss of weight, recent cough, or haemoptysis. Secondary brain abscess is suggested by a history of lung abscess or bronchiectasis; chronic otitic abscess by symptoms of cachexia and a discharging ear. Weight loss is always suspicious, as there is no wasting with primary cerebral tumour.

Clinical examination must include the general examination in search of primary disease.

Neurological examination of cranial nerves and nerve tracts may localise *where* a tumour is, but never indicates *what* it is.

Accessory investigations are essential. X-ray of the skull, x-ray of the chest, and the erythrocyte sedimentation rate must be taken in every case. A high E.S.R. is strongly suggestive of secondary tumour or abscess.

An x-ray of the chest may reveal an unsuspected bronchial carcinoma. Thirty per cent of bronchial carcinomas present with cerebral symptoms before any chest symptoms have occurred.

An x-ray of the skull may show that a tumour is present:

(1) By pressure changes including: (*a*) *Most important*—erosion of the posterior clinoid processes, a very valuable sign. (*b*) Separation of sutures in young subjects, (*c*) A beaten silver appearance of the vault from the pressure of tight convolutions (sometimes normal in thin skulls).

(2) By lateral displacement of a calcified pineal shadow indicating the side of the tumour.

(3) By characteristic intracranial calcification produced by astrocytomas, angiomas, 50% of craniopharyngiomas, and some meningiomas and tuberculomas (fig. 421).

(4) By alteration in skull vascular markings in meningioma, including converging diploic channels, and an increase in the size of the meningeal groove (fig. 417).

(5) By changes in the skull bones, including meningioma hyperostosis, local expansion at the site of a cyst, and bone destruction in secondary tumours.

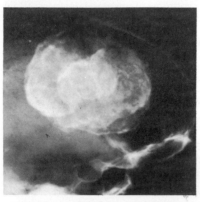

FIG. 421.—Calcified meningioma.

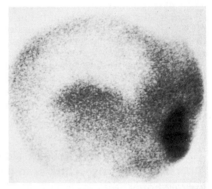

FIG. 422.—Isotope scan showing large sphenoidal meningioma.

Electroencephalogram.—Characteristic wave-forms indicate the site or presence of focal or deep-seated tumours, and distinguish between epileptic seizures produced by focal lesions and idiopathic epilepsy.

Isotope scan is a valuable method of investigation for supratentorial tumours (fig. 422).

CT scanning (see p. 455), when available, provides reliable information concerning the presence of a tumour, and ventricular displacement or distension. It is possible to distinguish the type of tumour, especially by the appearance after *intravenous contrast enhancement*. Thus, meningiomas, Schwannomas and some pituitary adenomas enhance vividly. Gliomas show variable patterns of enhancement and low density which do not necessarily indicate the degree of malignancy. (figs. 423, 424, 425). However, certain differentiation between malignant growth and abscess may not be possible.

Invasive Methods of Investigation. Although CT scanning has largely replaced them, ventriculography and carotid arteriography may still be of value. Ventriculography with ventricular draining may be life-saving in acute hydrocephalus.

Magnetic resonance imaging (**MRI**) is becoming a powerful tool for the surgeon. Nuclei of atoms when placed in a magnetic field and subjected to radiofrequency electromagnetic radiation will absorb energy. A signal is produced by perturbating these atomic nuclei. There are marked differences in the frequencies at which different nuclei absorb energy and much smaller but distinguishable differences caused by the local environment

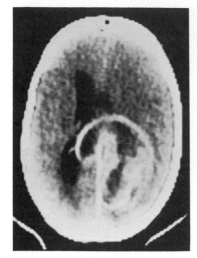

FIG. 423.—CT scan showing necrotic malignant glioma.

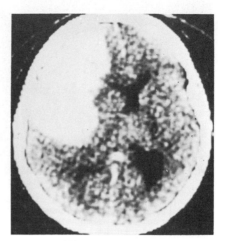

FIG. 424.—CT scan showing sphenoidal meningioma.

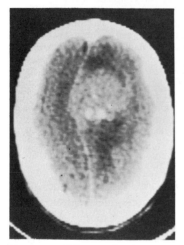

FIG. 425.—CT scan showing parasaggital meningioma with surrounding brain oedema.

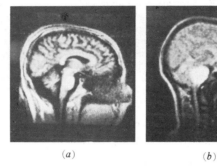

(a)   (b)

FIG. 426.—(a) Magnetic resonance head image of the T_1 property of protons. (b) Magnetic resonance head image of the T_2 property of protons showing a tumour (astrocytoma) of the brain stem distinguished by its natural contrast.
(*Professor J. Stewart Orr, Royal Postgraduate Medical School, London.*)

of the nuclei. Equipment for imaging special properties of protons, the nuclei of hydrogen atoms, can produce cross sectional clinical images showing normal and pathological tissue with excellent contrast and detail. Both the T_1 images (fig.426 (a)), with good demonstration of normal antomy, and the T_2 images (fig. 426 (b)), often more sensitive to pathological changes (Orr), reflects the state of cellular and tissue water, and of fat giving a discrimination of different tissue types. *In vivo* magnetic resonance spectroscopy of phosphorous-31 allows non-invasive study of metabolic energy pathways of tissues (e.g. in transplantation surgery).

Positron Emission Tomography (PET), using shortlife isotopes, is developing as an investigation of the function of the parts of the brain.

Arteriography was originated by Egas Moniz. Pathological tumour circulation is seen in meningioma and glioblastoma multiforme. Meningiomas produce a diffuse blush; glioblastomas produce a group of very primitive and imperfect vessels (fig. 427).

Investigation by Air Study.—Ventriculography was originated in 1918 by Walter

Antonio Caetano de Abreu Freire Egas Moniz, 1874-1955. Professor of Neurology, Lisbon. Introduced cerebral arteriography in 1927 and leucotomy in 1936.

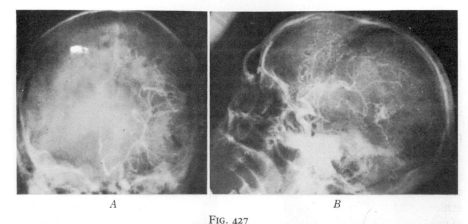

A

B

Fig. 427

(A) A.P. arteriogram showing inward displacement of the anterior and middle cerebral arteries and tumour circulation causing a blush in a meningioma at the outer third of the sphenoid ridge.

(B) Lateral arteriogram showing primitive glioblastoma vessels in posterior temporal region.

Dandy. Bilateral parietal burr holes are formed under local anaesthesia. A hollow ventricular cannula is inserted to a depth of up to 5 cm to puncture the vestibule of the ventricle. Available cerebrospinal fluid is removed and replaced with 10% less volume of air. Since air rises and fluid falls the patient is positioned in such a way that the portion of the ventricular system which is wished to fill with air is brought to the highest level during arteriography, films being taken in various planes to show displacement and distortion of the ventricle. The investigation is dangerous, as tapping of a displaced and expanded ventricle on the side opposite to the tumour may allow the brain to be pushed over. Arteriography is therefore preferable. However, when CT scanning is not available, *ventriculography* remains a valuable method of investigation for posterior fossa and third ventricle tumours when the lateral ventricles are dilated and there is no lateral displacement. In an emergency situation it can be performed with simple radiographic equipment.

Myodil ventriculogram in hydrocephalus will demonstrate the third and fourth ventricles and aqueduct after the injection of 5 ml of Myodil.

Further Management and Surgery

Having established on clinical grounds that there is evidence of raised intracranial pressure (see Abscess, p. 464), and having demonstrated radiologically the presence of a space occupying lesion the objects of further management are:

1. The relief of raised intracranial pressure.
2. Establishment of a pathological diagnosis.
3. Removal of benign tumours.
4. Operative and non-operative treatment of malignant tumours.

1. Relief of raised intracranial pressure.—Raised intracranial pressure may be responsible for distressing symptoms (*e.g.* severe headache, vomiting, failing visual acuity) and if pressure is not relieved the outcome is soon fatal. The degree of urgency of action depends upon the severity of the symptoms and signs of pressure, the most important being severe headache and deterioration in level of consciousness. Papilloedema is present in only 30% of patients with intracranial space occupying lesions and therefore absence of papilloedema never excludes such lesions. Although CT scanning has improved pre-operative pathological diagnosis, in most patients, this cannot be established without some form of surgery and therefore relief of pressure is essential unless a malignant (and untreatable) pathology has been proven.

Walter Edward Dandy, 1886-1946. Neurosurgeon, Johns Hopkins Hospital, Baltimore.

Pressure may be relieved by:

(*a*) Ventricular tap and drainage through a posterior-parietal burr hole when the lateral ventricles are symmetrically dilated as in posterior fossa and third ventricle tumours.

(*b*) Tapping of supratentorial cystic tumours and abscesses. If the lesion is solid needling will not lower pressure and may raise it further by provoking haemorrhage and oedema.

(*c*) Administration of mannitol (p. 456) which may produce *temporary* improvement.

(*d*) Urgent removal or partial removal of supratentorial tumours, so creating an 'internal decompression'.

(*e*) Dexamethasone in doses initially of up to 24 mg a day may bring relief of raised pressure and even of focal neurological deficit in patients with malignant tumours.

2. Establishment of a pathological diagnosis.——This is essential if further decisions about tumour removal are to be taken. Tissue for histology is obtained either by burr hole biopsy or by craniotomy and tumour removal, the latter achieving relief of intracranial pressure. Craniotomy is therefore safer. The choice of method depends upon many factors which include accessibility of the tumour, the likelihood of abscess, the anticipated quality of survival and the age of the patient. Whatever method is used it is essential to have facilities for immediate histological examination by frozen section.

3. Removal of benign tumours (see meningioma, p. 469).

4. Treatment of malignant tumours.——Much depends upon the histology and degree of malignancy of the tumour. For astrocytoma of grade 3 and 4 malignancy the outlook remains poor however extensive and 'complete' the removal may be, survival being between 3 and 18 months; on average radiotherapy improves survival by about 6 months. The results of chemotherapy are as yet inconclusive. Medulloblastoma responds more favourably to radiotherapy and chemotherapy.

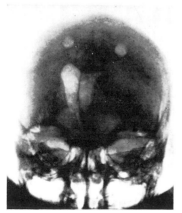

FIG. 428.—X-ray indicating dangers of ventriculography. Both ventricles are already on one side of the head. This is not unusual.

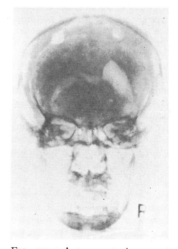

FIG. 429.—Antero-posterior ventriculogram showing flattening and downward displacement of left lateral ventricle by large parasaggital meningioma. The middle meningeal groove is enlarged on the left side.

Burr Hole Biopsy.——If investigation suggests the presence of an unfavourable lesion in which craniotomy is contraindicated, such as secondary carcinoma or malignant glioma, or if a cyst is suspected, a burr hole is fashioned over the tumour site and the tumour is aspirated by ventricular cannula.

The recent development of *CT-guided sterostactic biopsy* allows safer histological diagnosis of deeper tumours.

Operation must not be delayed if pressure is high, as sudden and unexpected collapse may occur. Improvement is neurosurgical technique permits a radical excision in many cases.

Principles of Supratentorial Craniotomy. Details can be found in neurosurgical texts. The placing of osteoplastic flaps is a specialised matter, depending upon the site and nature of the lesion to be dealt with. The scalp flap is based laterally, frontally or occipitally, the middle of the base being at least equal to the height of the flap in order to ensure an adequate blood supply to the margin of the flap. Incisions may be rectangular or rounded. Scalp haemostasis is achieved by applying a series of artery clips to the galea aponeurotica, the forceps being allowed to fall back over the margins of the scalp (*e.g.* fig. 395). The flap is then reflected at the relatively bloodless sub-galeal layer. The muscle and pericranium is then cut with diathermy in a form suitable to the scalp incision, the skull exposed in that line using a rougine or periosteal elevator.

Four or five burr holes are then made along the line of exposure of the skull. The underlying dura is separated from the bone with care using an elevator, and the burr holes, except those at the base of the flap, are joined by saw cuts using a Gigli wire saw. By narrowing the base of the bone flap, using nibblers, the bone flap will crack across its base as it is prised up, and it is hinged (*e.g.* on the temporal muscles); thereby the osteoblastic flap remains viable.

Dural openings are usually in the form of a flap based medially, so that the risk of damage to the cortical veins as they approach the superior sagittal sinus is reduced.

Closure is in layers, using interrupted black silk. A crucial step is the insertion of hitching stitches between the dura and the pericranium or muscle so that the dura is pulled up against the skull and a post-operative extradural haematoma avoided. The bone flap is replaced and secured by stitches through the pericranium and temporal fascia. The galea and finally the skin are brought together. Skin stitches are removed after two or three days.

Principles of Posterior Fossa Exploration. The procedures are even more specialised than above and should not be undertaken by those unfamiliar with the grave difficulties and complications that may occur. Prior to posterior fossa surgery a posterior parietal burr hole should be placed so that the lateral ventricle can be rapidly cannulated during or after the operation if need arises. Operations may be done with the patient prone, in the lateral position, or in the sitting position, the latter requiring special precautions because of the risk of air embolism. Incisions are either midline, extending from the external occipital protuberance to the vertebra prominens, or lateral (curved or straight). The bone of the suboccipital region and the margin of the foramen magnum are exposed by stripping off the suboccipital muscles on one or both sides. Exposure of the dura is usually by craniectomy and the dura is opened in a tri-radiate or cruciate fashion. Many hazards beset the unwary, including profuse haemorrhage from damage to the lateral sinus if the craniectomy is taken too high.

Closure of the dura is advisable, and the muscles and skin are closed carefully in layers without drainage.

Individual Tumours

Malignant Gliomas. The majority being supratentorial the approach is by that route. Ideally the pathology is established immediately by examination of frozen section or smear, after a small cortical incision and insertion of a brain cannula. Removal of tumour in lesions of higher grades of malignancy (grades 3 and 4) by suction and rongeur is limited to areas of obvious tumour, in order to achieve relief of pressure by creating an internal decompression without increasing the neurological deficit. In lower grade tumours (astrocytoma grade 2, oligodendroglioma) tumour removal may be more aggressive if the lesion is in a relatively 'silent' area. Tumours in the anterior part of the frontal or temporal lobe, or in the posterior part of the occipital lobe may be removed in the course of frontal, temporal or occipital lobectomy. Haemostasis is obtained by the application of tantalum clips to larger vessels, but packing, hydrogen peroxide, diathermy and above all, patience and waiting, will control most bleeding and cause least damage.

Metastases. These may be supra or infratentorial, single or multiple. The decision to operate depends on many factors including the general state of the disease and the prognosis, the nature of the intracranial symptoms, the site and multiplicity of the intracranial metastases and accessibility. Generally carcinoma of the breast and kidney, and the rarer lymphomas merit surgery, but results with bronchial carcinoma and melanoma are disappointing. The approach is smaller to that for the malignant gliomas, but metastases are often relatively well circumscribed and can be totally removed, at least macroscopically by suction, blunt dissection and rongeur.

Meningiomas. Specialised techniques are necessary. The general principles are: exposure of the lesion by a large craniotomy, definition of the plane of cleavage between tumour capsule and brain, painstaking clipping or diathermy of feeding vessels, reduction of the bulk of the tumour out of the cavity it has created within the brain, excision of the dura from which the tumour arose in order to prevent recurrence. The principles are most easily followed in the removal of cortical or convexity meningiomas. The parasagittal tumours create difficulties in removing the origin of the tumour which may involve the sagittal sinus. The basal tumours (suprasellar, cerebello-pontine angle, subfrontal) may involve the dura widely so that truly total removal is impossible.

Acoustic Schwannoma. These histologically benign tumours in the cerebello-pontine angle still present a formidable neurosurgical challenge in a highly specialised field. The approach is by posterior fossa craniectomy, the main steps being the opening of the basal cisterns, identification and protection of the lower cranial nerves (9, 10, 11), definition of the tumour, intracapsular reduction of its bulk, separation of the capsule from the brain stem, definition and attempted preservation of the facial nerve and, finally, the total removal of the tumour. The operating microscope is of great benefit, but the surgery is prolonged, difficult and hazardous. A trans-sphenoidal approach has also been used.

Haemangioblastoma and Benign Cystic Astrocytoma. These benign tumours are restricted to the cerebellum and may be totally removed, the astrocytoma occurring mainly in children or young adults. With cystic lesions the cyst is opened after exposure of the cerebellum by posterior fossa craniectomy, and the tumour usually presents as a small mural nodule. The nodule alone is completely excised.

TUMOURS OF THE PITUITARY BODY

Traditionally, pituitary adenomas were classified as chromophobe, eosinophil and basophil, depending on the predominant cell type and its endocrine activity or inactivity. However, although this classification has some convenience many adenomas do not fit this pattern, but show a mixture of cell types, and are better characterised by their endocrine status (see Adrenal tumours, Chapter 38).

Chromophobe adenomas occur most commonly in female patients between the ages of twenty and fifty. The tumour is solid and slow-growing and expands steadily to form a mass the size of a walnut in a period of several years. Spontaneous involution may occur with cessation of growth and cystic change (cf. adenoma of thyroid). Occasionally highly cellular rapidly growing tumours assume the characteristics of local malignancy invading laterally into the cavernous sinus or extending into the lobes of the brain. Three stages of development may be recognised:

(*a*) The stage of intrasellar development.

(*b*) The stage of suprasellar extension.

(*c*) The stage of massive intracranial extension.

(*a*) *Intrasellar Development.*—In the sella turcica, the expanding chromophobe cells, which possess no active secretion of their own, compress the acidophil and basophil cells of the pars anterior and inhibit their secretions which are concerned

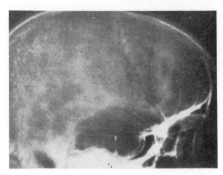

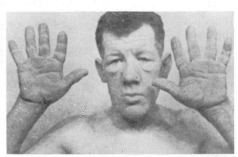

FIG. 430.—Typical x-ray appearances of enlarged sella in chromophobe adenoma.

FIG. 431.—Acromegaly.

with growth and sex functions. Since the tumour arises at an age when growth is complete, the effect is felt by the thyrotropic and gonadotropic hormones. The patient becomes fat and sluggish with a lowered metabolic rate, as in myxoedema, and amenorrhoea is invariable. Pressure on the diaphragma sellae causes severe headache. X-ray of the skull reveals enlargement of the pituitary fossa (fig. 430).

(b) *The Stage of Suprasellar Extension.*—The tumour breaks through the diaphragm at a weak point between the anterior clinoid processes and extends up in front of the pituitary stalk to press on the under aspect of the optic chiasma, and gradually bitemporal hemianopia is produced by stretching of the decussating fibres in the optic chiasma over the posterior border of the tumour. Stretching of the optic nerves anterior to the chiasma produces primary optic atrophy with pale white optic discs. The diagnosis is usually made at this stage and confirmed by CT scan or lumbar air encephalogram.

Acute infarction may rarely produce a sudden swelling of the tumour with rapidly increasing visual loss. Infarction may cause complete blindness and then be followed by atrophy and disappearance of the tumour.

(c) *The stage of massive intracranial extension* is rare. If the optic chiasma is in an abnormal position, either pre- or post-fixed, the tumour may slip by it without causing visual disturbance and enter the frontal lobe, or highly cellular rapidly growing tumours may spread laterally into the temporal lobe or upwards and backwards behind the chiasma into the third ventricle. These extensions will act as a space-occupying tumour and produce symptoms of raised pressure or epilepsy.

Differential Diagnosis.—The syndrome may be simulated by a meningioma of the dorsum sellae or an aneurysm of the anterior communicating or internal carotid artery. Arteriography is required in doubtful cases.

Treatment.—Few chromophobe tumours are radio-sensitive. Many alleged successes attributed to deep x-ray have been due to spontaneous cystic involution or an abnormality of the chiasma which allows the tumour to go on growing without serious visual loss developing. Years later the growth is found to have formed a massive intracranial extension.

Operation performed before the stage of massive extension has a mortality of 2 to 4%; after extension 30%, hence early operation is advisable. Pre- and post-operative treatment by steroids is advisable in order to prevent post-operative adrenal deficiency.

The objective of surgery is primarily relief of chiasmal or optic nerve compression. If the tumour and its suprasellar extension are restricted to the midline, the trans-sphenoidal route is generally favoured, with reduction of tumour mass from within the capsule. When the tumour is more extensive or there is doubt about the diagnosis, craniotomy and a sub-frontal approach is advisable.

Eosinophil (Acidophil) adenomas are small in size and rarely cause pressure on the optic chiasma. Normally the symptoms are due to excessive production of growth hormone by the acidophil cells.

In children the tumour causes gigantism, while patients whose epiphyses have united develop acromegaly (a term which implies enlargement of the extremities).

Acromegaly is characterised by thickening of the subcutaneous tissues of the scalp, lips, and tongue, the face, hands and feet, and overgrowth of the frontal sinuses, jaw, and distal phalanges. There is also overgrowth of hair and sebaceous glands. Asthenia causes slackening of ligaments with kyphosis, so that the enlarged hands hang below the knees. This combined with the atavistic appearance produced by the beetling brow, prognathous jaw, and overgrowth of hair on the chest, produces the 'ape man' of the circus. Fatty degeneration of the heart and herniae are associated conditions.

Treatment.—There is still uncertainty about the ideal treatment of acromegaly. Methods used have included bromocriptine, external radiotherapy, implantation of radio-active Yttrium, transfrontal surgery and trans-sphenoidal surgery. Currently the trans-sphenoidal route with micro-surgical removal of the adenoma is the method of choice.

BASOPHIL ADENOMAS AND CUSHING'S SYNDROME

Basophil adenomas are small, usually only a few millimetres across; their effects are produced by secretion of adreno-corticotrophic hormones.

Cushing described a syndrome associated with basophil adenomas, although a similar condition may be due to adrenal dysfunction (adreno-genital syndrome, Chapter 38). Females are more commonly affected. Fat accumulates on the trunk, neck, and face which becomes red and moonshaped but the limbs remain normal. Purple striae appear in considerable numbers on the skin, which is thin and atrophic. Hirsutism, arterial hypertension and glycosuria develop early. There is moderate polycythaemia and atrophic changes affect the bones of the os calcis and pubis. A psychotic state sometimes develops.

If endocrine studies indicate that the cause of the syndrome is due to over-production of pituitary hormones, trans-sphenoidal surgery may enable a secreting micro-adenoma to be removed. *Prolactin secreting adenomas* may be the cause of infertility and amenorrhoea.

CRANIOPHARYNGIOMAS

In structure, these growths form large masses in which cystic cavities lined with ciliated epithelium and containing cholesterol crystals are separated by areas of connective tissue. More than 50% of these growths are calcified and may form coral-like masses filling the inter-peduncular space and extending backwards to the pons. Since they are adherent to the basal arteries and adjacent nerves, they are irremovable. Occasionally single cysts are found in or above the sella, but the term suprasellar cyst describes only this one variety. In fact, these tumours are by no means always suprasellar, nor are they necessarily cystic.

Clinical Features.—The symptoms depend upon the site of the tumour and the age of the patient.

(1) Intrasellar craniopharyngioma cysts produce symptoms like the inert chromophobe tumour, but in young subjects they inhibit growth by compression of the acidophil cells as well as inhibiting sexual maturation. The result is a fat, impotent dwarf, who may subsequently develop bitemporal hemianopia from upward pressure on the chiasma (Frölich's syndrome).

Harvey Cushing, 1869–1939. See footnote, p. 470. Described this disease in 1932.
Alfred Frölich, 1871–1953. Formerly Professor of Pharmacology, University of Vienna, described his syndrome in 1901.

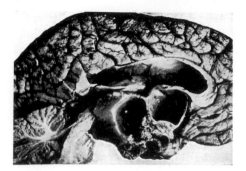

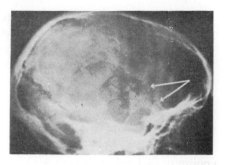

FIG. 432.—A large craniopharyngioma.

FIG. 433.—Arrows indicate suprasellar calcification in craniopharyngioma.

(2) Suprasellar craniopharyngiomas in young subjects, by downward pressure on the sella, also produce a Frölich's syndrome. Radiography may show suprasellar calcification.

Pressure on adjacent centres of the hypothalamus, which control sleep and water metabolism, produce pathological somnolence and diabetes insipidus, so that the subject is liable to fall asleep during the day, and to drink and pass abnormal quantities of fluid. Similar symptoms may occur at a later age in adults.

(3) Further upward extension of the tumour, or those which arise within the third ventricle, may cause hydrocephalus by obstructing the flow of CSF, and thereby raised intracranial pressure.

Treatment.—Cystic tumours in and above the sella may be evacuated by frontal craniotomy or by trans-sphenoidal surgery. When large masses block the third ventricle, the cerebrospinal fluid may be short-circuited to the cisterna magna by leading a catheter from the ventricle through a burr opening in the skull, thence under the skin and occipital muscles to drain into the cisterna magna, which has been exposed above the foramen magnum (Torkildsen's operation)—ventriculo-cisternostomy. More commonly, relief is by ventriculo-atrial shunt.

HYDROCEPHALUS

Hydrocephalus is usually spoken of as being congenital or acquired. Subdivision of these two groups is useful from a clinical point of view. When the obstruction is within the ventricular system or at the exit of the fourth ventricle, then the hydrocephalus is described as non-communicating. If the distended ventricles communicate freely with the subarachnoid space then the hydrocephalus is communicating.

Congenital hydrocephalus is often associated with other abnormalities of the neuraxis, such as spina bifida or myelomenigocele. It is produced by defective absorption of, or obstruction to, the cerebrospinal fluid. The commonest cause is failure of development of the CSF pathways in the basal cisterns or at the tentorial hiatus. In the Arnold-Chiari malformation, the fourth ventricle lies below the level of the foramen magnum and there is obstruction of the exit foramina and, at a higher level, congenital stenosis of the aqueduct of Sylvius.

Clinical Features.—The enlargement of the head may be pre-natal and constitute a rare cause of obstructed labour. After birth, rapid enlargement usually occurs. The scalp veins become distended, the fontanelles widen and are abnormally tense and the brow overhangs the roof of the orbits. Although the ventricles become enormously dilated and the cortex reduced to a mere shell, there are no motor symptoms. A certain minority of cases stabilise spontaneously, and intelligence is then preserved despite the enormous size of the head. Secondary

Arne Torkildsen, Contemporary. Neurosurgeon, Rikshospital, Oslo, Norway.
Julius Arnold, 1835–1915. Professor of Pathological Anatomy, Heidelberg University.
Hans Chiari, 1851–1916. Professor of Pathological Anatomy, Strasbourg University.
François de le Boe (or Fransciscus Sylvius, according to the Latinised form of his name), 1614–1672. Professor of Medicine, Leyden.

endocrine effects result from pressure of the distended third ventricle in the pituitary fossa. Congenital stenosis of the aqueduct may not produce serious symptoms until the age of six or much later. It then causes raised intracranial pressure which may be associated with secondary endocrine disturbances.

Acquired Hydrocephalus

Non-communicating hydrocephalus is produced by obstruction within the cerebrospinal fluid pathways either by a tumour or as the result of a previous inflammatory process. Inflammatory obstruction most commonly occurs at the points of anatomical narrowing (*vide supra*) and that part of the ventricular system cranial to the block dilates. Dilation may be unilateral in the case of obstruction of one foramen of Monro, or bilateral and symmetrical in the case of midline tumours, *e.g.* colloid cysts of the third ventricle, craniopharyngiomas, pineal and cerebellar tumours, and arachnoid cysts over the roof of the fourth ventricle. Communicating hydrocephalus is usually post-inflammatory in origin and complicates acute or chronic meningitis, or it may follow subarachnoid haemorrhage or trauma when blood in the CSF may produce defects of CSF absorbtion by the arachnoid villi.

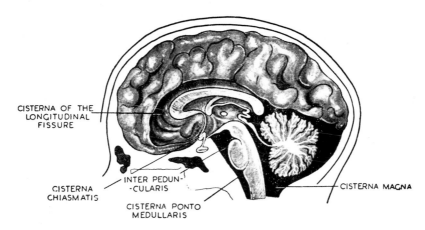

CISTERNA OF THE LONGITUDINAL FISSURE

CISTERNA CHIASMATIS

INTER PEDUN-
-CULARIS

CISTERNA PONTO
MEDULLARIS

CISTERNA MAGNA

FIG. 434.—The principal arachnoid cisterns.

In the above types of hydrocephalus the intra-ventricular pressure is usually very high. An interesting type of acquired communicating hydrocephalus is becoming increasingly recognised in which the ventricular pressure is either normal or low. This type of hydrocephalus, usually discovered during the course of investigations for dementia, appears to be a late effect of either trauma or previous haemorrhage, although in many cases the cause remains obscure.

Treatment.—Hydrocephalus is investigated by CT scan, ventriculography and air encephalography; isotope cisternography has been used. In cases of obstructive hydrocephalus the cause of the obstruction is removed if possible, *e.g.* tumour. In acute hydrocephalus with symptoms of severe raised intracranial pressure, urgent relief is achieved by tapping the lateral ventricles through posterior parietal or frontal burr holes, and setting up external drainage. The treatment of all forms of hydrocephalus has advanced considerably in the last few years. During this time various shunting procedures have been developed and refined and have now largely replaced the older operations of third ventriculostomy and ventriculo-cisternostomy.

The shunting procedures are of two general varieties:

Intracranial Shunts.—These connect the ventricles to other intracranial areas such as the basal cisterns. Ventriculocisternostomy, in which one or both lateral ventricles are connected to the cisterna magna by polythene catheters, was devised by Torkildsen for treating obstructive lesions in the region of the aqueduct of Sylvius (p. 482).

Ventricular or Lumbar Shunts.—The basic principle involved with this type of shunt is the diversion of the cerebrospinal fluid from the lateral ventricle into a body cavity or into the right side of the heart.

Shunts without valves into the pleural and peritoneal cavities have a part to play in the treatment of hydrocephalus but most surgeons now use the ventriculo-atrial shunt utilising one of the several valves now available for this purpose. All these valves have a similar function of promoting unidirectional flow of cerebrospinal fluid from the ventricles to the heart. The most popular of these are the Pudenz and Holter valves.

A tube passes from the ventricle of the brain to beneath the scalp where it connects with the valve. A further tube then passes down beneath the scalp and into the neck where it enters the common facial vein and thence into the internal jugular vein and right atrium.

The great disadvantage of these shunting procedures is that they necessitate the implantation of foreign material into the body and are liable to become blocked and infected. Despite these drawbacks the ventriculo-atrial shunt is a satisfactory treatment for hydrocephalus irrespective of its cause.

INTRACRANIAL ANEURYSM

Intracranial aneurysms may be considered in two main groups:

(1) *Subclinoid.*—On the carotid syphon of the internal carotid artery within the cavernous sinus.

(2) *Supraclinoid.*—On the main branch of the carotid above the cavernous sinus and on the circle of Willis.

Subclinoid Aneurysms

These are produced by weakening of the muscle coat of the internal carotid by uneven distension of its walls at the anterior and posterior curves of the carotid syphon leading to the protrusion of a saccular berry aneurysm. The condition is most common in women owing to the finer structure of their arteries, and in the elderly.

Because the aneurysms lie below the level of the dura and subarachnoid space they do not cause subarachnoid haemorrhage. Pressure upon adjacent structures in the wall of the cavernous sinus may produce pain in the trigeminal territory or defects of external ocular movements, and ptosis.

Treatment.—If pain is severe, common carotid artery ligation may bring relief, but in the elderly there is a risk of hemiplegia.

Arterio-venous fistula in the cavernous sinus may occur *spontaneously*, probably from rupture of an atheromatous plaque in the wall of the carotid artery in the elderly, or from the effects of *trauma* on the arterial walls in association with head injury. Acute back pressure in the veins draining into the cavernous sinus produces pulsating exophthalmos, distension of the orbital and supraorbital veins, and bone erosion and enlargement of the orbit. A few cases heal spontaneously. Usually, however, the condition will progress if untreated, and produce severe proptosis, chemosis and loss of vision.

Robert Harry Pudenz, Contemporary. Neurosurgeon, Huntington Memorial Hospital, Pasadena, California, U.S.A.
John W. Holter, Contemporary. Engineer, Holter Instrument Company, Bridgeport, Pennsylvania. The valve was first used by Fugris B.
Spitz, Neurosurgeon, Children's Hospital, Philadelphia, Pennsylvania, and is also known as a Spitz-Holter valve.
Thomas Willis, 1621–1675. Professor of Natural Philosophy, Oxford.

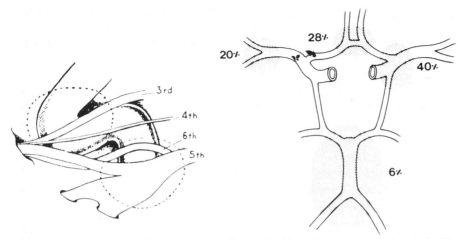

FIG. 435.—The relationship of aneurysmal sacs to structures in wall of the cavernous sinus.

FIG. 436.—Main sites of intracranial supraclinoid aneurysm.

Treatment.—The surgery of carotido-cavernous fistula is difficult and controversial. Common carotid artery ligation is usually ineffective and methods used include embolism of the fistula by a plug of muscle, closure of the fistula by a carotid balloon catheter and intracranial trapping procedures.

Supraclinoid Intracranial Aneurysms

Management of these intracranial aneurysms forms a large part of major neurosurgical practice. Aneurysms may cause:

1. Spontaneous intracranial haemorrhage (subarachnoid haemorrhage).
2. Pressure upon local structures.
3. Epilepsy—very rarely.

Pathology.—*Congenital 'berry' aneurysms* are caused by a weakness in the media of the major arteries at the base of the brain. They occur particularly at points of junction or division of the arteries and assume different forms which may be saccular, fusiform, multilocular, unilocular, the base of the aneurysm may be narrow or broad. About 20% of patients who present with subarachnoid haemorrhage have more than one aneurysm. The main sites of congenital aneurysm and their relative incidence are: Internal carotid artery (40%), Anterior communicating artery (28%), Middle cerebral artery (20%), Vertebrobasilar system (6%) (fig. 436).

Internal carotid artery aneurysms occur most commonly at the origin of the posterior communicating artery, and middle cerebral artery aneurysms at the trifurcation of that artery. Aneurysms on the vertebrobasilar system most commonly arise at the termination of the basilar artery.

Why aneurysms should rupture at a particular time is still uncertain but relevant factors are hypertension, the development of atheroma in the wall of the aneurysm, and ischaemia of the wall of the aneurysm which weakens it further. When rupture occurs there is usually a rapid discharge of blood into the basal cisterns, an acute rise in intracranial pressure which may be fatal, disturbance of blood flow in critical vessels (*e.g.* perforating arteries), and ischaemic changes which may be fatal. Disruption of nerve cells and fibres, and haematoma, may produce persisting focal neurological deficits. Haemorrhage is usually brief and is stemmed by the natural formation and organisation of clot over the tear in the wall of the aneurysm. However this clot is unstable and if lysis occurs, as is common, a second haemorrhage may prove fatal.

Mycotic aneurysms occur in association with bacteraemia, as in bacterial endocarditis, and are produced by infection within the wall of the cerebral vessels, most commonly peripheral branches of the middle cerebral artery.

Subarachnoid haemorrhage.—The term 'subarachnoid haemorrhage' is used loosely to indicate spontaneous intracranial haemorrhage which has occurred primarily into the subarachnoid space of the basal cisterns, the most likely cause being intracranial aneurysm. However, aneurysm may rupture and bleed initially into the ventricles (*e.g.* anterior communicating artery aneurysm) or into the brain substance producing an intracranial haematoma (*e.g.* middle cerebral artery aneurysm). The peak frequency for aneurysmal haemorrhage is between 50 and 54; in approximately 50% of patients who suffer a subarachnoid haemorrhage an aneurysm is the cause.

Clinical Presentation.—The characteristic features are:

1. Sudden onset of severe headache.

2. Sudden loss of consciousness from which the patient may not recover (approximately 25%).

3. Onset of focal neurological deficit due either to the acute disturbance of an eloquent part of the brain (*e.g.* hemiplegia, dysphasia) or to direct pressure of the aneurysm upon an adjacent structure (*e.g.* ptosis, dilated pupil and defect of elevation and adduction of one eye from compression of the oculo-motor nerve by a 'posterior communicating artery aneurysm'). The onset of such defects is not usually as abrupt as in an ischaemic 'stroke'. Sometimes the development of an oculo-motor nerve palsy may precede the haemorrhage, and is probably due to enlargement of the aneurysm prior to rupture.

4. Neck stiffness, photophobia and vomiting due to irritation of the meninges by blood. The blood pressure may rise and the ECG show changes similar to ischaemia.

5. In the majority of patients who survive the initial haemorrhage, the conscious level improves after some hours. However a secondary gradual deterioration over the ensueing days is most commonly due to *spasm* of the cerebral arteries as a reaction to the discharge of blood into the basal cisterns. This spasm may lead to irreversible and often fatal ischaemic damage. Less commonly the subsequent progressive deterioration is due to an intracranial haematoma and brain oedema.

6. A second fatal haemorrhage occurs in approximately 40% of patients within six weeks following the first haemorrhage.

Other causes of subarachnoid haemorrhage include: hypertension, arteriovenous malformation (angioma) (see below), blood dyscrasias, (especially leukaemia), anticoagulant drugs, malignant brain tumours, (especially metastases).

Management.—The objects of management are (1) to provide care to improve the chances of survival from the initial haemorrhage, and (2) to prevent by surgical treatment a second fatal haemorrhage from an aneurysm if it is shown to be the cause of the haemorrhage. The risks of dying from a second haemorrhage from an aneurysm rise to about 40% during the second to fifth weeks after haemorrhage and from the end of the sixth week remain between 10 and 20% over the ensuring years. The factors which determine the favourability of patients for aneurysm surgery are complex and include younger age, good neurological state and especially level of consciousness, interval since haemorrhage, absence of hypertension, absence of arterial spasm shown by arteriography, absence of significant cardiac and pulmonary disease, and the site, configuration and relationships of the responsible aneurysm. It is often a matter of weighing these factors against the natural history.

The usual steps in management after clinical assessment are:

1. **Lumbar puncture.**—It is important to take at least two consecutive specimens into separate containers for comparison. In subarachnoid haemorrhage from any cause the fluid is evenly blood stained, and the finding of xanthochromia in the supernatant fluid confirms the diagnosis. Although lumbar puncture in the presence of raised intracranial pressure, and especially intracerebral haematoma, may precipitate tentorial herniation (coning), lumbar puncture remains an important investigation especially if the differential diagnosis includes meningitis.

2. **CT Scan.**—This is of great value following spontaneous intracranial haemorrhage. As well as demonstrating significant compressing haematomas in patients whose condition is poor, it may also indicate the site of haemorrhage in patients who are relatively well. Thereby the extent of angiography may be limited, and the hazards of that investigation reduced. To give information of this type, CT scan needs to be done as soon as possible after haemorrhage. Thus in an ideal situation, a strong case can be made for doing a CT scan as soon as possible on all patients who on clinical grounds have sustained a spontaneous intracranial haemorrhage.

3. **Bilateral carotid and vertebral arteriography.**—The timing and indications for arteriography depend upon the exclusion of 'medical' causes of haemorrhage (see above), and the factors determining suitability for surgery. Therefore arteriography is usually deferred in patients who remain 'unconscious'.

4. **Surgery of intracranial anaeurysm.**—With improvements in the methods of selection of patients suitable for surgery, and in operative conditions, and above all with the use of the *operating microscope* the surgical treatment of intracranial aneurysm has become increasingly exposure of the neck of the aneurysm, careful dissection and preservation of adjacent and parent arteries, and then *obliteration of the aneurysm by the application of a metal clip.* Despite the technical problems this method is favoured for most aneurysms. If the configuration and arterial relationships of the aneurysm prevent clipping, the risks of haemorrhage may be reduced, but less effectively, by *wrapping* the aneurysm with gauze, muscle or plastic.

Internal carotid artery aneurysms have been treated by common carotid artery ligation, thereby reducing the overall mortality from further haemorrhage from about 30% to 8%. However there are significant risks of hemiplegia, and therefore the tendency now is for direct attack, the approach being through a fronto-temporal craniotomy.

Anterior communicating artery aneurysm may cause severe intellectual and emotional disturbances. Operation approach is by fronto-temporal craniotomy.

Middle cerebral artery aneurysms are approached through a fronto-temporal craniotomy, and entering the Sylvian fissure. These aneurysms may be fusiform dilatations of the trifurcation of the artery and in these circumstances are wrapped rather than clipped.

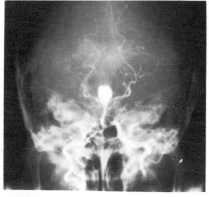

FIG. 437.—Vertebral arteriogram showing basilar artery aneurysm.

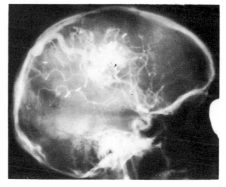

FIG. 438.—Carotid arteriogram showing parietal angioma and metal clips from surgery many years previously.

Vertebro-basilar aneurysms require either a fronto-temporal approach (terminal basil artery aneurysm) (fig. 437) or a posterior fossa craniectomy (vertebral artery aneurysm).

Local pressure effects of aneurysm.—These may produce symptoms and signs which occasionally precede rupture of the aneurysm, or more commonly persist without rupture. Aneurysms on the posterior branches of the circle, posterior cerebral and posterior communicating vessels, produce symptoms of third nerve palsy. Posterior cerebral aneurysms also cause hemianopia or pressure on the crus. Aneurysms of the anterior branches, such as the internal carotid bifurcation, anterior cerebral, and anterior communicating, produce pressure on the optic tracts, optic nerves, and chiasma respectively, producing hemianopia, monocular visual loss, or bi-temporal hemianopia and optic atrophy.

Prodromal symptoms are uncommon. There may be comparatively mild headache due to distension of the aneurysmal sac, lasting from a few hours to a few days before rupture. Unilateral supra-orbital pain, without tenderness or other signs of frontal sinusitis is suspicious of an enlarging posterior communicating aneurysm. Paraesthesia in a limb sometimes immediately precedes haemorrhage from a vascular malformation.

Prodromal Signs.—The most important of these is unilateral 3rd nerve palsy, presenting as ptosis. When accompanied by the supra-orbital pain mentioned above it is an urgent warning of enlargement of a posterior communicating aneurysm demanding confirmative angiography and treatment before it ruptures. Rapidly advancing hemianopia or unilateral blindness may indicate enlargement of an internal carotid aneurysm adjacent to the chiasma.

Vascular malformations involving arterio-venous shunts are similar to cirsoid aneurysms elsewhere. Arterialised varices burst into the substances of the brain and only secondarily into the subarachnoid pathways. An intracranial bruit may be audible by the patient or examiner, and occasionally, apart from rupture, they may be responsible for epilepsy or unilateral migraine (*vide infra*).

Intracranial angiomas are congenital malformations and not true tumours. Although an excess of blood passes through the large arterio-venous malformations, absence of a true capillary system causes defective nutrition of the affected area, with death of tissue, gliosis, and calcification. This may produce epilepsy and paralysis, often in adult life. Alternatively, the angioma may rupture spontaneously or following a minor trauma, producing apoplexy in young subjects.

Vascular malformations are treated by excision of that part of the lesion containing the actual arterio-venous shunt, including brain tissue immediately surrounding it. The risk of fatal recurrence from these lesions is much less than that from aneurysms, and treatment is neither so urgent nor so imperative.

Intracerebral Haemorrhage

The classical apoplexy, occurring typically in the ageing plethoric man with known hypertension and arteriosclerosis, is usually diagnosed correctly by the family doctor. Fatal cases present with sudden stupor, stertorous respirations and hemiplegia. In younger patients with no known arterial disease, rupture of an aneurysm is the commonest cause of such a picture. In both these cases only limited success may be hoped for from the removal of the blood clot from the brain, for much damage to neurones has already been done at that time of the haemorrhage, and removal of the mass, though it may save the patient from death due to raised intracranial pressure, is often disappointing as far as restoration of cerebral function is concerned.

The diagnosis of intracerebral haemorrhage is confirmed angiographically or by CT scan. Removal of the clot is done most effectively by craniotomy.

CHAPTER 27

THE SPINE
THE VERTEBRAL COLUMN AND SPINAL CORD

INJURIES TO THE VERTEBRAL COLUMN

Classification.—Essential to the rational treatment of an injury to the vertebral column is an accurate classification of the lesion which in turn depends on a recognition of the structures which have been damaged.

Fundamental to any classification system is the concept of stability. An unstable spine may be defined as one in such a condition, that, given routine hospital care, is nevertheless likely to undergo such a degree of further displacement as to jeopardise the spinal cord or result in unacceptable deformity. Once such a state of affairs has been recognised the implications for treatment are self evident, although it is important not to oversimplify the problem since intermediate degrees of instability can exist.

In recognising an unstable injury it is helpful to think of the spine, not as a single column but rather as three (fig. 439); an anterior consisting of the vertebral bodies joined by the discs and longitudinal ligaments, an intermediate column consisting of the facet joints and their ligaments and a posterior column which consists of the strong interspinous ligament interrupted by the spinous processes themselves. Clearly if all three columns are disrupted then the situation is anal-

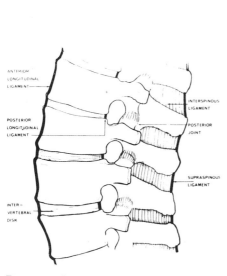

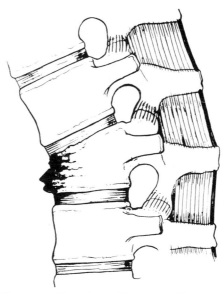

FIG. 439.—Anatomy of the normal spine showing the three columns of which it is composed.

FIG. 440.—Typical 'crush' fracture. The posterior interspinous ligament is intact.

ogous to the fracture of a long bone and is obviously extremely unstable. If only one column is interrupted on the other hand, as in a simple crush fracture, then conversely the spine may be regarded as stable and the anatomical situations giving rise to the intermediate situations can be readily envisaged.

STABLE INJURIES

These include appendicular fractures of the vertebrae, *e.g.* fractures of the transverse processes, and isolated fractures of spinous processes. These may arise either from a direct blow or indirectly from violent muscular action; the 'clay shoveller's' fracture of the spinous process of C.7. is an obvious example of the latter and it should be borne in mind that when multiple fractures of the lumbar transverse processes are seen the soft tissue injury is often more serious than the bony lesion suggests and usually implies a tear of the entire musculo-fascial plane in this region.

The commonest stable injury involving the vertebral body is the simple crush fracture (fig. 440). This is most commonly found in the dorsal region and usually follows a flexion injury; the posterior elements remain intact so that the force is expended on the front of the vertebral body which becomes depressed. Such fractures are of course commonly seen without a history of violence in osteoporosis.

Treatment.—No specific treatment is required for any of these injuries; relief of pain is the main objective since this may be considerable at first. For crush fractures a short period of bedrest together with suitable analgesics is usually all that is required, without the need for external supports or corsets.

UNSTABLE INJURIES

Although the same principles governing the recognition of instability apply to all regions of the vertebral column, these differ so greatly in their anatomical configuration that each must be considered separately.

Fractures of the Dorsi-Lumbar Spine

Fracture Dislocations.—Pure dislocations in this region are uncommon because of the orientation of the massive articular processes which are usually damaged themselves (fig. 441). Although these injuries can occur at any level in the lumbar spine 90% of them occur between T.12. and L.1. Classically the lesion results from a flexion and rotation force. In former times this was a characteristic injury which befell the kneeling miner following a fall of rock onto one side of the flexed spine but with improved underground safety it is now much more common among motor cyclists thrown into the air and landing on one shoulder.

Diagnosis.—This can often be made on clinical grounds alone with a characteristic history of injury, often with a tell-tale abrasion over the patient's scapula (fig. 442). However, the key to clinical diagnosis lies in the recognition of the ruptured interspinous ligament which is easily detected since it lies just beneath the skin. A boggy haematoma can be felt and usually the enlarged interval can

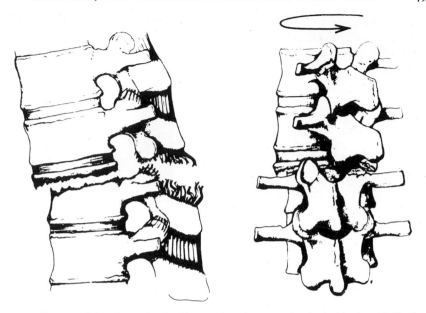

FIG. 441.—Fracture dislocation at the dorsi-lumbar junction, note the classical horizontal slice fracture of the vertebral body, the fracture dislocation of the facet joints and the complete rupture of the posterior interspinous ligament. The spine is effectively in two halves.

be defined between the relevant spinous processes by palpation of a characteristic 'gap' (fig. 442).

Radiologically the features may be equally characteristic. The classical appearance of the vertebral body is of a horizontal 'slice' fracture passing through the upper part of the body with forward displacement of the upper vertebra on

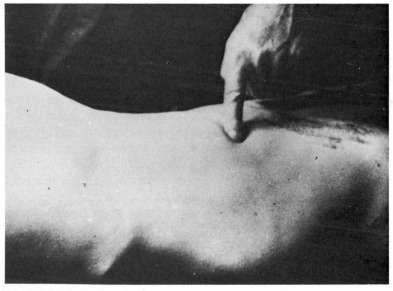

FIG. 442.—Fracture dislocation of the dorsi-lumbar spine. The examiner's finger is identifying the gap created by the torn interspinous ligament, note the characteristic abrasion over the scapula.

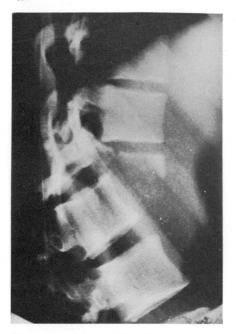

FIG. 443.—Fracture dislocation at the dorsi-lumbar junction, note the characteristic appearance of the fractured vertebral body.

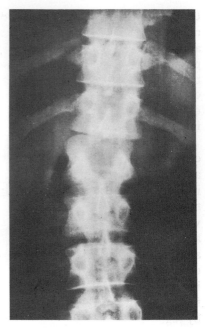

FIG. 444.—Fracture dislocation of the dorsi-lumbar spine. There is an abnormally large interval between the spine of T.12. and L.1. indicating rupture of the posterior interspinous ligament.

the lower (fig. 443). There are however many variants on this appearance. The intermediate facet column can be demonstrated by oblique radiography to show fractures and any overriding of the facets. Most important of all however, is the spacing of the spinous processes which may be recognised either on a low penetration lateral or an A.P. film showing an increased interval at the affected level indicating rupture of the interspinous ligament (fig. 444). It should be remembered that the amount of vertebral body displacement may be minimal at first making the diagnosis difficult but some degree of abnormal separation of the spinous processes is almost invariably present and is therefore the most reliable sign. The predilection of this injury for the dorsi-lumbar junction should also be remembered and indeed all fractures which involve the vertebral body in this region should be regarded as unstable until proved otherwise.

Treatment.—The majority of unstable injuries in this region are accompanied by damage to the spinal cord and nerve roots. In assessing this it is helpful to recall that the first sacral segment of the cord is approximately level with the T.12./L.1. interspace so that injury at this level can affect the cord only from the first sacral segment down. However, the lumbar nerve roots can also be damaged as they pass the lesion so that the classical neurological injury at this level consists of a lower motor neurone lesion of the lumbar segments and an upper motor neurone lesion of the sacral segments.

In such circumstances measures to mitigate any neurological damage would appear logical, but unfortunately there is little evidence that much can be done.

Unlike the situation in closed head injuries where damage may be caused by rising pressure which may be relieved, in spinal injuries most of the damage appears to be inflicted anatomically at the time of injury. Laminectomy, for the purposes of producing general decompression therefore is probably of little value but although statistical proof is lacking it would seem reasonable in the interests of promoting recovery, particularly of the nerve roots, to realign gross distortions of the spinal canal and possibly to remove large intruding fragments of bone or intervertebral disc.

Undoubtedly the most important aspect of treatment is the avoidance of the complications of the paraplegia itself (see below) but the fact that the patient has a serious fracture should not be forgotten. Even if the paralysis does not recover it is important that the fractured spine should unite in good alignment in order to maximise the patient's subsequent function. This subject is controversial but where the displacement is minimal and where skilled paraplegic nursing is available, as in special centres, alignment may be preserved by recumbency aided by strategically placed pillows and packs. Where displacement is significant on the other hand most surgeons would prefer to treat this by open reduction and internal fixation, thus converting an unstable lesion into a stable one. The internal fixation may consist of plates bolted to the spinous processes or by rods secured by segmental sublaminar wires (fig. 445). The latter technique, although more extensive has the advantage that the patient can be mobilised almost straight away.

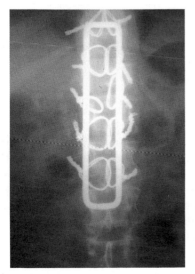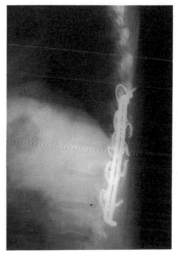

FIG. 445.—Technique of internal fixation of a fracture dislocation using sublaminar wiring.

'Burst' Fractures.—These fractures arise as a result of axial violence, usually due to a heavy fall on either the heels or the buttocks (fig. 446). In severe cases there can be damage to the posterior elements, therefore the spine should be assessed for instability in the same way as in a fracture dislocation.

Treatment.—In the majority of instances displacement is not great and the spinal cord undamaged and after a period of a few weeks recumbency, when the spine has become comfortable, the patient may be mobilised in some form of spinal jacket. Where there is

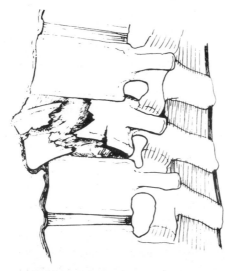

FIG. 446.—Burst fracture in the lumbar spine. The vertebral body is literally shattered. Neurological damage may result from the protrusion of bony fragments into the vertebral canal. In this particular instance the posterior elements are intact and the fracture is therefore *stable*, but this is not invariably so.

displacement of the vertebral column and evidence of posterior element damage internal fixation may be required and here the distracting effects of Harrington rods (Chapter 22) may be useful in producing re-alignment.

Where there is an unusually large protrusion into the spinal canal associated with neurological damage surgical removal may be indicated in the hope of promoting neurological recovery. This is most conveniently done by the anterior extra-peritoneal route, the fragments of the shattered vertebral body being removed and replaced by a bone graft taken from the iliac crest.

Fracture of the Dorsal Spine.—The majority of injuries in this region are stable due to the influence of the thoracic cage. Occasionally a powerful blow on the back will produce a shearing type of fracture dislocation which is usually accompanied by rib fractures or a fracture of the sternum. The spinal canal is very narrow at this point and its blood supply particularly vulnerable. Such injuries usually lead to a complete and irreversible paraplegia and surgery has little to offer in injuries in this region; the treatment is that of the paraplegia itself.

Dislocations and Fracture Dislocations—Cervical Region

While fracture dislocations are commonest in the dorsi-lumbar region, in the neck pure dislocations are the rule because of the sloping nature of the facet joints, and forward displacement of the upper vertebra usually, but not invariably, occurs through the disc itself (fig. 447). The mechanism of the injury is a combination of flexion violence together with restraint of the vertex so that most injuries arise from falls on the head with the neck in some flexion. Motorcycle accidents, diving and rugby football account for many of these injuries which unhappily almost all occur in schoolboys and young men.

Dislocations may involve one or both of the articular facets, the situation being revealed by oblique radiographs. If both facets are involved the forward displacement is usually more than half the diameter of the vertebral body (fig. 447) and *vice versa*. Serious neurological involvement may accompany either situation.

Pain is felt in the neck and may be referred along a local nerve root due to entrapment. Neck movements are limited and posterior tenderness is invariably present due to the rupture of the interspinous ligament which accompanies all dislocations.

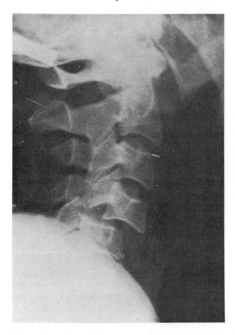

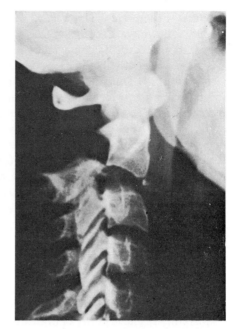

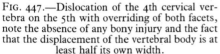

FIG. 447.—Dislocation of the 4th cervical vertebra on the 5th with overriding of both facets, note the absence of any bony injury and the fact that the displacement of the vertebral body is at least half its own width.

FIG. 448.—'Hangman' fracture of C.2. Note the fracture of the pars intra-articularis with forward displacement of the body while the posterior elements remain intact. As a result the diameter of the vertebral canal is increased.

Treatment.—Reduction of the dislocation should be carried out as soon as possible in all cases but *where there is evidence of cord involvement the situation constitutes an emergency.*

Skull traction should be instituted and under systemic analgesia the weight should be increased under radiological control with the neck in slight flexion. Weights of up to 40 pounds (18 kg) may have to be used. Once the facets have been seen to disengage the neck is slightly extended and the weights reduced to 8 or 10 pounds (4 kg). The facets should then settle back into their correct position. If this fails manipulation under anaesthesia may be attempted by a surgeon experienced in the technique. Otherwise the patient should be carefully turned into the prone position and open reduction carried out under direct vision. In a fresh case this is fairly easily accomplished by levering the facets carefully over one another. Extensive removal of facet bone should be avoided because subsequent stabilisation of the neck will be rendered more difficult. At the end of the operation it is usual to wire the relevant spinous processes together over a bone graft. Some form of firm supporting collar is then used until consolidation has occurred.

In cases where closed reduction has been successful light skull traction should be retained for three weeks at the end of which a lateral radiograph should be taken. If this shows early evidence of interbody fusion then immobilisation should be continued until this is consolidated. Otherwise fusion should be carried out either posteriorly as above, or by the anterior route.

'Burst' Fractures.—These occur from axial violence as in the lumbar region, usually following a fall on the head with the neck in the neutral position. The cord is more frequently damaged by these injuries than in the lumbar region and the prognosis is usually poor, particularly if paralysis is complete.

Treatment.—Light skull traction is usually applied until the fracture has consolidated in order to avoid the development of unacceptable deformity. In incomplete lesions the cord may be decompressed by removal of the damaged vertebral body from in front and replacing it with a massive bone graft. However, the neurological benefits from this procedure have not been unequivocally demonstrated and some recovery frequently follows conservative management. Laminectomy is contraindicated since it has not been shown to improve the neurological prognosis and it greatly increases the instability of the spine.

Fractures of the atlas and axis.—Because of the great anatomical differences in this region many of the above generalisations do not apply. A *burst fracture of the atlas* (the Jefferson fracture) may result from a fall on the vertex; the ring is often broken at several points but since the effect is to widen the vertebral canal there are usually no neurological sequelae. Light traction for a few weeks followed by a suitable supporting collar is all that is required.

Fractures of the odontoid may be accompanied by either forward or backward displacement. The majority of injuries are not accompanied by neurological damage since many with this complication do not survive. Most of these fractures will unite following immobilisation with light skull traction, the head being positioned so as to re-align the fracture. If however, union does not occur or the injury is diagnosed late, as is not infrequently the case, then the neck must be assessed for stability by flexion and extension views. If abnormal movement can be demonstrated there is a risk of late myelopathy and the lesion should be stabilised by fusing the axis to the atlas and/or the occiput.

The 'hangman' fracture as described by Wood-Jones (fig. 448), results from forcible hyperextension of the neck as in judicial hanging when the knot is placed beneath the chin. In clinical practice the hyperextension results in the same bony lesion with a fracture of the pars intra-articularis of C.2. and as the head comes forward again the body of C.2. displaces forward in what is effectively a traumatic spondylolisthesis. This actually increases the size of the spinal canal so that neurological damage is unlikely in the absence of a hangman's rope. The fracture although alarming is simply dealt with by light traction in recumbency when the fractured surfaces unite directly to one another without the need for surgical intervention.

ASSESSMENT AND MANAGEMENT OF SPINAL CORD INJURY

Spinal Concussion (Spinal Shock).—This may occur on its own as a result of an injury or be superimposed upon actual spinal cord damage. The effect is to abolish voluntary power, sensation and all reflex activity below the level of the lesion.

Recovery usually begins within 24 hours of injury, starting in the more distal cord. The failure of return of any cord activity within 48 hours of an apparently complete lesion is a very poor prognostic sign. Where there has been irreversible cord damage reflex activity will eventually return, again starting in the most distal segments with the peri-anal and bulbo-cavernosus reflexes which usually appear within a few days. Their manifestation without at the same time any evidence of

Sir Geoffrey Jefferson, 1886–1961. Professor of Neurosurgery, University of Manchester.
Frederic Wood Jones, 1879–1954. FRS, Professor of Anatomy, Universities of Adelaide and Melbourne, Australia, University of Manchester, England, Royal College of Surgeons of England and Conservator of the Hunterian Museum.

voluntary recovery is again a gloomy prognostic sign. The ankle jerks usually return within a matter of weeks but it may be several months before the knee jerks return. In some instances of course there may be total destruction of the cord distal to the lesion, especially in dorsi-lumbar injuries in which case the paralysis will remain flaccid.

Partial Spinal Cord Injury.—By demonstrating that the cord is in continuity the outlook is naturally rendered more hopeful and the majority of such cases do show some further improvement although this may not necessarily be of functional value. Although the pattern of these injuries can be infinitely varied there are a number of common presentations; the *anterior cord syndrome*, in which there is severe motor loss but the posterior columns are intact; the *posterior cord syndrome* in which the pattern is reversed and the *Brown-Séquard syndrome* indicating hemi-section of the cord is also common. In more severe injuries the distinction between a lesion which is incomplete and virtually complete is important because the prognosis in the former is not so hopeless. In this connection it is important to examine carefully the peri-anal region which is often spared in incomplete lesions and the presence of some preserved sensation here is, therefore, a reason for restrained optimism.

Central Cord Syndrome (so-called) requires special mention. This condition results not uncommonly from an extension injury of the neck and may result in some diagnostic confusion since there is no accompanying bony injury demonstrable on x-ray. Typically the patient is middle aged or elderly and usually has radiological evidence of degenerative change in the cervical spine. The mechanism of the cord damage is not known but is generally thought to have a vascular basis.

The clinical features of the condition are very distinct; there is an incomplete tetraparesis with a patchy sensory loss whose upper limit is often difficult to define accurately. Most characteristic of all is that the upper limbs are much more severely affected than the lower, indeed in some cases the latter are often overlooked. However, careful clinical examination will almost invariably reveal that the plantar responses are up-going and there is other evidence of spastic paresis.

Fortunately like other incomplete lesions the prognosis is reasonably good and substantial recovery may be looked for in the majority of instances although severe residual paralysis, particularly in the upper limbs, persists in a proportion of cases.

No specific treatment is indicated; a supporting collar may be required if the neck is painful. The liability of this type of patient to suffer this injury should be borne in mind when patients with cervical spondylosis are given general anaesthesia, particularly if the neck is extended for any reason.

Management of Spinal Cord Injury

First Aid Treatment.—Cervical injuries should be transported supine with the head supported between sandbags which may also be used to anchor a towel passed across the forehead. In moving the patient, flexion and particularly rotation of the neck should be avoided by an attendant who is made responsible

Charles Edouard Brown-Séquard, 1817–1894. Physician, National Hospital for Nervous Diseases, London (1860–1964), Professor of Medicine, Harvard University, Boston, Mass. (1864–1878) and College de France, Paris (1878–1894). Described this syndrome in 1851. He was a native of Mauritius.

for controlling this alone. With dorsal and lumbar injuries the patient should never be moved except by at least two attendants, one being responsible for the pelvis and the other for the shoulders; the two being kept parallel and the patient effectively rolled like a log. The patient may be transported either prone or supine, depending upon other injuries.

Clinical Examination.—Upon arrival at hospital the same precautions about moving the patient must be observed until the stability of the spine has been confirmed. Simple examination of the sensory, motor and reflex function will usually indicate the site of the lesion although there are a number of pitfalls. Loss of sensation from the nipples downwards is often attributed to a high dorsal injury but more often it is in fact the result of a much higher cervical injury and the sensation over the shoulders and upper chest is due to the innervation provided by the supra-clavicular nerves. Examination of the sensation of the ulnar border of the upper limbs will avoid this error together with a proper assessment of motor function in the hands.

If the neurological level does not correspond with the demonstrated vertebral lesion, suspect that a second lesion may be present and it should be sought at the site indicated by the neurological signs.

Nursing Care.—Nursing and general care is particularly directed to the avoidance of the complications of spinal cord injury, particularly the development of pressure sores, urinary infections and in the case of cervical injuries, chest infections. Pressure sores may develop within a few hours.

The regime of two hourly regularly turning should be begun as soon as the patient is admitted to hospital. This routine must be continued throughout the night and experience has shown that this is often difficult to maintain in a busy emergency ward. For that reason as soon as the patient is fit to travel and any surgery has been undertaken he should be transferred to a special Spinal Injuries Unit as soon as possible. Urinary retention is invariable and an indwelling catheter is used in the initial stages. The subsequent management of bladder problems is dealt with in Chapter 58.

Bowel paralysis is also present and the use of enemas and suppositories is usually essential. In most patients bowel movements are eventually managed in the long term by manual evacuation performed either by an attendant or the patient himself. Chest infections are a serious threat in tetraplegic patients, especially in the first two weeks and vigorous chest physiotherapy should be instituted immediately after admission.

Rehabilitation.—At the end of the 1914–18 war the life expectancy of a paraplegic was approximately two years and that short span was spent in progressive bedridden misery. Nowadays that expection has risen to around thirty years and the whole social outlook transformed.

Much of the credit for this must be given to the late Sir Ludwig Guttmann who realised that by grouping these patients into special units the lethal complications of bed sores and urinary infections could be most efficiently dealt with and better still, prevented on the lines indicated earlier. Given that the patient's bodily health could thus be preserved it became possible to take a more positive attitude to the resumption of the normal activities of daily living and, later on, to employment.

Sir Ludwig Guttmann, 1899–1980. Director of Research, National Spinal Injuries Centre, Stoke Mandeville Hospital, Bucks, England.

As a result most paraplegics and tetraplegics are able to live outside an institution provided it is available when complications develop, and many paraplegics and even some tetraplegics are gainfully employed.

The mainstays of rehabilitation are firstly the development of the unparalysed muscles where appropriate, the teaching of the techniques of transfer so important to independence, and even walking with the aid of suitable calipers. These activities lie in the province of the physiotherapist as does the prevention of contractures of joints and the development of secondary deformities in general. The occupational therapist on the other hand is responsible for modifications to the physical environment and the provision of special aids and appliances although there is obviously a great deal of overlap between the two and indeed the whole concept of rehabilitation is based on teamwork.

The surgeon also has a part to play at this stage; patients still develop pressure sores when living at home from time to time and a plastic surgeon may be required to treat these by the swinging of appropriate flaps. The orthopaedic surgeon on the other hand may be required to release severe joint contractures and in some instances to denervate the groups of muscles, which are over-acting, to reduce spasm (Chapter 25).

In selected tetraplegic patients tendon transfers in the hand may be extremely useful in improving function but such procedures must be considered very carefully since the loss of existing function can be all too easily precipitated.

The function of the Spinal Injuries Unit is to provide as many of these services as possible under one roof and to co-ordinate the very diverse types of expertise which may be required from time to time.

INFECTIVE CONDITIONS

Meningitis.—Acute infective meningitis is likely to follow a penetrating wound, or may be a complication of septicaemia. Severe constitutional disturbances follow with local and referred pain, hyperaesthesia, muscular spasms, and increased reflexes. Extension to the basal meninges is usual, and the only hope lies in an adequate course of antibiotics able to penetrate the blood/brain barrier (see Chapter 3).

Spinal Epidural Abscess.—Pus may collect in the extradural space of the cervical mid-dorsal or lumbar regions, to which infection has extended through the intervertebral foramina from adjacent sepsis, particularly from a perinephric abscess in the lumbar region. This produces a syndrome of progressive cord compression and meningeal irritation. The pus is evacuated by laminectomy.

SPINA BIFIDA

Embryology.—During the second week of intrauterine life a longitudinal furrow appears on the dorsum on the embryo, this groove being formed by infolding of the epiblast. The margins of the neural groove unite, so that it becomes converted into a tube from which the nervous system is developed. This epiblastic tube becomes separated from the surface by mesoblast, which grows over it from either side, and from which are developed the vertebrae, spinal muscles, membranes, *etc*. In each segment bars of cartilage appear on either side of the neural tube, and during the fourth month they fuse with each other to form the vertebral arches. Failure of fusion of these arches gives rise to spina bifida, with which is frequently associated mal-development of the spinal cord and membranes. The incidence of spina bifida, excluding spina bifida occulta, is 0·1%.

The types of spina bifida are as follows:

(1) *Spina bifida occulta* is due to failure of the neural arches to unite, but there is no protrusion of cord or membranes. Frequently only one vertebra is affected, most commonly in the lumbo-sacral region. A local patch of hair, a naevo-lipoma, or a depression in the skin are suggestive of underlying bony deficiency. A fibrous band, the *membrana*

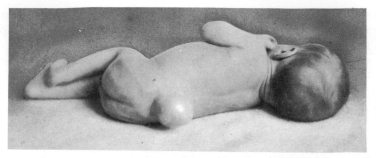

FIG. 449.—A typical meningocele which was excised successfully.

reuniens, connects the skin to the spinal theca. Growth of the body causes the membrana to pull on the theca and nerve roots. Foot-drop, nocturnal enuresis, or backache occur when the child is older or in adult life. Many cases are symptomless and are undiagnosed unless an x-ray is taken for some other reason.

(2) *Meningocele.*—This is a protrusion of meninges through a defect in the spino-laminar segment (fig. 449). It contains only cerebrospinal fluid.

(3) *Meningo-myelocele.*—The normally developed spinal cord or cauda equina lies in the sac, and may be adherent to the posterior aspect. The cord or nerves can be seen as dark shadows on transillumination.

(4) *Syringo-myelocele.*—The rarest type of spina bifida, in which the central canal of the cord is dilated, and the cord lies within the sac together with the nerves arising from it.

(5) *Myelocele* results from arrest of development at the time of closure of the neural furrow. An elliptical raw surface is seen, which represents the ununited groove. At the upper end the central canal opens on the surface and discharges cerebrospinal fluid.

With the exception of spina bifida occulta, myelocele is the most common type of spina bifida; many cases are stillborn. If the child is born alive, death ensues within a few days from infection of the cord and meninges. Gross talipes is obvious.

Meningocele and meningo-myelocele are distinguishable on transillumination. A depression in the skin is sometimes produced by adherent cord or nerves in a meningo-myelocele. Interference with the spinal cord or nerves may occur in either condition but is more severe in meningo-myelocele, in which condition bilateral talipes with trophic changes are common, and in advanced cases extensive paralysis of the legs and incontinence occur. In serious cases no surgical intervention is indicated.

Treatment.—Operation for meningocele or meningo-myelocele is advisable as soon as the surgeon is of the opinion that the child's strength and condition warrant the procedure (often within a few days of birth), otherwise the sac is liable to grow out of proportion to the growth of the child, and the overlying skin will become atrophic and ulcerate.Hydrocephalus may follow sac closure, and require relief by CSF shunting.

Operation.—The sac is opened and redundant membrane excised. If the cord or nerves are adherent, they are either freed by dissection, or separated with a strip of attached membrane, and replaced in the vertebral canal. Membranes are sutured over the cord, spinal muscles are approximated and the wound is reinforced with flaps of sheath from the erector spinae muscles. Those cases which survive with gross paralysis of one or both lower limbs either after operation or without operation, when the sac fails to rupture and develops some form of permanent coverage, may achieve some useful activity. However, the further care of these unfortunate children is life-long and complex, and may involve repeated orthopaedic, urological and abdominal surgery, and repeated revisions of CSF shunts for hydrocephalus. Therefore, in the early management of the totally paraplegic infant there is room for debate, often emotional, about the indications for skin closure over the myelomeningocele, and the preservation of life.

Operation for spina bifida occulta is required when neurological, urological or orthopaedic symptoms progress or appear after infancy. These symptoms are only rarely produced by traction from the membrana reuniens alone but are more likely to be due to compression of the cord by intra- or extradural lipomas or the effect of diastemato-myelia, a condition in which the cord is split in the mid-line by a bony spur which divides the neural canal beneath one laminae into two lateral compartments. These abnormalities are almost always associated with the presence of a hairy tuft on the overlying skin, which is an important warning sign.

Myelography is required in all cases prior to operation.

The extradural and intradural findings at operation are unpredictable and very variable, and it is often difficult to decide what is functioning neural tissue, and what can be sacrificed to relieve traction on the low spinal cord.

INFLAMMATORY DISEASES

Acute osteomyelitis occurs in the epiphysis of the body of a vertebra or, more rarely, one epiphysis of the neural arch. Severe constitutional disturbance is associated with local pain and tenderness. Pain may also be referred along an adjacent spinal nerve. If the disease commences in a neural arch, some local evidence of inflammation is often detected. Acute osteomyelitis of a vertebral body has been mistaken for spinal meningitis, acute appendicitis, acute pancreatitis, and other abdominal conditions.

As soon as the disease is suspected, penicillin is administered, supplemented by chemotherapy. X-rays assist in determining the progress of the disease, and evacuation of pus or sequestrectomy is performed if necessary.

Tuberculous Disease—Chapter 18.

Spondylitis—Chapter 19.

TUMOURS OF THE VERTEBRAL COLUMN

Innocent tumours are extremely rare and include chondromas, osteomas, and fibromas. Many cases previously described as chondromas were in reality protrusions of an intervertebral disc. These tumours produce a syndrome of spinal compression affecting the anterior surface of the cord associated with characteristic x-ray appearances.

Malignant tumours of the spine are primary or secondary. Primary sarcoma is most frequent in children and young adults. The neural arches are usually affected, a palpable swelling may be detected in the paravertebral muscles, or invading tumour is discovered at this site during laminectomy performed for spinal-cord compression. Operative removal is always incomplete. Deep x-ray therapy is seldom effective.

Secondary deposits in the spine are common and far outnumber primary spinal or spinal-cord tumours (see below). The majority are produced by bone metastasis chiefly derived from the breast, prostate, or bronchus, and commonly occur in the extradural space due to the rich venous plexuses at that site. Malignant ganglion neuroblastomas of the sympathetic chain may invade through the intervertebral foramen.

Clinical Features.—Bone deposits produce severe local pain which may be the only symptom for a variable period. Later, as nerves become involved, the pain becomes girdle in type and increases in intensity. It is aggravated by movement, so that the patient may remain crouched in a chair or huddled up in bed for hours at a time. If diagnosis is established at this stage, radiotherapy may prevent vertebral collapse and cord damage.

The sudden collapse of a vertebra in which a deposit has developed painlessly may lead to instantaneous paralysis and severe back pain as the first symptom. A similar disaster may occur if manipulation of the spine has been unwisely performed in an attempt to relieve the local pain produced by a vertebral deposit which has not been diagnosed. The diagnosis of secondary tumour should always be suspected when severe local pain is associated with a high ESR. Commonly, a period of local pain is gradually followed by the onset of paraplegia and spasticity with increased reflexes, but once paraplegia is established it may become complete (see below).

Treatment.—Secondary deposits from the prostate respond to treatment with stilboestrol, and those from the breast may regress with hormone therapy or adrenalectomy (Chapter 38). In other cases, treatment is limited to a support to the spine, analgesics, and deep x-ray therapy. Intrathecal phenol (5% in Myodil®) injections are a satisfactory method of relieving agonising pain.

TUMOURS OF THE SPINAL CANAL

Tumours of the spinal canal are either extradural or intradural. Intradural tumours are either extramedullary or intramedullary.

Extradural tumours.—As indicated above, the commonest extradural tumour is the spinal metastasis. The tumours lie in the extradural space, between the dura and the bone and ligamenta flava, where there is a rich venous plexus, which may account for the tumour's predilection for that particular site. Involvement of the laminae or vertebral bodies may or may not be present. As with other bony metastases the common sites of origin are: bronchus, breast, prostate, kidney and myeloma. Other rarer sites of origin are thyroid, alimentary tract, melanoma, and lymphoma. It is rare for the growth to transgress or infiltrate the dura, which it compresses and may encircle, causing compression of the spinal cord or cauda equina. Tumours may be multiple and at several levels, when there may be difficulties in clinical location and radiological demonstration.

Other extradural tumours are rare. They include primary bone tumours (sarcoma, aneurysmal bone cyst, osteoclastoma, chordoma), lipoma, angiolipoma and liposarcoma, and very rarely, extradural Schwannoma and meningioma.

Intradural tumours.—*Extramedullary* (75% of intradural tumours), are neurofibromas and meningiomas. Neurofibromas are commoner in males and usually arise from a posterior nerve root forming a fusiform tumour about 2·5 to 3·75 cm long present on the postero-lateral aspect of the cord. Occasionally there is an extradural dumb-bell extension through an enlarged intervertebral foramen. Meningiomas occur almost exclusively in women and usually form a small globular tumour the size of a grape attached to the dura and indenting the cord.

Intramedullary Tumours (25% of intradural tumours). Approximately half these are irremovable diffuse gliomas. The rest are ependymomas, a growth derived from the ependyma lining the central canal, forming either solid tumours like pencils which can be excised, or cysts which can be evacuated. Vascular malformations comprise 4%, and for these little can be done. More than half the intramedullary tumours lie in the cervical cord.

Clinical presentation

Because the space within the spinal canal is limited, enlargement of a mass will cause compression of the spinal cord, or cauda equina at a stage when the lesion is relatively small. This is in contrast to intracranial tumours which may reach a considerable size before producing any major symptoms. Furthermore the blood supply to the spinal cord is crucial and tenuous with poor longitudinal anastomoses especially in the thoracic region. Therefore, pressure on the anterior spinal artery by a compressing mass, or as a result of distortion of the spinal cord, may suddenly cause a critical reduction of the blood flow with infarction of the

Theodor Schwann, 1810–1882. Professor of Anatomy, Louvain.

cord. Thus, when cord compression is present, a relatively mild neurological deficit may, at any time, become severe and irreversible.

The clinical presentation of spinal cord or cauda equina compression will vary with the level of the lesion and its rate of growth. But if early clinical diagnosis and rapid relief of compression is to be achieved, the following general clinical features must be sought:

Symptoms of Spinal Cord or Cauda Equina Compression

1. Weakness of limbs
2. Numbness
3. Disturbance of micturition
4. Pain in the back

Signs of Spinal Cord or Cauda Equina Compression

1. Weakness of limbs
2. A sensory level
3. Changes in tendon reflexes
4. A distended bladder

Weakness of limbs.—Cervical lesions may produce quadriparesis (or plegia), thoracic or lumbar lesions paraparesis (or plegia). Lesions low in the cauda equina may produce little weakness in the lower limbs. Tumours arising on nerve roots in the cervical or lumbar regions (*e.g.* Schwannoma) may produce at first selective weakness in part of a limb before the stage of compression of the spinal cord or cauda equina. The weakness may progress very slowly or advance suddenly (see pathology), and its early detection may require no more than careful assessment of the history and observation of the patient's gait. The absence of overt weakness never excludes cord compression in the presence of other clinical features.

Sensory changes.—A history of numbness in the lower limbs, even in the absence of detectable sensory loss may be sufficient for the diagnosis of early thoracic cord or cauda equina compression. The pattern of sensory loss may vary with the type of the lesion (*e.g.* intramedullary lesions tend to produce dissociated loss, that is loss of pain and temperature and preservation of touch and position sense), but loss or impairment of pain (*e.g.* pin prick) is the most rapid and accurate method of detecting a sensory level. A sensory level is the most accurate guide to the level of the lesion and is crucial in planning investigation (see below).

Reflexes.—In cord compression (*i.e.* an upper motor neurone lesion) the tendon reflexes are usually increased, the plantar responses are extensor, and there may be spasticity. In lesions of the cauda equina or nerve roots at other levels (*i.e.* a lower motor neurone lesion), the tendon reflexes are reduced or absent. Tone may be diminished, and there may be muscle wasting and fasciculation. These signs may be helpful in clinical localisation of the lesion, but normal reflexes and plantar responses do not in themselves vitiate the diagnosis of compression. In very gradually advancing thoracic cord compression spasticity may proceed overt weakness by many months.

Micturition.—Pressure on the spinal cord or cauda equina will cause retention of urine, either through loss of bladder sensation, or through loss of detrusor control. With extramedullary lesions this is a relatively late effect. With intra-medullary lesions and with those affecting the conus medullaris or lower roots of the cauda equina, disorders of micturition occur relatively early. When the sensory disturbance is predominant, retention will be painless, an important point of distinction from prostatic obstruction. If compression of the conus or cauda equina is not relieved rapidly, loss of bladder function may become permanent.

Pain.—Pain in the back may be caused by bony lesions (*e.g.* metastases) or by pressure of a tumour upon the dura within the spinal canal. The severity of pain is variable and even with large tumours may be mild. With extramedullary tumours it tends to precede the neurological symptoms and signs. With intrame-dullary lesions it is less prominent. Tumours which involve nerve roots early (Schwannoma) may produce pain in a root distribution before the back pain. Thus in the thoracic region pain may radiate round the trunk in a band, and from the cauda equina the pain may radiate in the lower limb mimicking that produced by a prolapsed intervertebral disc.

Principles of Management

Relief of spinal cord or cauda equina compression, whatever its cause is a surgical emergency. If the compression is not relieved without delay, neurological deficit such as paraplegia and retention of urine may at any stage become irreversible. Even if there is widespread malignancy patients should be spared the distressing disability of paraplegia during their last months of life. To fail to relieve compression by a benign spinal tumour is a disaster and is usually due to a failure of simple clinical assessment. Therefore the objectives of management are: 1. Urgent relief of compression. 2. Establishment of pathology. 3. Removal of benign tumours. 4. Further treatment, such as radiotherapy.

Investigation.—The degree of urgency depends upon the speed of advance of the neurological deficit. With slow advance and a mild deficit, investigations should be done as soon as possible in normal working hours. If advance is rapid, investigation becomes an emergency because the prospects of neurological recovery depend upon the cord or cauda equina function which remains before decompression. Once the lesion is total, there is little prospect of any useful recovery.

Chest x-ray is done in all cases and may show a primary tumour or lung deposits. However, that does not diminish the need for urgent spinal decompression.

Plain radiographs of the spine may show destructive changes, especially vertebral body collapse or loss of pedicles, with metastases. However, plain radiographs may be normal in the presence of malignant or benign tumours. Conversely, Schwannomas may erode pedicles and enlarge intervertebral foramina especially in the cervical region, changes which are clearly seen if oblique views are taken.

Myelography is essential in all cases in which cord or cauda equina compression is suspected, however remote that possibility. It is dangerous practice to accept the diagnosis of acute myelitis (*e.g.* multiple sclerosis) unless a compressing lesion has first been excluded by myelography. Myelography should be done by the lumbar route, because although the clinical sensory level may indicate the upper level of a lesion the full extent of the lesion can only be demonstrated by myelography from below, and the actual level of the myelographic block.

Lumbar puncture, as an isolated procedure has no part to play and may be dangerous in the investigation of spinal tumours. It should only be done in the course of lumbar myelography. If there is no manometric block (*i.e.* there is a normal rise on jugular compression) this does not exclude a spinal tumour. However, the CSF below the block may be yellow and proteinaceous, the so-called Froin's syndrome. Although protein levels in the lumbar CSF are usually raised in the presence of spinal tumours, and especially with the intradural Schwannoma, *e.g.* up to 5000 mg/100 ml (normal 20–40mg/100ml), a normal protein level does not exclude the diagnosis of tumour.

Surgery.—The techniques of surgery for spinal tumours are described fully in neurosurgical texts. The principles are: the performance of a laminectomy of at least three vertebrae, the level of the incision being indicated by the level of the myelographic block and the accurate placing of a skin marker at the time of myelography. With tumours of the extradural space the laminectomy itself may be the most important part of the decompression. Metastatic tumour tissue may be peeled off the dura to improve the decompression, but a total removal is not usually possible and attempts to remove tumour lying anteriorly may damage the spinal cord. Histological diagnosis is essential.

The removal of intradural tumours is very specialised surgery, important points being the gradual separation of the extramedullary tumour from the spinal cord, the piecemeal reduction of the bulk of the tumour and the avoidance of retraction upon the spinal cord. The Schwannoma can usually be mobilised and then removed after division of the nerve root from which it arises. Careful dural closure is desirable.

PROLAPSE OF INTERVERTEBRAL DISC

Intravertebral discs are interposed between the vertebral bodies, and serve not only as shock absorbers for the column but also provided the normal mobility between the adjacent vertebrae. Each disc consists of a soft central portion of spongy material, the nucleus pulposus, containing a remnant of the notochord, which is surrounded by a tough fibrous ring, the annulus fibrosus, which is attached to the adjacent vertebral bodies, the whole being enclosed between fibrocartilaginous plates above and below.

During normal flexion of the spine the disc is deformed and the annulus fibrosus and nucleus bulges backwards slightly into the neural canal.

Intervertebral disc protrusion is produced by the effect of flexion-forces acting upon the most mobile portions of the spine. A sudden strain with the spine in an unguarded position will rupture the tough annulus, allowing portions of the torn annulus and soft nucleus to escape into the spinal canal and form either a central protrusion in the midline under the posterior common ligament of the vertebrae, or a lateral protrusion at the side of the posterior common ligament adjacent to the intervertebral foramen (fig. 450).

In 80% of cases the protrusion is traumatic in origin and there is either a history of sudden severe strain, or the patient's occupation is one in which flexion strain must be resisted, such as a packer, fireman, porter, *etc.* The condition is therefore more common in males.

In 20% of cases the condition is degenerative in origin. There is no history of injury. A small portion of the nucleus pulposus herniates through a weak area in the annulus without tearing that structure.

Since the mechanism demands the combination of stress and mobility, protrusions are most common in the most mobile portions of the spine which are subject to the greatest stress, hence approximately:

19% occur in the cervical region at the mobile C.5/6 and C.6/7 levels.

1 to 2% occur in the immobile dorsal spine.

80% occur in the lumbar regions, particularly at the mobile L.4/5 and L.5/S1 levels.

Georges Froin, 1874–1932. French Neurologist. Described this syndrome in 1903.

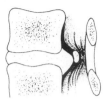

FIG. 450.—Intervertebral disc protrusion passing towards the intervertebral foramen, the posterior margin of which is constituted by the anterior edge of the subflavian ligament.

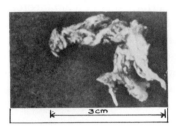

FIG. 452.—A typical portion of protruded disc removed at operation.

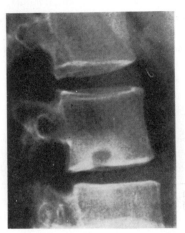

FIG. 451.—Schmorl's node in a lumbar vertebra (see text). Note also the narrowed disc space.

Escape of disc material leads to:

1. The narrowing of the invertebral joint space visible in x-ray in 50% of cases.

2. Slackening of the anterior common ligament of the vertebrae producing abnormal mobility between the vertebrae with local joint pain, and ultimately the development of intervertebral arthritis. Traction osteophytes form on the anterior aspect of the vertebrae and are visible in x-ray. Compensatory thickening of the ligamenta flava occurs in an attempt to check the abnormal mobility.

Massive protrusions may occur as a result of major cervical injuries (p. 508). Alternatively when the spinal ligaments are softened at the end of pregnancy the strain of labour may force out a massive protrusion in the lumbar region, giving rise to one form of obstetric paralysis.

A Schmorl's Node (fig. 451) is a radiological manifestation of an extrusion of the nucleus pulposus into the body of a vertebra. In itself, it has no clinical significance. As time goes by, the new bone activity which surrounds it condenses into a shell.

Lumbar Disc Protrusion.—In the lumbar region the roots of the cauda equina run obliquely over a number of intervertebral joint spaces, hence a lateral protrusion may press on two roots. The nerve root that issues from the corresponding intervertebral foramen may be compressed against the lateral margin of the disc, whilst the nerve root going to the intervertebral foramen next below is caught against its inner margin.

Clinical Features.—In all cases there is an initial period of low back pain resulting from injury to the disc. Later the pain will radiate to the leg when nerve roots become compressed. There is then root pain, accentuated by coughing, in the distribution of the affected nerve, paraesthesiae and pins and needles in the peripheral portion of that area, cramps, and tenderness in muscles supplied by the nerve, and a variable degree of sensory loss and motor weakness. Since the commonest roots to be involved are the first sacral and fifth lumbar, pain is usually in the back and side of the leg radiating to the sole of the foot and the big toe, and is called sciatica. Sensory loss is found on the sole and side of the foot and the ankle-jerk is lost. But in higher disc lesions the pain may be referred to the front of the thigh or leg.

In an endeavour to reduce pressure on the nerve root, the patient adopts a position of scoliosis and walks with a limping gait. Attempts to touch the toes or at straight-leg raising, or neck flexion with the legs raised, increases pain by pulling the nerve root against the protrusion.

In cases where nerve root compression is associated with pressure severe enough to cause paralysis of muscles or urinary retention immediate laminectomy is indicated.

Christian G. Schmorl, 1861-1932. Professor of Pathology, Dresden, Germany.

Root Involved	Pain and Sensory Loss	Motor Weakness	Reflex Change	
1st sacral root	Back of leg. Sole and side of foot.	Gastrocnemius, weak plantar flexion.	Absent A.-J.	
5th lumbar	Back of thigh. Most of lateral aspect of leg. Dorsum of foot to big toe.	Anterior tibials. Weak dorsiflexion.	Nil.	Often combined in L.4/5 disc. / Often combined in L.5/S.1 disc.
4th ,,	Side of thigh. Front of inner aspect of leg.	Quadriceps and anterior tibial, weak dorsiflexion and extension of knee.	Diminished K.-J.	
3rd ,,	Front of lower thigh.	Quadriceps.	Diminished K.-J.	
2nd ,,	Front of mid-thigh.	Quadriceps.	Diminished K.-J.	
1st ,,	Groin.	Nil.	Nil.	

A.-J. = ankle jerk.
K.-J. = knee jerk.

Physical Signs.—Pain is produced by friction of the nerve against the protrusion. Small protrusions only compress the nerve root slightly and the nerve is free to rub against the protrusion. *Small protrusions* thus cause very severe pain because there is maximum friction without much loss of conduction in the nerve. Since there is little impairment of conduction, physical signs are slight and limited to a small patch of sensory loss in the periphery of the skin area involved where long sensory fibres have been affected. *Larger protrusions* cause less pain because they lock the root more firmly so that there is less friction, while the conduction of the nerve is diminished. Since conduction is diminished the physical signs are more marked and sensory loss is extensive owing to involvement of short sensory fibres. *Massive protrusions* completely fix the root and cause no pain whatsoever, but produce the maximum sensory loss and motor paralysis (obstetric paralysis).

Treatment consists of confinement to bed until symptoms abate, which is usually a matter of two to four weeks. A plaster jacket is applied for two to three months, after which a spinal brace is worn for a further period. The majority of cases are cured by this routine. Operation is indicated if symptoms persist, if severe pain recurs, or if motor weakness is developing (see above).

The disc is removed by hemilaminectomy, removing the adjacent margins of two laminae and the subflavian ligament which obscures the view of the nerve root and disc protrusion until it has been excised (fig. 452). After removal of the subflavian ligament, the swollen root is seen overlying the protrusion by which it is displaced inwards. Loose disc material (looking like crab meat) is then grasped with forceps and extracted.

A full laminectomy is contraindicated as it encourages further weakness of the spine. Even after satisfactory removal of a prolapsed disc, symptoms or physical signs are not always alleviated. Two conditions may persist. Prolonged compression of the nerve may have resulted in interstitial neuritis producing sensory loss or motor weakness, or the intervertebral joint may be unstable or become affected by osteoarthritis. Intervertebral arthritis or instability is to be suspected when pain is not relieved by rest, but persists at night and wakes the patient when he turns over in bed. If this condition is present, spinal fusion should be performed when the disc is removed so as to afford complete rest to the affected segment of the spine.

Cervical disc protrusions are relatively uncommon. In many cases a diagnosis of cervical disc lesion is mistakenly applied in patients who are really suffering from referred pain arising from a cervical strain which has affected the interspinous ligaments, or lateral articulations following a flexion strain, or who are suffering from cervical spondylosis. As true cervical disc protrusions are uncommon, this diagnosis must only be accepted when there is definite evidence of compression of the spinal cord or nerve roots, and when the presence of a disc protrusion has been confirmed by demonstrating a lateral filling defect at myelography. In the cervical region the nerve roots run transversely and come into relation with one intervertebral disc only. Each nerve issues above the level of the corresponding vertebra.

Lateral protrusions press on the corresponding nerve and half the spinal cord, producing cervical rhizalgia with half-cord compression, a Brown-Séquard syndrome. They are never situated sufficiently far laterally to press upon the nerve root alone. Symptoms of brachial rhizalgia without cord compression are produced by intraforaminal osteophytes occurring in association with cervical spondylosis, which may, unlike a disc, affect multiple nerve roots. Each spinal root emerges above the corresponding vertebra, hence C.5/6 protrusion compresses the C.6 nerve root and half the cord (see Table below).

Root	Pain, Sensory Loss	Sensory Loss	Muscle Weakness and Reflex Change
C.6	Trapezius. Shoulder tip, outer border of upper arm. Dorsum of forearm.	Lateral border of upper arm. Dorsum of forearm and thumb.	Weakness of biceps, diminished biceps and supinator jerk.
C.7	Trapezius. Shoulder tip, back of upper arm, and dorsum of forearm.	Dorsum of forearm and all fingers except thumb.	Weakness of trapezius and extensors of the fingers. Diminished triceps jerk.

Mid-line protrusions compress the anterior part of the cord and affect the anterior spinal artery and the anterior spinal veins. Compression of the anterior spinal artery may affect the pyramidal and spinothalamic tracts and anterior horns. Compression of the veins which ascend on the front face of the cord produces stasis in the anterior horns below the level of the lesion.

The symptomatology varies on repeated examination as pressure on the vessels varies, and may simulate syringomyelia, disseminated sclerosis or primary lateral sclerosis. In time secondary atrophic changes produce an atrophy of the cord substance with permanent spastic paresis.

Acute mid-line protrusions occurring in cervical injuries may produce symptoms of a partial or complete cord lesion without bone displacement. High protrusions at the 4th cervical level may cause serious respiratory embarrassment.

Treatment.—If neurological symptoms and signs do not improve as the result of conservative treatment by support and immobilisation operation is required. Lateral protrusions are exposed by hemilaminectomy and removed by an extradural approach. Midline protrusions are treated by a full laminectomy of sufficient length to permit one to open the dura and divide the dentate ligaments for several segments above and below the protrusion in order to allow the cord to fall back and thus relieve pressure on the arteries and veins. Attempts to remove a mid-line protrusion may damage the anterior spinal artery and cause permanent paralysis.

CERVICAL SPONDYLOSIS

Cervical Spondylosis is a degenerative condition characterised by (1) degeneration of the intervertebral discs with the formation of bony ridges running across the anterior surface of the neural canal and (2) the formation of osteophytes from the neurocentral joints of Luschka which project backwards into the intervertebral foramen (fig. 453). The condition may be quite symptomless or may cause neurological symptoms.

(*a*) Sudden strains inflicted on the affected joints as, for example, in the violent forward lurch sustained in road traffic accidents, so called 'whip-lash' injuries, may give rise to referred pain in the occipital or post-auricular regions and in the upper portion of the trapezius, and between the shoulder blades. Persistent occipital and posterior auricular pain can be relieved by excision of the corresponding nerves. Since referred pain and muscle spasm in the lower cervical region is the result of movement in the painful joints, these symptoms are often relieved by wearing a collar, but if they become chronic they may be permanently relieved by the insertion of a paraspinal inlay to immobilise the affected joints or by anterior spinal fusion in which the vertebrae are approached anteriorly internal to be carotid sheath. A portion of the upper and lower surfaces of adjacent vertebrae are channelled out to form a prepared bed into which a small bone graft is inserted from in front. Great care is required to avoid penetration of the dura and damage to the closely adjacent spinal cord. (*b*) Bony ridges on the anterior surface of the cord may compress arteries and veins with consequent neurological symptoms and spasticity and ultimate cord atrophy simulating a mid-line disc lesion. This should be treated by

Hubert von Luschka, 1820–1875. Professor of Anatomy, Tübingen, Germany.

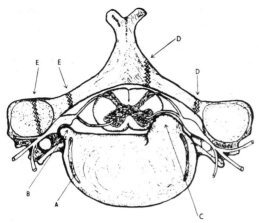

FIG. 453.—Diagrammatic cross-section of the cervical spine and cord showing the position of (A) the neurocentral joint of Luschka, (B) an intraforaminal osteophyte developing from the joint compressing the nerve root within the foramen, (C) a lateral disc protrusion compressing the cord and nerve root. Projection into the intervertebral foramen is prevented by the position of the joint of Luschka. (D-D) the section of bone removed in hemi-laminectomy giving access to a lateral disc protrusion. (E-E) The section of bone removed in hemi-facetectomy giving access to an intraforaminal osteophyte.

(*G. B. Northcroft, FRCS, London.*)

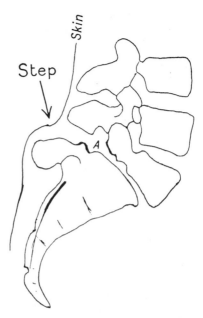

FIG. 454.—Spondylolisthesis at the level of L5-S1 disc. Note the defect at A and the step over S1 spine.

division of the dentate ligaments. (*c*) Intraforaminal compression by osteophytes may affect multiple nerve roots. The nerve roots may be decompressed by excision of the back of the intervertebral foramina by hemifacetectomy.

SPONDYLOLISTHESIS

Spondylolisthesis is a condition in which a lower lumbar vertebra, usually the fifth, slips forward through the plane of the intervertebral disc below it and so carries with it the whole of the upper portion of the spine. The essential lesion is a separation of the body of the vertebra from the posterior articulation, lamina, and spinous process as a result of a defect in the pedicles which hold these two parts of the vertebrae together (fig. 454). Because the lamina is left behind in its normal position, the forward displacement of the vertebral body does not narrow the spinal canal. The deformity can, however, cause root pressure which may manifest itself as sciatica.

In general, the main symptoms are usually those of long-standing low-back pain. On examination, in a mild case nothing will be found other than some excessive prominence of the first sacral spinous process. In a severe case, where the lumbar vertebra has become dislocated in front of the sacrum, there will be a severe lordosis and a rather characteristic shortening of the trunk, so that the lower ribs seem to rest on the brim of the pelvis.

Though trauma was frequently regarded in the past as a common cause of spondylolisthesis, accurate x-ray studies show that a congenital defect in the development of the pedicles is much the commonest explanation. X-ray studies often reveal a condition sometimes known as 'prespondylolisthesis', or 'spondylolysis', where slipping of the vertebrae is absent, or minimal, in the presence of defects in the pedicles.

The majority of these cases never require any special treatment other than simple placebos for backache, such as local heat and rest from time to time. A stiff lumbosacral corset will give relief to the majority, but a few will require lumbosacral fusion to abolish pain. As in the management of any case of 'low-back pain', it is unwise to alarm the patient with injudicious reports about the x-ray appearance. Many cases of severe spondylolisthesis go through life with nothing more than an occasional attack of 'lumbago'. Injudicious remarks can convert a mild case into a complete invalid!

CHAPTER 28

NERVES

CRANIAL NERVES

1. Olfactory Nerve.—Injured by fractures of the cribriform plate, resulting in partial loss of smell (hyposmia) or anosmia on the corresponding side. Olfactory filaments may be ruptured as a result of anterior displacement following blows on the back of the head (*contre-coup*, Chapter 26).

2. Optic Nerve.—Damaged by fractures involving the optic foramen or by contusion against the margin of the foramen. Involvement by tumours or aneurysms is not uncommon. Primary optic atrophy results in partial or complete blindness of the affected eye, but contraction of the pupil will occur if the opposite retina is stimulated[1]. The optic nerve is an outgrowth of the brain and gliomas arise in its substance, particularly in young children.

3. Third Nerve (Oculomotor).—Involved by tumours, trauma, or aneurysm in the skull, sphenoidal fissure, or orbit. Pressure on the nerve above the tentorium occurs in the early stages of midbrain pressure cone formation causing a dilated pupil. Partial lesions may only produce a dilated pupil, but in complete lesions the following features are noted.

(*a*) Ptosis of the upper eyelid, owing to paralysis of the levator palpebrae superioris.

(*b*) Proptosis, owing to paralysis of the majority of the ocular muscles, which normally exercise traction on the eyeball; this will be increased if an intraorbital tumour is also present.

(*c*) Mydriasis, as the sympathetic fibres are unopposed, and cause unhampered dilatation of the pupil.

(*d*) Loss of accommodation, owing to paralysis of the ciliary muscle.

(*e*) Diplopia and external strabismus, with a slight downward inclination of the eye-ball due to unopposed action of the external rectus and superior oblique muscles. Owing to their proximity, other nerves passing to the orbit are often affected.

4. Fourth Nerve (Trochlear).—Supplies the superior oblique muscle, and is rarely involved alone. Diplopia and deficient movement of the eye in a downward and outward direction may be observed.

5. Fifth Nerve (Trigeminal).—Sensory disturbances follow injury to its branches.

Trigeminal Neuralgia.—This distressing condition occurs predominantly in the middle-aged and elderly, in women more than men, and is characterised by sudden very severe pain in the distribution of the trigeminal nerve; it is usually restricted to one or two divisions. The pain is often precipitated by exposure to cold, touching certain points

---

[1] This reflex is transmitted through the ciliary ganglion.

on the face (trigger points), eating, talking and even walking. The pain is so severe that the patient 'screws up' the affected side of the face and the hand comes up in a protective gesture; hence the condition acquired the name 'tic douloureux'.

In the majority of patients no cause is found. Very rarely it may be symptomatic of a cerebello-pontine angle lesion (*e.g.* acoustic neuroma), and onset at a younger age is suggestive of multiple sclerosis.

Treatment is initially by drugs, of which carbamazepine (Tegretol) is currently the most effective. However if this fails surgery may be indicated. Prior to surgery it is essential to establish that the symptoms are those of true trigeminal neuralgia; in other types of facial pain surgery may well aggravate the condition. The methods used are:

1. *Peripheral neurectomy*—supra-orbital or infra-orbital.—These procedures rarely bring lasting relief.

2. *Open surgery.*—(*a*) *Middle fossa approach* (fig. 455). The Gasserian Ganglion is approached subtemporally either extra or intradurally. By differential section it is possible to spare the ophthalmic division and therefore avoid the complications of anaesthesia affecting the surface of the eye.

(*b*) *Posterior fossa approach.*——By this approach the sensory root of the fifth nerve is divided in the cerebello-pontine angle as it runs towards Meckel's cave. By microsurgical techniques it may be possible to preserve touch sensation but abolish pain.

Both these operative approaches are major procedures which will carry some element of risk particularly as many of these patients are very elderly.

3. *Trigeminal Ganglion Alcohol Injection.*—This long-established method involves the insertion of a needle 1 cm below the zygomatic notch upwards, backwards and inwards for 5-6 cm through the foramen ovale to enter the ganglion or the CSF surrounding the ganglion. The position of the needle is checked by radiography and a trial injection of local anaesthetic (resistance being felt if the needle is in the nerve and ganglion) causing loss of sensation in one or more of the sensory divisions. Then 4-5 ml absolute alcohol is injected. This method is effective, provided the patient will accept the consequent numbness and is able to take precautions for the care of eye, skin and mouth.

4. *Electro-coagulation of the trigeminal ganglion.*—In recent years the technique of inserting an electro-coagulating probe through the foramen ovale into the trigeminal ganglion has been developed. With this it is possible to produce a staged or restricted lesion in terms of the distribution of the sensory loss and the modalities involved.

6. Sixth Nerve (Abducent).

—Slender with a long intracranial course. It may be affected by fractures of the base of the skull or displacement of intracranial structures, or it may be involved in association with other ocular motor nerves by lesions in the cavernous sinus, sphenoid fissure, or orbit. The external rectus muscle is paralysed, and internal strabismus results.

7. Seventh Nerve (Facial).

—Involved by a variety of causes.

1. *Intracranial.*—Lesions within the brain are supranuclear, nuclear, or infranuclear. Supranuclear lesions involve only the lower half of the face, as the occipito-frontalis and orbicularis palpebrarum muscles enjoy bilateral innervation. In nuclear lesions the whole face and the sixth nerve on the same side are affected and also the opposite arm and leg, as the motor decussation takes place at a lower level. An infranuclear lesion occasionally results from pressure of a tumour, *e.g.* of the cerebello-pontine angle, in which case involvement of the auditory nerve is also evident.

2. *Cranial.*—The intraosseous portion of the facial nerve may be affected by fractures of the base (fig. 456) and middle ear disease. Following fracture paralysis may appear immediately as a result of direct injury to the nerve or within hours or days from haemorrhage within the nerve sheath, in which latter case recovery is possible. Paralysis occurring after some weeks is produced by the pressure of callus and is unlikely to recover. Facial paralysis is a complication of middle ear disease and may follow injury at operation on the mastoid antrum.

Johann Ludwig Gasser, died 1765. Professor of Anatomy, Vienna. His pupil, Raymond Balthasar Hirsch, discovered the ganglion and named it after his teacher.
Johann Friedrich Meckel (the elder) 1724-1774. Professor of Anatomy, Botany and Gynaecology, Berlin.

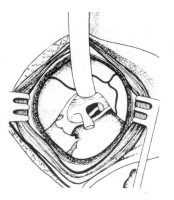

FIG. 455.—Fractional section of the lower and outer two-thirds of the trigeminal sensory root at the apex of the petrous. The motor root is visible behind the cut portion of the sensory root.

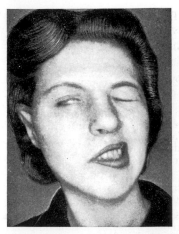

FIG. 456.—Right-sided facial paralysis following fracture through the middle fossa.

Compression within the aqueduct of Fallopius occasionally follows chronic inflammation.

3. *Extracranial.*—The facial nerve or its branches may be injured outside the skull. The nerve is commonly involved by Bell's palsy, which is due to herpetic neuritis and follows exposure to cold or draught. Swelling within the sheath of the nerve extends into stylomastoid foramen, and the nerve is compressed within the bony canal. Absorption of exudate usually occurs before the pressure has damaged the nerve permanently, but in about 3% of cases complete paralysis remains, and in 5 to 10% some degree of paralysis persists. Tetanus arising from a wound in the distribution of the facial nerve sometimes causes paralysis, the cause being similar to that described above. Malignant tumours of the parotid gland involve the facial nerve, and paralysis is an important diagnostic sign distinguishing simple from malignant tumours.

Branches of the facial nerve are injured either accidentally, *e.g.* by broken windscreens, or by ill-placed operation incisions. For operating on the parotid, the main trunk of the nerve must first be located and then branches followed forward.

The paralysed face is flat and expressionless. The eye cannot be closed, and attempts to do so result in the eyeball being turned upwards and outwards (fig. 456). Corneal ulceration may follow from exposure. Epiphora occurs owing to drooping of the lower eyelids. Whistling is impossible, as the cheek merely flaps, and food collects between the gums and cheek.

Treatment is directed to the cause. To promote recovery the angle of the mouth is supported by a malleable rod covered with rubber tubing, which is bent like an 'S' so that the upper curve will hook around the ear and the lower will elevate the angle of the mouth. Small strips of adhesive strapping applied under tension also form a very convenient method of preventing overstretching of the facial muscles. If considered advisable, an intra-oral splint can be fashioned from plastic material. Electrical treatment and massage are prescribed, and during recovery

Gabriel Fallopio, 1523-1563. Professor of Anatomy and Surgery, Padua, Italy.
Sir Charles Bell, 1774-1842. Surgeon, Middlesex Hospital, London (1812-1835). Professor of Surgery, Edinburgh (1836-1842).

the patient should practise facial movements with the aid of a mirror. Hypoglossal anastomosis may be considered in hopeless cases (p. 520). Repeated facial tic with spasmodic contracture of the facial muscles may be relieved by fractional division of the branches of the facial nerves which supply the affected muscles, these branches being exposed through a curved incision anterior to the lobe of the ear. (See also p. 571, ref. fascial slings.)

In cases of Bell's palsy early decompression of the nerve may be achieved by cortisone (60 mg daily for 3 days, then 20 mg for 3 days).

Facial tic.—An embarrassing condition in which repeated spasm of the facial muscles produces repeated winking or twitching of the face according to the muscles affected; may be relieved by partial section of branches of the facial nerve supplying the affected areas.

8. Eighth Nerve (Vestibulocochlear).—May be involved in fractures of the middle fossa, or compressed by a tumour, *e.g.* of the auditory nerve sheath, causing unilateral deafness (Chapter 33). Vestibular functions are sometimes impaired (see Menière's disease, Chapter 33).

9. Ninth Nerve (Glossopharyngeal).—Occasionally injured by a fractured base. Some dysphagia may occur from paresis of the constrictor muscles.

Glosso-pharyngeal neuralgia is characterised by severe explosions of pain either in the region of the tonsil or deeply in the ear. The 'trigger' zone is in the tonsillar area, and the diagnosis is clinched by the fact that cocainisation of the zone temporarily relieves the condition. In genuine cases the nerve must be divided. It is approached via the posterior fossa and severed as it enters the jugular foramen.

10. Tenth Nerve (Vagus).—May be damaged in association with a fractured base, or crushed by a ligature which includes it as well as the internal jugular vein or common carotid artery. In doubtful cases examination of the laryngeal muscles will reveal recurrent laryngeal nerve involvement.

The recurrent laryngeal nerve may be damaged in operations on the thyroid gland or on the ductus-arteriosus by traction or post-operative extravasation. Complete paralysis may follow division or inclusion by a ligature at operation, infiltration by neoplasm of the thyroid gland or secondary lymph nodes from carcinoma of the lung, and on the left side by pressure of an aneurysm of the aortic arch. Partial involvement affects the abduction fibres, which are more susceptible than those which supply the adductor muscles, and thus if partial involvement is bilateral, stridor results, and tracheostomy may be required. Complete involvement results in paralysis of both abductors and adductors, and consequent paralysis of the corresponding vocal cord in the half-way or 'cadaveric' position. The opposite vocal cord increases its range of mobility, so that it reaches across the mid-line and closes the glottis. The voice is adequate but somewhat monotonous (see Chapter 35).

Hysterical aphonia is emotional in origin and is distinguished from true paralysis by the fact that, although the patient can only whisper, coughing is readily performed on request.

11. Eleventh Nerve (Accessory).—Rarely damaged by fractures but is more commonly injured during high cervical dissections, particularly in the removal of tuberculous lymph nodes which often entirely surround it. The nerve passes downwards and backwards at right angles to the centre of a line connecting the angle of the jaw and the mastoid process, and emerges from the posterior border

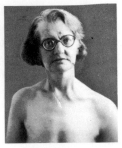

FIG. 457.—Drooping of the left shoulder and wasting of the trapezius muscle following division of the spinal accessory nerve.

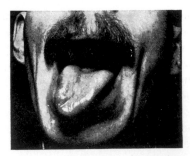

FIG. 458.—Hemiatrophy of the right side of the tongue following involvement of the hypoglossal nerve by syphilitic basal meningitis.

of the sternomastoid muscle at the junction of the upper third and lower two-thirds; it then passes across the posterior triangle, and disappears under cover of the trapezius muscle. Division of the nerve in the anterior triangle often produces complete paralysis of the sternomastoid muscle, but the motor supply contributed from the second and third cervical roots is sufficient in a third of the cases to prevent complete paralysis. Division will result in only a partial paralysis of the trapezius as the trapezius receives a sufficient additional supply from the third and fourth cervical nerves. If injury occurs in the posterior triangle, the trapezius alone is affected. On inspection, drooping of the shoulder is seen, and wasting of the trapezius is obvious (fig. 457). Contraction of the sternomastoid muscle is tested by asking the patient to turn his head to the side opposite to the muscle. Palpation detects the rigid band of muscle if contraction is normal. Injury of the nerves to the trapezius results in inability to continue elevation of the arm after it is abducted to a right angle by the deltoid muscle. If the branches to the muscle from the third and fourth cervical nerves are intact, about 20 degrees elevation from the right-angled position is possible.

If division of the spinal accessory nerve is recognised at operation, primary suture should be performed. Secondary suture is not successful on account of retraction of the ends and difficulty in identifying them in scar tissue.

12. Twelfth Nerve (Hypoglossal).—Escapes in fractures of the base of the skull, as the anterior condyloid foramen is protected by a bony ridge which diverts a fissure towards the foramen magnum. It may be injured in removal of the submandibular salivary gland. Hemiatrophy of the tongue occurs, the corresponding side of the tongue being shrivelled and wrinkled, the tongue being pushed towards the paralysed side on protrusion (fig. 458).

SPINAL (PERIPHERAL) NERVES

Injuries of nerves are classified according to the extent of the damage to the nerve fibres and sheath, as neurapraxia, axonotmesis and neurotmesis.

Neurapraxia

Neurapraxia is the equivalent of concussion. There is physiological paralysis of conduction in the intact nerve fibres as the result of stretching or distortion without any organic rupture. Neurapraxia is produced by minor stretch injuries, or by the concussion and vibratory effect of a high-velocity missile passing near a nerve without contacting it. Fibres remain intact within intact sheath. It produces sensory loss, paraesthesiae, and weakness of muscle groups lasting for days. During this time there is no reaction of degeneration in the muscles. There is no degeneration of the axons. When the power of conduction returns, all functions, motor and sensory, return together, sensation recovering in the whole limb within a period of hours. Recovery is complete.

Treatment consists of splinting the limb in a position of relaxation of the paralysed muscle groups until spontaneous recovery occurs.

Axonotmesis

Axonotmesis consists of the intrathecal rupture of nerve fibres within an intact sheath. According to the cause, the nerve fibres are damaged to a variable degree (see below). Wallerian degeneration occurs in the distal portion of the broken axons, leaving an empty tubule. Intraneural fibrosis occurs at the sites of axonal rupture and minute intraneural haemorrhages. Recovery takes place slowly by the proliferation and down-growth of axons into the distal tubules, the combined bulk of the proliferating axons and intraneural fibrosis producing a fusiform neuroma on the course of the nerve. There is some loss of nerve fibres owing to the blockage of the down-growing axons by the intraneural fibrosis, but since the relative position of axon and distal tubule is preserved by the intact sheath there is little maldistribution, hence the quality of regeneration is often good except in the case of progressive fibrosis. Recovery is delayed until the down-growing fibres reach their appropriate endings, and occurs first in the muscle groups nearest to the site of division and lastly in the peripheral skin areas, where the anaesthetic area begins to decrease steadily from the margin inwards. The length of time required for the recovery depends upon the level of the lesion. After an initial delay of approximately ten days, down-growing axons proceed distally at a rate of approximately 1 mm a day, and on arrival at their endings there is a further delay of three weeks before the end organs become activated. Partial or complete intrathecal rupture of fibres may complicate a single stress occurring in association with fractures or dislocations, or excessive vigour during attempted reduction of such injuries; it also accompanies traction injuries at birth and may be produced by clutching for support when falling, as in brachial plexus lesions. It may follow contusion of a nerve with extensive haemorrhage into its sheath or be the result of severe and acute compression by tourniquets, splints, or incorrect posture on the operating table.

Gradually increasing lesions are produced by progressive compression from crutches, splints, callus, and scar tissue or by repeated minor stretching of a nerve which becomes fixed near a mobile joint. The latter is seen when a nerve such as the external popliteal becomes fixed at the head of the fibula, or the ulnar nerve becomes fixed behind an arthritic elbow or stretched by cubitus valgus; in such cases movements of the joint pulling on the fixed nerve produce repeated minor ruptures at different levels, each of which is succeeded by a small degree of fibrosis, which gradually induces a progressive fibrosis and loss of function within the nerve.

Augustus Volney Waller, 1816-1870. General Practitioner, Kensington, London (1842-1851). Subsequently worked as a physiologist at Bonn, Paris, Birmingham and Geneva.

Clinical Features.—Following a severe stretch, there is an initial picture of neurapraxia with widespread loss of sensation, tone, power, and reflex activity in the limb; this is followed by an incomplete recovery. The resolution of concussion will restore sensation and movement to certain areas of the limb to which the nerve fibres remain intact. The numbness and paralysis will persist in those areas to which the fibres have actually ruptured. Usually the total area affected is less than the known anatomical distribution of the nerve as a proportion of fibres have escaped.

Secondary pathological changes accompanying nerve injury affect the skin, muscles, and joints. Impaired circulation consequent on disuse renders the part blue and cold. The skin becomes thin, the nails brittle, and so-called trophic changes occur as a consequence of minor unrecognised trauma. Those muscles which are paralysed and flaccid will be overstretched by unopposed action of antagonist groups. Within three weeks the reaction of degeneration appears. The muscle fibres no longer respond to the rapid make-and-break of faradic stimulation owing to an increase in the duration of chronaxie which accompanies paralysis, but they will still respond to the slow make-and-break of galvanism. The polarity also changes so that A.C.C.[1] becomes greater than K.C.C.[2]. If the muscle nutrition is not maintained by galvanic stimulation, muscle fibres degenerate and progressive fibrosis replaces inert fibres. Recovery is then impossible. Periarticular adhesions eventually form around the immobile joints and fix them in a contracted position. To combat these effects the part must be protected by warm padding to prevent injury, and splinted in a position of relaxation of the paralysed groups. The electric reactions of the muscles are recorded and muscle movement is maintained by regular galvanic simulation of all paralysed groups.

Treatment of Closed Injuries of Nerves

Treatment consists in maintaining the nutrition of the limb and combating, by suitable means, the secondary pathological changes which would otherwise follow nerve injury, in order to maintain the muscles and joints in good working order pending the arrival of down-growing axons.

All joints are put through full passive movements daily to prevent contraction. Movements and exercise of the paralysed muscles are best maintained by the use of elastic splints mounted on frames in positions corresponding to the paralysed tendons, so as to provide an elastic counter-pull to replace the normal contraction of the paralysed muscles against which the opponents can act. This not only ensures full normal movement of all joints, but will also permit partial use.

Considerable encouragement must be given to the patient during the long period of time required for restoration of function. Progress is carefully checked by taking regular records of the electrical reactions and skin sensitivity. Electrical reactions change back to normal in the proximal groups as the downgrowth of fibres proceeds. These changes must be recorded, together with diagrams of the skin sensation, in order to determine whether normal recovery is taking place. Failure to recover, or regression after the initial recovery, is an indication for the local exploration of the injured site. It is occasionally necessary to deal with a perineural scar or remove an intraneural fibroma.

Movements produced by unaffected muscles must not mislead the observer. Thus, in a case of radial paralysis, the fingers can be extended by the interosseous and lumbrical muscles, provided that the hand is supported. Also vicarious movements may be per-

---

[1] A.C.C. = Anodal Closing Contraction.
[2] K.C.C. = Kathodal Closing Contraction.

formed by adjacent muscles, *e.g.* in the case of division of the median nerve, the adductors of the thumb, acting in conjunction with the extensor ossis metacarpi pollicis, can produce opposition of the thumb.

H. J. Seddon *et al.* have endeavoured to calculate the rates of nerve regeneration, basing their results on the following clinical data:

(1) Tinel's sign—the course of the nerve is lightly percussed with a patella hammer, from below upwards. A tingling sensation is experienced when the level of regeneration is reached.

(2) Measurement of the rate at which pain and touch sensibility return.

(3) Observation of the times at which the function of muscles returns at different levels from the injury.

It appears that regeneration occurs initially at about 2 mm a day, but the rate diminishes as time passes, so that after about three months it has slowed down to about 1 mm a day. (Other factors which influence the results of suture are discussed on p. 518.)

Compression of a nerve.—Nerve entrapment.—The first symptoms usually consist of paraesthesiae, numbness, and tingling along the distribution of the nerve, associated with neuralgic pain. Complete paralysis and wasting of muscles are uncommon unless the initial compression has been prolonged and severe, but when the compressing cause is progressive, paralysis can occur later and may then necessitate operative measures.

Treatment is by removal of the cause, usually a tight splint or plaster, but may necessitate exploration of the nerve and the excision of perineural scar tissue, or mobilisation of the nerve from callus, following which a new bed is prepared for the nerve in adjacent muscles, the nerve itself being wrapped in a layer of tantalum foil. Sensory symptoms are satisfactorily relieved by these steps, but if intervention is delayed too long intraneural fibrosis may lead to persistent motor disability (see also ulnar neuritis (p. 526) and carpal tunnel syndrome (Chapter 24).

Progressive fibrosis produced by fixation of the nerve has to be treated by nerve transplantation; recovery may be complete or incomplete, according to the degree of fibrosis.

Neurotmesis

Neurotmesis is usually produced by penetrating wounds and results in partial or complete division of the nerve sheath and fibres. Very rarely, complete rupture of nerves may occur in major brachial plexus injuries (p. 520). In war and severe industrial injuries extensive soft tissue damage to muscle and skin, and associated fractures, greatly complicate the problems of repair.

Partial lesions produce a lateral neuroma of the nerve. Complete division produces a terminal neuroma on the end of the proximal segment. In the proximal portion of the divided axons, retrograde degeneration occurs as high as the first node of Ranvier. After an interval of ten days the axons begin to subdivide to produce an excess of end bulbs, which then commence to grow downwards. By this time, however, the gap between the divided nerve ends, which was at first filled with blood, has now been replaced by organising clot and fibrous tissue, which presents an almost impenetrable barrier to the down-growing axons. In the distal segment of the divided nerve, Wallerian degeneration of the axons occurs, but the cells of the sheaths of Schwann proliferate, forming a slight bulb at the commencement of the distal end from which sprouts of Schwann cells grow

Sir Herbert John Seddon, 1903-1977. Professor of Orthopaedic Surgery, Royal National Orthopaedic Hospital, London.
Jules Tinel, 1879-1952. Physician, Hôpital Beaujon, Paris.
Louis Antoine Ranvier, 1835-1922. French histologist and pathologist.
Theodor Schwann, 1810-1882. Professor of Anatomy, Louvain, 1839-48, and, thereafter at Liège. Original researches before the age of twenty-seven laid the foundation of Physiology of Nerve and Muscle. The first to deal with problems related to living matter on a purely physical and chemical basis, and to recognise the cell as the unit of living matter. Discoverer of pepsin, and rôle of living organisms in fermentation.

proximally into the plane of division, being drawn by chemotaxis towards the down-growing axons. A few axons may by this means succeed in entering the distal segment, producing there a deceptively encouraging Tinel's sign, but any spontaneous healing is minimal.

Even after accurate suture the quality of regeneration is less perfect than in cases of axonotmesis owing to the wastage of axons in the scar tissue at the suture line, and mal-distribution of those fibres which reach the distal segment. The density of scar tissue at the suture line is increased by local sepsis and inflammation, and by tension at the suture site.

Mal-distribution of fibres is greatest in the case of mixed motor and sensory nerves, for motor fibres may then unite with sensory endings. It is also greatest in those motor nerves which supply a large number of small muscles; hence the quality of recovery is best in the case of a pure motor nerve, such as the radial, which supplies a few groups of large muscles concerned in coarse movement, and is worst in mixed sensory and motor nerves supplying a large number of small muscles concerned in fine movement, such as the ulnar or median nerves at the wrist.

Treatment is by suture under suitable conditions, in the absence of sepsis and in the absence of tension, when the nerve can be placed in a suitable bed. In war injuries where there has been considerable loss of surface tissue, preliminary plastic operations such as pedicle grafting must precede attempted repair of the nerve in order to provide a suitable covering and bed at the suture site.

Open wounds (Chapter 1). In tidy clean incised wounds immediate primary suture is the ideal treatment for a divided nerve. In untidy contaminated wounds, the nerve suture should be postponed until three or four weeks after the injury. If a divided nerve is encountered during excision of such a wound, the ends are approximated by one stitch of fine silk, which prevents retraction during the period of delay. On no account should an attempt be made to identify or scrutinise a nerve in the vicinity. If only one end of a nerve is seen, then a suture should be inserted so as to fix it to adjacent muscle or fascia. The advantages of early secondary suture over immediate primary suture in untidy wounds are as follows:

(i) Primary suture usually requires enlargement of the wound by further incisions, so as to mobilise the nerve in order to allow approximation of the ends without tension. As the wound is potentially infected, exposure of previously uncontaminated tissues should be avoided.

(ii) The normal nerve sheath is a delicate structure, which is easily torn by the slightest tension, and accurate suturing is essential for the success of the operation. In addition, the sheath is often further weakened by longitudinal slits or tears. After about three weeks of the injury, epineural fibrosis occurs and the sheath becomes thicker and tougher, consequently the insertion of sutures and accurate coaptation of the nerve ends are greatly facilitated (an exception is brachial plexus injury—see p. 520).

NERVE SUTURE

The two ends of the nerve are identified, the incision being prolonged sufficiently to expose the nerve well above and below the seat of injury, in such a position that its normal anatomical relations are not obscured by scar tissue. The two ends of the nerve are freed and 'freshened' by means of a scalpel or a Bard-Parker knife. Scissors should not be used,

Bard-Parker Inc., Danbury, Connecticut, U.S.A.

as the nerve is crushed thereby. Slices are removed from the ends of the nerve until the projecting fibres are seen, and blood freely oozes from the cut surface. Apposition of the two ends is accomplished as follows:

(*a*) *Mobilisation.*—The two ends are dissected from surrounding structures, care being taken to preserve important motor branches. Branches can often be stripped from the parent nerve in order to facilitate mobilisation.

(*b*) *Posture.*—The limb being held in a relaxed position.

(*c*) *Transposition.*—The radial nerve is brought in front of the humerus, or the ulnar nerve in front of the internal condyle (p. 526).

(*d*) *Nerve Anchoring.*—If it is obvious that the two ends of a divided nerve cannot be brought together, on account of excessive loss of tissue or retraction, then the two untrimmed ends are approximated as closely as possible by tension stitches, the position of the limb being such that approximation is facilitated. Subsequently the nerve is stretched by gradually straightening the limb, and at a second operation the two ends are brought together. In some cases adequate suture can be performed while the limb is flexed, and extension is gradually regained.

(*e*) *Resection of Bone.*—This extensive procedure may be justifiable if nerve injury is associated with an ununited fracture, which also needs operative measures, *e.g.* in the case of the radial nerve and a fractured humerus.

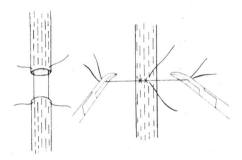

Fig. 459.—Primary nerve suture. Two sutures are passed through the sheath of the nerve in order to approximate the cut ends. The sheath is then sutured.

Approximation having been obtained by one of the above procedures, sutures are introduced through the nerve sheath (fig. 459). Non-irritating material is used, such as fine black silk or tantalum wire. Catgut encourages fibrosis of the nerve. The suture line can be further supported by painting with fibrin glue. Torsion of the nerve ends must be avoided, so that, as far as possible, proximal nerve fibres will join with their corresponding distal fibres. 'Shunting' is thus avoided, and delay due to re-education of groups of muscles is obviated. If adjacent tissues are fibrosed, a new path can be constructed for the sutured nerve by opening a muscle sheath, and embedding the nerve among the muscle fibres. Finally, a layer of tantalum foil is always wrapped round the nerve to prevent epineural fibrosis and the out-sprouting of axons from the suture line, which may produce a painful local lesion. The limb is placed in a suitable position to prevent any strain on the sutured nerve, and a plaster cast may be advisable for a few weeks to immobilise the limb.

Results of Nerve Suture

This depends on many factors:

1. **Pre-operative.**—(*a*) *The Nerve Affected.*—Mixed motor and sensory nerves, *e.g.* ulnar and median, are subject to a greater degree of mal-distribution of down-growing fibres than purely motor nerves supplying a small number of large muscles, *e.g.* radial.

(*b*) *Infection* may cause delay in performing suture at the appropriate time and increases scar tissue formation following suture.

(*c*) *Time.*—Early secondary suture (p. 518) yields the best results, and further delay is detrimental.

(*d*) *Pre-operative Management.*—If muscles and tendons have been allowed to stretch or if the tone of the muscles has not been maintained, then the chances of recovery are correspondingly diminished.

2. **Operative.**—This consists of attention to the details already mentioned, *e.g.* haemostasis, prevention of torsion and tension, preparation of suitable bed, and the use of non-irritating suture material.

3. **Post-operative.**—(*a*) *Absence of Infection.*—If the wound is already infected, or if infection supervenes, then little improvement is likely.

(*b*) *After-treatment* consists in continuance of the relaxation of paralysed muscles, massage, electrical treatment, and muscular effort gradually increased as muscles recover their power.

(*c*) *Co-operation of the patient.*—This important factor must receive due consideration and the patient given every encouragement during his rehabilitation.

(*d*) *Vicarious Movements.*—Although the physiological results of nerve suture may be poor, yet adjacent muscles often take upon themselves some of the functions of those which are paralysed, *e.g.* if the hamstrings are paralysed and flexion of the knee thereby affected, the sartorious and gracilis muscles hypertrophy, and partially compensate for this deficiency. Thus the functional result of a nerve injury is often more satisfactory than the physiological recovery would suggest.

Irremediable Injury.—If suture is impossible on account of loss of tissue or wide separation of the ends of a divided nerve, the following procedures may be considered:

(*a*) *Nerve anastomosis*, *e.g.* part of the hypoglossal nerve is united to the distal end of the facial nerve. This method often results in improvement, but 'successful' cases are sometimes associated with uncontrolled grimaces on movement of the tongue.

(*b*) *Nerve grafting* has produced encouraging results in selected cases, *e.g.* a gap in the facial nerve within its body channel may be bridged by insertion of an autograft from the external cutaneous nerve of the thigh. Grafting of peripheral nerves is disappointing.

(*c*) *Tendon transplanation*, *e.g.* in the case of radial paralysis, tendons and muscles of the forearm may be transplanted into the extensor group. However, if proper relaxation of the extensor muscles has been consistently maintained, drop wrist should not occur, as the extensor tendons will not be over-stretched.

(*d*) *Arthrodesis*, *e.g.* in the case of injury to the sciatic nerve, arthrodesis of the flail ankle joint will render it stable and rigid.

(*e*) *Amputation*, for persistent sores and ulcers on the foot, particularly if growth is impaired. Sympathectomy might first be tried (Chapter 14).

Incomplete division of a nerve gives rise to a central or lateral neuroma. Effects vary according to the extent of the injury. Fibres supplying certain muscles are often constant in position, and hence are more liable to injury if their position exposes them to trauma. Thus partial division of the great sciatic nerve affects the lateral popliteal portion nine times more commonly than the medial popliteal, which passes down on the inner and deeper aspect of the great sciatic nerve.

Partial lesion of the median or medial popliteal nerves, or injury to their branches, may give rise to the distressing condition of *causalgia* (see end of chapter).

Injection lesions are due to accidental injection of therapeutic agents. They are more common in tropical countries where amoebiasis, schistosomiasis, and malaria are treated by intramuscular injections. The sciatic and radial nerves are usually involved. Injections in the buttock should always be given into the upper and outer quadrant and in the case of the arm into the upper half of the deltoid muscle.

Cervical Plexus Lesions

Injuries of the Cervical Plexus are uncommon, although muscular branches, *e.g.* to the trapezius and sternomastoid muscles, are occasionally damaged.

Phrenic Nerve.—Arising from the third, fourth, and fifth cervical nerves. Paralysis of the diaphragm secondary to malignant disease in the thorax is equally frequent on the right and left sides and is often due to direct invasion of the phrenic nerve by adjacent growth. When phrenic paralysis is due to lymph node metastases, it is almost always due to involvement of a node which lies alongside the phrenic nerve at the level of the pulmonary artery at the upper region of the hilum.

Brachial Plexus Lesions.

Lesions of this plexus are due to 1. Trauma and 2. Other conditions in the area (see Brachial Neuralgia below).

1. **Trauma** to the plexus includes injury due to (*a*) Traction, (*b*) open, penetrating injuries by knife or missile (Chapter 2), (*c*) compression of the plexus (pall bearer's palsy,

haversack strap palsy) and (*d*) operation in the area (*e.g.* for cervical rib, during cervical sympathectomy, for removal of malignant lymph nodes).

Traction Injury.—Is particularly associated with road traffic accidents to motor-cyclists. Any component of the plexus (fig. 460) can be stretched and torn—Nerves (C5—DI), Trunks, Divisions, Cords, Branches. The anatomical location of the injury determines the prognosis. Thus, if the anterior and posterior primary rami (the roots) of a spinal nerve are avulsed from the spinal cord (*i.e.* a pre (supra) ganglionic injury) recovery cannot take place. Below this (a post (infra) ganglionic injury), if the sheath is intact (axonotmesis—see above) some spontaneous recovery is possible, but if there is complete severence of the neural tissue and sheath (neurotmesis) some recovery is only possible by operative exploration and some kind of interposed nerve graft. According to the degree of injury the paralysis varies from a completely flail and useless arm and hand to paralysis of groups of muscles (Table) and anaesthesia according to the roots affected (fig. 460). The common and distinct types of injury according to the different types of violent stretching are the *Upper Brachial Plexus Lesion (Erb-Duchenne)* and the *Lower Brachial Plexus Lesion (Klumpke)*.

Although the segmental innervation of the arm muscles is somewhat inconsistent, this table summarises a distribution which is commonly accepted:

Nerve		*Muscles*
C.v	.	Rhomboids, spinati, deltoid, teres minor, biceps, brachialis, brachio-radialis, supinator brevis.
C.vi	.	Pectoralis major (clavicular head) and minor, subscapularis, coraco-brachialis, latissimus dorsi, teres major, serratus anterior, triceps, pronator teres, pronator quadratus.
C.vii	.	The extensors of the fingers, extensor carpi ulnaris, and sternal part of the pectoralis major.
C.viii	.	The flexors of the wrist and fingers.
D.i	.	The small muscles of the hand.

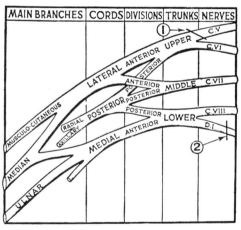

FIG. 460.—The brachial plexus, showing two classical sites for injury—see text.

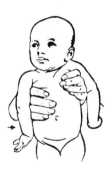

FIG. 461.—Erb's paralysis. The 'tip' position.

Upper Brachial Plexus Lesion (Erb-Duchenne, fig. 460 (1)). This injury is due to excessive displacement of the head, depression of the shoulder, or a combination of these two conditions. (It is also seen in infants (fig. 461) after a difficult confinement). The fifth and sometimes the sixth cervical roots are involved. In the former case the muscles affected are the biceps, brachialis, brachio-radialis, supinator brevis, spinati and deltoid, and thus the limb, internally rotated by the unopposed subscapularis, hangs by the side with the forearm pronated, in the well known 'tip position. Sensory changes are absent if the fifth nerve only is involved, but if the sixth nerve also suffers, an area of anaesthesia is present over the outer side of the arm. Innervation of the hand is preserved.

Wilhelm Erb, 1840–1821 Professor of Medicine, Heidelberg, Germany.
Guillaume Benjamin Amand Duchenne (Duchenne de Boulogne), 1806–1875. Neurologist, successively in Boulogne and Paris, but never held
* a hospital appointment.*
Madame Augusta Marie Dejerine-Klumpke, 1859–1927. Neurologist, Paris.

Lower Bracial Plexus Lesion (Klumpke, fig. 460 (2)).—This follows excessive hyper-extension accidents (e.g. arm trapped in moving machinery, skiiing injury). The inner portion of the plexus is involved, and wasting of all the small muscles of the hand occurs, together with sensory loss along the inner side of the forearm and the inner three and a half fingers, owing to involvement of fibres passing to the ulnar and inner head of the median nerves.

Concomitant Vascular Injury to the subclavian vessels can occur in association with the forces causing an upper plexus lesion, the clavicle being forced like a guillotine on to the edge of the first rib. The axillary vessels can be damaged by the violence causing other (*e.g.* lower) plexus lesions. If the injury is not recognised and treated adequately (Chapters 2 and 14) muscle ischaemia is followed by contractures (*e.g.* Volkmann's contracture, Chapter 15).

The Management of a Traction Injury includes careful history taking and clinical neurological examination in order to decide if surgical exploration is required. The criteria which indicate an inoperable avulsion from the cord (pre(supra)gan-glionic) injury include the presence of a complete C5—T1 (D1) injury, severe fracture of the cervical spine (shifting, dislocation, fractured transverse process), spasticity of the leg on the same side from damage to the pyramidal tract, Horner's syndrome (avulsion T1), vascular injury, paralysis of the thoracoscapular muscles, supraclavicular par- or an-aesthesia and severe pain in the anaesthetic arm. These features need to be backed up by electrical studies on sensory conduc-tion (sensory action potential) and by electromyography. Myelography can be misleading if the rent in the dura has become sealed to give a normal appearance. Postganglionic, mixed and vascular injuries are explored up to 3 days after injury, before the fibroblastic reaction of repair makes operation too difficult. Nerve grafting using sural and musculocutaneous nerves is performed, and vascularised ulnar nerve grafting can be employed when there is an irreparable injury of the lower plexus but a reparable injury to the upper plexus.

Subsequent management includes a period in a rehabilitation unit concentrat-ing on the prevention of joint stiffness and deformity (see paralysis Chapter 25), the use of splints, particularly functional splinting. Muscle and tendon transfer can also be considered (see paralysis Chapter 25). The control of pain can be a difficult problem even requiring transcutaneous electrical stimulation devices.

At least 2 years should be allowed for recovery to be completed.

Stab Wounds should be explored and any nerve injury repaired using sural or musculocutaneous nerve grafts.

2. Brachial Neuralgia.—This condition (*syn.* brachial neuritis) is comparable to sci-atica in the leg. The cutaneous distribution of the cervical nerves is illustrated in fig. 462, and the muscular innervation is summarised on p. 521. Some of the more important causes of brachial neuralgia are as follows:

Prolapsed intervertebral disc (Chapter 27) is often difficult to distinguish from osteo-arthritis, but localised pain in the neck, which often appears suddenly and which is aggravated by coughing, suggests a disc lesion.

Osteoarthritis of the cervical spine (*syn.* spondylitis) causes neuralgia either as a result of pressure on a spinal nerve by an osteophyte or from absorption of the disc and consquent compression of the spinal roots. The onset is gradual and symptoms intermittent, and radiography usually establishes the diagnosis.

Costo-clavicular syndromes are due to many conditions. Sagging of the shoulder girdle, especially in middle-aged females, is a common cause, quite apart from cervical rib. Exercises and physiotherapy directed to improving the tone of muscles which elevate the shoulder may relieve the symptoms in such cases.

Malignant infiltration at the base of the neck (e.g. Pancoast syndrome Chapter 40).

Friedrich Horner, 1831–1886. Professor of Ophthalmology, Zürich, described his syndrome in 1869.

Spinal Tumour (Chapter 27).—Evidence of pressure on the cord is usually present, and Queckenstedt's test is commonly positive.

Branches of the Brachial Plexus

Circumflex or Axillary Nerve.—This passes through the quadrilateral space, and winds around the shaft of the humerus about one finger's-breadth below the centre of the deltoid muscle. It is sometimes injured by a direct blow, or involved by a fracture or dislocation of the humerus.

The deltoid muscle is paralysed and wastes rapidly, and a patch of anaesthesia over the outer side of the arm distinguishes this condition from a partial lesion of the fifth cervical nerve. Paralysis of the teres minor is unrecognisable clinically.

Recovery commences in a few weeks if the cause of the compression is removed, provided that the arm has been supported in right-angled abduction.

Nerve to Serratus Anterior (Nerve of Bell).—It arises from the fifth, sixth and seventh cervical nerve roots. It may be injured by blows or carrying a heavy object on the shoulder, or during operation on the breast or chest wall, as it lies on the inner wall of the axilla. Paralysis of the serratus anterior allows 'winging' of the scapula, *i.e.* the vertebral border and inferior angle are unduly prominent (fig. 463). The 'lunge' stroke of fencing is dependent on the serratus anterior, and this and similar movements, such as pushing forward with the arm, are deficient. Owing to inability to rotate the scapula on the chest wall, difficulty is experienced in raising the arm above a right angle from a position in front of the body. Suture of the nerve is sometimes possible.

Radial or **musculospiral nerve.**—A nerve which is commonly injured. The classical sites are the axilla and the radial groove.

1. **Injury in the axilla** follows: (i) Crutch palsy: all crutches should have hand-grips, and their length should be carefully adjusted, especially if use is likely to be prolonged. Paresis has occurred after only four hours' use of crutches unsupplied with hand-grips.

(ii) Fractures and dislocations of the upper end of the humerus, or by attempts at their reduction.

(iii) Rarely by pressure of an aneurysm or new-growth.

Clinical Features.—(*a*) *Motor.*—The triceps and extensors of the wrist and fingers are paralysed, and consequently inability to extend the elbow, wrist, and fingers results, and wrist drop is present. If the hand is supported, as by supporting it upon the table, extension of the fingers can be produced by the action of the lumbricals and interossei, which are inserted into the extensor expansions. The supinator and brachio-radialis are also paralysed, but supination is ably performed by the biceps. The brachio-radialis muscle is tested readily by endeavouring to flex the semi-prone forearm against resistance. If the muscle is active, the contraction is visible, and the rigid muscle is easily palpable.

(*b*) *Sensory.*—Anaesthesia is present over the dorsum of the forearm and back of the hand where anesthesia is reduced to a patch over the base of the thumb and first interosseous space owing to overlap of the musculocutaneous and other adjacent nerves (fig. 464). In peripheral nerve injury when sensory function is not restored, the final sensory loss is less extensive than the anatomical distribution of the nerve owing to the overlap of adjacent sensory areas.

Hans Queckenstedt, 1876–1918. Chief of Medical Services, Hamburg, Germany, described the test in 1916. Killed by an army waggon on last day of 1914–18 War.
Sir Charles Bell, 1774–1842. (See footnote p. 512.)

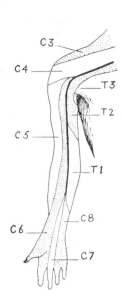

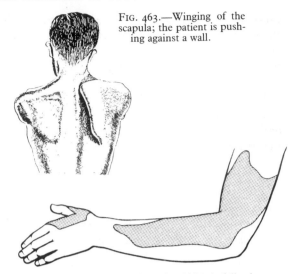

FIG. 463.—Winging of the scapula; the patient is pushing against a wall.

FIG. 462.—The dermatomes of the upper limb.

FIG. 464.—Areas of anaesthesia and anhidrosis following complete division of the radial nerve above the dorsal cutaneous nerve of the forearm and lower lateral cutaneous nerve of the arm. In lesions below the origin of the dorsal cutaneous nerve of the forearm the sensory loss is limited to the lower segment depicted over the dorsum of the base of the thumb and first interosseous space (the anatomical snuff-box).

(c) *Trophic.*—These are usually trivial.

2. Injury in the radial groove is due to:

(i) Pressure, *e.g.* of the arm on the edge of the operating table, especially in Trendelenburg's position, or as in 'Saturday night' paralysis, due to the enjoyment of a heavy sleep with the arm over the sharp back of a kitchen chair. Prolonged application of a tourniquet is especially liable to compress the radial nerve, as it lies close to the bone, and possibly the median and ulnar nerves as well. For this reason a sphygmomanometer should preferably be used on the arm.

(ii) Fracture of the shaft of the humerus when immediate injury of the nerve occurs in about 8% of cases. It is often overlooked owing to the more obvious fracture overshadowing the nerve injury.

(iii) The nerve being overstretched during operations on the humerus, *e.g.* in dealing with an ununited fracture.

(iv) 'Intramuscular' injections of drugs being given into the radial nerve.

Clinical Features.—(*a*) *Motor.*—These are similar to those following injury in the axilla, except that the triceps and anconeus muscles escape.

(*b*) *Sensory.*—If the external cutaneous branch escapes, anaesthesia will be limited to a patch over the ball of the thumb. Division of the radial nerve in the upper third of the forearm is symptomless. Below this position the musculocutaneous nerve joins the radial, and division then causes anaesthesia over the ball of the thumb.

(*c*) *Trophic.*—These are slight.

The *posterior interosseous nerve* may be injured as a result of fracture or dislo-

Friedrich Trendelenburg, 1844–1924. See footnote Chapter 5. Described this position for pelvic operations in 1890.

cation of the upper end of the radius, or in operations performed to deal with these conditions. Paralysis of the long extensors of the fingers results. The upper end of the nerve has been sutured with excellent results. If nerve repair is impracticable, good results are obtained by a tendon and muscle transplant.

Median Nerve.— Is classically injured at the elbow or wrist.

1. Injuries at the elbow are due to fractures of the lower end of the humerus or dislocations of the elbow joint. A tourniquet endangers the nerve at any level in the arm, in which case other nerves, particularly the radial, will also be involved.

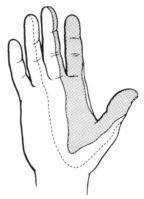

FIG. 465   Median Nerve Injury.—Area of persistent sensory loss in a complete median nerve injury above the wrist showing, in broken line, the distribution of the median nerve and, in stipple, the reduced area of anaesthesia, anhidrosis and analgesia finally persisting after injury owing to overlap of adjacent nerves. The ulnar nerve overlaps the ulnar side of the third finger.

Clinical Features.—(a) *Motor.*—The pronators of the forearm and flexors of the wrist and fingers, with the exception of the flexor carpi ulnaris and the inner part of the flexor profundus digitorum, will be paralysed. As a result of paralysis of the flexor carpi radialis, the hand deviates to the ulnar side when flexed against resistance. The index fingers cannot be flexed at the phalangeal joints—the 'pointing index'—but flexion of the other fingers is performed by that portion of the flexor profundus digitorum which is supplied by the ulnar nerve. Flexion of the terminal phalanx of the thumb is impossible,owing to paralysis of the flexor longus pollicis. The muscles of the thenar eminence are wasted and paralysed, and on inspection the eminence is flattened, so that the metacarpal bone of the thumb is apparently on the same plane as the other metacarpal bones—the so-called 'simian' or 'ape-like' hand. Paralysis of the two outer lumbricals is unrecognisable.

(b) *Sensory.*—Appreciation of touch is at first lost over the thumb and radial two and a half fingers in front, and posteriorly as far proximally as the middle of the proximal phalanges. Loss of response to pin-prick affects the terminal phalanges of the index and middle fingers, but sometimes a larger area is involved. Deep sensibility is lost over the terminal phalanges of the index and middle fingers. Later this area is reduced to overlap from adjacent nerves.

(c) *Trophic.*—Obvious trophic changes are usually seen in the hand and affected fingers, particularly the index finger. Causalgia may complicate partial injuries (see end of chapter).

2. Injuries at the wrist are comparatively common, and are due to cuts from a variety of causes. Fractures of the lower end of the radius or dislocation of the semilunar bone sometimes cause injury to the median nerve.

Clinical Features.—(*a*) *Motor.*—The muscles of the thenar eminence are paralysed and wasted. The hand is 'simian', and abduction and opposition of the thumb are lost. Attempts to oppose the tip of the thumb to the tip of the little finger result in flexion and adduction of the thumb, as the patient is unable to swing it across the palm.

(*b*) *Sensory.*—Sensory losses resemble those following an injury at the elbow. Muscular sense is not impaired if tendons are not served. Thus, as no striking muscular deficiency occurs, and as no part of the hand is complete anaesthetic, a divided median nerve at the wrist is readily overlooked, particularly in those who use refinements of sensation but little, *e.g.* a horny-handed labourer.

(*c*) *Trophic.*—These occur, as with an injury at the elbow.

The poor prognosis of a divided median nerve is rendered even more gloomy if tendons are also severed.

Median compression occasionally occurs as the nerve passes through the carpal tunnel (*entrapment neuropathy*). Paraesthesia, followed by wasting of the thenar muscles, suggests the diagnosis. A description is to be found in Chapter 24.

Ulnar Nerve.—Also classically injured at the elbow and wrist.

1. Injuries at the elbow are due to the following causes:

(i) Fractures in the region of the internal condyle.

(ii) Excision of the elbow joint.

(iii) Cubitus valgus, due to old injury of the humerus and increase of the 'carrying angle'. Hence the nerve is unduly stretched, and friction occurs as the groove on the internal condyle becomes a pulley, and this continuous friction results in interstitial neuritis. This condition may occur many years after the original injury, and transposition of the nerve is required.

(iv) Fixation of the nerve in the groove due to adhesions complicating osteoarthritis may lead to traction with resulting rupture of axons and progressive interstitial neuritis requiring transposition of the nerve (*entrapment neuropathy*) (see below).

Clinical Features.—(*a*) *Motor.*—The flexor carpi ulnaris and inner portion of the flexor profundus digitorum are paralysed. Normally, on flexion of the wrist, the tendon of the flexor carpi ulnaris is readily palpable just above its insertion into the pisiform bone, but when the muscle is paralysed the tendon is impalpable, and wasting causes flattening of the inner border of the forearm. Weakness of the flexor profundus digitorum results in hyperextension of the little, ring, and slightly of the middle fingers at the metacarpophalangeal joints.

Paralysis of the small muscles of the hand also results, with the exception of the thenar muscles and outer two lumbricals. Inability to abduct and adduct the fingers results, and the patient cannot grip a piece of paper placed between the fingers (fig. 466). If the patient pinches a piece of paper between his thumb and fingers the terminal phalanx of the thumb assumes a flexed position, as weakness of the adductor pollicis permits overaction of the long flexor of the thumb (Froment's sign) (fig. 467). Considerable wasting occurs, which is obvious in the interosseous spaces and along the inner border of the hand, the normal curve being lost.

(*b*) *Sensory.*—The appreciation of light touch is at first lost over the inner one

Jules Froment, 1878–1946. Professor of Clinical Medicine, Lyons, France

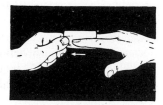

FIG. 466.—Ulnar Nerve Injury.
Test for weakness of the interosseous muscles.

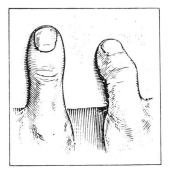

FIG. 467.—Froment's sign for
right ulnar paresis.

and a half fingers in front and behind. Response to pin-prick is lost over the little finger and ulnar border of the palm (fig. 468). Later this area will be reduced by overlap from adjacent nerves.

(c) *Trophic.*—These changes are usually well marked.

Anterior transposition of the ulnar nerve is sometimes required for friction (axonotmesis), following fracture of the internal condyle, pressure by an osteophyte, recurrent dislocation of the nerve, or injury which results in loss of substance, so that approximation is thus rendered possible. The nerve is exposed by a curved incision with the concavity forwards, and the humeral head of the flexor carpi ulnaris is divided. Careful dissection is necessary so as to avoid injury to motor branches, and the internal intermuscular septum should be divided or excised, otherwise the nerve may be kinked by this structure when it is displaced forwards. A bed is then prepared in the flexor group of muscles and the nerve buried therein.

2. Injury at the wrist is due to the same causes as those enumerated in connection with the median nerve. The ulnar nerve passes in front of the anterior annular ligament, and is damaged by more superficial injuries.

Clinical Features.—(*a*) *Motor.*—Paralysis and wasting of small muscles of the hand, as described above.

(*b*) *Sensory.*—The dorsal cutaneous branch of the ulnar nerve leaves the main trunk about 6·3 cm above the styloid process of the ulna. Sensation is therefore lost only on the anterior aspect of the inner one and a half fingers.

(*c*) *Trophic.*—Correspond to the area of sensory loss.

FIG. 468.—Ulnar Nerve Injury. Persistent sensory loss in a complete ulnar nerve injury showing, in broken line, the anatomical distribution of the ulnar and, in stipple, the reduced area of persistent anaesthesia finally resulting.

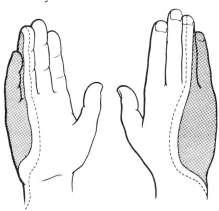

Twelfth Dorsal Nerve.—As in the case of the intercostal nerves this is sometimes implicated by severe neuralgia, which may be associated with herpes zoster. More commonly the nerve is caught up by a suture during a kidney operation, or by subsequent scar tissue.

Ilio-inguinal Nerve.—A nerve often damaged on the right side in a gridiron incision for appendicectomy, although with care the nerve should be avoided. If drainage tubes are inserted through this incision, the resulting scar tissue may implicate the nerve. On the left side, injury to the nerve may follow iliac colostomy. Weakness of the conjoined tendon results, with consequent predisposition to the formation of an inguinal hernia.

External Cutaneous Nerve of thigh.—Occasionally compressed as it passes through the deep fascia of the thigh, especially in muscular subjects, *e.g.* oarsmen. The neuralgia so caused is termed *meralgia paraesthetica*, and resection of part of the nerve is sometimes necessary to rid the patient of pain.

Sciatic Nerve.—It is occasionally injured by wounds, fractures, or 'intramuscular' injection of drugs. The component nerves in the pelvis may be involved by fracture, tumour, or aneurysm. Injury in the upper part of the thigh sometimes complicates deep wounds or posterior dislocation of the hip joint. If the lesion is above the origin of branches to the hamstrings, the following features will be present:

(*a*) *Motor.*—The flexors of the knee are paralysed, but some degree of flexion is possible owing to the action of the sartorius and gracilis muscles. Complete paralysis exists below the knee, and the pull of gravity therefore causes foot drop.

(*b*) *Sensory.*—Complete loss below the knee, with the exception of the skin supplied by the long saphenous nerve, *i.e.* a strip along the inner side of the leg extending along the inner border of the foot to the ball of the big toe.

(*c*) *Trophic.*—Especially on the sole of the foot and toes.

(*d*) Causalgia may complicate partial lesions (see end of chapter).

Partial involvement of the sciatic nerve affects the lateral popliteal portion nine times as commonly as the medial popliteal.

Common Peroneal (Lateral Popliteal) Nerve.—Tends to be injured:

(i) With fracture or excision of the upper end of the fibula.

(ii) By pressure from plasters or splinters.

(iii) In operations for multiple ligation of varicose veins.

(iv) By pressure within the origin of the peroneus longus from the fibula (*entrapment neuropathy*).

(v) During subcutaneous tenotomy of the biceps tendon.

Clinical Features.—Complete lesions will cause:

(*a*) *Motor.*—Complete paralysis of the extensor and peroneal groups of muscles, with resulting talipes equino-varus.

(*b*) *Sensory.*—Anaesthesia of the outer side of the leg in its lower two-thirds, and of the dorsal aspects of all the toes, with the exception of the outer side of the little toe, which is supplied by the external saphenous (sural) nerve, as one contributory branch—the sural communicating from the medial popliteal nerve—escapes.

(*c*) *Trophic.*—Corresponding to the sensory loss. Moderate degrees of pressure will cause ill defined pain and variable degree of weakness or sensory loss.

Tibeal (Medial Popliteal) Nerve.—A nerve rarely injured because of its protected position. The calf muscles and muscles of the sole are paralysed, and talipes calcaneovalgus may result. The sole is anaesthetic, and trophic changes are usually severe. Causalgia (see below) occasionally follows a partial injury of the nerve.

AUTONOMIC NERVOUS SYSTEM

Hyperhidrosis (excessive sweating) can be very distressing both at work and socially. Sweating of the hands responds promptly to cervico-dorsal sympathectomy (Chapter 14). Sodden, offensive feet, the skin of which is cracked and painful, may be a genuine disability for which lumbar sympathectomy is justified. If the axilla is troublesome, relief follows the excision of that area of axillary skin which contains apocrine sweat glands. The area can be mapped out by applying a sweat-sensitive starch and iodine dusting powder. Alternatively these glands can be destroyed by curettage or excision by careful snipping away of all subcutaneous fat, inverting the skin through axillary incisions.

Causalgia is a condition in which paroxysmal attacks of pain follow an incomplete nerve injury, especially of the brachial plexus, sciatic or median nerves. In more than half the cases symptoms supervene immediately after the injury, in the remainder symptoms are deferred for any length of time up to two or three months. The incomplete lesion on the nerve, usually a lateral neuroma, gives rise to antidromic impulses which pass peripherally to the sensory nerve endings where stimuli give rise by the production of histamine-like substance (H substance) similar to that liberated to the posterior nerve root vasodilators. The accumulation of H substance causes vasodilation and renders the part red and engorged, the affected area also sweats profusely and is exquisitely painful and hyperaesthetic owing to the increased pressure. The skin is often thin as the result of trophic changes. Sooner or later the patient loses his morale and becomes introspective and uncooperative. The condition is often so distressing that surgical alleviation is desirable.

Treatment.—Paravertebral block (either D.2 and 3, or L.1, 2 and 3) relieves the pain for a short time, and confirms the necessity for operation (Chapter 14). Thoracic sympathetic trunk section or lumbar sympathectomy is the treatment of choice.

Visceral Pain.—*Pancreas.*—The wearying pain from recurring pancreatitis and carcinoma may respond to injection of the coeliac and related sympathetic ganglia.

CHAPTER 29

THE EYE AND ORBIT

PERIORBITAL AND ORBITAL SWELLINGS

A. Swellings Related to the Supraorbital Margin (fig. 469)

Dermoid cysts are usually external angular cysts but may occur medially. They often cause a bony depression by their pressure, and may have a dumbbell extension into the orbit. They can also erode the orbital plate of the frontal bone, to become attached to dura, and for this reason it is important to x-ray the area prior to excision.

Neurofibromatosis may also produce swellings above the eye. The diagnosis can usually be confirmed by an examination of the whole body, as there are multiple lesions.

B. Swellings of the Lids

Meibomian cysts (chalazion).—The commonest lid swelling. It is a chronic granulomatous inflammation of a meibomian gland. It may occur on either upper or lower lids, and presents as a smooth painless swelling. It can be felt by rolling the cyst on the tarsal plate. It is distinguished from a *stye (Hordeolum)* which is an infection of a hair follicle, usually painful. Meibomian cysts are treated by incision and curettage from the conjunctival surface. Styes are treated by antibiotics and local heat.

Basal cell carcinomas (Rodent ulcers).—This is the commonest malignant tumour of the eyelids. It is locally malignant, is more common on the lower lids, and usually starts as a small pimple which ulcerates, and has raised edges. It is easily excised in the early stages, and can be treated with local radiotherapy if too big to be excised.

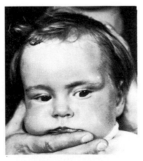

FIG. 469.—External angular dermoid.

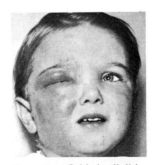

FIG. 470.—Orbital cellulitis.

Other lid swellings can occur, but are less common. These include sebaceous cysts, papillomas, keratoacanthosis, and molluscum contagiosum. When the latter occurs on the lid margin they can give rise to a mild keratoconjunctivitis, and they should be curetted. Carcinoma of the meibomian glands, and rhabdomyosarcomas are rare lesions, and need to be treated radically.

C. Swellings of the Lacrimal System

Lacrimal sac mucocele.—This occurs from obstruction of the lacrimal gland beyond the sac, and results in a fluctuant swelling which bulges out just below the medial canthus. It can become infected to give rise to a painful tense swelling (acute dacryocystitis). If untreated it may give rise to a fistula. Treatment is by performing a bypass operation between the lacrimal sac and the nose (a dacryocystorhinostomy (D.C.R.)).

Lacrimal gland tumours.—Pathologically these resemble parotid tumours (Chapter 31). These are swellings of the gland which lies in the upper lateral aspect of the orbit, and eventually they lead to impairment of ocular movements, and displacement of the globe forwards, downwards, and inwards.

Watering of the eye can be caused by eversion of the lower lid (*ectropion*) which everts the lower lid punctum through which 95% of the tears drain away from the eye. Treatment is by local cautery to invert the lid by scarring, or by lid surgery if the ectropion is more marked.

Orbital Swellings

If these reach any size they result in displacement of the globe, and limitation of movement. A full description of these is outside the realm of this text, but some of the commonest causes are listed.

1. *Pseudoproptosis.*—Due to a large eyeball as seen in congenital glaucoma or high myopia.
2. *Orbital inflammatory conditions* as in orbital cellulitis (fig. 470).
3. *Haemorrhagic lesions* in the orbit after trauma or retrobulbar injections.
4. *Neoplasia* affecting the lacrimal gland, the optic nerve, the nasal sinuses, glioma, (Neurofibromatosis (fig. 471)) meningioma and osteoma (fig. 472).
5. *Dysthyroid Exophthalmos* (fig. 473).—A condition which often starts after thyroidectomy, and may need urgent tarsorrhaphy, or even orbital decompression, if the eyeball is threatened by exposure. This is best and most easily done into the nasal sinuses (see Chapter 37).
6. *Pseudotumour*, or malignant lymphoma.
7. *Haemangiomas* of the orbit (fig. 474).
8. *Secondaries.*—These are rare. In children they usually come from neuroblastomas of the adrenal gland, while in adults, the oesophagus, stomach, breast, and prostate can be sites for primary lesions.

Diagnostic aids include: X-ray, Tomogram, Orbital venogram, Ultra-sound, and CT scans.

Treatment is directed to the cause of the lesion if at all possible, taking care to prevent exposure of the eye, and discomfort from diplopia.

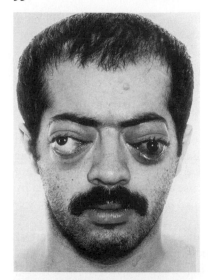

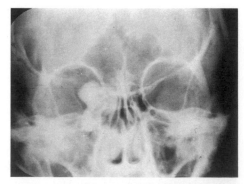

FIG. 472.—X-ray showing an osteoma on the nasal side of the orbit giving rise to proptosis.

FIG. 471.—Neurofibroma in the orbit with proptosis, and also similar lesion in the forehead.

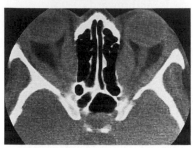

FIG. 473.—CT scan of orbit in Dysthyroid Exophthalmos showing swollen muscles
(Dr. Glyn Lloyd.)

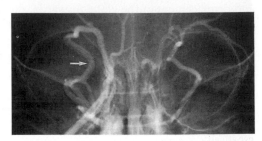

FIG. 474.—Capillary haemangioma in a child. Orbital venogram demonstrates displacement of the second part of the superior ophthalmic vein.
(Dr. Glyn Lloyd.)

INTRAOCULAR TUMOURS

Children.—**Retinoblastoma** is a multicentric malignant tumour of the retina, which can be bilateral. Some are sporadic, but many are hereditary. It is often not spotted until the tumour fills the globe, and presents as a white reflex in the pupil (fig. 475). Differential diagnosis is from retinopathy of prematurity, primary hyperplastic vitreous, and intraocular infections.

Adults.—**Malignant melanoma** is the commonest tumour, and it originates in the pigment cells of the choroid ciliary body (fig. 476), or iris. It can present as a reduction in vision, a vitreous haemorrhage, or by the chance finding of an elevated pigmented lesion in the eye. Growth can be rapid or fairly slow, and as a general rule the more posterior the lesion the more malignant it is likely to be. Malignancy is ultimately related to the cell type. Spread is often delayed for many years, and often goes to the liver, hence the advice 'beware of the patient with a glass eye, and an enlarged liver' (fig. 477). Treatment is by light, or laser coagulation, cobalt plaques, enucleation, or in selected cases, local excision using hypotensive anaesthesia. *Note.*—A blind painful eye may hide a malignant melanoma.

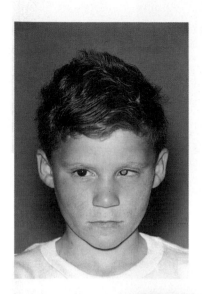

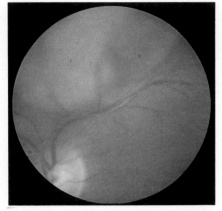

FIG. 476.—Choroidal melanoma.

FIG. 475.—Retinoblastoma giving rise to a white pupillary reflex. This child was first seen with a convergent squint and discharged without a fundus examination. He was next seen many years later with a 'white reflex' and died soon after diagnosis.
(M. A. Bedford, FRCS)

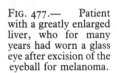

FIG. 477.— Patient with a greatly enlarged liver, who for many years had worn a glass eye after excision of the eyeball for melanoma.

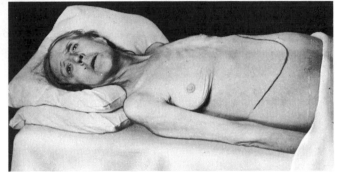

INJURIES INVOLVING THE EYE AND ADJACENT STRUCTURES

Corneal abrasions and ulceration.—The cornea is frequently damaged by trauma and foreign bodies. Ulceration can occur with infection, or after damage to the facial nerve (Chapter 28). Post-herpetic ulceration is common and serious if not treated. Fluorescein instillation can show up corneal ulceration at an early stage. Treatment is by protection (by eye pads or tarsorrhaphy) and antibiotics topically and systemically: 1% chloramphenicol eye drops are commonly used. In Eastern countries chronic infection with trachoma can cause corneal opacification and blindness. Corneal grafting is the only cure for an opaque cornea.

Blunt injuries to the eye and orbit.—The floor of the orbit is its weakest wall, and in blunt trauma such as fist injuries, it is often fractured without fractures of the other walls. This is called a 'Blow-out' fracture. Clinical signs are enophthalmos, bruising around the orbit, and limitation of upward gaze with diplopia. This occurs when the extraocular muscles become trapped in the fracture, and can be identified as a soft tissue mass in the antrum on x-ray (fig. 478),

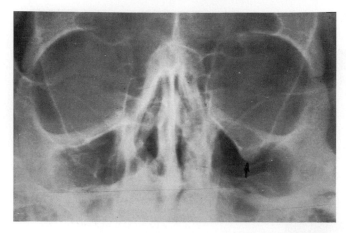

FIG. 478.— X-ray showing a 'Blow out' fracture of the orbit (lt) with soft tissue in the antrum.
(*Dr. Glyn Lloyd.*)

although tomograms may be necessary. Surgical repair of the orbital floor with freeing of the trapped contents may be necessary if troublesome diplopia persists. If an orbital haemorrhage is too extensive to examine the eye, then it may be necessary to give a short anaesthetic, as there may be a hidden perforation of the globe.

Concussional injuries of the eye can give rise to several problems, which include:

1. *Hyphaema* (blood in the anterior chamber) (fig. 479). Bed rest and sedation are advised, as the main danger in this condition is secondary bleeding, giving rise to an acute rise in intraocular pressure, and blood staining of the cornea. The use of anti-fibrinolytic agents (aminocaproic acid) has been advocated, and, if the pressure rises, surgery to wash out the blood may be necessary.
2. *Subluxation of the lens* can be suspected if the iris, or part of the iris 'wobbles' on movement (iridodonesis).
3. *Secondary glaucoma* often associated with recession of the angle.
4. *Retinal and macular haemorrhages.*
5. *Retinal dialysis* which may lead to a retinal detachment, and permanent damage to vision.

Penetrating eye injuries.—These occur when the globe is penetrated, often after road traffic, and other major accidents (fig. 480), and also injuries from sharp instruments. The seat belt law has reduced this type of eye injury by up to

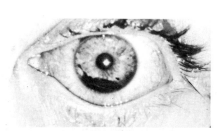

FIG. 479.—Hyphaema—blood in anterior chamber after blunt injury.

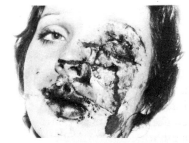

FIG. 480.—Facial lacerations from windscreen injury: beware of a perforating eye injury.

73% in some series. The presence of an irregular pupil, or prolapse of the iris, and other intraocular contents should arouse the suspicion of a penetrating injury. Treatment is immediate surgery to restore the integrity of the globe. If a perforation is suspected, extensive examination should not be attempted before anaesthesia as this may lead to further extrusion of the intraocular contents. In severe corneal, and intraocular injuries, primary corneal grafting, lensectomy and vitrectomy have considerably improved the visual prognosis; these must be done by an experienced eye surgeon. Injuries to the optic nerves must also be excluded in severe accidents.

Intraocular foreign bodies must always be excluded when patients attend the accident and emergency department with a history of working with a hammer and chisel. *X-ray of the orbit should always be performed, and ferrous and copper foreign bodies should always be removed.* Beta Scan ultrasonography can also assist in localising foreign bodies when a vitreous haemorrhage is present.

Burns. 1. *Radiational after arc welding.* These cause intense pain and photophobia due to a keratitis, which may start some hours after exposure. Mydriatic and local steroid drops ease the condition, and healing usually occurs after 36 hours.

2. *Thermal burns.* If these involve the full thickness of the lids, corneal scarring may occur, and immediate skin grafting to the lids is necessary. A splash of molten metal may cause marked local necrosis, and may lead to permanent corneal scarring. Treatment is to remove any debris by irrigation, and to instil local atropine and antibiotics and steroids, to prevent superadded infection and scarring.

3. *Chemical burns.* Especially alkali burns can be serious, as ocular penetration occurs quickly, and ischaemic necrosis can result. Immediate irrigation will ensure that the chemical is diluted as much as possible, and all particles should be removed from the fornices. Treatment can then be continued as with thermal burns.

DIFFERENTIAL DIAGNOSIS OF THE ACUTE RED EYE

The importance of this is in the management of minor ocular complaints, and the recognition of conditions requiring expert attention. Possible causes of the acute red eye can be divided into:

1. Conjunctivitis.
2. Keratitis.
3. Uveitis.
4. Episcleritis and Scleritis.
5. Acute glaucoma.

1. **Conjunctivitis.**—Symptoms are grittiness, redness and discharge. Causes are infective, viral or allergic. In the newborn it can be serious, and gonococcal infection must be excluded. Vernal conjunctivitis (fig. 481) is a form of allergic conjunctivitis, usually worse in the Spring and early Summer, and often associated with other allergic problems such as hayfever. Clinically, most signs are under the upper lid which may have a cobblestone appearance instead of a smooth surface. A similar condition may be seen in soft contact lens wearers. Viral

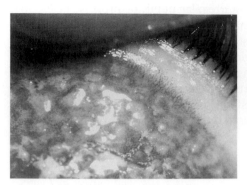

FIG. 481.—Vernal conjunctivitis (Spring catarrh) showing cobblestone appearance under the upper lid.

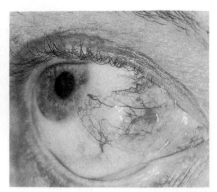

FIG. 482.—Episcleritis

conjunctivitis has become much more common. Chlamydia and adenovirus infections must be considered.

Vision is not affected in conjunctivitis, but with some virus infections a keratitis may be present, and result in visual loss. All the other conditions are painful, and usually affect vision.

2. Keratitis (Inflammation of the cornea).—Herpes Simplex infection is the most serious, and presents itself as a dendritic (branching) ulcer, shown easily by staining with fluorescein or Bengal Rose.

Corneal ulceration may occur due to ingrowing lashes, or corneal foreign bodies, which can be removed, or marginal ulceration, and infected ulcers. The latter can occur in patients wearing soft contact lenses. *Herpes zoster* (shingles) when it affects the ophthalmic division of the Vth nerve, can give rise to a keratitis and uveitis. It is important to exclude the use of steroid drops until a diagnosis has been made.

3. Uveitis.—This can be anterior (iritis) or posterior. In anterior uveitis the pupil will be small, there is circumcorneal injection, and there may be keratin precipitates (KP) present on the posterior surface of the cornea. Pain, photophobia, and some visual loss are usually present.

4. Episcleritis and Scleritis. Episcleritis or inflammation of the episcleral tissue often occurs as an allergic reaction following an eye infection (fig. 482). Scleritis is a more serious condition in which the deeper sclera is involved. There is often an associated uveitis and thinning of the sclera. It may require the use of systemic steroids in order to treat adequately.

5. Acute glaucoma.—This usually occurs in older, often hypermetropic patients. The cornea becomes hazy, the pupil oval and dilated, the vision very poor, and the eye feels rock hard. In severe cases the pain may be accompanied by vomiting, and the case can be mistaken for one of an acute abdomen. In doubtful cases the use of the tonometer to measure the intraocular pressure is a useful diagnostic procedure.

Except for a simple conjunctivitis which is self limiting, these conditions require expert treatment, and a specialist opinion should be sought.

PAINLESS LOSS OF VISION

This may occur in one or both eyes, and the visual loss may be transient or permanent. Possible causes are:

1. Obstruction of the central retinal artery.
2. Obstruction of the central retinal vein.
3. Cranial arteritis.
4. Ischaemic papillitis.
5. Migraine and other vascular causes.
6. Retrobulbar neuritis and papillitis.
7. Vitreous haemorrhage.
8. Retinal detachment.
9. Macular hole, cyst, or haemorrhage.
10. Hysterical blindness.

Specialist help should be sought in any case of loss of vision. An ESR should be done immediately if cranial arteritis is suspected, and the carotid system should be examined for bruit and other signs of arteriosclerosis in cases of ischaemic papillitis, and central retinal artery occlusion. Glaucoma and hypertension should be looked for in cases of central vein thrombosis.

RECENT DEVELOPMENTS IN EYE SURGERY

In the last few years eye surgery has changed to become a microsurgical speciality. Cataract surgery has been transformed by intraocular implants. The power of the implant to be used can be accurately measured by A-Scan ultrasonography. Vitrectomy instruments have enabled membranes to be peeled off the retina.

Paralytic squints can be treated more accurately by the use of adjustable sutures, or injection of Botulinus toxin into the overacting muscles. Surgery for myopia (radial keratometry) can be done, and lasers are used for many conditions.

The Argon laser is used as a coagulator, mostly for proliferative diabetic retinopathy and also to treat glaucoma. The YAG laser (Yittrum Aluminium Garnet) is used as a Q-switch cutting laser for posterior capsulotomies, iridectomies, and cutting vitreous bands. Tunable dye lasers and excimer lasers are also being developed.

Excision of an Eyeball

Indications include a blind painful eye, a blind cosmetically poor eye, intraocular neoplasm, and in cadavers for use in corneal grafting.

The operation.—The speculum is introduced between the lids, and opened. The conjunctiva is picked up with toothed forceps and divided completely all round as near as possible to the cornea, Tenon's capsule is entered, and each of the rectus tendons is hooked up on a strabismus hook and divided close to the sclera. The speculum is now pressed backwards and the eyeball projects forward. Blunt scissors, curved on the flat, are insinuated on the inner side of the globe, and these are used to sever the optic nerve. The eyeball can now be drawn forward with the forceps and the oblique muscles, together with any other strands of tissue which are still attaching the globe to the orbit, are divided. A swab moistened with hot water and pressed into the orbit will control the haemorrhage. If an orbital implant is inserted to give better eye movement, the muscles are sutured to the implant at the appropriate sites.

Evisceration of the eyeball

Owing to the danger of opening up lymphatic spaces at the back of the globe, and thus favouring meningitis, evisceration is to be preferred to excision in panophthalmitis. The sclera is transfixed with a pointed knife a little behind the corneo-sclerotic junction, and the cornea is removed entirely by completing the encircling incision in the sclera. The contents of the globe are then removed with a curette, care being exercised to remove all the uveal tract. At the end of the operation the interior must appear perfectly white.

Jacques Rene Tenon, 1724–1816. Surgeon, La Salpetriere, Paris.

AIDS and the eye (see HIV:Chapter 4)

Kaposi's Sarcomas, purplish or brown nonpruritic nodules or macules, are a frequent early manifestation of AIDS. Commonly affecting the face, especially the tip of the nose, the lesions may involve the eyelids and the conjunctiva, and are mostly seen in male homosexual AIDS sufferers.

Fundus Lesions are divided into 'Non-infective' and 'Infective' categories. 'Non-infective' changes consist of 'cotton wool' spots, retinal haemorrhages and vascular sheathing. 'Infective' lesions are a typical retinitis, the usual cause being a cytomegalovirus infection, which has been described as 'Tomato Ketchup and Salad Cream retinopathy.'

Neuro-ophthalmological complications in AIDS have been reported, most frequently as nerve palsies associated with intracranial infections with cryptococcus and toxoplasmosis, or as a manifestation of an intracranial lymphoma.

CHAPTER 30

FACE, PALATE, LIPS,
MAXILLO-FACIAL INJURIES

EMBRYOLOGY OF THE FACE

The buccopharyngeal membrane lies between the forebrain and the developing heart in the pericardial sac. Bending of the brain at the midbrain flexure brings the anterior end of the neural crest above the buccopharyngeal membrane and ectomesenchyme migrates downwards beneath the epithelium and over the forebrain to form a prominence, the frontonasal process. Further neural crest cells migrate by a longer route between the buccopharyngeal membrane and the heart to form a series of ridges, the first two of which are substantial and form the mandibular and hyoid arches. Ectomesenchyme from the dorsal end of the mandibular arches migrates forwards subepithelially to raise prominences, the maxillary processes, on either side of the buccopharyngeal membrane which, as a result, lies at the bottom of a pit, the stomatodeum. At this stage the buccopharyngeal membrane perforates.

The epithelium on the lateral aspects of the frontonasal process thickens to form the olfactory placodes and frontonasal ectomesenchyme proliferates to raise a horseshoe-shaped ridge medial to, above and lateral to the placode. The medial part of the ridge is called the medial nasal process and the lateral part the lateral nasal process. Mandibular arch mesenchyme on each side proliferates medially merging in the mid-line to smooth out the notch between the two sides and establish a single complete arch.

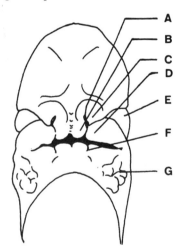

FIG. 483.—The head of a human embryo at five weeks.

A. Olfactory pit.
B. Median nasal process.
C. Lateral nasal process.
D. Maxillary process.
E. Eye.
F. Lateral groove in mandibular arch.
G. Hyomandibular cleft with auricular tubercles.

During the sixth week the medial nasal processes enlarge, bulging down between the maxillary processes and towards one another (fig. 483). They merge in the mid-line smoothing the furrow between them. The maxillary elevations also enlarge substantially, maintaining a relationship with the medial nasal processes also advancing medially below the lateral nasal processes and the olfactory pits. As the olfactory placodes sink below the surface they maintain contact with the epithelium between maxillary and medial nasal mesenchyme which, at this stage, cannot mingle.

The maxillary and medial nasal processes bulge forward together and the epithelium on their surfaces fuse to form a sheet, the nasal fin. Subsequently this breaks down and maxillary and medial nasal mesenchyme intermingle. The epithelial fins behind this fusion are stretched laterally to form the bucconasal membranes and break down to form the nasal choanae connecting the nasal pits and the stomatodaeum. The tissues below the nasal pits now form the primary palate or intermaxillary segment. The posterior part will form the premaxillary part of the definitive palate, the intermediate zone the premaxillary alveolar process and teeth and the anterior zone the medial portion of the upper lip.

During the seventh week shelf-like processes grow medially and downwards from the maxillary processes, which form the sides of the stomatodaeum, so as to embrace the developing tongue. The tongue disengages itself from between them from before backwards, they reorientate medially, their edges touch in the mid-line and the covering epithelium adheres, fuses and then breaks down. These processes forming the secondary palate also fuse with the primary palate.

The nasal choanae are stretched upwards by growth of the surrounding tissues and a nasal septum appears in the roof of the stomatodaeum behind them and grows downwards. Both frontonasal and maxillary mesenchyme via tectoseptal extensions contribute to the septum. It fuses with the palatine shelves soon after they unite.

CONGENITAL ABNORMALITIES

Cleft lip and palate

These are two separate entities. Cleft lip (fig. 484) results from abnormal development of the medial nasal and maxillary processes at the time that they

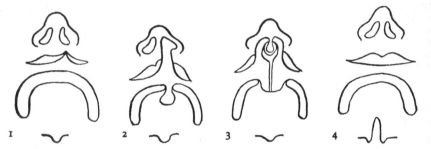

FIG. 484.—1. Partial cleft lip. 2. Complete cleft of lip and alveolus (see fig. 487). 3. Double cleft of lip and alveolus. 4. Cleft soft palate.
(After Kernahan and Starke.)

bulge downwards in front of and below the nasal pit and when their surfaces should touch, the epithelium over them fuse and then break down. (In experimental animals such as the rat the lateral nasal processes rather than the maxillary processes are involved.) In minor degrees of clefting the deficiency appears to be mainly of tissue from the medial nasal process. More severe degrees are deficient on both sides and the cleft involves the alveolar process, between the primary and secondary palates. The presence of a cleft lip appears to interfere with dislocation of the tongue from between the palatal shelves so producing the combined cleft lip and palate deformity. Cleft palate (fig. 485) results from a failure of fusion of the two palatine processes or, in the case of the soft palate, of a merging process to carry the union backwards from the site of initial fusion.

Bilateral cleft lip and alveolar process may occur on its own, or again in combination with a cleft of the secondary palate. When this happens the palatal cleft is often wide and the nasal septum not attached to either side.

A failure of merging of the medial nasal processes can lead to a median cleft lip, with sometimes, in addition, a deficiency of the nasal tip. Various deficiencies

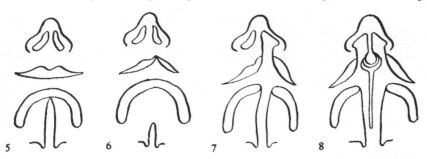

FIG. 485.—5. Cleft soft and hard palate. 6. Partial cleft of palate and lip. 7. Complete cleft of lip, alveolus and palate. 8. Double complete cleft of lip, alveolus, and palate (see fig. 489).
(After Kernahan and Starke.)

of frontonasal development can lead to an absence of the premaxilla (but not necessarily a median cleft of the lip), absence of the nose, or cyclopia (which is not compatable with life).

Experimentally, a variety of insults to the embryo can result in the production of a cleft lip or cleft palate depending upon the timing of the event. There is little evidence to link specific aetiological factors with these deformities when they occur spontaneously. There are likely to be a variety of aetiologies and several mechanisms which can result in one or the other of these defects. For example, cleft palate could result from a failure of the tongue to dislocate from between the palatal shelves at the appropriate time, a failure of reorientation of the palatal shelves, a failure of the rapid medial growth which usually precedes fusion, or a failure of the fusion process itself.

In a proportion of cases, which varies with the closeness of the relationship, a family incidence of clefting is found. Cleft lip and cleft lip and palate occur with increased frequency among relatives and isolated cleft palate similarly, but as a separate relationship.

Caucasians have a higher incidence of cleft lip than Negroes, and Japanese than Europeans. Certain communities such as in Iceland have a high incidence.

After a study of records of 703 Danish patients, P. Fogh-Anderson found a relative incidence as follows:

Cleft lip alone	25%	(60% males)
Cleft palate alone	25%	(59% females)
Cleft lip and cleft palate combined	50%	(70% males)

In 75% of patients the cleft was unilateral.

In most series of unilateral cleft lip the cleft is on the left side in 60% of cases.

Classification of Cleft Lip and Palate Defects

A classification based on those of Kernahan and Starke is simple and generally useful:

1. Clefts of Primary Palate only

UNILATERAL (right or left)	MEDIAN	BILATERAL
(a) Complete	(a) Complete (premaxilla absent)	(a) Complete
(b) Incomplete	(b) Incomplete (premaxilla rudimentary)	(b) Incomplete

2. Clefts of Secondary Palate

(a) Complete	(b) Incomplete	(c) Submucous

Poul Fogh-Andersen. Plastic Surgeon, Deaconess Hospital, Copenhagen, Denmark.
D. A. Kernahan, Contemporary. St. Luke's Hospital, New York.
R. B. Starke, Contemporary. St. Luke's Hospital, New York.

3. *Clefts of both Primary and Secondary Palates*

UNILATERAL (right or left)	MEDIAN	BILATERAL
(*a*) Complete	(*a*) Complete	(*a*) Complete
(*b*) Incomplete	(*b*) Incomplete	(*b*) Incomplete

In addition, where clefts of the secondary plate are involved the nasal septum may or may not be attached to one of the palatal shelves and where the cleft is incomplete the cleft may involve only the soft palate.

Effect upon Function

Sucking and eating.—Because the infant takes a substantial part of the areola as well as the nipple into its mouth, sucking is not greatly affected by a cleft lip. Where bottle feeding is used the hole in the teat may have to be enlarged with a hot needle. Cleft palate babies have been successfully fed with a spoon, but a special plate which covers the cleft facilitates bottle feeding. It would be assumed that an unrepaired cleft palate was incompatible with successful eating, but from time to time adults are seen, often with quite large clefts who have grown up in places where surgery was not available and who are well nourished. A denture with a special extension can be made to occlude the cleft, even that between the soft palate.

Speech.—A person with a cleft palate is unable to make the consonant sounds B.D.K.P.T. and the hard G. Various arguments are advanced about the optimum time at which palatal repair should be effected, and the degree to which early surgery reduces the growth potential of the maxilla. However, closure before serious attempts are made by the child to speak is an important consideration. Speech therapy is almost always needed after surgery for the best results. Unfortunately once nasal speech has developed as a result of delayed closure, a nasal intonation may persist despite speech training. The aim of surgery is a long, flexible soft palate which can be elevated to seal off the nasopharynx. Even if this is not managed surprisingly good speech can be achieved by dedicated speech therapy. Because the child mimicks the parents, a mother or father with cleft palate speech is a hindrance to the development of good speech in the child.

The teeth.—The alveolar cleft interferes with the dental lamina and the upper lateral incisor may be small, absent or even duplicated with a supernumerary lateral incisor on the canine side of the cleft. All the incisors in bilateral cleft cases may be badly displaced. The maxilla tends to be smaller than average, particularly the lesser segment and the latter is often at a higher level at the anterior end than the canine region on the other side. The teeth, particularly the adult ones, therefore tend to be crowded and the maxilla retroposed, giving a relative mandibular prognathism. In the past unskilful surgery damaged the unerupted teeth. Orthodontic treatment is required to ensure correctly aligned arches.

The nose.—The upper respiratory mucous membranes are contaminated with oral organisms through a cleft palate or via a residual defect after repair. The nostril and ala on the cleft side are inadequately supported by a defective anterior bony aperture to the nose.

Hearing.—If a palatal repair is not attempted and sometimes even if a good palatal repair is achieved, acute and chronic otitis media, 'glue' ear and hearing

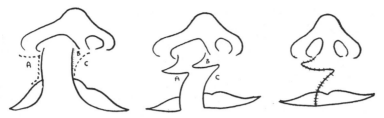

FIG. 486.—Repair of cleft-lip (after Millard).

problems ensue. Inflammatory oedema of pharyngeal mucosa and defective muscular activity impede the ventilation and drainage of the middle ear via the Eustachian tube with retention of inflammatory exudate and deafness.

Treatment

Aims.—The aims are a normal appearance, swallowing without nasal regurgitation, normal sounding speech, well aligned teeth in normal occlusion and no loss of hearing.

A normal appearance.—An infant with a cleft lip, even a unilateral one, appears grotesque to the parents (fig. 489). Much trouble should be taken to reassure them and particularly the mother and to establish a normal parent-child bonding. Fortunately lip repair soon creates a normal looking face (fig. 487 and 488). A

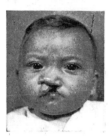

FIG. 487.—Cleft lip.

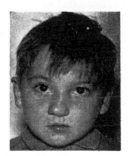

FIG. 488.—Same case as fig. 487 four years after repair.

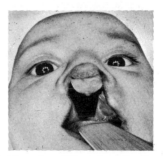

FIG. 489.—Bilateral cleft lip associated with an unfused pre-maxilla and cleft palate.

cleft palate baby requires intensive pre-surgical treatment and presents feeding problems which need to be overcome. These put an additional strain on the parents. After the primary surgical treatment (fig. 486), revision to deal with various aesthetic problems is required as growth proceeds. If the maxilla is hypoplastic and retroposed a maxillary osteotomy may be required as soon as skeletal growth has ceased to advance the mid face downwards and forwards. The level at which this is effected depends upon the degree to which the nose and infraorbital rims also are hypoplastic. Even where the facial skeleton is generally well formed secondary procedures to produce symmetrical nostrils and alae are often required in early adolescence: sometimes with lengthening of the columella to raise the nasal tip. Revision of lip scars at the same time may be needed. If there is a genuine inequality of size between upper and lower lip and not just a postural

David Ralph Millard, Jr. Contemporary. Plastic Surgeon, Miami, Florida. U.S.A.
Bartolommeo Eustachi (Eustachius), ?1520–1574. Professor of Anatomy, Rome.

effect due to a small maxilla, an Abbe flap may be needed to reduce the lower lip size and increase that of the upper.

Well aligned teeth.—Orthodontic help is required to achieve this once the adult dentition starts to erupt. Tooth movement, preceded sometimes by extractions to balance tooth size and arch size is usually started around age 10 or 11. Minor inequalities of jaw size between maxilla and mandible may be disguised. Where greater discrepancies are likely to appear in adolescence future corrective surgery must be borne in mind. Crowning of unsightly upper incisors is sometimes needed in the late teens.

Sucking and swallowing.—Sound surgical repair of the palatal cleft, or of the alveolar cleft and labial sulcus fistula if only an alveolar cleft is present is the definitive answer to feeding problems.

Normal sounding speech.—Again the solution is a functional soft palate repair and good speech therapy. Well aligned teeth are helpful.

Normal hearing.—Supervision by an ENT surgeon from an early age is needed.

It is obvious that many specialists are involved in a team effort from birth until perhaps 20 years of age if the best results are to be obtained. The detailed problems are many and special texts should be consulted about them. Where possible these children should be cared for by those who have a special interest in this work and who have had special training.

An outline of the sequence of treatment.—Soon after birth the cleft palate child should be seen by an orthodontist or paedodontist experienced in cleft palate work. A plate is constructed which will cover the cleft to facilitate feeding and which will mould the parts of the palate into the optimum position for surgical repair. Fresh plates will be constructed at intervals to continue the moulding until the alveolar processes are aligned and related correctly in space to the lower arch. If there is a bilateral cleft lip, facial strapping will be applied to the outside of the lip and premaxilla which is usually markedly displaced forwards under the tip of the nose, so as to mould it back into place.

The lip is normally repaired at about 10 weeks after birth. The repair should be relatively simple and sacrifice the minimum of tissue. The aim should be a long scar that will not contract and create a notch, accurate alignment of the mucocutaneous junction, conservation of a cupid's bow, correction of the shape of the nostril and repair of the nasal floor. Above all the two parts of the orbicularis oris must be joined together. In cleft lip patients the ends of the muscle are inserted into the adjacent bone and have to be mobilised before a complete oral sphincter can be achieved. If necessary, closure of the alveolar cleft can be left to a subsequent occasion. Bone grafting of the alveolar cleft in infants is probably not beneficial. Bilateral cleft lips are repaired one side at a time so that tension created by the closure of one side helps to reposition the premaxilla.

Repair of the palatal cleft is usually undertaken between the ages of 12–18 months (figs. 490 and 491). The soft palate is closed in layers, first separating the abnormal insertions

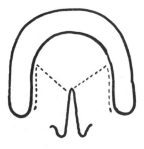

FIG. 490.—V-Y Repair of cleft palate.

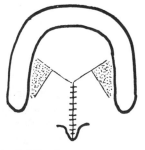

FIG. 491.—Four-flap method.

of the tensor palati into the back edge of the hard palate; rotating the ends medially and sewing them together in the mid-line. Flaps should be raised gently and with precision to avoid unnecessary damage to growing tissues. Repeated operations lead to scarring, bony deformity and poor soft palate function.

Speech therapy, ENT and orthodontic supervision follow. Around age 10–11 bone grafts are sometimes placed in the alveolar cleft to permit movement of the permanent canine into a good position. During the teenage period the need for and timing of further orthodontics, surgery of the facial skeleton, revision of lip scars and correction of residual nasal deformity are considered.

OTHER DEVELOPMENTAL ABNORMALITIES

Preauricular sinus.—The auricle develops from the fusion of six tubercles grouped around the external auditory canal. Failure of successful merging of the anterior tubercles leads to the formation of one or more narrow, blind pits. The opening leading into a preauricular sinus may become occluded, whereupon a cyst forms. If the cyst becomes infected and bursts or is incised a preauricular ulcer may follow. The ulcer refuses to heal as the infection is maintained from the sinus. The treatment is complete excision of the sinus.

Periauricular dermoid cyst.—These dermoid cysts extend out from under the pinna as a fluctuant swelling, usually posteriorly. They should be differentiated from a post-auricular sebaceous cyst. They result from inclusion of epithelium as two adjacent auricular tubercles merge (fig. 494).

Large upper labial frenum

In the child the deciduous maxillary central incisors are often separated from one another by a diastema and the labial frenum extends between them to the palatine papilla. With the eruption of the permanent incisors the diastema usually closes and a normal adult frenum is established. In some children the frenum remains thick and fleshy between the centrals and the diastema cannot be closed (fig. 492). The palatal extension of the frenum is dissected out from between the incisors and advanced up the labial side of the alveolar process as a V-Y procedure. Following this, orthodontic treatment to approximate the incisors may be successful.

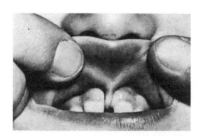

FIG. 492.—Large labial frenum.
(The late Patrick Clarkson, FRCS, London.)

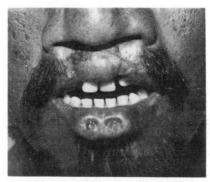

FIG. 493.—Sinuses of the lower lip. Note also the repaired cleft lip (Van der Woude's syndrome).
(John C. Nicholls, FRCS, London.)

Sinuses of the lower lip.—Demarquay described a pair of developmental sinuses, one either side of the mid-line of the lower lip. A mucoid material from adjacent mucous glands may discharge through them. Van der Woude drew attention to a familial syndrome in which lower lip sinuses are associated with a cleft upper lip and palate (fig. 493). It is suggested that the sinuses may develop from transient paramedian grooves in the developing lower lip. The sinuses may be excised with a wedge of lip but the wound must be closed in eversion to prevent notching.

Prolapse of the mucous membrane of the upper lip.—This produces a condition

Anne van der Woude, Contemporary. Institute of Human Biology, University of Michigan, Ann Arbor, U.S.A. Described this syndrome in 1954.

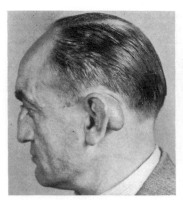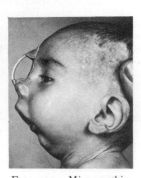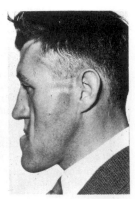

FIG. 494.—Peri-auricular dermoid
cyst.

FIG. 495.—Micrognathia.
An endotracheal tube has
been passed.
(*The late Sir Alan Moncrieff, London.*)

FIG. 496.—Mandibular
prognathism.
(*J. H. Hovell, FDS, RCS, London.*)

described as double lip. The patient may also have a sagging of the chin and of the upper eyelids and a non-toxic goitre (Ascher syndrome).

Micrognathism.—Relative mandibular retrognathism is common but in some instances the mandible is excessively small (fig. 495). Pierre Robin was interested in such cases and devised a monoblock orthodontic appliance to try to correct the small mandible. He drew attention to the respiratory obstruction which can affect neonates with micrognathism because the deformity results in backwards displacement of the tongue. Lenstrup reported three cases which all had cleft palates. It is suggested that dislocation of the tongue from between the palatal shelves is prevented because the mandible, and therefore the oral cavity is so small. In some instances the mandible is simply compressed in utero and may, to a degree, subsequently 'catch up' in size postnatally. Special airway plates prevent obstruction and now make unnecessary the sewing of the tip of the tongue to the lower lip as a temporary manoeuvre to pull it forward.

Hemifacial microsomia.—Haemorrhage near the developing ear in the foetus leads to varying degrees of tissue destruction producing the so-called first and second branchial arch syndrome. There may be a degree of hypoplasia or absence of the condyle and ramus of the mandible, the masticatory muscles, and external, middle and inner ear producing degrees of unilateral facial hypoplasia. Rarely both sides are affected, but if so the deformity is not symmetrical.

Treacher Collins syndrome.—Mandibulo-facial dysostosis results from a symmetrical loss of neural crest cells destined to migrate by the longer posterior route into the face (Poswillo). There is hypoplasia of the zygomatic bone and a deficiency or absence of the arch. As a result there is an antimongoloid slant to the palpebral fissure. There may be a colomboma of the lower eyelid with absence of lashes lateral to the notch and hypoplasia of the mandible resulting in a lack of chin and an anterior open bite. The ears are set low and the auricles and middle ear structures may be deficient in severe cases. The abnormality tends to run in families.

Mandibular prognathism.—The mandible may be larger than average producing a true mandibular prognathism (fig. 496) or the maxilla may be hypoplastic producing a relative mandibular prognathism. Conditions which interfere with growth at the spheno-occipital synchondrosis will also produce a retroposed maxilla. Enlargement of one side of the mandible can result from unilateral condylar hyperplasia.

Surgical correction of deformity of the facial skeleton.—Many abnormalities may now be corrected or improved by a variety of osteotomy procedures. The mandible may be lengthened or shortened, as appropriate, and the chin increased or reduced in size by a genioplasty. Segments of alveolar process such as the premaxilla may be moved to correct, for example, prominence of the upper incisors. The maxilla may be advanced at various levels; just the teeth, alveolar process and palate by an osteotomy at a Le Fort I level (see page 552), the maxilla including the nose and infra orbital rims (Le Fort II level osteotomy), or including also the lateral orbital rim and zygomatic bone (Le Fort III level osteotomy). The palate and upper alveolar process may be raised by a Le Fort I osteotomy

Pierre Robin, 1867–1950. French histologist and stomatologist.
Edward Treacher Collins, 1862–1932. Surgeon, Moorfields Eye Hospital, London.
David E. Poswillo, Contemporary. Professor of Oral Surgery, The United Medical & Dental Schools (Guys Hospital Dental School), London. Formerly Professor of Terratology, Royal College of Surgeons of England.

to correct the 'long face' appearance in which the whole upper alveolar process is exposed when the patient smiles and the mandible is prevented from rotating up into a normal position as it gags on the posterior teeth.

Craniofacial surgery.—Paul Tessier established a major advance by carrying similar corrective surgery inside the cranial cavity to mobilise the orbits. Many severe facial deformities involving maxilla, orbits and cranial vault are now treated by combined intra-cranial and extracranial operations.

LESIONS OF THE PALATE

Swellings of the palate may be mid-line or lateral.

A mid-line swelling:

(*a*) just behind the incisive papilla may be a cyst of the papilla or, beneath the papilla and in the bone, of the incisive canal (nasopalatine cyst);

(*b*) a bony hard swelling in the centre of the hard palate is likely to be a torus palatinus, a developmental bony excrescence;

(*c*) a diamond shaped group of miniature white cysts seen at the junction of the hard and soft palate in infants which are called Epstein's pearls. They are cell rests at the line of fusion of the palatal shelves and disappear spontaneously.

A lateral swelling:

(*a*) behind an upper lateral incisor is likely to be an abscess or apical cyst arising from that tooth;

(*b*) opposite the molars a periodontal abscess or cyst from an upper molar;

(*c*) medial to the tuberosity and extending back towards the soft palate a salivary neoplasm arising in palatal salivary glands or more rarely a neurofibroma of the greater palatine nerve;

(*d*) a malignant neoplasm of the maxillary sinus extending downwards, usually in the region of the tuberosity;

(*e*) primary squamous cell carcinoma of the palate, usually of the soft palate.

Perforations of the palate may also be mid-line or lateral.

A mid-line perforation:

(*a*) a gumma producing first a swelling and then a perforation in the centre of the palate is rarely seen these days, a complication of congenital rather than acquired syphilis;

(*b*) suckers on the fitting surface of an upper denture causing ulceration and eventual perforation of the palate either at the rim of the rubber sucker or over the metal retaining stud. These perforations too are now rarely seen.

A lateral perforation:

(*a*) may be created during the removal of a malignant neoplasm or may occur as a result of necrosis of a malignant neoplasm;

(*b*) may rarely occur through the socket of a palatally misplaced tooth.

Palatal perforations may be covered by a denture or if conditions are favourable, repaired by flaps based on one or both palatine arteries; raised if necessary as island flaps.

LESIONS OF THE LIPS

Pigmentation of the lips and buccal mucous membranes.—Blotchy brown pigmentation of the oral mucous membranes is usually racial and of no importance. A more uniform pigmentation is seen in Addison's disease. Accidentally

Paul Louis Tessier, Contemporary. Head of Department of Plastic Surgery, Foch Hospital, Suresnes, Paris, France.
Alois Epstein, 1849–1918. Director of Children's Clinic and Professor of Pediatrics, Prague. Described Epstein's pearls 1880.
Thomas Addison, 1793–1860. Physician, Guy's Hospital, London.

implanted dental amalgam will produce a dark bluish spot. Small bluish black spots on the lips, on the skin about the eyes and on the buccal and palatal mucous membranes is seen in Peutz-Jeghers syndrome. The condition is inherited as an autosomal dominant and includes adenomatous polyps of the small bowel. These may cause intussusception or intestinal colic, but rarely undergo malignant change.

Macrocheilia.—Recurrent, chronic or persistent swelling of the upper lip may be due to the Melkersson-Rosenthal syndrome. A Bell's palsy may precede or accompany the swelling. Granular hyperplasia of palatal and cheek tissues similar to that associated with oral Crohn's disease may be seen. Cavernous haemangioma and less often lymphangioma can produce enlargement of the lips.

Cracked lips.—An indolent crack in the mid-line of the lower lip can occur as a result of exposure to cold weather. A patent lip salve ointment and protection of the lip is advised. Cracks at the angles of the mouth are described in Chapter 32.

Herpes simplex infections (see Chapter 32).—Doctors, dentists and nurses should protect their hands while touching these lesions to avoid herpetic whitloes and should particularly avoid transferring the virus to their eyes. A preparation containing 'acyclovir' promises to bring speedy relief if applied early.

Chancre of the lip presents as a painless ulcer with a dull red, clean base. As in other sites there is a sufficient local inflammatory infiltrate to produce a button like sensation to the gloved fingers. The regional lymph nodes are substantially enlarged, unlike the situation with genital chancres.

Neoplasms of the lip

Salivary neoplasms arise in minor mucous glands, usually of the upper lip. Firm, slow growing, lobulated, mobile tumours may be excised *in toto* on the assumption that they are pleomorphic adenomas. Less well defined, fixed or rapidly enlarging tumours should be biopsied by the shortest route of access, which is usually through the mucous membrane. Treatment is determined by the type of neoplasm.

Carcinoma of the lip tends to occur in older individuals and typically in men who follow an outdoor occupation (fig. 497). The lower lip is involved in over 90% of cases and it is believed that exposure to sunlight is an important aetiological factor. The lip first develops a whitish tinge then suffers repeated cracking and desquamation to form erosions (actinic cheilitis). Initially the carcinoma may appear as a persistance of an erosion at a particular site. A dry, red granular appearance with whitish flecks then replaces the yellowish crusting of exuded serum. As the tumour develops the centre becomes ulcerated and the margin everted. With deeper invasion of the lip the skin over the tumour becomes red and vascular, then breaks down here and there over areas of necrosis. The unwary at this stage may mistake the lesion for a carbuncle.

Some smokers develop a hyperkeratotic patch where a cigarette is held habitually between the lips at one place and may develop a carcinoma at this site. Metastasis is often first to the submental nodes which, as they are buried in fatty fibrous tissue, are less easy to feel than nodes elsewhere in the neck.

John Law Augustine Peutz, 1886–1957. Chief Specialist for Internal Medicine, St. John's Hospital, The Hague, Holland.
Harold Jos Jeghers. Professor of Internal Medicine, New Jersey College of Medicine and Dentistry, Jersey City, U.S.A.
Sir Charles Bell, 1774–1842. Surgeon, The Middlesex Hospital, London.
Burrill Bernard Crohn, Contemporary. Gastroenterologist, Mount Sinai Hospital, New York, U.S.A.

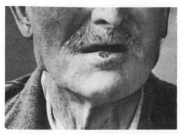

FIG. 497.—Carcinoma of the lower lip.

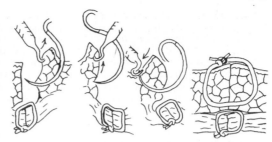

FIG. 498.—Facial wound. Method of skin closure avoiding inversion of the wound edges. The skin stitch embraces a greater width of deep tissue than at the surface.

Because the early ulcer may resemble a herpetic lesion or other chronic infective lesion a biopsy should be performed for any indolent ulcer slow to show signs of healing. Excision biopsy is not advised as it is unlikely that an adequate curative margin will be taken unless the operator knows the diagnosis for certain.

Around 5% of squamous cell carcinomas of the lip occur on the upper lip and 2% involve the angle of the mouth. These are usually an extension of a carcinoma arising in speckled leucoplacia affecting the mucosal aspect of the cheek and consequently are often more extensive when first seen. Both commissures are usually affected by speckled leucoplacia and bilateral squamous cell carcinomas are not unusual. Not only is the prognosis less good because the lesion is larger at diagnosis, but metastasis to both sub-mental and sub-mandibular nodes may occur.

As the site is easily seen, patients with carcinoma of the lower lip tend to notice the ulcer at an early stage and seek treatment. The tumour tends to be well differentiated and whether treated by surgery or radiotherapy the prognosis is better than average with a five-year survival of 70%. Carcinoma of the lip must be distinguished from a kerato-acanthoma or molluscum sebaceum described in Chapter 10.

Treatment by Radiotherapy.—If the lesion is less than 2 cm in diameter a high rate of cure may be expected. With larger lesions a substantial regression can be expected even if complete disappearance of the tumour is not achieved. External beam irradiation is usually employed, delivering 5500 rads in fractionated doses over four weeks.

Treatment by surgery.—The classical mode of excision is to resect a wedge of lower lip which includes the carcinoma. If the whole red margin shows evidence of pre-malignant change the affected mucosa should be included in the specimen as a 'lip shave' and the mucosa of the inner aspect of the lip undermined and advanced up to the cutaneous edge. Care should be taken to plot out with a marking pen the extent of the intended margins to avoid an inadequate excision. Compression of the lip on either side by an assistant will control haemorrhage from the labial arteries until they can be clamped and tied. The defect is closed in layers; first the mucosa, then the muscle and finally the red margin and skin, being careful to align the mucocutaneous junctions. The red margin should be heaped up a little so that a notch does not form as healing occurs.

If a large wedge needs to be removed the deficiency can be shared with the upper lip by rotating an Estlander flap into the excision site. A wedge shaped flap based on one side on the upper labial artery and half the width of the lower lip defect is rotated down. The pedicle is divided after three weeks and the flap set in.

Jakob August Estlander, 1831–1881. Finnish Surgeon.

Large rectangular defects may be closed by advancing local flaps from the lower cheek. Textbooks of plastic surgery should be consulted for details. Large tumours soon involve the bone of the chin and their excision involves difficult reconstructive surgery.

Lymph node spread is initially to the sub-mental nodes. Beyond these, spread may be to either side and often direct to nodes beneath the lower half of the sternomastoid. If there is a large carcinoma distinctly involving one side of the lower lip a full block excision on that side, including the submental nodes is indicated. The neck incision should be extended well round to the other side for adequate access. If nodes appear on the other side subsequently and are not fixed, consideration is given to a conservative block, retaining the accessory nerve down to the trapezius and the internal jugular. The sternomastoid is divided between the upper two thirds and the lower third. It too may be preserved and repaired afterwards, provided an adequate clearance is possible. Where there are only suspicous submental nodes and a tumour close to the mid-line, a submental block alone may be appropriate.

To remove the submental nodes a skin flap is raised from an incision over the hyoid bone, from one digastric tendon to the digastric tendon on the other side. Skin and subcutaneous tissue with the anterior parts of the platysma muscles are raised from the submental fat. The submental tissues are separated along the *posterior* margins of both anterior bellies of the digastric muscles and dissected off the anterior bellies and then off the mylohyoid towards the mid-line. The muscles should be left clean from hyoid to mandible.

Where, because of the advanced nature of the primary, or the general state of the patient, surgery is not appropriate, mega voltage radiotherapy provides a satisfactory alternative and may well control neck metastases. Preoperative radiotherapy with surgery 6 weeks later or post operative radiotherapy not more than 4–6 weeks after a neck dissection reduces the chance of local tumour recurrence. Radiotherapy can be combined with chemotherapy (Mitomycin-C) for advanced cases beyond surgical care.

MAXILLO-FACIAL INJURIES

Injuries to the face are extremely common and may involve no more than black eyes or small lacerations over bony prominences. They are often due to sports injuries, domestic accidents or fights. In more severe injuries, such as result from road traffic accidents, trauma to the face and facial skeleton occurs in at least 30% of cases. The unrestrained front seat passenger in a car is thrown forward, the head striking, or passing through the windscreen or hitting the dashboard. Once through the windscreen the face may encounter the crumpling rear end of the bonnet. Toughened glass windscreens shatter on impact causing many lacerations. Fragments of glass may be found in the wounds and conjunctival sacs. Impacts at surprisingly low speed can cause such injuries. Seat belts, now worn compulsorily, reduce the incidence of such injuries. Head restraints reduce whip lash neck injuries from rear impact, but not from frontal impact accidents.

First aid.—The immediate danger to patients with severe injuries of the face is respiratory obstruction, caused by the inhalation of blood, accumulation of clot in the airway, or the falling back of the tongue as a result of bilateral fractures of the body of the mandible. The unconscious person slumped forwards in the car with the face down is safer, as blood will drain out of the mouth, in this position than if removed and laid flat on his back! Such patients should be placed in the semi-prone, tonsil position with the head supported on the bent arm. Great care should be taken not to flex or extend the neck in case there is an unstable fracture of the cervical spine. Bleeding may be brisk but is rarely dangerous and can be controlled by local pressure with pads. Profoundly shocked patients usually have other injuries to account for the blood loss (bleeding into the tissues from a fractured femur or pelvis or rupture of spleen, liver or kidneys if there is no external severe haemorrhage).

Examination of the injuries

The vault of the skull, supra-orbital ridges, nasal bridge, infra-orbital rims and zygomas, condyles via the external auditory meati and the posterior and lower border of the mandible should be palpated in turn for (*a*) asymmetry, (*b*) step deformity, (*c*) localised tenderness, or (*d*) a localised firm swelling due to haematoma. Fractures of the zygoma are often missed because soft tissue swelling disguises the deformity. So also are fractures of the orbital floor. The ill effects of these can include diplopia which may be difficult to correct if appropriate measures are not undertaken early on.

All road traffic accident patients, including pedestrians, hit perhaps from behind by a vehicle, and who have substantial facial damage should be examined from head to toe, back and front, lest the startling appearance of the facial wounds (Chapter 1, figs 3 and 480) causes other injuries to be overlooked. Detailed inspection of the facial injuries may not be possible until the patient is examined in the operating theatre under an anaesthetic.

Soft tissue injuries.—The facial soft tissues have a good blood supply and usually heal well after injury. Only heavily traumatised and obviously dead tissue needs to be excised from wound edges. Normally, even irregular wound margins can be pieced together. Nearly all wounds can be treated by primary suture, even when treatment has been delayed for as long as 24 hours. The major exception is high velocity missile wounds (see Chapter 2).

Great care is taken accurately to replace tissues where they belong, to align cosmetically important landmarks like the mucocutaneous junction of the lips and to avoid ugly stitch marks so preventing unnecessary additional disfigurement for the patient. Rarely can a wide band of deeply cut-in stitchmarks be eradicated by further surgery. Lacerations caused by toughened glass are likely to contain pieces of glass. Tiny fragments of glass may enter the conjunctival fornix and must be irrigated out. Surprisingly large fragments of plastic trim may escape notice as they are radiolucent. If the chin of an unseated motorcyclist hits the ground it may be degloved, scooping up gravel into the interval between the soft tissues and the mandible. Fractured tooth crowns may be embedded in the lips. All wounds should be diligently but gently explored under an anaesthetic and all dirt and foreign bodies removed. Once healed in they may be difficult to locate unless suppuration ensues. Infected wounds tend to produce hypertrophic scars. Dirt embedded in grazes must be removed by gentle, persistent scrubbing as any left behind will cause permanent ugly tattooing. Copious irrigation with sterile isotonic saline solution should precede closure. All layers are carefully reconstituted, mucosa and muscle with 4/0 (2 metric) chromic catgut sutures and skin with 4/0 or 6/0 (1·5 and 0·7 metric) black silk. Sutures should be set close to the wound edge and numerous narrow gauge sutures are better than a few, widely spaced, thick ones (fig. 498). Careful haemostasis should precede closure. Large wounds should be drained with vacuum drains and a firm dressing applied for 24 hours. After that skin wounds need no dressing and should be left open (fig. 1). Often alternate sutures may be removed from clean dry wounds at 48 hours. Sutures in the nose should be removed at 5 days or permanent stitch marks may remain. Usually, elsewhere sutures can be removed at 7 days.

Facial nerve injury.—Primary repair may be indicated (depending on other injuries, the availability of good skin cover and the general state of the patient). Locating divided branches in oedematous tissues suffused with blood is likely to be difficult and time consuming. Flaps may need to be raised forward and backwards from the laceration over the surface of the deep fascia until normal looking tissues are reached and the branches identified and traced towards the injury. No easy task even for surgeons familiar with the surgical anatomy of the nerve. Substantial recovery may occur without definitive repair over a period of 8-12 months. Attempts at late secondary repair are rarely satisfactory.

Parotid duct.—A divided duct is often easier to suture than expected. A fine polythene cannula is introduced into the orifice in the mouth and threaded back along the distal segment. Approximation of the laceration will indicate where to look for the proximal cut end. The outer side of the distal end and the inner of the proximal are slit up for 2–3 mm and the ends anastomosed side to side to avoid stricture formation. The cannula is left in for 14 days to drain the anastomosis. If the distal end cannot be found the proximal end can be ligated in the hope of gland atrophy. Accumulations of saliva in the tissues post-operatively should be aspirated at intervals of several days and a pressure dressing applied until they dry up.

Lacrimal apparatus.—Suturing of the lid is performed in layers after cannulating both ends of the injured canaliculus with a fine nylon thread, the distal end of which is passed into the lacrimal sac. This thread is kept in for as long as possible (up to 3 months). Scarred duct systems are best referred to plastic or ophthalmic surgeons for secondary procedures.

Injuries to the Facial Bones and Jaws

Fractured nose.—This is the simplest type of maxillo-facial injury and like other fractures in this region may be missed as the soft tissue swelling may disguise the deformity. Fractures involving the nasal bones and septum and even the frontal processes of the maxillae can be reduced by manipulation and immobilised by fairly simple measures. Delay in treatment of five to seven days may not be a disadvantage. In the face of great swelling a delay of a few days until it subsides may be sensible. A neglected simple nasal fracture can usually be corrected by plastic surgery. Where the nasal bones, often with fragments from the lower part of the frontal bone, are driven into the ethmoids the consequent traumatic telecanthus needs open operative correction and reattachment of the medial canthal ligaments. Delay until partial union or neglect until complete union has occurred will leave the patient permanently deformed.

A lateral injury results in the impaction of one nasal bone under the other. Reduction cannot be effected unless the side away from the impact is elevated first. A frontal injury hinges the nasal bones on a fracture in the region of naso-frontal suture with crumpling of the underlying septum. The nasal bones splay out. Additional force fractures the frontal processes of the maxilla and then impacts the whole into the ethmoids.

Treatment.—Reduction is best undertaken using a general anaesthetic and pharyngeal pack. If there are no other facial injuries an oral tube is used. If there is a fractured maxilla or mandible a nasal endotracheal tube is necessary, but tends to displace the nose after reduction. For a laterally displaced nose Walsham's forceps are used first (fig. 499). The external blade is covered with thin, soft, rubber tube to avoid damage to the skin. The nasal bones are rotated first laterally to disimpact them and then medially to realign them. Next the nasal septum is straightened with Asch's forceps (fig. 500). The crumpled nose resulting from a frontal injury is lifted with Asch's forceps and again the septum ironed out and reseated in the groove of the nasal crest and vomer. While gently compressing the nasal bones below the bridge Vaseline® ribbon gauze is packed lightly up between the nasal bone and the septum on one side. The ribbon gauze is cut off at a suitable length and the other end packed beneath the other nasal bone so that the gauze loops around the collumella. It should not occlude the inferior meatus. A nasal plaster may be applied for 14 days (fig. 501) but the pack removed after 7 days. Where the reduction is unstable trans-nasal wires may be passed and tied over lead plates.

Fractures of the maxilla are classified according to Le Fort[1] (fig. 502):

A Le Fort I level fracture (or Guerin fracture) passes through the thin antral walls, including the lateral wall of the nose below the inferior concha, and across the nasal

---

[1] René Le Fort, Surgeon, Paris, defined these fractures as early as 1901 by macabre research in which he dropped rocks and other heavy objects on the faces of cadavers.

William Johnson Walsham, 1847–1903. Surgeon, St. Bartholomew's Hospital, London.
Morris Joseph Asch, 1833–1902. Surgeon, New York Eye and Ear Hospital, New York, U.S.A.

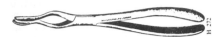

FIG. 499.—Walsham's forceps.

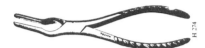

FIG. 500.—Asch's forceps.

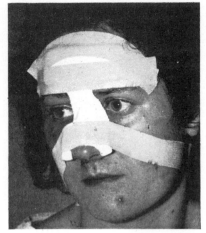

FIG. 501.—Reduced nasal fracture. Position may be maintained by P.O.P. cast (see text).
(E. Melmed, FRCS, Dallas, U.S.A.)

septum. It results in bony separation of the hard plate and upper alveolar process from the rest of the maxilla. Often the fragment is not impacted, tends to drop down until suspended by the sulcus tissues and 'floats' when the patient bites together or the examining clinician manipulates it.

A Le Fort II fracture (or pyramidal fracture) passes obliquely across the maxilla on each side from the zygomatic process of the maxilla, upwards and medially to the infraorbital margin near the infraorbital foramen and then, either across the root of the nose, or downwards to the articulation of the nasal bones with the frontal process of the maxilla at the anterior bony aperture of the nose. Fracture lines run backwards through the ethmoids and across to the inferior-orbital fissure. Frequently this central block of bone is driven backwards between the zygomatic bones and downwards, fracturing the pterygoid plates. Both maxillary sinuses are filled with blood and radiographically opaque. The fractures are usually well seen in an occipitomental radiograph at the infraorbital margins. Misalignment above and below the fracture through the posterior walls of the maxillary sinuses should be looked for in a lateral sinuses radiograph as well as possible dysjunction at the frontonasal suture.

Le Fort III fractures across the root of the nose, join the supra-orbital fissures and pass laterally through the zygomaticofrontal sutures. These high level fractures often involve the cribriform plate and result in CSF rhinorrhoea.

Gross oedema of the face, circumocular ecchymosis, subconjunctival haemorrhage, haemorrhage from the nose, gagging on the back teeth, bruising and a palpable fracture through the zygomatic buttress in the upper buccal sulcus, diplopia due to entrapment of external ocular muscles in the fractured floor of the orbit and anaesthesia of the cheek are a few of the signs of a fractured maxilla.

Treatment is best carried out at a maxillo-facial injuries centre. Prophylaxis with sulphadiazine together with ampicillin and flucloxacillin should be given in case there is an injury to the cribriform plate. A tracheostomy may be required particularly if there is also an injury to the chest or coma due to a cranial injury. Where neurosurgery is required, careful coordination of surgery is important.

Broadly speaking fractured zygomas are disimpacted first, then an impacted central block is mobilised and drawn forward with Norman Rowe disimpaction forceps. Finally the nasal complex is reduced.

Norman Lester Rowe, Contemporary. Formerly Consultant in Oral and Maxillo-Facial Surgery, Queen Mary's Hospital, Roehampton and Westminster Hospital, London.

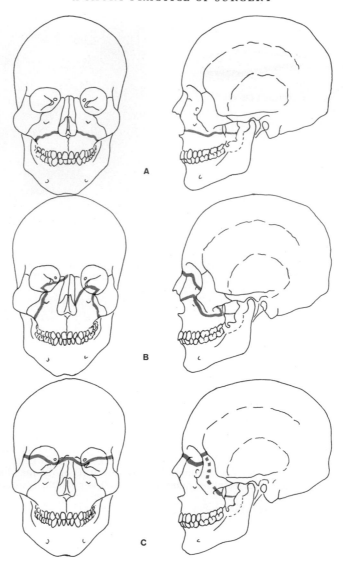

FIG. 502.—Maxillary fractures as classified by Le Fort. A. Le Fort I fracture. B. Le Fort II fracture. C. Le Fort III fracture.

Open reduction and direct wiring of the zygomatical frontal suture, the infraorbital rim and the frontonasal region and medial canthal ligaments may be needed. Fixation of the teeth in occlusion by means of eyelet wires, arch bars or silver cap splints, joined by intermaxillary wires helps to immobilise the bone fragments in the correct position and ensures proper articulation of the teeth. Once reduced, the fractured bones of the facial skeleton must be immobilised against the underside of the cranial base. This may be done by wires passed through the soft tissues from holes drilled in the zygomatic process of the frontal bone or the infraorbital rim, or wires looped over the zygomatic arches. These wires are attached at the lower end to arch bars or splints on the upper teeth. Alternatively they are attached to splints or arch bars on the lower teeth so that the maxilla is sandwiched between the mandible and the base of the skull. Screw pins may be driven into the lateral ends of the supra-orbital ridges and the body of the mandible on each side and joined by rods and universal joints again holding the fractured maxilla between mandible and skull.

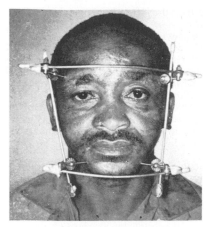

FIG. 503.—Extra-oral rods maintaining position of jaw in facio-maxillary injury (Le Fort II).
(E. Melmed, FRCS, Dallas, U.S.A.)

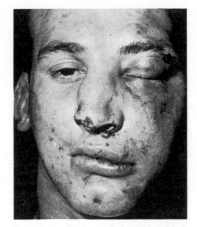

FIG. 504.—Depressed fracture of left zygomatic arch. Motor cycle accident.
(T. McNair, FRCS, Edinburgh.)

This is called a Mount Vernon box frame (fig. 503). If silver cap splints are used the upper jaw may be fixed to the skull by means of system of rods joined to a band of metal or halo which attaches to the outer table of the skull by four pins which engage firmly on the surface of the bone.

The Zygomatic bone and Zygomatic Arch form a prominence on the side of the face and are fractured by heavy, laterally directed blows. There is swelling of the cheek, of both upper and lower eyelids, usually with bruising (fig. 504), and a subconjunctival haemorrhage lateral and below the cornea. If the eye is directed medially the posterior limit of the subconjunctival haemorrhage cannot be seen. The arch should be palpated and compared with the uninjured side while looking at the head from above in order to detect depression. The depressed bone obstructs the coronoid and prevents proper opening of the mouth. There may be diplopia on looking upwards and laterally due to trapping of the inferior oblique muscle in the fractured orbital floor (sometimes this happens with a 'blow out' fracture of the orbital floor in the absence of a fractured zygoma. A compressing injury of the orbit forces the contents against the thin floor and pushes it downwards). There will be haemorrhage from the nostril. Sometimes the coronoid process is fractured. An occipitomental and a 30° occipitomental radiograph will demonstrate the injury.

Failure to reduce a depression of the arch results in a dimple over the injury. Failure to elevate a depressed zygomatic bone results in a flat cheek, enophthalmos, 'hooding' of the upper eyelid with lowering of the lateral canthus, infraorbital anaesthesia, which may be permanent or replaced by painful paraesthesia, and obstruction to full jaw opening.

Treatment.—(i) *Elevation.*—An incision is made at 45° to the arch anterior to the upper part of the pinna and within the (shaved) hair line. It is deepened to the temporal fascia which is incised. A Bristow's periosteal elevator may be used to elevate the bones but must not be levered against the temporal bone as a fulcrum. If available a Kilner elevator is preferred. This is hinged like a nutcracker permitting a direct upwards pull. The instrument is passed through the incision in the fascia over the surface of the temporalis muscle and down under the arch. A lateral elevation lifts the arch and a forwards and lateral elevation lifts the zygomatic bone. A thumb on the infraorbital margin will feel the fractured bone click back into place.

(ii) *Fixation.*—Simple fractures will be stable provided the patient takes care not to press on the injured side for three weeks. If the bones tend to sag down the zygomatico-frontal suture should be wired with 0·35 mm stainless steel wire. A depressed orbital rim may be wired through an infraorbital incision. If there is trapping of the inferior rectus the orbital floor is explored, the muscle released and the damaged floor repaired with either a thin sheet of silastic or a shaped piece of inner cortex of ilium. If the walls of the antrum are badly comminuted and the zygomatic bone collapsed inwards the antrum is packed through a Caldwell-Luc incision with one inch ribbon gauze. A finger is inserted to mould the fragments back into place, then, while an assistant holds the zygomatic bone out in place with an elevator, the gauze, soaked in Whitehead's antiseptic varnish, is packed in. The pack is removed after one month.

Just occasionally, either as a result of the original injury or during reduction, there will be a *haemorrhage* at the back of the orbit which will cause the eye to be proptosed. The optic stalk is stretched and the retinal artery goes into spasm. The light reflex is lost and the pupil dilates. The situation requires urgent action to decompress the back of the orbit or the sight of the eye will be lost. Drainage of the haematoma may be achieved either through a short incision in the lower lid, close to the orbital rim, or through the roof of the antrum.

Fractures of the mandible

The mandible tends to fracture at one of three situations (fig. 505).

1. At the neck of the condyle as this is the weakest part of the bone. Almost always the fracture is an indirect one. A blow to the canine-premolar region can cause a fracture of the condyle neck on the opposite side, a blow to the chin may fracture one or both condyle necks. The condyle is displaced forwards and medially by the pull of the lateral pterygoid and may be dislocated medially. Pain is felt in front of the ear when the jaw is moved, the chin deviates towards the side of the injury as the mouth opens and closure may be impeded by gagging on the molar teeth.

2. At the angle where the abrupt curvature concentrates the force of the blow. If an impacted third molar is present the deeply placed socket constitutes a line of weakness. Fracture lines which are across the upwards, forwards and inwards pull of the muscles are described as favourable as the fragments are little displaced. Fracture lines parallel to the direction of pull are unfavourable and permit considerable displacement. For these, open reduction and either direct wiring or plating of the fragments is usually necessary.

3. In the body of the mandible and often through the canine socket, again because this is a place of marked curvature and where there is a deep tooth socket. A bilateral fracture in this situation may permit the digastric muscles and geniohyoid muscles to pull the chin fragment and the attached tongue backwards, impairing the airway.

Most fractures involving the tooth bearing portions of the mandible are compound into the mouth because the mucoperiosteum is firmly attached to the bone and tears over the injury. There is swelling and bruising over the bony injury and importantly a haematoma in the floor of the mouth if the body of the mandible is fractured (Coleman's sign). There is tenderness where the fracture reaches the lower border and sometimes a palpable step in the bone. Speech and swallowing may be impaired and a local disturbance in the line of the teeth may mark the upper end of the fracture. Where the inferior dental canal is involved, anaesthesia of the lower lip is likely.

George Walter Caldwell, 1866–1946. Otolaryngologist, New York, U.S.A.
Henri Luc, 1855–1925. Otolaryngologist, Paris.
Walter Whitehead, 1840–1913. Surgeon, Manchester Royal Infirmary, Manchester, England.
Alfred Coleman, 1828–1902. First dentally qualified doctor to pass the FRCS. Dental Surgeon to St. Bartholomews and Royal Dental
*   Hospital. Inventor of the mouth gag, commonly known as Mason's.*

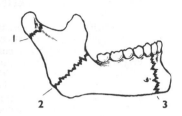

FIG. 505.—Lower Jaw.
1. Neck of condyle.
2. Through the angle or ascending ramus.
3. Anterior to the mental foramen, through the canine fossa.

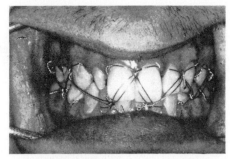

FIG. 506.—Interdental wiring for fractured mandible.
(E. Melmed, FRCS, Dallas, U.S.A.)

Principles of treatment.—With lack of proper function the mouth quickly becomes dirty and delay in reduction and fixation leads to infection since so often the fracture is compound into the mouth. Chronically infected teeth close to the fracture are also a source of infection and should be extracted. The apical blood vessels of a previously healthy tooth may be torn if a fracture passes through the socket and such teeth also may need to be extracted (unless valuable aesthetically or functionally) to immobilise the fracture. If the bone ends protrude into the mouth infection and necrosis may follow. Early reduction and the covering of bare bone with mucosa is important. Gun shot wounds overlying comminuted bone fragments need copious irrigation in preparation for surgical debridement and closure. Mandibular fractures may be immobilised in several ways:

1. By using the teeth both to reduce the fragments and to immobilise them; fixing the mandibular teeth in correct occlusion with those in the maxilla. This may be achieved by (*a*) direct wiring in which short lengths of 0·45 mm soft stainless steel wire are threaded twice around the necks of the teeth in the form of a clove hitch and twisted tight. The twisted ends of wires around upper and lower teeth are twisted together in pairs. (*b*) eyelet wiring in which a small loop is twisted in the centre of a length of wire which is threaded between and around a pair of teeth. After eyelets have been applied to most of the upper and lower teeth connecting wires are threaded through the loops to join the jaws together (fig. 506). (*c*) by means of arch bars. These may be prefabricated lengths of stiff steel tape with hooks on, or rigid half round German silver bar bent to fit on a model. An arch bar is wired to the teeth in each arch and then the bars wired together to effect inter-maxillary fixation. (*d*) by silver alloy or plastic cap splints which are cemented to the teeth. Hooks on the splints enable them to be joined together by wires or elastic bands. Even if other means of fixation are also used, intermaxillary fixation ensures proper occlusion of the teeth and prevents stress at the fracture lines.

2. By directly fixing the fragments at the fracture lines at open operation using wires or bone plates.

3. By bone pins inserted firmly in pairs into cortical bone on either side of fracture lines and joined with rods and universal joints.

The edentulous mandible may be immobilised by wiring either the patient's own denture or Gunning's splints to the jaws. Gunning's splints are like dental plates, but with plastic bite blocks instead of teeth. Circumferential wires are passed around the mandible and the lower splint. The upper plate may be fixed to the upper jaw by per alveolar wires or circumzygomatic wires. The two plates are wired together or joined with hooks and elastic bands.

Antibiotics are given from admission and until all soft tissue wounds are healed. The mouth is kept clean by irrigation and by the use of a small tooth brush and toothpaste on accessible tooth and splint surfaces. A fluid diet is required. Except for comminuted or infected fractures immobilisation for four to six weeks is sufficient.

Thomas Brian Gunning, 1813–1889. Dentist, New York, U.S.A. Invented a vulcanite jaw splint. Noted for his successful treatment of the fractured jaw of William H. Seward, President Lincoln's Secretary of State.

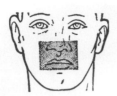

FIG. 507.—The 'danger'
area of the face.

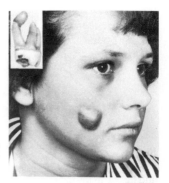

FIG. 508.—Subacute subcutaneous abscess arising from a
chronically infected upper first molar. Inset, molar tooth
with apical granuloma.
(D. C. Bodenham, FRCS, (Edin.) Bristol.)

Mandibular dislocation

Instead of fracturing, the mandible may be dislocated at the mandibulo-temporal joint, especially after a blow to the chin with the mouth open. Occasionally, spontaneous dislocation after yawning has been described, and is usually bilateral. Reduction is difficult if trismus has set in and a general anaesthetic with a relaxant may be required. If mandibular fractures are also present, an open reduction of the dislocation may be necessary, and the accompanying fractures can be wired at the same time. The aim should be to restore a 'perfect bite' because misalignment of the temporo-mandibular joint leads to a 'clicking' joint and premature changes of osteoarthritis.

SPECIAL INFECTIONS OF THE FACE

Boils and pimples in the region of the danger area around the upper lip and nasolabial fold (fig. 507) should never be squeezed or pricked with a needle, for by so doing the infection may be spread via venous connections to the cavernous sinus causing cavernous sinus thrombosis.

Subcutaneous abscess of dental origin.—A subacute periapical abscess may present as a painless, hemispherical, fluctuant, subcutaneous swelling which may be mistaken for a sebaceous cyst (fig. 508). If it is incised, pus is released, not the pasty contents of a sebaceous cyst and no dissectable lining is found. Unless the tooth of origin is extracted a chronic sinus will result (see Chapter 33).

Anthrax (Chapter 4).

Lupus (Chapter 10).

Leprosy (Chapter 4).

NEOPLASMS OF THE FACE

Benign and malignant neoplasms of the skin of the face are considered in Chapter 10.

CHAPTER 31

THE SALIVARY GLANDS

Surgical Anatomy of the Parotid Salivary Gland

Facial Nerve.—The trunk of the facial nerve emerges from the stylomastoid foramen and lies deeply beneath the surface in the angle between the bony external auditory meatus and the mastoid process. It passes forwards around the neck of the condyle of the mandible and rapidly becomes superficial. As it does so, it divides; first into an upper *temporofacial division* and a lower *cervicofacial division* and then subsequently into a varying number of branches, some of which may be interconnected (Pes Anserinus[1]) (figs. 509 and 510).

The Parts of the Gland.—Because the branches of the facial nerve lie, broadly speaking, in the same plane, the gland is described as being composed of a *superficial part* or lobe

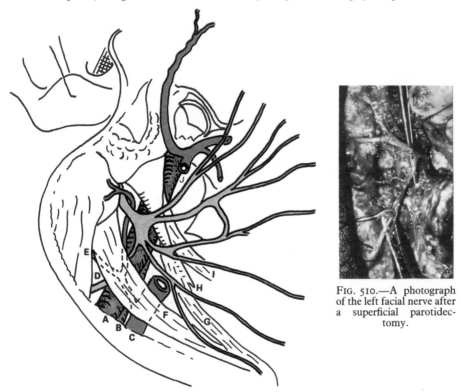

Fig. 510.—A photograph of the left facial nerve after a superficial parotidectomy.

FIG. 509.—Structures related to the deep aspect of the parotid gland. An arrangement of the branches of the facial nerve is also shown. A. Internal jugular vein; B. Internal carotid artery; C. External carotid artery (divided where it passes through the parotid gland); D. Accessory nerve; E. Sternomastoid muscle and occipital artery; F. Posterior belly of the digastric muscle; G. Stylohyoid muscle; H. Styloid process; I. Styloglossus muscle; J. The dangerous triangle at the base of the skull where a carcinoma can spread around the internal jugular and internal carotid.

---

[1]Pes Anserinus = Like the foot of a goose.

and a *deep part* or lobe. The superficial part overlies the posterior border of the ramus of the mandible and the masseter muscle. A prolongation immediately above the parotid duct is called the *accessory parotid* (or socia parotidis), but only rarely is the latter separated from the rest of the gland. The size of the deep part is less obvious as it is tightly wedged into the space behind the mandible and medial pterygoid muscle. It embraces the lateral surface of the styloid process and the muscles attached thereto and insinuates itself into every adjacent crevice.

The Duct.—The parotid (Stensen's) duct is 2–3 mm in diameter. Beginning deep to and behind the angle of the mandible it curves upwards and forwards through the gland receiving interlobular ducts as it goes. The last three interlobular ducts join it from above, the final one being that from the accessory parotid. At its termination it turns inwards between the fibres of the buccinator muscle and then forwards submucosally to open into the mouth via a small papilla on the inside of the cheek, opposite the second upper molar tooth.

Surgical Anatomy of the Submandibular Gland

The gland is composed of a superficial part and a deep part.

The superficial part lies in the submandibular triangle, above and between the two bellies of the digastric muscle. It is superficial to the sloping undersurface of the mylohyoid muscle and superficial to the hyoglossus. One-third to half its bulk lies below the lower border of the mandible and one half to two-thirds above. The upper part lies in the concavity of the submandibular fossa on the medial aspect of the mandible.

The deep part varies in volume with the size of the posterior sublingual glands and lies below and lateral to the line of the submandibular duct, in the floor of the mouth, and above and deep to the mylohyoid (fig. 511).

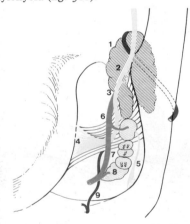

FIG. 511.—Diagram of the relations of the submandibular gland and lingual nerve from above (i.e. through the floor of the mouth, between the tongue and the mandible).

1. The path of the facial artery as it passes upwards in a deep groove in the gland, or through the gland, to reach its lateral surface.

2. The lingual nerve is enclosed in the fascial sheath of the gland at its upper pole. The submandibular ganglion is attached to the nerve at this point and is also within the sheath of the gland.

3. The submandibular duct lies beneath the lingual nerve as it emerges from the upper pole of the gland.

4. The lingual nerve lies first between the duct and the deep part of the gland, then crosses medially beneath the duct to ascend on the hyoglossus to supply the tongue.

5. The lingual nerve gives off a sublingual branch which lies deep in the interval between the sublingual glands and the mandible. It supplies the lingual alveolar mucosa and lateral part of the floor of the mouth.

6. In some subjects a posterior sublingual gland drains into the submandibular duct.

7. Minor sublingual glands drain individually into the plica sublingualis.

8. Bartholin's major sublingual gland may drain via a single duct into the submandibular duct or by a separate opening close to the submandibular papilla.

9. The sublingual artery emerges from deep to the anterior border of the hyoglossus and enters with its fellow of the other side into a small foramen in the mandible, in the midline above the genial tubercles. The artery and sublingual veins lie medial to the submandibular duct.

Niels Stensen, 1638–1686. Professor of Anatomy, Copenhagen. He abandoned medicine for the church on being appointed Bishop of Titiopolis. He is also regarded as 'The Father of Geology'.

The duct (Wharton's duct), about 5 cm long, runs forward from the deep part of the gland to enter the floor of the mouth on a papilla beside the frenum of the tongue. The sublingual veins lie lateral and the sublingual artery medial to the duct, more anteriorly.

The lingual nerve is attached to the upper pole of the gland (superficial part) by the fascial sheath of the gland. The sublingual (submandibular) ganglion may be seen attached by two roots to the lower side of the nerve at this point. The nerve passes forwards and downwards between the duct and the deep part of the gland before passing medially under the duct opposite the first lower molar. While still lateral to the duct it gives off its sublingual branch, which runs close to the mandible, lateral to the sublingual glands.

The facial artery emerges from under the stylohyoid muscle and either enters the gland substance towards the posterior aspect of its deep surface or deeply grooves the gland. It passes upwards to gain the lateral surface of the gland deep in the lower border of the mandible, around which it curls to enter the face. It lies behind the duct and is at risk from incisions into the upper pole of the gland. Small vessels also enter the gland from the posterior border of the mylohyoid muscle which is firmly attached to the corresponding groove in the gland between the superficial and deep parts.

The venous drainage is into both the anterior facial vein and into the venae comitantes of the lingual artery.

Sialography

A suitable radio-opaque liquid such as Hypaque® (sodium diatrizoate) or Lipiodol® is introduced into the duct system of the parotid or submandibular gland as appropriate and a radiograph taken (fig. 514). One-half to two ml of solution, depending on the gland, is introduced either through a fine polythene catheter, or a blunt metal cannula which is inserted into the orifice of the duct. The radiograph records the outline of the lumen of the duct system. By this means radiolucent obstructions, and dilation and narrowing of the duct may be shown. The position and size of a salivary neoplasm, or even an extraglandular mass may be determined because the related ducts will be displaced by the expanding lesion. Fistulae and abscess cavities can be displayed.

INFLAMMATIONS

Acute Parotitis

May be due to a virus, a non-specific bacterial infection or more rarely actinomycosis or tuberculosis. Mumps is the usual virus infection but other viruses such as the Coxsackie A virus may produce a similar illness. A tuberculous infection of a salivary gland is usually as a result of spread from a tuberculous lymph node.

Bacterial infections mostly reach the gland by ascending the duct from the oral cavity. There are two possible predisposing factors—either a reduction in salivary flow or partial obstruction to the duct with retention of secretions. Salivary flow may be reduced:

Following Major Surgical Operations.—Acute parotitis as a complication of major surgery is less common now that the fluid and electolyte balance is better controlled. Care should be taken to maintain a high standard of oral hygiene during the postoperative period, and patients with neglected mouths should have dental treatment pre-operatively. Serious acute infections in the dehydrated patient are usually due to *Staphylococcus aureus*, as are the rare metastatic abscesses of the parotid gland. Some infections secondary to obstruction of the duct also may be due to staphylococci but more often are due to *Streptococcus viridans* or pneumococci.

Thomas Wharton, 1616–1675. Physician, St. Thomas's Hospital, London. Said to have remained on duty during the Great Plague.

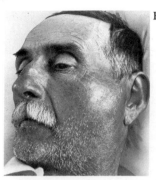

Fig. 512.—Acute parotitis.

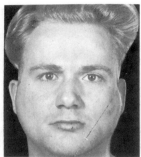

Fig. 513.—Sjögren's syndrome with superimposed bilateral chronic bacterial parotitis.

During debilitating illness, especially those like typhoid fever and cholera, where the patient may become dehydrated, even while under medical care.

Following radiotherapy where one or more of the major salivary glands are within the field of irradiation. Usually the suppression of salivation following radiotherapy is temporary, but may be permanent.

In Sjögren's Syndrome where the gland substance is destroyed by auto-antibodies (p. 572).

Clinical Features.—There is a brawny swelling of the side of the face (fig. 512). In the case of a virus parotitis or early suppurative parotitis the swelling corresponds to the shape of the gland and raises the lobe of the ear. As suppurative parotitis progresses, widespread cellulitis is seen and the overlying skin becomes dusky red. Pus can be expressed from the parotid duct, and a swab should be taken for culture, identification of the organism, and antibiotic sensitivity tests. The temperature is usually well over 37·8C. Fluctuation will be elicited only after pus has penetrated the dense fascia of the parotid sheath.

Treatment.—Everything should be done to improve the general state of the patient, and antibiotics are administered. Meticulous oral hygiene should be practised with toothbrush and paste where teeth are present and with sodium bicarbonate mouthwashes for the edentulous patient. Dentures should be left out except at meal times. A soft diet is prescribed as chewing is difficult. The gland can be massaged gently at regular intervals to express pus. If pus ceases to drain through the duct, and improvement in the general and local condition is not seen within 48 hours of the start of treatment, drainage of the gland should be considered. Drainage is essential if the dusky redness becomes localised to the lower pole because an abscess here might drain spontaneously into the external auditory meatus.

Drainage of Suppurating Parotitis.—The line of the incision runs vertically in the crease in front of the tragus, curves under the lobe of the ear and curves forward again over the mastoid process and around the posterior aspect of the lower pole of the gland. The transverse incisions in the capsule traditionally used to decompress the gland are rarely necessary. Mosquito artery forceps can be thrust through the fascia and opened within the gland at several levels to effect drainage. Both the extent of the incision and the drainage depend on the severity of the case. A corrugated drain is inserted. When the swelling reduces and drainage ceases the wound in front of the ear may be sutured under local anaesthesia.

Henrik Samuel Conrad Sjögren, Contemporary. Professor in Ophthalmology, Jönköping, Sweden.

Acute Suppurative Sialoadenitis of the Submandibular Gland

Is usually secondary to an obstruction to Wharton's duct. The organism is frequently sensitive to penicillin and incision and drainage rarely required, unless suppuration of the adjacent lymph nodes supervenes.

Recurrent Subacute and Chronic Sialoadenitis

These inflammations are always secondary to a pre-existing condition such as an obstruction of the duct or autoimmune disease (fig. 513). The recurrent attacks of pain and swelling are accompanied by the discharge of flecks of pus in the saliva. The infection should be controlled by antibiotics and then a sialogram performed. If the sialographic changes are confined to the side affected by infection then an obstructive cause is most likely (fig. 514). Where changes are present on both sides Sjögren's syndrome is the more likely predisposing cause even if the attacks of pain and swelling are only unilateral. However, calculi can be a complication of the reduced salivary flow of Sjögren's syndrome and this possibility should be borne in mind (p. 572).

Recurrent Subacute Parotitis of Childhood

The patient may present at any age between 3 months and 10 years with swelling of one of the parotid glands. Both pain and constitutional symptoms are mild. There may have been one or more previous episodes each lasting 10-14 days and affecting either gland. The first attack may have been mistaken for mumps. A sialogram reveals an appearance of multiple, small, proximal dilatations—like a snowstorm. The appearance is called punctate sialectasis. While characteristic of this particular condition, punctate sialectasis may also be seen in Sjögren's syndrome, or after irradiation of the gland.

Katzen has found that the condition remits spontaneously by age 15. His biopsy material shows an appearance suggestive of an autoimmune cause and similar to that seen in Sjögren's, but there is no evidence that the childhood condition precedes, or progresses to, adult Sjögren's. More than one child in the family and the children of more than one generation may be affected, suggesting a congenital predisposition to the condition. Antibiotics will control the acute episodes, but a sialogram will often cut short the attacks.

Children who combine recurrent parotid swelling with the upper respiratory allergic condition may benefit from regular doses of an anti-histamine mixture.

Obstruction to the Duct of a Major Salivary Gland

The characteristic symptom is recurrent painful swelling of the affected gland at meal times (fig. 515), but the first indication may be an acute or subacute infection as described above.

Proximal to a site of chronic obstruction the duct will be dilated with retention of secretions and chronic infection. Causes of obstruction include salivary calculi, strictures of the duct wall, oedema or fibrosis of the papilla, pressure on the duct due to an adjacent mass, or invasion of the duct by a malignant neoplasm.

Papillary Stenosis.—Ulceration of the papilla of either the submandibular or parotid duct may follow trauma from a denture. Ulceration of the parotid papilla may also follow irritation from a sharp tooth, or a bite of the cheek. The obstruction and recurrent swelling will subside as the ulcer heals. Repeated trauma

Michael Katzen, Contemporary. Surgeon, Transvaal Memorial Hospital for Children and Department of Pediatric Surgery, University of Witwatersrand, Johannesburg, South Africa.

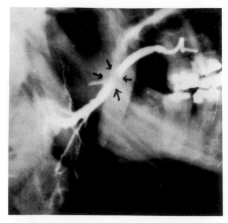

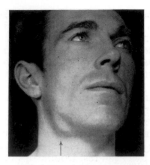

FIG. 515.—Enlargement of the sub-mandibular salivary gland due to a calculus in Wharton's duct.

FIG. 514.—A parotid sialogram showing an oval filling defect due to a calculus.

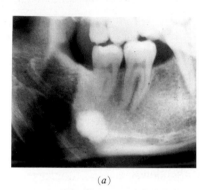

(a)

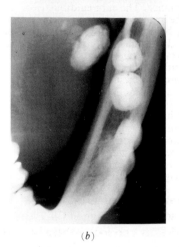

(b)

FIG. 516.—(a) An oblique lateral radiograph demonstrating a submandibular calculus, but the image of the stone is superimposed on the mandible. (b) A posterior oblique occlusal view which reveals the stone, medial to the mandible and without bony superimposition. A small calculus at this site in the upper pole of the submandibular gland is best shown by a posterior oblique occlusal.

results in fibrosis which is only relieved by papillotomy with suture of the duct lining to the oral mucosa.

Salivary Calculi.—*Submandibular calculi* are by far the most common and are relatively easy to demonstrate by plain radiography (fig. 516). *Calculi within the duct* may be removed via the floor of the mouth, although those near to the gland require special experience. For calculi anteriorly in the floor of the mouth a stitch is passed under the duct proximal to the stone to stop the stone slipping backwards. An incision is made in the mucosa over the duct and the latter mobilised. A stay suture is passed under the duct to bring it up into the top of the wound and to control it while the wall is incised to release the stone. *Where the calculus is within the intraglandular* part of the duct (fig. 516), or the gland severely damaged by chronic infection, then excision of the gland is indicated.

Excision of the submandibular gland proceeds as follows.—The gland is removed through an incision in a skin crease over the lower third of the gland and about 5 cm long. The tissues are divided down to the platysma muscle and the subcutaneous tissues separated from the surface of the muscle by pressure with a swab (gauze sponge) to facilitate closure of the wound in layers. The muscle is divided to expose the deep fascia which is opened with care to avoid damage to the facial nerve. The marginal mandibular branch of the facial nerve is sought beneath the deep fascia and retracted upwards. The anterior facial vein is found within the fat superficial to the gland. If the anterior facial vein is divided over the gland and below the marginal mandibular branch it may be retracted upwards, drawing the nerve upwards and out of the operative field, because the nerve passes superficial to the vein. The lower pole of the gland is freed keeping close to the surface of the gland, grasped with Allis' tissue forceps and turned upwards and forwards. The posterior belly of the digastric and the stylohyoid muscles are identified and retracted backwards with a Langenbeck's retractor. The facial artery with its veni comitantes will be seen emerging from deep to the muscles and entering the deep surface of the gland. It is ligated three times using an aneurysm needle and divided between the distal two ligatures. Double ligation of the proximal end is advisable as the artery retracts beneath the muscles once it is cut and a slipped ligature results in troublesome haemor-rhage. The facial artery is divided again at the lower border of the mandible and the gland drawn down and separated from the lower border of the jaw dissecting close to the gland substance. The submandibular branch of the facial artery will be divided as this is done. If the lower pole is now retracted backwards the posterior border of the mylohyoid muscle may be separated with scissors from the groove between the superficial and deep parts of the gland. Small arteries entering the gland from the muscle should be sealed with dia-thermy. A finger is passed around the gland separating loose connective tissue around the capsule and the gland drawn down to bring the lingual nerve into view. The nerve is within the fascial sheath of the gland at the upper pole and will be drawn into a V shape by traction on the gland. The nerve is separated under direct vision after which the duct may be drawn down through the loop of the nerve. The duct should be clamped, divided and ligated well forward to leave only a short stump. If the dissection keeps close to the under surface of the gland the hypoglossal nerve should remain covered with loose connective tissue and should not be at risk. Sometimes veins from the gland drain into the veni comitantes of the hypoglossal nerve or lingual artery and will be divided as the gland is separated. They must be clamped and ligated with care or the nerve will be damaged. The wound is closed in layers with vacuum drainage.

Parotid calculi are not infrequent, but only the larger ones can be seen against the soft tissue image of the cheek in plain radiographs. Sialograms are necessary to identify and locate them but even these are not always easy to interpret.

Parotid calculi anterior to the accessory parotid can be reached via the oral cavity. A ≺ shaped incision is made around the parotid papilla and a flap raised which includes the submucosal part of the duct. The duct is mobilised for a distance out into the cheek and drawn as a loop into the mouth so that the calculus can be reached. Calculi in the intraglandular part of the duct are approached through a pre-auricular incision as for parotidectomy. The duct is identified at the anterior border of the gland and traced backwards until the calculus is uncovered. Care is taken to identify and conserve related branches of the facial nerve.

Strictures and Fistulas

If a duct ulcerates around a calculus a characteristic short stricture will form after the calculus has been removed. There will then be a recurrence of mealtime swelling. Removal of the stricture or excision of the gland will be required. Fortunately the submandibular duct is the one most often affected. A stricture anterior to the second molar region may be circumvented by transecting the duct behind the obstruction, slitting the end to increase the size of the opening and implanting it in the floor of the mouth.

Some submandibular calculi ulcerate directly into the mouth and an internal fistula is formed. Unless there is also a stricture present this is of no consequence.

Bilateral strictures affecting sizeable lengths of the parotid ducts are seen. The ducts proximal to the stricture dilate and both recurrent obstructive swellings and recurrent infective swellings are experienced by the patient. Mostly these patients do not have positive tests for autoimmune antibodies, nor do they suffer from rheumatoid arthritis, and they lack the characteristic histological changes as seen in labial salivary gland biopsies in Sjögren's syndrome. Dilatation of the stricture with Neoplex filiform bougies lubricated with lignocaine gel will often relieve symptoms temporarily.

Oscar Huntingdon Allis, 1836–1921. American Surgeon.
Bernard Rudolph Konrad von Langenbeck, 1810–1887. German Surgeon.

Partial excision or a laceration of the parotid gland may be followed by an accumulation of saliva in the tissues. Aspiration of the pool of saliva through an oblique needle track, followed by the application of a firm pressure dressing, and repeated as necessary will cure this, but may take some weeks or months. Incisional drainage of such a collection of saliva, or of pus in a parotid abscess can result in an external parotid fistula as can a laceration involving Wharton's duct.

Management of Fistulas.—Fistulas from divided gland substance usually granulate and heal. Duct fistulas need to be explored because quantities of saliva pour out on to the face each meal time, and even the amount which leaks out between meals is sufficient to keep the skin and a dressing moist. Following a pre-operative sialogram a flexible bougie is passed into the duct from the mouth, to mark the distal segment. A pre-auricular flap is raised and the proximal end is sought. If repair without tension is possible the ends of the divided duct are slit longitudinally so that they may be joined by an oblique suture line which will not contract to a stricture.

If the distal part has been destroyed, or if a stricture obliterates part of the distal 2 cm of duct, continuity can be restored using a rectangular pedicle flap of mucosa from the inner aspect of the cheek which is rolled into a tube and anastomosed to the duct end (fig. 517). If no reconstructive procedure is possible the gland is excised.

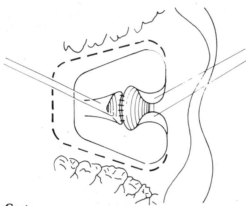

FIG. 517.—The technique of using a flap of cheek mucosa to repair a damaged parotid duct. The mucosa is tubed and sutured to the proximal segment of duct. In the case of a stricture the obstructed segment is excised prior to the anastomosis.

Cysts

As a rare entity a cyst lined with epithelium may be found in the parotid gland and behind the angle of the mandible. The origin of such cysts is uncertain, they may be related to the developmental preauricular sinuses occasionally seen in front of the ear, or they may be related to the branchial cleft cysts which more typically are found beneath the upper third of the sternomastoid muscle. A lateral dermoid cyst of the floor of the mouth which develops from the first branchial cleft can enlarge backwards until the submandibular salivary gland is spread out over its surface. It will then present as a fluctuant swelling both in the floor of the mouth and in the submandibular triangle. The treatment of these cysts is enucleation.

NEOPLASMS

The International Classification of Salivary Gland Tumours is recommended and reproduced below.

I. EPITHELIAL TUMOURS

A. Adenomas
   1. Pleomorphic[1] adenoma (mixed tumour)
   2. Monomorphic adenomas
     (a) Adenolymphoma
     (b) Oxyphilic adenoma
     (c) Other types
B. Mucoepidermoid tumours

C. Acinic cell tumour
D. Carcinoma
   1. Adenoid cystic carcinoma
   2. Adenocarcinoma
   3. Epidermoid carcinoma
   4. Undifferentiated carcinoma
   5. Carcinoma in pleomorphic adenoma

II. NON-EPITHELIAL TUMOURS

[1]Pleomorphic=many forms.

Many salivary neoplasms are distinctly rare and of interest only to the specialist surgeon and pathologist. Only those which are common enough to be of general interest will be described.

Incidence.—Approximately 75% of all salivary neoplasms arise in the parotid gland. Of these some 80% are benign and 80% of the benign tumours are pleomorphic adenomas.

Approximately 15% of salivary neoplasms arise in the submandibular salivary gland. Of these 60% are benign and 95% of the benign tumours are pleomorphic adenomas.

Approximately 10% of salivary neoplasms arise in the minor salivary glands of palate, lip and cheek and in the sublingual glands; with the site incidence decreasing in that order. Only 40% of these are benign but virtually all the benign tumours are pleomorphic adenomas.

Pleomorphic Adenomas.—Epithelial cells proliferate in strands and some take on a duct like arrangement. Other cells, probably of myoepithelial origin, proliferate in sheets. In parts of the tumour a mucoid material is produced which separates the cells producing a myxomatous appearance and then an appearance resembling cartilage in histological sections. On occasions sufficient mucoid material may accumulate to produce a cystic part to the swelling. In general the tumour is slow growing and forms a firm or elastic, lobulated mass (figs. 518 and 519). The pleomorphic adenoma is classed as benign, but strands of tumour cells

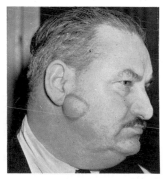

Fig. 518.—Pleomorphic adenoma of parotid gland, typical location.

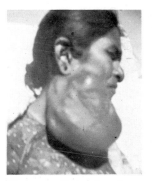

Fig. 519.—Unusually large pleomorphic adenoma of the submandibular salivary gland. It weighed 1.2 kg.
(*M. K. Rana, MS, Mandvi-Kutch, India.*)

tend to penetrate the thin capsule of compressed gland substance and connective tissue which surrounds it. Further, lobules of tumour attached only by a narrow neck of tissue may extend beyond the main limits of the mass. For these reasons, simple enucleation will leave residual neoplasm behind and result in multicentric recurrence. After perhaps 10, 20 or 30 years a few pleomorphic adenomas will exhibit rapid growth and clinical signs of malignancy. This is described as a carcinoma arising in pleomorphic adenoma.

Adenolymphoma or Warthin's Tumour.—A benign neoplasm composed of a double-layered epithelium which lines spaces which are frequently cystic. The

Aldred Scott Warthin, 1866–1931. Professor of Pathology, University of Michigan, Ann Arbor, U.S.A.

epithelium is markedly eosinophilic and the inner cells are columnar. It tends to be folded inwards into the cavities to produce a papillary appearance in section. Characteristically the stroma contains lymphoid tissue, including lymph follicles.

Clinically it presents as a slowly enlarging soft, sometimes fluctuant swelling, usually towards the lower pole of the parotid gland in the middle aged or elderly male. More than one tumour may be found at times, either on one side, or bilaterally. Adenolymphomas form 10% of parotid tumours, are rare in the submandibular gland, and found only exceptionally in the minor glands. Unlike all other neoplasms which form a 'cold' spot, the adenolymphoma produces a 'hot' spot in a $^{99}Tc^m$ Pertechnetate 'scan' so that a firm pre-operative diagnosis is possible without biopsy. Other types of monomorphic adenoma are rare. Again, they are found in older people and may be bilateral.

Muco-epidermoid Tumour.—Is composed of sheets and masses of epidermoid cells and clefts and cystic spaces lined by mucous secreting cells. The cartilage-like appearance and myxoid appearance characteristic of the pleomorphic adenoma is not seen.

These tumours are of varying degrees of differentiation and speed of growth. Mostly they are slow growing and invade local tissues to a limited degree and only occasionally metastasise to lymph nodes, lungs or skin. Some grow rapidly and are aggressive. Clincially they are usually hard; noticeably harder than a typical pleomorphic adenoma, yet become fixed only when large. Mostly they do not cause facial paralysis when they occur in the parotid gland.

Acinic Cell Tumour.—Almost all acinic cell tumours occur in the parotid gland. They are composed of cells resembling those of serous acini. They occur in women more often than in men. This comparatively rare and usually slow growing neoplasm is important in that like the muco-epidermoid carcinoma it is invasive, though, if slow growing, to a limited extent. Again, like the muco-epidermoid carcinoma, those with a relatively benign appearance may metastasise unexpectedly. Acinic cell tumours tend to be soft and occasionally cystic.

Adenoid cystic carcinoma consists of myoepithelial cells and duct epithelium cells. The former form sheets of cells within which a basophilic material accumulates in blobs to give them a cribriform, or lace-like appearance. Duct epithelium cells form strands and cords, but tend also to form duct-like structures and microcysts in which an eosinophilic material accumulates. These also add to the cribriform appearance.

Many adenoid cystic carcinomas are comparatively slow growing and difficult to differentiate clinically from the previously described tumours. However, sooner or later pain, areas of anaesthesia of the skin and paralysis of muscles appear due to involvement of related nerves. Unlike the previously described neoplasms, however, the chance of eradicating an adenoid cystic carcinoma is poor because it infiltrates for long distances in the perineural tissues of adjacent nerves and may invade medullary bone for many centimetres or travel over the periosteum before inducing significant bone resorption. Thus, the tumour is always more extensive than the physical signs or radiographic appearances suggest. The percentage incidence increases from parotid to submandibular to minor salivary glands. The adenoid cystic carcinoma tends to be both hard and fixed.

Adenocarcinomas, Epidermoid Carcinomas and Undifferentiated Carcinomas.—Some salivary carcinoma cells and cell arrangements resemble the various glandular elements seen in salivary glands. These are the adenocarcinomas. Some specialist pathologists subdivide these according to the predominant cell type, but their subdivisions are not of clinical importance. Epidermoid and undifferentiated carcinomas resemble those seen at other sites.

All these neoplasms tend, at an early stage, to produce obvious clinical signs of malignancy. These are fixation, resorption of adjacent bone, pain, anaesthesia of skin or mucous membrane and paralysis of muscles. In the case of the parotid gland, facial nerve irritability occurs first and muscle spasm can be produced if the tissues over the nerve are tapped. Later this gives way to facial paralysis. Limitation of mandibular movement results from invasion of the jaw and masticatory muscles.

Treatment of Salivary Tumours

Treatment of Slow Growing Salivary Neoplasms.—Slow growing *parotid* neoplasms are assessed clinically and are *not biopsied* (p. 570). Warthin's tumours and pleomorphic adenomas are usually recognisable with reasonable certainty. Both are excised by partial parotidectomy with conservation of the facial nerve

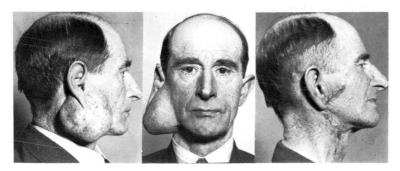

FIG. 520.—Mixed parotid tumour of over twenty years' duration, latterly increasing rapidly in size. Complete parotidectomy with preliminary ligation of the external carotid artery. The facial nerve was preserved. The patient was free from recurrence twelve years later.

(fig. 520). The main trunk is identified proximal to the gland and each branch is traced out in turn (fig. 521). A margin of normal gland and if necessary masseter muscle, is taken with a pleomorphic adenoma. The connective tissue sheath of the nerve is adequate margin at this site and only the occasional branches actually penetrating the tumour need be sacrificed and replaced by a graft. Unusually hard and fixed, slow growing, neoplasms are treated similarly, but a larger margin is taken with a greater readiness to sacrifice nerve branches. Further treatment depends on the histological report and adequacy of the excision. Most mucoepidermoid carcinomas will be effectively managed this way.

Slow-growing *submandibular* gland neoplasms not fixed to the mandible are treated by excising the whole gland with the adjacent connective tissue, but conserving lingual and hypoglossal nerves. To prevent rupture and seeding of the neoplasm the gland must not be grasped with tissue forceps or other instruments, nor biopsied.

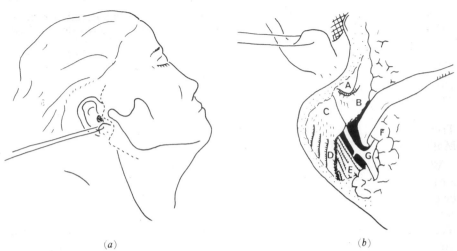

(a)   (b)

FIG. 521.—**Parotidectomy.** (a) The dotted line outlines the pre-auricular incision through which the parotid gland is explored. It starts within the hair line, uses the edge of the tragus, turns underneath the lobe of the ear and then turns again over the mastoid process to follow a skin crease in the neck. The whole or part of this line is used for an incision as indicated.

(b) The main trunk of the facial nerve (G) and the two main divisions as exposed at the beginning of a superficial parotidectomy. Each division and branch is traced out in turn to permit excision of the gland. The important landmarks for finding the nerve are:
(A) the pointed lower end of the tragal cartilage,
(B) the bony external auditory meatus,
(C) the mastoid process,
(D) the sternomastoid muscle,
(E) the posterior belly of the digastric,
(F) the retracted lower pole of the parotid gland.

Palatal pleomorphic adenomas, after a pre-operative biopsy, are circumscribed with an incision well wide of the obvious swelling as the tumour here is flattened and dish-shaped rather than spherical. The periosteum is raised from the bone, the greater palatine vessels mobilised and drawn down until they can be clamped, divided, and diathermised beyond the tumour. The wound is packed and heals by granulation. Palatal bone need be sacrificed only if obviously invaded clinically or radiographically.

Biopsy?—Salivary neoplasms shed cells if they are incised and will 'seed' readily giving rise to recurrence. Biopsy of the parotid also carries the risk of damage to the facial nerve. Pre-operative biopsy is largely confined to tumours of the sublingual, palatal and minor glands, as these carry the greatest likelihood of being malignant.

Dumb-bell Parotid Tumours.—Some parotid neoplasms arising in the deep part of the gland produce virtually no visible or palpable swelling in the pre-auricular region. The tumour enlarges medially, passing between the styloid process and the mandible to present as a swelling of the soft palate, lateral wall of pharynx and posterior pillar of the fauces. Computerised axial tomography will demonstrate the size and anatomical relations of the mass (fig. 522).

If, on examination under anaesthesia, a lump with a history suggestive of slow growth is palpably lobulated and the lateral pharyngeal wall moves freely over it, the assumption may be made that it is a pleomorphic adenoma and no biopsy performed. Other tumours should be biopsied through a limited incision in the posterior pillar of the fauces and the biopsy site removed with the tumour.

The surgical approach is through a parotidectomy incision with a submandibular extension. After mobilising the facial nerve and its branches from the parotid gland the mandible is divided anterior to the mental foramen and the angle retracted upwards. Division of the styloid process between the origin of the stylopharyngeus and the styloglossus and stylohyoid muscles completes access to the tumour for dissection under direct vision. The parotid gland and the tumour, with a covering of connective tissue, are removed together. The mandible and styloid process are repaired and the wound closed with vacuum drainage.

Treatment of Neoplasms which present with Clinical Signs of Malignancy

Where the neoplasm presents the clinical signs of malignancy, a radical excision is carried out. In the case of the parotid gland the facial nerve is sacrificed, but may be grafted using the great auricular nerve. Such other structures are sacrificed as are both surgically reasonable and necessary. A specimen can be taken for frozen section during the operation and before any irrevocable or mutilating step is carried out. Depending on the pathologist's report on the type of neoplasm and the adequacy of the surgical excision, postoperative radiotherapy is arranged. Unfortunately most salivary neoplasms are relatively radioresistant.

Radical excision of a parotid neoplasm is limited by the internal carotid artery on its deep aspect and the cranial cavity posteriorly. Excision of the parotid including the mandible is straightforward, but inclusion of the temporal bone requires special surgical expertise.

A similar management is followed for the submandibular gland with fewer anatomical restraints. Radical excision of the submandibular gland with, if necessary, the adjacent mandible and tongue and in continuity with a neck node dissection presents no special problems.

In the case of the minor salivary glands a biopsy is made pre-operatively (fig. 523). Excision with a wide margin is carried out. In the case of palatal neoplasms this means a maxillectomy. The cavity in the upper jaw is lined with a split skin graft held in place by a gutta percha bung on a dental plate which is wired to the remaining facial skeleton. Most adenoid cystic carcinomas require post-operative radiotherapy irrespective of their site of origin.

Post-operative Persistent Facial Paralysis

Where nerve grafting is not possible or proves unsuccessful following radical surgery, consideration can be given to transposing the hypoglossal nerve and anastomosing it to the peripheral branches. Fascial slings may also be used to support facial tissues and mask the deformity (fig. 524).

Non-epithelial Tumours

Haemangiomas, lymphangiomas and neurofibromas may involve the parotid salivary gland. Haemangiomas most often present during childhood and account for almost half of the hamartomatous and neoplastic parotid lesions seen in this age group. Excision requires special care, not only because of the problems of haemorrhage, but because the facial nerve is not so deeply placed in the child.

THE AURICULO-TEMPORAL SYNDROME (FREY'S SYNDROME)

In this condition there is flushing and sweating of the skin innervated by the auriculotemporal nerve whenever salivation is stimulated. The condition follows surgery in the region of the parotid gland or temporomandibular joint, but may follow accidental injury of the parotid gland or joint. Some cases are congenital and possibly due to birth trauma. It is thought that following injury to the auriculotemporal nerve, postganglionic parasympathetic fibres from the otic ganglion become united to sympathetic nerves from the

Luiji Frey, 1889–1944. Physician, Neurological Clinic, Warsaw, Poland.

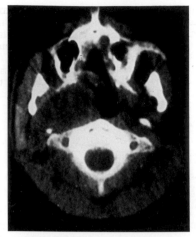

FIG. 522.—CT scan of a large deep lobe dumb-bell tumour of the parotid.

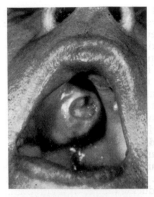

FIG. 523.—Ulcerating salivary gland neoplasm of palatal mucous salivary glands. A neoplasm presenting like this is likely to be a muco-epidermoid carcinoma or an adenocystic carcinoma.

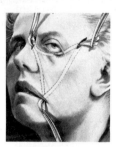

FIG. 524.—A strip of fascia lata inserted subcutaneously as shown helps to overcome the deformity of facial palsy.
(After W. O. Lodge.)

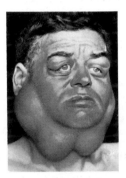

FIG. 525.—Mikulicz disease.
(C. Fischer.)

superior cervical ganglion destined to supply the vessels and sweat glands of the skin. Mostly the condition is an inconvenience rather than a real disability. Only in severe cases is an intra-tympanic para-sympathetic neurecomy considered. This involves division of the tympanic branch of the glossopharyngeal nerve below the round window in the middle ear.

SJÖGREN'S SYNDROME

Sjögren's syndrome is the clinical triad of dry eyes (keratoconjunctivitis sicca), dry mouth (xerostomia) and rheumatoid arthritis. More recently other connective tissue diseases such as systemic lupus erythematosis or scleroderma have been recognised as a possible third component. Such patients are regarded as having secondary Sjögren's syndrome. If only the dry eye and dry mouth aspects of the condition are present the patient is said to have the sicca syndrome or primary Sjögren's syndrome. In these patients the salivary and lacrimal glands are infiltrated with lymphocytes and the acini progressively destroyed. The epithelium of the ducts becomes hyperplastic, forming casts within the lumen and blocking smaller ducts. Mucous gland metaplasia of the duct epithelium leads to the formation of a gelatinous saliva in some patients. Strictures, duct dilatations and ascending infection complicate the picture. The histological changes can be seen in biopsies of the labial mucous salivary glands. Hypergamma-globulinaemia may be detected in an electrophoretic strip and autoantibodies such as rheumatoid factor, antinuclear factor

Henrik Samuel Conrad Sjögren, Contemporary. Professor of Opthalmology, Jönköping, Sweden, described this syndrome in 1933.
Johann von Mikulicz-Radecki, 1850–1905. Polish Surgeon. Described this disease in 1892.

and salivary duct antibody may be demonstrated in the serum. The lack of lacrimal secretion can be shown by the Schirmer test and the keratitis by Rose Bengal and fluorescein staining. Salivary secretion studies are conducted by collecting saliva under standard conditions using small cups applied by a vacuum ring over the parotid papillae. Gland function can also be quantified by $^{99}Tc^m$ Pertechnetate scans.

The effect of the disease in the salivary glands is a progressively more severe dryness of the mouth. Rampant, uncontrollable caries of the teeth follows. After the loss of the natural teeth, dentures are almost unwearable and lips, tongue and palate stick together. The tongue becomes cracked and attacks of monilia stomatitis occur.

Intense infiltration of the glands with lymphocytes can result in diffuse enlargment or the formation of localised nodules, which must be distinguished from neoplasms.

Mikulicz Disease.—Mikulicz described his triad which constituted (1) Symmetrical enlargement of all the salivary glands (2) Narrowing of the palpebral fissures due to enlargement of the lacrimal glands and (3) Parchment-like dryness of the mouth (fig. 525). Subsequently Mikulicz disease and Mikulicz syndrome were recognised, both producing the same clinical picture. Mikulicz syndrome is the enlargement of the salivary and lacrimal glands due to leukaemia or some other generalised disease resulting in infiltration of the glands with round cells. Mikulicz disease is due to an autoimmune process in the glands themselves and is generally looked upon as a clinical variant of Sjögren's syndrome.

Treatment.—The dry eyes can be treated by diathermy obliteration of the lacrimal punctum and the instillation of artificial tears composed of methyl cellulose drops. Meticulous oral hygiene with toothbrush and fluoride toothpaste, dental floss and a special 1% chlorhexidine gluconate preparation will help control the caries and periodontal disease and delay tooth loss. Methyl cellulose mouth washes help to keep the mouth moist, but are less successful than artificial tears.

Steroids and immunosuppressive agents will generally alter the course of the disease, but their use is rarely warranted in view of their side effects. In addition, such treatment increases the risk of ascending infection. Radiotherapy will reduce the enlargement of Mikulicz disease, but increases both the dryness of the mouth and any tendency to attacks of infection.

Patients with Sjögren's syndrome are at greater risk than the rest of the population from the development of reticulum-cell sarcoma, either in the glands, or in the related lymph nodes.

Other Causes of Salivary Gland Enlargement

A variety of drugs will cause enlargement of the salivary glands in a percentage of patients, notably those used in the treatment of thyrotoxicosis. Many other drugs reduce the salivary flow, cause dryness of the mouth, and predispose to ascending infection of the salivary glands.

Sialosis is enlargement of the salivary glands for metabolic reasons. It is seen in certain hormonal disturbances such as diabetes and acromegaly, in patients who stick to bizarre diets, and in patients who are overweight. In the case of the latter the glands may be infiltrated with fat. The condition is important in drawing attention to an underlying cause or in the differential diagnosis from other causes of salivary gland enlargement.

CHAPTER 32

THE MOUTH. THE CHEEK. THE TONGUE

Stomatitis

Stomatitis is a general term applied to inflammatory, erosive and ulcerative conditions widely affecting the mucous membranes which line the oral cavity. Gingivitis (Chapter 33) refers to inflammatory, erosive and ulcerative conditions which are confined to the mucoperiosteum (gums) covering the alveolar processes. Some inflammatory conditions of the gums may spread to involve other parts of the oral mucous membrane, in which case the term gingivostomatitis is used.

The mucous membrane which covers the alveolar process, the retromolar region and the hard palate is keratinised, firmly attached to the underlying periosteum and bone and is relatively resistant to injury. It is described as the masticatory mucosa. The papillated mucosa of the dorsum of the tongue is also keratinised and tough and firmly attached to the underlying muscle. Certain diseases have a characteristic distribution in relation to the different types of mucosa lining the oral cavity.

Infecting Organisms.—Many organisms are to be found in the oral cavity where, under normal circumstances, the majority are harmless to the individual. The number of such organisms is controlled, and their ability to cause harm is reduced, by a variety of factors such as:

1. The regular desquamation and replacement of surface cells. By this means microscopic damage to the surface is repaired and many organisms are carried away on the shed cells.
2. The constant washing of the oral cavity by saliva so that organisms are swallowed and destroyed in the stomach.
3. The mild antibacterial activity of the saliva.
4. The health and integrity of the lining epithelium. Certain oral commensals are *facultative pathogens* and will take advantage of any weakness in the defences of the oral mucosa to produce a localised or generalised infection of the mouth. Certain other organisms produce specific infections and are *true pathogens*.

The surface of an ulcer in the oral cavity, irrespective of its cause, is soon colonised by facultative pathogens such as oral streptococci, staphylococci and occasionally Vincent's organisms. There is a resultant non-specific, acute, inflammatory reaction in the tissues forming the floor of the ulcer. For this reason a microbiological examination of swabs from oral ulcers and a biopsy is not often helpful as a means of establishing the diagnosis. Where necessary, secondary infection of oral ulcers may be treated by an 0·2% aqueous solution of chlorhexidine gluconate which is used as a mouthwash four times a day.

Predisposing Factors.—1. *The patient's general health and nutrition* are reflected in the state of the oral mucosa. Anaemia associated with vitamin B_{12}, folic acid and iron deficiency all lead to thin, atrophic, epithelia and loss of the papillae from the dorsum of the tongue. The mucosae are easily damaged during mastication so that the patient suffers from recurrent ulceration of the insides of the lips and cheek. Lack of several other B vitamins can lead to loss of the papillae on the dorsum of the tongue. All such patients may present with a complaint of a red, burning tongue and angular cheilitis. Both the sore tongue and the angular cheilitis are due to secondary infection by candida albicans. Severe vitamin C deficiency ('scurvy') also causes ulceration of gums and buccal mucosae by interfering with collagen synthesis. A similar condition of the mouth is seen in severe protein deficiency

Jean Hyacinthe Vincent, 1862–1950. Professor of Epidemiology, Val-de-Grace Military Hospital, Paris.

(kwashiorkor[1]) and in sprue. Cancrum oris is another serious condition associated with malnutrition.

2. *Other factors affecting the health and efficiency of the epithelium* may lead to recurrent ulceration, or chronic candida infection. Several inherited conditions, such as epidermolysis bullosa result in abnormalities of both skin and oral mucous membrane. Epidermolysis bullosa leads to bullae which, in the moist environment of the mouth, soon rupture to form ulcers. In severe forms, gross scarring occurs with adhesions which obliterate the sulci. Hyperkeratotic patches, due to any cause, may be invaded by candida albicans. Cytotoxic drugs affect the ability of the epithelial cells to reproduce so that the epithelium is abnormally thin and easily damaged. Repair is also slow because epithelialisation of the resultant ulcers is delayed.

3. *A reduced ability to deal with secondary infection* may lead to recurrent ulceration or the persistence of ulceration of the oral mucosa which is the result of minor trauma. Cyclical leucopaenia, agranulocytosis, aplastic anaemia and hypogamma-globulinaemia are conditions which predispose to recurrent oral ulceration in this way. Patients who are taking adrenal cortical steroid drugs tend to develop thrush.

4. *An immune or auto-immune mechanism* is believed to underlie a variety of conditions affecting the oral mucous membranes. Damage to epithelial cells can result in a slough which separates to form an ulcer. Such a mechanism has been invoked to explain recurrent aphthous ulcers. Damage to cell membranes and intercellular cement substance can lead to intra-epithelial bullae as in pemphigus. If the basement membrane is damaged subepithelial bullae or blood blisters may result as in benign mucous membrane pemphigoid. Damage to submucosal vessels leads to thrombosis and a deep-penetrating ulcer as in *Behçet's disease*. Indirect immunofluorescent studies with serum from patients with pemphigus may demonstrate antibodies in the intercellular region in the epithelium of tagged monkey oesophagus. Direct immunofluorescence studies on biopsy material will demonstrate antibody on the basement membrane in benign mucous membrane pemphigoid.

If a biopsy is used in the diagnosis of these conditions a specimen should be taken which includes the adjacent mucous membrane. The fragment of tissue should be handled with particular care as the epithelium will separate readily from the underlying tissues, rendering it useless to the histopathologist.

Lichen planus, for which an auto-immune mechanism forms a less certain explanation, may also produce widespread oral erosions, submucosal bullae and frank ulceration in addition to the more familiar lace-like hyperkeratotic lesions.

An immune reaction often in response to a drug such as sulphonamide or phenobarbitone underlies the severe bullous and ulcerative stomatitis which is seen in erythema multiforme and usually occurs in association with the characteristic target-like skin lesions.

5. *Certain chemicals* predispose to, or give rise to, a stomatitis. Inhalation of mercury vapour results in mercury poisoning, the ill effects of which include redness and swelling of the gums, and loosening of the teeth. Necrosis of the bone may follow. Chronic lead poisoning results in the appearance of a blue-black line at the gingival margin due to the depositon of lead sulphide in the tissues. The sulphur which reacts with the circulating lead to form the insoluble sulphide comes from bacterial activity in food debris at the gingival margin. Now bismuth is not used to treat syphilis, the similar black or purple bismuth line is no longer seen. In each of these conditions a secondary Vincent's gingivitis is prone to arise. The excessive ingestion of iodides leads to a sore mouth and excessive salivation.

Particular Types of Stomatitis

Aphthous Stomatitis.—This term is now applied to three specific entities: recurrent minor aphthous ulceration, recurrent major apthous ulceration and herpetiform aphthous ulceration.

Minor aphthae appear as crops of between one and many ulcers on a cyclical basis. The ulcers are up to 0·5 cm across, round or oval in shape, with a yellow base and a red erythematous margin (fig. 526). They are distinctly painful, occur

---

[1]The name means 'the red boy' or 'the disease the child gets when the next baby is born' in the language of Ghana.

Hulusi Behçet, 1889–1948. Dermatologist, Istanbul, Turkey.

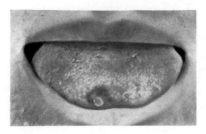

FIG. 526.—Aphthous ulcer of the tongue.

in the unkeratinised mucosa of the cheek, lips, soft palate and floor of the mouth and normally heal within 10–14 days. The frequency of the ulcerative episodes varies considerably. They occur more frequently in women than men and may then coincide with the second half of the menstrual cycle.

Major aphthae are in many ways similar, but are usually larger and deeper. As a consequence they may enlarge to involve the keratinised mucosae, take longer to heal and do so with scarring.

A chlorhexidine gluconate mouthwash will help many sufferers. Major aphthae can be coated, after the use of the mouthwash, with triamcinolone acetonide (Adcortyl in Orabase); a pectin material which adheres to the moist surface of the ulcer and protects it. Choline salicylate gel can be applied to minor ulcers to relieve pain. The disappearance of pain from the ulcers heralds rapid healing.

If the patient has genital and conjunctival lesions as well as severe oral ulcers, the possibility of *Behçet's syndrome* should be considered. In *Reiter's syndrome* there is urethritis, arthritis, periarteritis nodosa, conjunctivitis and oral ulcers. The latter may either resemble minor aphthae or the erosions seen in bullous lichen planus. They are noticeably less painful than aphthous ulcers and respond to tetracycline.

Herpetiform aphthous ulcers are quite small; only 1–2 mm in diameter. They occur in crops of many ulcers. They are probably of a different aetiology to minor and major aphthous ulcers. Despite their name they are *not* caused by the herpes simplex virus. 0·2% chlorhexidine or a tetracycline mouthwash will lead to rapid healing.

Herpes Simplex Infections

For most individuals the primary infection with the herpes simplex virus is subclinical. In others it results in a marked gingivostomatitis which usually occurs in infancy or childhood, but may also occur during adolescence or early adult life. Many small vesicles appear and rapidly break down to form small, yellow ulcers with bright red margins. They occur on the gingivae, cheeks, lips and tongue. Lesions may also occur around the nostrils and even on the skin of the cheek. The patient is unwell, febrile and has markedly swollen submandibular lymph nodes. A soft diet, plenty to drink, an analgesic elixir and the gentle swabbing of the ulcers with 0·2% aqueous chlorhexidine is all that usefully can be done until the child recovers naturally in about 10-14 days.

Herpes labialis, which appears in response to cold winds, bright sunlight, or febrile illnesses is due to periodic reactivation of the virus. Parents who suffer from herpes labialis should avoid kissing their children when they have active

Hans Reiter, 1861–1969. President of the Health Service and Honorary Professor of Hygiene, Berlin.

lesions for obvious reasons. Doctors, dentists and nurses should be careful how they handle the lips and mouths of affected patients, lest they develop a herpetic whitlow or transfer the virus to their eyes to produce a herpetic keratitis.

Other Virus Infections.—Intraoral bullae and painful ulceration can occur in herpes zoster. Small bullae and ulcers also appear in the mouth, though mainly on the soft palate, in chicken pox. Ulceration of the soft palate and fauces occurs in both herpangina (due to coxsackie group A3 virus) and hand, foot and mouth disease (coxsackie group A16 virus) but the latter is not to be confused with the foot and mouth disease of cattle which only rarely affects humans. Small bullae are also found on the palms of hands, soles of the feet and gingivae in hand, foot and mouth disease which tends to occur in localised outbreaks affecting several individuals. A large sloughing ulcer on the faucial tonsil or posterior third of the tongue may be an early cause of complaint in glandular fever.

Monilial Stomatitis.—Several clinical forms are seen of oral infection with candida albicans.

Acute pseudomembranous candidiasis or thrush occurs classically in debilitated infants. Small, thin, soft, moist, creamy-white plaques form on the mucous membrane, looking like adherent curds of milk. If the white patch is wiped off a bleeding erosion is revealed. Thrush may be seen also in the chronically ill, the elderly, or at any age during treatment with adrenocortical steroids or cytotoxic agents. 1% aqueous gentian violet applied direct to the lesions is the best treatment for the very young and amphotericin B lozenges to dissolve in the mouth four times a day for older patients.

Acute hypertrophic or hyperplastic candidiasis resembles the acute pseudomembranous form except that the tongue is usually involved and a thick, confluent, white mass of mycelia and keratin coats the dorsum.

Acute atrophic candidiasis is most often seen as a complication of treatment with broad spectrum antibiotics. Again it is the tongue which is most affected. The lateral part of the dorsum is smooth and red and the patient complains of a burning sensation.

Chronic atrophic candidiasis or denture sore mouth, produces a red oedematous mucosa over the area covered by an upper denture. Sometimes there is a papillary hyperplasia of the mucosa of the hard palate. Despite the name 'denture sore mouth', it is usually painless. The patient's denture hygiene is usually poor and needs to be improved. Further, the patients are often wearing the dentures at night, and this they should not do. Amphotericin B lozenges are sucked to get rid of the candida in the palatal epithelium, or Nystatin cream may be applied to the inside of the dentures before they are worn.

Chronic Hypertrophic or Hyperplastic Candidiasis and Speckled Leucoplacia (see candida leucoplacia p. 586).

Angular Cheilosis (Syn: Angular Stomatitis).—There are moist, infected and crusting cracks at the angles of the mouth. The cause is a leak of saliva at the corners of the mouth and the moist skin becomes infected by candida and staphylococci. It may be seen in children who suck a finger, when it is called *perleche*, or in the middle-aged and elderly (fig. 527). In the older patient the face sags and wrinkles to produce a moist fold. A similar deepening of the crease at the angle of the mouth tends to occur in the edentulous person, particularly where atrophy of the ridges under the dentures permits overclosure. Loss of the canine eminence also permits the angles of the mouth to sag. The local infection can be treated with nystatin cream and fusidate ointment, or alternatively miconazole cream, which is effective against both candida and staphylococci. The denture wearer should go to the dentist for new dentures to correct the overclosure of the jaws. Any atrophic candidiasis under the upper denture should be treated at the same time.

Vincent's Acute Ulcerative Gingivitis and Stomatitis (Syn: acute ulceromembranous stomatitis).— The *Borrelia vincentii* and the *Fusiformis fusiformis* are always to be found in large numbers in smears from slough over the lesions in these conditions. On this evidence they are likely to be the aetiological agents.

However, experiments in which material from the surface of active lesions has been packed into the interdental spaces of volunteers have failed to produce the disease. The *Borrelia vincentii* is a mobile spirochaete with three to four loose spirals while *Fusiformis fusiformis* is a large rod-shaped organism with pointed ends. They are both anaerobic and Gram negative. They may be demonstrated in smears of slough from the lesions stained with carbol fuchsin, but are very difficult to culture. Acute ulcerative gingivitis starts on the crests of the interdental papillae and progresses to form a deep crater covered with a greenish grey slough which is composed largely of necrotic tissue. The organisms are found only in the slough and do not penetrate into the underlying tissue.

In some patients the infection starts around a partly erupted widsom tooth and in others in the crypts of the tonsils. Tonsillar infection is called Vincent's angina. In severe cases it may spread over the adjacent tissues. The ulcers bleed readily and the patient may complain of spontaneous gingival haemorrhage. In developed countries the disease is not seen in young children, but is not uncommon in adolescents and young adults. It does not affect the edentulous mouth. There is a characteristic musty foetor oris.

In acute cases the patient is unwell, has a pyrexia, complains of a persistent, severe ache in the affected part and salivation. However, subacute infections may also occur with little constitutional disturbance. The incidence increases during the winter months and during war time, so that other intercurrent illnesses, or a mild degree of malnutrition may be important factors in the occurrence of the disease. The Vincent's organisms are sensitive to both penicillin and metronidazole, but treatment with antibiotics alone is insufficient to eradicate the gingival or pericoronal infection. Various local factors also need to be treated by the patient's dental surgeon. Unless the disease is controlled, severe damage to the attachment of the teeth can result.

The organisms may also infect deep human bites where anaerobic conditions exist in the depths of the wound.

Cancrum oris is a severe form of the disease affecting young, poorly nourished children and occurs as a complication of measles and other childhood illnesses. Malnutrition is a predisposing cause and the presence of erupted teeth appears necessary for the onset. Vincent's ulceration start on the gingivae and spreads over and into the bone of the jaw. From the gum it spreads on to the inside of the cheek and then through to the skin surface, producing a large area of full thickness tissue loss.

Unless treatment is prompt the child is likely to die. The treatment is systemic penicillin and metronidazole, local wound irrigation and the introduction of a high-protein, vitamin-rich diet with a nasogastric tube. Healing results but with gross scarring which prevents movement of the mandible and, of course, there is often a large hole through the cheek. All scarred tissue should be excised and the defect repaired with a lined, tubed pedicle flap which is inset with the mouth wide open.

Rhagades occur at the corners of the mouth in congenital syphilis which, when they heal, leave radiating scars and furrows. These usually extend further round the lips than the lesions of perleche for the latter condition rarely causes scarring.

AIDS (Acquired Immune Deficiency Syndrome) may be the cause of oral lesions and a patient with AIDS may first present with these. Kaposi sarcoma is rare outside Africa but may occur in AIDS; when these lesions appear in the mouth they present as reddish or purple pedunculated lumps, sessile or only slightly raised swellings. The palate is a not infrequent site. Leucoplacia or chronic hypertrophic candidiasis should also raise suspicions if they occur in a young adult.

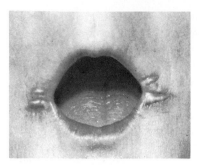

FIG. 527.—Angular stomatitis.
(*Professor Charles Wells, Liverpool.*)

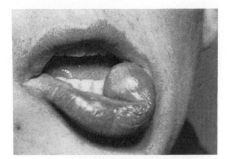

FIG. 528.—Extravasation cyst of a labial
mucous gland.

Burns

Burns and scalds from hot food and drink may cause blistering, but rarely severe injury. Children occasionally put the spout of a kettle in the mouth and this causes more severe scalding. Hydrocortisone cream and chlorhexidine mouth washes may help but little else is possible for the acute injury. Small electrical connections from a mains electric plug to portable radios and razors *etc.* may be placed in the mouth by a small child to produce severe electrical burns. The lips particularly are damaged, resulting in complete loss of skin and mucous membrane. Subsequent surgical correction of microstomia may be required; however a dentist is sometimes able to construct an appliance to keep the raw surface stretched until secondary epithelialisation occurs. Chemical burns are also seen occasionally. The commonest type is the aspirin burn. The patient places a tablet of aspirin in the sulcus against a painful tooth, where it produces a white, soggy, sloughing lesion.

The Single Oral Ulcer

The most frequent cause of a single ulcer in the oral cavity is acute or chronic trauma. Toothbrush abrasions produce linear ulcers in the sulcus. The flange of a denture which has been over extended, or which is too deep because the ridge has atrophied, will produce recurrent acute or chronic linear ulcerations also in the sulcus. Thinly epithelialised scars of healed ulcers may be seen. The tongue is an inquisitive organ and once it has discovered a sharp point or edge on a tooth, a cavity in a tooth, or a projection on a dental appliance it will constantly seek it out and explore it until an ulcer results. Such ulcers may persist for weeks or months, in which case the possibility that a malignant neoplasm is the cause must not be overlooked.

Any obvious source of irritation should be dealt with, but a biopsy is necessary if rapid healing does not follow. In some benign ulcers biopsy provokes healing, perhaps because the surgical lesion is painful and deters the patient from rubbing his tongue over it.

Tuberculosis, syphilis and various fungi can produce chronic ulcers which require biopsy, or special microbiological examinations to find the cause. Wegner's granuloma, eosinophil granuloma and reticulum cell sarcoma may all

Friedrich Rudolf Georg Wegner, 1843– . German Pathologist.

produce chronic, slowly progressive ulcers. Because of the effects of secondary infection the diagnosis may not be readily apparent, even in a biopsy.

Salivary Mucus Extravasation and Retention Cysts

Mucus cysts of minor salivary glands produce pinkish, bluish, or yellowish, globular, soft swellings up to 1·5 cm in diameter on the inner aspect of lips or cheeks (fig. 528). A few are retention cysts behind minute calculi. The majority are extravasation cysts. Mucus escapes into the tissues following rupture of the duct. The cyst and the associated minor gland from which the saliva is leaking should be excised together.

Ranula.[1]—Ranulas are extravasation cysts arising from a damaged sublingual gland. If the saliva distends the floor of the mouth a translucent bluish swelling is formed with prominent blood vessels running over its surface (fig. 529). If mucus is escaping from a posterior sublingual gland it may flow over the posterior margin of the mylohyoid and down into the neck to form a *plunging ranula*.

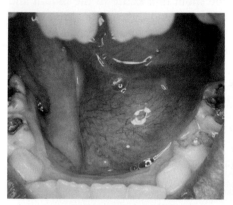
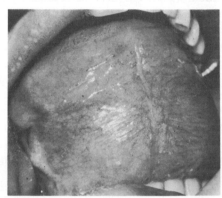

FIG. 529.—A simple ranula.
(R. N. Baird, FRCS, Bristol.)

FIG. 530.—Large median sublingual dermoid cyst. The tongue is pushed upward by it.

The wall of a ranula is composed of a delicate capsule of fibrous tissue and is lined by a layer of macrophages. Many ranulas rupture and discharge. Some fail to refill, but many will recur. Gentle dissection to identify the sublingual gland from which the swelling is arising permits the offending gland mass to be removed. It is unnecessary to explore the neck for a plunging ranula. All that is required is to remove the entire mass of sublingual glands on the same side and to pass a drain from the floor of the mouth down into the neck cavity.

Lingual and Sublingual Dermoids

Dermoid cysts produce an opaque swelling. They may be lined by stratified squamous epithelium, with, or without, dermal appendages. Such cysts are filled with a doughy mass of keratin. Others are lined by ciliated, mucus secreting epithelium and filled with mucus. These are fluctuant. Dermoid cysts may be

---

[1] So named because of the likeness of the swelling to the belly of a little frog (Latin, *ranula*, diminutive of *rana* = a frog).

found in the midline of the tongue, or in the floor of the mouth, either in the midline or laterally in the sublingual region.

Median sublingual dermoids are seen more often than the other types (fig. 530). They are probably derived from epithelial rests left as the two contributions to the tongue from the back of the mandibular arch merge together, they enlarge backwards between the genial muscles, into the tongue and down towards the hyoid. They lie above the mylohoid muscle, but bulge downwards towards the submental region as the mouth is closed and the oral swelling is compressed by the tongue. Their removal is best effected via an incision which extends vertically in the midline from the tip of the tongue to the attachment of the lingual frenum to the mandible.

Lateral sublingual dermoid cysts develop below the submandibular duct and lingual nerve, and anterior to the stylohyoid ligament; that is, from the region of the first branchial pouch. They displace the submandibular salivary gland backwards as they enlarge. Small ones are removed through the floor of the mouth and large ones through a submandibular incision.

TUMOURS OF THE CHEEK AND THE FLOOR OF THE MOUTH

A miscellaneous variety of abnormal lumps may be found within the substance of the cheek or floor of mouth or arising from their surface. Some are benign neoplasms, some are hamartomas and others are inflammatory hyperplasias. A few of the more common examples are:

Fibro-epithelial Polyp (fig. 531).—If the cheek is repeatedly traumatised at one place a thickened, submucous scar is formed which may be pulled out on to a stalk by the suction of deglutition. A lump of cheek may be sucked by a similar mechanism into a gap where a tooth is missing. The result is a soft, rounded, pedunculated, fibrous swelling. Fibro-epithelial polyps are excised through the base of the pedicle.

Denture-induced Granuloma.—Fusiform, fibrous masses arising from a linear pedicle are formed in edentulous individuals in the buccal or lingual sulci; sometimes singly and sometimes several together parallel to one another. These granulomatous masses arise as a result of chronic irritation and ulceration from the flange of an ill-fitting denture.

Papilloma.—Papillomas may occur on the cheek, alveolar mucosa, palate or floor of the mouth (fig. 532). They may be solitary or multiple. Some are a mass of tiny, close-set, finger-like processes, others have a knobbly surface like a cauliflower. They are covered with keratinised epithelium which is white in the moist environment of the mouth. Some patients have multiple papillomas in their mouth and may have viral warts else-

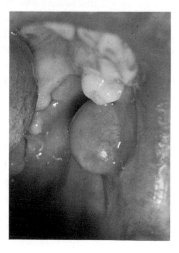

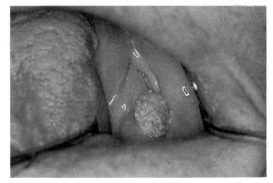

FIG. 532.—Papilloma of the floor of the mouth in an elderly lady.

FIG. 531.—Fibro-epithelial polyp of the cheek opposite an endentulous space in the dental arch.

where. In children, such other warts may be on the knuckles. In adults the lesions may be genital warts.

Haemangiomas.—May occur in the cheek and floor of the mouth. Small cavernous haemangiomas up to 0·5 cm in diameter may be found on the inside of the cheek opposite the occlusal plane and arise as a result of a bite which damages a submucosal vessel. More massive haemangiomas surround the buccal pad of fat in the buccal space.

Lipomas.—Produce yellowish submucosal swellings in the cheek and floor of mouth.

Neurofibromas.—Most often produce a diffuse thickening of the gums spreading out into cheek or floor of mouth. Occasionally a single, fusiform, soft, fibrous mass is found along the line of a nerve, such as the lingual nerve. Others may produce pedunculated swellings.

Lymphangiomas.—Tend to occur posteriorly in the cheek over the coronoid process and look like brownish frog spawn.

Salivary Tumours.—Pleomorphic adenomas, muco-epidermoid carcinomas, adenoid-cystic carcinomas, and more rarely other salivary neoplasms, may arise in buccal, retromolar, labial and sublingual salivary glands (see Chapter 31).

Facial Lymph Node.—Some individuals have a lymph node which is an outlying member of the submandibular nodes; it is found lying over the body of the mandible along the path of the facial artery as it goes towards the angle of the mouth. When enlarged it may produce a palpable lump in the cheek or lower buccal sulcus (Chapter 33).

Carcinoma of Cheek

While adenocarcinomas may arise in a minor salivary gland, these are uncommon. The majority of carcinomas of the mucosal aspect of the cheek are squamous cell in nature. In members of Western races they are more common among those who smoke heavily and drink spirits. Some arise in candida-infected speckled leucoplacia. Carcinoma of the cheek is specially common where betel nut is chewed and the 'pan'or plug stored in the cheek pouch. It is also a complication of submucous fibrosis. An exuberant papilliferous tumour may be produced by a verrucous carcinoma.

Treatment of Carcinoma of Cheek.—The best results from the point of view of function and appearance are achieved by radiotherapy. Interstitial radiation may be delivered by [137]Caesium needles or by [192]Iridium wire. The latter can be afterloaded into nylon tubes which may be placed accurately without risk to the operator and the position checked by radiography with non-active wires in position. Alternatively external beam treatment with megavoltage machines may be used.

Surgery is required for residual or recurrent tumour or where radiotherapy is not available. Post-irradiation surgery may also be advisable for large tumours involving the adjacent jaw. A small or superficial tumour can be excised and the resultant wound grafted with split skin applied on a polyurethane foam pad which is sutured in place for 10 days. Larger tumours require full thickness resection of the cheek and repair. A deltopectoral flap, previously raised and lined with split skin, may be used, or a combination of a forehead flap on the inside and a deltopectoral flap on the outside of the cheek. Adequate size of flaps should be used to recreate buccal sulci so as to permit movement of the mandible.

Neck nodes are treated by pre-operative radiotherapy to 4000 rad and then block dissection of the neck 6–8 weeks later.

THE TONGUE

Developmental Anomalies

Tongue-tie.—The lingual frenum is short, often thicker than normal and fibrous. It holds the top of the tongue close to incisal edges of the lower central incisors (fig. 533). Attempts to raise or protrude the tongue result in eversion of the lateral margin and a heaping up of the mid-portion of the dorsum. More often than not the deformity causes no disability and no action is required. However, it may result in lisping. The patient can

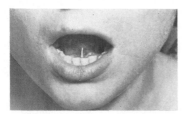

FIG. 533.—Short frenum linguae.

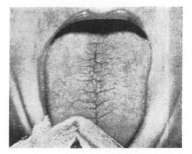

FIG. 534.—Congenital fissured tongue. Note the transverse direction of the fissures.

also have difficulty in cleaning the backs of the lower front teeth. Where division is necessary a small quantity of local anaesthetic solution is injected with a fine needle. A traction suture is passed through the tip of the tongue and the frenum divided with scissors just below the undersurface of the tongue until adequate mobility of the tip is achieved. The wound takes on a linear shape in a vertical direction if the tip of the tongue is raised and may be closed with fine, plain catgut.

Congenital Fissured Tongue.—Fissures of varying depth run laterally from a median groove, but the surface between is covered with normal papillae (fig. 534). Sometimes the fissures become infected with candida albicans (the syphilitic tongue tends to be bald and with longitudinal fissures).

Lingual Thyroid.—Produces a reddish lobulated mass behind the foramen caecum (Chapter 37).

Median Rhomboid Glossitis

A smooth, lobulated, oval, or triangular patch immediately anterior to the foramen caecum. The mucosa may be of a rather deeper colour than the rest of the tongue and firm. Chronic infection of the fissures between the lobules with candida albicans is not uncommon. The condition may be mistaken for carcinoma which is rare in the midline of the tongue.

Geographic Tongue (Glossitis migrans)

Small red patches develop with a white, furred margin. The patches spread and recede in an irregular fashion and fresh patches appear (figs. 535–538). Keratinised epithelium and inflammatory cells accumulate on the filiform papillae to form the white margin and are then shed. The condition is quite benign but the real aetiology is unknown. It is more common in patients with congenital heart defects. It is also seen in those with acute gastrointestinal problems.

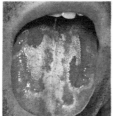 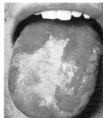 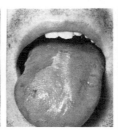 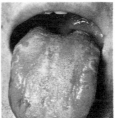

FIG. 535.—March 5th. FIG. 536.—March 7th. FIG. 537.—March 9th. FIG. 538.— March 12th, patient making satisfactory recovery.

FIG. 535-538.—Glossitis migrans—this patient had a partial gastrectomy on March 1st, followed by paralytic ileus and pulmonary collapse which was treated by tetracycline.

Macroglossia

A variety of developmental conditions and hamartomas can result in a persistent, painless, enlargement of the tongue. The tongue may be of normal structure, but large in proportion to the oral cavity. The patient can usually retract it into the mouth, but is able to protrude it to a surprising degree. Neurofibromatosis may be a cause of macroglossia, but often one side only is affected. Cavernous haemangiomas also tend to produce unilateral enlargement while lymphangiomas tend to occur bilaterally and produce a thick and cumbersome tongue which prevents closure of lips and jaws. All developmentally enlarged tongues exert continuous pressure on the teeth and alveolar process resulting in spacing of the teeth and proclination of the incisors (fig. 539).

Elongation of the tongue may be corrected by wedge resection from the midline of the anterior third or more. Vertical thickening may be reduced by wedge-shaped slices removed from the lateral margins. Care should be taken not to damage the nerve supply or the major branches of the lingual artery. While the tongue is a very vascular organ, damage to both lingual arteries can lead to problems with wound healing.

Acquired Causes of Enlarged Tongue

Acromegaly..—The tongue enlarges in a similar fashion to the lips, nose, liver *etc.*

Amyloidosis.—Deposits of amyloid in the tongue in primary amyloidosis may cause macroglossia.

Cretinism.—In long-standing hypothyroidism the tongue is enlarged as a result of an accumulation of a mucoproteinous material in the tissues.

Laceration of the Tongue

Lacerations most commonly arise as a result of the patient biting his tongue. Epileptics may do this during the clonic convulsive phase of a grand mal attack unless a suitable pad, gag or rubber ring is placed between the posterior teeth. Fractured jaws sustained during road traffic accidents may also be associated with a laceration of the tongue if this organ lies between the teeth during the accident. A blow on the face or a fall while the patient is smoking a pipe can result in the stem breaking and lacerating the tongue. In an unconscious patient the brisk haemorrhage which follows such an injury can endanger the airway.

Severe haemorrhage as a result of damage to the lingual artery can be controlled by hooking the tongue forward with a finger and compressing the tongue against the mandible and between the fingers and a thumb in the submental region. Fortunately the tongue has such a good blood supply that quite extensive lacerations may be sutured with every hope of sound healing.

A *closed injury* of the tongue or a fracture of the mandible in an elderly patient can result in a haematoma which spreads in the tongue and floor of mouth, eventually producing respiratory embarrassment so that a tracheostomy may be required.

Inflammation of the Tongue

Pyogenic infections of the tongue are extremely rare. There may be some oedema of the tongue associated with a cellulitis of the sublingual space and in *Ludwig's angina* the infection spreads backwards between the hyoglossus and genial muscles, but not often into the tongue proper. The tongue of course is raised and protruded from the mouth in these conditions because of the swelling of the floor of the mouth.

Great swelling of the tongue can follow a *wasp sting*. Classically this occurs when a holiday-maker drinks from a beer bottle which has been left open.

Wilhelm von Ludwig, 1790–1865. Professor of Surgery and Midwifery, Tübingen, Germany.

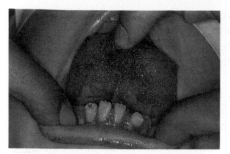

FIG. 539..—Haemangio-lymphangioma of tongue.

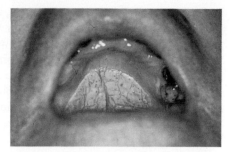

FIG. 540..—Smoker's keratosis of the soft palate. The mucosa of the hard palate has been protected by the upper denture. Notice the prominent openings of the ducts of the mucous glands. A pipe smoker.

Angioneurotic oedema, or hereditary angio-oedema may affect the tongue to produce life-threatening swelling. The insertion of a nasopharyngeal airway is the quickest way to establish an airway behind a swollen tongue, but in some circumstances a tracheostomy may be required.

Tuberculosis can affect the tongue in two ways: to produce shallow, oval, indolent, painful ulcers with overhung margins, or to produce a circumscribed, interstitial tuberculoma. Both types of lesion only occur in advanced, untreated tuberculosis.

Syphilis may produce lesions of the tongue at each stage of the disease.

Primary syphilis of the tongue. An extragenital chancre can occur on the tongue. The submaxillary and submental lymph nodes become greatly enlarged, as in the case of a similar lesion on the lip. There is a comparative lack of pain compared with other ulcers of the tongue.

Secondary Syphilis

1. Multiple shallow ('snail track') ulcers may be present on the sides and undersurface of the tongue.

2. Mucous patches occur on the tongue and on the fauces.

3. Hutchinson's wart, really a condyloma, is always found in the midline.

Tertiary Syphilis

1. The, now rare, gumma starts as a slowly enlarging, non-tender, midline swelling. Following necrosis of the overlying tissues the wash-leather slough separates to leave a deep, crater-like ulcer. Two features distinguish the gummatous ulcer from a carcinoma: firstly, carcinomas very rarely arise in the midline of the tongue and secondly there is no tethering of the tongue with a large gumma.

2. Multiple small gummas heal with scarring to produce fissures.

3. Chronic superficial glossitis causes a loss of papillae on a tongue which is also fissured due to the underlying interstitial glossitis. The result is a bald, lobulated tongue. The epithelium becomes hyperkeratotic and squamous cell carcinoma tends to arise in the resultant leucoplacia. There is a reduced blood supply to the syphilitic tongue due to endarteritis, and radiotherapy may be contraindicated as a treatment of carcinoma arising in a tongue affected by chronic superficial glossitis. The increased ischaemia which follows the radiotherapy may lead to necrosis.

Hyperkeratosis and Leucoplacia

In the mouth, a hyperkeratotic epithelium is kept moist by the saliva and appears white. The term 'keratosis' is usually used where the aetiological factor is readily recognised and where withdrawal of the irritant tends, in time, to regression of the white patch; for example, a friction keratosis, or a smoker's keratosis. Leucoplacia is also used as a descriptive term for a white, hyperkeratotic patch in the mouth, or on certain other mucous membranes. It is used

Sir Jonathan Hutchinson, 1828–1913. Surgeon, The London Hospital.

in different ways by different clinicians, but in general is used where the aetiological agent is not recognised or known or where the lesion has become established to a point where it no longer regresses when the causative irritant is withdrawn. Some pathologists require that the epithelium should exhibit dyskeratosis on histological examination of a biopsy.

Tradition has it that Smoking, Syphilis, Sepsis, the Sharp edge of a tooth (chronic frictional irritation), Spirits and Spices are the causes of leucoplacia (the Six Ss). There is more than a grain of truth in this tradition and to this list should be added *candidiasis*.

The majority of ulcers caused by broken, carious teeth or dentures are innocent, but from time to time hyperkeratosis and a carcinoma is found just where the sharp edge rubs against the tongue. Syphilis, as was described above, causes chronic superficial glossitis in which leucoplakia develops, again with malignant change a likelihood.

Smoking causes hyperkeratosis of the hard and soft palate (fig. 540). The mucous gland ducts, plugged with keratin, stand up as prominent points. Hyperkeratosis also develops on the cheek behind the commissure of the lips, on the floor of the mouth, where chemical-laden saliva flows, and on the lips where a cigarette or cigar is held. A white patch may also develop on the tongue opposite the end of the cigar or pipe stem. Leucoplacia and squamous cell carcinoma are most likely to develop if spirit drinking is added to smoking, but mainly of tongue or floor of mouth. Carcinoma rarely arises in the palatal smokers' keratosis.

The classical 'spice' is betel nut. Areca (betel) nut mixed with tobacco, spices and slaked lime is wrapped in a betel leaf (from the plant *Piper betle*). Leucoplacia develops adjacent to where the 'pan' is normally held in the mouth, usually on the cheek and the side of the tongue. Another leaf, Qat, is chewed in the Yemen.

The relationship of candida albicans to leucoplacia is incompletely understood. Leucoplacia appears to arise following long-standing candida infection (*chronic hypertrophic candidiasis*). In other instances the candida seems to be a secondary invader of the hypertrophic epithelium. The clinical appearance may be speckled white on a pink background rather than a uniform white.

Speckled leucoplacia is particularly prone to develop a carcinoma. Initially in the development of leucoplacia there is a hyperkeratosis with a small increase in the prominence of the rete pegs. Lymphocytes and plasma cells accumulate in the dermal papillae. At this stage there is a milky blush on the mucosal surface. Later there is a marked increase in the thickness of the epithelium, the rete pegs elongate (acanthosis) and the round cell infiltration becomes quite dense (fig. 541). Mitoses increase in number among the basal cells. Clinically there is now a distinct, paint-like, smooth, white patch which is dry and rough to the touch. Finally mitoses appear in the cells above the basal layer and some cells become keratinised before reaching the surface (dyskeratosis). The leucoplacia is then only a step away from carcinoma *in situ* and the development of a frank squamous cell or verrucous carcinoma. At the dyskeratotic stage patchy loss of the keratinised layer tends to occur to give a patch-work appearance of red and white (fig. 542). A warty appearance of the surface heralds the development of a carcinoma.

Opinions vary as to the risk of carcinomatous change and what is advised depends partly on the extent of the lesion and partly on the judgement of an

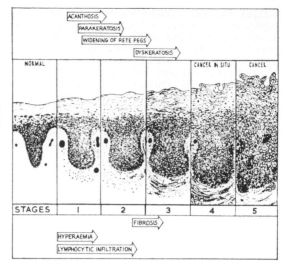

FIG. 541.—Leucoplacia. Diagram of the histological stages of leucoplacia leading to carcinoma.

experienced clinician. The patient should be councilled to give up identified irritants, then early lesions may disappear after some months but will return promptly if the old habits are resumed. Small white patches may be excised and large ones biopsied. A prolonged treatment with local nystatin or amphotericin B should be tried if candida are present. Hyperkeratotic lesions without premalignant change should be watched and monitored by exfoliative cytological examinations from time to time.

Dyskeratotic lesions and carcinoma *in situ* should be excised and the area grafted.

Where there is a likelihood of malignant change, this may not be confined to the obvious white patches however. In some months the whole of the mucosal surface is unstable and at risk. Atrophic red areas are as likely to undergo malignant change as the white patches.

Radiotherapy will get rid of the leucoplacia, though the hyperkeratosis tends to reappear after months or years. Unfortunately there is evidence that radiotherapy increases the likelihood of malignant change.

Other Hyperkeratotic Lesions.—Other conditions which produce white patches are: *lichen planus*, which characteristically produces a striated and lace-like appearance, but may form a plaque. White patches are sometimes seen in *discoid lupus erythematosis*. The *white sponge naevus* has a folded appearance and covers both cheeks and the floor of the mouth. It is inherited in some cases.

The symmetrical white patch of the underside of the tongue and sublingual region is also considered to be a developmental lesion, but can give rise to a squamous cell carcinoma.

Leucokeratosis mucosae oris is another congenital abnormality in which all the oral mucous membranes have a filmy white appearance.

Submucous Fibrosis.—Submucous fibrosis produces a mottled or marbled pallor of the mucosa of cheeks, palate, tongue and gingivae, but in this case the pallor is due to collagen deposited in the submucosa. The lips and cheeks become stiff and lose their elasticity. Bands of fibrous tissues develop beneath the mucosa and limit jaw movement so that opening of the mouth becomes greatly restricted. It is thought that the condition results from a hypersensitivity to chilli. Some of the chemical constituents of the betel nut chew (Pan) also may be causative (see leucoplacia). Squamous cell carcinoma is a not infrequent complication.

Hairy Tongue.—The keratinised layer fails to desquamate normally from the filiform papillae and becomes greatly elongated to resemble a coating of hair. The 'hair' may take on various colours due to the presence of chromogenic organisms to produce a black or brown hairy tongue. Sometimes, following the use of antibiotics, the normal filiform papillae becomes slightly lengthened by keratin and coloured black by antibiotic-resistant organisms such as fungi. This form of black hairy tongue clears up soon after the use of the antibiotic ceases. True hairy tongue is more intractable, but can be kept under control by mechanical scraping. Both conditions must not be confused with the normal furring of the tongue in an ill patient. Dehydration and lack of mechanical cleaning in a patient who is not eating normally combine to let keratinised cells accumulate on the filiform papillae. Bacteria and food debris accumulate among the papillae. Heavy smoking increases the keratinisation of the papillae and stains the fur black and brown to make it more obvious.

Ulcers of the Tongue

It is advisable at this stage to review the more common types of ulcers of the tongue, as their differential diagnosis is so important.

Dental Ulcers.—Mostly occur at the side of the tongue and an obvious cause will be seen. This may be a carious and broken tooth, or a broken denture. Usually the ulcer lies in relation to the sharp object at rest so the relationship is not apparent when the tongue is protruded for inspection. More extensive oval ulcers may occur to one side of the upper surface in relation to a sharp palatal cusp of an upper tooth, or even close to the midline and related to a rough or fractured surface of an upper denture. The dorsum of tongue is reasonably tough but once a rough surface is discovered the patient may explore it and habitually run the tongue against it.

If the ulcer does not heal promptly when the apparent cause is removed, or if there are features suggestive of carcinoma, it *must* be biopsied. Often a biopsy will provoke an indolent, innocent ulcer to heal.

Post-pertussis ulcers occur on the upper part of the lingual frenum and the undersurface of the tip in patients who protrude the tongue over the lower incisors during bouts of coughing; typically with whooping cough.

Aphthous ulcers (p. 575).

Ulcers in lichen planus, pemphigus, erythema multiforme *etc.* (p. 575).

Syphilitic ulcers (p. 585) occur typically in the midline.

Tuberculous ulcers (p. 585) occur on the dorsum, towards the midline or near the tip and irregular with undermined margins. Pale, indolent, granulations in the floor, sometimes with a thin slough.

Malignant ulcer (p. 590).—This is usually a squamous cell carcinoma, but may be a salivary adenocarcinoma or a lympho-epithelioma when the ulcer is on the posterior third.

Neurological Lesions of the Tongue

Common sites of surgical damage to the *lingual nerve* are at the upper pole of the submandibular salivary gland, beneath the mucoperiosteum lingual to the third molar and where the nerve crosses beneath Wharton's duct (Chapter 31) in the floor of the mouth. Return of sensation may be imperfect (paraesthesia) or accompanied by causalgic pain. Another cause of lingual neuralgia is as an aftermath of herpes zoster. Pain and anaesthesia, often with referred pain to the ear, result from invasion by a malignant neoplasm.

Hemiatrophy follows damage to the *hypoglossal nerve*, either during the extracapsular removal of the submandibular gland, or as the carotids are approached, high in the neck

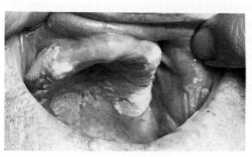
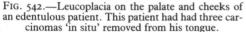

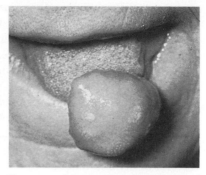

FIG. 542.—Leucoplacia on the palate and cheeks of an edentulous patient. This patient had had three carcinomas 'in situ' removed from his tongue.

FIG. 543.—A large pedunculated lipoma of the tongue.

during a block dissection. In the former location the nerve is accompanied by easily damaged *veni comitantes* and the nerve can be included in hastily applied artery forceps. Paralysis of the musculature on the same side and deviation towards the affected side on protrusion are seen.

Glossodynia occurs typically in middle-aged and elderly women. Often no cause can be found. Sometimes there is an atrophic candidiasis. Sjögren's syndrome (Chapter 31) and diabetes are two possible underlying conditions which should be considered if this is so. Some middle-aged patients complain of an unpleasant change in taste. The abnormal sensation can be confirmed by appropriate taste tests. The cause is unknown.

BENIGN NEOPLASMS

Benign neoplasms are uncommon, compared with squamous cell carcinoma.

Papilloma (p. 581) must be distinguished from the rare Hutchinson's wart (p. 585) which resembles a pinkish, soft, cauliflower-shaped papilloma. Papillomas are readily excised, or if multiple can be treated with a small cryoprobe.

Fibro-epithelial polyps (p. 581), usually small and opposite a source of mild, chronic irritation such as a gap between the lower incisor teeth.

Pregnancy tumour (Chapter 33), usually found on the gum, but can occur on the tongue.

Haemangioma and lymphangioma (p. 582).

Plexiform neuroma and neurofibroma (p. 582).

Lipoma is another uncommon entity recognised by its softness and yellow colour. Rarely gets large before advice is sought, but see fig. 543.

Osteoma of the tongue is a clinical curiosity. A hard swelling found beneath the foramen caecum or in the posterior third of tongue.

Sublingual varicosities should not be confused with a cavernous haemangioma. The sublingual veins are greatly dilated and tortuous in this condition. Initially small veins enlarge to produce a caviare appearance, then the larger ones. Not uncommon in the elderly. Reputed to indicate chronic heart failure, but this is not so.

Granular cell myoblastoma produces a firm mass in a mobile tongue. The overlying mucous membrane is smooth and often hyperkeratotic. A biopsy of the epithelium alone reveals pseudo-epitheliomatous hyperplasia which may be mistaken for carcinoma. A deeper biopsy reveals the eosinophilic granular cells. A benign, but not encapsulated lesion which is cured by conservative local excision.

Juvenile fibroma produces a softer, central, slowly enlarging lump. At operation this benign tumour has no readily discerned margin from the adjacent muscle, consequently is not easy to remove, particularly as it tends to occur in the small tongues of young children.

CARCINOMA OF THE TONGUE

Since 1910 there has been a decreasing incidence of carcinoma of the tongue in *males*. Possible factors bringing this about are: more efficient treatment of syphilis so that while this disease is still common, the late effects are rare; the passing of the clay pipe, improved standards of oral hygiene and oral health, and possibly a decrease in the consumption of spirits. While the reduction of the incidence in males is gratifying, there has been an increase in females (Russell), possibly related to an increase in female smokers, so that the sex incidence is now equal.

Clinical Features. As in carcinoma in other situations, early stages of the disease are virtually symptomless. Observant and fastidious patients may seek advice for a comparatively small lesion. Others may mention it in passing to doctor or dentist. Because the mouth is so easily examined, doctors should inspect the oral cavity and tongue whenever the fauces need to be examined. Dentists likewise should be on the look out for suspicious lesions when they examine a patient.

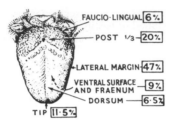

FIG. 544.—Relative frequency of the seat of carcinoma of the tongue.
(*Birmingham United Hospitals' Statistics.*)

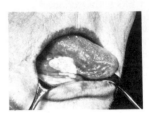

FIG. 545.—Carcinomatous ulcer of the tongue.
(*Denis Bodenham, FRCS, Bristol.*)

Carcinoma of Tongue may Present as:

1. An oval, raised, papillated plaque with white keratin flecks on the surface.
2. An ulcer with sloughing from an indurated base and with everted margins (fig. 545).
3. A deep, often infected, fissure with surrounding induration.
4. A lobulated, indurated mass, possibly with seemingly normal mucosa over it, sometimes with yellow patches of submucosal necrosis which appear like pointing abscesses.

Many patients seem to disregard the lesion in its early stages or are too frightened to seek help until a large and offensive tumour is present. These more advanced cases present with:

1. *Pain in the tongue*, which is initially due to infection and ulceration but later is due to involvement of the lingual nerve. Once the lingual nerve is involved there may be referred *pain in the ear*. Pain on swallowing or pain in the back of the tongue may mean a carcinoma of the posterior third. In such cases careful inspection of tongue and vallecula in the conscious patient with a laryngeal mirror, or direct examination with a laryngoscope with the patient under anesthesia, is essential. The posterior third can be palpated, but induration due to neoplasm is not easily appreciated because of the lumpiness of the lingual tonsils.

2. *Salivation.*—Pain promotes salivation and a stiff, lumpy, partially fixed tongue makes swallowing difficult. The elderly man sitting in outpatients and spitting into a handkerchief may well have a carcinoma of tongue.

Marion H. Russell, 1907–1966. Medical Statistician, Christie Hospital, Manchester, England.

3. *Ankyloglossia.*—Inability to protrude the tongue or deviation to one side means it is fixed by extensive infiltration of the floor of the mouth.

4. *Dysphagia.*—Difficulty in swallowing may occur with any advanced lingual carcinoma, but is more pronounced when the growth is in the posterior third.

5. *Inability to articulate clearly.*

6. *Foetor.*—Once necrosis occurs the lesion becomes grossly infected and highly offensive.

7. *A lump in the neck* due to secondary deposits in the draining lymph nodes.

8. *Alteration in the voice* may be a first indication of a carcinoma of the posterior third. In this inacessible situation a tumour may escape notice. Such tumours are more often anaplastic than those of the anterior third and a large tumour with nodes in the neck may be present by the time the diagnosis is made.

Spread of the Disease

Local Spread.—Carcinoma of the anterior two-thirds usually starts on the lateral margin and frequently reaches the floor of the mouth before it extends across the midline. At the junction of anterior two-thirds and posterior third it may invade the mandible. Carcinoma of the posterior third spreads laterally into the tonsil, side of the pharynx and cervical spine and up into the soft palate, posteriorly into the epiglottis and downwards towards the larynx, and across to the other side of the tongue.

Lymphatic Spread.—Metastasis to the submandibular nodes, particularly if the floor of the mouth is involved, means that tumour is already present close to the periosteum of the mandible and resection of the relevant segment of the mandible may be necessary to ensure surgical clearance. Once the anterior part of the floor of the mouth is involved bilateral spread to neck nodes is common.

Blood Stream Spread.—Death tends to occur as a result of uncontrollable primary tumour or lymphatic spread so that distant metastasis rarely manifests itself. Metastasis by the blood stream is more likely from posterior third than anterior two-thirds tumours.

Terminal Events

Death from an uncontrolled primary tumour occurs as a result of:

(i) Inhalation bronchopneumonia as a result of inhalation of infected material from necrotic neoplasm.

(ii) Haemorrhage from erosion of the lingual artery, or in the case of a carcinoma of the posterior third, erosion of the internal carotid.

(iii) Combined cancerous cachexia and starvation due to the pain and difficulty of attempting to swallow where a large tumour replaces the tongue, or where there is compression of pharynx or oesophagus by metastatic deposits in lymph nodes.

(iv) Asphyxia, which is most often due to pressure on the air passages from enlarged and fixed carcinomatous lymph nodes. Sometimes obstruction is due to oedema of the glottis.

Treatment

Surgery or radiotherapy or a combination of the two. The most appropriate use of chemotherapy in relation to the main methods of treatment is not yet settled.

Establishment of the Diagnosis.—An adequate biopsy must precede treatment. But there is no place for the so-called excision biopsy. Only rarely will such an excision be generous enough to avoid incomplete removal and local recurrence. Indeed should the lesion prove not to be malignant, unnecessary mutilation will have been inflicted by such an excision.

Preliminary Preparation.—Teeth are scaled and polished and oral hygiene established. Where the surface of the lesion is necrotic or infected, frequent irrigation with eusol is required. Any teeth which will be in a field of substantial irradiation should be extracted.

Tests for syphilis should be carried out and treatment initiated if necessary. In some cases a diagnosis of syphilis will mean that radiotherapy is not advised.

Definitive Treatment

1. *Carcinoma in situ* may be excised with a 1 cm margin and to a depth of about 0·5 cm. Excision wounds on the lateral border may be closed by undermining and advancing mucosa from the floor of the mouth. Larger defects are grafted with split skin.

2. *Lesions less than 2 cm* are treated primarily with radiotherapy, because if treatment is successful there is virtually no functional disability. For lesions of the anterior two-thirds of the tongue of this size, and where there are no palpable lymph nodes, interstitial irradiation with ^{137}Caesium needles or ^{192}Iridium wire is used. A close watch is kept upon the patient, with follow-up appointments at monthly intervals. If regression is incomplete, or recurrence occurs, or neck nodes become suspiciously palpable, surgery is added.

3. *A small carcinoma confined to the lateral border* may be removed by local excision with a generous 1·5 cm of margin beyond visible and palpable disease. The configuration of the resection depends upon the site of the tumour, but approximates to a hemiglossectomy. The success of the operation depends upon the care with which the excision is carried laterally below the neoplasm for it is here that the operator may fail to maintain an adequate margin.

If there are palpable nodes a block dissection of neck is required. Advantage should be taken to tie the lingual artery before the primary lesion is resected as bleeding will be reduced and surgical precision increased. An in-continuity resection facilitates an adequate margin on the deep aspect of the primary tumour.

If a block dissection becomes necessary resection of the primary site should be considered even if it is apparently controlled by previous radiotherapy. Pre-operative irradiation of the neck to between 4000 and 4500 rad may be advisable.

4. *Primary lesions larger than 2 cm* are usually irradiated by external beam irradiation. The submandibular nodes may be included in the field of irradiation even if no nodes are palpable. Great care is required with follow up to avoid extensive spread occurring should the treatment fail to achieve healing. Large tumours require a submandibular dissection to enable adequate excision. Because this makes a subsequent block dissection difficult a prophylactic neck dissection should be considered if local control is not achieved, even if no nodes are palpable.

5. *If there is a large tumour with palpable nodes* both primary and the neck are irradiated to 4500 rad then, 6–8 weeks later, an in-continuity resection is carried out. (Surgery should be undertaken within three months of the irradiation but after the reaction has subsided.) Where the tumour extends on to the floor of the mouth, or up to the anterior pillar of the fauces, the mandible should be included in the specimen.

6. *Tumours which involve the tip of the tongue* may metastasise to the submental nodes. Tumours which involve the anterior part of the floor of the mouth are likely to metastasise to both sides of the neck. Prophylactic irradiation of the second side should be considered, even if nodes are not palpable.

7. *Bilateral neck nodes* may be dealt with by various strategies without sacrifice of both

internal jugulars. Resection of both internal jugulars is to be avoided because of the high mortality due to post-operative cerebral venous engorgement and oedema of the head and face should the patient survive.

(i) Bilateral block dissections may be carried out, but the internal jugular left on the least involved side. The operation should be completed first on the side in which the vein is to be retained.

(ii) Alternatively low-dose pre-operative irradiation should be given to the worst side followed by a block dissection and a therapeutic dose given to the other side. Contrary to previous opinion, squamous cell carcinoma metastases in lymph nodes will respond to megavoltage irradiation. The problem is that recurrence of tumour after irradiation of nodes is often not amenable to salvage surgery.

(iii) A full block on one side and a suprahyoid block on the other is another possible form of treatment.

Pre-operative irradiation of the neck reduces the incidence of diffuse, local recurrence of tumour whch is difficult to differentiate from post-operative induration.

8. *Posterior extension of the carcinoma* requires division of the lower lip and section of the mandible for access. The incision should be vertical through the lip, curved around the chin pad, and then broken into a **Z** until the hyoid crease is reached. Posterior third primary tumours are treated almost entirely by external beam irradiation as they are rarely amenable to surgery.

Where the anterior part of the mandible is sacrificed with a carcinoma involving the floor of the mouth, a Bowerman-Conroy implant is inserted and the hyoid and tongue suspended from it (Wilson).

Repair.—The tip of the tongue may be repaired by suture. Small lateral defects can be closed by advancing floor of mouth mucosa (fig. 546).

There are two ways in which mobile raw surfaces in the mouth, like those resulting from section of the tongue, can be covered with a Thiersch graft (Chapter 10); by quilting on the graft (McGregor) and by use of a foam plastic pad (Seward). In McGregor's method small, plain, interrupted, catgut sutures are placed at the corners of squares across the graft after suture of the periphery. Tiny stab incisions are made in the centres of the square to let out any exudate or haematoma. Alternatively (Seward), a pad of 1 cm thick polyurethane foam is cut slightly larger than the defect, and the Thiersch graft is draped over it, wrapped round, and sutured to the outer surface. A suture transfixes the centre of the pad, picks up the centre of the defect and passed back through the pad and is tied. The margins of the pad are then sewn to the margins of the defect (fig. 547).

Where there is a sizeable loss of tongue a forehead flap makes an excellent repair. The forehead flap is brought into the mouth deep to the zygomatic arch. Adequate space to bring it through may be created by resecting the coronoid process, by sectioning the zygomatic bone or by resection of the anterior part of the temporalis muscle (fig. 548).

For very large defects of tongue and floor of mouth a delto-pectoral flap must be brought in via the submandibular wound. It can be de-epithelialised over a strip to enable the oral wound to be sealed by a suture line. Where a block dissection of neck has been performed a pectoral myocutaneous flap may be brought up to repair the tongue. The pedicle, composed of a strip of pectoralis major muscle and vessels can be used to cover the carotids under the neck skin flaps.

Palliation.—Where there is a large, unresectable primary tumour or where there are already fixed nodes in the neck a full dose of therapeutic irradiation should be delivered to the tongue. Where irradiation has been used already and either primary or the nodes are unresectable, resection of the primary alone may make the patient more comfortable. Necrotic lingual carcinoma is difficult to tolerate for the patients, the relatives or the attendants. Irrigation of the mouth with eusol and hydrogen peroxide can reduce the local infection and the foul smell.

In some patients chemotherapy with the Price-Hill regimen may be helpful and indeed, in some patients, of substantial benefit. This treatment involves the administration of a carefully selected list of cytotoxic drugs to a precise schedule. In 1975 Price and others reported a trial involving the use of the following drugs in the treatment of oral squamous

John Ernest Bowerman, Contemporary. Oral Surgeon, Westminster Hospital and Queen Mary's Hospital, Roehampton, London.
B. Conroy, Contemporary. Senior Chief Maxillo-Facial Technician, Queen Mary's Hospital, Roehampton, London.
John Samuel Pattison Wilson, Contemporary. Plastic Surgeon, Westminster and St. George's Hospital, London.
Ian Alexander McGregor, Contemporary. Consultant Plastic Surgeon, Canniesburn Hospital, Glasgow.
Gordon Robert Seward, Contemporary. Professor of Oral Surgery, The London Hospital, London.
Leonard Anthony Price, Contemporary. The Institute of Cancer Research and the Royal Marsden Hospital, and Bridget T. Hill, Contemporary. Imperial Cancer Research Fund.

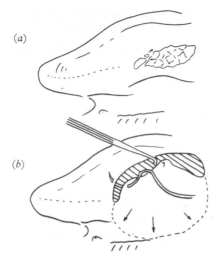

FIG. 546.—(*a*) and (*b*) An intraepithelial carcinoma (carcinoma *in situ*) on the lateral border of the tongue may be excised and the adjacent mucosa of the floor of the mouth undermined and advanced to cover the defect. The undermining must not involve the sublingual plica.

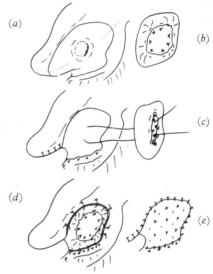

FIG. 547.—(*a*) A diagram of a small squamous cell carcinoma on the lateral margin of the tongue. The outline of the tissue to be excised is shown. Excision with a margin of about 1·5 cm around the palpable extent of the neoplasm with particular care to achieve a proper margin on the deep aspect. (*b*) A pad of soft, polyurethane foam has been cut and a Thiersch graft wrapped round and sewn on to it. (*c*) A transfixing suture has been placed. The tip of the tongue is repaired with sutures and (*d*) the pad and skin graft sewn to the lateral defect. Inset (*e*) shows how a Thiersch graft can be applied by McGregor's quilting technique.

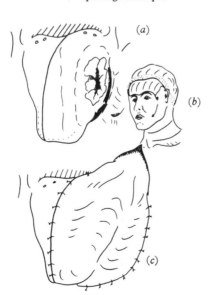

FIG. 548.—(*a*) A diagram of a large squamous cell carcinoma of lateral border of tongue. Excision with a 2 cm margin requires removal of a substantial part of the tongue, floor of mouth and mandible on that side. (*b*) A forehead flap is raised, based on the superficial temporal artery of the same side. A radical neck dissection will be required and the primary tumour should be excised in continuity. (*c*) The flap is brought into the mouth beneath the zygomatic arch, sectioning the zygoma if necessary. The flap is sewn on to the wound margins, folding it to reconstitute the shape of the tongue and lingual sulcus.

cell carcinoma, including cases of carcinoma of the tongue: Vincristine, Adriamycin, Bleomycin, Methotrexate, Fluorouracil, Hydroxyurea and Mercaptopurine.

Rapid advances are being made in this field, and clinicians intending to use this form of treatment would be advised to make themselves familiar with the most recent papers and with the pharmacology and toxic effects of these highly potent drugs. Strict adherence to the chosen advocated regimen is necessary if unexpected problems are to be avoided. Great care must be taken also in the preparation and administration of these substances to avoid dangers to the staff involved.

Difficulty with swallowing may require the patient to be fed via a nasogastric tube and respiratory obstruction may require a tracheostomy. Adequate analgesia and sedation with morphine, or the 'Brompton cocktail', should be used to control pain and apprehension (Chapter 63).

Prognosis.—Despite advances in the treatment of cancer and significant improvement in the functional results achieved for patients with carcinoma of tongue, the overall mortality at 5 years has remained surprisingly constant. The prognosis for women is better than men and approaches 50% survival at 5 years while no more than 25% of men are alive at the end of 5 years.

Sarcoma of the tongue is rare and usually fatal. **Malignant melanoma** of the tongue is also rare and has a bad prognosis, although vigorous local treatment may eradicate the primary tumour and permit a less distressing death from metastases.

CHAPTER 33

THE TEETH AND GUMS, JAWS, NOSE, EAR

CONGENITAL AND DEVELOPMENTAL ANOMALIES OF THE TEETH

Abnormalities of number and size.—One or more teeth may fail to develop. The ones most often absent are the third molars and the upper lateral incisors. Many teeth may be missing from both the primary and secondary dentition in partial anodontia or all may fail to develop in total anodontia. Such individuals may also lack adult hair, sebaceous and sweat glands, and are suffering from ectodermal dysplasia.

Supernumerary teeth may be either smaller and more simple in form than normal, often conical, or resemble the adjacent teeth of the normal series; so called supplemental teeth. Supernumerary teeth between or behind the upper central incisors (mesiodens) are often conical, those in the lower premolar region tend to resemble normal premolars. Fourth molars may develop behind the lower third molar or behind or lateral to the upper ones. Teeth of the normal series may be smaller or larger than normal and with fewer or extra cusps or roots.

Odontomes and Odontogenic Tumours

The more severe developmental abnormalities of tooth form are called odontomes. Dentine and enamel may be invaginated into the pulp chamber and root canal to produce invaginated odontomes like the dens en dente and the dilated odontome (fig. 549).

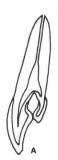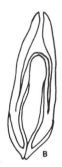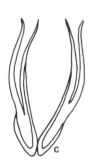

FIG. 549.—Invaginated odontomes of varying degrees of severity. Diagramatic sections longitudinally through the tooth. A. a cingulum invagination; B. a dens en dente malformation; C. a dilated odontome.

Invaginated odontomes are important as their pulps may become infected and the source of an abscess. A compound odontome is a hamartoma composed of an encapsulated cluster of small denticles, many of which are minute so that when the tumour is dissected out a surprising number of denticles are uncovered. A complex odontome is composed of an irregular mass of prismatic enamel, tubular dentine and pulp. Many other hamartomas and benign or even malignant neoplasms of dental tissues, the odontogenic tumours, are recognised. Most are uncommon or very rare and require the opinion of clinicians and pathologists expert in this field for their identification, and management. Only the ameloblastoma and odontogenic myxoma will be described here.

Ameloblastoma.—This neoplasm develops from the dental lamina. Typically, cords of odontogenic epithelium ramify in a cellular connective tissue. Follicles are formed with stellate reticulum-like cells within and a single layer of columnar ameloblast-like cells at the periphery. These cells undergo reversal of polarity but neither induce the formation of odontoblasts nor deposit enamel. Cysts may form either in the stellate reticulum (epithelium lined cysts) or within the stroma. Thus, this neoplasm may form a solid, soft tissue tumour, a single large cyst with a small solid component, or a multilocular cystic

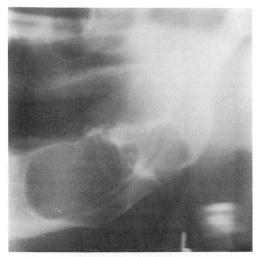

FIG. 550.—Rotational tomogram of an ameloblastoma of the mandible. Note the characteristic cluster of small cysts in the centre of the lesion.

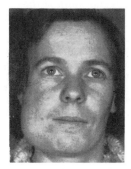

FIG. 551.—Ameloblastoma of right ramus and angle of mandible.
(A. H. London, FRCS, Adelaide.)

mass which is the typical type (fig. 550). It may enclose the crown of an unerupted tooth and resemble a dentigerous cyst. Many involve the third molar region extending into the coronoid process, angle and body of the mandible (fig. 551). Less frequently the anterior part of the mandible is involved and rarely the maxilla. Patients may present at any age from around 11 years upwards, but most present in the 4th and 5th decade. It is slow growing and painless unless infected. This neoplasm is locally invasive within medullary bone and soft tissues and should be excised with about a 1 cm margin at these sites. Subperiosteal excision is satisfactory where the overlying bone is intact and of reasonable thickness. There is evidence that the tumour cells implant readily and it should not be cut into or fragmented at operation. If an ulcerated surface is handled, gloves should be changed. It does not metastasise to lymph nodes, but will do so to the lungs, usually after incomplete local excision. Long standing tumours can reach a large size. It is usually possible to reconstruct the mandible with an iliac crest bone graft at the time of resection. Diagnosis of histologically typical lesions from a biopsy is not difficult but there are cases presenting problems which require special expertise. Local recurrence can follow enucleation or currettage and has been reported as long as 15–20 years after the initial operation. Recurrence involving the base of the skull or tissue planes of the neck may occur after inappropriate surgery. These neoplasms are not radiosensitive.

Odontogenic Myxoma.—These comparatively uncommon jaw tumours also have a predilection for the angle of the mandible though they may be encountered more anteriorly in the mandible or maxilla. They are composed of stellate connective tissue cells in a myxomatous stoma. They are lobulated and produce a bone cavity which radiographically has a well defined polyarcuate periphery and which is crossed by straight ridges or septa. Like the ameloblastoma it can penetrate the adjacent medullary spaces and once it involves the surrounding soft tissues either during natural growth or as a result of fragmenting surgery can be next to impossible to eliminate. If incorrectly handled on the first occasion the patient usually suffers multiple operations for recurrence over many years. These neoplasms also are not radiosensitive.

Abnormalities of Structure

Acute infections during childhood may affect the deposition of enamel and dentine, especially those which disturb nutrition. Enamel defects are seen as hypoplastic pits in the crowns of all teeth which are developing at that time. They form a line across the crown corresponding to the stage of development of the enamel at the relevant age. The condition is called linear hypoplasia. A special abnormality results from congenital syphilis which, while rarely seen these days, remains diagnostically important. The width of the incisal edge of the upper central incisors and often one or more of the lower incisors is less than normal to produce a screwdriver or barrel shape. The enamel in the centre of the incisal edges may be defective, so forming a notch. The notched incisor with a narrow incisal edge is called a Hutchinson's incisor. It must be distinguished with care from acquired notching of an otherwise normal incisor, due for example, to biting cottons to cut the thread. Hutchinson's incisors may be recognised radiographically before eruption. The length and width of the occlusal surface of the first molars is also less than average so that the cusps are closer together, forming the bud molar. If the enamel is also pitted with hypoplastic pits the teeth are described as mulberry molars.

If water which contains 1 part per million of fluoride is drunk during the time of tooth development, enamel is laid down which is less readily attacked by the acid produced by plaque organisms. This amount of fluoride does not affect the appearance of the enamel, but does reduce the incidence of dental caries. Drinking water containing significantly greater concentrations of fluoride during the development of the crowns of the adult dentition produces a whitish enamel with a rough surface which takes up brown stains to produce an unsightly mottled appearance.

Ingesting additional fluoride as well as fluoridated water may produce minor degrees of mottling. Topical fluoride applied to the enamel as fluoridated toothpaste or as solutions or gels by dentists also reduces the incidence of caries and may aid the recalcification of the initial lesions of caries in the enamel.

There are a variety of inherited abnormalities of structure of the enamel or forms of amelogenesis imperfecta or of the dentine; dentinogenesis imperfecta. For example the enamel may be hypocalcified, but of normal thickness or pitted, or consist of no more than a thin layer. The latter form may accompany severe epidermolysis bullosa. In dentinogenesis imperfecta the enamel tends to separate from the dentine which in its inner layer has relatively few dentinal tubules. The pulp chamber and root canals are greatly narrowed even before the apices are fully formed. A similar abnormality of the dentine is seen in osteogenesis imperfecta.

Impacted and Unerupted Teeth

If there is insufficient room in the arch for a tooth, or if it is tilted, impaction may occur. Those teeth which erupt after their neighbours such as canines, premolars and third molars tend to become impacted. Supernumerary teeth may impede the eruption of adjacent teeth of the normal series, notably the upper central incisors, or may themselves fail to erupt. Failure of eruption may result from severe crowding and impaction or from a disturbance of the eruption mechanism such as a failure of alveolar bone growth. Both tooth development and eruption are arrested at a chronological stage of development, corresponding to the onset of the disease, in hypoparathyroidism and a failure of many teeth to erupt in both the primary and secondary dentitions is typical of cleido-cranio-dysostosis.

The most frequent tooth to be impacted is the lower third molar (fig. 553). Partially erupted lower third molars cause problems in two age groups: either in teenagers and young adults or in the edentulous or partially edentulous elderly when previously buried teeth are uncovered as a result of alveolar atrophy. Impacted lower third molars may be the site of a pericoronal infection (fig. 552). Caries either of the wisdom itself or of the second molar at the point where the tooth is impacted against it may result from food stagnation and result in alveolar abscess formation. Several types of cyst (see below) or odontogenic tumour such as the ameloblastoma (see above) are associated with lower third molars. Impacted wisdoms also create a weakness in the jaw so that during accidents fractures tend to occur which involve their sockets.

Pericoronitis

Once an erupting tooth has penetrated the overlying tissues a potential cleft exists between the enamel surface and the adjacent follicular soft tissues. In the majority of cases the epithelial attachment remains intact and eruption is completed quite rapidly so as to achieve a normal gingival crevice. If this process is disturbed an actual cleft can be established around the crown of almost any tooth which potentially can become infected, though in practice pericoronitis is virtually confined to third molars and lower third molars in particular.

If the lower alveolar process is too short to contain the third molar, or if it becomes impacted, a gum flap or operculum partially covers the incompletely erupted tooth. An

Sir Jonathan Hutchinson, 1828–1913. Surgeon, The London Hospital.

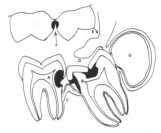

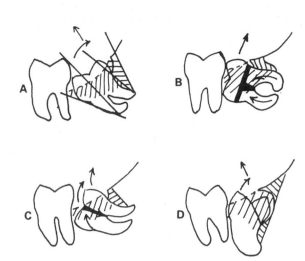

FIG. 552.—A diagram illustrating some of the complications of an impacted lower third molar: A. Caries distally in the second molar; B. Caries mesially in the third molar; C. Periodontal pocketing distally to the second molar; D. Periocoronitis and occlusal caries; E. Trauma to the gum flap from an over-erupted upper third molar; F. An open contact point between the upper second and third molar, as the third is over erupted, with approximal caries and food packing; G. A lateral dentigerous cyst.

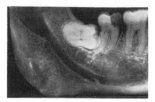

FIG. 553.—Radiograph showing horizontal impaction of third molar.

(*Dr Sydney Blackman, London.*)

FIG. 554.—Diagrams illustrating how some impacted lower third molars may be removed. A. A mesio-angular tooth with favourable root pattern. The crown and upper part of the roots exposed and a trough cut distally to permit the tooth to be tilted into an upright position and dislocated from the socket. B. A horizontal tooth with unfavourable roots. After exposing the crown and distal root, the crown is cut off and the roots separated and removed individually. C. A horizontal tooth with favourable roots. Such a tooth is uncovered and split longitudinally with an osteotome permitting each half to be extracted separately. D. A distoangular tooth. The crown is uncovered and the distal half of the crown split off giving access for the operator to cut a trough down the back of the root. The tooth is tilted backwards, then dislocated from the socket. (Note mesial means the aspect towards the mid-line of the dental arch, distal, the aspect away from the mid-line of the dental arch.)

acute or subacute infection can involve this hood of gum. Such an infection may be suppurative so that pus oozes from under the flap. A pericoronal abscess can form which may track forward along the buccinator origin to discharge into the buccal sulcus opposite the lower first molar. More seriously the infection may spread into the adjacent tissue spaces such as the buccal space laterally, or the pterygoid and parapharyngeal spaces medially. If it reaches the submasseteric space it may form a submasseteric abscess and cause a superficial osteomyelitis of the ramus of the mandible. Should infection spread to the submandibular lymph nodes these in turn may suppurate and produce a submandibular abscess. Fulminating infections of these spaces are dangerous, particularly a parapharyngeal abscess. If a submandibular infection spreads via the sublingual spaces to the submandibular space on the other side and also from the sublingual spaces backwards medial to the hyoglossus to the epiglottis a Ludwig's angina results. Both parapharyngeal infections and Ludwig's angina threaten to obstruct the airway and can cause the death of the patient.

Vincent's acute ulcerative gingivitis may start under a pericoronal gum flap (ulcerative pericoronitis) (see Chapter 32).

Patients with acute pericoronitis present with soreness in the lower third molar region, with pain which often radiates to the ear, swelling of the cheek, limitation of jaw opening and enlarged and tender submandibular lymph nodes. The severity of the illness varies between wide limits.

Treatment of pericoronitis.—Mild infections may respond to irrigation under the gum

Wilhelm von Ludwig, 1790–1865. Professor of Surgery and Midwifery, Tübingen, Germany.
Jean Hyacinthe Vincent, 1862–1950 (see footnote p. 574).

flap with Eusol and the introduction of Povidone iodine under the flap. Treatment is repeated daily together with the frequent use of hot salt water mouth washes. Where there is persistent pain, cheek swelling, lymph node enlargement or limitation of opening, amoxycillin, metronidazole or tetracycline should be given for five to seven days. If there is a pericoronal abscess the flap is incised lateral to the third molar to establish drainage. Often the upper third molar bites on the gum flap. If it does it should be extracted. Extraction of the lower third molar, and certainly one needing surgical removal is deferred until the acute infection has completely subsided. A Vincent's acute ulcerative pericoronitis is treated with metronidazole.

Alveolar abscess on a lower third molar

If the wisdom can be extracted without the surgical removal of bone this should be done straight away. If there is an abscess pointing it is incised. Removal of a third molar which can be accomplished only by bone surgery should be deferred and the infection controlled by an antibiotic such as amoxycillin. If the infection is spreading into the soft tissues antibiotics should be added even if the tooth can be extracted without difficulty.

Removal of lower third molars.—Where the bone around the tooth is young and elastic it may be removed with chisels, making use of a predictable direction of split. This requires skill and practice. The bone may be removed precisely in all age groups with No. 10 and No.6 round dental burs in a straight dental handpiece. An incision is made *over the external oblique ridge* behind the third molar and a short vertical relieving incision added lateral to the second molar. Mucoperiosteal flaps are elevated buccally and lingually to the tooth and a Howarth's rougine is placed under the lingual periosteum to protect the lingual nerve. Bone is cut away, buccally and behind the third molar and, if necessary, lingually until the greatest diameter of the crown is uncovered. A trough is cut lateral to the tooth down to the bifurcation of the roots. Another trough may be cut behind to create space into which the tooth can be tilted to disimpact it. If the crown of a horizontally placed tooth presses tightly against the second molar in front it is cut off using a No. 6 fissure burr. If the roots lock the tooth in place the crown is cut off and the roots separated with a fissure burr so that they can be dislodged individually. All cutting with a burr is done under a trickle of sterile saline applied with a syringe. Impacted teeth may be elevated out as shown in the diagram (fig.554). The socket is washed with saline and the flaps sewn together.

DENTAL CARIES

Certain oral organisms proliferate on the surface of the teeth and their adhesion is aided by the precipitation of sticky dextrans to form plaque. If sucrose, or refined carbohydrates which are readily converted to sugar by ptyaline are eaten they are metabolised by plaque organisms to produce high local concentrations of lactic acid. The underlying enamel is attacked and eventually penetrated to the dentine. The dentine is invaded by organisms capable of proteolysis which reduce it to a brown, soft, crumbly consistency. The process spreads laterally under the enamel until the force of mastication causes the overlying enamel to fracture, producing an obvious cavity. It also spreads inwards, following the dental tubules until the organisms reach and destroy the pulp. Pulp necrosis may also follow trauma to a sound tooth, mostly a front tooth, either because the crown is fractured or because the blow jerks the tooth and tears the apical vessels. Infection may also reach the pulp via imperfections in enamel in the depths of invaginated odontomes. The latter are rare, but minor degrees of invagination at the cingulum are relatively common in upper lateral incisions.

Periodontal disease.—Where it is in contact with the gingival margin, toxins from organisms in plaque can cause inflammation which, by a process which also involves certain immune reactions, results in damage to the epithelial attachment. The underlying periodontal membrane fibres and then the alveolar bone are also

W. G. Howarth, 1879–1962. London otolaryngologist.

attacked. First a chronic marginal gingivitis results and then a pocket between gum and tooth as the periodontal membrane is progressively destroyed. The deeper layers of the plaque become calcified by calcium salts found in solution in saliva to form calculus. A bacteraemia results whenever teeth affected by periodontal disease are chewed upon. Organisms from the pockets are also forced into the blood stream as an affected tooth is extracted.

ALVEOLAR ABSCESS

Alveolar abscesses may result from the spread of infection from a necrotic pulp into the periapical tissues to produce a periapical abscess. Resorption of the overlying cortical bone occurs to permit the pus to escape into the adjacent soft tissues and mostly to point in the adjacent buccal or labial sulcus (fig. 555(a)) On occasions organisms produce an abscess apical to the bottom of a periodontal pocket. Such a periodontal abscess forms another type of alveolar abscess which may discharge through the pocket or through the overlying alveolar tissues so as to point on the side of the alveolar process (fig. 555(b)).

FIG. 555.—A. A diagram of apical abscesses on a carious upper right first molar. Pus usually points buccally and most often on the oral side of the buccinator origin, and into the buccal sulcus. It may escape above the buccinator and into the buccal space. From the palatal root an abscess may point palatally. B. A periodontal abscess starting apical to a periodontal pocket and pointing through the buccal mucosa. Calculus is shown on the tooth at the top of the pocket.

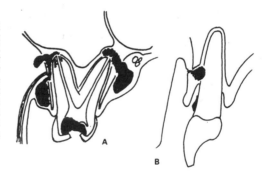

Emergency treatment of toothache.—Dental caries is not obvious in the early stages as the breach in the enamel, which occurs either in the depths of an occlusal fissure or where one tooth is in contact with the next, is quite small. Not until a large dentinal lesion is close to the pulp and where the overlying enamel has broken away does the cavity cause pain and then only when hot, cold or sweet food is in contact with the cavity stimulating the pulp. Such pain passes within a minute or two.

With a double ended enamel chisel, weak enamel around the cavity opening can be chipped away to enlarge it. The soft carious dentine can be scraped out gently with a spoon excavator and a dressing inserted. Zinc oxide powder is mixed with one or two drops of eugenol or oil of cloves using a small knife as a spatula to form a stiff paste and a lump pressed into the cavity.

If the pain resulting from pulp stimulation persists or comes on spontaneously the pulp is likely to be inflamed. After gently excavating caries a soft dressing can be pressed in, made by mixing zinc oxide with carbolized resin and a few fibres of cotton wool. This may well relieve the pain until expert help is available. If the patient has a throbbing pain an antibiotic is prescribed. Should an abscess point in the sulcus it should be incised and drained for which little operation a topical spray with ethyl chloride to freeze the gum will provide sufficient anaesthesia. Analgesic tablets are prescribed for the pain.

Spreading Infection from an Alveolar Abscess

Strangely osteomyelitis of the jaws is an unusual complication of a periapical abscess (see below), but the infection may well spread in the surrounding soft tissues rather than point in the adjacent sulcus. Infection from lower teeth spreading lingually may cause a cellulitis of the sublingual space. From apical abscesses on second and third molars perforation of the lingual plate occurs below the mylohyoid muscle with spread into the submandibular space. Buccal spread from molars in either jaw can involve the buccal space and posterior spread to the pterygoid space between the pterygoid muscles and the medial side of the ramus. Upwards spread from the pterygoid fossa carries the infection into the infratemporal fossa and then by way of emissary veins to the cavernous sinus. Posterior spread from an abscess on a lower molar may also result in a parapharyngeal abscess with swelling of the lateral pharyngeal wall and soft palate. There is difficulty in swallowing and later in breathing. Respiratory obstruction may threaten in neglected cases or the infection may spread via the carotid sheath to the mediastinum. Bilateral sublingual and submandibular space infections constitute Ludwig's angina. Backward spread around the sublingual vessels results in oedema of the epiglottis and respiratory obstruction. Abscesses from upper canines discharging into the cheek beneath the levator labii superioris travel up to point below the medial corner of the eye. If neglected, the infection can cause thrombophlebitis of the angular vein and cavernous sinus thrombosis. The apex of the upper lateral incisor is closer to the palatal than the labial cortex and causes a palatal abscess while pus from a lower third molar may travel back beneath the masseter as a submasseteric abscess. It strips the periosteum from the bone and results in necrosis and even sequestration of the outer cortex of the ramus. The swelling of a submasseteric abscess does not raise the lobe of the ear and results in complete limitation of opening; features which distinguish it from a suppurative parotitis. Lymphatic spread carries infection from the lower incisors and canines or a sublingual cellulitis to the submental lymph nodes where secondary suppuration can produce a submental abscess. Infection from all the other teeth drains to the submandibular nodes where lymph node suppuration can result in a submandibular abscess.

Signs, Symptoms and Treatment.—An early pulpitis causes a sharp pain exacerbated by hot or cold food or drink. The pain becomes throbbing and then subsides as the pulp necroses.

With the onset of an acute alveolar abscess a deep, boring, throbbing pain develops with a soft, puffy swelling of the overlying lip or cheek (collateral oedema) (fig. 556). The causative tooth becomes acutely tender to percussion and mobile. As pus nears the surface of the bone the periosteum and parosteal tissues become oedematous, firm and tender and there is redness of the sulcus mucosa. When pus bursts into the soft tissues the pain eases for a while but returns as an abscess forms in the sulcus. The overlying soft tissues become

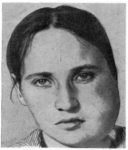

FIG. 556.—Extensive facial oedema from an alveolar abscess.

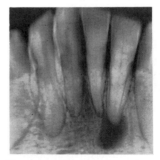

FIG. 557.—Periapical bone destruction due to a granuloma at the apex of pulpless $\overline{2}$. $\overline{1}$ has a narrowed root canal and pulp chamber. The cause of these changes is probably trauma to $\overline{12}$.

more swollen and the skin a pinkish red. If a sinus forms, the pus discharges and the acute symptoms subside (fig. 558). Many pulps necrose without symptoms and a chronic periapical granuloma forms about the apex with local destruction of bone apparent in an x-ray (fig. 557). An acute exacerbation of a previous chronic infection results in the early onset of throbbing pain and swelling.

If a cellulitis supervenes in the overlying tissues the swelling becomes more severe and indurated with the skin a brighter red colour, the lymph nodes become more swollen and tender and severe constitutional symptoms appear. The change to a dusky redness of the overlying skin in the centre of the swelling, the appearance of localised increased tenderness and pitting oedema, together with a sharp rise in temperature herald the formation of pus beneath the deep fascia. Incision and drainage should be undertaken at this stage and should not await the appearance of a fluctuant swelling beneath the skin. Amoxycillin, flucloxacillin, tetracycline and metronidazole are antibiotics to which the organisms are likely to be sensitive.

Where there is a swelling of the floor of the mouth, which raises the tongue, or a parapharyngeal swelling, the induction of general anaesthesia should be undertaken by an expert because of the risk of respiratory obstruction, and intubation and drainage are conducted in the head down position. Sublingual abscesses are incised lateral to the sublingual plica and pointing parapharyngeal ones may be opened without general anaesthesia. A dental mouth prop is inserted between the teeth, the tongue sprayed with topical anaesthetic and depressed with an angled spatula, the mucosa immediately over the swelling is injected twice with 0·5 ml 2% lignocaine with 1:80,000 adrenaline and the abscess opened with a No. 11 scalpel blade and the pus immediately sucked away. In the case of genuine Ludwig's angina a tracheostomy should be undertaken under local anaesthetic before respiratory obstruction threatens. The traditional deep incisions dividing the muscles of the upper neck are damaging and do not help the outcome. Incisions made in both submandibular regions permit the submandibular, sublingual and parapharyngeal spaces on both sides to be drained as necessary by appropriately directed sinus forceps using Hilton's method. Long corrugated rubber drains are inserted. Submental pus requires a separate transverse skin incision between hyoid and chin.

The causative tooth should always be dealt with unless bone surgery is necessary for its removal. Incised abscesses will continue to drain until the source of the infection has been removed. Chronic apical abscesses may be dealt with by tooth extraction or root canal therapy.

Where the tooth is valuable a dentist may drain an acute apical abscess via the root canal and subsequently root treat and fill the tooth. Attempts to save the tooth should be abandoned if a spreading infection supervenes. Most sizeable periodontal abscesses require the extraction of the involved tooth.

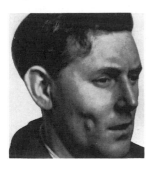

FIG. 558.—Chronic sinus from an alveolar abscess which burst spontaneously.

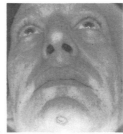

FIG. 559.—Median mental sinus.

Poultices and sinuses.—Poultices do not benefit most face and neck infections and by inducing skin redness and oedema may make the recognition of the signs of pus formation difficult. They are helpful where enlarged lymph nodes associated with an acute infection are slow to resolve despite the continued administration of an antibiotic which controls the pyrexia and constitutional symptoms. Pus should never be permitted to discharge through the skin spontaneously or an ugly scar will result (fig. 558). Where a spontaneous skin sinus has appeared and drained before the patient is seen the relationship to a particular tooth may not be obvious as the facial muscles determine the site at which it points. Often the sinus track can be felt as a fibrous cord beneath the sulcus and leading to the

John Hilton, 1804–1878. Surgeon, Guy's Hospital, London.

bone. Pus from the lower incisors can breach the bone below the origin of the mentalis muscle. If so the abscess reaches the surface between the two muscles and drains via a sinus in the midline of the chin (fig. 559). Curiously the source of this lesion is often not recognised and it may be mistaken for an infected sebaceous cyst or even a skin malignancy. Concern is heightened as local excision is always followed by its reappearance. Extraction or root treatment of the offending incisor results in the sinus drying up and healing.

An ugly, chronic, facial sinus scar should not be excised for six months after the causative tooth has been dealt with. Many will improve and be more cosmetically acceptable in this time. Those that do not, need skilful excision if the surgical scar is to be an improvement upon the sinus scar. An elipse of skin around the sinus is removed in the line of skin creases. The fibrous cord is cored out and the track closed with deep sutures. The skin is undermined and closed carefully in layers.

If there is obvious periapical bone destruction due to a chronic abscess or granuloma to be seen in a radiograph, this may enable the causative tooth to be identified. Periapical films are best for this but oblique lateral views may suffice. Failure to identify the tooth by this means does not exclude a tooth as a cause. Tests for pulp vitality or removal of existing restorations may be needed to find the culprit.

SURGICALLY IMPORTANT COMPLICATIONS OF DENTAL DISEASE

Loose or grossly carious teeth which may be dislodged or fractured, should an anaesthetist use a laryngoscope, are best removed before an operation and, if the socket is sutured, need not delay it. Once such an accident has happened it may be difficult to prove the extent of the disease which made dislodgement of the tooth likely. Patients should always be questioned about crowns and bridges and the anaesthetist warned of their presence. Replacement of damaged crowns and bridges can be costly.

The need, where appropriate, to introduce Povidone iodine solutions into gingival crevices or pockets and for the administration of antibiotics for the prophylaxis of infective endocarditis is well known. Artificial heart valves may become infected by a bacteraemia not only after extractions but by mastication upon teeth involved by periodontal disease. As well as the risk of infection of a valve post-operatively there is the need to manage extractions in an anticoagulated patient should an alveolar abscess occur at this time. Diseased teeth therefore should be dealt with pre-operatively before heart valve replacement. Similar risks of haematogenous infection are present where joint replacement has been undertaken and again are best anticipated.

If any patient presents for elective surgery an inspection of the oral cavity may reduce the risk of future problems, particularly if a prolonged anaesthetic will be necessary. Patients with generally dirty mouths and much calculus should be advised to visit a dentist for a scale and polish and to improve their oral hygiene. Those with many carious teeth and marked periodontal disease should be told to seek treatment before they are admitted.

Post extraction bleeding occasions considerable alarm on behalf of the patient. Mostly the haemorrhage is reactionary in nature, starting two to three hours after the extractions. Occasionally it is secondary and occurs several days later, perhaps as an accompaniment of a Vincent's ulcerative gingivitis. In certain instances it is not the socket which is bleeding but an incision in the sulcus, made to drain an alveolar abscess. The mouth is carefully cleaned of clot with gauze swabs and the site of the haemorrhage identified. A folded gauze swab or a roll of gauze bandage is placed accurately on the bleeding socket and the patient instructed to bite upon it continuously for 15 minutes.

During this time an enquiry is made of relatives, if present, for any evidence suggesting a major defect in the haemostatic mechanism. It is not unknown for haemophiliacs in pain to conceal their problem and persuade a dentist to extract a tooth! Mostly the cause is local, not general. 3/0 (3 metric) black silk on a 22 mm half circle cutting needle or similar suture material, is put out, a syringe and needle and 2% lignocaine containing 1:100,000 adrenaline, a needle holder and stitch scissors. If at the end of 15 minutes haemostasis is not complete, and the clot stable, the socket should be sutured. 0·5 ml of local anaesthetic solution is injected into the sulcus laterally and into the floor of the mouth or palate medial to the socket. The adrenaline will reduce the haemorrhage temporarily and the anaesthesia permits deliberate unhurried suturing. A bite of labial or buccal gum and then of lingual gum is taken and the suture tied with a surgeon's knot. The two turns in the first throw will prevent the knot slipping and enable the suture to be tied tightly. Each bleeding socket is sutured in turn and then the patient bites on a swab again. Failure of haemostasis after suturing is rare. Should it happen a small amount of resorbable oxydised cellulose can be inserted in the socket under the suture.

Some patients experience great pain starting in a socket around the third day after an extraction. The gum margin around the socket is red and swollen and the socket empty of clot or filled with debris. The clot has been lost either as a result of infection or by the action of plasmin to produce a 'dry socket'. Daily irrigation of the socket with eusol, a prescription for metronidazole and one for an analgesic is effective though the patient's dentist can provide more rapid relief with socket pastes.

There are some patients in which the maxillary sinus dips down between the roots of the upper premolars and molars. Granulation tissue about diseased teeth may destroy bone between the tooth and the antrum such that a fistula results when the tooth is removed. Sometimes the tooth mechanically grips the adjacent bone which fractures away as the tooth is extracted. In other cases as bone is removed to expose a retained root the sinus is uncovered. If this is noticed the opening will be closed at the time but infection in the antrum may lead to break-down of the repair. In the first instance the exodontist may not be aware of the opening until the clot in the socket breaks down. Infection in the maxillary sinus must be controlled then one of a variety of small repair operations is performed dependent upon the defect.

Occasionally a tooth root is displaced into the antrum. Usually the dentist is aware of the accident and takes measures to retrieve it. In certain circumstances he may not know this has happened and the root can be a cause of chronic sinus infection.

Osteomyelitis of the jaws

Despite how often periapical abscesses occur, osteomyelitis of the jaws is not common, and it is the mandible which is usually involved. In the majority of cases, infection spread from a local focus directly into the bone but metastatic spread from osteomyelitis or an abscess elsewhere in the body is not unknown. There is usually some local or general factor which tips the balance. For example, acute osteomyelitis affecting large segments of the mandible is seen more often in members of malnourished communities. Extraction of the offending tooth is the most effective way to both decompress an intra-bony periapical abscess and also to remove the source of infection. Failure effectively to treat an apical abscess on a lower molar tooth can lead to involvement of the mandibular neurovascular bundle interfering with the blood supply to the medullary bone. That this is a factor leading to osteomyelitis of the mandible is suggested by the frequency with which the onset of anaesthesia of the lip marks the change from a localised to a spreading bony infection. A traumatic extraction in the face of an acute infection may also result in osteomyelitis. If a fracture of the mandible, compound into the mouth, is not immobilised at an early stage and the mucosa closed over the bone end, infected saliva is sucked into the wound whenever the bone ends move relative to one another. Infection of the bone

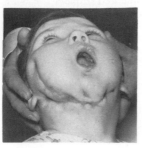 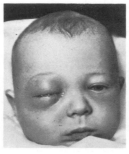 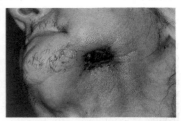

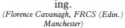

FIG. 560.—Osteomyelitis of the lower jaw shortly after a very large sequestrum had been removed.

FIG. 561.—Acute osteomyelitis of the maxilla in infancy showing characteristic periorbital swelling.

(Florence Cavanagh, FRCS (Edin.) Manchester)

FIG. 562.—Radionecrosis of mandible. Necrotic left side of mandible is ulcerating through the skin.

ends soon follows. Gunshot wounds produce many devitalised fragments of bone which, if not removed and the adjacent viable ones covered with soft tissue, soon became grossly infected.

Chronic osteomyelitis occurs where there is bone sclerosis. Sclerosis may develop at the periphery of a segment of mandible affected by acute osteomyelitis. The local reduction in blood supply impedes the natural defences of the body and also the ingress of systemic antibiotics. Some diseases such as Paget's disease result in the production of patches of sclerosed bone which if exposed at the bottom of a tooth socket may become infected. Incurable osteomyelitis of the mandible can follow tooth extraction in marble bone disease.

The course of osteomyelitis of the mandible is similar to that in other bones. Acute osteomyelitis is accompanied by swelling of the overlying soft tissues, a boring, throbbing pain, malaise and pyrexia. The gum over the affected segment is swollen and the contained teeth become mobile and tender. Pus may reach the surface via sinuses which penetrate the cortex and the overlying subperiosteal new bone which forms the involucrum and discharges on to the face or into the mouth. It may also point via the periodontal membranes of the teeth. Once pus has discharged the disease enters a less painful, chronic phase when the patient is comparatively well except during flare ups in the infection. Infection involving sclerotic bone masses is often chronic from the start. Sequestra composed largely of cortical bone may be discharged spontaneously, but often require surgical removal (fig. 560).

Management.—Provided effective antibiotic therapy is started early, for example as soon as mental anaesthesia appears, frank osteomyelitis involving large parts of the mandible will not develop. Amoxycillin and flucloxacillin in combination are given and persisted with for 4-6 weeks unless investigation of the pus, once it is available, indicates another antibiotic.

Subperiosteal abscesses should be drained and loose teeth surrounded by pus, or grossly carious teeth which might be a source of infection should be extracted if this can be easily accomplished. Later, once sequestra have separated, they are surgically removed. Chronic osteomyelitis may require saucerisation of the affected bone back to healthy bleeding medulla or the removal of sclerotic bone masses; preferably once they have been demarcated by bone resorption.

Acute osteomyelitis of the maxilla of infancy is a well recognised entity (fig. 561). It starts in the neonate in the first few weeks of life and produces gross swelling of the eyelids so that it may be mistaken for orbital cellulitis. Antibiotics should be given promptly. If pus points it is likely to be below the medial corner of the eye or over the as yet unerupted second deciduous molar tooth germ. A small incision should be made to effect drainage. No attempt should be made to remove infected bone surgically unless an obvious sequestrum presents. Bone surgery will lead to unnecessary later deformity. Hypoplasia of the enamel of the related primary teeth may be seen when they erupt and the maxilla may fail to reach the size of the unaffected side. Osteomyelitis of either jaw may be seen in childhood mainly in the poorly nourished and is accompanied by the formation of masses of subperiosteal new bone.

Florence Cavanagh, Contemporary. Honorary Clinical Lecturer in Child Health, University of Manchester.

Therapeutic irradiation damages the blood vessels within bone and impairs the bone cells' ability to divide and effect a repair in the event of injury. Extraction of teeth from a part of the jaw previously irradiated to therapeutic levels carries the risk of post irradiation osteomyelitis; so called radionecrosis (fig. 562). There is also a risk if the soft tissues are stripped from part of the bone, or if bone is left bare after an injury.

Following irradiation of a tumour of the perioral tissues there is a fibrinoid reaction and ulceration of the mucous membrane in the irradiated field. The patient finds tooth cleaning difficult and the natural cleansing due to chewing is reduced as mastication is painful. Salivary flow is also reduced, sometimes permanently. There is periodontal tissue atrophy and the vulnerable necks of the teeth are exposed. As a result even patients with previously well cared for mouths can suffer rampant caries. Where this is likely extraction of the teeth in parts of the jaws which will be heavily irradiated is advised before treatment begins. Tuberculous and actinomycotic osteomyelitis and gummas involving bone are conditions rarely seen these days.

Infection of the Temporo Mandibular Joints.—Suppurative arthritis may occur as a complication of acute osteomyelitis of the mandible, of acute mastoiditis where the air cells involve the eminentia articularis or where middle ear infection, sometimes as a complication of measles, discharges between the cartilaginous and bony meatus into the joint. Much of the growth in length of the mandible occurs in the region of the condyle and infection of the condyle in childhood can lead to restriction in growth of that side of the mandible.

LUMPS ON THE GUM

Gingival enlargement may be *generalised* (hyperplastic, hypertrophic gingivitis) or *localised*. Discrete lumps on the gums are known by the traditional name of epulides. Where the upper alveolar process is prominent and the upper lip short the patient may keep the lips apart at rest. The exposed gingival margin becomes dry and chronically inflamed. A pocket is formed between the swollen gum and the enamel of the tooth crown (false pocketing). With time a degree of fibrosis occurs rendering the enlargement permanent. Hormonal changes during adolescence may play a part in the onset of hyperplastic gingivitis. Phenytoin prescribed to control epilepsy will produce generalised gingival hyperplasia though there is some evidence that this does not occur if meticulous oral hygiene can be maintained. Nifedipine, a coronary artery vasodilator, also may cause the condition.

Pale, swollen gums, often with purple patches where there has been submucosal haemorrhage may be the presenting complaint in cases of acute lcukaemia. The most dramatic hypertrophy is seen in the familial condition, fibromatosis gingivae where the enlargement may be so gross that the teeth, though fully erupted from the bone are buried in the enlarged gums.

Provided the cause of the gingival enlargement can be controlled or treated the excess tissue can be removed, the false pockets eliminated and the gum recontoured by the operation of gingivectomy (fig. 563A). (Marked improvement may occur following the elimination of causative factors and the establishment of effective oral hygiene so gingivectomy should be delayed until no further improvement occurs.) As well as abolishing the pockets, a bevelled gum margin is re-established. The raw wound surface is covered by a special protective paste (Coepack®). A gingivectomy may be used to treat false pocketing or cases of periodontal disease with moderate pocketing. Where bony recontouring is also necessary flap procedures with apical repositioning of the mucoperiosteum to eliminate the pockets is used (fig. 563B and C).

The fibrous epulis is a localised inflammatory hyperplasia of gum. It arises in response to local irritation, from the sharp margin of a carious cavity or the presence of sub-gingival calculus. It often arises from an interdental papilla. At

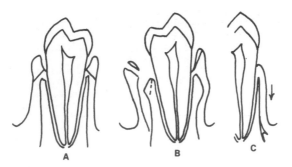

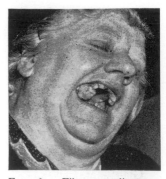

FIG. 563.—Periodontal surgery. A. A gingivectomy to excise moderately deep pockets. B. and C. A flap operation. A reverse bevel excises the epithelium on the pocket aspect of the gum. A mucoperiosteal flap is reflected and the alveolar bone recontoured. The flap is advanced apically and sutured against the bone to eliminate the pocket.

FIG. 564.—Fibrous epulis upper first molar region.

first it is soft and red, but becomes firm and pink as more collagen is deposited in the central mass. It is often pedunculated though the pedicle may be so short that at first sight the epulis appears sessile. The majority of fibrous epulides cease to enlarge after attaining about 1 cm diameter. A few become considerably larger, ulcerate as a result of trauma during mastication and can resemble a malignant neoplasm at first sight (fig. 564). Simple excision, local gingival recontouring and the application of a gingival pack is curative provided the source of irritation is also dealt with; otherwise the epulis will recur.

Pregnancy Epulis and Pyogenic Granuloma (figs. 565 and 566).—In adolescence, during pregnancy and sometimes in older individuals of both sexes soft, rapidly enlarging lumps appear on the gums. Like the fibrous epulis they arise at sites of local irritation, are generally pedunculated and usually start as an enlargement of an interdental papilla. In children they may be related to small, sharp fragments remaining after a primary tooth has been shed. Unlike the fibrous epulis they remain soft, pink and vascular. In pregnant women the irritant may be relatively insignificant deposits of calculus and the unusual response is thought to be conditioned by the hormonal changes in pregnancy. These inflammatory hyperplastic tumours are termed pregnancy epulis or pregnancy

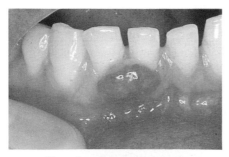

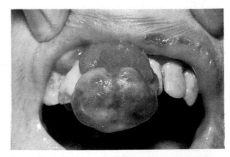

FIG. 565.—Pregnancy tumour.

FIG. 566.—Pyogenic granuloma of the gingivae of a middle aged lady. The tumour is ulcerated and has been bleeding, hence the pallor of the lips.

tumours. Indeed the gum margins may be generally red and swollen and, as a result, bleed easily during the last months of pregnancy. The patient should be encouraged to see her dental surgeon and to improve rather than neglect her oral hygiene if she develops a pregnancy gingivitis. Similar tumours occurring in males and non-pregnant women are called pyogenic granulomas. Histologically all these lesions are composed of a cellular, vascular connective tissue and if ulcerated many inflammatory cells are present. Pregnancy tumours tend to regress after the child is born. Because they are vascular and haemorrhage after excision can be troublesome, their removal may best be undertaken with a special dental diathermy machine with a unipolar cutting electrode.

Giant Cell Epulis.—These purple, pedunculated tumours are also probably inflammatory hyperplasias. They are less common than the fibrous epulis or the pyogenic granuloma and may arise adjacent to an infected socket or the site of a shed primary tooth. For these epulides local excision should include curettage of the bone surface. Any local irritant must be dealt with. Histologically they resemble the intrabony giant cell granuloma (p. 613).

Denture Induced Granuloma.—(See page 581.)

Fibrous hyperplasia of the Tuberosities.—The mucoperiosteum of the tuberosities is thickened particularly on the palatal aspect. The enlargement may be considerable so that the sessile hemispherical masses almost meet in the midline.

CYSTS OF THE JAW (fig. 567)

A variety of cysts occur in the jaws and those which are likely to be encountered by general surgeons will be described. In most instances the cyst is composed of a fibrous capsule covered on the inner aspect by epithelium. The two layers are together referred to as the lining of the cyst.

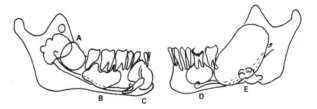

FIG. 567.—Diagrams of some jaw cysts. A. a multilocular keratocyst with daughter cysts; B. a solitary bone cyst; C. an extrafollicular dentigerous cyst; D. a periapical cyst (dental cyst or radicular cyst); E. a dentigerous cyst.

Periapical, Radicular or Dental Cysts.—These develop at the apices of teeth with necrotic pulps. They are lined by stratified squamous epithelium derived from the epithelial debris of Mallassez. Once formed these cysts enlarge slowly causing resorption of the adjacent bone and then expansion of the jaw. If left untreated they can become large, involving the greater part of the body of the mandible, or most of one side, including the ramus. In the maxilla they tend to enlarge to fill the maxillary sinus and inferior meatus of the nose before causing visible expansion and radiographically must be distinguished from carcinoma of the antrum.

Dentigerous Cyst.—Dentigerous cysts arise as a result of separation of the reduced enamel epithelium from the surface of the crown of an unerupted tooth and the accumulation of fluid in the interval. They enlarge in a similar manner to periapical cysts except that they displace the teeth to which they are attached.

Louis Charles Mallassez, 1862–1910. Parisian surgeon and pathologist. Described epithelial rests in the periodontal membrane in 1885.

The tooth is normally displaced deeper into the jaw and prevented from erupting by the cyst. The cyst lining is usually attached around the neck of the tooth so that the crown protrudes into the cyst cavity. Sometimes only the side of the crown is adjacent to the cyst cavity. Unerupted upper third molars seen in a radiograph displaced up to the orbital floor are usually involved in dentigerous cysts.

Treatment.—Both periapical and dentigerous cysts may be treated either by enucleation of the lining from the bony cavity and primary closure of the surgical wound or marsupialisation. If the cyst is marsupialised a sizeable opening is made in both the thin bone covering the cyst and the lining and the surgical flap of oral mucosa turned in to meet the cut edge of the lining. Initially the cavity is packed. Later a special plug may be needed to keep the opening patent. Once decompressed the cavity will fill in. Large maxillary cysts occupying much of the maxillary sinus can be treated by stripping out the cyst lining and removing the partition between the bony cavity and the antrum. The oral wound is closed carefully.

In the case of periapical cysts the causative dead tooth must be dealt with either by extraction or root treatment. Sometimes it is possible to retain the tooth involved in a dentigerous cyst and encourage it to erupt. There are a substantial number of technical details relating to these procedures with which the operator should be familiar to ensure success.

Keratocysts.—Keratocysts have a thin layer of keratinised epithelium on their inner aspect. The lining has a number of distinctive features recognised by the specialist histopathologist. These cysts arise from residual strands of epithelium from the dental lamina. Some arise between standing teeth and others posterior to the third molar, in the base of the coronoid process. Cysts in these locations are also called primordial cysts. Others arise from the epithelial debris of Serres (i.e. dental lamina remnants immediately above the crown of the tooth) and envelop the tooth as they enlarge and so are radiographically indistinguishable from a dentigerous cyst. However, these cysts remain separated from the crown of the tooth by the tooth follicle so are called extrafollicular dentigerous cysts. Keratocysts may arise singly or from multiple foci of dental lamina. They may do this in a group to form a multilocular cyst or individually in several places in both jaws. In just under half there are proliferations of the lining epithelium into the fibrous capsule and daughter cysts may form in this way. There is a tendency for these cysts to recur after operation in about 40% of cases. The lining is often very delicate, easily torn and any left behind will start a new cyst. A daughter cyst may be retained (particularly if microscopic) or new cysts may form from the epithelial rests of an adjacent or another part of the dental lamina. Painstaking enucleation to avoid damage to the lining and to ensure its complete removal reduces the recurrence rate and careful conservative treatment is usually adequate. Any recurrences or new cysts arising in patients afflicted with multiple cysts are dealt with in the same way. Occasionally a patient with a large cluster of keratocysts is seen. Such highly multilocular cysts are not easily dealt with conservatively and resection of the involved segment of jaw and its replacement by a bone graft is to be preferred. Care must be taken not to fragment the specimen as recurrence in bone grafts has been reported, probably from particles of lining which have seeded in the wound.

Multiple cyst-basal cell naevus syndrome.—There is a syndrome affecting several systems and which is often inherited in which the first presenting com-

Etienne Reynaud Augustin Serres, 1786–1868. Professor of Anatomy and Natural History at Jardin des Plantes, Paris.

plaint may be of keratocysts of the jaws which start to appear as the adult dentition erupts. Palmar and plantar pits, milia around the eyelids, basal cell naevi and true basal cell carcinomas develop in the skin during later life. Multiple subcutaneous epidermoid cysts may also appear. A short skull base, a prognathic mandible, bridging of the sella turcica, calcification of the falx, cervical spina-bifida and bifid ribs are some of the skeletal anomalies which may be found. Many other defects have been reported as occasional features.

Naso-palatine cysts.—These cysts develop in the incisive canals to cause a spherical bone cavity behind the upper central incisors (fig. 568). They are com-

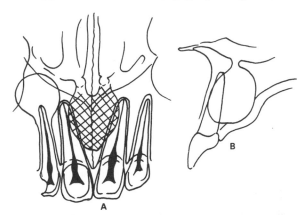

FIG. 568.—A. Diagram of the radiographic appearance of a nasopalatine (incisive canal) cyst. A periapical cyst is shown on the upper right lateral incisor. B. A section through the premaxilla showing the relationship of a nasopalatine cyst to the incisors, the palate and the incisive canals.

posed of a fibrous capsule lined on its inner aspect with epithelium, but while in some this is stratified squamous epithelium in others it is respiratory in nature, with columnar cells, mucus secreting cells and ciliated cells. Nasopalatine cysts rarely achieve a large size but may get big enough to produce a swelling in the midline of the palate or bulge the labial alveolar plate. They arise from epithelium of the nasopalatine ducts. They are treated by reflecting a palatal flap and stripping out the lining.

Naso-labial cysts.—Arise outside the bone of the maxilla but may cause a depression in its surface. They lift the ala of the nose, flatten the upper part of the naso-labial fold, form a fluctuant swelling in the labial sulcus and bulge into the inferior meatus of the nose. They may arise from the upper part of the epithelial fin or from epithelium trapped between lateral nasal and maxillary elevations as they merge. Like the nasopalatine cysts they tend to be lined by respiratory epithelium and often contain a mucoid liquid. The sac of a nasolabial cyst is dissected out through an incision in the mucosa of the upper buccal sulcus.

Solitary Bone Cyst.—These resemble the solitary bone cysts of long bones. Most occur in the mandible and in the premolar-molar region rather than the incisor region or ramus. Initially the bone cavity is round or oval, but it bulges outwards in a lobulated fashion, leaving ridges on the walls. In particular it loops up between the roots of adjacent teeth (fig. 569). Expansion of the jaw occurs late on with the covering sub-periosteal bone also exhibiting ridges on the cavity surface. There is no dissectable lining, but a thin layer of connective tissue over the cavity surface of the bone. Histological examination of this reveals limited bone resorption and even bone deposition. Haemorrhage readily occurs from the

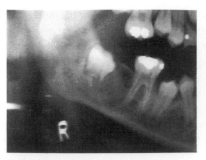 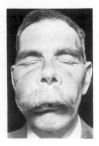 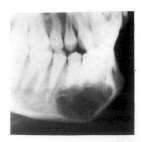

FIG. 569.—A solitary bone cyst displacing   FIG. 570.—Paget's   FIG. 571.—Radiograph show
the developing lower second molar.   disease of the max- ing a giant-celled reparative
                                            illae.   granuloma of the mandible.
                                                                 (Dr H. L. Jaffe, New York.)

thin walled vessels in the wall if aspiration is attempted. Careful aspiration of
large examples while a second needle admits air reveals a yellow fluid containing
high bilirubin levels. If blood is aspirated and centrifuged the supernatant fluid
will be yellow with bilirubin. Unlike the fluid from other jaw cysts it will clot.
Removing part of the bony wall and suturing the soft tissue flap back into place
will stimulate these cysts to heal in adults, but they may recur during childhood
or early adolescence. They may represent a local aberration of bone growth.

Cyst fluids.—Aspirations can help to differentiate jaw cysts. Periapical and dentigerous
cysts contain a clear or brownish fluid containing cholesterol crystals. Keratocyst fluid is
creamy white like pus, but odourless, while that from nasopalatine and nasolabial cysts
may be glary or mucoid.

Complications of Jaw Cysts.—A swelling of the face or of the jaw inside the mouth will
occur as the cyst enlarges. Pressure against the roots of adjacent teeth displaces them
sideways. Dentigerous and extrafollicular dentigerous cysts prevent the eruption of the
involved tooth, but the eruption of adjacent unerupted teeth may be obstructed by any
cyst which develops in the jaws of a young person. The cyst contents may become infected
and if the cyst is large this can be potentially serious. Obviously a large cyst weakens the
mandible and pathological fracture may occur.

FIBRO-OSSEOUS JAW TUMOURS

A variety of conditions which produce enlargement of one or other jaw show the histological appearance called 'osteitis fibrosa'. Histological examination reveals replacement
of the bone by a cellular osteogenic fibrous tissue. Woven bone is deposited in the fibrous
tissue in a three dimensional spongework. Radiographically this has a ground glass, finger
print or orange peel pattern, but in histological sections irregular, thin trabecula are seen
likened to Chinese figures. More mature lesions often contain lamellar bone, others a
concentrically laminated, basophilic calcified tissue resembling cementum. A thin layer
of sub-periosteal new bone covers the lesion where it expands the jaw.

Fibrous dysplasia of bone can affect the bones of the jaw as a monostotic lesion, as
part of polyostotic fibrous dysplasia, or as a component of Albright's syndrome. The
swelling may enlarge rapidly during the adolescent growth spurt and the resulting deformity cause concern. Surgery at this age may result in recurrence and an enhanced speed of
growth. Enlargement usually slows down once skeletal growth is complete when trimming
will produce an acceptable result. If surgery becomes essential during adolescence subperiosteal resection of the lesion should be the aim with immediate reconstruction with a
bone graft. Some examples of fibrous dysplasia in young patients contain scanty deposits
of woven bone and present as a lobulated, largely radiolucent lesion in the bone, with
ridges on the inner aspect of the surrounding bone giving it a coarsely trabeculated
appearance. Diagnosis prior to biopsy may be difficult as this radiographic appearance is
common to a variety of jaw tumours.

Fuller Albright, 1900–1969. Physician, Massachusetts General Hospital, Boston, Mass., U.S.A.
Sir James Paget, 1814–1899. Surgeon, St. Bartholomew's Hospital, London.
Henry Lewis Jaffe, Contemporary. Formerly Director of Laboratories, Hospital for Joint Diseases, New York, U.S.A.

Ossifying and cementifying fibromas.—Fibrous dysplasia responds to some of the normal controls of bone growth, and normally has an ill defined periphery radiographically in the jaws, except in the case of the markedly radiolucent form. The ossifying fibroma is a benign neoplasm which can resemble fibrous dysplasia histologically or may feature the spherical cementum-like clumps of tissue described above. These lesions remain circumscribed but enlarge progressively. The cementifying variant particularly can reach a large size but is usually easily enucleated, though care may be required to maintain continuity of the jaw.

Paget's disease can affect the jaws. Most often it is the maxilla which is involved (fig. 570). In the early stages both the histological and radiographical features of osteitis fibrosa are seen. In more mature lesions the typical cotton wool sclerotic patches appear. These are of more mature lamellar bone and histologically show the mosaic pattern characteristic of the disorder. Hypercementosis of the teeth makes them difficult to extract. The bone is very vascular and a brisk haemorrhage follows surgery, including tooth extraction. As mentioned above dry sockets and infection of the adjacent sclerosed bone, which is only slowly sequestrated, is a complication. Facial deformity and difficulty in the wearing of dentures due to enlargement of the ridges can require trimming operations. These benefit the patient for a while but enlargement often recurs. When the maxilla is affected, the lesion progresses through the face into the vault of the skull. Paget's disease of the mandible is less common than of the maxilla and the mandible can be the only bone affected for many years. Paget's disease affecting both jaws is rare. Benign giant cell granuloma-like lesions (see below) and osteosarcoma are other rare but important complicatons.

Giant Cell lesions of the Jaws

The giant cell granuloma.—Histologically this lesion bears some resemblance to the osteoclastoma of long bones, but is quite benign. The tumour has a stroma of plump, connective tissue cells, scanty collagen, many thin walled blood vessels and a considerable number of osteoclast-like giant cells. Many histocytes can be found, scattered through the lesion. Histologically therefore it resembles the giant cell epulis and the brown tumour of hyperparathyroidism. For the most part the giant cell granuloma occurs centrally in the jaw, either in the mandible or in the maxilla. It forms a lobulated tumour which consequently produces a ridged cavity within the bone (fig. 571). Where it erodes through the cortex it is covered by a thin layer of sub-periosteal new bone which, in the occlusal radiograph outlines the lobulated surface, distinguishing the condition radiographically from a cyst which would produce a hemispherical expansion. The roots of adjacent teeth are displaced, or often markedly resorbed. A subperiosteal variant of the giant cell granuloma is seen in children (fig. 572). A biopsy will distinguish it from a malignant neoplasm which often is the first impression of the clinician. It must not be confused with a giant cell epulis as the underlying bone involvement is often greater than at first appears. Removal of the superficial soft tissue mass only will leave much of the tumour behind.

Because a giant cell granuloma is indistinguishable fom the brown tumour of hyperparathyroidism and as the latter may develop before the more generalised bone changes are obvious, this diagnosis should be excluded before local surgery is undertaken. Rapid and alarming enlargement of a giant cell granuloma may take place during pregnancy. Careful enucleation of a giant cell granuloma with primary closure of the mucosal flap will

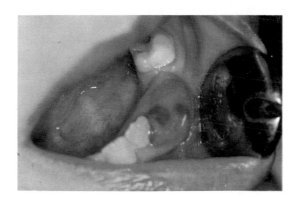

FIG. 572.—Subperiosteal giant cell granuloma of the left alveolar process in a child. It destroys the cortex and the underlying cancellous bone, but from an early stage produces a sinister looking, sessile soft tissue mass.

normally effect a cure. Gentle curettage of the cancellous bone of the cavity wall will ensure no peripheral lobules are left behind. Unnecessary damage to unerupted teeth should be avoided during curettage of the subperiosteal type.

Osteoclastoma.—A malignant osteoclastoma occurs only rarely in the jaws. Diagnosis rests mainly on the histological features. Rapid enlargement and substantial destruction of the jaw can occur both with the giant cell granuloma and brown tumour of hyperparathyroidism.

Aneurysmal bone cyst.—Presents with a similar clinical and radiographic appearance to the giant cell granuloma. It forms a soft, sponge-like tumour centrally in the jaw which oozes blood until enucleation is complete. A cellular fibrous stroma forms septa around blood filled spaces with groups of giant cells here and there in the tissue.

Cherubism is inherited as a dominant gene with variable penetration. The lesions of cherubism contain many osteoclast-like giant cells and in early childhood resemble the giant cell granuloma. Later they become tough and fibrous, with a gradual reduction in the number of giant cells, then spicules of woven bone appear. Typically, lesions appear bilaterally in the angles of the mandible during the first year of life. In the more severe cases further lesions appear both anteriorly in the mandible and in the posterior part of the maxilla. Both jaws may be diffusely involved and substantially enlarged. The bulging cheeks pull down the lower lids to show the sclera below the cornea, so the child appears to look upwards, hence the name of the condition. During adolescence the maxillary lesions regress and the mandibular ones follow suit by the mid-twenties. Cosmetic trimming only is required. Extensive lesions interfere with tooth development and eruption and even erupted teeth may be lost early.

Endosteal Haemangioma not to be confused with aneurysmal bone cyst. Both endosteal cavernous haemangioma and arterio-venous malformations can be encountered. They may produce no more than local gigantism of the affected bone, or a distinct intra bony tumour, which on account of the radiographic appearance may be mistaken for a cyst or giant cell granuloma. Large examples are dangerous and catastrophic haemorrhage can follow extraction of overlying teeth or surgical exploration.

Tumours of Bone

Osteomas normally present as pedunculated, rounded lumps on the surface of the jaws. Both cancellous and ivory osteomas are encountered. Multiple osteomas of the mandible, particularly at the angles, are a feature of Gardner's syndrome which is inherited as a dominant gene. Other features include: osteomas of the frontal bone, multiple polyposis of the colon and rectum in middle age with malignant change, leiomyoma of the stomach and desmoid tumours in surgical scars.

Symmetrical rounded sessile exostoses on the lingual side of the mandible in the premolar region and in the mid line of the palate are called mandibular and palatal tori and do not usually enlarge further in adult life; they are developmental rather than neoplastic.

Osteogenic sarcoma rarely affects the jaws. A full therapeutic dose of irradiation followed by radical resection is the treatment and carries a better prognosis than osteogenic sarcoma of the long bones.

Chondrosarcoma of the jaws is also rare and tends to be misdiagnosed as a chondroma so that the chance of cure by radical surgery is allowed to slip by.

MALIGNANT TUMOURS OF THE MANDIBLE

Squamous cell carcinoma is the commonest malignant neoplasm to involve the mandible. It may arise in the mucosa covering the alveolar process when it almost immediately invades the underlying bone. Alternatively advanced carcinoma of the floor of the mouth, cheek or tongue may spread to involve the adjacent bone. Rarely intra bony primary squamous cell carcinoma may develop from cell rests of the dental lamina or the lining of cysts.

The treatment of squamous cell carcinoma when involving the mandible used to be entirely surgical because bone reduces the local dose of ortho voltage irradiation below an effective level because high doses give a risk of radionecrosis of the jaw. Mega voltage irradiation however is now much more effective in controlling

E. J. Gardner, Comtemporary. American geneticist.

carcinoma invading bone, and in skilled hands there is a lower incidence of bone necrosis. For large tumours, combined radiotherapy and surgery is used and surgery alone, of course, for recurrence after radiotherapy.

Surgical Procedures.—When carcinoma spreads from an adjacent tissue to involve the mandible superficially, the opposite cortex can be conserved to maintain continuity of the jaw. Once the cancellous bone is substantially involved segmental resection is necessary. In general it must be assumed that spread along the inferior dental canal has occurred and the bone from proximal to the mandibular foramen to beyond the mental foramen should be excised. Medial spread via the periosteum and mylohyoid muscle can occur so the latter needs to be removed down to the hyoid. Generous removal of soft tissues around the ulcer is essential and a block dissection of neck added if nodes are palpable.

It is not essential to replace the mandible for resections short of the mid-line, but soft tissue repair with appropriate flaps is necessary for acceptable function and appearance. Delto-pectoral (DP) and pectoralis major myocutaneous flaps are often used, sometimes with a de-epithelialised strip to permit repair of both the inside of the mouth and the skin surface. A forehead flap can be combined with a DP flap to repair both surfaces. Where the mental region also is excised replacement of the mandible either by a temporary implant or by bone is essential to permit suspension of the larynx. Free flaps anastomosed by microvascular techniques to local arteries and veins can be used to replace soft tissues and as compound flaps, both soft tissues and vascularised bone.

Secondary neoplasms, such as carcinoma from other sites, or in children from adrenal medullary neuroblastoma are occasionally seen. Lymphomas, 'histocytosis X' and myeloma may present as central mandibular tumours. Osteogenic and other sarcomas are seen, though not very frequently, as also as a rare occurrence, are malignant odontomes. Treated vigorously with radiotherapy and radical surgery, osteogenic sarcoma has a better prognosis than in the long bones.

MALIGNANT TUMOURS OF THE MAXILLA

Tumours of the upper jaw are rare in the UK. They include the following pathological types:

1. Squamous carcinoma.

2. Adenocarcinoma. This may occur as an occupational disease in woodworkers.

3. Miscellaneous tumours such as transitional cell carcinoma, tumours of salivary gland origin, sarcoma and melanoma. Burkitt's lymphoma presents as a rapidly growing tumour of the maxilla and mandible (Chapter 9).

Clinical features. Initially the carcinoma is symptomless. Obstruction to the ostium and infection of secretions or ulceration of the neoplasm leads to symptoms suggestive of chronic sinusitis. Epistaxis may be an early symptom. In radiographs at this time thickening of the lining is seen, but often no evidence of bone destruction and the seriousness of the case not appreciated. A histological diagnosis can be obtained by intranasal antrostomy or a Caldwell-Luc operation (see maxillary infections below), and all surgical specimens from these procedures must be examined histologically even if the clinical evidence suggests chronic inflammatory disease.

Once the bony walls are breached the clinical presentation depends upon the direction of growth:

1. *Downwards through the floor.* Pain in the related teeth due to involvement of nerves and the loosening of teeth due to destruction of their supporting bone is followed by expansion of the alveolar process, and the fit of dentures may be upset. Necrosis of the tumour leads first to ulceration and then a large sloughing antro-oral fistula.

2. *Medial enlargement* results in fungation into the nose. A blood-stained mucoid or foul smelling, purulent discharge results. Obstruction of the ostia of the other nasal sinuses leads to a unilateral pansinusitis. Obstruction to the naso-lacrimal duct leads to epiphora. All polypoid growths in the nose must be histo-logically examined to avoid missing a malignancy.

3. *Antero-lateral spread* leads to pain in the cheek with anaesthesia of the cheek and anterior teeth and gums. An obvious swelling of the cheek occurs with ultimate ulceration and fungation of the tumour through the skin.

4. *Superior spread* results in pain and possibly epiphora. Involvement of the external occular muscles causes diplopia and gross invasion of the orbit results in proptosis.

5. *Posterior spread.* This is the most sinister as significant symptoms may not occur until invasion of the base of the skull has occurred. Limitation of mandibu-lar movement due to involvement of the pterygoid muscles (trismus), pain and anaesthesia of cheek, tongue and lower lip, from invasion of the maxillary, lingual and inferior dental nerves and ultimately a bloody post-nasal discharge from ulceration into the nasopharynx all indicate advanced disease.

Metastasis to the regional lymph nodes occurs comparatively late on. Either the sub-mandibular or upper deep cervical nodes or both are usually involved.

CT scanning. Tomography.—Once the bony walls are invaded bone destruction will be seen on x-ray but CT scans in two planes will demonstrate more clearly the actual extent of the tumour. Where CT scanning is not available conventional tomography should be used.

Treatment.—Where curative treatment is the aim, preoperative megavoltage radiotherapy is given in full dose. Four to six weeks later, when tissue reaction has subsided, operation is performed.

Surgical Procedures (specialist journals should be referred to for detail).—If the tumour is free of the palate and is mainly antroethmoidal it may be successfully removed by a lateral rhinotomy approach. Involvement of the palate or walls of the antrum require a maxillectomy. If the growth extends into the orbit or anterior cranial fossa, an extended procedure is required such as a craniofacial resection (with good cure rates).

Lateral rhinotomy (fig. 601).—A vertical incision down the side of the nose exposes the nasal bones and the medial aspect of the maxilla. Removal of the lateral wall of the nose gives excellent exposure of the antrum and ethmoids allowing good clearance of tumours not involving the palate. If the tumour is found to involve the orbit or anterior fossa additional exposure via the anterior fossa allows en-bloc (craniofacial) resection.

Maxillectomy.—The maxilla is exposed by raising a facial skin flap along the lower lid margin, down the side of the nose and through the middle of the upper lip and then along the upper buccal sulcus. The intra-oral incision is completed along the midline of the palate and then laterally to separate the hard and soft palates. The maxilla is then freed with osteotomies from the skull base. Medially the hard palate is split in the midline, the frontal process of the maxilla and the lamina papyracea is divided. Laterally the osteotomy through the zygoma extends to the interior orbital fissure. The final osteotomy is made posteriorly detaching the pterygoid plates. The incision is closed and the defect left by the removal of the maxilla is filled with an immediate dental obturator. This results in surprising little deformity either cosmetically or functionally for such a radical resection.

Palliation following maxillectomy can often be prolonged by use of cryosurgery or laser ablation to suspect areas.

Spread to Lymph Nodes in the Neck.—Where lymph nodes in the neck are invaded a block dissection is required. If the subcutaneous tissues of the cheek are invaded to any degree it may be wise to include a triangle of soft tissues down to the submandibular nodes, so as to include the lymphatics around the facial vessels (see p. 658).

INFECTION OF THE MAXILLARY ANTRUM

Surgical Anatomy.—The maxillary antrum (of Highmore) is rudimentary at birth and attains full development by the age of twelve years. Lined with ciliated epithelium, it communicates with the middle meatus of the nose by a small ostium situated high on its medial wall. The apices of the roots of the second premolar and the first and second molar teeth are in close apposition to the floor of the antrum being separated only by periosteum and mucous membrane. Rarely, the first premolar and the canine teeth are related similarly.

Maxillary Sinusitis may be unilateral or, much less frequently, bilateral. Infection occurs as an extension from the nose. One epidemic of acute respiratory infection (common 'cold') brings as an aftermath many cases of infection of the accessory nasal sinuses, of which the maxillary antrum always heads the list; while another epidemic, in all other respects similar, is free from this complication. A less frequent cause is penetration of the floor of the antrum by bacteria from a periodontal abscess connected with a carious tooth; also entry of infected water during swimming.

Acute Sinusitis.—As a rule the general symptoms are severe, especially when the pus is confined by occlusion of the natural ostium. Pain and tenderness are present over the affected maxilla; sometimes the pain is referred along one of the divisions of the trigeminal nerve. Breathing through the nostril on the side of the lesion is impaired and often obstructed. If the ostium is patent, which is unusual in acute cases, a flow of pus can be obtained when the head is held downwards and forwards with the affected side uppermost.

Transillumination of the antrum and a radiograph (fig. 573) are likely to reveal a relative opacity of the affected antrum.

Treatment.—This includes bed rest, analgesics, ephedrine 1% in saline by a nebulizer, menthol inhalations, and systemic chemotherapy if the temperature is over 38°C. Puncturing the antrum is for diagnostic and therapeutic purposes. An antral trocar and cannula punctures the antrum beneath the inferior turbinate bone after application of surface anaesthesia. Pus is aspirated and washouts are performed with isotonic saline.

Chronic Sinusitis.—Pain and swelling are often absent, and frequently the only symptom is an intermittent discharge and facial discomfort or headache. Diagnosis is established by x-ray or by fibreoptic examination through a small

Nathaniel Highmore, 1613–1685. General Practitioner, Sherborne, Dorset, England. Published a treatise on anatomy in 1651.

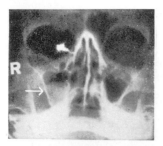

FIG. 573.—Radiograph showing pus in the right antrum of
Highmore.

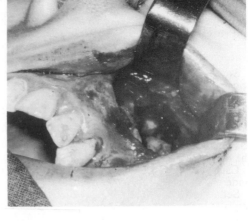

FIG. 574.—Caldwell-Luc
operation (see text).
(*H. Holden, FRCS, London.*)

trocar punch opening either under the inferior turbinate or sublabially in the anterior wall using local anaesthesia.

Treatment.—Chronic infection does not respond to antibiotic therapy and needs surgical drainage by an intranasal antrostomy or a Caldwell-Luc operation.

Intranasal antrostomy.—Under general anaesthesia the inferior turbinate is slightly elevated and a window created in the medial wall of the antrum in the inferior meatus of the nose.

Caldwell-Luc Operation.—This is a good standard procedure, though not advocated in children as dentition may be affected. Under general anaesthesia, with oral intubation and packing, an intra-oral incision 2·5 cm long is made in the buccolabial sulcus, centred over the canine fossa. The muco-periosteum is elevated and a gouge is used to make an opening about 12 mm in diameter through the anterior wall of the antrum (fig. 574). All the mucous membrane is removed with Luc's forceps (fig. 575) and any diseased ethmoid cells can be exenterated. An intra-nasal antrostomy completes the procedure, allowing post-operative washouts.

Nasal Polypi.—Nasal polypi (oedematous ethmoid sinus mucosa) are usually multiple and are seen to prolapse from the ethmoid cells in the region of the middle turbinate. They are recognised by their glistening gelatinous appearance when light is focused upon them.

They are practically confined to adults, and patients complain of nasal obstruction, nasal discharge, and some loss of smell. Many of the sufferers are allergic to dusts and pollens which may initiate attacks of sneezing and rhinorrhoea.

Treatment.—Single polypi are removed under local surface anaesthesia with a snare and appropriate forceps (fig. 575). Multiple polypi usually require a

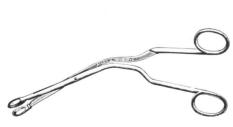

FIG. 575.—Luc's ethmoidal forceps.

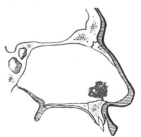

FIG. 576.—Little's area.

George Walter Caldwell, 1866–1946. Otolaryngologist who practised successively in New York, San Francisco and Los Angeles. Described his operation for treating suppuration of the maxillary antrum in 1893.
Henri Luc, 1855–1925. Otolaryngologist, Paris. Described his operation in 1889.
James Lawrence Little, 1836–1885. Professor of Surgery, University of Vermont, Burlington, Vermont, U.S.A.

general anaesthetic for more complete removal. Associated ethmoidal or antral procedures can be then undertaken at the same time. Antihistamines or topical steroids should be used after removal, since recurrence is common.

EPISTAXIS

Source and Cause of the Bleeding.—The bleeding may be arterial or venous. In 90% of cases it comes from a plexus of veins (sometimes varicose) situated in Little's area (fig. 576) on the antero-inferior portion of the septum. The most frequent cause is nose-picking—epistaxis digitorum. Other causes include trauma, nasal infection, neoplasms, hypertension, blood dyscrasias, acute specific fevers, nephritis and uraemia.

Treatment.—Sit the patient up so that blood does not run down the throat. Blow nose to remove clots. Pinch the nose for ten minutes. An ice-pack or cold sponge applied to the nose is often helpful.

Cauterising the bleeding-point with trichloracetic acid, 50%, or electric cautery, is undertaken if the bleeding-point can be seen.

Sedation with diazepam or Omnopon and admission to hospital are necessary if bleeding is uncontrolled. Blood transfusion may be required.

Packing: *Anterior Packing.*—After anaesthetising the mucous membrane with 4% xylocaine, ribbon gauze coated with B.I.P.P. (Bismuth Iodoform Paraffin Paste) is inserted so as to fill the nasal cavity, and if the bleeding is from the septum the nasal cavity of the opposite side is packed also. Antibiotics are given to combat infection.

Posterior Packing.—The insertion of a cone-shaped gauze tampon moistened with B.I.P.P. is the most satisfactory, although a quick method is to insert a Foley-type catheter as far as possible to the back of the nasal cavity and inflate the balloon. The pack can be left in for five days if an antibiotic is administered.

Arterial Ligation.—When the above methods fail, or profuse haemorrahge recurs, it is likely that the source of the bleeding is more posterior. Ligation of the anterior ethmoidal artery in the orbit is indicated, particularly in traumatic cases (fig. 577). Transantral ligation of the internal maxillary artery and ligation of the external carotid artery are other methods which are sometimes called upon.

DEFLECTED NASAL SEPTUM

Although the majority of adults do not have a completely straight septum, it is only the grosser deflections causing symptoms which require correction. Septal deformities are caused either by trauma or by disproportionate growth during development. They may produce nasal obstruction or headaches in the region of the nasion.

The submucous resection (S.M.R.) operation consists of the removal of cartilaginous and bony spurs from between the two coverings of mucoperichondrium and mucoperiosteum. This allows the septum to take a more midline position.

Nasal Bone Fractures (Chapter 30).

THE EAR

Now follows a brief presentation of well-known afflictions of the ear. The reader is referred to the appropriate text-books for fuller accounts and descriptions of operative surgery.

Surgical Anatomy (fig. 578).—The ear consists of four parts: (1) Pinna, (2) External auditory canal, (3) Middle ear, (4) Inner ear and Eighth nerve track.

The pinna is cartilaginous, covered by stratified squamous epithelium. The external auditory canal is in two parts: the outer cartilaginous part, which is lined by similar epithelium, tapers to its narrowest part where it joins the bony external auditory canal. This is lined by a thin stratified epithelium containing no glands or hair follicles, and widens medially until closed off by the tympanic membrane at an angle of 60° to the vertical.

The middle ear is part of the mastoid bone. Above, is the attic connected by the aditus to the mastoid antrum and variable air cells. Below, it communicates with the nasopharynx via the Eustachian tube. It contains (*a*) three ossicles: malleus, incus, and stapes; (*b*) two muscles—tensor tympani and stapedius; (*c*) two windows—oval and round; (*d*) one

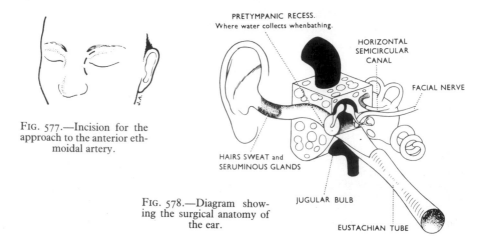

FIG. 577.—Incision for the approach to the anterior ethmoidal artery.

FIG. 578.—Diagram showing the surgical anatomy of the ear.

nerve—chorda tympani. The facial nerve traverses the superior and posterior wall in its bony canal. The horizontal semi-circular canal lies in the attic.

Congenital Abnormalities.—These are: partial or complete absence of pinna; partial or complete occlusion of external auditory canal; partial or complete absence of middle ear—the stapes is nearly always present. Treatment is surgical reconstruction when the child is old enough for the precise hearing level of each ear to be established.

EXTERNAL EAR

Wax.—This is best removed by syringing with warm water and bicarbonate of soda solution (1%) after appropriate oily drops have been introduced for the previous two nights. An aural syringe with a small nozzle must be used, and directed upwards and backwards. An intact drum is unlikely to rupture if these rules are followed.

Foreign bodies easily become wedged in the narrow part of the meatus, whence they can be removed using a hook, sucker or fine forceps under indirect lighting or under the surgical microscope[1]. This should be done by someone familiar with such procedures, especially in children. In difficult cases, a general anaesthetic may be required.

Inflammation.—Inflammation of the external canal may be localised (furuncle) or widespread (external otitis).

Furuncles are staphylococcal in origin, and produce pain, pyrexia, periauricular swelling and, characteristically, a painful pinna on movement.

Treatment.—Decongestive drops or wicks (*e.g.* glycerine and icthyol or antibiotic hydrocortisone cream). If symptoms are severe or generalised (pyrexia), broad spectrum antibiotics are required.

External otitis (*syn.* telephonist's ear, Singapore ear) is often fungal in origin and may start as a dry scaly eczema. Irritation, discharge, and minimal deafness are the symptoms—secondary bacterial infection introduced by scratching the ear leads to further discharge and pain. Antifungal preparations combined with a local antibiotic either as drops or cream are indicated. The primary cause,

---

[1] Celsus (see Chapter 3) recommended tying the patient on a wooden plank with the affected ear downwards and hitting the plank with a hammer.

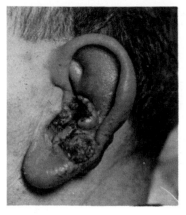

FIG. 579.—Carcinoma of the pinna.

FIG. 580.—Bony exostoses of the deep meatus produce a bizarre appearance seen through the auroscope. Only if the remaining chink is very small is removal indicated to alleviate deafness. They are removed by elevating the meatal skin and drilling away the bony exostosis. There is potential danger to the facial nerve.

scalp or toes, must be treated at the same time and the ears kept dry. Mild sedation, *e.g.* Phenergan 25 mg may be advisable.

Carcinoma of the Pinna (fig. 579) is of the squamous-celled type, and the condition is often comparatively advanced before the patient seeks relief. However, if treated early, favourable results accrue from excision of a part, or the whole of the pinna. Acrylic and rubber prostheses effectively replace the lost part.

Bony Exostoses.[1]—See fig. 580.

MIDDLE EAR

Note: glue ear and acute otitis media in children are conditions which are encountered very commonly.

'**Glue ear**', more correctly called seromucinous otitis media, has become an increasingly common disorder in children. It usually affects those with recurrent otitis media and often enlarged infected adenoids, presumably because of poor Eustachian tube function. It is especially common in children with cleft palate (even after repair) as the muscles which open the tube have lost their insertion into the middle of the palate and atrophied. Inadequate antibiotics for acute infections is another possible cause. 'Glue ear' is painless, and simply causes conduction deafness, of which it is the commonest cause in childhood. The appearances of the eardrum may be striking (gross retraction, yellow or grey/blue discoloration, increased vascularity), but more often are not. The condition must therefore be suspected from the history.

Treatment.—An antihistamine/decongestant mixture is usually tried first, but if this fails to clear the condition, adenoidectomy, myringotomy (fig. 581) and grommet insertion (fig. 582) are advised. In cleft palate cases the adenoids are never removed, however, lest nasal air escape during speech be worsened.

Acute otitis media is secondary to an upper respiratory infection, and presents as severe prolonged earache with pyrexia and systemic illness. In some very acute cases, pus may discharge through a perforation before treatment can be started.

---

[1] Supposed to afflict those who indulge in under-water swimming.

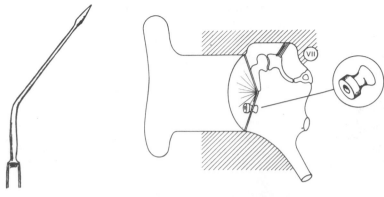

FIG. 581.—Myringotomy knife.

FIG. 582.—Grommet tube positioned in the anterior-inferior quadrant of drum.

More usually, the eardrum is reddened in appearance. Vomiting may be a presenting symptom.

Treatment.—Antibiotics are given in full dosage for five days; nasal decongestants may be added. Early antibiotic treatment has meant that myringotomy (incision of the eardrum) is rarely required nowadays.

Complications.—Acute mastoiditis and intracranial complications have become rare since the widespread use of antibiotics.

Recurrent otitis media.—Frequent attacks of otitis media in childhood are an indication for adenoidectomy.

Acute Mastoiditis (now rare)—The symptoms are pain deep in the ear, periauricular swelling, pyrexia. The pinna is not painful on movement (as distinct from a furuncle). Conduction deafness is marked.

Treatment.—Pus must be let out. Therefore a simple mastoidectomy is performed, with an adequate course of antibiotics in support.

The operation entails the removal of the infected air-cells through a posterior auricular incision. The middle ear is not disturbed. The wound is drained for twenty-four hours.

Complications are lateral sinus thrombosis, extradural abscess, meningitis, cerebral or cerebellar abscess, facial palsy, and, rarely, labyrinthitis.

Chronic Otitis Media.—This term simply means that there is a perforation of the eardrum. If the ear is constantly discharging scanty offensive pus through a posterior or superior perforation ('unsafe type', fig. 583 right upper and lower

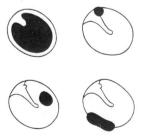

FIG. 583.—Types of perforation of tympanic membrane in chronic otitis media.

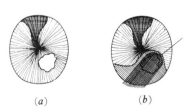

(a)   (b)

FIG. 584.—Myringoplasty. (a) Central perforation. (b) Epithelium elevated and fascial graft inserted to cover perforation. The epithelium is then replaced over fascia.

diagrams), modified radical mastoidectomy may be required, especially if chole-steatoma is present (see below).

A dry central perforation ('safe type', fig. 583 left upper and lower diagrams) which discharges intermittently with colds or swimming, is treated by antibiotic/steroid drops when wet, and may be repaired when dry by grafting of the eardrum (myringoplasty, fig. 584) if necessary with reconstruction of the ossicular chain (tympanoplasty).

Tympanoplasty (fig. 585).—Operations and procedures under this group are designed to repair or reconstruct the tympanic membrane and ossicular chain of the middle ear. Various tissues have been used including homografts from cadavers and animals but the most widely accepted are autogenous fascia with repositioned ossicles or shaped bone chips.

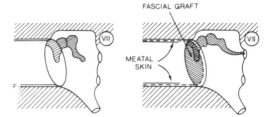

FIG. 585.—Tympanoplasty (*a*) Sub-total perforation with erosion of ossicles and loss of stapes. (*b*) Repair with fascia and ossicular continuity re-established by incus repositioning.

Complications.—Conduction deafness with ossicular chain destruction, labyr-inthitis, facial palsy, cerebral meningitis, cerebral and cerebellar abscess. A *chole-steatoma* (skinball), whose origin is debatable, produces otorrhoea and the above complications by pressure necrosis.

Treatment is surgical by (modified) radical mastoidectomy.

Ruptured drum is due to trauma, *e.g.* hard slap on ear or syringing. There is sudden pain and deafness, with tinnitus and bloodstained discharge.

Treatment.—Do not touch. No eardrops. No antibiotics required.

Otosclerosis produces bilateral conduction deafness. Common in females, it is often hereditary, and may be exacerbated by pregnancy.

Treatment by hearing aid or operation—stapedectomy with Teflon (or wire) strut and vein (or fat) graft (fig. 586). This produces improvement permanently in 90% and it has replaced the fenestration operation.

Serous Otitis Media is usually found in adults and, in contrast with 'glue ear', the middle ear effusion is thin and watery; like 'glue ear', however, it causes conduction deafness. It may result from viral upper respiratory infection or from nasopharyngeal

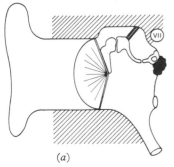
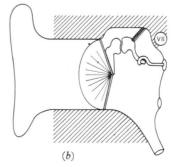

(*a*)   (*b*)

FIG. 586.—Stapedectomy. (*a*) Condition prior to removal of stapes and footplate. (*b*) After removal of stapes; sound conduction restored by a Teflon prosthesis.

carcinoma (causes of Eustachian tube obstruction), or from barotrauma (sudden change in atmospheric pressure produced by flying or diving). Treatment is by decongestants and, if persistent, by myringotomy and grommet insertion (fig. 582).

Malignant Tumours.—Excluding the pinna (fig. 579), **squamous-celled carcinoma**, though uncommon, can arise in the middle ear or mastoid cells. There is pain and otorrhoea (which may be long-standing), becoming bloodstained. Deafness is variable. Biopsy will confirm. Treatment is by combined surgery and radiotherapy, but the prognosis is poor.

Glomus jugulare tumours are rare but of special interest as they resemble carotid body tumours (Chapter 36). Slow growing and locally invasive, they are highly vascular, with nests of epithelioid cells and fibrous tissue. Early signs are seventh nerve palsy, pulsatile tinnitus, and free bleeding. Radiotherapy diminishes both size and vascularity. Cryosurgery is effective for small tumours.

THE INNER EAR

Presbyacusis[1].—High-tone bilateral perception deafness gradually affects lower tones with advancing years. It is often associated with atherosclerosis. Treatment is by a hearing aid.

Cochlear Concussion.—Hearing at 4000 Hz is commonly affected, but if concussion is repeated daily (*e.g.* gunfire, road-driller, or aircraft pilot not using ear defender), the loss spreads up and down. Failure to hear the telephone bell is often the first symptom.

Menière's syndrome is unilateral perception deafness, intermittent true rotational vertigo associated with nausea and tinnitus. It may be associated with hyper- or hypo-tension, intracranial lesions, syphilis, or disseminated sclerosis. But if all these are excluded, and labyrinthine function tests show loss of function on one side, it is true Menière's disease.

Treatment may be (*a*) medical—Tab. nicotinic acid 100 mg, t.d.s. (vasodilator), Avomine, Stemetil, or (*b*) surgical.—1. Operations to reduce endolymphatic pressure by a surgical approach to the endolymphatic sac for drainage can prove satisfactory. Also relatively minor procedures such as ultra-sound or cryosurgery applied to the labyrinth may indirectly produce a similar result.

2. Labyrinthine destruction. A labyrinthectomy may be indicated in cases where the hearing is severely impaired and the patient is getting vertigo symptoms not controlled by other means.

Congenital Deafness.—This is due to intrauterine viral toxins in the first three months of pregnancy (*e.g.* rubella, influenza, *etc.*).

RECENT ADVANCES

1. *Surgery for acoustic neuroma*, formerly the province of the neurosurgeon, is now often a team operation by otologist and neurosurgeon, using a translabyrinthine or posterior cranial fossa approach.

2. *Middle cranial fossa approaches* to the temporal bone, mainly to decompress or to repair the facial nerve, or to section the vestibular nerve are practised in a few centres.

3. *Cochlear implantation*, for electrical stimulation of the inner ear in total deafness is still at an experimental stage.

---

[1] Presbys (Gr.) = old.

Prosper Menière, 1799–1862. Physician, Institute for the Deaf and Dumb, Paris. Described this condition in 1861.

CHAPTER 34

THE PHARYNX

TONSILS AND ADENOIDS

Surgical Anatomy.—The lymphadenoid tissue of the nasopharynx is Nature's barrier to bacterial invasion and antigen recognition in early life. The aetiology of certain cervical inflammations can be better understood if Waldeyer's inner and outer rings (fig. 587) are studied. *The faucial tonsils* are the largest and most important moieties of the inner ring. The tonsils contain tortuous crypts, which extend throughout the tonsillar substance to the external capsule. These crypts can harbour pus and micro-organisms. Clothing the lateral two-thirds of each tonsil is the capsule, a well-defined structure composed of fibrous and elastic tissue, and muscle fibres. The medial third of the tonsil lies between the pillars of the fauces and, being bereft of covering, is accessible to clinical examination. The tonsil has an exceptionally good blood supply (fig. 589). It is well to bear in mind that a tortuous *facial artery* may be closely related to the lower pole. A vein unaccompanied by an artery— the paratonsillar vein—is often a source of serious venous bleeding following tonsillectomy. When divided, the bleeding end retracts into the upper part of the tonsillar fossa, and must be found and ligated before the patient leaves the theatre.

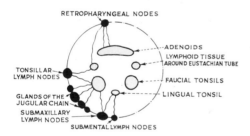

FIG. 587.—Waldeyer's rings. Inner ring—first barrier to infection; outer ring—second barrier.

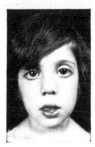

FIG. 588.— The adenoidal facies. Tonsillar hypertrophy is a usual accompaniment.

Examination of the nasopharynx, pharynx and larynx.—Fibre-optic techniques are now available for examination of nasopharynx, pharynx and larynx. The fibrescopes for this purpose may be rigid or flexible. Surface anaesthesia only is required (as for bronchoscopy). Although in many cases a good fibre-optic examination obviates the necessity of giving a general anaesthetic for direct endoscopy, should there be any doubt or if a specific lesion is apparent, then direct endoscopy must be undertaken. This also permits biopsy material to be taken.

ENLARGEMENT OF THE TONSILS AND ADENOIDS

Enlarged tonsils are not necessarily infected; a certain amount of hypertrophy is common in early childhood. As adult life approaches, the tonsils, together with other lymphoid tissues, tend to atrophy. Excessive hypertrophy is often bilateral. Occasionally, the tonsils are so large that they almost meet in the mid-line.

Heinrich Wilhelm Gottfried Waldeyer-Hartz, 1836–1921. Professor of Pathological Anatomy, Berlin.

Enlarged Adenoids.[1]—The 'nasopharyngeal tonsil' is present at birth but undergoes atrophy at puberty, although remnants of it often persist into adult life. The most common period for hypertrophy is between the ages of four and fourteen, and a damp climate favours the development. Enlarged adenoids consist of masses of lymphoid tissue covered by ciliated epithelium and supported by a delicate framework of fibrous tissue.

Considerable adenoid hypertrophy causes the patient to snore loudly at night and to breathe through the open mouth, giving that well-known vacant expression (fig. 588). Added to this, hearing is impaired by the hypertrophied lymph-adenoid tissue obstructing the orifices of the Eustachian tubes, and infections of the middle ear and upper respiratory tract occur frequently.

Acute follicular tonsillitis is a common condition characterised by pyrexia associated with a sore throat. The cervical lymph nodes are enlarged and tender. Pain occasionally radiates up to the ears. The most usual cause is *Streptococcus pyogenes*. On examination the tonsils are swollen, and yellow spots, due to pus exuding from the tonsillar crypts, can often be discerned. The condition can be distinguished from diphtheria by a rapid bacteriological examination of a smear.

Treatment.—Aspirin is administered to relieve pain and gargles of glycerol-thymol are soothing. If the symptoms persist after 24 hours, a throat swab should be taken for culture and penicillin is given until antibiotic sensitivities are known.

Chronic tonsillitis is sometimes associated with hypertrophy. During early childhood chronically inflamed tonsils are usually soft, but by the time puberty has been reached they have frequently become indurated and adherent, due to recurrent attacks of inflammation and subsequent fibrosis. The tonsillar lymph node of the jugular chain is usually palpable. Sometimes pus and debris can be expressed from infected tonsillar crypts to enable a bacteriological examination to be made.

TONSILLECTOMY[2]

Indications.—1. A history of recurrent attacks of acute tonsillitis

2. One attack of peritonsillar abscess.

3. Chronic tonsillitis (especially if associated with cardiac, renal or rheumatic problems).

4. Biopsy for suspected malignancy.

Removal of the tonsils may also be considered in the treatment of tuberculous and non-tuberculous cervical adenitis.

Operation.[3]—Tonsils are removed by dissection. If there has been a recent infection or if an associated arthritic, renal or cardiac lesion is suspected, it is wise to cover the procedure with penicillin to prevent bacteraemia and aid local healing.

Either local or general anaesthesia can be employed. The mouth is kept open and the tongue depressed with a Davis's gag. The tonsil is seized with vulsellum forceps. An

---

[1] To be exact—there is only one adenoid.

[2] Should a recently tonsillectomised patient contract poliomyelitis, he is liable to develop the more lethal bulbar type. Tonsillectomy is therefore contraindicated during an epidemic of this disease. The British Association of Otolaryngologists recommend inoculation against poliomyelitis before tonsillectomy is undertaken. The child should have had at least two inoculations before the operation.

[3] Suggested pre-op. drugs for children—Quinalbarbitone 6mg/kg (max. 100 mg). Atropine 20 micrograms/kg (max 600 micrograms).

Bartolommeo Eustachi (Eustachius), ?1520–1574. Professor of Anatomy, Rome.
The original Davis's gag was invented by Dr. Davis, of Boston, Mass. Henry Edmund Gaskin Boyle, 1875–1941, anaesthetist, St. Bartholomew's Hospital, London, improved it.

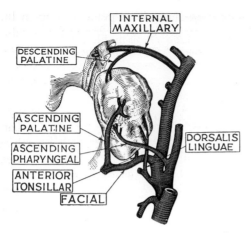

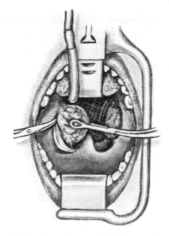

FIG. 589.—The arterial supply of the tonsil from branches of the external carotid.
(*After R. H. Fowler.*)

FIG. 590.—Removal of the tonsils by dissection. Davis's gag in place.

incision is made through the mucous membrane (fig. 590), and the capsule of the tonsil is exposed. The tonsil is removed by dissection, starting at the upper (palatal) pole. When the pedicle is defined, it is severed by a wire snare. Bleeding can be accurately stopped by ligating any bleeding vessels, arteries or veins, so that the patient does not leave the operating table until all bleeding has ceased. Until the patient has recovered consciousness he should be kept with his head low and well over to one side (fig. 591). *On no account should he be permitted to lie on his back or be left unattended.*

Complications after tonsillectomy

1. *Obstruction of the airway*, e.g. blood clot or the tongue falling back.
2. *Inhalation of foreign material*, e.g. blood, vomitus, broken teeth.
3. *Haemorrhage.* Reactionary haemorrhage occurs within the first few hours. It may be recognised by blood appearing from the corner of the mouth or nostrils, a rising pulse rate, generalised irritability. Immediate measures to be taken are: (1) Removal of clot from the tonsillar bed. (2) The application of pressure by means of a swab on a holder.

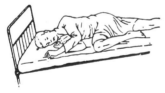

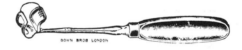

FIG. 592.—St. Clair Thomson's adenoid curette.

FIG. 591.—Position of patient after tonsillectomy.

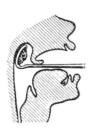

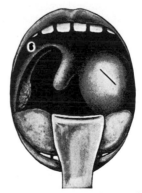

FIG. 593.—Curettage of adenoids.

FIG. 594.—Peritonsillar abscess, showing site of incision.

Sir St. Clair Thomson, 1859–1943. Surgeon, Ear, Nose and Throat Department, King's College Hospital, London.

If bleeding persists in spite of these measures, an intravenous infusion must be set up and blood taken for grouping and cross-matching (Chapter 5). The patient should be returned to the operating theatre, and under general anaesthesia the bleeding point sought and ligated. When the bleeding-point cannot be found, coaptation of the pillars of fauces with sutures will arrest the haemorrhage.[1]

ADENOIDECTOMY

Indications.—Hypertrophic adenoids associated with: (*a*) Recurrent otitis media. (*b*) Post-nasal obstruction. (*c*) Post-nasal discharge. (*d*) Recurrent sinusitis. Adenoids can be removed alone or in conjunction with tonsillectomy.

Removal of Adenoids.—Adenoids are removed with a guarded curette (fig. 592) pressed against the roof of the nasopharynx (fig. 593) and then carried backward and downward with a firm sweeping movement. The after-treatment is similar to that described above. Reactionary haemorrhage may be stopped by sitting the patient bolt upright. As a last resort, the nasopharynx may have to be packed (Chapter 33).

MALIGNANT TUMOURS OF THE TONSIL

Both carcinoma and lymphoma occur in the tonsil. The diagnosis in many instances is not easy. Any unilateral enlargement of the tonsil occurring in adult life should be regarded with suspicion. A biopsy is often required to confirm the diagnosis.

Carcinoma of the Tonsil (85%).—The patient is commonly an elderly man and pain is the leading symptom. The pain is severe and radiates to the ear, and, unlike that of tonsillitis, is unilateral. The breath is foul. Later, bleeding occurs, and as the ulcer deepens the loss of blood may be copious.

Lymphosarcoma of the tonsil (15%) has the reputation of being very malignant. While this is true if it is allowed to grow beyond the peritonsillar bed, the condition is by no means hopeless in its early stages. The patient is usually between fifty and sixty years of age, complains of a lump in the throat, which in the early stages is painless. Thick speech is a common symptom, and the tonsil appears large and pale. Later, the growth spreads, and often forms a swelling of the palate, which may be mistaken for a peritonsillar abscess, and incised. Once the barrier formed by the capsule of the tonsil has been breached, the growth extends rapidly into the neck, often forming a swelling behind the angle of the mandible. While the cervical lymph nodes soon become involved, a swelling in this position is likely to be an extension of the primary growth. Eventually bleeding, dysphagia, and dyspnoea foretell that the end is not far distant.

Treatment of both these conditions is similar. Following biopsy or excision biopsy the patient is given a course of external irradiation to cover the primary site as far as the clavicle to include the cervical lymph nodes. Should there be any residual tumour or suspicion of recurrence, energetic radical surgery must be undertaken with skin-flap and mandibular repair as required. These measures have vastly improved the 5 year survival rate to about 50%.

QUINSY (PERITONSILLAR ABSCESS)

As a rule the abscess is unilateral, but it is not uncommon for the contralateral side to become involved a few days later. The condition is rare in children, the incidence being highest in adult males. Extreme pain is experienced in the tonsillar region, radiating to the ear and to the side of the neck. Swallowing is so painful that saliva dribbles from the mouth; speech is thick and muffled. As the patient can open the mouth only to a slight extent, examination is often difficult. With good illumination, a diffuse swelling of the soft palate, mainly near the superior border of the affected tonsil, will be seen. The swelling displaces the oedematous uvula to the contralateral side.

---

[1] Morphine must not be given to children suffering from post-operative haemorrhage. It is a factor in tonsillectomy deaths.

Treatment, in the early stages, is the same as that for acute follicular tonsillitis (p. 626). If suppuration occurs, evacuation of pus in the following manner should not be delayed.

A small scalpel is modified by winding a strip of strapping around the blade so that only 1 cm of the tip projects. Except in small children, no general anaesthetic is used.[1] The patient sits upright. An incision is made in the position shown in fig. 594, which is usually described as midway between the base of the uvula and the third upper molar tooth. Dressing forceps are now pushed firmly *directly backwards*. As soon as pus is encountered, the forceps are opened widely and withdrawn.

Parapharyngeal abscess is similar to the above, but the maximum swelling is behind the posterior faucial pillar, and there is little or no oedema of the palate. The abscess is opened with a really blunt instrument, such as a tongue depressor. Often the gloved finger will suffice.

RETROPHARYNGEAL ABSCESSES

Acute retropharyngeal abscess is due to suppuration of the prevertebral lymph nodes. It is seen most commonly in children and 50% of cases occur under one year of age. The portal of entry is the tonsils, the nasopharynx, or the oropharynx. The condition may be accompanied by rigors, convulsions and vomiting. The neck is held rigidly, usually on one side, saliva dribbles from the child's mouth, and feeds are regurgitated. A croupy cough is common. The cry may resemble a 'squawk'. *Difficulty in breathing is the leading symptom* and this should always be the signal to examine a child's throat. The posterior wall of the pharynx is swollen. On digital examination a localised soft cushion-like protection can be felt on the posterior pharyngeal wall. The only condition with which acute retropharyngeal abscess may be confused is laryngeal diphtheria. A less acute form is seen in older children as a complication of otitis media.

Treatment.—No anaesthetic is used for infants, who must be placed in the prone position, with the head low. A pair of dressing forceps guided by the finger is thrust into the abscess cavity, the contents of which are evacuated. Suction must be available. Suitable antibiotic therapy is prescribed.

Chronic retropharyngeal abscess now rare, and sometimes due to an extension of tuberculosis of a cervical vertebra, presents with both a retropharyngeal swelling and a fullness behind the sternomastoid on one side. A chronic retropharyngeal abscess must never be opened into the mouth, for such a procedure will lead to secondary infection. The pus should be evacuated by an incision in front of the sternomastoid, to lead into the plane between the carotid sheath and the thyroid gland. The dissection towards the retropharyngeal space is conducted carefully until the abscess is opened. The cavity is then mopped dry and the wound closed. Suitable treatment of the underlying tuberculous lesion must then be instituted (Chapter 3).

DIVERTICULUM OF THE PHARYNX

Pharyngeal Pouch

Aetiology.—The pouch is a protrusion through Killian's dehiscence, that weak area of the posterior pharyngeal wall between the oblique fibres (thyropharyngeus) and the sphincter-like transverse fibres (cricopharyngeus) of the inferior constrictor muscle (fig. 595). Continued imperfect relaxation of the cricopharyngeus on swallowing and therefore repeated moments of high pressure as a bolus of food is propelled on its way to the oesophagus initiate the pouch. As it enlarges the resistance of the vertebral column behind causes it to turn outwards, usually to the left.

Clinical Features.—Patients suffering from this condition are usually elderly, and it is twice as common in men as in women.

There are three stages in the development of symptoms.

Stage 1.—There is a small diverticulum directed towards the vertebral column. Usually it is symptomless, and the finding of it is incidental during the course of a barium swallow. Occasionally it gives rise to symptoms identical with those of a foreign body in the throat. At this stage the diverticulum can be ignored.

Stage 2.—The diverticulum is larger and more globular, but its mouth still lies in the vertical plane. Regurgitation of undigested food at an unpredictable time after a meal, during the swallowing of the next meal, or after turning from one side to the other at

---

[1] In adult patients surface anaesthesia (5% cocaine on a pledget of wool) is the safest.

Gustav Killian, 1860–1921. Professor of Laryngo-rhinology, Berlin.

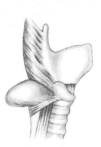

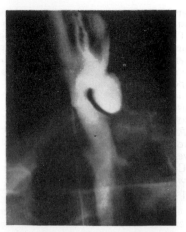

Fig. 595.—Pharyngeal pouch protruding between the thyropharyngeal
and cricopharyageal portions of the
inferior constrictor of the pharynx.
(After Sir Victor Negus.)

Fig. 596.—Semi-lateral radiograph
of a pouch after barium has been swallowed.

night, is the chief complaint. Sometimes the patient is awakened from sleep by a feeling of suffocation, followed by a violent fit of coughing. Infrequently an abscess of the lung results from food inspired from the pouch. Removal of the pouch is indicated.

Stage 3.—The pouch has become larger, and what is so important is that its mouth looks horizontally upwards. The fundus of the pouch has become dependent, and conse-quently when the pouch is full it compresses the oesophagus. The symptoms of the second stage persist; in addition, there are gurgling noises in the neck, especially when the patient swallows. In about one-third of cases, the pouch is large enough to form a visible swelling in the neck: sometimes such a pouch can be seen to enlarge when the patient drinks. Nevertheless, when this stage has been reached the symptom that transcends all others is increasing dysphagia, and in a large number of instances it is this symptom alone that compels the patient to seek relief. Eventually there is progressive loss of weight due to semi-starvation, and cachexia is sometimes extreme.

Radiography.—If a pharyngeal pouch is suspected, a very thin emulsion of barium should be used for the barium swallow; a thick mixture often requires much washing through a tube to remove the barium from the pouch. Quite often the fundus of the sac will be seen invading the superior mediastinum. Radiologically, the antero-posterior appearance of a barium-filled pouch can be simulated closely by a partial septum obstruct-ing the commencement of the oesophagus. Therefore, if this mistake is to be avoided a semi-lateral view (fig. 596) also must be taken. In this view the overflow of barium emul-sion into the oesophagus often can be seen to come from the top of the pouch—not from the bottom, as is the case with an oesophageal web. X-ray of the chest may reveal aspiration pneumonitis.

Oesophagoscopy or bouginage is unnecessary for diagnosis, and may be dangerous. On many occasions the tip of the instrument has entered the pouch and has perforated its fundus, which is thin and fragile, and mediastinitis has resulted.

Treatment.—When the pouch is of a considerable size, operation is strongly advised, because progressive symptoms are inevitable. When emaciation is extreme a preliminary temporary 'feeding' gastrostomy or jejunostomy may be required.

The operation is performed in one stage. To prevent mediastinitis, antibiotics should be given before and after operation.

Operation.—Prior to skin preparation, the surgeon should inspect the pouch endoscop-ically, and gently pack it with ribbon gauze. At the same time a stomach tube is carefully passed into the oesophagus. These will act as helpful guides in determining the position of the sac during the dissection. The pouch is approached through either a transverse incision at the level of the cricoid cartilage, or, as many prefer, an oblique incision follow-ing the anterior border of the left sternomastoid. The first step is to mobilise the superior pole of the lateral lobe of the thyroid gland, therefore it is necessary to ligate and divide the middle thyroid veins, and sometimes the inferior thyroid artery. The lateral lobe and

Sir Victor Ewings Negus, 1887–1974. Surgeon, Ear, Nose and Throat Department, King's College Hospital, London.

thyroid cartilage are rotated forwards by means of a hook retractor placed under the posterior border of the thyroid lamina; this exposes the sac.

The walls of the sac vary in thickness; in some cases they are so thin that great care must be taken not to tear them. Having freed the pouch completely, a cuff of the outer layer of the pouch is dissected from the mucous membrane. This permits the closure of the neck of the sac, which must be performed very accurately in two layers. It is very important not to narrow the upper end of the oesophagus at the point where the pouch is removed. In all cases a cricopharyngeal myotomy dividing the hypertrophied circular muscle must be performed (cf. Heller's operation, Chapter 43). The wound is closed with drainage.

After-treatment.—The patient is fed through an in-dwelling transnasal gastric tube for three days. Fluids only are permitted for the next three days. After this, semi-solids are given, and the diet is then increased gradually.

Complications.—1. *Infection.*—Severe infection of the wound and the mediastinum is now infrequent. 2. *Pharyngeal Fistula.*—Usually the fistula closes spontaneously if the upper end of the oesophagus has not been narrowed.

NEOPLASMS OF THE PHARYNX

Surgical Anatomy.—Concerning neoplasms of the pharynx, the clinico-anatomical division into three component parts (fig. 597) is of practical importance.

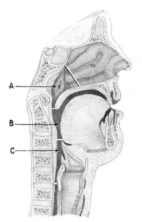

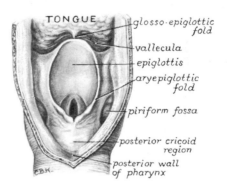

FIG. 597.—The component parts of the pharynx. A. Nasopharynx. B. Oropharynx. C. Laryngopharynx.

FIG. 598.—The epilarynx: the valleculae are shown also. In, or on, all the structures labelled a carcinoma can arise.

The **nasopharynx** (*syn.* post-nasal space, epipharynx) is that portion of the pharynx lying above the level of the soft palate which forms its incomplete floor. With the exception of this floor, the nasopharynx has rigid, immovable walls. Each Eustachian tube opens into the antero-lateral wall of the nasopharynx just behind the posterior end of the inferior turbinate. Above and behind this orifice is a depression termed the supratonsillar fossa of Rosenmüller.

The **oropharynx** (*syn.* the mesopharynx) extends from the inferior border of the soft palate to the lingual surface of the epiglottis. In the sulcus between the back of the tongue and the anterior (lingual) surface of the epiglottis lie a median glosso-epiglottic and a right and left pharyngo-epiglottic fold. The corresponding depression on either side of the glosso-epiglottic fold is known as the vallecula (fig. 598).

The **laryngopharynx** is the longest of the three divisions of the pharynx and it diminishes in width from above downwards. it extends from the tip of the epiglottis to the inferior border of the cricoid cartilage opposite the body of the sixth cervical vertebra, where it is continuous with the oesophagus. It is convenient to subdivide the laryngopharynx into (i) posterolateral pharyngeal walls, (ii) the pyriform fossae and (iii) the postcricoid region (fig. 598).

Johann Christian Rosenmüller, 1771–1820. Professor of Anatomy and Surgery, Leipzig, Germany.

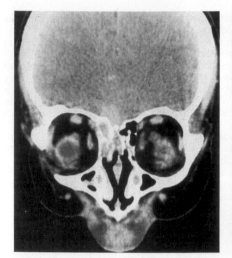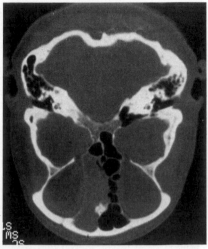

FIG. 599.—CT scans of right side tumour (angio-fibroma) of nasopharynx.
(Institute of Laryngology and Otology.)

TUMOURS OF THE NASOPHARYNX

Benign

Angio-fibroma.[1]—Although its local behaviour is the antithesis of benignity, this tumour is not malignant, for it never metastasises, neither does it infiltrate tissues. However, on account of its ability to send tentacles into first one and then the other nasal fossa, and thence into the accessory nasal sinuses, and above all because of its power to cause pressure necrosis of bone, it is a *highly destructive* tumour. As a result of these intrusions the tumour expands the nose, may fill the antra and in turn expand the cheek, and cause the palate to bulge, and at times invades the ethmoid and produces a 'frog face' appearance.

Nasopharyngeal angio-fibroma is a reddish, firm tumour covered with normal mucous membrane. Ulceration seldom occurs unless the tumour is traumatised. Histologically it is composed of immature fibroblasts and blood-vessels; in the early stages cavernous blood-vessels predominate. In long-standing cases fibrous tissue is more plentiful.

Clinical Features.—This tumour is almost confined to juvenile male patients.

Appearing at the age of puberty, the tumour usually regresses in the early twenties, provided that no secondary complications occur. Although nasophyaryngeal angiofibroma is rare, when a boy presents with progressive nasal obstruction, recurrent epistaxis, a purulent nasal discharge and a firm mass in the nasopharynx, this clinical entity should spring to mind.

Investigation.—CT scan will demonstrate the extent of the tumour (fig. 599). *Biopsy should be avoided* unless there are compelling reasons for undertaking it, when matched blood must be in readiness and the surgeon must be prepared to deal with haemorrhage.

Treatment.—Surgical resection requires an adequate exposure of the entire region,

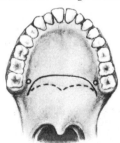

FIG. 600.—Incision for transpalatal approach to the nasopharynx.
(After the late C. P. Wilson, FRCS.)

---

[1] Formerly called 'nasopharyngeal tumour', which is ambiguous.

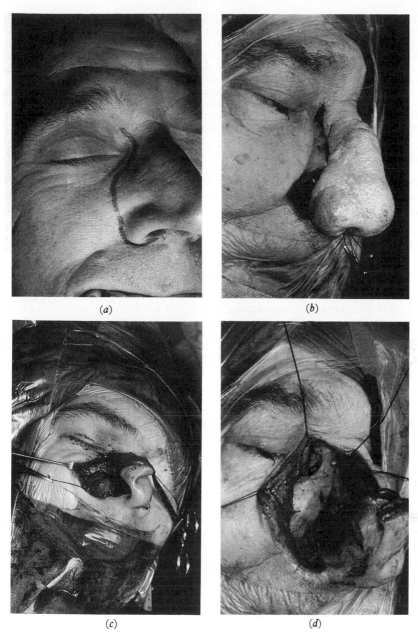

(a)   (b)

(c)   (d)

FIG. 601.—Lateral rhinotomy (see also Chapter 33). (a) Skin marking. (b) Incision. (c) Exposure of tumour (angio-fibroma). (d) Tumour removed.

(Institute of Laryngology and Otology, Professor D. F. N. Harrison, FRCS.)

and although small localised tumours can be removed by the transpalatal approach (fig. 600), for more extensive tumours a transfacial or lateral rhinotomy gives a safer exposure allowing lateral ligation of the feeding maxillary artery (fig. 601).

Operation.—The transpalatal route (fig. 600) is used. The tumour is excised with diathermy and the soft palate is replaced and sutured to the mucoperiosteum of the hard palate. Hypotensive anaesthesia and cryosurgical techniques have facilitated the procedure. Alternatively, in order that early recurrence may be seen, and destroyed by diathermy, a permanent palatal fenestra can be made. The fenestra is closed by an obturator attached to a denture. The patient can then talk and eat quite normally.

A choanal polypus may give rise to difficulty in differential diagnosis. Aetiologically it belongs to nasal polypi, originating either in the ethmoid region or in the maxillary antrum. If large, it may descend through the posterior nares into the nasopharynx and present behind the soft palate. A choanal polypus may be distinguished from angiofibroma by its mobility due to the long pedicle by which it is attached, avascularity and an elastic rather than firm consistency. It can be easily removed with a snare, although the corresponding sinus may have to be opened for complete removal.

Malignant

In China, Japan and Malaysia malignant tumours are more common in the nasopharynx than in any other part of the body save the cervix uteri, a possible cause being the use of smoky kerosene lamps in these countries. The majority are carcinomas (70%), followed by lymphoma (15%), lympho-epithelioma[1] (10%), while the remainder include mixed salivary tumour. Fifty per cent of these growths arise in the lateral wall of the nasopharynx, mostly in the supratonsillar fossa of Rosenmüller; the remainder are divided equally between the roof and the posterior wall.

Clinical Features.—These depend mainly on whether the growth is obstructive (lymphoma), or infiltrating (carcinoma). Usually the *first* symptoms for which advice is sought fall into four groups:

1. *The Nasal Group.*—Slight, intermittent epistaxis and nasal speech are early nasal symptoms; other nasal symptoms, *viz.* a feeling of obstruction to the airway and a post-nasal discharge, usually are delayed.

2. *Aural Group.*—Unilateral deafness, with pain in the ear, is the usual complaint. Obstruction of the pharyngeal orifice of the Eustachian tube by a growth leads to a collection of sero-sanguinous fluid within the middle ear. The deafness that results is relieved by paracentesis of the tympanic membrane and suction, but a fresh accumulation soon occurs. Bleeding on Eustachian catheterisation is a sign of the utmost importance.

3. *Enlarged Cervical Lymph Nodes.*—By the time the diagnosis is established, 70% of patients with a malignant tumour of the nasopharynx have enlarged cervical lymph nodes, and 40% present on account of the cervical swelling. The swelling is in the upper jugular chain and the nodes are firm, rather than hard, and may be mistaken for tuberculous adenitis.

Unlike carcinoma of the tongue, metastases more distant than the neck occur eventually in about a quarter of cases.

4. *Cranial Nerve Involvement.*—In Far Eastern patients this is the most common presenting symptom; in British patients 30% have some cranial nerve involvement when first seen. All suffer implication by the growth either at their exit through their respective foramina at the base of the skull, or, less frequently, by intracranial extension of the growth. Pain of trigeminal distribution is an important feature in this group. X-ray of the base of the skull may show destruction of bone by the tumour, but it is not unusual for patients to develop root pains without x-ray changes.

---

[1] A tumour containing many lymphoid elements in addition to carcinomatous elements.

Trotter's Triad.—The three cardinal symptoms of a locally invasive tumour can be summarised as follows: (i) Conductive deafness, (ii) Elevation and immobility of the homolateral soft palate—due to direct infiltration. (iii) Pain in the side of the head—due to involvement of the fifth cranial nerve from infiltration via the foramen lacerum.

Biopsy is necessary to ascertain the histological characteristics of the tumour. Inspection of the nasopharynx is facilitated if a soft rubber catheter is passed through the nose, and withdrawn through the mouth. Gentle traction displaces and immobilises the soft palate, and thereby an uninterrupted view is obtained. If more detailed inspection is desirable. Wilson's approach (fig. 600) through the junction of the hard and soft palate should be used.

Treatment.—Present practice favours supervoltage external irradiation, given to the primary tumour and to the lymph node fields on both sides of the neck at least as far down as the clavicles. Lymphoma, undifferentiated carcinoma, and lympho-epithelioma are very radio-sensitive. If the primary responds satisfactorily, it is feasible to perform a cervical block dissection of the enlarged lymph nodes.

Prognosis.—Owing to their secluded position and consequent late diagnosis, and the inaccessibility of the nasopharynx, the prognosis is poor. The five-year survival rate is about 40% for the lymphoma group and under 20% in the case of carcinoma.

NEOPLASMS OF THE OROPHARYNX

Benign

Diffuse cavernous angioma involving the pharynx, fauces, and often extending into the neck (where it forms a swelling) has been treated successfully by injecting into the bluish mass in the pharynx 0·5 ml of 1·4 solution of ferrous chloride in sterile water. The injected area immediately turns bright red, remains swollen for a few days, and then cicatrizes. Further injections may be required. Later, if necessary, abnormal tissue is removed by diathermy, with practically no bleeding. Cryosurgery can be effective in dealing with these lesions.

Malignant

Usually carcinoma of the oropharynx is of the ulcerative type. The commonest site of origin is the tonsillo-lingual sulcus. There is discomfort at the back of the throat, foetor, and blood-stained sputum. Pain is absent until the growth is far advanced.

Treatment.—The management is identical to tumours of the nasopharynx of similar histological picture.

Operation.—Although the long-term results are far from good, when possible, extirpation of the growth and the regional lymph nodes holds out a better prospect of success than irradiation.

Lateral pharyngotomy with partial pharyngectomy is performed as follows. A tracheostomy is usually performed as the first step. Then a block dissection of the cervical and retropharyngeal lymph nodes is carried out. The lateral lobe of the thyroid is then mobilised and displaced forwards. The inferior constrictor muscle is detached from the thyroid and cricoid cartilages. The great cornu of the hyoid bone and the posterior two-thirds of the ala of the thyroid cartilage are removed without opening the mucous lining.

Should the growth be situated on the lateral wall and have invaded the tonsillar region, the cervical operation is halted at this stage, and through the widely open mouth an incision is made at least 2·5 cm distant from the accessible margins of the neoplasm

---

Wilfred Batten Lewis Trotter, 1872–1939. Professor of Surgery, University College Hospital, London.
Charles Paul Wilson, 1900–1970. Surgeon, Ear, Nose and Throat Department, Middlesex Hospital, London.

with a diathermy knife, the internal carotid artery being held aside in the neck (Raven). Returning to the neck, the pharynx is opened longitudinally and that portion of the pharyngeal wall containing the growth and a wide margin of healthy tissue is removed in continuity with its lymphatics.

When the loss of the pharyngeal wall is not great the pharynx is closed. A portion of the upper part of the posterior skin flap is anchored by stitches to the prevertebral fascia, thus providing free exit to infected matter should leakage occur. The remainder of the cervical wound is closed with drainage at its lower end.

After-treatment includes transnasal intragastric feeding and antibiotic therapy.

When it is known beforehand that the defect in the pharyngeal wall is likely to be a large one, the operation is performed through a rectangular skin flap, and after partial pharyngectomy has been performed, the first stage of the plastic procedure is carried out as shown in fig. 602. In the early post-operative period, the patient is fed by a tube passed into the stomach through the fistula.

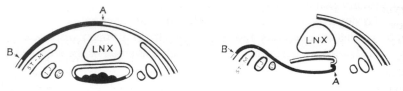

FIG. 602.—Trotter's method of reconstructing the pharynx from a flap of skin (A–B) of the neck after excision of an extensive pharyngeal carcinoma.

In both the procedures just described the resulting cervical fistula will require closure; this is undertaken after a short convalescence.

Growths situated in the vallecula, unless very advanced, must be treated by pharyngolaryngectomy with, if necessary, excision of a portion of the back of the tongue.

NEOPLASMS OF THE LARYNGOPHARYNX

In accordance with their site of origin, it is customary to subdivide malignant tumours of this part of the pharynx into four groups:

1. Epilaryngeal (20%).—Nearly always the patient is a man between fifty and sixty years of age. The lesion is situated on an aryepiglottic fold, extending to the epiglottis or the corresponding arytenoid cartilage, and is either of the ulcerative or the papillary type. It may be symptomless in the early stages. The earliest symptom is a slightly sore throat. A muffled voice and increasing dysphagia occur later. Real hoarseness indicates involvement of the interior of the larynx, *i.e.* the vocal cord. Later there are attacks of dyspnoea associated with blood-stained sputum. The diagnosis is made by indirect laryngoscopy.

2. Sinus Piriformis[1] (40%).—Again, this group occurs chiefly in men about fifty years of age, and the lesion is notoriously silent. Often its first intimation is an enlarged lymph node behind the angle of the jaw. Frequently this is not heeded in its early stages. Exceptionally, the patient presents himself at an earlier stage, because of slight difficulty in swallowing saliva, as opposed to food. Pain is absent until the growth has involved the superior laryngeal nerve. The pain is referred to the ear. Carcinoma of the piriform fossa is nearly always of the ulcerative type. The growth may be seen with a laryngeal mirror, but sometimes its extent cannot be determined without direct laryngoscopy.

3. Lateral Wall (12%).—Once again men are attacked much more often than women. Contrary to the sinus piriformis, the growth is often papillary.

---

[1] Piriformis—Latin, *pirum* = a pear.

Ronald William Raven, Contemporary. Consulting Surgeon, The Royal Marsden Hospital, London.

A lateral radiograph of the neck, with air inflation of the pharynx, is often more informative than a barium swallow in the demonstration of a neoplasm in this and nearby situations.

4. Post cricoid (28%) occurs on the anterior wall of the hypopharynx at the level of the cricoid cartilage. The patient is nearly always a woman of over forty years of age, who gives a history of increasing dysphagia.

The higher incidence in women is possibly due to their ability to swallow hotter fluids and food than men can tolerate. Many of these neoplasms are secondary to the Plummer-Vinson syndrome.[1] Indirect laryngoscopy seldom reveals the growth, which lies hidden beneath a pool of mucus. Radiographic examination after a barium swallow is often helpful in determining the site of the lesion. Direct pharyngoscopy is the most informative, and allows a portion of the growth to be removed for biopsy.

Treatment of Carcinoma of the Laryngopharynx.—The condition is notoriously difficult to treat successfully. Surgery, often the treatment of choice, involves the major operation of laryngo-pharyngectomy, combined with block dissection of the neck, the establishment of a permanent tracheostomy, and the plastic reconstruction of the pharynx. About 20% of patients survive five years.

External irradiation is the alternative method of treatment and is advised for those patients who are considered unsuitable for such a major procedure, either because of their poor general condition, or because it is thought that they will not be able to adjust themselves to a life without a larynx.

Types of Operation.—Operations which combine excision and reconstruction of the gullet in one stage are preferable to staged procedures. The following is an example of a one-stage operation, in which the stomach is used to replace the pharynx:

Two teams are used. The first team performs the pharyngo-laryngectomy, the block dissection of the lymph nodes of the neck on the side of the tumour, and establishes the tracheostomy. The larynx and pharynx are excised from above the level of the hyoid bone down to the level of the third or fourth tracheal ring, and including the whole of the cervical oesophagus. The stump of the oesophagus is closed by inverting sutures and allowed to slide into the thorax. The thyroid gland is included in the excision. A block dissection of lymph nodes on the less involved side may be undertaken, but the sternomastoid muscle and the internal jugular vein are usually spared.

Stomach pull-up.—At the same time as the larynx, pharynx and oesophagus are mobilised in the neck, the stomach is moblised via a left upper paramedian incision. The left gastric artery is divided, but the blood supply from the marginal branch of the right gastro-epiploic artery is preserved when the omentum is freed from the greater curvature of the stomach. A pyloromyotomy is necessary to allow adequate drainage. The oesophagus is then mobilised in the posterior mediastinum by blunt finger dissection from both the upper and lower ends with especial care to prevent damage to the posterior wall of the trachea. The stomach is then pulled up through the posterior mediastinum by gentle traction on the oesophagus which is then resected and the fundus of the stomach is anastomosed to the pharyngeal stump. A large suction drain is placed in the chest, but the bleeding from the azygos veins is controlled by pressure from the bulk of the stomach.

The patient is allowed to swallow fluids the following day and to eat normal foods within two weeks. Should recurrence of the neoplasm occur, radiotherapy can be given with little risk of damage to the artificial gullet and hence little interference with the patient's swallowing.

Chemotherapy

Cytotoxic drugs have a limited value as an adjunct to surgery and radiotherapy in patients who have not responded, or who have recurrent growths. Before deciding to give

---

1 Also widely known as the Paterson-Brown Kelly syndrome.

Henry Stanley Plummer, 1874–1937. Physician, Mayo Clinic, Rochester, Minnesota, U.S.A.
Porter Paisley Vinson, 1890–1959. Physician, Mayo Clinic, Rochester, Minnesota, U.S.A.
Donald Rose Paterson, 1862–1939. Surgeon, Ear, Nose and Throat Department, Royal Infirmary, Cardiff, Wales.
Adam Brown Kelly, 1865–1941. Surgeon, Ear, Nose and Throat Department, Victoria Infirmary, Glasgow, Scotland.

chemotherapy, one must balance the prognosis of the disease against the expected relief and possible toxic side-effects and then consider the types of agent required and the most suitable method of administration. The regimen to follow has been discussed in Chapter 32 and Chapter 10.

CRYOSURGERY

Cryosurgery[1] is a technique in which tissues are exposed to extreme cold in order to produce irreversible cell damage. Alternate rapid freezing and thawing to a temperature of at least—10°C. causes multiple intra-cellular ice crystals to form which will be lethal to the cell. Its main use in appropriately trained hands would seem to be, 1. destruction of benign vascular lesions of the head and neck (*e.g.* haemangioma, angiofibroma), 2. palliation and relief of pain in uncontrolled or recurrent accessible cancers (*e.g.* carcinoma of nasopharynx), 3. a large number of ophthalmological procedures, including fixation of detached retina.

Technique.—Modern equipment consists of a hollow probe refrigerated by liquid nitrogen or pressurised nitrous oxide. Incorporated in the probe is a rewarming device, thus tissue can be rapidly frozen and thawed as required. The probe is applied to the tissue and freezing started, and when a 'tissue ice-ball' has formed in the area to be treated, it is then immediately allowed to thaw. The process must be repeated 2 or 3 times to achieve maximum destruction.

---

1 The idea of 'freezing surgery' is not new; a Dr. James Arnott in 1851 at the Middlesex Hospital described the beneficial effects of a salt-ice mixture at –20°C. in the treatment of various superficial cancers.

James Moncrieff Arnott, 1794–1885. Surgeon, Middlesex Hospital, London.

CHAPTER 35

THE LARYNX

FOREIGN BODY IN THE LARYNX

Impaction of foreign bodies is more likely to occur in children than in adults. Cardiac arrest and death may occur.

Treatment.—If the foreign body cannot be dislodged by hooking it out with a finger, or by inverting the child and slapping its back, immediate tracheostomy is necessary in urgent cases with obstructive symptoms. In less urgent cases radiography is useful when the foreign body is radio-opaque. By the aid of direct laryngoscopy the object can be seized and removed.

ACUTE OEDEMA OF THE GLOTTIS (EPIGLOTTIS)

Pathology.—Strictly speaking, the oedema is not of the glottis (the chink between the vocal cords) but of the aryepiglottic folds and the epiglottis, but this ancient and inaccurate term is difficult to displace.

Aetiology.—1. Extension of acute inflammation, especially acute streptococcal and haemophilus influenzal laryngitis or tonsillitis, diphtheria, acute parenchymatous gloss-itis, and Ludwig's angina.

2. Angioneurotic oedema.

3. Irradiation either with or without perichondritis.

4. Trauma (*e.g.* car accidents).

5. Indirect irritants such as corrosives, scalds or noxious gases.

6. Extension of an adjacent carcinoma.

7. Local dropsy (renal or heart failure).

The patient's voice is reduced to a hoarse whisper and some dysphagia may be present. Increasing dyspnoea occurs and frequently the oedema is sufficient to cause urgent stridor. If laryngoscopic examination is possible, the entrance to the larynx can be seen resembling the appearance of the cervix uteri.

Treatment.—Inhalation of steam and spraying with a dilute solution of adrenaline afford relief in early and mild cases. Systemic antihistamines (*e.g.* Phenergan) or cortisone are valuable.[1] When dyspnoea is urgent, intubation or tracheostomy must be performed forthwith.

TRACHEOSTOMY

The indications are as follows:

(*a*) **To relieve obstruction of the upper air passages due to:**

1. Impaction of a foreign body.

2. Acute infections such as: acute laryngo-tracheo-bronchitis of children, acute epiglottis of influenzal or virus origin. Laryngeal diphtheria.

3. Oedema of the glottis.

4. Bilateral abductor paralysis of the vocal cords following injury to the recurrent laryngeal nerves during thyroidectomy.

---

[1] In cases of laryngeal obstruction, never give morphine. A patient under the influence of morphine stops fighting for breath, seems peaceful, and not infrequently the nurse returns to find him dead (Chevalier Jackson).

Chevalier, L. Jackson, 1900–1961. Professor of Laryngology and Broncho-Oesophagoscopy, Temple University, Philadelphia, Pennsylvania, U.S.A.

Wilhelm von Ludwig, 1790–1865. Professor of Surgery and Midwifery, University of Tübingen, Germany.

5. Tumours, particularly carcinoma of the larynx.

6. Chronic stenosis following tuberculosis or scalding.

7. Congenital webs or atresias.

8. Cut throat.

(*b*) **To improve respiratory function**, by reducing the anatomical dead space, and also enabling effective aspiration of bronchial secretions to be done in:

1. Fulminating bronchopneumonia.

2. Chronic bronchitis with severe emphysema.

3. Chest injuries, particularly 'flail' chest.

(*c*) **Respiratory Paralysis.**—It allows assisted or positive pressure respiration to be performed. Also secretions or inhaled foreign material (*e.g.* vomitus) can be aspirated. Causes:

1. Unconsciousness associated with head or facio-maxillary injuries.

2. Coma from other causes persisting for more than a few hours where there is difficulty in maintaining a free airway, *e.g.* barbiturate poisoning.

3. Bulbar type of poliomyelitis.

4. Tetanus. Many of these patients are, of necessity, heavily sedated, have trismus, and are in mortal danger because of inability to expectorate.

(*d*) **As a preliminary to certain operations on the upper airway.**

In cases of dire emergency the operation has been performed successfully with nothing available except a penknife. If at all possible, intubation even with a small intratracheal tube, should be attempted. If successful, a general anaesthetic can be administered and a hurried procedure transformed into a deliberate, calm operation. Intubation brings the abnormally low intrapleural tension to normal and prevents the occurrence of surgical emphysema and possibly pneumothorax, especially in children (see Mediastinal emphysema, p. 641). Insertion of an intratracheal tube also permits aspiration of secretions which have accumulated below the laryngeal obstruction. Intubation will also prevent spasm of the glottis.

Operation.—If a skilled anaesthetist is unavailable, local anaesthesia is employed, but in desperate cases none is required. The patient may be pinned in a blanket so that a sudden movement of the arms may not embarass the surgeon. When preparations are complete, a rolled towel or a small sandbag is inserted beneath the shoulders, and an assistant keeps the head extended strictly in the midline (fig. 603)

The surgeon, standing at the right side of the patient, places his left index finger on the upper border of the cricoid cartilage, with the thumb and the second finger on either side

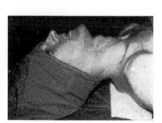

FIG. 603.—The position for tracheostomy.

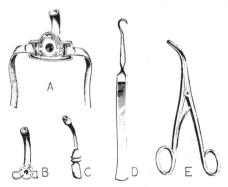

FIG. 604.—Instruments for tracheostomy (excluding scalpel and haemostats).
A. Outer tube with tapes attached. B. Inner tube. C. Pilot. D. Cricoid hook. E. Tracheal dilator.

of the trachea, and makes an incision vertically downwards for 2.5 to 3.75 cm, dividing skin, fascia, platysma, pretracheal fascia, and passing between the infrahyoid muscles. (When circumstances permit, a horizontal skin incision midway between the cricoid and the suprasternal notch should be used, as subsequent healing is far more satisfactory.) If seen, the isthmus of the thyroid gland is divided between haemostats. In an emergency, haemorrhage is ignored. A cricoid hook (fig. 604) is then inserted under the cricoid cartilage and grasped in the left hand. The hook steadies the trachea and brings it to the surface of the wound. The trachea is incised with a scalpel, the second, third, and often the fourth rings being divided: the lower the tracheostomy, the less will be the liability to laryngeal stenosis. A tracheal dilator is inserted through the tracheostoma, the cricoid hook removed, and the edges of the tracheal wound are separated gently. In the case of diphtheria the surgeon places a swab over the wound so that the violent expiratory efforts which follow do not spray membrane, infected mucus, and blood over himself and his assistants. When respiratory efforts have become less violent, a tracheostomy tube on a pilot (fig. 604) is inserted into the trachea, the dilator is removed, and the surgeon keeps his finger on the tube while the assistant ties the attached tapes around the patient's neck. The inner tube[1] is then fixed in position, and one or two nylon or silk stitches are introduced if necessary.

In the case of a less urgent tracheostomy all bleeding is stopped before the trachea is opened. The injection of a few drops of 2% Xylocaine before the trachea is incised prevents the bout of coughing that follows the insertion of the tube. When the operation is performed on an adolescent or an adult, the isthmus of the thyroid gland is divided. The tracheostomy opening should be circular in shape (not just a vertical slit), by excising the edges of the incision with a scalpel strong enough to cut cartilage. A circular stoma facilitates the introduction and later changing of the tracheostomy tube, and heals well after eventual removal of the tube.

If a patient is unable to breathe unaided, an *inflatable rubber or polyethylene cufftube* is introduced through the tracheostomy opening in order to seal off the air passage. The airway must be kept clear by frequent aspiration, assisted by postural drainage.

After-treatment.—Beside the bed is placed a trolley containing a tracheal dilator, duplicate cannulae and introducer, retractors, and dressings. Oxygen is at hand. For the first few days a special nurse must be in constant attendance. A mechanical humidifier is essential in order to render the secretion less viscid. A sucker with a catheter attached should be at hand to keep the tracheo-bronchial tree free from secretions. The catheter must be kept sterile on a special tray covered by a sterile towel. The introduction of the catheter must be carried out under aseptic precautions by all concerned (nurses and physiotherapists). Unless these precautions are observed, secondary broncho-pneumonial infection is inevitable. When mucus is very tenacious, and consequently difficult to aspirate, isotonic saline or a detergent such as Alevaire® (Bayer Products Ltd.) is administered through the tracheostomy by a fine nebuliser.

The inner tube is removed and washed in sodium bicarbonate solution every four hours, more if necessary. Before removal the patient should be able to sleep with the tube occluded.

Complications:

1. *Crusting in the trachea* or main bronchi can seriously embarrass the airway; it can be cleaned by the aid of a bronchoscope passed through the tracheostoma.

2. *Surgical emphysema* in the neck is a complication and may occur if the skin is too tightly sutured around the tube, or if the tube slips into the tissues of the neck (fig. 605).

3. *Mediastinal Emphysema.*—The cause is an abnormally low intrapleural tension—air is sucked into the tissue planes during the operation before the trachea is opened, causing

---

[1] The inner tube is longer than the outer tube, so that the latter cannot remain obstructed when the inner tube is removed for cleaning. To carry out suction effectively, the inner tube must be of such a diameter that it will not be occluded by the passage of a No.3 or 4 rubber catheter.

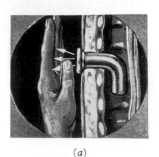
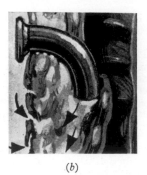

FIG. 605.—(a) Tracheostomy tube in the correct position. Testing for a free airway. (b) The tube has slipped, or has been incorrectly positioned, so causing surgical emphysema.

(a)   (b)

subsequent dyspnoea and cyanosis. In severe examples the air in the mediastinum causes the mediastinal pleura to rupture, and a pneumothorax results. The diagnosis can be confirmed by radiography. Apart from oxygen therapy in high concentration, there is no specific treatment. The extravasated air is slowly absorbed.

4. *Tracheal Stenosis* is described later.

Endotracheal catheterisation is a substitute for tracheostomy (mainly cases in group (c), p. 640), but it is usually less desirable, for two reasons:

(a) Repeated bronchial tree toilet is performed more easily by a nurse through a tracheostomy. (b) Intubation granuloma of the vocal cords (p. 644) and subsequent stricture may occur.

LARYNGEAL PARALYSIS

The muscles of the larynx are innervated by the recurrent laryngeal nerves, with the exception of the crico-thyroid muscle which is supplied by the superior laryngeal nerve. Lesions of the recurrent laryngeal nerve cause the vocal cord on the affected side to lie in the paramedian position: this is due to the unopposed tensing and adducting action of the crico-thyroid. Lesions of the vagus nerve above the origin of the superior laryngeal nerve will cause complete vocal cord paralysis on the affected side. The cord will be flaccid and lie midway between abduction and adduction, which is the state and position of the vocal cords soon after death.

Aetiology.—The lesion may be central, cervical, or mediastinal. Of over-riding importance is the relation of a goitre, and especially of thyroidectomy, to recurrent laryngeal paralysis. Routine laryngoscopic examination must be made before thyroidectomy, as 3 to 5% of patients are found to have paresis or paralysis of one vocal cord, possibly due to neuritis following exanthemata during childhood, although no symptoms point to such a lesion. Pre-operative laryngoscopy is especially necessary when operating on a case of recurrent goitre. If pre-operative paralysis of a vocal cord is found, this fact *must* be recorded in the patient's notes in order to protect the surgeon from possible litigation. Pre-operative paralysis of a vocal cord with symptoms, *e.g.* a recent husky voice, is highly suggestive that the goitre is carcinomatous. Other causes of recurrent laryngeal paralysis are a central lesion (*e.g.* tabes), carcinoma of the upper oesophagus, carcinoma of the bronchus, malignant disease of the mediastinal lymph nodes, aneurysm of the arch of the aorta (always left-sided), and peripheral neuritis. Thirty per cent of cases are idiopathic.

Clinical Features.—Unilateral recurrent laryngeal palsy of sudden onset produces a whispering voice and occasionally some slight difficulty in swallowing fluids, due to paralysis of the crico-pharyngeus on the affected side. These symptoms are short-lived and the voice may return to normal within a few weeks as the muscles in the opposite cord compensate and move it across the midline to meet the paralysed cord. Owing to this efficient compensation, in slowly progressive lesions, the patient may only experience slight weakness of the voice towards the end of the day.

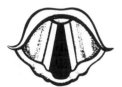 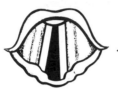 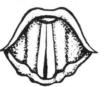 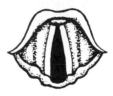

FIG. 606.— Normal larynx on inspiration. Indirect laryngoscopy.

FIG. 607.—Left recurrent nerve laryngeal palsy.

FIG. 608.— Bilateral recurrent nerve laryngeal palsy.

FIG. 609.—Bilateral flaccid paralysis of the vocal cords. The cadaveric position.

Bilateral recurrent laryngeal nerve palsy is an occasional and very serious complication of thyroidectomy. Acute dyspnoea occurs due to the paramedian position of the cords which tend to get sucked together on inspiration. Unless tracheostomy or intubation is carried out forthwith, death from asphyxia is probable.

Unilateral complete laryngeal paralysis causes a hoarse voice in which compensation does not readily occur owing to the flaccid state of the vocal cord and its lateral position. The healthy vocal cord has difficulty in meeting it.

Bilateral complete laryngeal palsy is an uncommon condition which occurs in lesions of the brain stem. It is usually associated with other cranial nerve lesions.

Treatment.—Tracheostomy should be performed in all cases of bilateral lesions, even when the paralysis is flaccid, for it is far better to provide the patient with a free airway than to permit him to suffer from chronic dyspnoea and its attendant evils, chief of which is the risk of asphyxia. The use of a tracheostomy tube with a speaking valve allows the patient to speak: the delicate valve opens on inspiration and closes on expiration. The expired air passes through the vocal cords so that the patient has an audible voice. With an ordinary tracheostomy tube the inspired and expired air by-passes the larynx and the patient's voice amounts only to a whisper. In cases following thyroidectomy where the patient is otherwise in good health, the next step is to wait up to a year in the hope that one or both of the nerves will recover, otherwise arytenoidectomy either by endoscopic laser resection or by an external approach may be considered. It gives permanent relief of stridor at the expense of a good voice.

SIMPLE SWELLINGS OF THE LARYNX

1. **Vocal Cord Polypus.—**This is the most common of the simple swellings in the larynx and must be distinguished from true benign neoplasms. It originates in the sub-epithelial space within the vocal cord. Initial congestion is followed by localised areas of

oedema and hyalinisation; a soft, pearly grey often pedunculated mass is formed. It is easily removed endoscopically with cupped forceps or by laser.

2. **Intubation granuloma** may arise as a rare complication following the use of endotracheal anaesthetic tubes.

3. **Laryngocele.**[1]—A laryngocele is a unilateral (occasionally bilateral) narrow-necked, air-containing diverticulum resulting from a herniation of laryngeal mucosa. It originates in the laryngeal sacculus, situated in the anterior third of the laryngeal ventricle, and ascending between the false cords and the ala of the thyroid cartilage, and it herniates through the thyrohyoid membrane, and when distended forms a visible, often resonant, swelling in the neck.

The symptoms, due to a recrudescence of infection, come in attacks when the swelling, which often appears when the patient blows his nose, does not abate completely for hours or days; the explanation being that the neck of the sac becomes obstructed by mucopus. The attack often terminates with a gurgling noise and discharge of mucus into the pharynx. The sac should be excised and the neck, which is crushed, ligated, and divided, is invaginated like the stump of a vermiform appendix.

TUMOURS OF THE LARYNX

Benign.—**Papilloma** is the commonest benign tumour of the larynx.

In an adult a papilloma is usually single, and its pedicle is attached to one of the true or false vocal cords. The symptoms to which it gives rise are similar to those of carcinoma of the larynx, from which it must be distinguished. The diagnosis is made by laryngoscopic examination. Rarely, a papilloma becomes malignant; therefore the papilloma should be removed and submitted to microscopical examination.

In a child the growth is relatively common: it is usually more vascular and softer than a papilloma appearing during adult life. Moreover, implantation growths soon appear in the vicinity and may obstruct the glottis. There is a marked tendency to recurrence after removal, and the papillomas may spread to almost any site in the larynx, pharynx, or trachea.

Treatment.—Chevalier Jackson's warning was not to be too radical in the treatment of multiple papillomas for fear of damaging the vocal cords. 'Laryngeal papilloma,' he said, 'is a self-limiting disease and disappears spontaneously in early adult life provided the patient can be carried through until that time.'

Endoscopic removal with cupped forceps is the usual method of treatment but if a laser is available the long-term results are better.

Micro-surgery of the Larynx.—This is a technique whereby the vocal cords can be inspected under magnification and benign lesions more carefully and accurately removed (Kleinsasser). The operating microscope is used with a special laryngoscope which is inserted and fixed to a clamp for stability. Healing of the cords and the post-operative voice are generally much better than after ordinary laryngoscopy.

Angiofibroma is always single, and is distinguished from a papilloma by its smooth contour (fig. 610). Except that occasionally it gives rise to haemoptysis, it resembles a papilloma in symptomatology. In appropriate cases the condition must be distinguished from *singer's nodules*, which are nearly always bilateral. The latter condition, which produces a pearly-white nodule on the free edge of the vocal cord, is not a neoplasm, but an epithelial hypertrophy, and should, if possible, always be treated by prolonged voice rest (which is sometimes successful) before resorting to operation. On the other hand, an angiofibroma should be removed endoscopically with cupped forceps or cryosurgery.

---

[1] Cervical air-pouches are present in many mammals, and can be inflated voluntarily; they are exceptionally well developed in South American monkeys that utilise them for howling (howling pouches). The condition, therefore, can be looked upon as partly atavistic but mainly acquired, for it occurs in professional trumpet-players, glass-blowers, and in persons with chronic cough.

Oskar Kleinsasser, Contemporary. Associate Professor, Ear, Nose and Throat Clinic, Cologne, Germany.

FIG. 610.—Angiofibroma of the left vocal cord. It seldom becomes much larger than depicted here.

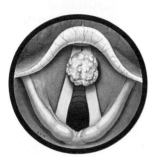

FIG. 611.—Carcinoma of a true vocal cord.

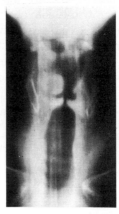

FIG. 612.—Tomogram of larynx showing tumour of the right false vocal cord encroaching on the laryngeal ventricle. The vocal cords are not affected.

Great precision is necessary, because if normal tissue is removed the speaking voice will be impaired and the singing voice ruined.

Malignant.—Squamous-cell Carcinoma is more common than an innocent tumour of the larynx. It usually occurs between forty and sixty years of age, and men are ten times more often attacked than women. Smoking is by far the most important aetiological factor.

There are three varieties of laryngeal carcinoma:

1. *Glottic* (70% of growth), arising from the true vocal cord, which is relatively common and the most favourable type.

2. *Subglottic* (10%), below the vocal cords, with a worse prognosis.

3. *Supraglottic* (20%), originating from the ventricular bands (false vocal cords), laryngeal ventricles or the root of the epiglottis. This group has the worst prognosis.

1. Carcinoma of a vocal cord (glottic) usually arises from the anterior half of one of the true vocal cords. Most frequently it is of the papillary variety (fig. 611), occasionally it is flattened, rarely it is ulcerative. Due to the paucity or absence of lymphatic vessels of the vocal cords, this type of carcinoma of the larynx remains locally malignant for a long period.

The first symptom is huskiness of the voice. The huskiness is progressive, and the patient can speak only in a low whisper, which finally gives place to aphonia. About this time the growth breaks through its confines, and metastases occur in the cervical lymph nodes and elsewhere.

The diagnosis is made by laryngoscopy examination and biopsy, and every patient with hoarseness persisting for more than three weeks should be submitted to this form of examination. According to the length of time the growth has been present, *four stages* of the disease are recognised:

i. The growth is confined to a *still mobile* vocal cord.

ii. Infiltration impairing mobility of the cord. Extension to other cord.

iii. Fixation of the cord. The growth has entered adjoining part of larynx. Isolated involved lymph nodes.

iv. Extension to the pharynx or skin. Lymph node metastases with fixation.

2. **Subglottic carcinoma** is a less common variety that occurs beneath the vocal cords. In this site the neoplasm grows steadily and silently, until dyspnoea develops. The paratracheal and lower deep cervical nodes, and even the thyroid gland may be involved.

3. **Supraglottic Carcinoma.**—The initial symptom is often a sense of discomfort in the larynx. Pain and hoarseness come relatively late. In 60% of cases there is cervical lymph node involvement at the time of presentation.

Tomograms are very helpful to determine the extent of the growth (fig. 612).

Treatment.—Supraglottic tumours metastasise early into the cervical lymph nodes, whereas tumours of the true vocal cords remain locally malignant for many months. For early (stage 1 and 2) carcinoma of the true vocal cord, the results of irradiation are as good as those of surgery and the voice is better. Therefore, where adequate facilities exist, irradiation (supra voltage x-ray therapy, or telecobalt) is preferable to surgery. Although in the stage 1 growths there is an 80% five years' survival rate, every effort should be made to have a careful follow up. If recurrences occur, or where the cervical lymph nodes are involved by metastatic deposits of squamous-celled carcinoma, laryngectomy, with block dissection of the lymph nodes in continuity, gives results superior to irradiation.

Laryngo-fissure and Excision of the Growth.—The vocal cord must be still mobile. After preliminary tracheostomy, the thyroid cartilage is bisected and the whole vocal cord is removed. The tracheostomy tube is removed after a few days. As the vocal cord becomes replaced by fibrous tissue, the patient tends to have a gruff voice.

Total laryngectomy (fig. 613) is performed for carcinoma of the vocal cord which is already *fixed* by infiltration, when radiotherapy fails to destroy the growth or where the growth recurs after radiotherapy.

Anaesthesia.—General anaesthesia is given through an endotracheal tube inserted via the nose. This is changed by the surgeon during the later stages of the operation after delivery of the larynx.

Incision.—A variety of incisions is used. A satisfactory exposure is shown in fig. 613A. This may be modified if a block dissection is necessary.

Dissection.—The laryngeal cartilages and trachea are exposed by division of the thyroid isthmus. The strap muscles are divided and the inferior constrictor is carefully dissected off the thyroid cartilage. The hyoid is freed. The pharynx is opened by incisions above the hyoid bone. After changing the anaesthetic tube, the hyoid is drawn forward and the mucous membrane incised down each pyriform fossa, to meet along the back of the arytenoids. A nasal feeding tube is passed into the oesophagus and the defect in the pharynx is closed by interrupted sutures, and reinforced by suturing the inferior constrictors together anteriorly.

The trachea is divided between the second and third rings. A laryngectomy stoma is fashioned by suturing the trachea to the cut edges of the wound in the suprasternal notch.

For supraglottic carcinoma, subglottic tumours, and in cases where cervical lymph nodes are obviously the sites of secondary deposits, block dissection of the lymph nodes must be combined with the laryngectomy. If the carcinoma extends into a lobe of the thyroid gland, this lobe is also removed.

Speech after laryngectomy. Prior to operation the patient should have already met and been assessed by a speech therapist so that as soon as the neck and pharynx have healed the therapist can commence teaching oesophageal voice. In many cases the patient becomes quite proficient in its use and should at least communicate to some extent.

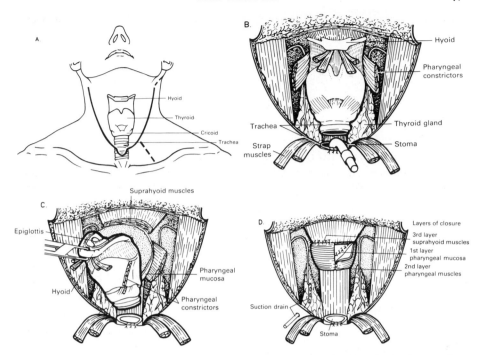

FIG. 613.—Total laryngectomy. A. Incision. B. Larynx exposed and endotracheal tube moved to new position. C. Larynx mobilised. D. Pharynx repaired. Tracheostoma formed.

However, should the patient not acquire a reasonable competence, one of the following methods can be used to create communication:

1. *Surgical rehabilitation of the voice* is now possible by means of a valve placed in a small fistula which is formed between the upper part of the trachea near the tracheostome and the pharynx. During expiration the patient occludes the tracheostome with his thumb so that the column of air is diverted through the valve into the pharynx. As the column of air passes up the irregular contours of the pharynx it creates a primary vibration which is then modified by the tongue and lips to create a very credible and satisfactory voice. The shape of the valve prevents ingested material passing from the pharynx into the trachea.

2. *The use of an electrically operated vibrator sound* (so called artificial larynx) which is applied to the side of the neck creating a primary sound while the patient articulates to produce the words.

CHAPTER 36

THE NECK

THE BRANCHIAL APPARATUS AND ITS ABNORMALITIES

In a foetus approximately thirty-five days old, four grooves can be seen on each side of the neck. These are the branchial clefts, which resemble the gills of a fish; the intervening bars are the branchial arches. Each arch contains a central cartilage. The clefts in human embryos are composed of grooves on the outside and pouches on the inside (pharynx). The first cleft persists as the external auditory meatus; the second, third, and fourth clefts normally disappear. The whole, or a portion, of one of the clefts that normally disappear may persist. Alternatively, a portion can become sequestrated.

Branchial Cyst.—From the vestigial remnants of the second branchial cleft the cyst is usually lined by squamous epithelium, and its contents are either clear fluid or like toothpaste. It appears in young adults, sometimes in later life. It protrudes from beneath the anterior border of the upper third of the sternomastoid as a fluctuant swelling which may transilluminate. If infection has occurred, it may be difficult to differentiate from a tuberculous abscess. If the aspirated fluid contains cholesterol crystals, the diagnosis is made.

A rare variety of branchial cyst is found lying closely related to the pharynx. It is lined by columnar epithelium, and filled with mucus. Occasionally small symptomless cysts of this type are discovered at necropsy.

Treatment.—A branchial cyst should be excised. Through an incision parallel to the skin creases the anterior wall of the cyst is exposed and some of the content is aspirated. This procedure permits the wall of the cyst to be grasped in suitable forceps, and assists materially in a dissection which, in some instances, entails following a track that passes through the fork of the common carotid artery as far as the pharyngeal wall. It passes superficial to the hypoglossal and glossopharyngeal nerves but deep to the posterior belly of the digastric. The hypoglossal and the spinal accessory nerve may be in danger and should be recognised and protected. If the specimen is examined microscopically, the wall of the cyst is often found to be surrounded by a layer of lymphadenoid tissue. This suggests that the cyst arose as a result of branchial epithelium becoming entrapped within a lymph node during development. It also explains why branchial cysts become inflamed: the lymphadenoid shell participates in regional lymphadentis.

Branchial fistula may be unilateral or bilateral (fig. 614) and it is highly probable that the fistula represents a persistent second branchial cleft, the occluding membrane of which has broken down. Nearly always the external orifice of the fistula is situated in the lower third of the neck near the anterior border of the sternomastoid muscle.

The internal orifice is located on the anterior aspect of the posterior pillar of the fauces, just behind the tonsil (Wilson), but more often than not the track ends blindly on the lateral pharyngeal wall, the condition then being a sinus rather than a fistula. The track is clothed with muscle and lined by ciliated columnar epithelium until destroyed by recurrent attacks of inflammation. The discharge is mucus or muco-pus. The condition may also be secondary to an incision in an infected branchial cyst.

Treatment.—When causing troublesome symptoms, *e.g.* by a discharge of mucus, branchial fistulae should be excised.

Operation.—A ureteric catheter or a probe is passed up the track via the orifice, so that by means of an incision higher in the neck the track may easily be identified and dissected as it passes through the fork of the common carotid artery towards the pharyngeal wall.

Charles Paul Wilson, 1900–1970. Surgeon, Ear, Nose and Throat Department, Middlesex Hospital, London.

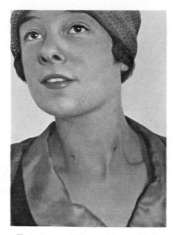

FIG. 614.—Bilateral branchial
fistulas; left side inflamed.

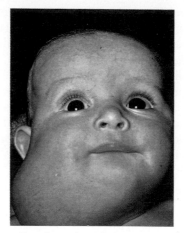

FIG. 615.—A cystic hygroma.
(Harold William Rodgers, FRCS.)

When the upper dissection is completed the orifice below is freed by a small elliptical incision and the whole of the lower part of the track can be eased out of the upper wound (Small).

Branchial Cartilage.—A small piece of cartilage, connected to the deep surface of a cutaneous dimple in the position of an external orifice of a branchial fistula, is occasionally encountered.

Cervical Auricle.—So named because of its morphological significance, this cutaneous projection is found almost invariably in the position of the external orifice of a branchial fistula. Cervical auricles were recognised in the days of the Roman Empire, and are represented in some of the statuary of that period.

Pharyngeal Pouch (Chapter 34).

Laryngocele (Chapter 35) are possibly derived from the branchial apparatus.

Branchiogenic carcinoma is very rare; such a diagnosis is unjustifiable until every possible source of a primary growth in the mouth, pharynx and external auditory meatus has been excluded.

Cystic Hygroma (Cavernous Lymphangioma)

About the sixth week of embryonic life the primitive lymph sacs develop in mesoblast, the principal pair being situated in the neck between the jugular and subclavian veins; these, which correspond to the lymph hearts of lower animals, are known as the jugular lymph sacs. Sequestration of a portion of a jugular lymph sac from the lymphatic system accounts for the appearance of these swellings.

Of all the swellings of the neck, cystic hygroma rivals, and at times surpasses, sternomastoid 'tumour' as the earliest to appear: usually it manifests itself during early infancy, occasionally it is present at birth, and exceptionally it is so large as to obstruct labour. Typically, the swelling occupies the lower third of the neck, and as it enlarges it passes upwards towards the ear (fig. 615); often it is the posterior triangle of the neck that is mainly involved. Due to intercommunication of its many compartments, the swelling is softly cystic and is partially compressible; it visibly increases in size when the child coughs or cries, but *the* characteristic that distinguishes it from all other cervical swellings is that it is brilliantly translucent.

The cheek and the axilla are other, though less frequent, sites for a cystic hygroma. Another infrequent, though striking dual lesion is that of a cystic

Hugh Alan Dugleby Small, 1910–1981. Formerly Surgeon, The Royal Northern Hospital, London.

hygroma and a lymphangiogenetic macroglossia. Exceptionally a cystic hygroma occurs in the groin or in the mediastinum. When situated wholly within the thorax (Chapter 40), it cannot be differentiated, prior to operation, from other benign neoplasms.

Clinical Course.—The behaviour of cystic hygromas during infancy is so uncertain that it is impossible at that age to prognosticate as to what will happen. Sometimes growth is extremely rapid and occasionally respiratory difficulty ensues, a contingency that demands immediate aspiration of much of the contents of the cysts and possible tracheostomy. At other times, as a result of nasopharyngeal infection, the swelling becomes inflamed and spontaneous regression of the cysts may then occur.

Pathology.—The swelling consists of an aggregation of cysts like a mass of soap bubbles. The larger cysts are near the surface, while the smaller ones lie deeply and tend to infiltrate muscle planes. Each cyst is filled with clear lymph and is lined by a single layer of endothelium having the appearance of mosaic.

Treatment.—Excision of all the cysts at an early age is the treatment of election. It is often helpful to give preliminary injections, at weekly intervals, of sclerosing solutions or even boiling water into the cysts. The swelling will then slowly reduce in size and the cysts walls become more fibrous. Dissection is thus facilitated.

CERVICAL RIB AND THE SCALENE SYNDROME

By mass radiography it has been ascertained that a rib arising from the seventh cervical vertebra occurs in 0·46% of persons. In a little more than half of these the cervical rib is unilateral, and somewhat more frequent on the right side. It is paradoxical that a cervical rib or ribs found in the course of routine x-ray examination hardly ever gives rise to symptoms, whereas more often than not, when a radiograph of the cervical region is requested on account of nerve-pressure symptoms, no such rib is demonstrable.

Usually extra ribs spring from the seventh cervical vertebra and may be associated with spinal anomalies elsewhere.

Four main varieties of cervical rib are recognised (fig. 616).

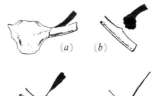

(a) A complete rib, often containing a false joint in its length, articulates anteriorly with the manubrium or the first rib.

(c) A rib ending in a tapering point, which is connected by a fibrous band to the scalene tubercle of the first rib.

(b) The free end of rib expands into a large bony mass.

(d) A fibrous band closely applied to, or incorporated in, the scalenus medius alone is present. This not infrequent variety, of course, cannot be demonstrated radiologically.

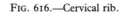

FIG. 616.—Cervical rib.

At their exit from the neck, the brachial plexus and the subclavian artery pass through a narrow triangle (fig. 617). It is to the *base* of the triangle that attention must be focused.

Pathology.—Should the base of the triangle be raised the height of one vertebra by the interposition of a cervical rib, the subclavian artery and the first dorsal nerve are bound to be angulated, if not compressed, as they pass over the new floor, *i.e.* that formed by the cervical rib, instead of the first thoracic rib.

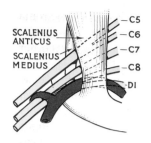

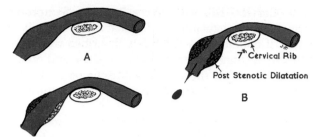

FIG. 617.—The anatomy of the parts concerned.
(After the late Professor Lambert Rogers, F.R.C.S., Cardiff.)

FIG. 618.—A, showing the narrowing and post-stenotic dilatation of the vessel, with early thrombus formation; B, an embolus has been detached.

Pathology of the Vascular Symptoms.—Owing to the angulation over the cervical rib, the lumen of the artery at this site becomes constricted. *Pari passu* with the formation of the constriction, fusiform dilatation of the first 2 to 4 cm of the artery occurs distal to the constriction (fig. 618). Within the post-stenotic dilatation (or possibly at the site of the constriction) clotting occurs on the intima. Portions of this mural thrombus may become detached, and give rise to an embolus (fig. 618) or emboli. Also proximal extension of the thrombus can occur so that the vertebral artery may be involved and cerebrovascular embolic episodes occur[1] (Shucksmith)

Three clinical types are encountered:

1. **Cervical Rib with Local Symptoms.**—From time to time a patient presents on account of a lump in the lower part of the neck which may be visible, or, more commonly, because of the tenderness in the supraclavicular fossa. On palpation the lump is found to be bony hard and totally fixed. Type (*b*) is most likely to give rise to these signs.

2. **Cervical Rib with Vascular Symptoms.**—*Vascular symptoms* occur only when a cervical rib is complete.

Pain is the prevailing symptom. It is located in the forearm, but in some instances it radiates to the upper arm. What is so characteristic is that the pain is brought on by use of the arm: should the arm be in a raised position at the time of exercising it, the onset of the pain is accelerated. The pain is relieved by rest. Without doubt, this pain is ischaemic muscle pain, comparable to intermittent claudication in the leg.

Temperature and Colour Changes.—The hand on the affected side tends to (*a*) be colder than its fellow, (*b*) become unduly pale when held aloft and (*c*) become unduly blue when it is dependent for any length of time.

The Radial Pulse.—Sometimes it is as full as that of the other side; sometimes it is absent, and at others it is feeble, depending upon whether the collateral circulation is good, bad or indifferent. The distal part of the subclavian artery should be auscultated; a systolic bruit is significant.

Numbness of the fingers may be complained of, and ulceration or, more rarely, gangrene may occur.

Treatment is timely extraperiosteal excision of the cervical rib, together with any bony prominence of the first rib. At the same time it is advisable to perform sympathetic denervation of the upper limb.

---

[1]Described by Sir Charles Symonds in 1927.

Henry Samuel Shucksmith, Contemporary. Formerly Surgeon, General Infirmary, Leeds, England.

3. **Cervical Rib with Nerve-Pressure Symptoms.**—Nerve-pressure symptoms, due to angulation of the first dorsal nerve is of doubtful occurrence and most, if not all, cases previously described were due to cervical spondylosis or the carpal tunnel syndrome. Only if these and other localised nerve lesions are excluded, should the scalene syndrome be considered as the cause of pain and tingling in the hand and forearm, whether wasting or the thenar and hypothenar muscles is present or not.

Differential Diagnosis.—Many of the nerve-pressure symptoms formerly attributed to a cervical rib can be, and are, produced by pressure on the cervical roots in the region of the intervertebral foramina by lateral protrusion of intervertebral discs. Secondly, paraesthesia and wasting of the thenar eminence are often due to carpal tunnel syndrome. Thirdly, hypothenar wasting can also arise from angulation of the ulnar nerve behind the elbow (Griffiths). Other conditions to be considered include motor neurone disease and syringomyelia.

Treatment.—In mild cases the use of a sling and exercises aimed at strengthening the muscles of the shoulder girdle may alleviate the symptoms, at least temporarily. In about 70% of cases even if a cervical rib cannot be recognised, the symptoms are relieved by dividing the scalenus anterior (scalenotomy). Other surgeons remove the cervical rib or the corresponding band in addition, and in this way reduce the number of unsatisfactory results. When a cervical rib is excised, it is essential to remove it with its periosteum or it will regenerate. Care must be exercised to avoid damage to the branchial plexus and phrenic nerves.

INJURIES

Cut Throat.—In more than half the cases of cut throat that reach surgical aid the wound does not involve any vital structure—only the skin, platysma, and perhaps the sternomastoid or other muscles are severed.

Wounds above the Hyoid Bone.—The cavity of the mouth may have been entered. The epiglottis is often partially divided near its base. This should be repaired with catgut sutures. The mucosa of the pharynx is trimmed and united and the skin wound is closed.

Wounds of the Thyrohyoid Membrane.—Again the epiglottis is often damaged. The severed thyrohyoid membrane can usually be sutured. If there is respiratory distress, it is advisable to perform tracheostomy.

Wounds of the Thyroid or Cricoid Cartilage.—A tracheostomy well below the larynx is usually indicated. The laryngeal skeleton is then fully exposed and the damaged cartilages repositioned and sutured. An indwelling stent or 'keel' is moulded to fit within the lumen and also shaped with a narrow waist to lie between the vocal cords. This stent is held by a wire or nylon retaining suture through the neck. In 2–3 weeks the stent is removed endoscopically after cutting the retaining suture. The tracheostomy is then closed.

Division of the Trachea.—Wounds of the trachea are comparatively rare. In order to obtain adequate exposure it is usually necessary to divide the thyroid isthmus between haemostats. In most instances it is advisable to perform tracheostomy below the wound, and then to proceed to repair the latter with sutures.

Injury to Nerves.—It is remarkable how rarely important nerves are injured in self-inflicted wounds. In stab wounds any nerve may be involved. In one of our patients, a sailor, the most inaccessible nerve in the neck, the cervical sympathetic, was divided in this way, the assailant's weapon being a small penknife (and see fig. 204).

Complications of Cut Throat.—Haemorrhagic shock can be severe and blood transfusion is necessary. Venous air embolism is a likely cause of death. Infection of the wound is common and, if cellulitis supervenes, it may spread downwards to cause mediastinitis. Pneumonia also is common. Rare complications include surgical emphysema due to the omission of a tracheostomy, and aerial fistula between the air passages and the exterior, which can be prevented or treated by the stent or 'keel' operation described above. Oeso-

David Lloyd Griffiths, Contemporary. Director, University Department of Orthopaedic Surgery, Royal Infirmary, Manchester, England.

phageal or pharyngeal fistula usually heals by itself. Aphonia or dysphonia may follow injury to the vocal cords or division of a recurrent laryngeal nerve, while stenosis of the trachea or larynx due to scarring may necessitate permanent tracheostomy.

WOUNDS OF THE CERVICAL PORTION OF THE THORACIC DUCT

Wounds of the thoracic duct are rare, and usually occur during dissection of lymph nodes in the left supraclavicular fossa. When the accident is not recognised at the time, chyle pours from the wound—as much as 1 to 1·5 litre in twenty-four hours—and, as a result, the patient wastes rapidly.

Treatment.—Should the accident be recognised during an operation, the proximal end of the duct must be ligated with fine silk. Ligation of the duct is not harmful, for there are a number of anastomotic channels between the lymphatic and the venous systems in the neighbourhood. Usually the first intimation of a severed thoracic duct is a copious chylous discharge from the wound on the day following the operation. That the fluid *is* chyle is substantiated if it has a specific gravity of over 1·012 and if fat can be extracted from it with ether. Firm pressure by a pad and bandage should be applied, but this simple expedient may not be successful. More often the wound must be reopened. It the patient is given cream to drink an hour before the operation, more especially if the cream is coloured with confectioners' green dye (D-C 6), there is seldom any difficulty in locating a cut thoracic duct, which is about the size of a straw and an immediate external relation of the last 3·75 cm of the left internal jugular vein. If the duct is found, it should be ligated, but in any case the wound should be packed firmly and allowed to heal by granulation. Thanks to subsidiary anastomotic channels, these measures are regularly satisfactory.

INFLAMMATORY CONDITIONS

Acute cellulitis is either superficial or deep to the deep cervical fascia.

Superficial cellulitis is common, and methods of treating it follow that of cellulitis elsewhere. When, however, it occurs above the level of the hyoid bone it is especially dangerous, because sudden asphyxia from oedema of the glottis is an ever-present possibility.

Deep cellulitis in the lower third of the neck, on the other hand, is free from this danger. Consequently, it can be treated by antibiotic therapy with every confidence, and should an abscess develop, it is opened.

Ludwig's Angina.—Ludwig described a clinical entity characterised by a brawny swelling of the submandibular region combined with inflammatory oedema of the mouth. It is these *combined* cervical and intrabuccal signs that constitute the characteristic feature of the lesion. The cause is a virulent (usually streptococcal) infection of the cellular tissues surrounding the submandibular salivary gland. It may be a complication of advanced carcinoma of the floor of the mouth.

Clinical Course.—Unless the infection is controlled, these cases may rapidly assume a grave aspect. The swollen tongue is pushed towards the palate and forwards through the open mouth, while the cellulitis extends down the neck in that most dangerous plane—deep to the deep fascia.

Ludwig's angina is an infection of a closed fascial space, and, untreated, the inflammatory exudate often passes via the tunnel occupied by the stylohyoid to the submucosa of the glottis, in which event the patient is in imminent danger of death from oedema of the glottis (Chapter 35).

Treatment.—When the condition is diagnosed early, the results of antibiotic therapy are sometimes dramatic. In cases where the swelling, both cervical and intrabuccal, does not subside rapidly with such treatment, a curved incision beneath the jaw is made. The incision is deepened, and after displacing the superficial lobe of the submandibular salivary gland, the mylohyoid muscles are divided. This decompresses the closed fascial space

Wilhelm von Ludwig, 1790–1865. Professor of Surgery and Midwifery, Tübingen, Germany.

referred to. The wound is lightly sutured and drained. The operation can be conducted with the greatest safety under local anaesthesia. Thiopentone anaesthesia usually precipitates laryngeal spasm and asphyxia.

Infection of the Pharyngo-maxillary Space (*Parapharyngeal Abscess*).—The pharyngo-maxillary space is a potential cone-shaped space, base uppermost. The base is formed by the base of the skull; the apex abuts the great cornu of the hyoid bone; the medial wall consists of the superior constrictor muscle; the lateral wall, from above downwards, is composed of the fascia covering the internal pterygoid muscle, the mandible about its angle, and the submandibular salivary gland, below which the apex of the space becomes relatively superficial. Usually infection of this space originates in the tonsil, and may occur after tonsillectomy, especially when the operation has been performed under local anaesthesia.

Clinical Features.—Every posterior peritonsillar abscess is a potential pharyngomaxillary space infection, the general reaction of which is greater than that accompanying peritonsillar abscess. There is often *slight* trismus, and swelling over the lower part of the parotid gland; this is never present in quinsy. Tenderness, and later swelling below the angle of the mandible, appears when the apex of the space is involved. As the carotid sheath runs through the space, the dreaded complications of thrombophlebitis of the internal jugular vein and/or erosion of an artery, usually the internal carotid, may occur if the space is not adequately drained. Sometimes the abscess bursts spontaneously between the cartilaginous plates of the external auditory canal, but obviously such an eventuality is a fortunate escape from death, for which the patient's medical advisers can take no credit.

Treatment.—As soon as the diagnosis is strongly suspected an incision should be made below and behind the angle of the mandible, on a line towards the hyoid bone. A finger is passed upwards, medial to the mandible and the distended space is entered by rupturing its wall. The space is drained with a large soft wick drain.

CERVICAL LYMPHADENITIS

There are approximately 800 lymph nodes in the body; no fewer than 300 of them lie in the neck. Inflammation of the lymph nodes of the neck is exceedingly common. Infection occurs from the oral and nasal cavities, the ear, the scalp, and face. The source of infection must be sought for systematically.

Acute Lymphadenitis.—The affected lymph nodes are enlarged and tender, and there is a varying degree of pyrexia. The treatment, in the first instance, is directed to the general condition and to the focus of infection, the neck itself being simply protected by a bandage over wool. If, in spite of antibiotic therapy, pain continues or certain lymph nodes appear to be getting larger, fomentations are applied locally. Abscess formation calls for adequate drainage.

Chronic Lymphadenitis.—In the early stages it is extremely difficult to distinguish tuberculous adenitis from chronic non-tuberculous adenitis, but clinical experience shows that chronically inflamed lymph nodes which do not resolve in the space of three or four weeks are nearly always tuberculous.

Tuberculous adenitis (Chapter 9)

The majority of patients affected are children or young adults, but the condition can occur for the first time at any age. Usually one group of cervical nodes is first infected (fig. 619), most frequently those of the upper jugular chain. More rarely there is widespread cervical lymphadenitis, and in these cases especially, periadenitis or matting of the lymph nodes is evident.

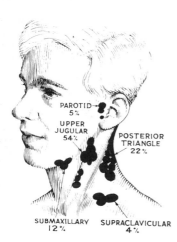

FIG. 619.—Groups of cervical lymph nodes infected by tuberculosis, founded on 372 consecutive cases. The 3% not labelled are divided between the mid-jugular group (shown) and the submental group (not shown).

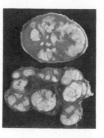

FIG. 620.—Caseating tuberculous lymph nodes.

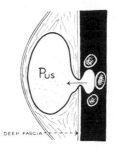

FIG. 621.—Showing the abscess and the source of the pus beneath the deep fascia.

Source of Infection.—In the majority of instances tubercle bacilli gain entrance through the tonsil of the corresponding side. The nodes of the posterior triangle are infected in 22% of cases, probably stemming from adenoidal infection.

Contrary to what is believed, it is the human,[1] and not the bovine, bacillus that is responsible for tuberculous cervical adenitis in about 70% of cases. In fully 80% of cases the tuberculous process is virtually limited to the clinically affected group of lymph nodes; nevertheless, a primary focus in the lungs must be suspected. Renal tuberculosis may co-exist and the urine should be examined for this organism.

In the event of the patient developing a natural resistance to the infection or (more often) as a result of appropriate general treatment, fibrosis or calcification may occur. In other circumstances the caseating material (fig. 620) liquefies, breaks through the capsules of the lymph nodes, and a 'cold abscess' forms. The pus is at first confined by the *deep* cervical fascia. In a few weeks this dense sheet becomes eroded at one point, and the pus flows through the small opening into that more commodious space beneath the *superficial* fascia. The process has now reached the well-known stage of collar-stud abscess (fig. 621 and Chapter 9). The superficial abscess enlarges steadily, and unless suitable treatment is adopted, the skin will soon become reddened over the centre of the fluctuating swelling, and before long a discharging sinus, with its attendant evils, is at hand.[2]

---

[1]The human bacillus is responsible for 100% of cases among the Bantu-speaking urban population of South Africa (Keen).

[2]For 600 years the King's touch was believed to cure this prevalent disease. Charles II touched on an average 10,000 sufferers a year. In addition, he presented each with half a sovereign. The condition was known as the King's Evil.

Paul Keen, Contemporary. Formerly Senior Surgeon, Non-European Hospital, Johannesburg, South Africa.

DIFFERENTIAL DIAGNOSIS

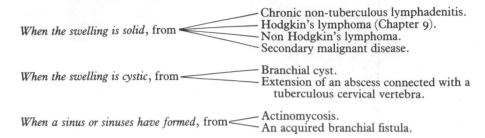

When the swelling is solid, from — Chronic non-tuberculous lymphadenitis.
— Hodgkin's lymphoma (Chapter 9).
— Non Hodgkin's lymphoma.
— Secondary malignant disease.

When the swelling is cystic, from — Branchial cyst.
— Extension of an abscess connected with a tuberculous cervical vertebra.

When a sinus or sinuses have formed, from — Actinomycosis.
— An acquired branchial fistula.

TREATMENT OF TUBERCULOUS LYMPHADENITIS

The patient should be treated by general measures and appropriate chemo-therapy (Chapter 4). If abscess is present it should be aspirated and an attempt should be made to grow the tubercle bacillus and find out its sensitivity to the anti-tuberculous drugs. Repeated aspiration of a collar-stud abscess cannot be recommended because this predisposes to sinus formation and secondary infec-tion.

Operation for Collar-stud Abscess.—After an incision in line with the skin creases, the pus in the superficial compartment is mopped away, and the hole in the deep fascia is enlarged to admit a small curette, so that the caseating lymph node can be scraped out and the cavity packed with iodoform gauze. This is brought out through the edge of the wound which is closed by careful primary suture. It is removed after 24 hours, but the sutures are left for 10 days.

Excision of Lymph Nodes.—This becomes necessary when there is no local response to chemotherapy and if a sinus persists. When there is active tuberculosis of another system, *e.g.* pulmonary tuberculosis, removal of tuberculous lymph nodes in the neck is, of course, illogical.

An oblique incision conforming with the skin creases, gives satisfactory access. If the nodes are related to the internal jugular vein this structure should be identified first and then the nodes can be dissected away from it.

To minimise unnecessary injury to large veins, no tissue should be divided when stretched taut. Should the internal jugular vein prove to be involved to such an extent that freeing it is difficult or impossible, this great vessel can be ligated, or a portion of it can be resected, without any untoward effect at any age (cf. block dissection of the neck).

There is no contraindication to dividing the sternomastoid muscle if, as is frequently the case, such a step facilitates access to the diseased nodes and enables the operator to visualise the spinal accessory nerve more easily. The divided muscle is subsequently reunited.

During the dissection of cervical lymph nodes every effort must be made to preserve: the spinal accessory nerve; the mandibular branch of the facial nerve; the hypoglossal nerve; which are the nerves most likely to be injured.

Actinomycosis of the Neck (See Chapter 4).

PRIMARY MALIGNANT TUMOURS OF THE NECK

Carotid Body Tumour ('Potato' Tumour).—The carotid body, which is situ-ated at the bifurcation of the carotid artery, is the most important moiety of the chemoreceptor system (fig. 622). The cells of this system are sensitive to changes in the pH and temperature of the blood. Hence a tumour is called a chemodec-toma, though it is classified histologically as a non-chromaffin para-ganglioma. It will remain localised for years but regional metastases will occur in about 20% of cases and distant metastases less frequently.

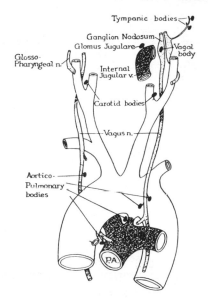

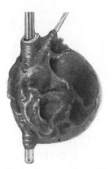

Fig. 623. — Carotid body tumour removed successfully.

Fig. 622.—Sites where chemodectomas are known to occur. In addition, they have been found in the orbit, along the course of the inferior alveolar artery, and in proximity to the femoral artery.
(After S. O. Burman.)

Clinical Features.—Usually unilateral, it becomes apparent in middle life, but occasionally earlier. The diagnosis is suggested by a long history and a lump at the carotid bifurcation which moves from side to side but not vertically, and usually a pulsating vessel overlies its outer surface (Westbury).

Arteriography is valuable and shows the carotid fork to be splayed and a 'blush' outlining the abnormal tumour vessels.

The Special Danger of Excision of a Carotid Body Tumour is due to its vascularity and the way it is blended with the carotid bifurcation. Therefore:

1. There is considerable danger of torrential haemorrhage occurring if a biopsy is attempted in the erroneous belief that the lump is an infected or neoplastic lymph node. Control of this bleeding by artery forceps inevitably results in occlusion of the carotid artery with hemiplegia or death occurring in at least 33% of cases.

2. If extirpation is to be attempted it is essential to have ready a length of silicone bypass tubing in case carotid occlusion becomes necessary, otherwise a similar tragedy is likely.

In some cases it is possible to dissect the tumour away from the fork of the carotid (fig. 624). But when the tumour is large and inseparable from the vessels resection will be necessary (fig. 623) and a bypass is essential while a vein autograft is being inserted to restore arterial continuity.

Recurrence after complete removal is unusual.

In the old and enfeebled it may be decided that it is best to let Nature take its course. Hardly any of the tumours are radiosensitive.

Lymphomas (Chapter 9).

SECONDARY CARCINOMA OF THE NECK

Secondary carcinomatous infiltration of the cervical lymph nodes is only too common. When a patient presents with enlargement of cervical lymph nodes that

Gerald Westbury, Contemporary. Professor of Surgery, Royal Marsden Hospital, London.

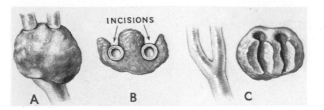

FIG. 624.—The tumour is split in the manner shown, so that it can be dissected from the arteries it envelops.
(After T. Farrar et al.)

are suspiciously indurated, search for a primary growth is imperative and must be made *before* a node is removed for biopsy. Often the primary growth lies within the nasopharynx; when this is not the case, the search must continue. Among the sites that are prone to be overlooked are the base of tongue (vallecula), laryngo-pharynx, paranasal sinuses, and less commonly, distant sites (bronchus, breast, stomach, testis).

Management.—The management of involved cervical nodes depends on the overall treatment regime: 1. If primary surgery is used and the cervical nodes are palpable, they must be excised *en-bloc* with the primary; 2. If radiotherapy is used initially and there is resolution of the primary but persistence of the metastatic nodes, they can be resected subsequently by a cervical block dissection; 3. Should lymph node metastasis develop subsequent to the successful treatment of the primary, a block dissection can often be curative.

Types of Neck Dissection.—1. Classic Radical Neck Dissection (Crile). The classic operation involves resection of the cervical lymphatics and those structures closely associated such as the internal jugular vein, the accessory nerve, the submandibular gland and the sternomastoid muscle. A variety of incisions have been described but it is important in the irradiated case that the incision line does not pass over the carotid bulb, because if wound breakdown occurs a fatal carotid blowout may ensue. The main disability that follows the operation is the drooping of the shoulder due to paralysis of the accessory muscle.

2. Conservative (Functional) Neck Dissection. In selected cases the classic operation is modified to preserve one or other of the associated structures. It may be used in those cases needing bilateral neck dissection (to prevent excessive venous congestion of the head if both internal jugulars are divided or resected). It may be used when the metastasis has not spread beyond the capsule of the lymph node, especially in early cases of carcinoma of the tongue, floor of the mouth or the lower lip. This modified procedure preserves the accessory nerve, the jugular vein and the sternomastoid muscle. However, it must be emphasised that this conservative dissection should only be used if it does *not* compromise the complete exenteration of the carcinoma.

Procedure for Crile dissection.—The skin flaps having been dissected up (fig. 625), the sternomastoid is divided about 2·5 cm above the clavicle. The muscle is freed and retracted upwards. Next, the internal jugular vein is divided between ligatures low down in the neck. The dissection proceeds upwards methodically and the muscle, fascia, fat, lymph nodes, the internal jugular vein, together with the salivary gland, are dissected and removed *en bloc*. Attention must be directed to clearing the space between the parotid and the great vessels, and also the submental triangle between the hyoglossi, for it is in these areas that a lymph node can easily be overlooked. Bleeding vessels are ligated as they occur; finally the upper end of the internal jugular vein is ligated by transfixion, and divided. When the dissection has been completed, the carotid artery is laid bare, and lying

George Washington Crile, 1864–1943. Professor of Surgery, Western Reserve University, and one of the Founders of the Cleveland Clinic, Cleveland, Ohio, U.S.A.

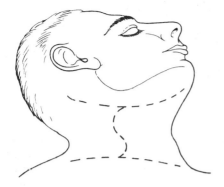

FIG. 625.—An incision for block dissection of the neck.

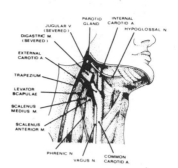

FIG. 626.—Crile's block dissection of the neck.

with it is the vagus nerve, which has been carefully preserved. The operation aims at removing the whole of the lymphatic-bearing tissues on the affected side of the neck (fig.626). The skin flaps are approximated and the wound is drained. Surprisingly little deformity follows this extensive dissection, but the neck is stiff and there is drooping of the corner of the mouth. (The cervical branch of the facial nerve is severed.) When *bilateral* block dissection is required it must be undertaken, not simultaneously, but consecutively with an interval of about three weeks. Removal of both internal jugular veins can be attended by obstructed cerebral circulation and brain swelling (see above and Chapter 26).

Postoperative Care.—Suction drainage is essential where there are such large skin flaps in order to prevent subcutaneous collections of blood or serum. If the pharynx or oral cavity has been opened by the dissection the patient should be given antibiotics (including metronidazole) prophylactically. Blood and fluid replacement and nutrition should be as required (Chapters 5, 6, 7).

Head and Neck Reconstruction

Over the last decade, the major advance in head and neck surgery has been the advent of immediate reconstruction, minimising surgical mutilation, both cosmetic and functional. The use of local flaps has been superceded by regional or myocutaneous flaps. In certain cases free microvascular flaps are valuable.

Regional flaps usually derive their blood supply from an axial artery running along the length of the flap.

Forehead Flap.—This is supplied by the superficial temporal artery and is used to provide a lining for the oral cavity and pharynx. A second stage may be necessary to divide the pedicle.

Deltopectoral Flap.—This versatile flap from the upper chest was popularised by Bakamjian and is supplied by the perforating branches of the internal mammary artery. It is used to provide both lining and cover in may sites of the head and neck. A two-stage operation is usually needed.

Myocutaneous flaps derive their blood supply from the underlying muscle included in the flap, consequently they can be used with an island of skin enabling a one stage reconstruction to be performed. The usual donor sites are the pectoralis major muscle and the latissimus dorsi muscle and a 'paddle' of overlying skin.

A variety of *free microvascular flaps* often with bone are also used.

CHAPTER 37

THE THYROID GLAND AND THE THYROGLOSSAL TRACT

SURGICAL ANATOMY AND PHYSIOLOGY

Embryology.—The thyroid gland is developed from the median bud of the pharynx (the thyroglossal duct) which passes from the foramen caecum at the base of the tongue to the isthmus of the thyroid. The ultimo-branchial body which arises from a diverticulum of the fourth pharyngeal pouch of each side amalgamates with the corresponding lateral lobe. Parafollicular cells (C-cells) are derived from the neural crest and reach the thyroid via the ultimo-branchial body. Recently, consideration has been given to the possibility that some C-cells are of endodermal rather than neural crest origin. It is doubtful whether the branchial apparatus itself contributes to the thyroid follicular cells.

Surgical Anatomy.—The normal gland weighs 20–25 g. The functioning unit is the lobule supplied by a single arteriole and consisting of 20–40 follicles which are lined by cubical epithelium. The resting follicle contains colloid in which thyroglobulin is stored. The arterial supply is rich, and extensive anastomoses occur between the main thyroid arteries and branches of tracheal and oesophageal arteries (figs 627 and 628). There is an extensive lymphatic network within the gland. Although some lymph channels pass directly to the deep cervical nodes, the subcapsular plexus drains principally to the juxta-thyroid nodes—*i.e.* pretracheal (Delphic)[1] and paratracheal nodes, and nodes on the

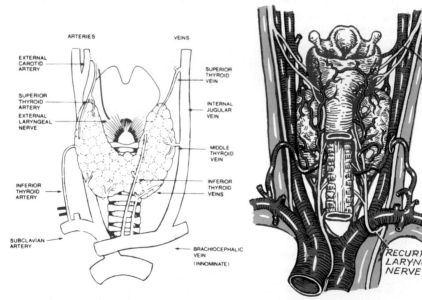

FIG. 627.—The thyroid gland from the front.

FIG. 628.—The thyroid gland from behind, showing the laryngeal nerves and the four para-thyroids.
(After Martin Norland.)

---

[1] Pythia, the snake-woman oracle of Delphi, sat on her tripod, clutching the ribbons of the monolithic 'omphalos' of the world. She inhaled sulphurous fumes and laurel, and uttered a meaningless jargon which was interpreted equivocally by the attendant priests for those who came to consult her. Formerly, the meaning of these lymph nodes was uncertain and they were therefore called 'Delphic'.

superior and inferior thyroid veins, and thence to the deep cervical and mediastinal group of nodes.

Physiology.

The hormones tri-iodo-thyronine (T3) and thyroxine (T4)[1,2] are bound to thyroglobulin within the colloid. Synthesis within the thyroglobulin complex is controlled by several enzymes, in distinct steps: (1) Trapping of inorganic iodide from the blood. (2) Oxidation of iodide to iodine, and binding of iodine with tyrosine to form iodotyrosines. (3) Coupling of mono-iodotyrosines and di-iodotyrosines to form T3 and T4. (4) When hormones are required the complex is resorbed into the cell and thyroglobulin broken down; T3 and T4 are liberated and enter the blood where they are bound to serum proteins. A small amount of hormone remains free in the serum in equilibrium with the protein bound hormone and is biologically active. The principal metabolic effects of the thyroid hormones are due to unbound free T4 and T3 (0·03–0·04% and 0·2–0·5% of the total circulating hormones respectively). T3 is quick acting (within a few hours) whilst T4 acts more slowly (4–14 days). T3 is the more important physiological hormone and is also produced in the periphery by conversion from T4. Reversed T3 is an inactive form of T3 found in varying concentrations in the serum.

Thyrocalcitonin.—(see calcitonin, Chapter 38)

The Pituitary Thyroid Axis.—Synthesis and liberation of thyroid hormones from the thyroid is controlled by thyroid stimulating hormone (T.S.H.) from the anterior pituitary. Secretion of T.S.H. depends upon the level of circulating thyroid hormones and is modified in a classic negative feedback manner. In hyperthyroidism where hormone levels in the blood are high, T.S.H. production is suppressed whilst in hypothyroidism it is stimulated. Regulation of T.S.H. secretion also results from the action of thyrotrophin releasing hormone (T.R.H.) produced in the hypothalamus.

Thyroid Stimulating Antibodies.—These are a family of IgG immunoglobulins each of which acts as a stimulating antibody probably to the T.S.H. receptor on the thyroid cell membrane. L.A.T.S.[3] is one of these IgG immunoglobulins with an action on the thyroid cell similar to T.S.H. but a duration of stimulation more prolonged. It is estimated to produce its maximum effect after 16–24 hours as compared with 1·5-3 hours for T.S.H. Another abnormal thyroid stimulator specific for human thyroid tissue is L.A.T.S. protector, also called Human Specific Thyroid Stimulator.

These Thyroid Stimulating Immunoglobulins (T.S.I.) are often referred to as Thyroid Stimulating Antibodies (TsAb) and are now thought to be responsible for all cases of hyperthyroidism not due to autonomous toxic nodules.

The concentration of these immunoglobulins in the plasma is small and measurement is difficult. Methods of measurement include mouse bioassay, receptor assay and in vitro slice assay.

TESTS OF THYROID FUNCTION

The principal value of these tests is in asssessing the thyroid status when the clinical picture is equivocal. However, even if the clinical diagnosis appears quite certain, it is valuable to have confirmatory evidence to look back upon should doubt as to the diagnosis arise at a later date. Several parameters[4] should be obtained because no single test is conclusive.

1. Measurement of Thyroid Hormones in the Serum

  (a) Total Serum Thyroxin (T4) (Normal range 55–150 nmol/l)
  (b) Total Tri-iodothyronine (T3) (Normal range 1·2–3·1 nmol/l)
  (c) Free Serum Thyroxine (T4) (Normal range 8–26 pmol/l)
  (d) Free Serum Tri-iodothyronine (T3) (Normal range 3–9 pmol/l)

The iodine containing hormones T3 and T4 are transported in the plasma mainly by specific binding proteins, Thyroxine Binding Globulin (T.B.G.) and Thyroxine Binding

---

[1] Extracted by E. C. Kendall in 1916.
[2] Therapeutic Notes—L-thyroxine (T4) is the official name; trade name Eltroxin; tablet size 0·1 mg and 0·05 mg. Tri-iodothyronine (T3), official name lio-thyronine, trade names, Cynomel, Tertroxin. Tablet size 20 μg.
[3] L.A.T.S. = lung-activity thyroid stimulator.
[4] A parameter is any yard-stick or independent variable.

Edward Calvin Kendall, 1886–1972. Professor of Physiological Chemistry, Mayo Clinic, Rochester, Minnesota, U.S.A.

Prealbumin. As only a small amount of T3 and T4 are free in the blood estimation of the serum Protein Bound Iodine (P.B.I.) was used for many years as representing total circulating thyroid hormone. This estimation was rather unreliable and is now rarely employed in the assessment of thyroid function.

The Total Serum T4 and Total Serum T3 represent the total protein bound thyroxine and tri-iodothyronine and are not measurements of the free active hormone. These measurements are influenced by changes in the level of thyroxine binding proteins in the serum. False high results are seen in pregnancy and in individuals on oral contraceptives. False low results are seen in hypoproteinemic states such as the nephrotic syndrome. Drugs which are protein bound such as salicylates and penicillin compete with T4 and T3 for protein binding. Measurement of the free hormones (T4 and T3) by radioimmuno assay is in theory more representative of the level of hormones available to the individual body cells and is thought to give a more precise estimate of either the euthyroid state or abnormalities of thyroid function. With the advent of commercial kit assays estimation is now becoming generally available. Estimation of T3 is essential if T3 toxicosis is suspected.

2. **Measurement of Free (unoccupied) binding sites for thyroid hormones in the blood.**—In the T uptake test radio-active T3 is incubated with the patient's serum so that it becomes fixed to any thyroid binding protein not already carrying T3 or T4. The amount so fixed can be measured and from this can be estimated the number of binding sites in the serum which are unoccupied. In hyperthyroidism the number of free binding sites is low because few are not already carrying hormone. In hypothyroidism and myxoedema, however, the number of free sites is high. Using the Thyopac method and taking 100% as the mean normal value for free binding sites, a figure of 85% or less suggests hyperthyroidism and a figure of 120% or more suggests hypothyroidism. This is not a very accurate test in itself, but in conjunction with Total Serum T4 the Free Thyroxin Index (F.T4I.) can be calculated from the formula F.T4I. = Serum T4 × 100/T3 uptake per cent. Similarly, the Free Tri-iodo-thyronine Index (F.T3I.) can be calculated. The euthyroid range of the F.T4I. is 55–145: and that of the F.T3I. is 1·4–3·7. These indices give close approximations to Free Serum T4 and Free Serum T3 and are the best parameters of thyroid hormone levels generally available at present.

THYROID ¹²³I UPTAKE

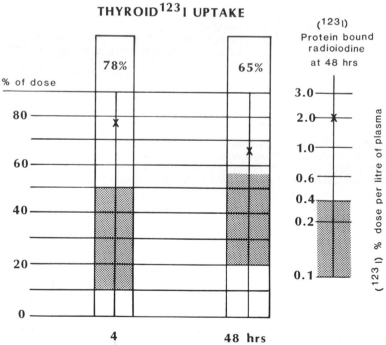

FIG. 629.—Radio-iodine uptake test. Thyroid uptake at 4 hours and 48 hours after administration of ¹²³I and serum protein bound ¹²³I in a typical case of diffuse toxic goitre. Stippled areas represent the euthyroid range.

3. **Measurement of Serum T.S.H.**—The estimation of the level of Serum T.S.H. is now routinely available; the normal range is up to 5 mU/l. Levels over 40 mU/l are present in gross thyroid insufficiency. Sensitivity of the standard assay in the range 0–5 mU/l is poor. The test, however, is invaluable in the early detection of the mild (but disabling) degrees of hypothyroidism so frequently seen after the treatment of thyrotoxicosis by surgery or by radioiodine. New and more accurate assays are now available with sensitivity in the 0–5 mU/l range. Estimation of these low concentrations should aid the distinction of hyperthyroidism from euthyroidism.[1]

4. **The T.R.H. Test.**—Thyrotrophic Releasing Hormone (T.R.H.) which arises from the hypothalamus stimulates T.S.H. secretion by the Anterior Pituitary. When Thyroid Hormone levels are high—as in Hyperthyroidism—T.S.H. secretion is suppressed and the intravenous injection of T.R.H. does not result in a rise in serum T.S.H. When Thyroid hormone levels are normal or low, injection of T.R.H. does increase the serum T.S.H.

Serum T.S.H. is estimated at the beginning of the test and again 20 minutes and 60 minutes after the injection of 200 μg of T.R.H. In thyrotoxicosis and when a full suppressive dose of exogenous T3 or T4 is being given, Serum T.S.H. levels remain at below 2·5 m units/l throughout the test. In the euthyroid patient the 20 minute and 60 minute T.S.H. levels rise above the basal level but in the hypothyroid patient there is an exaggerated response.

This test is generally available because T.S.H. estimations are now freely available, but the test is time consuming and only occasionally gives information not obtained from routine tests of thyroid function. In particular, this test will be outmoded by the newer, more sensitive T.S.H. assays.

5. **In vivo tests of uptake and discharge of 123 I by the thyroid gland.**—(a) *Radioactive iodine uptake test* (fig. 629). The thyroid treats radio-active isotopes of iodine exactly as it treats inorganic iodine (^{127}I). When a tracer dose of ^{123}I is given (5 microcuries[2] is the usual dose) it is rapidly absorbed from the small bowel into the blood, and the thyroid and kidneys compete for it. In hyperthyroidism the thyroid uptake is rapid and little is excreted in the urine. Ultimately the isotope—now incorporated into the T3 and T4 molecules—passes back into the serum and can be measured as protein bound ^{123}I (P.B. ^{123}I.) A rapid uptake of ^{123}I (high counting rate over the thyroid at four hours) and a rapid turnover (high serum P.B. ^{123}I at 24 or 48 hours) are typical of hyperthyroidism. This can, however, occur when the mass of functioning thyroid tissue has been reduced so that radio-iodine studies after surgery or radio-iodine therapy must be interpreted with caution. ^{123}I is almost the ideal diagnostic tracer as it has a short half life (13 hours as opposed to the 8 days of ^{131}I). Because the radio-active dose is low it can be used on children, for serial tests and in pregnancy. Technetium 99 pertechnetate (^{99}Tc^m) can be used as an alternative agent for scanning but is not organified in the gland in the same way as iodine.

(b) *Thyroid Scanning* (fig. 630). Scanning of the thyroid after a tracer dose of ^{123}I shows which parts of the gland are functioning or functionless (hot or cold).[3] Whilst scanning is sometimes helpful in cases of thyroid carcinoma, its principal value is in the diagnosis of an autonomous toxic nodule—either as a solitary toxic nodule or as part of a toxic multinodular goitre.

Whole body scanning can also be used to demonstrate metastases but the patient must have no normal functioning thyroid tissue when the isotope is given because thyroid cancer can only very rarely compete with normal thyroid tissue in the uptake of iodine.

6. **Miscellaneous Tests.**—These comprise the T3 suppression test, B.M.R.[4], E.C.G., serum cholesterol and measurement of tendon reflexes. Some clinicians use the ankle reflex as a measurement of hypothyroidism but otherwise these tests are of little value today.

---

[1] Euthyroid—Euthyroidism = the state of normal thyroid function.
[2] Microcurie = a millionth part of a Curie (μCi)
Millicurie = a thousandth part of a Curie (mCi)
The new SI unit of activity is one nuclear transition per second and is called a becquerel (Bq). This activity is very small and therefore megabecquerels are frequently used in practice. (Mbq = 10^6 Bq).
1 curie (Ci) = 3·7 × 10^{10} Bq
1 millicurie (Ci) = 37 Mbq
[3] Technetium (^{99}Tc^m), taken up exactly like ^{123}I is also used for scanning.
[4] B.M.R. = basal metabolic rate.

Pierre Curie, 1859–1906, and Marie Sklodowska Curie, 1867–1934. Co-discoverers of radium. Madam Curie succeeded her husband as Professor of Physics at the Sorbonne, Paris.

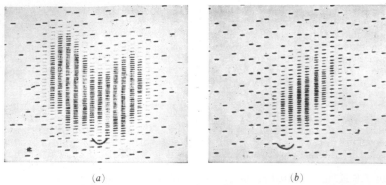

(a)   (b)

FIG. 630.—(a) Thyroid scan of a normal gland. The position of the sternal notch is indicated. (b) Thyroid scan showing autonomous 'hot' thyrotoxic nodule in the left lobe.
(Dr. A. W. H. Goolden, London.)

Routine Tests of Thyroid Function.—These will vary in individual laboratories. The following tests are suggested:

1. Thyroid Profile. This comprises estimation of Total Serum T4 and Total Serum T3 and the Thyopac test for unoccupied binding sites. From these tests the F.T4I and F.T3I are calculated.

2. Estimation of Free T4 and Free T3 if available.

3. ^{123}I uptake tests with uptake at 4 hours and 48 hours together with P.B.^{123}I. at 48 hours if hyperthyroidism is suspected.

4. Serum T.S.H. estimation is automatically done if the Total Serum T4 is below 60 nmol/l or Free T4 below 14 pmol/l.

5. T.R.H.[1] Test if the thyroid status is still doubtful.

HYPOTHYROIDISM

CLASSIFICATION OF HYPOTHYROIDISM

1. **Failure of Thyroid Development**—(a) Complete (Sporadic Cretinism), (b) Partial.
2. **Endemic Cretinism** (often goitrous).
3. **Iatrogenic**—(a) After thyroidectomy, (b) After radio-iodine therapy, (c) After pituitary ablation, (d) Drug induced.[2]
4. **Auto-immune thyroiditis**—(a) Non-goitrous (Primary myxoedema), (b) Goitrous (Hashimoto goitre).
5. **Dyshormonogenesis.**
6. **Goitrogens.**
7. **Vascular damage to anterior pituitary.**

Cretinism (Foetal or Infantile Hypothyroidism (figs 631 and 632)). Sporadic cretinism is due to complete or near complete failure of thyroid development (partial failure causes juvenile myxoedema): the parents and other children may be perfectly normal. In endemic areas goitrous cretinism is common, and is due to maternal and foetal iodine deficiency. Immediate diagnosis and treatment with thyroxine within a few days of birth are essential if physical and mental development are to be normal, or if further deterioration is to be prevented when damage has already occurred in utero. Hypothyroidism occurs in 1 in 4,000 live births and for this reason, in the U.K. there is routine biochemical screening of neonates for hypothyroidism using T.S.H. assay on a simple heel-prick blood sample. Women under treatment with antithyroid drugs may give birth to a hypothyroid infant.

Adult Hypothyroidism

Myxoedema is a very advanced form of adult hypothyroidism and this term should never be applied to the milder degree seen much more frequently after

---

[1] T.R.H. = Thyrotrophic releasing hormone secreted by the Hypothalamus.
[2] Antithyroid drugs, P.A.S., and iodides in excess.

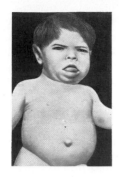

FIG. 631.—An infant cretin with pot belly, umbilical hernia, protruding tongue and pale puffy face.
(The late Professor de Quervain, Berne.)

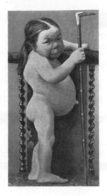

FIG. 632.—A cretin girl aged twenty-two, mentally and physically retarded with dry wrinkled skin and supra-clavicular pads of fat.

thyroidectomy and ^{131}I therapy, and with Autoimmune Thyroiditis. Significant early symptoms are tiredness, mental lethargy, cold intolerance, increase in weight, constipation, menstrual disturbance and a carpal tunnel syndrome due to increased tissue fluid deep to the flexor retinaculum (Hubble). Significant physical signs are a slow pulse rate, dry skin and hair, cold extremities, periorbital puffiness, hoarse voice, slow movements and slow relation of the ankle jerks. Comparison of the facial appearance with a previous photograph is helpful.

Tests of Thyroid Function—The Serum T4 is below 55 nmol/l (Free T4 below 8 pmol/l). Radio-iodine studies show reduced thyroid uptake[1] and increased renal excretion. In an E.C.G. the voltage is reduced and the T wave flattened or even inverted. Serum T.S.H. values are raised and in doubtful cases a T.R.H. test will be helpful.

Treatment.—The hormone l-thyroxine is curative. A full replacement dose is 0·15–0·2 mg a day and because of its slow action, it can be given in a single dose. In the elderly or those with myocardial insufficiency, the initial dose must be as low as 0·05 mg a day and cautiously increased. If a rapid or short-lived response is essential, tri-iodothyronine is used.

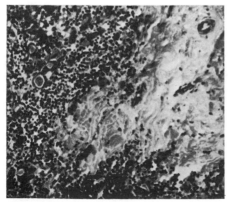

FIG. 633.—Myxoedema. Histology × 100. Gross fibrosis, lymphocytic infiltration and atrophy of acini. Compare with normal histology fig. 643.
(Dr. Bernard Fox, London.)

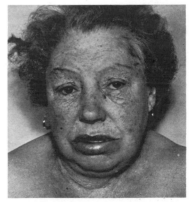

FIG. 634.—Myxoedema: note the bloated look, the pouting lips, and the dull expression.
(Dr. V. K. Summers, Liverpool.)

[1] Thyroid ^{123}I uptake of less than 12% at 24 hours is diagnostic.

Sir Douglas Vernon Hubble, 1900–1981. Professor of Paediatrics and Child Health, University of Birmingham, England.

Myxoedema.—The signs and symptoms of hypothyroidism are accentuated. The facial appearance (fig. 634) is typical, and there is often supraclavicular puffiness, a malar flush, and a yellow tinge to the skin. Myxoedema coma occurs in neglected cases and carries a high mortality: the body temperature is low and the patient must be warmed slowly: 1 g of intravenous hydrocortisone should be given daily, and intravenous tri-iodo-thyronine in slowly increasing doses.

Auto-immune Thyroiditis.—The so-called primary or atrophic myxoedema is now considered an autoimmune disease similar to Hashimoto thyroiditis (p. 690) but without goitre formation from T.S.H. stimulation. Because of the delay in diagnosis the hypothyroidism is usually much more severe than in goitrous auto-immune thyroiditis.

Dyshormonogenesis and Goitrogens.—Genetically determined deficiencies in the enzymes controlling the synthesis of thyroid hormones, if severe, are responsible for goitre formation with hypothyroidism. If of moderate degree, a simple (euthyroid) goitre results.[1-3] Similarly goitrogens may produce a goitre with, or without, hypothyroidism.

GOITRES

A goitre[4] is an enlarged thyroid gland.

CLASSIFICATION OF GOITRES

Simple Goitre (Endemic[5] or sporadic[6]) (Euthyroid)
— Diffuse hyperplastic goitre.
— Nodular goitre.

Toxic Goitre
— Diffuse toxic goitre (Graves' disease).
— Toxic nodular goitre.
— Toxic nodule.

Neoplastic Goitre
— Benign.
— Malignant.

Thyroiditis
— Granulomatous thyroiditis. (de Quervain's disease)
— Auto-immune thyroiditis.
— Riedel's thyroiditis.

Other Rare Goitres
— Acute bacterial thyroiditis.
— Chronic bacterial thyroiditis (Tuberculosis and Syphilis).
— Amyloid Goitre.

---

[1] A number of non-endemic goitrous cretins have been born to a group of itinerant tinkers living in Scotland who inter-marry (Hutchison). This was due to a deficiency of the enzyme dehalogenase. When thyroglobulin is broken down uncoupled iodotyrosines are liberated as well as T3 and T4. They are broken down by the enzyme dehalogenase and the iodine retained within the thyroid. If dehalogenase is deficient, iodothyrosines pass into the blood, are excreted in the urine and this may result in iodine deficiency and goitre formation.

[2] Another classical example of dyshormonogenesis is Pendred's Syndrome, where goitre is associated with congenital deafness. This is due to a deficiency of peroxidase, the enzyme responsible for organification of trapped iodines. A perchlorate discharge test will confirm the diagnosis.

[3] Defects in thyroglobulin synthesis are also being recognised in dyshormonogenesis.

[4] Goitre-Latin, guttur = the throat.

[5] Endemic = prevalent in a people or a district.

[6] Sporadic = haphazard occurrence.

Sir William Withey Gull, 1816–1890. Physician, Guy's Hospital, London. Wrote the first account of Myxoedema in 1873.
James Holmes Hutchison, Contemporary. Professor of Child Health, Glasgow, Scotland.
Vaughan Pendred, 1869–1946. General Practitioner, East Sheen, Surrey, England. Described this Syndrome in 1896 when practising in Durham City.

SIMPLE GOITRE

Simple goitre is due to stimulation of the thyroid gland by the anterior pituitary (*i.e.* by increased levels of circulating T.S.H.). T.S.H. secretion is increased by low levels of circulating thyroid hormones. Any factor, therefore, that maintains a persistently low level of circulating thyroid hormones can be responsible for a simple goitre. The most important factor is iodine deficiency, but defects in hormone synthesis may be responsible.

1. **Iodine Deficiency.** The daily requirement of iodine is about 100–125 μg. In nearly all districts where simple goitre is endemic there is a very low iodide content in the water and food. Endemic areas are in the mountainous ranges, such as the Rocky Mountains, the Alps, the Andes and the Himalayas. In Great Britain endemic goitre is found in the Mendips, Chilterns, Cotswolds and the Pennine Chain of Derbyshire and Yorkshire. Endemic goitre is also found in lowland areas where the soil lacks iodide or the water supply comes from far away mountain ranges, *e.g.* the Great Lakes of North America, the Plains of Lombardy, the Struma Valley,[1] the Nile Valley and the Congo. Calcium is also goitrogenic and goitre is common in low iodine areas on chalk or limestone, *e.g.* Derbyshire and Southern Ireland. Although iodides in food and water may be adequate, failure of intestinal absorption may produce iodine deficiency (McCarrison).

2. **Defects in Synthesis of Thyroid Hormones.** (*a*) Enzyme deficiency within the thyroid gland. (*b*) Goitrogens.

It is probable that enzyme deficiencies of varying degree of severity are responsible for many sporadic goitres (*i.e.* in non-endemic areas), and there is often a family history of goitre in these cases suggesting a genetic defect. If the iodine intake is very high an enzyme deficiency may be overcome, *e.g.* in Iceland where goitre is practically unknown. Enzyme deficiency is often associated with a low iodine intake, *e.g.* a dislike of sea-fish.

Well known goitrogens are vegetables of the brassica family (cabbage, kale and rape) which contain thiocyanate, drugs such as P.A.S. and, of course, the antithyroid drugs.[2]

Surprisingly enough, iodides in large quantities are goitrogenic as they inhibit the organic binding of iodine and give an iodide goitre.[3]

The Natural History of Simple Goitre. This has been investigated by autoradiographs of slices of goitre from patients who have received a pre-operative tracer dose of [131]I. Blackening of an x-ray film takes place in areas where colloid contains iodine, and the autoradiographs are compared with histological sections of the same slice. In any single lobule all follicles behave uniformly. Active follicles are small, lined by tall cells and their colloid contains iodine. Inactive follicles are three times larger, lined by flattened cells and contain colloid without iodine (Taylor).

Stages in goitre formation are:

1. Persistent T.S.H. stimulation causes diffuse hyperplasia; all lobules are composed of active follicles and iodine uptake is uniform. This is a diffuse hyperplastic goitre which may persist for a long time but is reversible if T.S.H. stimulation ceases.

2. Later, as a result of fluctuating T.S.H. levels, a mixed pattern develops with areas of active lobules and areas of inactive lobules.

3. Active lobules become more vascular and hyperplastic until haemorrhage occurs causing central necrosis and leaving only a surrounding rind of active follicles.

4. Necrotic lobules coalesce to form nodules filled either with iodine-free colloid or a mass of new but inactive follicles.

5. Continual repetition of this process results in a nodular goitre. Most nodules are inactive and active follicles are present only in the internodular tissue.

6. There are likely to be other thyroid growth factors in addition to T.S.H. responsible for the growth and development of nodular goitre. These factors include growth stimulating immunoglobulins (Studer). It is thought that chronic thyroid stimulation may affect

---

[1] Struma. In the mountains of Bulgaria arises the River Struma that flows into the Aegean Sea. Along its banks, and those of its tributaries, dwell persons of several nationalities among whom endemic goitre has long been prevalent. Struma is a continental term for a goitre.

[2] Antithyroid drugs—Thiocyanates and perchlorates interfere with iodide trapping, Carbimazole and Thiouracil Compounds interfere with the oxidation of iodide and the binding of iodine to tyrosin.

[3] Iodide goitre is usually seen in asthmatics who have taken proprietary preparations containing iodides (*e.g.* Felsol) over a prolonged period.

Sir Robert McCarrison, 1878–1960. Indian Medical Service. Director of the Nutrition Research Laboratories, Coonoor, Madras, India.
Selwyn Francis Taylor, Contemporary. Formerly Surgeon, Royal Postgraduate Medical School, London.
Hugo Studer, Contemporary. Inselspital, Berne, Switzerland.

particularly sensitive cells which are derived from growth prone cell clones. One of the hallmarks of such nodular goitres is the heterogeneity of structure and function often between adjacent follicles of the same gland.

CLINICAL TYPES OF SIMPLE GOITRE

1. Diffuse Hyperplastic Goitre

Diffuse hyperplasia corresponds to the first stages of the natural history. The goitre appears in childhood in endemic areas but in sporadic cases it usually occurs at puberty when metabolic demands are high—Puberty Goitre (fig. 640). If T.S.H. stimulation ceases the goitre may regress, but tends to recur later at times of stress such as pregnancy. The goitre is soft, diffuse and may become large enough to cause discomfort. A colloid goitre is a late stage of diffuse hyperplasia when T.S.H. stimulation has fallen off and when many follicles are inactive and full of colloid (fig. 641).

2. Nodular Goitre

Persistent fluctuating T.S.H. stimulation results inevitably in progressive nodule formation. Nodules are usually multiple, forming a multinodular goitre. Occasionally, only one macroscopic nodule is found, but microscopic changes will be present throughout the gland: this is one form of a clinically solitary nodule. Nodules may be colloid or cellular, and cystic degeneration and haemorrhage are common, as is subsequent calcification. Nodules appear early in endemic goitre and later (between 20 and 30 years) in sporadic goitre, although the patient herself may be unaware of the goitre until the late forties or fifties. All types of simple goitre are far more common in the female than in the male. It is of interest that recently oestrogen receptors have been identified in normal thyroid tissue and also in nodular goitre.

Diagnosis is usually straightforward. The patient is euthyroid: the nodules are palpable and often visible; they are smooth, usually firm and not hard, and the goitre is painless and moves freely on swallowing. Hardness and irregularity, due to calcification, may simulate carcinoma. A painful nodule, sudden appearance, or rapid enlargement of a nodule, raises suspicion of carcinoma, but is usually due to haemorrhage into a simple nodule. Differential diagnosis from a Hashimoto goitre in a euthyroid patient is often difficult.

Investigations.—Tests of thyroid function may be necessary to exclude mild hyperthyroidism, and the estimation of titres of thyroid antibodies to differentiate from Hashimoto goitre. Plain x-rays may show calcification and tracheal deviation or compression (fig. 635).

Complications.—(i). *Tracheal obstruction*—due to gross lateral displacement, or compression in a lateral or antero-posterior plane. Acute respiratory obstruction may follow haemorrhage into a nodule impacted in the thoracic inlet.

(ii). *Secondary Thyrotoxicosis*—many patients with nodular goitres develop hyperthyroidism sooner or later. The incidence is difficult to estimate, but figures as high as 30% have been suggested.

(iii). *Carcinoma*—which is usually of follicular pattern. It is uncommon but an increased incidence has been reported from endemic areas.

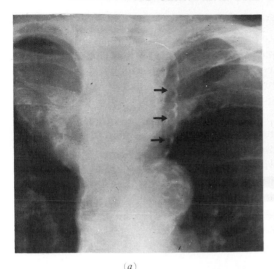
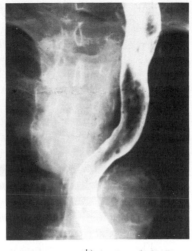

(a)   (b)

FIG. 635.—Restrosternal goitre causing deviation of (a) the trachea and (b) oesophagus, by barium swallow.

Prevention and Treatment of Simple Goitre.—All table salt should be iodised (potassium iodide 1 part in 10,000) although in the U.K. this is not the practice. In endemic areas (e.g. Switzerland, parts of the U.S.A. and Argentina) the incidence of goitre has been strikingly reduced by this prophylactic measure.

In the early stages a hyperplastic goitre is reversible if l-thyroxine is given in maximum doses—0·2 mg a day for several months—and then very slowly tailed off to 0·1 mg a day which should be continued for many years. If regression does not occur, thyroidectomy may be indicated for cosmetic reasons or pressure symptoms.

The nodular stage of simple goitre is irreversible. A multinodular goitre is often uncomfortable and unsightly and, in view of the possible complications, subtotal thyroidectomy is advisable unless the expectation of life is short. Resection aims at removing nodules and leaving up to 8 g of relatively normal tissue in each remnant. The technique is essentially the same as described for toxic goitre as are the post-operative complications. Occasionally the multinodular change is asymmetrically distributed with one lobe significantly involved with perhaps only minimal micronodularity in the opposite lobe. Under these circumstances, a unilateral total lobectomy on the affected side is the appropriate management. In many cases the causative factors persist and recurrence is likely, particularly in the younger patient, unless further T.S.H. stimulation is prevented. 0·1 mg of l-thyroxine a day should be given post-operatively to all patients until after the menopause. Some clinicians give 0·2 mg a day and consider that it should be given indefinitely. If one thyroid lobe appears normal in size and consistency at operation, it is justifiable not to resect it, but post-operative thyroxine is more than ever essential.

3. The Problem of the Clinically Solitary Nodule

The clinically solitary nodule may be defined as 'A goitre which, on clinical examination, appears to be a single nodule in an otherwise normal gland'.

Clinically solitary nodules fall into two categories. In the first are those in which there is a certainty or grave suspicion of malignancy; in these exploration is essential. In the second and far larger category, there is a smooth, firm, mobile nodule which is probably benign but carries a small but significant risk of being a carcinoma. In this category about 50% prove to be simple multinodular goitres when explored.

The thyroid status of these patients must be established by clinical examination and by laboratory tests. Isotope scanning is essential if there is hyperthyroidism but is of limited diagnostic value with respect to malignancy. These tests should divide the patients into three categories:

(i) Hyperthyroid with a hot (overactive) nodule.[1]
(ii) Euthyroid with a warm (active) nodule.[2]
(iii) Euthyroid with a cold (inactive) nodule.[3]

(i) The solitary toxic nodule is never malignant, it is a toxic adenoma: it is treated by excision or radio-iodine.

(ii) The euthyroid warm nodule is a functioning adenoma or a simple nodule with some active thyroid tissue in it. Very rarely, a well differentiated carcinoma will take up isotope. For this reason, and because a functioning adenoma may develop into an overactive adenoma, it should be excised.

(iii) The euthyroid cold nodule is suspect, because a carcinoma so rarely takes up isotope if normal thyroid tissue is present. It should be excised.

Resection entails taking a wide margin of healthy thyroid tissue and this should be achieved by a total lobectomy on the side of the lesion with inclusion of the thyroid isthmus. Subtotal lobectomy is rarely appropriate and should only be performed when the nodule is small, anteriorly situated and has been shown on thin needle cytology to be likely to be benign. Incisional biopsy is absolutely contraindicated. It could result in seeding of malignant cells.

Other investigations which may be undertaken are:
(i) **Needle biopsy.**—Needle biopsy of the thyroid gland is a valuable technique which can aid diagnosis of the solitary thyroid nodule and influence its subsequent management. There are two quite distinct types of needle biopsy:
    1. Trucut large needle
    2. Thin needle aspiration biopsy cytology (ABC)
The former produces a core of tissue for histological examination and the latter yields a cellular aspirate to be smeared for cytological examination. *Trucut large bore biopsy* has a high diagnostic accuracy *but* has poor patient compliance and may be associated with complications such as pain, bleeding, tracheal damage and recurrent laryngeal nerve palsy.

Thin needle ABC has excellent patient compliance, is simple and quick to perform in the out patient department, is readily repeated and in experienced hands has a high diagnostic accuracy. This technique has been popular in Scandinavia for more than 25 years but has only gained popularity in the USA and UK in recent years. More than 20,000 aspirations have been performed at the Karolinska Hospital in Stockholm with no complications. Tumour implantation and seeding does not occur.

Thyroid conditions which can be diagnosed by thin needle cytology include colloid nodules (fig. 636), thyroiditis, papillary carcinoma (fig. 637), medullary carcinoma,

---

[1] A hot nodule is one that takes up isotope, whilst the surrounding thyroid tissue does not. Here the surrounding thyroid tissue is inactive because the nodule is producing such high levels of thyroid hormones that T.S.H. secretion is suppressed.
[2] A warm nodule takes up isotope and so does normal thyroid tissue about it.
[3] A cold nodule takes up no isotope.

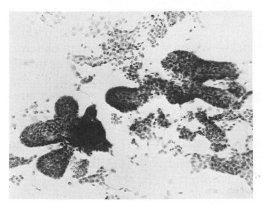

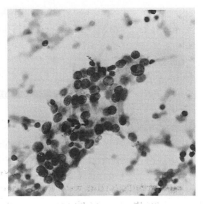

FIG. 636.—Needle biopsy.—Colloid goitre with large follicular sheets and haemosiderin containing macrophages.
(*N. Dallimore, Cardiff.*)

FIG. 637.—Needle biopsy.—Papillary carcinoma with typical papillary architecture and nuclear inclusions.
(*N. Dallimore, Cardiff.*)

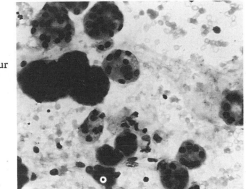

FIG. 638.—Needle biopsy.—Follicular tumour with uniform small follicles.
(*N. Dallimore, Cardiff.*)

anaplastic carcinoma and lymphoma. ABC cannot distinguish between a benign follicular adenoma (fig. 638) and follicular carcinoma as this distinction is dependant not on cytology but on histological criteria which include capsular and vascular invasion.

Using the technique at the Karolinska Hospital, Löwhagen and his colleagues recorded no false positives with respect to malignancy and a false negative rate of 2·2% which later fell to zero. These workers believe that nearly 80% of patients with thyroid nodules can be spared surgical exploration as a result of this diagnostic technique.

Thyroid cysts can be aspirated and the aspirate examined cytologically. There is however a need for caution as many cysts occur in malignancies. After aspirating a cyst a check must be made for any residual thyroid mass and ideally a further sample taken from the cyst wall for cytology. Any cyst which re-accumulates after initial aspiration must be subjected to surgery.

(ii) **Ultrasound.**—This is of limited value in the diagnosis of malignancy but should differentiate between solid and cystic nodules and will often detect other impalpable nodules, *i.e.* demonstrate that the goitre is multinodular.

(iii) **C.T. and M.R.I.**—The sophisticated newer scanning techniques of CT (Computed Axial Tomography) and M.R.I. (Magnetic Resonance Imaging) probably have only a small role to play in the day to day management of thyroid disorders and are still undergoing evaluation.

(iv) **Fluorescent Scanning.**—This comparatively new technique permits an in vivo determination of thyroid gland iodine content. Fluorescent scanning requires a collimated source of photon radiation (^{241}Am) which results in the characteristic 28·5 KeV x-ray emission from any iodine atoms in the field. The number of x-rays detected is proportional to the amount of iodine present. It has been shown that in a cold solitary nodule the ratio

Torsten Löwhagen, Contemporary. Associate Head Division of Cytology, Department of Tumour Pathology, Karolinska Hospital, Stockholm, Sweden.

of iodine content in the nodule to that in the corresponding area of the contralateral lobe may be used to distinguish benign from malignant lesions. This technique is still being evaluated and it remains to be seen what its precise role will ultimately be in the management of thyroid nodules.

Note.—The clinically solitary nodule presents a diagnostic problem when the nodule is smooth, firm and mobile in a euthyroid patient. Scanning, needle biopsy and ultrasound may increase or decrease the suspicion of malignancy, but there is only one certain diagnostic procedure and that is excisional biopsy.

4. Retrosternal Goitre

A very few retrosternal goitres arise from ectopic thyroid tissue, but most arise from the lower pole of a nodular goitre. If the neck is short and the pretracheal muscles are strong, as in men, the negative intrathoracic pressure tends to draw these nodules into the superior mediastinum. The degree of descent varies accounting for—(a) *Substernal type*—when the nodule is palpable. (b) *Plunging type*—when an intrathoracic goitre is occasionally forced into the neck by increased intrathoracic pressure. (c) *Intrathoracic goitre*.

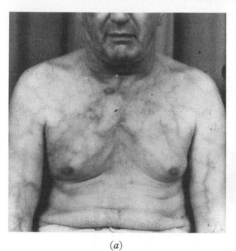 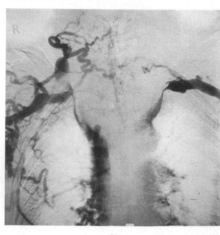

(a)   (b)

FIG. 639.—(a) Infra-red photograph of patient with enormous retrosternal goitre producing superior vena cava obstruction. Dilated superior veins seen on trunk and arms. (b) Venogram showing obstruction of superior vena cava.

Clinical Features.—A history of a previous cervical goitre which had disappeared is not uncommon. A retrosternal goitre maybe symptomless or produce severe symptoms; (a) Dyspnoea, particularly at night, cough and stridor.[1] Many of these patients may attend a chest clinic with a diagnosis of asthma before the true nature of the problem is discovered. (b) Dysphagia. (c) Engorgement of neck veins and superficial veins on the chest wall. In severe cases, there may be obstruction of the superior vena cava (fig. 639). (d) Recurrent nerve paralysis is rare. The goitre may also be malignant or toxic.

X-rays show a soft tissue shadow in the superior mediastinum—sometimes with calcification—and often causing deviation and compression of the trachea

---

[1] Stridor = harsh sound on inspiration.

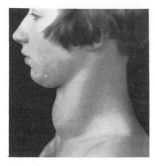

FIG. 640.—Physiological hyper-plasia of the thyroid gland (goitre of puberty).

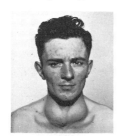

FIG. 641.—Colloid goitre.

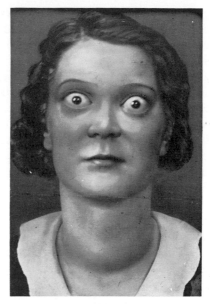

FIG. 642.—Primary toxic goitre.
(*Professor E. J. Wayne, Glasgow.*)

(fig. 635). A ^{123}I scan may help to distinguish a retrosternal goitre from a mediastinal tumour.

Treatment.—If obstructive symptoms are present it is unwise to treat a retrosternal goitre with antithyroid drugs or radio-iodine as these may enlarge the goitre. Resection can almost always be carried out from the neck and a midline sternotomy is hardly ever necessary. The cervical part of the goitre should first be mobilised by ligation and division of the superior thyroid vessels and by ligature and division of the middle thyroid veins and the inferior thyroid artery. The retrosternal goitre can then be delivered by traction and finger mobilisation. Haemorrhage is rarely a problem because the goitre takes its blood supply with it from the neck. The recurrent laryngeal nerve should be identified if possible before delivering the retrosternal goitre, as it is particularly vulnerable to injury from traction or tearing. If a large multinodular goitre cannot be delivered intact from the retrosternal position it may be broken with the fingers and delivered piecemeal but this should never be done if the lesion is solitary and there is the possibility of carcinoma.

TOXIC GOITRE

Thyrotoxicosis (Hyperthyroidism)

The term thyrotoxicosis is retained because hyperthyroidism, *i.e.* symptoms due to a raised level of circulating thyroid hormones, is not responsible for all manifestations of the disease.

Clinical Types. 1. Diffuse toxic goitre. (Graves' disease.[1]) 2. Toxic nodular goitre. 3. Toxic nodule. 4. Hyperthyroidism due to rarer causes.

1. **Diffuse Toxic Goitre.**—Graves' disease—a diffuse vascular goitre appearing at the same time as the hyperthyroidism, usually in the younger woman and

---

[1] First noted in 1786 by Caleb Hillier Parry, 1755–1822, Physician, General Hospital, Bath, England. His account was published posthumously in 1825.

Robert James Graves, 1796–1853. Physician, Meath Hospital, Dublin. Published his account of exophthalmic goitre in 1835.

frequently associated with eye signs. The syndrome is that of primary thyrotoxicosis (fig. 642). The whole of the functioning thyroid tissue is involved, and the hypertrophy and hyperplasia are due to abnormal thyroid stimulating antibodies (TsAb).

2. **Toxic Nodular Goitre.**—A simple nodular goitre is present for a long time before the hyperthyroidism, usually in the middle aged or elderly and very infrequently associated with severe eye signs. The syndrome is that of secondary thyrotoxicosis.

In many cases of toxic nodular goitre, the nodules are inactive, and it is the internodular thyroid tissue that is overactive. This is Graves' disease in a background nodular goitre. However, in some toxic nodular goitres one or more nodules are overactive and here the hyperthyroidism is due to autonomous thyroid tissue as in the toxic nodule.

3. **Toxic Nodule.**—A solitary overactive nodule. It is autonomous and its hypertrophy and hyperplasia are not due to thyroid stimulating antibodies (TsAb). *Because T.S.H. secretion is suppressed by the high level of circulating thyroid hormones, the normal thyroid tissue surrounding the nodule is itself suppressed and inactive.*

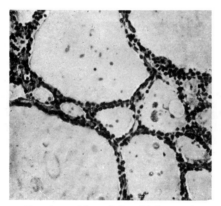 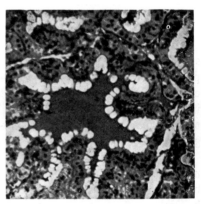

Fig. 643.—Normal thyroid (see text).   Fig. 644.—Thyrotoxicosis (see text).
× 100.   × 100.
(Dr. Bernard Fox, London.)

Histology. The normal thyroid gland (fig. 643) consists of acini lined by flattened cuboidal epithelium and filled with homogenous colloid. In hyperthyroidism (fig. 644) there is hyperplasia of acini which are lined by high columnar epithelium. Many of them are empty, and others contain vacuolated colloid.

Symptomatology.—Thyrotoxicosis is 8 times commoner in females than in males. It may occur at any age. Wayne's clinical diagnostic index gives all the important symptoms and signs of thyrotoxicosis and indicates by their score the relative importance of each. The most significant symptoms are loss of weight in spite of a good appetite, a recent preference for cold, and palpitations. The most significant signs are the excitability of the patient, the presence of a goitre, exophthalmos, and tachycardia or cardiac arrhythmia.

Sir Edward Johnson Wayne, Contemporary. Formerly Regius Professor of Medicine, Glasgow, Scotland.

WAYNE'S CLINICAL DIAGNOSTIC INDEX

Symptom score + Sign score = Diagnostic Index

INDEX—Under 11 = Non-Toxic
11–19 = Equivocal
over 19 = Toxic

Symptoms of Recent Onset and/or Increased Severity	Present Score	Score
Dyspnœa on effort	+1	
Palpitations	+2	
Tiredness	+2	
Preference for heat (irrespective of duration)		−5
Preference for cold	+5	
Indifferent to temperature	0	
Excessive sweating	+3	
Nervousness	+2	
Appetite increased	+3	
,,　　decreased		−3
Weight increased		−3
,,　　decreased	+3	

Signs	Present Score	Absent Score
Palpable thyroid	+3	−3
Bruit over thyroid	+2	−2
Exophthalmos	+2	
Lid retraction	+2	
Lid lag	+1	
Hyperkinetic movements	+4	−2
Fine finger tremor	+1	
Hands		
Hot	+2	−2
Moist	+1	−1
Casual pulse rate:		
Atrial fibrillation	+4	
Regular rates:		
80 per minute		−3
80 to 90 per minute	0	
90 per minute	+3	

The goitre in primary thyrotoxicosis is diffuse and vascular, it may be large or small, firm or soft, and a thrill and a bruit may be present, usually at the upper poles over the superior thyroid arteries. The onset is abrupt, but remissions and exacerbations are not infrequent. Hyperthyroidism is usually more severe than in secondary thyrotoxicosis but cardiac failure is rare. Manifestations of thyrotoxicosis not due to hyperthyroidism *per se*, *e.g.* orbital proptosis, ophthalmoplegia and pretibial myxoedema may occur in primary thyrotoxicosis.

In secondary thyrotoxicosis the goitre is nodular. The onset is insidious and may present with cardiac failure or atrial fibrillation. It is characteristic that the hyperthyroidism is not severe. Eye signs other than lid lag and lid spasm (due to hyperthyroidism) are very rare.

Cardiac rhythm.—A fast heart rate, which persists during sleep, is characteristic. Cardiac arrhythmias are superimposed on the sinus tachycardia as the disease progresses, and they are commoner in older patients with thyrotoxicosis because of the prevalence of coincidental heart disease. Stages of development of thyrotoxic arrhythmias are:

(1) Multiple extrasystoles. (2) Paroxysmal atrial tachycardia. (3) Paroxysmal atrial fibrillation. (4) Persistent atrial fibrillation, not responsive to digoxin.

Myopathy.—Weakness of the proximal limb muscles is commonly found if looked for. Severe muscular weakness (Thyrotoxic myopathy) resembling myaesthenia gravis, occurs occasionally. Recovery occurs as hyperthyroidism is controlled.

Exophthalmos.—Some degree of exophthalmos is common. It may be unilateral. True exophthalmos is a proptosis of the eye, caused by infiltration of the retrobulbar tissues with fluid and round cells, with a varying degree of retraction

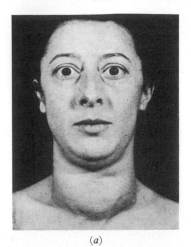 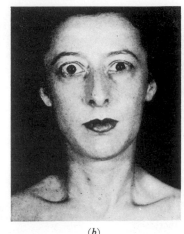

(a)   (b)

FIG. 645.—(a) Prior to sub-total thyroidectomy following preparation with carbimazole and potassium iodide; note lid retraction, which is more marked on the right. (b) Relapse of thyrotoxicosis. Weight loss; a bilateral partial tarsorrhaphy has been performed because of early exposure keratitis.
(Dr. Bruce Fowler, London.)

or spasm[1] of the upper eyelid. This results in widening of the palpebral fissure (the inner and outer canthus) so that the sclera can be seen clearly above the upper margin of the iris and cornea (above the 'limbus').

Spasm and retraction usually disappear when the hyperthyroidism is controlled. They may be improved by ß-adrenergic blocking drugs, e.g. Guanethidine eye drops. The condition is aggravated by compression of the ophthalmic veins.

The proptosis can be measured with an exophthalmometer. Oedema of the eyelids, conjunctival injection and chemosis are aggravated by compression of the ophthalmic veins. Weakness of the extra-ocular muscles, particularly the elevators (interior oblique), results in diplopia. In severe cases papilloedema and corneal ulceration occur. When severe and progressive it is known as malignant exophthalmos (fig. 646) and the eye may be destroyed. It is postulated that Graves' ophthalmopathy is an autoimmune disease in which there are antibody mediated affects on the ocular muscles.

Exophthalmos is usually self-limiting and may even regress a little. Sleeping propped up and lateral tarsorrhaphy will help to protect the eye but will not prevent progression. Hypothyroidism increases proptosis by a few millimetres and must be avoided.

Improvement has been reported with massive doses of prednisone. Intra-orbital injection of steroids is dangerous because of the venous congestion, and total thyroid ablation has not proved effective. When the eye is in danger, orbital decompression may be required (see Dysthyroid Exophthalmos, p. 531 and fig. 473).

Pretibial Myxoedema (fig. 647) is a thickening of the skin by a mucin-like deposit, nearly always associated with true exophthalmos, past or present hyperthyroidism, and high levels of thyroid stimulating antibodies (TsAb).

---

[1] Lid spasm occurs because the levator palpebrae superioris muscle is partly innervated by sympathetic fibres.

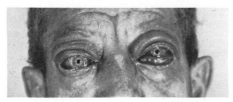

FIG. 646.—Progressive (malignant) exophthalmos, with chemosis and exophthalmic ophthalmoplegia.
(The Lahey Clinic, Mass., U.S.A.)

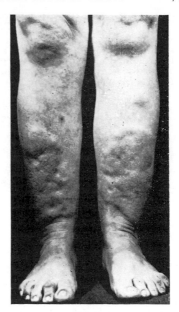

FIG. 647.—Pretibial myxoedema. It is usually symmetrical, and minor degrees are not uncommon but are easily missed. The earliest stage is a shiny red plaque of thickened skin with coarse hair, which may be cyanotic when cold. In severe cases the skin of the whole leg below the knee is involved, together with that of the foot and ankle and there may be clubbing of the fingers and toes. (Thyroid Acropachy.)

Diagnosis of Thyrotoxicosis.—Most cases are diagnosed clinically and the Wayne diagnostic index is an excellent discipline. Difficulty is most likely to arise in the differentiation of mild hyperthyroidism from an anxiety state when a goitre is present. In these cases the thyroid status is determined by the diagnostic tests described earlier. If there is still doubt after a routine Thyroid Profile and a ^{123}I uptake test, than a T.R.H. test should be done.

T^3 thyrotoxicosis is diagnosed by estimating the Free T^3. It should be suspected if the clinical picture is suggestive, but routine tests of thyroid function are within the normal range. A thyroid scan is essential in the diagnosis of an autonomous toxic nodule.

Thyrotoxicosis should always be considered in: (a) children with a growth spurt, behaviour problems or myopathy. (b) Tachycardia or arrhythmia in the elderly. (c) Unexplained diarrhoea. (d) Loss of weight.

Principles of the Treatment of Thyrotoxicosis.—Non-specific measures are rest and sedation, and in established thyrotixicosis should be used only in conjunction with specific measures which are the use of anti-thyroid drugs, surgery and radio-iodine.

Antithyroid Drugs.—Those in common use are Carbimazole and Propylthiouracil. Beta adrenergic blockers such as Propranolol may also be used. Iodides, once thought to reduce the vascularity of the thyroid, should only be used as immediate preoperative preparation in the ten days prior to surgery. Antithyroid drugs are used to restore the patient to a euthyroid state and to maintain this for a prolonged period in the hope that a permanent remission will occur (i.e. that production of Thyroid Stimulating Antibodies (TsAb) will diminished or cease). It should be noted that antithyroid drugs cannot cure a toxic nodule. The overactive thyroid tissue is autonomous and recurrence of the hyperthyroidism is certain when the drug is discontinued.

Advantages.—No surgery and no use of radio-active materials.

Disadvantages.—(a) Treatment is prolonged and the failure rate after a course of 1½–2 years is at least 50%. Recently, there has been a trend towards the use of shorter courses (6 months) of these drugs. (b) It is impossible to predict which patient is likely to go into a remission.[1] (c) Some goitres enlarge and become very vascular during treatment[2]—even if thyroxine is given at the same time. (d) Very rarely there is a dangerous drug reaction, *e.g.* agranulocytosis[3] or aplastic anaemia.

Initially, 10 mg of Carbimazole[4] are given three or four times a day, and there is a latent interval of 7–14 days before any clinical improvement is apparent. It is most important to maintain a high concentration of the drug throughout the 24 hours by spacing the doses at 8 or 6 hourly intervals. When the patient becomes euthyroid a maintenance dose of 5 mg two or three times a day is given for another 12–18 months. If Tri-iodo-thyronine—20 µg to 4 times daily, or Thyroxine— 0·1 mg daily, are given in conjunction with antithyroid drugs, there is less danger of producing iatrogenic thyroid insufficiency or an increase in the size of the goitre.

Surgery.—In diffuse toxic goitre and toxic nodular goitre with overactive inter-nodular tissue, surgery cures by reducing the mass of overactive tissue. It seems that a cure is probable if the thyroid tissue can be reduced below a critical mass.[5] In the autonomous toxic nodule, and in toxic nodular goitre with overactive autonomous toxic nodules, surgery cures by removing all the overactive thyroid tissue: this allows the suppressed normal tissue to function again.

Advantages.—The goitre is removed, the cure is rapid, and the cure rate is high if surgery has been adequate.

Disadvantages.—(a) A recurrence of thyrotoxicosis occurs in less than 5% of cases. (b) Every operation carries a morbidity but with suitable preparation and an experienced surgeon the mortality is negligible. (c) Although post-operative thyroid insufficiency occurs in 20–45% of cases, this is rarely due to the operation itself. (d) Parathyroid insufficiency should occur in less than 0·5%.

Radio-iodine.—Radio-iodine[6] destroys thyroid cells and, as in thyroidectomy, reduces the mass of functioning thyroid tissue to below a critical level.

Advantages.—No surgery and no prolonged drug therapy.

Disadvantages.—(a) Isotope facilities must be available. (b) There is a high and progress-ive incidence of thyroid insufficiency which may reach 75–80% after 10 years.[7] (c) An indefinite follow-up is essential.

There is no convincing evidence that radio-iodine has been responsible for genetic damage, leukaemia, damage to the foetus if given inadvertently in early pregnancy, or carcinoma in the adult. In some North American Clinics radio-

---

[1] Attempts have been made to predict which patients might relapse after a six month course of antithyroid drugs on the basis of H.L.A. status and the presence of TsAb (Thyroid Stimulating Antibody production).

[2] This is probably due to TsAb stimulation during the prolonged course of treatment and not a direct effect of the drug.

[3] Agranulocytosis—The patient should be instructed to discontinue treatment if she develops a sore throat until the white cell count has been checked.

[4] Carbimazole = propriatary name Neomercazole, 5 mg tablets. This agent also has an immuno-supressive action on Thyroid Stimulating Antibody production.

[5] This may result in a reduction of TsAb or it may be that the circulating TsAb, however high its level, can only produce limited hypertrophy and hyperplasia when the mass of thyroid tissue is small.

[6] Radio-active iodine was first used in the treatment of thyrotoxicosis by Hertz and Roberts in 1942. Isotope—Greek, *isos* = equal, *topos* = place.

[7] This is due to sublethal damage to those cells not actually destroyed by the initial treatment and this eventually causes failure of cellular reproduction.

Saul Hertz, Contemporary. Director of Radioactive Isotope Research Institute, Boston, Mass., U.S.A.
A. Roberts, Contemporary. Isotope Department, Massachusetts Institute of Technology, Boston, Mass., U.S.A.

iodine is given to almost all patients over the age of 25—when development is complete.[1] In this country, on account of the real and potential risks, most clinicians are unwilling to advise it under the age of 45. The dose of radio-iodine varies with the size of the goitre and a suggested dose is 160 μCi per 1 g of thyroid tissue (5·9 MBq). Thus, for a gland estimated at 60 g between 9 and 10 mCi (360 MBq) would be prescribed.[2] Response is slow, but a substantial improvement is to be expected in 8 to 12 weeks. Accurate dosage is difficult and, should there be no clinical improvement after 12 weeks, a further dose is given (Mcgregor). Two or more doses are necessary in 20–30% of cases.

The Choice of Therapeutic Agent.—Each case must be considered individually. Below are listed guiding principles as to the most satisfactory treatment for a particular toxic goitre at a particular age: these must however be modified according to the facilities available and the personality, intelligence and wishes of the individual patient, her business or family commitments and any other co-existent medical or surgical condition.

1. *Diffuse Toxic Goitre.*—Over 45—Radio-iodine. Under 45—Surgery for the large goitre—Antithyroid drugs for the small goitre.
Large goitres are uncomfortable and remission with antithyroid drugs is less likely than in the small goitre.
2. *Toxic Nodular Goitre.*—Surgery.
Toxic nodular goitre does not respond as well or as rapidly to radio-iodine or antithyroid drugs as does a diffuse toxic goitre, and the goitre itself is often large and uncomfortable and enlarges still further with antithyroid drugs.
3. *Toxic Nodule.*—Surgery or Radio-iodine.
Resection is easy, certain and without morbidity. Radio-iodine is, however, the treatment of choice over the age of 45 because the suppressed thyroid tissue does not take up iodine and there is thus no risk of delayed thyroid insufficiency.
4. *Recurrent Thyrotoxicosis after adequate surgery.*—Over 45—radio-iodine. Under 45—antithyroid drugs.
5. *Failure of previous treatment with antithyroid drugs or radio-iodine.*—Surgery or thyroid ablation with [123]I.

In advising treatment, the age of 45 must not be taken as a rigid dividing line. Intelligence is important: unintelligent patients cannot be trusted to take drugs regularly if they feel well, and are unlikely to attend follow-up clinics indefinitely, which is essential after radio-iodine therapy.

Special Problems in Treatment
1. **Pregnancy.**—Radio-iodine is absolutely contraindicated because of the risk to the foetus. The danger of surgery is miscarriage; and that of antithyroid drugs is of inducing thyroid insufficiency in the mother, and because both T.S.H. and anti-thyroid drugs cross the placenta, of the baby being born goitrous (fig. 648) and hypothyroid. The risk of either surgery in the second trimester, in competent hands, or careful administration of antithyroid drugs, is very small and the choice is exactly as in the uncomplicated case.
2. **Post-partum Hyperthyroidism.**—Pregnancy may lead to an exacerbation of a variety of auto-immune diseases in the post-partum period. Post-partum hyperthyroidism may be a problem in a patient previously diagnosed with hyperthyroidism or may occur in a patient without any previous history of thyroid disease.
3. **Children.**—Radio-iodine is absolutely contraindicated because of the risk of inducing thyroid carcinoma. There is an increased risk of recurrence after thyroidectomy

---

[1] In some North American centres a total ablative dose of radio-iodine is administered followed by routine replacement treatment with thyroxine.
[2] A more sophisticated method is to give a dose of 7500 rad, calculated from the peak uptake of ^{123}I in the thyroid and the length of time the ^{123}I remains in the gland.

Alastair Goold Macgregor, 1919–1972. Regius Professor of Materia Medica and Therapeutics, Aberdeen, Scotland.

because thyroid cells are highly active in the young. It is probably best to treat children and adolescents with antithyroid drugs until the late teens. If thyroidectomy is to be undertaken it must be very radical.

4. **The Thyro-cardiac.**—This is a patient with severe cardiac damage due wholly or partly to hyperthyroidism. The patient is usually middle aged or elderly with secondary thyrotoxicosis and the hyperthyroidism is not very severe. The cardiac condition is far more significant than the hyperthyroidism, but this must be rapidly controlled to prevent further cardiac damage. B-blockade (Propanolol) can assist rapid control of cardiac effects.

Thyroidectomy is the treatment of choice after control of the cardiac condition. In the elderly, however, or when the operative risk is unacceptable, radio-iodine is given, and treatment with antithyroid drugs is started 48 hours later and continued until the radio-iodine has had effect (usually six weeks).

5. **High Pre-operative Titres of Thyroid Antibodies.**—Their presence indicates lymphatic infiltration of the goitre—i.e. a diffuse or focal thyroiditis—and a liability to thyroid insufficiency after thyroidectomy. These patients are best treated conservatively unless the goitre is large, vascular and uncomfortable. Steroids can help to reduce pain and swelling.

6. **Proptosis of Recent onset.**—It is considered unwise to terminate thyrotoxicosis abruptly by thyroidectomy or radio-iodine if proptosis is recent, because malignant exophthalmos may be induced. There is no real proof of this, but it is advisable to treat these patients with antithyroid drugs, and until the proptosis has been static for six months.

Hyperthyroidism due to other causes

1. *Thyrotoxicosis factitia.*[1] Hyperthyroidism can be induced by taking l-thyroxine, but only if the dosage exceeds the normal requirements of 0·2–0·3 mg a day. Doses below the normal requirements simply suppress normal hormone production by the thyroid.

2. *Jod-Basedow[2] Thyrotoxicosis.* Large doses of iodide given to a hyperplastic endemic goitre which is iodine avid may produce temporary hyperthyroidism, and very occasionally a persistent hyperthyroidism.

3. *In subacute or acute forms of autoimmune thyroiditis or of de Quervain's thyroiditis* (p. 690), mild hyperthyroidism may occur in the early stages due to liberation of thyroid hormones from damaged tissue.

4. *A large mass of secondary carcinoma* will rarely produce sufficient hormone to induce mild hyperhyroidism.

5. *Neonatal thyrotoxicosis* occurs in babies born to hyperthyroid mothers or to euthyroid mothers who have had thyrotoxicosis. High TsAb titres are present in both mother and child because TsAb can cross the placental barrier. The hyperthyroidism gradually subsides in 3 to 4 weeks' time as the TsAb titres fall in the baby's serum.

Surgery for Thyrotoxicosis

Pre-operative Preparation (fig. 649).—The patient must be euthyroid or near euthyroid at operation. The thyroid state is determined by clinical assessment, *i.e.* by improvement in previous symptoms and by objective signs such as gain in weight and lowering of the pulse rate, and by serial estimations of the thyroid profile.

Preparation is as an outpatient and only rarely is admission to hospital necessary on account of severe symptoms at presentation, or failure to control the hyperthyroidism. Failure to control with antithyroid drugs is unusual but may be due to uneven dosage—*i.e.* not taking the drug at 6 or 8 hourly intervals.

Carbimazole[3] 30–40 mg a day is the drug of choice for preparation. When

---

[1] Usually seen in health cranks or those given thyroid extract as 'a tonic'.

[2] Jod = German for iodine + Basedow. In European countries Diffuse Toxic Goitre is often called Basedow's disease.

[3] Potassium perchlorate—200 mg 6 hourly may be used pre-operatively but Lugol's iodine cannot be used with it, as perchlorate interferes with the trapping of iodide. To stop potassium perchlorate and give iodides is highly dangerous and may promote thyroid crisis at operation.

Carl Adolph von Basedow, 1799–1854. General Practitioner, Merseburg, Germany. Published his account of exophthalmic goitre in 1840.

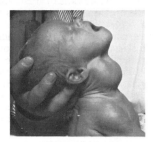

Fig. 648.—Transmitted thiouracil goitre.[1]

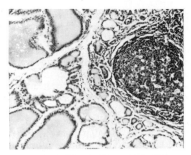

Fig. 649.—'Prepared' thyrotoxicosis with acini lined by low cuboidal epithelium, with more colloid. Compare figs 643, 644. The lymphocytic infiltration with lymph follicle formation is a feature. × 100.

(Dr. Bernard Fox, London.)

euthyroid—after 8–12 weeks—the dose may be reduced to 5 mg 8 hourly and the addition of thyroxine can facilitate maintenance of the euthyroid state. The last dose of Carbimazole can be given on the evening prior to surgery. Iodides[2] are now very rarely used alone because if the patient needs pre-operative treatment a more effective drug should be given. Iodides may be given with Carbimazole for 10–14 days immediately prior to operation but their use is of doubtful value and has been given up in many centres.

Propranolol 40 mg t.d.s. is used by some to prepare less severe cases. It is a betablocker[3] which acts on the target organs and not on the gland itself. It does not interfere with synthesis of thyroid hormones, so that hormone levels remain high during treatment and for some days after thyroidectomy. It is, therefore, important to continue to give the drug for 7 days post-operatively.

Propranolol controls symptoms very rapidly so that its principal value is in combination with Carbimazole in the immediate treatment of patients with very severe hyperhyroidism.

Subtotal Thyroidectomy.—Pre-operative investigations to be carried out and recorded are—(a) Indirect laryngoscopy—a symptomless cord paralysis is present in 3% of cases, without any previous thyroid surgery. (b) Thyroid antibodies. (c) Serum calcium estimation. (d) A scan prior to pre-operative preparation is essential in patients with toxic nodular goitre. The surgeon should know which nodules, if any, are autonomous and active in order to ensure their resection. A scan is of no value in diffuse toxic goitre when uptake, for practical purposes, is uniform. The diagnosis of a single toxic nodule can only be made by demonstrating that the nodule is active and the remaining thyroid tissue suppressed.

---

[1] This does not occur if T3 is given with antithyroid as it too crosses the placenta.

[2] Lugol's Iodine—Dose 30 minims (drops) t.d.s. It is helpful to the patient to prescribe in the old-fashioned minims as one minim = 1 drop. It is claimed that iodides reduce the vascularity of the goitre and make it softer and easier to handle. Potassium iodide tablets N.F. 60 mg t.d.s. may be used instead of Lugol's iodine.

[3] Propranolol inhibits the peripheral conversion of T4 to T3. Long-acting betablockers are now also available and can be administered once daily.

Jean Guillaume Auguste Lugol, 1786–1851. Physician, Hôpital Saint-Louis, Paris.
Henry Stanley Plummer, 1874–1937, Physician, Mayo Clinic, Rochester, U.S.A. was the first to use iodine for preparing thyrotoxic patients for operation.

Technique.—General anaesthesia is administered by an endotracheal tube and good muscle relaxation obtained. The patient is supine on the operating table with the table tilted 15° at the head end in order to reduce venous engorgement. A sandbag pillow is placed in the interscapular region and neck extended (with care particularly in the elderly) in order to make the thyroid gland more prominent. A skin crease incision is made and the flaps of skin, subcutaneous tissue and platysma are raised upwards to the superior thyroid notch and downwards to the suprasternal notch. Adequate exposure entails mobilisation of the sterno-mastoid muscles by incising the fascia along their medial border and midline incision of the cervical fascia. The pre-tracheal strap muscles are not divided as a routine but may be if greater exposure is required. Safe ligation of the superior thyroid vessels in a large vascular Graves' goitre may certainly be facilitated by strap muscle division. The thyroid lobes are mobilised by division between ligatures of the middle thyroid veins, the superior thyroid vessels, and inferior thyroid veins. The inferior thyroid arteries are ligated in continuity or divided between ligatures. The recurrent laryngeal nerve should be identified in its course in the operative field. It should first be sought below the level of the inferior thyroid artery as it passes obliquely upwards and forwards. This course (fig. 650), oblique to the trachea and oesophagus, is accentuated by mobilis-

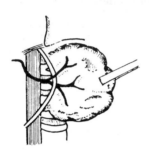

FIG. 650.—Identification of the recurrent laryngeal nerve (see text).

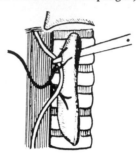

FIG. 651.—On obtaining haemostasis special care should be exercised on the medial side of the thyroid remnant as the nerve can easily be damaged.

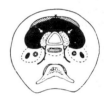

FIG. 652 .— Tension haematoma deep to pretracheal muscles.
(After V. H. Riddell, F.R.C.S., London.)

ation of the thyroid lobe: only rarely does the nerve lie in the groove between the trachea and oesophagus. The nerve often lies between the branches of the inferior thyroid artery so that identification is helped by traction of a ligature on the trunk of the artery, and if not seen it can frequently be palpated as a taut strand. The nerve passes into the larynx immediately behind the inferior cornu of the thyroid cartilage which is therefore a very important landmark. If the right nerve cannot be found in its usual course, an anomalous nerve, present in 1% of cases, should be suspected: this arises from the vagus trunk and usually passes from behind the carotid sheath curving medially, forwards, and upwards and may be mistaken for the inferior thyroid artery. The parathyroid glands are protected by careful inspection of the goitre before resection and by avoiding ligatures and sutures close to the hilum of identified glands. The use of diathermy in this area should be avoided as heat conduction may devascularise the parathyroids or damage the recurrent laryngeal nerves. If a parathyroid gland is inadvertently excised or devascularised it should be autotransplanted into a pocket fashioned within the sternomastoid muscle. Subtotal resection of each lobe is carried out leaving a remnant of 4 to 5 g on each side. Absolute haemostasis is secured by ligation of individual vessels and by suture of the thyroid remnants to the tracheal fascia (fig. 651). The pretracheal muscles and cervical fascia are sutured and the wound closed with suction drainage to the deep cervical space.

Post-operative Complications

1. **Haemorrhage.**—A tension haematoma deep to the cervical fascia (fig. 652) is usually due to slipping of a ligature on the superior thyroid artery: occasionally haemorrhage from a thyroid remnant or a thyroid vein may be responsible. It may be necessary to open the wound in the ward in order to relieve tension before taking the patient to theatre to

evacuate the haematoma and to tie off a bleeding vessel if one can be found. A small subcutaneous haematoma or collection of serum may form and should be evacuated or aspirated.

2. **Respiratory Obstruction.**—Is very rarely due to collapse or kinking of the trachea. Most cases are due to laryngeal oedema. The most important cause of laryngeal oedema is a tension haematoma. However, trauma to the larynx by anaesthetic intubation and surgical manipulation are important contributory factors—particularly if the goitre is very vascular—and may cause laryngeal oedema without a tension haematoma. Unilateral or bilateral recurrent nerve paralysis will not cause immediate postoperative respiratory obstruction unless laryngeal oedema is also present, but they will aggravate the obstruction.

If releasing the tension haematoma does not immediately relieve airway obstruction, the trachea should be intubated at once. An endotracheal tube can be left in place for several days; steroids are given to reduce oedema and a tracheostomy is rarely necessary. Intubation in the presence of laryngeal oedema may be very difficult and should be carried out by an experienced anaesthetist; repeated unsuccessful attempts may increase obstruction and cause serious cerebral anoxia (Wade). In an emergency it is far safer for the inexperienced surgeon to perform a needle tracheostomy as a temporary measure, a Medicut 12G needle (diameter 2·3 mm) is highly satisfactory.

3. **Recurrent Laryngeal Nerve Paralysis** may be unilateral or bilateral, transient or permanent (Chapter 35). Transient paralysis occurs in about 3% of nerves at risk and recovers in 3 weeks to 3 months. Permanent paralysis is extremely rare if the nerve has been identified at operation.

4. **Thyroid Insufficiency.**—This usually occurs within two years, but it is sometimes delayed for 5 years or more. It is often very insidious and difficult to recognise. The incidence is considerably higher than used to be thought and figures of 20–45% have been reported after operations on diffuse toxic goitres and toxic nodular goitres with internodular hyperplasia. It represents a change in the auto-immune response from stimulation to destruction of thyroid cells and is only rarely a result of operative removal of too much thyroid tissue. Thyroid insufficiency is rare after surgery for a toxic adenoma, because there is no auto-immune disease present.

5. **Parathyroid Insufficiency.**[1]—The incidence of this condition should be less than 0·5% and most cases present dramatically 2–5 days after operation but very rarely the onset is delayed for 2–3 weeks or a patient with marked hypocalcaemia is asymptomatic.

6. **Thyrotoxic Crisis (Storm)** is an acute exacerbation of hyperthyroidism. It occurs if a thyrotoxic patient has been inadequately prepared for thyroidectomy, and is now extremely rare.[2] Very rarely, a thyrotoxic patient presents in a crisis and this may follow an unrelated operation. Symptomatic and supportive treatment is for dehydration, hyperpyrexia and restlessness. This requires the administration of intravenous fluids, cooling the patient with ice packs, administration of oxygen, digoxin when there is cardiac failure, sedation and intravenous hydrocortisone. Specific treatment is by Carbimazole 15–20 mg 6 hourly, Lugol's iodine 10 drops 8 hourly by mouth or sodium iodide 1 g I.V. Propranolol 40 mg 6 hourly orally will block adverse beta adrenergic effects. This agent can be given by careful intravenous administration (1–2 mg) under precise electrocardiographic control.

7. **Wound Infection.**—A subcutaneous or deep cervical abscess should be drained.

8. **Keloid Scar** is more likely to form if the incision overlies the sternum. Intradermal injections of corticosteroid should be given at once and repeated monthly if necessary.

9. **Stitch Granuloma.**—This may occur with or without sinus formation and is seen after the use of non-absorbable suture material. Absorbable ligatures and sutures (either Dexon or Vicryl) should be used throughout thyroid surgery except for skin closure where silk is still appropriate.

Post-operative Follow-up

(1) Indirect laryngoscopy should be carried out routinely before leaving hospital.

(2) Screening for parathyroid insufficiency by serum calcium estimation at 6 weeks.

(3) Observation at 6 monthly and then yearly intervals for recurrence of hyperthyroidism—which occurs in 5–10% of cases.

---

[1] Parathyroid insufficiency is due to removal of parathyroid glands, or infarction through damage to the parathyroid end-artery: often both factors occur together. Vascular injury is probably far more important than inadvertent removal.

[2] Very rarely a thyrotoxic patient presents in a crisis and this may follow an unrelated operation.

James Stanley Hilary Wade, M.C. Contemporary. Formerly Consultant Surgeon, University Hospital of Wales, Cardiff.

(4) Observation at 6 monthly and then yearly intervals for delayed thyroid insufficiency, particularly if the resected goitre showed lymphocytic infiltration or if pre-operative thyroid antibody titres were high. Follow up should be for life.

(5) Once a stable situation has been achieved, follow-up after thyroid surgery can be carried out by an automated computer activated system. Such a system in Wales (Welsh Automated Follow-Up Register) has been shown to be extremely cost effective and dramatically reduces the number of patient attendances at the thyroid clinic.

NEOPLASMS OF THE THYROID

Classification of Thyroid Neoplasms

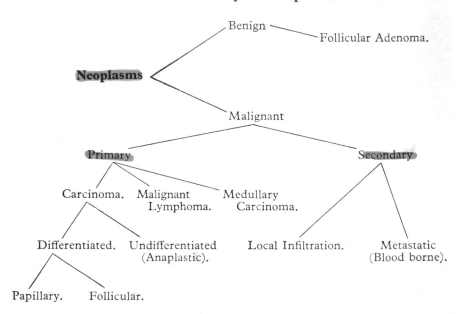

Benign Tumours.—Follicular adenomas present as clinically solitary nodules and frequently the distinction between a follicular carcinoma and an adenoma can only be made by histological examination: in the adenoma there is no invasion of the capsule or of pericapsular blood vessels. Treatment is, therefore, by wide excision—preferably a lobectomy. The remaining thyroid tissue is normal so that prolonged follow-up is unnecessary. It is doubtful if there is such an entity as a papillary adenoma and all papillary tumours should be considered as malignant even if encapsulated.

Malignant Tumours.—Secondary growths are rare. Blood-borne metastases occur from primary carcinomas of breast, colon, kidney and from melanomas. The vast majority of primary growths are carcinomas (fig. 653). Dunhill classified them histologically as differentiated and undifferentiated: we now subdivide the differentiated carcinomas into follicular and papillary. Clinico-pathological studies have demonstrated a pattern of behaviour according to histological type, which has an important bearing on treatment.

Papillary Carcinoma.—Most papillary tumours contain a mixture of papillary and colloid-filled follicles, and in some the follicular structure predominates.

Sir Thomas Peel Dunhill, 1876–1957. Surgeon, St. Bartholomew's Hospital, London.

Relative Incidence	(%)
Papillary Carcinoma	60
Follicular Carcinoma	17
Anaplastic Carcinoma	13
Medullary Carcinoma	6
Malignant Lymphoma	4

FIG. 653.—Relative incidence of primary malignant tumours of the thyroid gland.

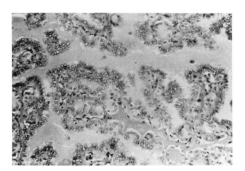

FIG. 654.—Histology of papillary carcinoma showing typical papillary projections.
(*Professor E. D. Williams, Cardiff.*)

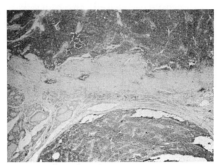

FIG. 655.—Histology of frankly invasive follicular carcinoma showing adjacent vascular channel containing tumour.
(*Professor E. D. Williams, Cardiff.*)

Nevertheless, if any papillary structure is present, the tumour will behave in a predictable fashion as a papillary carcinoma (fig. 654).

Woolner has divided papillary tumours into three subgroups according to their size and extent (fig. 656). Multiple foci may occur in the same lobe as the primary tumour or, less commonly, in both lobes. They are probably due to lymphatic spread in the rich intrathyroidal lymph plexus, rather than to multicentric growth. Spread to the lymph nodes is common but blood-borne metastases are most unusual unless the tumour is extrathyroidal.[1]

The primary aim of treatment is to eradicate the growth. The secondary aim is to prevent local recurrence, because a long and comfortable life is possible, even when metastases are present, provided the trachea and larynx are not involved. Because of the high incidence of multiple foci, a total thyroidectomy should be

CLASSIFICATION BY SIZE AND INFILTRATION.

	A Occult < 1·5 cm	B Intrathyroidal	C Extrathyroidal
Incidence	31%	53%	15%
Encapsulation	Rare	—	60%
Lymph spread	33%	55%	60%
Blood spread	—	—	Late
Death due to growth	Nil/240	9/354	10/68

FIG. 656.—Subgroups of papillary carcinoma and their behaviour.
(*after Woolner.*)

---

[1] The term extrathyroidal indicates that the primary tumour has infiltrated through the capsule of the thyroid gland.

Lewis B. Woolner, Contemporary. Pathologist, The Mayo Clinic, Rochester, Minnesota, U.S.A.

carried out[1] and, in the extrathyroidal tumours, this may entail resection of part of the trachea or a laryngectomy. Because of the high incidence of lymph metastases, even in occult tumours, the pretracheal and paratracheal nodes on the side of the primary tumour should be resected: any other involved nodes should be removed individually and only rarely is any form of block dissection necessary. After operation T.S.H. production must be suppressed by full doses of thyroxin—0·2–0·3 mg daily. A T.R.H. test may be used to monitor the adequacy of T.S.H. suppression by this treatment.

If properly treated, prognosis is extremely good. The presence of lymphatic metatases is of no significance, and only in the extrathyroidal tumours and in those which present over the age of 40 is the expectation of life lower than in a control group.

Follicular Carcinoma.—These appear to be macroscopically encapsulated but microscopically there is invasion of the capsule and of the vascular spaces in the capsular region (fig. 655). Follicular tumours in which invasion is minimal are termed 'non-invasive' and those in which invasion is moderate or marked are termed 'invasive' (fig. 657). The prognosis depends on the histological picture. 'Non-invasive' cases have as good a prognosis as the intrathyroidal papillary tumours. On the other hand, 50% of patients with 'invasive' tumours develop a local recurrence or secondaries in bone or lung, and have a mean survival time after surgery of six years.

	A Non-invasive	B Invasive
Incidence	50%	50%
Apparent encapsulation	All	Most
Lymph spread	V. rare	Uncommon
Blood spread	Uncommon	Common
Death due to growth within 6 years	3/104	51/104

FIG. 657.—Subgroups of follicular carcinoma and their behaviour.
(after Woolner.)

Although multiple foci are rare the surgical procedure of choice for follicular carcinoma is total thyroidectomy. Lymph nodes rarely require excision as lymphatic spread is uncommon and although this tumour is not particularly hormone-dependant, full doses of thyroxine should be given post-operatively. A whole body scan is advisable after surgery if the tumour is of the invasive type because blood-borne metastases are likely and if detected treatment can be undertaken at an early stage. A total thyroidectomy permits post-operative radio-active iodine scanning by removing all cervical tissue competing for iodine uptake.

---

[1] Less radical surgeons perform a total lobectomy on the side of the lesion with a subtotal lobectomy leaving approximately 1–2 grams of thyroid tissue on the opposite side. Some surgeons think that intrathyroidal papillary carcinoma in the young is a relatively innocuous cancer with a good long term survival rate after conservative surgery. They therefore advocate performing a lobectomy with excision of the isthmus and pyramidal lobe providing that the opposite lobe is normal in appearance and on palpation, and that there is no gross involvement of cervical lymph nodes. The rare encapsulated papillary thyroid cancer is also suitable for this less radical procedure. These relatively conservative procedures may reduce the risk of damage to recurrent laryngeal nerves and parathyroid glands.

Isolated secondaries can be irradiated directly, but ^{131}I therapy offers the only prospect of success when metastases are multiple. All normal thyroid tissue must have been ablated by surgery or by radio-iodine and the patient must be hypothyroid when the isotope is given, usually some 6 weeks after thyroidectomy. If metastases have been treated, the scan should be repeated within 1 year and further therapeutic doses of ^{131}I given as necessary. Re-scanning may then be necessary at regular intervals and it will be necessary to discontinue any thyroxine therapy for a 6 week period prior to these investigations. In order to avoid symptoms of hypothyroidism the patient can be changed to T3 medication and this drug stopped just 10 days before rescanning.

The measurement of serum thyroglobulin is of value in the follow-up and in the detection of metastatic disease in patients who have undergone surgery for differentiated thyroid cancer. This measurement may obviate the need for serial radio-active iodine scanning but when a rise occurs a scan will be indicated to confirm and locate the metastatic disease.

Anaplastic Carcinoma.—Local infiltration is an early feature of these tumours with spread by lymphatics and by the blood stream. They are extremely lethal tumours and survival for more than four years after presentation is most unusual. In most cases death occurs within months rather than within years. An attempt at curative resection is only justified if there is no infiltration through the thyroid capsule and no evidence of metastases. Radiotherapy should be given in all cases and may provide a worthwhile period of palliation as may multiple chemotherapy (including Adriamycin).

Medullary Carcinoma.—These are tumours of the parafollicular (C-cells) derived from the neural crest and not from the cells of the thyroid follicle as are other primary thyroid carcinomas. The cells are not unlike those of a carcinoid tumour and there is a characteristic amyloid stroma (fig. 658). High levels of serum calcitonin[1] are produced by many medullary tumours. These levels fall after resection of a tumour and will rise again if the tumour recurs. This is an extremely valuable tumour marker in the follow-up of patients with this disease.

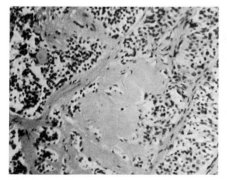

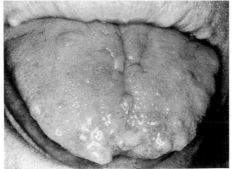

FIG. 658.—Histology of medullary carcinoma—nests of small cells in amyloid stroma.
(Professor E. D. Williams, Cardiff.)

FIG. 659.—Typical appearance of tongue and lips in patient with M.E.N. IIb syndrome showing projecting ganglioneuromas.
(Professor E. D. Williams, Cardiff.)

---

[1] Calcitonin, undetectable in the serum of most normal individuals, is never above 0·08 ng/l.

Diarrhoea is a feature in 30% of cases and this may be due to 5HT or prostaglandins produced by the tumour cells.

Some tumours are familial and may account for 10–20% of all cases. In these cases the tumour is invariably bilateral with a background of C-cell hyperplasia. Medullary carcinoma can occur in combination with adrenal phaeochromocytoma and hyperparathyroidism (usually due to hyperplasia) in the syndrome known as multiple endocrine neoplasia type IIa (M.E.N. IIa). The familiar form of the disease frequently affects children and young adults whereas the sporadic cases occur at any age with no sex predominance. When the familial form is associated with prominent mucosal neuromas involving the lips, tongue (fig. 659) and inner aspect of the eyelids, with occasionally a marfanoid habitus, the syndrome is referred to as the M.E.N. type IIb.

Involvement of lymph nodes occurs in 50-60% of cases of medullary carcinoma and blood-borne metastases are common. As would be expected tumours are not hormone dependent and do not take up radio-active iodine. The course of the tumour is unpredicatble; in general life expectancy is good as long as metastases are confined to the cervical lymph nodes and poor once blood-borne metastases are present. *Treatment* is by total thyroidectomy and resection of involved lymph nodes with either a radical or modified radical neck dissection.

Because calcitonin is a marker for this tumour, close relatives of patients who have medullary carcinoma should be screened by estimating serum calcitonin levels. This can be determined in the basal state and after stimulation by either calcium or pentagastrin. A rise in calcitonin levels under these circumstances should lead to a prophylactic thyroidectomy even though the disease may be at the pre-invasive C-cell hyperplasia stage.

Phaeochromocytoma must be excluded by measurement of urinary V.M.A. and metanephrine levels in these cases before embarking upon thyroid surgery in order to avoid the potential physiological hazards associated with this condition.

Malignant Lymphoma.—In the past many malignant lymphomas were diagnosed as small round cell anaplastic carcinomas. Response to irradiation is good and radical surgery is unnecessary once the diagnosis is established by biopsy either open or A.B.C. (p. 670). The prognosis is good if there is no involvement of cervical lymph nodes. Rarely is the tumour part of widespread malignant lymphoma disease and the prognosis in these cases is worse.

Aetiology of Malignant Thyroid Tumours.—Differentiated thyroid carcinoma, particularly papillary, has frequently followed accidental irradiation of the thyroid in childhood. The incidence of follicular carcinoma is high in endemic goitrous areas, possibly due to T.S.H. stimulation. Malignant lymphomas sometimes develop in auto-immune thyroiditis, so that the lymphocytic infiltration in the auto-immune process may be an aetiological factor. Some workers believe that all lymphomas of thyroid arise in a gland previously the site of such thyroiditis.

Clinical Features.—The annual incidence is about 3·7 per one hundred thousand of the population[1] and the sex ratio 3 females to 1 male. The commonest presenting symptom is a goitre and a 5-year history is far from uncommon in

---

[1] In the Annual Report of the Chief Medical Officer, Ministry of Health (1965), thyroid carcinoma accounted for 298 female and 86 male deaths. As a registered cause of death the incidence is approximately that of carcinoma of the tongue and of ulcerative colitis.

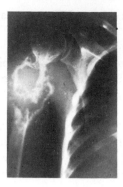

FIG. 660.— Metastasis from a carcinoma of the thyroid in a humerus.
(*D. S. Devadatta, Vellore, South India.*)

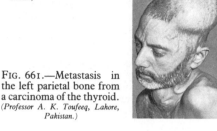

FIG. 661.—Metastasis in the left parietal bone from a carcinoma of the thyroid.
(*Professor A. K. Toufeeq, Lahore, Pakistan.*)

differentiated growths. Recurrent nerve paralysis, enlarged cervical lymph nodes, pathological fractures (fig. 660), or a pulsating bone tumour (fig. 661), may also be presenting features.

Anaplastic growths are usually hard, irregular and infiltrating. A differentiated carcinoma is usually suspiciously firm and irregular, but may resemble a simple nodule. Small papillary tumours may be impalpable—even when lymph metastases are present.[1] Pain, often referred to the ear, is frequent in infiltrating growths.

Diagnosis.—Diagnosis is obvious on clinical examination in most cases of anaplastic carcinoma, although Riedel's thyroiditis (p. 692) is almost indistinguishable. The localised forms of granulomatous thyroiditis and lymphadenoid goitre may stimulate carcinoma. It is not always easy to exclude a carcinoma in a multinodular goitre, and solitary nodules, particularly in the young male, are always suspect. Failure to take up radio-iodine is characteristic of almost all thyroid carcinomas,[2] but occurs also in degenerating nodules and all forms of thyroiditis. Thyroid antibody titres are often raised in carcinoma. The role of A.B.C. in preoperative diagnosis has already been discussed (p. 670). No diagnostic test is absolutely certain, and exploration with excisional biopsy and frozen section is essential when in doubt. Incisional biopsy may cause seeding of cells and local recurrence, and is most inadvisable in a resectable carcinoma. In an anaplastic and obviously irremovable carcinoma, however, incisional or needle biopsy is justified.

Histological Surprise.—Not infrequently a differentiated carcinoma of the thyroid is unsuspected until the histological report on the nodule is received several days after thyroidectomy. If the tumour is a follicular carcinoma of the minimally invasive type then further surgery is rarely necessary if the nodule has been excised by means of a total lobectomy including the isthmus. However, frankly invasive follicular carcinoma should be treated by total thyroidectomy in order to facilitate subsequent iodine scanning and therefore re-operation will be necessary to remove the remaining thyroid lobe. If the definitive histological picture shows the lesion to be a papillary carcinoma then re-exploration is again necessary with total thyroidectomy and excision of juxta-thyroid lymph nodes particularly if multiple foci are present in the resected lobe, because their presence indicates intrathyroidal lymphatic spread and the likelihood of foci in the opposite lobe. If the growth is truly solitary and small (occult), conservative treatment may be justified

---

[1] So called Lateral Aberrant Thyroid.

[2] Only very rarely will differentiated carcinoma (primary or secondary) take up ^{123}I in the presence of normal thyroid tissue.

as the risk of local recurrence can be accepted providing that a careful follow-up is carried out. In all cases long-term observation and full replacement doses of thyroxine are essential.

Local Recurrence of Differentiated Carcinoma.—This may be due to— 1. Tumour foci in the thyroid remnant if total thyroidectomy was not performed. 2. Tumour in affected juxta-thyroid nodes not cleared at the initial operation. 3. Spillage of cells from an ill-advised incisional biopsy.

Recurrence may occur 10 or more years after the initial operation.

Total Thyroidectomy.—This procedure if performed meticulously by an experienced surgeon can be performed safely with very little risk of post-operative complications such as recurrent nerve injury and parathyroid insufficiency. It is unnecessary to ligate the main trunks of the inferior thyroid arteries in this procedure as this may lead to devascularisation of the parathyroids. Instead the individual arterial branches supplying the thyroid gland should be ligated close to the thyroid, leaving the blood supply to the parathyroids intact. Both recurrent laryngeal nerves must be clearly identified. The nerves are particularly vulnerable close to the point of entry into the larynx where they may be angulated and pass through Berry's ligament.

SUMMARY OF SURGERY OF THE THYROID

A summary of the surgical procedures carried out on the thyroid and the indications for their use appears in Fig. 662.

	Procedure	Indications
(i)	Unilateral lobectomy— including isthmus	Almost all solitary nodules Multinodular disease in one lobe only
(ii)	Unilateral subtotal lobectomy	Small anteriorly placed nodules (A.B.C. or Thin needle cytology-benign) Solitary toxic autonomous nodule
(iii)	Bilateral subtotal lobectomy	Diffuse toxic goitre (Graves) Bilateral toxic multinodular goitre Bilateral non-toxic multinodular goitre Hashimoto's thyroiditis (sometimes)
(iv)	Bilateral total lobectomy (Total thyroidectomy)	Most cases of papillary, follicular and medullary carcinoma; modified neck node dissection if node sampling positive
(v)	Excision of isthmus	Anaplastic carcinoma and lymphoma—to free airway and obtain tissue diagnosis Riedel's thyroiditis

FIG. 662.—Surgery of the thyroid.

THYROIDITIS

1. **Granulomatous Thyroiditis** (Subacute Thyroiditis—de Quervain's Thyroiditis). This is due to a virus infection.[1] In a typical subacute presentation there is pain in the neck, fever, malaise and a firm, irregular enlargement of one or both thyroid lobes. There is a raised E.S.R., absent thyroid antibodies, the serum T4 is a high normal or slightly raised, and the ^{123}I uptake of the gland is low. The condition is self-limiting and in a few months the goitre has subsided: subsequent hypothyroidism is rare. In 10% of cases the onset is acute, the goitre very painful and tender and there may be symptoms of hyperthyroidism. 35% of cases are asymptomatic but for the presence of the goitre. If diagnosis is in doubt, it can be confirmed by the rapid symptomatic response to prednisone: but if symptomless a biopsy may be necessary. The specific treatment for the acute case with severe pain is to give prednisone—10 to 20 mg daily—for seven days and the dose is then gradually reduced over the next month.

2. **Auto-immune Thyroiditis.**—This is much more common than was previously thought. It is usually associated with raised titres of thyroid antibodies (see table) and not infrequently there is a family history of other auto-immune diseases, e.g. pernicious anaemia, auto-immune gastritis, vitiligo and thyrotoxicosis.

Classification.—1. Focal thyroiditis. 2. Diffuse non-goitrous thyroiditis (Primary Myxoedema, p. 666). 3. Diffuse goitrous thyroiditis (Hashimoto's disease).[2]

---

[1] An epidemic reported from Israel was due to a mumps virus.

[2] The concept of Hashimoto's disease as an auto-immune thyroiditis was first defined by Roitt and his co-workers in 1956.

Fritz de Quervain, 1868–1940. Professor of Surgery, Berne, Switzerland. Described this form of thyroiditis in 1902.
Hakaru Hashimoto, 1881–1934. Director of the Hashimoto Hospital, Mie, Japan. Described this disease in 1912.
Ivan Maurice Roitt, Contemporary. Professor of Immunology, Middlesex Hospital, London.

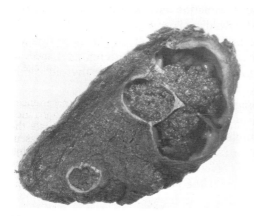

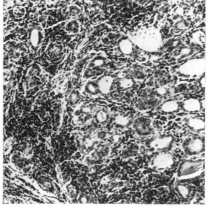

FIG. 663.—Papilliferous carcinoma of the thyroid, showing an intra-glandular seedling. This specimen demonstrates how necessary it is to remove the whole lobe, if not the whole gland (see p. 686).

(F. F. Rundle, FRCS, Sydney, Australia.)

FIG. 664.—Hashimoto's disease (struma lymphomatosa). × 100. Intense lymphocytic-plasma cell infiltration, acinar destruction, and fibrosis. Compare with the normal histology (fig. 643).

(Dr. Bernard Fox, London.)

Focal Thyroiditis is commonly seen on histological examination in association with other thyroid disease—notably toxic goitre. Its presence is a warning that postoperative hypothyroidism is likely.

Diffuse Goitrous Thyroiditis.—The histological picture is of interfollicular plasma cell and lymphocytic infiltration, lymph follicles, a varied epithelial change—ranging from destruction to hyperplasia, and a tendency to eventual fibrosis.

THYROID ANTIBODIES

Site of Antigen	Antibody	Test
Thyroid cytoplasm	Microsomal antibody	1. Complement Fixation (CFT) 2. Immunofluorescent.
Thyroid colloid	1. Thyroglobulin antibody	Tanned Red Cell (TRC)
	2. Second colloid antibody.	Immunofluorescent

Thyroid antibodies may be present in normal persons and in those with goitres of all varieties including malignancy. Tests normally available are CFT, TRC and IMF.

Clinical Features.—As might be expected from the varied histological picture (above), the onset, the thyroid status and the type of goitre vary profoundly from case to case. The onset may be insidious and asymptomatic, or so sudden and painful that it resembles the acute form of granulomatous thyroiditis. Mild hyperthyroidism may be present initially, but hypothyroidism is inevitable and may develop rapidly or extremely slowly. The goitre is usually lobulated, and may be diffuse or localised to one lobe. It may be large or small, and soft, rubbery or firm in consistency—depending upon the cellularity and the degree of fibrosis. The disease is commonest in women at the menopause, but may occur at any age. Papillary carcinoma and malignant lymphoma are very occasionally associated with Hashimoto goitre.

Diagnosis.—Chemical tests of thyroid function vary with the thyroid status and are of diagnostic value only if hypothyroidism is present. A radioactive iodine uptake test is often helpful.[1] Significantly raised titres of one or more thyroid antibodies are present in over 85% of cases. Nevertheless, differential diagnosis from nodular goitre, carcinoma and malignant lymphoma of the thyroid is not always easy and needle or open biopsy may be necessary (fig. 664).

Treatment.—Full replacement dosage of thyroxine should be given in every case, because eventual hypothyroidism is inevitable, and because some early Hashimoto goitres (under T.S.H. stimulation) may subside with hormone therapy. Occasionally a Hashimoto goitre increases in spite of hormone treatment and in these circumstances there may be a favourable response to steroid therapy. Subtotal thyroidectomy may be necessary if the goitre is large and causes discomfort. The clinician must, however, be cautious when a Hashimoto goitre increases in size and becomes unresponsive to thyroxine as this may be due to the development of malignant lymphoma.

3. Riedel's Thyroiditis

This is very rare, accounting for 0·5% of goitres. Thyroid tissue is replaced by cellular fibrous tissue which infiltrates through the capsule into adjacent muscles, paratracheal connective tissue and carotid sheath. It may occur in association with retroperitoneal and mediastinal fibrosis and is most probably a collagen disease. The goitre may be unilateral or bilateral and is very hard and fixed. The thyroid profile and radio-iodine uptake are within normal limits and the scan shows no uptake. The differential diagnosis from anaplastic carcinoma can only be made with certainty by biopsy when a wedge of the isthmus should also be removed to free the trachea. If unilateral, the other lobe is usually involved later and subsequent hypothyroidism is common.

ECTOPIC THYROID AND ANOMALIES OF THE THYROGLOSSAL TRACT

Some residual thyroid tissue along the course of the thyroglossal tract is not uncommon, and may be lingual, cervical or intra-thoracic. Very rarely the whole gland is ectopic.

Lingual Thyroid.—Forms a rounded swelling at the back of the tongue at the foramen caecum (fig. 665) and it may represent the only thyroid tissue present. It may cause

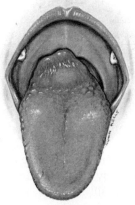

FIG. 665.—Lingual thyroid.
(*H. Wapshaw, FRCS, Glasgow.*)

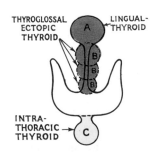

FIG. 666.—Ectopic and aberrant thyroids. A and B are ectopic thyroids, C intrathoracic aberrant thyroid (nearly always acquired).

---

[1] A low uptake by the thyroid at 4 hours and 48 hours together with a high 48 hour P.B. ^{123}I in the absence of a previous thyroidectomy or treatment with radio-active iodine is very suggestive.

Bernhard Moritz Carl Ludwig Riedel, 1846–1916. Professor of Surgery, Jena, Germany. Described this form of thyroiditis in 1896.

dysphagia, impairment of speech, respiratory obstruction or haemorrhage. It is best treated by full replacement with l-thyroxin when it should get smaller, but excision or ablation with radio-iodine is sometimes necessary.

Median (Thyro-glossal) Ectopic Thyroid.—Forms a swelling in the upper part of the neck (fig. 666B) and is usually mistaken for a thyroglossal cyst. Again, this may be the only normal thyroid tissue present.

Lateral Aberrant Thyroid.—There is no evidence that aberrant thyroid tissue ever occurs in a lateral position (Willis). 'Normal Thyroid Tissue' found laterally, separate from the thyroid gland, must be considered and treated as a metastasis in a cervical lymph node from an occult thyroid carcinoma, almost invariably of papillary type.

Struma Ovarii.—Is not ectopic thyroid tissue, but part of an ovarian teratoma. Very rarely carcinogenic change occurs or hyperthyroidism develops.

Thyroglossal Cyst.—May be present in any part of the thyroglossal tract (fig. 667). The common situations, in order of frequency, are beneath the hyoid, in the region of the thyroid cartilage, and above the hyoid bone. Such a cyst occupies the middle line, except in the region of the thyroid cartilage, where the thyroglossal tract is pushed to one side, usually to the left. It is to be remembered that the swelling moves upwards on protrusion of the tongue as well as on swallowing (because of the attachment of the tract to the foramen caecum).

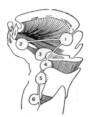

FIG. 667.—Possible sites of a thyroglossal cyst: (1) Beneath the foramen caecum. (2) In the floor of the mouth. (3) Suprahyoid. (4) Subhyoid. (5) On the thyroid cartilage. (6) At the level of the cricoid cartilage.

A thyroglossal cyst should be excised because infection is inevitable due to the fact that the wall contains nodules of lymphatic tissue which communicate by lymphatics with the lymph nodes of the neck. An infected cyst is often mistaken for an abscess and incised, which is one way in which a thyroglossal fistula arises.

Thyroglossal Fistula.—Is never congenital: it follows infection or inadequate removal of a thyroglossal cyst. Long-standing fistulas are inclined to be situated low down in the neck. A thyroglossal fistula is lined by columnar epithelium, discharges mucus, and is the seat of recurrent attacks of inflammation.

Treatment.—Because the thyroglossal tract is so closely related to the body of the hyoid bone, this central part must be excised, together with the cyst or fistula, or recurrence is certain. If the thyroglossal tract can be traced upwards towards the foramen caecum, it must be excised with a central core of lingual muscle (Sistrunk's operation).

Rupert Allan Willis, 1898–1980. Professor of Pathology, Leeds, England.
Walter Ellis Sistrunk, Jr., 1880–1933. Professor of Clinical Surgery, Baylor University College of Medicine, Dallas, Texas, U.S.A.

CHAPTER 38

THE PARATHYROID AND ADRENAL GLANDS

THE PARATHYROID GLANDS

Anatomy and Physiology.—The parathyroid glands, 4 in number, are small, oval in shape, about 0·5 to 1·0 cm in size, yellowish-brown in colour and arranged in pairs—closely applied to the thyroid gland, but outside its capsule. The upper pair are fairly constant in position and found on the posterolateral border of the thyroid immediately above the point of entry of the inferior thyroid artery. The lower pair, more variable in position, are usually found at the lower pole of the thyroid, but may be found anywhere along a line from this situation downwards to the upper pole of the thymus (fig. 668). Approximately 5% of parathyroid glands are found within the upper anterior mediastinum. Each gland has a smooth capsule and is supplied by a single leash of blood vessels which can be clearly seen running in the subcapsular plane (fig. 669).

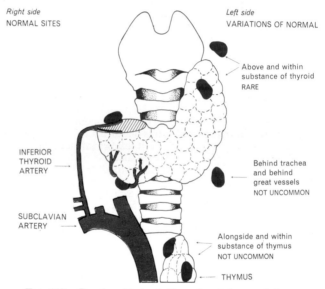

FIG. 668.—Parathyroid gland. Normal and abnormal sites.

Histology.—The stroma consists of a rich sinusoidal capillary network with islands of secretory cells interspersed with fat cells. The glandular cells are of two types. The 'chief' or 'principal' cells are small with vesicular nuclei and poorly staining cytoplasm. 'Water-clear' cells, derived from the chief cells, are found in the hyperplastic and neoplastic glands. The 'oxyphil' cells are less numerous and larger, with granular cytoplasm and deeply staining nuclei.

Function.—The chief cells of the parathyroids produce parathormone, the hormone being released directly into the blood-stream. The circulating level of parathormone can be measured by radio-immuno-assay. It is sufficiently reliable to distinguish between high and low levels. Facilities for obtaining the estimation are available everywhere in the United Kingdom through the Supra-Regional Assay Service.

Parathormone.—(i) Stimulates osteoclastic activity, thereby increasing bone resorption by mobilizing calcium and phosphate.

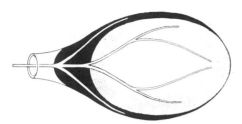
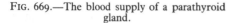

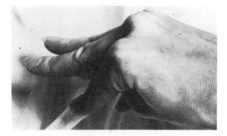

FIG. 669.—The blood supply of a parathyroid gland.

FIG. 670.—The 'obstetrician's hand' seen in parathyroid tetany.

(ii) Increases the re-absorption of calcium by the renal tubules, thus reducing the urinary excretion of calcium.

(iii) Augments the absorption of calcium from the gut.

(iv) Reduces the renal tubular re-absorption of phosphate, thus promoting phosphaturia.

Calcitonin (Copp) is secreted by the parafollicular cells of the thyroid (Thyrocalcitonin). It lowers the serum calcium and effects calcium storage in bones; quite the opposite action to parathormone. A second potent calcium lowering peptide (katacalcin) may be involved in both calcium regulation and skeletal maintenance. It does not duplicate the effect of calcitonin as it has no effect on plasma phosphate; indeed the effect may be additive.

HYPOPARATHYROIDISM

Parathyroid tetany, due to hypocalcaemia, is a rare complication of subtotal thyroidectomy (less than 1%). At this operation some of the parathyroid glands may be removed or have their blood supply temporarily embarrassed. Also it may occur after surgery to the parathyroids themselves. Symptoms usually appear on the second or third postoperative day, and are temporary. Milder forms of hypoparathyroidism have been described in the follow-up of thyroidectomised patients. Permanent hypoparathyroidism, most commonly encountered following radical thyroidectomy for cancer, requires constant supervision and treatment. Tetany in the new-born may occur within the first few days of life in the child born of a mother with undiagnosed hypoparathyroidism. Profound hypocalcaemia also occurs in patients with severe bone disease associated with impaired renal function.

Clinical Features.—The first symptoms are tingling and numbness in the face, fingers and toes. In extreme cases cramps in the hands and feet are very painful; the extended fingers are flexed at their metacarpophalangeal joints, with the thumb strongly adducted. The toes are plantar flexed and the ankle joints extended—the so-called carpopedal spasm. Spasm of the muscles of respiration not only results in pain and stridor, but dread of suffocation. In infancy, the symptoms of tetany may be mistaken for epilepsy, though there is no loss of consciousness.

Latent tetany may be demonstrated by:

(i) *Chvostek's sign.*—Tapping over the branches of the facial nerve at the angle of the jaw will produce twitching at the corner of the mouth, the ala of the nose and the eyelids.

(ii) *Trousseau's sign.*—A sphygmomanometer-cuff applied to the arm and

Douglas Harold Copp, Contemporary. Professor of Physiology, University of British Columbia, Vancouver, B.C., Canada.
Frantisek Chvostek, 1835–1884. Physician, Josefsakademie, Vienna.
Armand Trousseau, 1801–1867. Physician, Hôtel Dieu, Paris.

inflated above the systolic blood pressure for not more than two minutes will produce carpal spasm (fig. 670).

Treatment.—In acute cases the symptoms can be relieved speedily by the slow intravenous injection of 10–20 ml of a 10% solution of calcium gluconate. This can be repeated until the patient's circulating calcium level has been stabilised. For longer term management the absorption of calcium is enhanced by oral administration of the most active metabolite of vitamin D—1,25 dihydroxychole-calciferol (1,25(OH)$_2$D3). Its major action is on the gut, promoting active absorption of calcium and phosphorus, raising calcium levels to normal within one week. Magnesium supplements may occasionally be needed. Serum calcium levels must be estimated daily and the dosage adjusted as appropriate.

HYPERPARATHYROIDISM

Hyperparathyroidism is associated with an increased secretion of parathyroid hormone. This occurs in:

Primary Hyperparathyroidism, which is an unstimulated and inappropriately high parathyroid hormone secretion for the concentration of plasma ionised calcium and is due to adenoma or hyperplasia, and very rarely carcinoma.

Secondary Hyperparathyroidism is associated with chronic renal failure or malabsorption syndromes. The stimulus for the hyperplasia is chronic hypocalcaemia. All four glands are involved.

Tertiary Hyperparathyroidism is a further stage in the development of reactive hyperplasia where autonomy occurs as the parathyroids no longer respond to physiological stimuli.

A single adenoma is the commonest finding (multiple in 6%). The whole gland is usually considerably enlarged, darker in colour, firmer and more vascular than normal; in some a rim of normal parathyroid tissue can be seen surrounding the adenoma. The histological appearances are the same as in hyperplasia, with a predominance of chief and water-clear cells. ABO (H) cell surface antigens are lost from the parathyroid cell surface in adenoma and carcinoma, but not in hyperplasia. Carcinoma of the parathyroids is extremely rare, less than 1%. It tends to invade locally and recur after operation. Bloodborne metastases have been described.

Clinical Features.—Hyperparathyroidism, rarely found in the first decade of life, is commoner in women than men, and most commonly found between the ages of 20 and 60 years. The clinical features vary enormously, even when the biochemical changes are similar.

Asymptomatic cases. The most common presentation is the detection of unsuspected and asymptomatic hypercalcaemia by routine biochemical screening.

'Bones, stones, abdominal groans and psychic moans.' Only 50 % of the patients suffer from any of these (see below).

Non-specific symptoms include muscle weakness, thirst, polyuria, anorexia, and weight loss—a challenge to the astute clinician!

Bone Disease.—There may be generalised decalcification of the skeleton, as in osteitis fibrosa cystica (von Recklinghausen's disease), single or multiple cysts, or pseudotumours of any bone. The latter are particularly common in the jaw bones. Early x-ray changes first appear in the skull and in the phalanges, with loss of density and subperiosteal erosions. Many patients presenting with vague pains in the bones and joints are mistakenly diagnosed as rheumatic.

Renal Stones.—Hyperparathyroidism must be considered in every patient presenting with renal tract stone or nephrocalcinosis (fig. 671), and even in those cases of renal colic where no stone can be demonstrated.

Friedrich Daniel von Recklinghausen, 1833–1910. Professor of Pathology, Strasbourg, France.

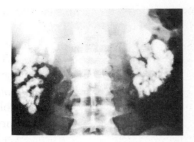

FIG. 671.—Nephrocalcinosis.

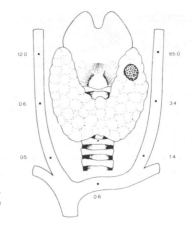

FIG. 672.—Selective venous sampling of parathormone levels to detect site of tumour.

Dyspeptic Cases.—Patients with nausea, vomiting and anorexia are relatively common. Peptic ulcer and pancreatitis are not infrequently found in association with hyperparathyroidism, but the relationship is not as yet fully understood.

Psychiatric Cases.—Are not uncommon; women, complaining of tiredness, listlessness and with obvious personality changes, are often wrongly labelled 'neurotic' or 'menopausal'. Patients have been admitted to mental institutions because of irrational behaviour.

Acute Hyperparathyroidism.—This diagnosis is difficult and only too often made after death. Nausea and abdominal pain is followed by severe vomiting, dehydration, oliguria, and finally coma. The serum calcium is very high, up to 17 mg/100 ml (4·2 mmol/l) or more. Treatment is urgent after rehydration. Clodronate sodium is a specific inhibitor of bone resorption and if given orally (1·0–3·2 g daily) may be valuable in the pre-operative short term medical management of hypercalcaemia in primary hyperparathyroidism.

Clinical Examination and Investigation.—Except in severe bone cases with skeletal deformities, swellings or pathological fractures, clinical examination is usually negative. The diagnosis is confirmed with the following biochemical findings:

(i) Elevation of serum calcium (upper limit of normal 10·9 mg/100 ml (2·6 mmol/l)).[1]
(ii) Diminution of serum phosphorus (lower limit of normal 3·0 mg/100 ml (0·8 mmol/l)).
(iii) Increased excretion of calcium in the urine (upper limit of normal 250 mg (62 mmol) per 24 hours for females, 300 mg (75 mmol) for males).
(iv) Elevation of the serum alkaline phosphatase in bone cases.
(v) Elevation of serum parathyroid hormone concentration (upper limit of normal 0·5 µg/l). Note that parathyroid hormone is always detectable in patients with hyperparathyroidism, in many normal people it is undetectable.

Preoperative Localisation.—A parathyroid tumour is rarely palpable in the neck and so pre-operative localisation is of great value!
(i) A video film barium swallow may identify one in five glands larger than 2·5 cm.
(ii) An ultrasound static B scan may be of value but results vary according to the skill and experience of the investigator.

---

[1] Serum calcium occurs as calcium ions complexed to citrate and bound to albumin. Therefore the serum albumin concentration should be known in order to apply a correction factor: Corrected serum calcium (mmol/l) = Measured serum Ca (mmol/l) + (40 − A) × 0·02, where A = serum albumin (g/l).

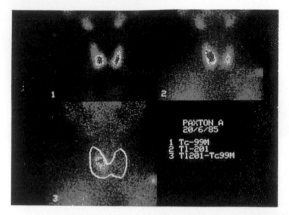

FIG. 673.—The pre-operative localisation of a parathyroid adenoma by
thallium-201 and technetium–99^M
subtraction scintigraphy. The technique is first to outline the thyroid
with technetium-99^M and then to
administer an isotope such as thalli-
um-201 which is taken up by both
thyroid and parathyroid tissue. The
two images are captured by a gamma
camera, and by computer subtraction
of the two images the enlarged parathyroid remains as a 'hot spot'.

(iii) CT scanning is of most value in localising a lesion in the mediastinum rather than the neck.

(iv) Selective venous sampling (fig. 672) may be difficult because of the variable venous drainage of the neck but is of value in up to 60% of cases of recurrent disease.

(v) A thallium-technetium isotope subtraction scan may locate up to 95% of parathyroid adenomas before surgery (fig. 673).

Differential Diagnosis.—Other cases of hypercalcaemia must be remembered and excluded. They are:

(i) Secondary cancer in bone (breast, prostate, bronchus, kidney and thyroid).

(ii) Carcinoma with endocrine secretion (bronchus, kidney and ovary).

(iii) Multiple myeloma.

(iv) Vitamin D intoxication.

(v) Sarcoidosis.

(vi) Thyrotoxicosis.

The differential diagnosis presents *no* problem if the parathyroid hormone level is estimated. In none of the above-mentioned conditions will parathyroid hormone be detectable in the blood.

Treatment.—The only corrective treatment is surgical removal of the overactive gland or glands.

Pre-operative treatment is not usually necessary. In acute cases, rapid correction of dehydration and electrolyte imbalance is necessary, with a careful daily check on the serum calcium. Post-operative calcium and vitamin D supplements may be required for several weeks to prevent tetany.

As there is no pre-operative method for determining the likely pathology, the surgeon at operation must identify all 4 glands, study each carefully, both macroscopically, and, if need be, microscopically after biopsy. Adenomas, single or multiple, are removed.

In approximately 10% of cases even the most experienced surgeon in this field may find difficulty in locating a parathyroid adenoma.

Parathyroid tissue can be successfully autotransplanted into the arm, a useful technique to avoid repeated potentially difficult explorations of the neck. The indications are parathyroid hyperplasia, tertiary hyperparathyroidism in patients undergoing chronic renal dialysis, and recurrent hyperparathyroidism. The technique is to excise all the parathyroid tissue from the neck and to implant eight 1 mm³ fragments into a pocket in the forearm muscle mass marking the site with black silk sutures. Post-operative vitamin D and calcium replacement therapy is required for varying periods. Recurrent hypercalcaemia is an indication for exploration of the implantation site and to further excise parathyroid tissue.

Prognosis.—With successful surgery, bones will recalcify and pseudo-tumours resolve. Renal stones will not disappear, but the incidence of recurrence after surgical removal is reduced, and deterioration in renal function is prevented. Psychiatric patients show an early, and often remarkable, recovery. In a small minority of cases hyperparathyroidism recurs after several years, and may warrant further surgery.

Hypertension associated with hyperparathyroidism is common, but the mechanism is unclear, and the hypertension may not improve after surgery to the parathyroid glands.

Parathyroid Carcinoma.—Parathyroid carcinoma is a rare condition to be considered when a high serum calcium is associated with a palpable lump in the neck. At operation it has a characteristic grey-white colour and is adherent because of local invasion of adjacent soft tissue (Dudley). The best results are obtained by early recognition, avoiding rupture of the tumour capsule and aggressive surgical management including ipsilateral thyroid lobectomy. Surgical clips should be used to outline the tumour bed for post-operative radiotherapy.

Multiple Endocrine Neoplasia Syndromes—APUD cells

Always consider that a patient with hyperparathyroidism may also have multiple endocrine adenomas. The cells involved irrespective of the site have the common chemical characteristics of **A**mine **P**recursor **U**ptake and **D**ecarboxylation and are thus known as 'APUD' cells. The disorder is inherited as an autosomal dominant, the manifestations in any one family tend to be similar and all members of the family should be investigated.

Type I. This most common variant involves the parathyroid glands (90%), pancreatic islets (80%), pituitary (65%), thyroid and adrenal cortex. There is hyperplasia of the parathyroid glands, a chromophobe adenoma of the pituitary which may result in increased prolactic production or acromegaly. The pancreatic tumour may produce gastrin (the Zollinger-Ellison syndrome) or insulin, glucagon, somatostatin or vasointestinal peptide (VIP) causing watery diarrhoea. Treatment is surgical excision.

Type IIa. 50% have parathyroid hyperplasia. The associated lesions may be a medullary carcinoma of thyroid, which produces calcitonin, and a phaeochromocytoma. The latter should be excluded or be the first priority for treatment before exploration of the neck.

Type IIb. This is differentiated from Type II because of additional neurological abnormalities. Mucosal neuroma produce 'lumpy and bumpy' lips or eyelids and there is a characteristic marfanoid facial appearance. Megacolon and ganlioneuromatosis are also found.

THE ADRENAL GLANDS

Surgical Anatomy.—At birth, the adrenal glands have attained nearly adult proportions. Fully developed, each weighs about 4 g, but the left is a little larger than the right. A deeper yellow colour and a firmer consistency enables the gland to be distinguished from the adjacent fat. Each rests on the superior, anterior, and medial aspects

Nicholas Eric Dudley, Contemporary. Consultant Surgeon John Radcliffe Hospital, Oxford.
Robert Milton Zollinger, Contemporary. Professor of Surgery, Ohio State University, Columbus, Ohio, U.S.A.
Edwin Holmer Ellison, Contemporary. Professor of Surgery, Marquette University, Milwaukee, Wisconsin, U.S.A.
Antonin Bernard Jean Marfan, 1858–1942. Professor of Paediatrics, Paris, France.

of the superior pole of the corresponding kidney, and presents the appearance of a French Liberty cap worn at a rakish angle.

Although intimately related anatomically, the adrenal cortex and the adrenal medulla are quite separate internal secretory glands.

The adrenal glands are supplied by several adrenal arteries, rendering them remarkably vascular, but only one vein drains each gland. On the right side the adrenal vein is short and enters the inferior vena cava just distal to the hepatic vein, while on the left it empties into the left renal vein (which communicates through the azygos vein with the left intercostal internal mammary, and vertebral veins (Anson)). This dissimilarity of the right and left venous flow determines, to some extent, the location of metastases from malignant tumours of these glands.

Diagnostic Radiology

(i) Non-invasive methods of detecting adrenal swellings are isotope scanning and CT scanning. CT scanning detects tumours larger than 2 cm diameter.

(ii) An IVU may show downward displacement of the kidney and rotation of the upper pole when the adrenal gland is enlarged. Skull radiographs may show enlargement of the pituitary fossa in Cushing's syndrome (p. 704).

(iii) Invasive techniques include selective retrograde venography (especially for left-sided tumours) and selective arteriography.

(iv) *Calcification* in an adrenal gland is difficult to interpret in a radiograph. It is liable to be confused with a renal calculus. Areas of calcification in the adrenal glands may be present in Addison's disease (p. 702).

THE ADRENAL CORTEX

The adrenal cortex is made up of the following layers from without inwards; the zona glomerulosa, the zona fasciculata, and the zona reticularis.

Physiology.—At least fifty steroid compounds have been isolated from the adrenal cortex. These hormones exhibit various types of activity which, for practical purposes, can be arranged in three groups.

1. **Salt Regulating Hormones** which are concerned in the maintenance of water and electrolytic balance. A deficiency of these hormones produces sodium diuresis, potassium retention and dehydration; an excess results in hypertension, oedema, cardiac dilatation, and hypokalaemia. **Aldosterone** is the most important of these 'salt regulating' hormones (see Conn's syndrome, p. 706).

2. **The cortisones** are concerned with the metabolism of proteins and carbohydrates, favouring the formation of the latter from the body's storehouse of the former. This conversion is known as gluconeogenesis. Consequently hormones belonging to this group are called glucocorticoids. The best known of these are **hydrocortisone** (also known as **cortisol**), and **cortisone** (which is converted in the body to hydrocortisone). The therapeutic application of these hormones falls into two headings:

(a) *In Endocrine Deficiencies.*—Cortisone is the logical need in adrenocortical insufficiency and after bilateral adrenalectomy.

(b) *In Non-endocrine Disease.*—Cortisone is used in the treatment of a diversity of diseases, including allergic conditions, granulomatous disorders, blood diseases and the collagenoses. Hydrocortisone is used in the treatment of hypocorticism and shock (Chapter 4) and is an effective anti-allergic agent in a number of skin diseases and eye conditions.

3. **Sex Hormones.**—Androgenic and oestrogenic hormones are produced by the adrenal cortex. Excessive secretion of androgens due to hydroxylase or hydrogenase deficiences causes virilism in females or, rarely, excessive secretion of oestrogens brings about effeminacy in males.

Inter-hormonic Action.—The anterior lobe of the pituitary gland secretes adrenocorticotropic hormone (ACTH) which stimulates the adrenal cortex, whereas the cortisol of the adrenal cortex inhibits the secretion of ACTH.

Tests of Adrenocortical Activity

The tests are of two types, those which confirm the presence of a change in cortisol production and those which indicate a cause. No tests should be interpreted in isolation but all the results of the investigations considered together.

Barry J. Anson, Contemporary. Research Professor, Department of Otolaryngology and Maxillofacial Surgery College of Medicine, University of Iowa, Iowa City, U.S.A.

1. **Plasma Electrolytes.**—Sodium levels are raised and potassium low in a hyperfunctioning adrenocortical lesion with the opposite in Addison's disease (p. 702).

2. **Water Excretion Test.**—After an eight hour fast a volume of water is drunk and the urine collected over four hours. Cortisol has a diuretic effect and 90% of the water volume will be excreted at this time, but in Addison's disease less than 55% is excreted.

3. **Plasma Cortisol Levels.**—Diurnal variation with a maximum value at 8.00 a.m. may be lost in both Cushing's syndrome where all levels are high and in insufficiency when levels are low (the normal range is 55–230 µg/l in the morning and 11–85 µg/l at midnight).

4. **Plasma ACTH Levels.**—Low plasma levels are found with adrenal tumours and high levels with a pituitary lesion or ectopic ACTH production. Normal range at 8.00 a.m. is 9–24 ng/litre. The ratio ACTH to related peptides such as β lipotrophin may facilitate the distinction between pituitary Cushing's and ectopic ACTH production.

5. **Plasma Aldosterone Levels.**—The concentration of aldosterone is only one thousandth that of cortisol, and both dietary sodium and posture may change the value. A recumbent subject on an unrestricted sodium diet has a normal range of 32–116 µg/l.

6. **Urinary Steroid Excretion.**—(a) *Cortisol Secretion Rate*. The daily output of cortisol is a precise measure of adrenocortical activity. Adult levels are reached by eighteen years of age and after forty years fall gradually to be halved by seventy years of age. The average excretion is higher in caucasian males. The daily output may be determined by the administration of a small amount of radioactive labelled cortisol which is metabolised and excreted, and the urinary radioactivity measured. The normal range is 5–28 mg per 24 hours, with high levels in Cushing's syndrome and low levels in adrenal insufficiency.

(b) *Total 17 Oxogenic Steroids*. These are cortisol, cortisone, their derivatives and pregnanetriol. Normal range for males 17–70 µmol per 24 hours and females 14–49 µmol per 24 hours.

(c) *The Free 11-Hydroxycorticosteroids*. These are mainly cortisol and are a specific index of cortisol secretion. Normal range 70–340 µg per 24 hours. Unlike plasma cortisol they are not raised in patients taking oral contraceptives. A normal result effectively excludes Cushing's syndrome. High levels are obtained in Cushing's syndrome.

(d) *17 Oxosteroids*. Reflect androgen output. In males the testes contribute one-third of the measured levels, but in females the sole contribution is from the adrenal glands. High levels are found in virilising syndromes and in Cushing's disease due to a carcinoma of the adrenal gland.

7. **The Dexamethasone Test.**—Dexamethasone is twenty-five times more potent than cortisol. 0·5 mg of dexamethasone is administered six hourly for two days and causes a marked decrease in urinary steroid excretion by inhibiting ACTH production, and thus cortisol, without contributing greatly to the total urinary steroid output. In Cushing's syndrome no effect is produced by the dose. Larger doses of up to 2 mg six hourly will, over several days, reduce urinary steroid excretion if the overactivity is secondary to bilateral adrenal hyperplasia, but not with an adrenal tumour, which is autonomous.

8. **The Metyrapone Test.**—This differentiates between excess ACTH production and a lesion in the adrenal cortex causing Cushing's syndrome. Metyrapone inhibits the biosynthesis of cortisol so plasma levels fall. If the pituitary adrenal axis is intact this results in an increase in ACTH production and stimulation of the adrenal cortex. The basal levels of 17 oxogenic and 17 hydroxysteroids in the urine are measured for two days, 750 mg of Metyrapone is given per four hours and a twenty-four hour urine collection completed. A normal response is a two to four fold increase in the urinary steroids over basal levels. A diminished response in Cushing's syndrome indicates a primary adrenal lesion.

9. **The Synacthen Test.**—250 µgm of Synacthen is given intramucularly and blood cortisol measured at 30 and 60 minutes. In normal subjects the basal plasma cortisol should be greater than 60 µg/litre and by at least 70µg/litre after stimulation. In Addison's disease the response is impaired.

DISORDERS OF ADRENOCORTICAL FUNCTION

Acute Hypocorticism:

1. **Adrenal Apoplexy in the Newborn.**—Extensive haemorrhage into one or both adrenals can be a cause of death in infants within the first few days of birth. The condition may occur after long and difficult labour, and particularly when resuscitative procedures

have to be employed to combat asphyxia neonatorum. The haemorrhage into the adrenals follows necrosis of the innermost layer of the cortex, which always occurs at birth, possibly as a result of sudden withdrawal of the female sex hormone (oestrogen). Adrenal crisis in the newborn produces signs of profound shock. A mass may be palpable in one or both renal regions. Intravenous fluid therapy with hydrocortisone, or, failing the latter, cortisone intramuscularly, offers the only hope.

2. **Waterhouse-Friderichsen Syndrome.**—Massive bilateral adrenal cortical haemorrhage, occurs in cases of fulminating meningococcal septicaemia and in some cases streptococcal, staphylococcal, or pneumococcal septicaemia. Most cases occur in infants and young children, but it can happen in adults with severe haemorrhage or burns. The onset is catastrophic, with rigors, hyperpyrexia, cyanosis, and vomiting. Petechial haemorrhages into the skin which coalesce rapidly into purpuric blotches are a constant feature. Profound shock follows, and before long the patient passes into coma. The condition is one of overwhelming sepsis that pursues a galloping course, death occurring in most cases within forty-eight hours of the onset of symptoms unless correct treatment is given without delay.

Unilateral haemorrhage causing a lesser degree of systemic upset and not associated with infections has been described. This type of case resembles a perinephric abscess or other upper abdominal acute condition.

Confirming the Diagnosis.—It is futile to await the result of a blood culture. Bilateral tenderness 5 cm below the costal margin, clear urine (oliguria is often present), and an absence of signs in the lungs help to call attention to the adrenal glands. In meningococcal infection the diplococcus can be demonstrated by smears obtained from a punctured petechial spot in the skin.

Treatment.—Antibiotic therapy must be given intensively by the intravenous route. 100 mg hydrocortisone sodium succinate is given i.v. or i.m. if venous access is difficult. Up to 400 mg hydrocortisone may be required in the first 24 hours. No mineralocorticoid is needed as the weak intrinsic salt retaining action of cortisone suffices at this dosage. Oral medication may be commenced after the first day and then over about 4 days reduced to a maintenance level. Oxygen should also be administered. Following such treatment, improvement often sets in within three hours, and a number of patients have recovered.

3. **Crises of Infantile Hypercorticism** (p. 703).

4. **Following Bilateral Adrenalectomy.**—If precautions are taken acute hypocorticism is unusual in the post-operative period. Treatment is to give 300 mg hydrocortisone on the first day and this may be increased as required. Most patients achieve a maintenance dose of 30 mg/day. After about three weeks 0·1 mg fludrocortisone may be given.

5. **Postoperative Adrenal Haemorrhage**.—Adrenal haemorrhage can be an unexpected cause of deterioration and sudden death in the postoperative period. In some cases the left adrenal gland is damaged during radical gastrectomy for carcinoma (Fox). In other cases when adrenal haemorrhage is bilateral, there is no evidence of operative injury, they are usually associated with intra-abdominal sepsis, pneumonia, coagulation defects and cancer. Thrombosis of the adrenal veins is the cause of infarction of glands.

The diagnosis of postoperative adrenal haemorrhage is difficult. It should be suspected when there is sudden collapse, with hypotension, particularly if associated with upper abdominal pain and tenderness. Other evidence of acute adrenal failure are vomiting, diarrhoea and mental confusion. The most useful laboratory finding is a low plasma cortisol, although unexplained blood eosinophilia is very suggestive of adrenal failure. The classical changes of hyperkalaemia and hyponatraemia often take several days to appear and may be obscured by intravenous therapy. If the diagnosis is suspected, then treatment should not be withheld for lack of laboratory confirmation.

Treatment.—A therapeutic trial of at least 100 mg of intravenous hydrocortisone hemisuccinate in 500 ml of isotonic saline as quickly as possible, and repeated in about an hour, is indicated. If there is a positive response then hydrocortisone (50 mg every 6 hours) should be given. When the patient's condition has sufficiently improved, then treatment with a synthetic oral steroid should be substituted. Occasionally there may be a deficiency in mineral corticoids so that treatment with fludrocortisone is necessary. Adrenal haemorrhage may result in chronic adrenal insufficiency (see below).

Chronic Hypocorticism (Addison's disease)

This is due to adreno-cortical insufficiency consequent upon progressive destruction with lymphocytic infiltration of the zona reticularis, the zona fasciculata,

Rupert Waterhouse, 1873–1958. Clinical Pathologist and Physician, Royal United Hospital, Bath, England. Described this syndrome in 1911.
Carl Friderichsen, 1886–. Formerly Medical Superintendent, Children's Department, Sundby Hospital, Copenhagen. Wrote his account of this syndrome in 1918.
Bernard Fox, Contemporary. Pathologist, Charing Cross Hospital, London.
Thomas Addison, 1793–1860. Physician, Guy's Hospital, London. Described the effects of disease of the suprarenal capsules in 1849.

the zona glomerulosa, and the medulla of the adrenal glands, in that order. In about 60% of cases the condition is believed to be due to an autoimmune disease, sometimes in association with Hashimoto goitre (Chapter 37) and pernicious anaemia. Tuberculosis, metastatic carcinoma and amyloidosis account for the remaining 40%.

Clinical Features.—Addison's disease usually commences in the third or fourth decade. Sometimes it is the terminal event in cases of adrenogenital hyperplasia. The sex distribution is about equal. The leading features are muscular weakness and a low blood pressure. Irregular dusky pigmentation of the skin, due to deposits of melanin, appears at points of pressure (*e.g.* garter, belt) and in the flexion creases. Pigmentation of mucous membranes, particularly of the mouth, is often striking. When fully established, the course of the disease is punctuated by crises of acute adrenocortical insufficiency (see above).

Treatment is medical. In long term management most patients require 20–30 mg cortisone in divided doses, with 0·05 mg fludrocortisone daily as mineralocorticoid replacement. Signs of overtreatment include hypertension, hyperkalaemia and oedema; those of undertreatment fatigue and hypotension. Where relevant, chemotherapy is mandatory for tuberculosis (Chapter 3).

Prognosis.—By the use of cortisone, the expectation of life of a patient suffering from Addison's disease has been extended from up to three years to at least seven years.

Hypercorticism

The various forms of adrenal cortical hyperfunction are classified according to the age of onset. (1) Infantile. (2) Pre-pubertal. (3) Adult, otherwise known as Cushing's syndrome—the commonest type. (4) Post-menopausal. (5) Primary aldosteronism (Conn's syndrome) can occur at any age.

1. **Infantile Hypercorticism.**—Androgenic excess during intrauterine life is one form of pseudo-hermaphrodism in the *female child*. The condition is present at birth, sometimes the enlarged clitoris and a varying degree of hypospadias make it difficult to determine the infant's sex. The 17-ketosteroid content of the urine may be sufficiently elevated to substantiate a diagnosis of a female with adrenal hyperfunction. If this is not the case, it is justifiable to perform sex determination by a skin biopsy before the age of one year. Female pseudohermaphrodism with virilism is invariably associated with disease of the adrenal cortex, usually bilateral hyperplasia of the cortex. Hormonal studies have shown that there is a congenital failure of the adrenal glands to synthesise gluco-corticoids. Due to this lack, these infants are liable to acute phases of adrenal insufficiency during stress or infection, or to suffer from periodic hypoglycaemic attacks. They need cortisone, not only in the emergency, but as long-term therapy, thereby inhibiting the secretion of excessive androgens. In the absence of such treatment the epiphyses join early, the patients are dwarfed, menstruation does not occur, and the breasts do not develop. These tendences are corrected by cortisone given orally, 25 mg or more daily, the dose being determined by 17-ketosteroid estimations (Leonard Simpson). Hirsutism is moderated, but not necessarily abolished. The treatment should be commmenced early if good results are to be obtained.

2. **Pre-pubertal Hypercorticism.**—There is never any doubt as to the sex of the infant at birth, and during the very early years of life the child is normal. The symptoms commence about the age of five or six years.

In the Female.—Pubic and axillary hair appear, but there is no gross enlargement of the clitoris. The child is short in stature, the legs being especially stunted, but she looks much older than she is. Puberty is often precocious, menstruation, if it occurs, being scanty. There is a deepening of the voice at this time.

Samuel Leonard Simpson, 1900–1983. Consulting Endocrinologist, St. Mary's Hospital, London.

In the Male.—The term 'infant Hercules' is descriptive. He is extremely short, muscular, and hirsute. The genitalia assume adult proportions, and spermatozoa are often present in the seminal fluid.

In both sexes, 17-ketosteroid content of the urine is increased. A very high reading supports the diagnosis of an adrenocortical tumour, which must always be excluded. In both males and females, with a later onset or the passage of time, the features of Cushing's syndrome becomes super-added.

Treatment.—This is identical with that of Cushing's syndrome.

3. **Post pubertal or Adult Hypercorticism (Cushing's syndrome)** is due to an excessive endogenous production of glucocorticoids, mainly hydrocortisone. It is an uncommon condition, often suspected but seldom confirmed. Pituitary-dependent Cushing's syndrome is the commonest form of endogenous hypercorticism accounting for up to two thirds of all cases. An adrenal adenoma accounts for 20% and carcinoma (which can be bilateral) in 5%. In the remainder there is no discernible structural alteration in the glands and the condition is due to an ectopic source of an ACTH-like substance being secreted by an undifferentiated carcinoma of the bronchus, or a tumour of the thymus or ovary. Alcoholism also must be considered.

In its most typical form, Cushing's syndrome is exogenous and is seen in patients treated with large doses of cortisone over long periods of non-endocrine diseases, particularly rheumatoid arthritis, and in patients receiving transplants.

Clinical Features.—The female: male ratio is at least 3 : 1. The great majority of cases (excluding those iinduced by cortisone therapy) occur in females between fifteen and thirty years of age, in whom it produces highly characteristic features. Although the patient's weight is not necessarily increased, there is a deposition of fat in certain situations. The face becomes rubicund, rounded like a full moon, and the lips are pursed. The abdomen becomes protuberant, the neck thick, the supraclavicular fossae obliterated, and a roll of fat appears over the region of the vertebra prominens (buffalo hump). The arms, and especially the legs, are relatively thin, the muscular development is poor, and the patient complains of increasing weakness. As the disease progresses, so the general contour becomes more and more that of a 'lemon on match-sticks' (fig. 675). Consequent upon the inhibitory effect of the hypercorticism on fibrous tissue, the skin becomes of tissue-paper consistency, and inelastic. Exceedingly characteristic are purple-red striae distentiae, mostly on the abdomen (fig. 674), of a texture that can be likened to an over-stretched garter. Ecchymoses are frequent and bruising occurs on the slightest trauma. Acne is common and there is a low resistance to skin infections. Often there is increased growth of lanugo hair, but hirsutism is usually absent. Amenorrhoea is usual or, in the male, impotence. Due to a negative calcium balance, the matrix of bone becomes thin, and severe osteoporosis results. Pathological fractures, particularly compression fracture of a vertebra, are common, and this is sometimes the first reason for the patient seeking advice. Mild glycosuria is often present. Hypertension is frequent, and eventually congestive heart failure supervenes. In about 60% of cases various psychoses occur.

Cushing's syndrome is rare in children; when it occurs, the patient is nearly always a female and an adrenal tumour is usually the cause.

A sub-group, probably due to an excessive secretion of adrenal androgens (*adreno-genital syndrome*), commences between the ages of fifteen and twenty-five

Hercules, one of the most famous of the heroes of Greek mythology, was noted for his prodigious strength.
Harvey Cushing, 1869–1939. Professor of Surgery, Harvard University, Boston, Mass. U.S.A. (1912–1932), (see footnote, p. 60). Described this syndrome in 1932.

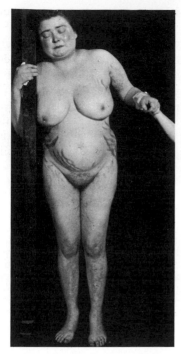

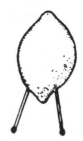

FIG. 675.— Cushing syndrome contour— lemon on match-sticks.

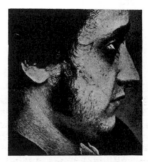

FIG. 674.—Cushing's syndrome in a woman aged twenty-three years. Adrenal hyperplasia.
(*Dr. Leonard Simpson, London.*)

FIG. 676.—Adrenogenital syndrome in a woman of twenty-eight.
(*Dr. Leonard Simpson, London.*)

and is confined to females. One of the first indications of its onset is amenorrhoea or oligo-menorrhoea. There follows an excessive growth of hair on the face (fig. 676), acne, atrophy of the breasts, alteration in bodily contour and muscular development, deepening of the voice, and enlargement of the clitoris. Jewish and Spanish women are more prone to this affliction than those of other races.

Arrhenoblastoma of the ovary.—This rare condition occurs between puberty and the menopause and also causes hirsutism. It may also arise in a suprarenal 'rest'.

Laboratory Findings.—Polycythaemia, lymphopaenia, and eosinopaenia are common. A fasting eosinophil count over 30 per mm³ of blood is good evidence against the diagnosis. The basal metabolic rate is low and the serum cholesterol is elevated. The dextrose tolerance is impaired, and the insulin tolerance test reveals a resistance to the action of insulin. Urinary steroids are above normal levels. There is a negative calcium balance and radiography of the skeleton reveals osteoporosis, most marked in the spine and pelvis. *Ultrasound, CT or MRI* are of help in the localisation of a lesion. Indocholesterol uptake scanning or adrenal venous sampling may also be employed.

Treatment.—Selective pituitary microadenomectomy is of value for small pituitary lesions, while low dosage external pituitary irradiation or radioactive yitrium-90 implant are also to be considered. In cases of cortical hyperplasia, total adrenalectomy on one side and resection of seven-eighths of the adrenal gland on the other side (usually after an interval) is the best course. Obviously the only treatment for neoplastic cases is excision of the adrenal gland bearing the tumour.

If a pituitary tumour causes oculomotor symptoms or enlargement of the pituitary fossa as seen on x-ray, it should be removed surgically.

Prognosis.—Most patients are alive 20 years after successful resection of an adrenal adenoma, but survival beyond five years is rare with a carcinoma (Welbourn). 50% of all patients with a treated pituitary lesion causing adrenal hyperplasia are alive after 20 years.

Very rarely, the *adreno-genital syndrome* appears in youths and men. Owing to excessive production of oestrogenic hormones by the adrenal cortex, gynaecomastia, atrophy of the testicles, and psychic signs of effeminacy appear (Adrenal Feminism).

4. **Post-menopausal hypercorticism** is usually characterised by the growth of a beard (the bearded woman of the circus), and is often accompanied by mental aberration. A lesser degree of hirsutism is almost a natural accompaniment of the aging process, particularly in dark-haired females, and it is difficult to draw the line between the normal and the pathological. Thus it is that operative treatment is usually disappointing.

Primary aldosteronism (Conn's syndrome) is due to a rare adreno-cortical tumour producing aldosterone. Excess of this leads to sodium retention and a fall in serum potassium. The latter causes the typical features of the syndrome, namely episodes of muscular weakness associated with polyuria and polydipsia. Hypertension may occur. The plasma sodium is high and the potassium is low, but simple administration of potassium does not relieve the condition. Renin and angiotensin levels are depressed. Effective treatment involves removal of the causative tumour, but there is the usual difficulty in ascertaining on which side it lies (see under operation).

Secondary aldosteronism is associated with cirrhosis of the liver, and renal artery stenosis with high levels of renin and angiotensin.

ADRENALECTOMY FOR HYPERCORTICISM

It is essential that all patients who are to be subjected to extirpation of adrenal cortical tissue be prepared adequately for the operation, and supported postoperatively by adrenocortical hormone replacement therapy, irrespective of the extent of adrenal resection.

Cortisone Therapy

Pre-operative	Cortisone acetate, 100 mg intramuscularly twice a day for two days. One dose is given two hours before operation.
During the Operation and Immediate Post-operative Period	Hydrocortisone, 100 mg slowly by intravenous drip. Then a similar quantity during the subsequent twelve hours, to be followed by cortisone 50 mg intramuscularly six-hourly. If the blood-pressure remains below 100 systolic, then blood-transfusion is given.
Post-operative	Day 1.—Cortisone 50 mg intramuscularly six-hourly. Days 2 and 3.—Cortisone 50 mg intramuscularly eight-hourly. Days 4 and 5.—Cortisone 50 mg intramuscularly every twelve hours. Days 6 and 7.—Cortisone 25 mg by mouth every eight hours.

Thenceforward cortisone by mouth should be reduced slowly to maintenance level in cases of total adrenalectomy, or to zero in subtotal adrenalectomy. Fludrocortisone 0·1 mg daily (replacing aldosterone) may be necessary to regulate fluid and salt balance.

After total adrenalectomy the patient should always carry a card stating the dosage of cortisone she is receiving. Any stress (a further operation or infection) is an indication to increase the dosage.

Operation: (*a*) When an adrenal tumour has been demonstrated preoperat-

Richard Burkewood Welbourn, Contemporary. Professor of Surgical Endocrinology, Royal Postgraduate Medical School, London.
Jerome W. Conn, Contemporary. Professor of Internal Medicine, University of Michigan, Ann Arbor, Michigan, U.S.A.

ively, excision of that adrenal gland alone is carried out. (*b*). If a tumour has not been demonstrated, the patient is prepared for bilateral exploration.

Because the difficulties are usually less on the left than on the right side, exploration of the left adrenal gland is undertaken first. If a tumour is found, adrenalectomy is carried out. If the left gland is found to be atrophic, it is highly probable that there is a tumour on the right side, which should be explored forthwith. Should the gland be hyperplastic or normal, subtotal (90%) adrenalectomy is indicated. If, after this has been performed, it is apparent that the patient will not tolerate a bilateral operation well, exploration of the contralateral side should be postponed.

Posterior Approach.—An ample postero-lateral incision, such as is used for nephrectomy (Chapter 57), is employed. After subperiosteal resection of the twelfth rib the lower border of the pleura is defined and protected. The incision is extended through the bed of the twelfth rib to reveal the perinephric fat, within which the adrenal gland is identified, as described below. Sometimes an approach through the bed of the eleventh rib, reflecting the pleura upwards is preferred. (See also the abdominal approach, below.)

On the right side the suprarenal vein is short and may be torn from the vena cava if it is not identified and ligated at an early stage of the dissection. By finger and gauze dissection, keeping close to the gland, the gland is freed from below and behind, upwards, ligating and dividing bleeding vessels as they are encountered, until it suspended only by its main vascular pedicle near its apex. If subtotal adrenalectomy is to be performed, the gland is cut across with scissors so as to leave a small triangular fragment of the apex well supplied with blood-vessels. Bleeding should be controlled by swab pressure, as diathermy coagulation leads to necrosis.

Anterior Approach.—The adrenal glands are approached through either a curved transverse incision or a long paramedian incision. *The left adrenal gland* is approached first by cutting along the lateral leaf of the lieno-renal ligament and then curving downwards and medially, so as to enable a wide peritoneal flap to be reflected. By retracting the spleen downwards and medially, the adrenal gland comes into view. The fascia over its lateral border is incised, and by gauze dissection the blood-vessels of the gland are defined, ligated, and divided, thus freeing the gland, which is removed. Alternative approaches can be made by an 'up and under' dissection of the mesocolon and pancreas, or through the lesser sac. *The right adrenal gland* is more deeply situated. The peritoneum is incised lateral to the duodenum and above the upper pole of the kidney. The flap of peritoneum is raised to expose the anterior surface of the adrenal gland as it lies against the bare surface of the liver. The fascia covering the lateral surface of the gland is incised. A finger can then be inserted above the upper pole of the gland into the space between the two layers of fascia enclosing the gland (fig. 677). This prevents the gland from becoming displaced upwards, which otherwise it is prone to do. The anterior fascial layer is then incised transversely and the gland can be dissected under vision, as on the left side. After removal, each gland should be inspected to check its completeness, and each adrenal bed must be searched for the presence of accessory adrenal tissue, which is present in 32% of cases. If this important step is omitted, failure of the operation is not unlikely. The abdomen is closed with small drainage tubes passing to the adrenal fossae on either side.

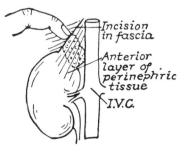

FIG. 677.—Incision in the fascia lateral to the right adrenal gland. Insertion of the finger into the space above the gland prevents its upward displacement.
(*After J. C. McKeown and A. Ganguli.*)

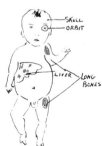

FIG. 678.—The common sites for metastases from neuroblastoma of the adrenal. Bones are involved more frequently than the liver.

THE ADRENAL MEDULLA

The medulla of the adrenal glands (chromaffin tissue), which is developed, together with sympathetic nerves, from ectoderm, is grey in colour and connected intimately, both anatomically and functionally, with splanchnic nerves. Chromaffin tissue is so-called because the large polyhedral cells of which it is composed contain granules that stain yellow with chromic acid. These granules are the internal secretion of the adrenal medulla itself, for they can be observed being extruded *in toto* into radicles of the adrenal vein. The secretion consists of the catecholamines[1], adrenaline and noradrenaline. In health, 80% of the output is adrenaline, and 20% is noradrenaline. However, in hyperfunctioning medullary tumour (phaeochromocytoma) this ratio is completely reversed. Fear, anger, pain, and effort give rise to an increased output in response to the stimuli received via the splanchnic nerves.

EFFECTS OF CATECHOLAMINES MEDIATED BY ALPHA- AND BETA-ADRENERGIC RECEPTORS

Effect on	Alpha Receptor	Beta Receptor
Cardiac output	Nil	Increase
Heart rate	Nil	Increase
Force of myocardial contraction	Nil	Increase
Myocardial excitability	Increase	Increase++
Blood pressure-systolic	Increase	Nil
Blood pressure-diastolic	Increase	Decrease
Blood vessels—in skin	Constrict	Dilate
Blood vessles—in muscle	Constrict	Dilate
Smooth muscle—in bronchi	Nil	Relax
Smooth muscle—in intestine	Relax	Relax
Smooth muscle—in bladder	Relax	Relax
Smooth muscle—in sphincters	Constrict	Constrict

Actions of Catecholamines. Catecholamines exert their effects through specific cell surface receptors, alpha receptors and beta receptors (see table). These mediate the actions of the endogenously released catecholamines, noradrenaline and adrenaline, and some of the actions of dopamine. The receptors have quite different pharmacological properties and an organ may have more than one type. The complex actions of catecholamines include altering enzyme activity, metabolic pathways, and the permeability of cell membranes to ions.

Pharmacological inhibitors of alpha stimulation (alpha blockers), include the long acting phenoxybenzamine (Dibenyline) and short acting phentolamine (Rogitine). Beta blockers include propanolol (Inderal) and practolol (Eraldin).

TUMOURS OF THE ADRENAL MEDULLA

Neoplasms of the sympathetic neurones
- Ganglioneuroma
- Neuroblastoma (sympatheticoblastoma)

Neoplasm of chromaffin cells = Phaeochromocytoma

Those occurring at any age:

A ganglioneuroma is relatively benign. This neoplasm is symptomless, grows to a large size, and constitutes one of the varieties of retroperitoneal 'sarcoma' (Chapter 49). Only 15% involve the adrenal, the remainder occurring in any position along the sympathetic chain. If removed completely at a comparatively early stage, a cure can be expected.

---

[1] Synthesis of catecholamines: Tyrosine→3·4 Dihydrophenylamine (DOPA)→3·4 Dihydroxyphenylethylamine (Dopamine)→Noradrenaline→Adrenaline.

Those occurring in infants and children:

Neuroblastoma of the adrenal medulla is a reddish-grey tumour that is highly malignant. It soon breaks its confines and invades neighbouring organs, *e.g.* the kidney and the pancreas, and metastasises by lymphatics, and even more frequently by the blood-stream. 5% of these tumours secrete catecholamines and, if diarrhoea is a symptom, vaso-active intestinal peptide (VIP).

Clinical Features.—Distributed equally between the sexes, 80% of these comparatively rare tumours occur below the age of five years. Usually the child is brought on account of an abdominal swelling. Pallor and loss of appetite are frequent accompaniments. The knobbly contour of an adrenal neuroblastoma helps to differentiate it from a Wilms' tumour (Chapter 57), which remains smooth even after it has attained a great size. Although unilateral, the growth, as it enlarges, extends across the middle line. About 60% of patients have metastases by the time they are seen (fig. 678).

Pepper's type of the disease.—The primary and secondaries are on the right side, with large liver metastases. In *Hutchison's type*, a left-sided primary spreads upwards by lymphatics and deposits are found in the orbit and skull. Metastases in the skull mimic the spicular osteogenic sarcoma; those in the long bones resemble Ewing's tumours. Chapter 19).

Investigations should include a complete radiographic examination of the skeleton (skeletal survey).

Treatment.—Unless there are secondary deposits, exploration (before or after radiotherapy) should be undertaken; in comparatively early cases the tumour can be removed completely. When total removal is not feasible, as much as possible of the neoplasm should be excised, followed later by a course of deep radiotherapy.

If complete excision is possible, the prognosis is enhanced, but an extraordinary feature of these cases is that from time to time a patient survives when the tumour is found to be so advanced that only a piece is removed for section, and no treatment of any kind is given; sometimes even secondary deposits disappear. There is some evidence that cases which are histologically borderline between ganglioneuroma and neuroblastoma become converted to the former with high doses of *folic acid* with subsequent betterment of the prognosis. With *operation*, followed by *x-ray therapy*, about 25% of the patients recover, and if they are free from recurrence by the end of one year, it is almost certain that they are cured permanently (Gross).

Those occurring in adults (rare in children):

Phaeochromocytoma is a soft brownish benign tumour, usually less than 5 cm in diameter, composed of large differentiated sympathetic ganglion cells, and a few fibres enclosed in a delicate capsule. It owes its name to the presence of chromaffin granules. In about 15% of cases the tumour is bilateral. This tumour occurs in both sexes, usually during early adult life or middle age. It produces, either intermittently or continuously, an excess of adrenaline, and especially of noradrenaline: the ratio of the latter to the former often being as high as 20:1 causing *hypertension* which is either *paroxysmal* or *persistent*. The latter predominates statistically and probably indicates a late stage of the disease. Consequently all patients under sixty years of age who suffer from sustained arterial hypertension deserve routine tests to confirm or exclude a phaeochromocytoma. While not more than 0·5% of cases of hypertension are caused by a phaeochromocytoma, at the Mayo Clinic, where routine diagnostic procedures are undertaken to confirm or exclude the presence of this tumour in all cases of hypertension, the percentage has been stated to be nearly 3%. Untreated, it progresses to a fatal termination from cardiac dysrhythmia or cerebral haemorrhage.

Clinical Features.—A typical complaint is that of fear—'I thought I was going to die.' The most common symptoms, in order of frequency are: headache (55%), palpitation, vomiting, sweating, dyspnoea, weakness, pallor—*i.e.* the symptoms

William Pepper (Junior), 1874–1947. Dean, University of Pennsylvania School of Medicine, Philadelphia, Pennsylvania, U.S.A.
Sir Robert Hutchison, 1871–1960. Physician, The London Hospital.
James Ewing, 1866–1943. Professor of Pathology, Cornell University, New York, U.S.A.
Robert Edward Gross, Contemporary. Ladd Professor of Children's Surgery, Harvard University, Boston, Massachusetts, U.S.A.
The Mayo Clinic, Rochester, Minnesota, U.S.A. was founded in 1889 by William Worrall Mayo (1819–1911) and his two sons William James Mayo (1861–1939) and Charles Horace Mayo (1865–1939).

of adrenal overdosage. The paroxysmal attack may vary from a few minutes to some hours. The blood pressure may be very high and hyperglycaemia present. The symptoms may be mistaken for hyperthyroidism, hypocalcaemia, an acute anxiety state, paroxysmal atrial tachycardia and carcinoid syndrome. The main obstacle to the diagnosis of a phaeochromocytoma is the failure to think of it as a cause of the observed symptoms.

Diagnostic Tests.—(i) *Vanillyl Mandelic Acid (VMA)* estimations on three consecutive 24-hour urine collections in a hypertensive phase. Normal excretion—less than 7 mg/24 h. False positive values occur with the use of vasodilator drugs such as hydralazine, in severe heart failure, carcinoid, hypoglycaemia, intracranial lesions and Guillain-Barré syndrome. Rarely drugs such as L-Dopa may interfere with the estimation of VMA in the urine. Another method is the 24 hour meta-adrenaline excretion (see Table).

(ii) *Radiology.*—An IVU may show displacement of the kidney by the tumour. Ultrasound and CT scanning delineate up to 80% of lesions and selective venous sampling 95%. Arteriography also reveals the vascular state and size of the kidneys. If a vascular 'blush' at the tumour site is not seen but one kidney is diseased, that is the likely explanation of the hypertension. Iodine labelled meta-iodobenzylguannidine, a guanethedine analogue, is structurally similar to nor-adrenaline and taken up by adrenergic storage vesicles after I.V. injection. Images may be obtained using a gamma camera.

DIAGNOSTIC TESTS IN RELATION TO METABOLISM OF CATECHOLAMINES

ADRENALINE		METADRENALINE	Monoamine Oxidase	VANILLYL
&	$\longrightarrow$	&	$\longrightarrow$	MANDELIC
NORADRENALINE		NORMETADRENALINE		ACID (VMA)

Any metabolite may be estimated in blood or urine and are greatly elevated in the presence of a phaeochromocytoma. Urinary normetadrenaline or VMA are most commonly measured.

Operation.—Catecholamine secreting tumours are a challenge to both the surgeon and anaesthetist. A patient with phaeochromocytoma is hypovolaemic because of the contraction of the vascular bed by excess circulating catecholamines. During surgery handling of the tumour can increase circulating catecholamine levels up to 600 fold causing large swings in blood pressure and cardiac arrhythmias. Severe hypotension may follow removal of the tumour. These dangers can be minimised by careful pre-operative preparation. Initially, the plasma volume is measured four days before surgery and the patient must have complete bed rest for three pre-operative days plus the following regimen:

A. *Pre-Operative Day 3.*—Infuse the alpha blocker Phenoxybenzamine 1 mg/kg body weight over two hours to give a recumbent blood pressure of 110/70 mm Hg. Give a beta blocking agent if the pulse rate rises above 120/min, and give extra I.V. fluids.

B. *Pre-Operative Day 2.*—Phenoxybenzamine infusion if the diastolic blood pressure is above 80 mm Hg. Give a beta blocking agent if the heart rate is above 100/min. Continue extra I.V. fluids.

C. *Day Before Operation.*—Infuse 2 mg/kg of Phenoxybenzamine over two hours if the diastolic blood pressure remains above 80 mm HG. Re-estimate the plasma volume. Continue extra I.V. fluids.

D. *Day of Operation.*—The supine blood pressure should be about 110/70 mm Hg and a pulse rate less than 90/min. At least ten units of whole blood should be available.

During surgery intravenous infusion of alpha and beta blocking drugs are given, if required, as determined by the blood pressure, pulse rate and central venous pressure. The hazardous phases in the operation are: during the induction of anaesthesia, positioning of the patient on the operating table, when the tumour is manipulated and immediately after removal of the tumour. With an intravenous drip of infusion of dextrose saline running the operation is commenced. Exploration via the anterior route is preferred, particularly if there is uncertainty about the tumour site; some 10% of phaeochromocytomas are ectopic.

With these precautions, the earlier operative mortality has been lowered. If symptoms persist after unilateral adrenalectomy, a tumour in the contralateral gland is highly prob-

Georges Guillain, 1876—. French Neurologist.
Jean Alexandre Barré, 1880—. French Neurologist.

able. In this instance the second tumour, which is usually well-defined, must be resected. Some consider this to be the better technique for all cases, particularly because these tumours are almost always benign and the operation is curative.

The excised specimen, when fixed in bichromate solution, stains brown.

Hyperplasia of the adrenal medulla, although often more in evidence on one side than the other, is usually bilateral. Paroxysmal hypertension, clinically identical with that produced by a phaeochromocytoma, is present. Unilateral adrenalectomy brings about amelioration, but for a cure of the condition, the remaining adrenal should be removed.

CHAPTER 39

THE BREAST

Comparative and Surgical Anatomy.—Mammals are distinguished and so-called because they are provided with mammary glands. The cow, sheep, goat, mare and the elephant have an udder surmounted by teats, while other animals are furnished with breasts, the number of pairs of which vary with the species, and is related to the average number of offspring in each litter. Thus the sow has six to nine pairs, rodents six or seven pairs, while, like man, the anthropoid apes, the lioness, the sea-cow and, as John Hunter first noted, the whale, have but a single pair.

In anatomical works the protuberant part of the human breast is generally described as overlying the second to the sixth ribs, and extending from the lateral border of the sternum to the anterior axillary line. Actually a thin layer of mammary tissue extends considerably farther on all sides, *viz.* to the clavicle above, to the seventh or eighth ribs below, to the mid-line medially, and to the edge of the latissimus dorsi posteriorly. This fact is of importance when he seeks to remove the whole breast. The full extent of the breast is apparent in cases of milk engorgement.

The axillary tail of the breast is of considerable surgical importance. In some normal cases it is palpable, and in a few it can be seen in the pre-menstrual phase and during lactation. A well-developed axillary tail is sometimes mistaken for a mass of enlarged lymph nodes or a lipoma.

The lobule is the basic structural unit of the mammary gland. In the human breast the number and size of the lobules vary exceedingly: they are largest and most numerous during early womanhood. From ten to more than a hundred lobules empty by means of ductules into a lactiferous duct, of which there are from fifteen to twenty. Each lactiferous duct is lined by a spiral arrangement of contractile myoepithelial cells and is provided with a terminal ampulla—a little reservoir for milk or abnormal discharges.

The ligaments of Cooper are hollow conical projections of fibrous tissue filled with breast tissue, the apices of the cones being attached firmly to the superficial fascia and thereby to the skin overlying the breast. These ligaments account for the dimpling of the skin overlying a scirrhous carcinoma, or other lesions of the breast accompanied by fibrosis.

The Areola.—The subcutaneous tissue contains involuntary muscle arranged in concentric rings as well as radially. The areolar epithelium contains numerous glands of three kinds—sweat glands, sebaceous glands, and accessory mammary glands. The sebaceous glands (known as the glands of Montgomery) enlarge strikingly during pregnancy and serve to lubricate the nipple during lactation. The accessory mammary glands are minute, inconstant, and possess ducts that open on the areola.

The Nipple is covered by a thick and rather crinkled skin. Near its apex, and very difficult to see because of the cutaneous corrugations, lie the orifices of the lactiferous ducts. The nipple and the areola of a nullipara are pink; with succeeding pregnancies they become pigmented by deposits of melanin. The nipple contains smooth muscle fibres arranged concentrically and longitudinally; thus it is an erectile structure and, for the convenience of the infant in arms, points forwards and *outwards*.

Lymphatics.—Lymphatic vessels of the breast drain into the axillary and the internal mammary lymph nodes. The axillary nodes receive approximately 75% of the drainage and are arranged in the following groups: (*a*) lateral, along the axillary vein; (*b*) anterior, along the lateral thoracic vessels; (*c*) posterior, along the subscapular vessels; (*d*) central embedded in fat in the centre of the axilla; (*e*) interpectoral, a few nodes lying between the pectoralis major and minor muscles; (*f*) apical, which lie above the level of the pectoralis minor tendon in continuity with the lateral nodes and receive the efferents of all the other groups. The apical nodes are also in continuity with the lateral lower deep cervical (supra-clavicular) nodes and drain into the subclavian lymph trunk which enters the great veins directly or via the thoracic duct or jugular trunk.

The internal mammary nodes are fewer in number and lie along the internal mammary

John Hunter, 1728–1793. Surgeon, St. George's Hospital, London.
Sir Astley Paston Cooper, 1768–1841. Surgeon, Guy's Hospital, London.
William Fetherston-Haugh Montgomery, 1797–1859. Obstetrician, Dublin.

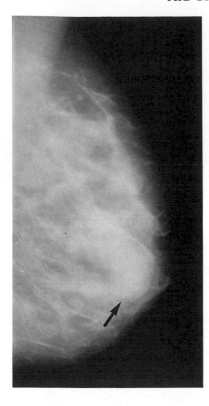

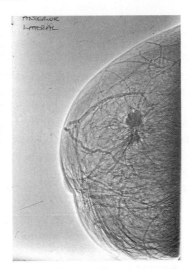

Fig. 680.—Xeromammogram. Note irregular density and distortion of breast tissue indicating carcinoma.

Fig. 679.—Mammogram showing smooth, well-defined opacity of a cyst.

vessels deep to the plane of the costal cartilages. They also drain into the great veins either directly or via one of the major lymphatic ducts.

Investigation of the Breast.—Although an accurate history and clinical examination are still the most important methods of detecting breast disease there are a number of investigations which can assist in the diagnosis:

Mammography (figs 679 & 680).—Soft tissue x-rays are taken by placing the breast in direct contact with ultrasensitive film and exposing it to low voltage, high amperage x-rays. *Xeromammography (xerography)* refers to an alternative x-ray technique using a photo-conductor which produces a final image on paper rather than film. The two methods are equally accurate in demonstrating the soft tissue architecture of the breast, but should always be combined with clinical examination.

Ductography (galactography).—Duct anatomy and pathology can be displayed by x-rays following injection of radio-opaque contrast medium into a major lacteal duct. It is seldom used nowadays.

Thermography.—A technique by which the heat emission from the surface of the breast in the form of infra-red radiation can be recorded. The information is usually displayed on a photographic plate or a cathode tube comparable to a television screen. The heat intensity varies with the vascularity and metabolism of the tissues and is increased in inflammatory conditions and some cancers. Unfortunately thermography lacks sensitivity and specificity and is therefore of little clinical value.

Ultrasound.—With appropriate experience, modern ultrasound equipment can be useful in distinguishing cystic from solid masses.

Needle biopsy.—This is of two types. In one, a high speed drill or a specially designed needle of trucut type produces a thin core of tissue for standard histological section. In the other, a fine needle aspirates tissue fluid which is smeared on a slide and examined cytologically. Either method achieves a high degree of accuracy in skilled hands but a negative result may be due to sampling error and must accordingly be interpreted with great caution.

THE NIPPLE

Absence of the nipple is rare, and usually associated with amazia.

Supernumerary nipples occasionally occur along a line extending from the anterior fold of the axilla to the fold of the groin. This constitutes the milk line of lower mammals.

Retraction of the nipple is of two important varieties: (*a*) that occurring at puberty (remote), and (*b*) that occurring during womanhood (recent).

(*a*) **Retraction Occurring at Puberty** is also known as simple inversion of the nipple, which, for some unknown reason, does not develop *pari passu* with the breast. In about one-quarter of the cases the condition is bilateral.

Non-protuberance of the nipple hinders an infant suckling at the breast. Clinical experience shows that a breast with long-standing retraction of its nipple is prone to local excoriation by the retained sebaceous gland secretion and, especially during lactation, to infection and abscess formation.

Treatment.—During and soon after puberty: if the patient draws out the nipple between finger and thumb daily for about three weeks the condition is usually remedied.

(*b*) **Recent Retraction.**—The importance of long-standing retraction of the nipple is dwarfed by the sometimes ominous significance of recent retraction, which may be caused by a scirrhous carcinoma. Therefore the all-important question to put to the patient is: 'How long has this nipple been retracted?'

Cracked Nipple.—Want of care in the preparation for lactation and neglect of the hygiene of the nipple during lactation are the chief causes of this not uncommon condition. Its main importance lies in the fact that the crack may be a forerunner of acute infective mastitis.

Prophylaxis.—During the last two months of pregnancy the nipples and their areolae should be washed, dried, and anointed with a little lanoline each day. The same routine may be continued, with advantage, after suckling.[1]

Treatment.—At the first sign of soreness the nipple is rested for twenty-four to forty-eight hours and the breast emptied with a breast-pump, as necessary. The nipple is washed and a mild antiseptic cream applied. When the soreness ceases, the baby is put to the breast for one minute at first and normal feeding is gradually resumed.

Papilloma of the nipple (fig. 681) presents the features of a cutaneous papilloma. Sometimes it grows to the size of a cherry, but the pedicle is always narrow. The treatment is excision together with a tiny disc of the skin from which it grows.

Retention Cyst of a Gland of Montgomery.—These glands, situated in the areola, secrete sebum and, as a result of an orifice of one of the glands becoming blocked, a sebaceous cyst forms.

Chancre of the Nipple.—The majority of chancres of the nipple occur by infection from a syphilitic buccal mucous patch in the mouth of a member of the opposite sex. Although wet-nurses are now seldom, if ever, employed in this country, when this form of infant feeding was used the nipple was sometimes infected from the mouth of a syphilitic baby. The mother of such an infant is immune to re-infection from her own child.

Eczema of the nipples is a rare condition and is bilateral, and presents features common to eczema elsewhere.

Paget's disease of the nipple (p. 728) must be distinguished from the foregoing.

ABNORMAL DISCHARGES FROM THE NIPPLE

The discharge occurs from one (rarely more) of the lactiferous ducts. The management depends on the presence of a lump, or of occult blood, or whether

---

[1] In some maternity hospitals the nipple is cleansed before and after suckling by wiping it with a sponge removed from 70% alcohol solution kept in a jar labelled with the patient's name.

it is localised to one duct. Mammography is usually unhelpful except to identify a grossly distended duct or a circumscribed tumour. Expert cytology may reveal the presence of malignant cells but a negative result does not exclude carcinoma.

A clear serous discharge is associated usually with a retention cyst, consequent upon mammary dysplasia, but may signify an underlying carcinoma.

A blood-stained discharge may be caused by duct papilloma, less commonly duct carcinoma or duct ectasia. It also occurs sometimes in the engorged breasts of pregnancy.

A black or green discharge may be due to altered blood from the foregoing, but is much more frequently an accompaniment of ductal changes and the secondary retention cysts of fibroadenosis. In cases of extensive dirty green discharge, the breast is usually riddled with cysts containing the same material.

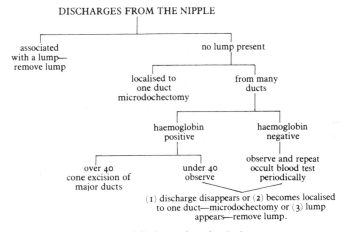

Scheme for management of discharges from the nipple.
(After Sir Hedley Atkins, Past P.R.C.S., London.)

Important causes of discharge are *Duct Papilloma, Mammillary Fistula* and *Duct Ectasia*.

Duct Ectasia.[1]—A primary dilatation of the major ducts of the breasts which is commonly associated with discharge from the nipple in middle aged women. The ducts become distended with amorphous debris and crystalline material probably lipid in nature and the discharge is of similar composition. As the condition progresses there is an associated periductal inflammation with lymphocytes and plasma cells at which stage there may be local pain and tenderness and ultimately a hard mass with local skin tethering and nipple retraction (Plasma cell mastitis). The condition is benign but may be mistaken for either cancer or an abscess (Haagensen, Hadfield). Provided a tumour can be excluded the treatment should be conservative but symptomatic relief can be gained by local removal of the affected ducts.

THE BREAST

CONGENITAL ABNORMALITIES

Amazia.—Congenital absence of the breast may occur on one (fig. 682) or both sides. It is sometimes associated with an absence of the sternal portion of the pectoralis major. Amazia, which is rare, is more common in males.

---

[1] John Birkett, 1815–1904, surgeon to Guy's Hospital gave an early account of this curious condition in 1850. He was a founder member of the Pathological Society of London.

Cushman D. Haagensen, Contemporary. Surgeon, Columbia University College of Physicians and Surgeons, New York, U.S.A.
Geoffrey John Hadfield, Contemporary. Surgeon, Stoke Mandeville Hospital, Aylesbury, England.

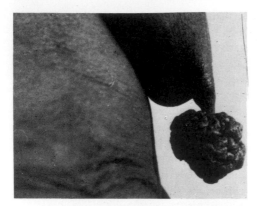

FIG. 681.—Papilloma of the nipple.
(R. R. Deshnukh, MS, Dhantoli, Nagpur, India.)

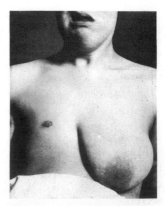

FIG. 682.—Congenital absence of the right breast.

Polymazia.—Accessory breasts have been recorded in the axilla, groin, buttock, and thigh, the most frequent site being the axilla. They have been known to function during lactation (fig. 683).

DIFFUSE HYPERTROPHY

Diffuse hypertrophy of the breasts occurs sporadically in otherwise healthy girls at puberty and, much less often, during the first pregnancy. The breasts attain enormous dimensions (fig. 684), and may reach below the knees when the patient is sitting. This tremendous overgrowth of the mammary glands is due, appparently, to their extreme sensitivity to oestrogenic hormone. Sometimes the hypertrophy is unilateral.[1] Unilateral hypertrophy may be easily mistaken for a breast which is pushed forward by a large lipoma or other tumour of the retromammary area. If diffuse hypertrophy causes real distress, a plastic procedure in the form of a reduction mammoplasty is indicated.

INJURIES OF THE BREAST

Injuries of the breast were rare until the introduction of the diagonal motor car seat belt but are comparatively unimportant.

Haematoma, particularly a resolving haematoma, gives rise to a lump which, in the absence of overlying bruising, is difficult, if not impossible, to diagnose correctly until an exploratory incision has been made.

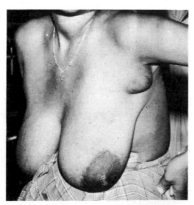

FIG. 683.—Functioning axillary breast.
(M. Kumar, F.R.C.S., Calicut, S. India.)

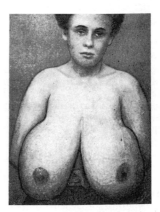

FIG. 684.—Diffuse hypertrophy (virginal).

[1] In tropical countries this must be distinguished from filarial elephantiasis of the breast.

Traumatic fat necrosis may be acute or chronic, and usually occurs in stout, middle-aged women. Following a blow, or even indirect violence (*e.g.* contraction of the pectoralis major), a lump, often painless, appears. In the absence of a definite lead, the swelling, which is often attached to the skin, is usually diagnosed as a carcinoma, and biopsy is required for diagnosis. A definite history of injury should bring the condition to the clinician's mind. On incising the lump a chalky white area of necrotic fat is found resembling necrosis seen in cases of subsiding acute pancreatitis.

ACUTE AND SUBACUTE INFLAMMATIONS OF THE BREAST

Mastitis of infants is at least as common in the male as in the female. On the third or fourth day of life, if a breast of an infant is pressed lightly, a drop of colourless fluid can be expressed; a few days later there is often a slight milky secretion, which finally disappears during the third week. This is popularly known as 'witch's milk'. The explanation of this phenomenon is that the hormone which stimulates the mother's breast reacts also upon the mammary tissue of the foetus. Thus it is essentially physiological.

Mastitis of puberty is encountered rather frequently, usually in males. The patient, aged about fourteen, complains of pain and swelling in the breast. In 80% the condition is unilateral but the opposite breast may be affected later. The breast is enlarged, tender and slightly indurated. Suppuration never occurs. The tenderness subsides in fourteen days or so, but induration often persists for several weeks. In some instances enlarged tender breasts may persist in males for a prolonged period even up to years. In such circumstances it may be justifiable to recommend local mastectomy, conserving the nipple.

Mastitis of mumps is usually unilateral, and more common in females.

Mastitis from milk engorgement is liable to occur about weaning time; and sometimes in the early days of lactation when one of the lactiferous ducts becomes blocked with epithelial debris. In the latter instance a sector only of the breast becomes indurated and tender.

Bacterial mastitis, which is by far the most common variety of mastitis, nearly always commences acutely. Although often referred to as mastitis of lactation, it is incorrect to assume that acute mastitis in women is necessarily lactational. Of a hundred consecutive cases of breast abscess, thirty-two occurred in women who were not lactating (De Jode); probably some were due to infection of a haematoma. In almost every case the infecting organism is a staphylococcus. In cases where the infection is acquired in hospital no less than 90% of the infecting staphylococci are insensitive to penicillin.

Aetiology.—Mastitis of lactation is seen far less frequently than in former years. Usually the intermediary is the infant; after the second day of life 50% of infants harbour staphylococci in the nasopharynx.

'Cleansing the baby's mouth' with a swab is also an aetiological factor. The delicate buccal mucosa is excoriated by the process; it becomes infected, and organisms in the infant's saliva are inoculated on to the mother's nipple.

There seems little doubt that in the great majority of cases the precursor of intramammary mastitis is failure of secretion to escape because one (rarely more) of the lactiferous ducts becomes blocked with epithelial debris—a hypothesis that is strengthened by the fact that, whether they are lactating or not, intramammary mastitis and abscess of the breast are relatively frequent in women with a retracted nipple. While stasis in some part of the lactiferous tree is a major factor in the production of this condition, undoubtedly the older hypothesis—ascending infection from a sore or an infected cracked nipple—

Louis Rene Julien De Jode, 1926–1982. Surgeon, Whipps Cross Hospital, Leytonstone, London.

must not be spurned. Once within the ampulla of the duct, staphylococci cause clotting of milk. Within the clot organisms multiply rapidly.

Clinical Features.—The affected breast, or more usually mainly one part of it, presents the classical signs of acute inflammation, and what is aptly called 'the cellulitic stage' of a breast abscess has been reached.

Treatment during the Cellulitic Stage.—The patient should rest in bed and, pending the results of bacterial culture of her milk, be given an antibiotic appropriate for a penicillin resistant staphylococcus, *e.g.* cloxacillin or flucloxacillin. Support to the breast and local heat will help to relieve the pain and permit examination of the inflamed breast daily, which is essential.

Unless there is some strong reason to continue breast feeding it is better to wean. Suppression of lactation usually follows naturally upon the cessation of suckling but if necessary bromocriptine can be given, 2·5 mg bd for 14 days. Stilboestrol is no longer used for this purpose.

If the mother insists on continuing breast feeding it is safer to use the uninfected breast only and to *empty the infected breast of milk*, which may have a high bacterial content, by means of a breast pump. Boiling or pasteurisation of expressed milk not only destroys its content of antibodies but also greatly reduces its nutritional value to the infant.

Formation of an 'Antibioma'.—It is absolutely essential that an antibiotic should *not* be given in the presence of undrained pus. In such circumstances, if an antibiotic is given the pus in the abscess frequently becomes sterile and a large brawny oedematous swelling remains in the breast and takes many weeks to resolve. Sometimes there is excessive fibrosis and this, with the absence of tenderness, had led to the mistaken diagnosis of carcinoma. It is better to explore the mass with a wide-bore aspirating needle than to cause an 'antibioma' with its attendant pain, chronicity, and ill health. Most 'antibiomas' are due to late, inadequate, and ineffective antibiotics.

Indications for Operation.—The breast should be incised when, after emptying, an area of tense induration is felt and/or when oedema of the overlying skin is found. In contrast to the majority of localised infections, fluctuation is a late sign and incision must not be delayed until it appears. Usually the area of induration is sector-shaped, and in early cases about one-quarter of the breast is involved (fig. 685); in many later cases the area is more extensive (fig. 686).

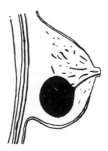

FIG. 685.—Intramammary breast abscess.

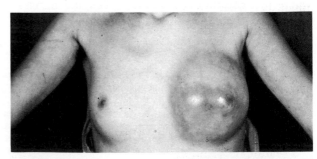

FIG. 686.—Intramammary breast abscess. The abscess should always be drained before it becomes subcutaneous.
(T. A. Boucher-Hayes, FRCSI, Dublin.)

Drainage of an Intramammary Abscess.—The usual incision is sited in a radial direction over the affected segment. One parallel with the cutaneo-areolar margin has a better cosmetic value and does permit access to the affected area. The incision passes through the skin and the superficial fascia. A long haemostat is then inserted into the abscess cavity. Every part of the abscess is palpated against the point of the haemostat and its jaws are opened. All loculi that can be felt are entered. Finally, the haemostat having been withdrawn, a finger is introduced and any remaining septa are disrupted. Unless the abscess cavity is situated at the very highest sector of the breast a counter-incision should be made at the most dependent part of the breast and a drainage tube inserted. In this, almost more than any part in the body, *dependent* drainage is essential.

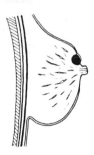

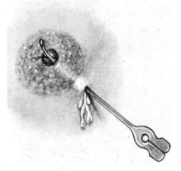

FIG. 687.—Subareolar abscess.

FIG. 688.—Milk-fistula originating in a chronic subareolar abscess.

FIG. 689.—Slitting up a chronic subareolar abscess. In this case the patient has a retracted nipple of long standing.
(After H. T. Caswell and A. W. E. Burnett.)

Subareolar mastitis is not a true mastitis but results from an infected (sebaceous) gland of Montgomery, or from a furuncle on or near the areola. The inflammation develops insidiously, usually without constitutional symptoms. When the patient presents early, there is often an area of induration no larger than a pea. No matter how small, if a lump can be felt, pus is present (fig. 687), and the abscess should be drained without delay. Spontaneous rupture, if allowed to occur, does not cure the condition; it merely results in recrudescence or chronicity.

Chronic intramammary abscess which follows inadequate drainage or injudicious antibiotic treatment is often a very difficult condition to diagnose: when encapsulated within a thick wall of fibrous tissue, the condition cannot be distinguished from carcinoma without the histological evidence from a biopsy.

Chronic Subareolar Abscess (leading to a *Mammillary fistula*).—A recurrent subacute or a chronic abscess may occur apart from lactation in women of the child-bearing age. The condition is a frequent complication of long-standing retraction of the nipple the infection being restricted to a single obstructed duct system. The abscess ruptures and subsides, only to repeat the cycle over and over again at intervals of a few months when it forms a chronic mammillary fistula (fig. 688). A non-infective inflammation such as duct ectasia may also result in fistula formation.

Treatment.—Antibiotic therapy followed by incision and drainage is useless. The fistula must be treated in the same way as a fistula-in-ano, *i.e.* the track is laid open and saucerised (fig. 689).

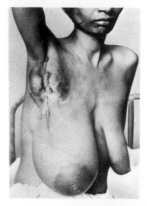

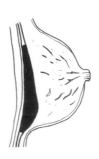

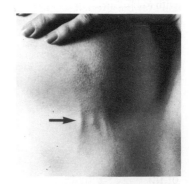

FIG. 690.—Tuberculosis of
the breast with secondary
suppurating axillary lymph
nodes.
*(Professor A. K. Toufeeq, Lahore,
Pakistan.)*

FIG. 691.—Retro-
mammary abscess.

FIG. 692.—Mondor's disease, under
the right breast.

Tuberculosis of the breast, which is comparatively rare among Western races but more common in Asia and some other parts of the world, is, as a rule, associated with active pulmonary tuberculosis, or tuberculous cervical adenitis.[1]

Tuberculosis of the breast (fig. 690) occurs more often in women who have borne one or more children and usually takes the form of multiple chronic abscesses with multiple sinuses and a typical bluish attenuated appearance of the surrounding skin. The diagnosis rests on bacteriological and histological examination. Treatment with antituberculous chemotherapy should be given. Healing is usual though often delayed, and mastectomy should be restricted to patients with persistent residual infection.

Actinomycosis of the breast is rarer still, except among peasant women who work in the fields of Europe. The lesions present the essential characteristics of facio-cervical actinomycosis (Chapter 4). If healing does not occur as a result of the systemic treatment of actinomycosis recommended, the affected breast should be amputated.

Syphilis of the Breast.—A primary chancre of the nipple has been referred to (above). Secondary lesions of syphilis include diffuse syphilitic mastitis.

Retromammary Abscess (fig. 691).—Here the pus is situated in the cellular tissues behind the breast, and in the great majority of cases the abscess has no connection with the breast proper. Usually a retromammary abscess originates from a tuberculous rib, infected haematoma, or possibly from a chronic empyema (Chapter 40), and treatment must be directed to the relief of these conditions. A submammary incision allows the breast to be retracted as necessary from the field of operation.

MONDOR'S DISEASE

Mondor's disease is thrombophlebitis of the superficial veins of the breast and anterior chest wall (fig. 692) though it has also been encountered in the arm.

In the absence of injury or infection, the cause of the thrombophlebitis—like that of spontaneous thrombophletis in other sites—is obscure. The essential characteristic physical sign is an indurated subcutaneous thrombophlebitic cord about 3 mm in diameter, of varying length, situated in the subcutis of the breast. Usually it is attached to the skin, and of a consistency that has been likened to that of the vas deferens. When the skin over the breast is stretched by raising the arm, a narrow, shallow subcutaneous groove alongside

---

[1] In 1829 Sir Astley Cooper, Surgeon to Guy's Hospital, London, described scrofulous swellings in the bosoms of young women, most of whom suffered from tuberculous cervical adenitis.

Henri Mondor, 1885–1962. Surgeon, Paris.

the cord becomes apparent. The great importance of the condition is that those unfamiliar with Mondor's disease are likely to diagnose the condition as one of lymphatic permeation from an occult carcinoma of the breast. The only treatment required is restricted arm movements, and in any case the condition subsides within a few months without recurrence, complications, or deformity.

MAMMARY DYSPLASIA[1]

Aetiology.—Mammary dysplasia is an aberration of the physiological changes that occur in mammary tissue at puberty (evolution) and at the menopause (involution). Although it is called an 'aberration' it may be nothing more than a variation on the normal theme of cyclic proliferation and regression. Some women, however, worry about the lumps or the pain which it sometimes causes and thus it has become a disease 'entity'. Many women are affected without being aware of it.

Pathology.—When sectioned with a knife the affected areas in the breast are white or yellow and of india-rubber consistency, but they never present the grey tones and hard gritty texture of carcinoma. Microscopically the disease consists essentially of five features which vary in extent and degree in any one breast— there are:

1. *Cyst Formation.*—Cysts are almost inevitable and vary much in size. They contain dark mucoid material.

2. *Adenosis.*—There is a budding and multiplication of acini and an overall increase in glandular tissue.

3. *Fibrosis.*—Fat and elastic tissue disappears and is replaced by dense white fibrous trabeculae. This fibrous tissue compresses the ducts and leads to cyst formation. The interstitial tissue is infiltrated with chronic inflammatory cells.

4. *Epitheliosis.*—Hyperplasia of epithelium in the lining of the ducts and acini may occur.

5. *Papillomatosis.*—The epithelial hyperplasia may be so extensive that it results in papillomatous overgrowth within the ducts.

After decades of discussion there is still no agreement among surgeons and pathologists as to whether mammary dysplasia is a premalignant condition. The majority are of the opinion that it is not, while others are equally emphatic that the epithelial hyperplasia when florid is undoubtedly premalignant. Both mammary dysplasia and carcinoma of the breast are common conditions; by coincidence, they can coexist.

Clinical Features.—Premenstrual pain and tenderness, usually bilateral and often associated with fine nodularity of the breast, occurs frequently. In some young women the discomfort may be disabling in its severity and may be so prolonged as to lose its cyclic pattern. There are minimal abnormal changes in the breast tissue of these patients and the symptoms are self-limiting requiring no active treatment. Pregnancy and lactation nearly always produce permanent relief. The contraceptive pill will also produce a reduction in symptoms in most women although in others, previously asymptomatic, the pill may stimulate discomfort. True mammary dysplasia, though it may occur at any age after puberty, is most prevalent between the ages of forty and fifty-five. Spinsters, childless

---

[1] Many alternative terms have been applied to this condition. Fibrocystic Disease, Fibroadenosis and Chronic Mastitis are in common use. Mastopathy is also used.

married women, and multiparous women who have not suckled their children are the usual sufferers. This suggests that the condition is prone to appear in breasts that have been denied their intended function. The patient usually complains of pain in *one* breast, worse before menstruation, or after using the arm. On examination both breasts are inclined to be nodular—the nodules being about the size of rice grains. As a rule it possible to define the saucer-like edge of the periphery of the breast. When the breast complained of is examined between finger and thumb its texture is unusually firm, more often than not an indefinite lump can be made out, but with the flat of the hand this can be felt only vaguely. The lump is neither adherent to the pectoral fascia nor to the skin. There is no recent retraction of the nipple, but occasionally there is a serous or dark-green discharge therefrom. The condition is sometimes more in evidence in one quadrant of the breast than in the remainder. The presence of a palpable cyst or cysts is complementary to the more general clinical findings of mammary dysplasia *per se*. Frequently the axillary lymph nodes are slightly enlarged; they are not hard but are often tender.

Treatment.—Reassurance is probably the most important part of treatment. It must be explained that these changes occur at this stage of life, that they are not precancerous and a certain amount of pain is to be expected.

Support for the breast by a firm brassière worn day and night is helpful. Diuretics administered during the time of greatest discomfort may reduce local tension pain but simple analgesia is usually the most effective management. for persistent, severe pain the antihormonal drugs Danazol®, or bromocriptine, given in a 3–6 months course are often of benefit. When the menopause is complete the pain will cease and the lumps disappear. From the surgeon's point of view it is important to confirm that the palpable lump is not a carcinoma. Mammography and needle biopsy may be helpful but an excision biopsy of the local lesion is necessary in doubtful cases.

Indications for Surgery in Mammary Dysplasia.—Apart from excision biopsy, surgery is only indicated when the patient is persistently disabled by intolerable pain or pathological anxiety, or when epitheliosis is so florid as to suggest the risk that malignancy may supervene. Such patients can be considered for the operation of subcutaneous mastectomy and replacement of the breast form with a synthetic prosthesis.

CLASSIFICATION OF CYSTIC SWELLINGS

Cysts of the breast are related to either the ducts or the stroma.

Ducts—Fibroadenosis < Solitary. / Multiple.

Intracystic papilliferous carcinoma.
Galactocele.
Papillary Cystadenoma.
Serocystic disease of Brodie.
Stroma—Colloid degeneration of carcinoma.
Lymphatic cyst.
Hydatid.

(*a*) *Simple Solitary Mammary Cyst.*—The size of the cyst varies widely, the seat of election being the upper and outer quadrant. Macroscopically the solitary

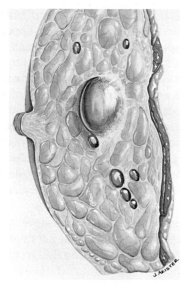

FIG. 693.—The blue-domed cyst of
Bloodgood.
(After C. F. Geschickter.)

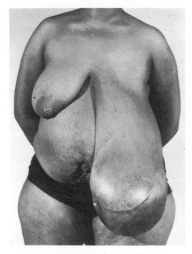

FIG. 694.—Galactocele. A 27-year-
old multipara (3) with progressive
breast enlargement following confinement.
*(O. O. Ajayi, FRCS, and O. Adekunle, FRCS,
Ibadan, Nigeria.)*

variety (fig. 693) presents as a blue-domed fluctuant mass (Bloodgood), the colour
being due to its fluid content. Although, clinically, the condition is a solitary
cyst, as a rule the breast parenchyma contains a number of tiny satellite cysts.
That the swelling is a cyst may sometimes be confirmed by transillumination;
aspiration is required to establish the diagnosis.

(*b*) *Multiple Cysts.*—This is the commonest type; the cysts are usually several
in number. Sometimes one sector of the breast is affected alone. If a main duct
near the nipple is obstructed, a duct papilloma should be suspected.

Treatment.—*To aspirate or not to aspirate? That is the question!*

Aspiration has its dangers as an intracystic neoplasm may be missed. It is only
safe if (1) the cyst does not refill, (2) the fluid withdrawn is not blood stained, (3)
there is no residual lump after aspiration (Patey), (4) the cytological examination
of the aspirated fluid shows no evidence of malignant cells. If any of these criteria
is not fulfilled, biopsy excision must be done. A solitary cyst can be excised
through a circumferentially orientated incision over the swelling.

Galactocele, which is extremely rare, usually presents as a solitary, subareolar cyst,
and always dates from lactation. It contains milk, liquid or inspissated, and in long-
standing cases its walls tend to calcify. It can become enormous (fig. 694).

Lymphatic cyst is a curiosity and its pathology is similar to the more common lymphatic
cyst of the neck (Chapter 36).

BENIGN NEOPLASMS OF THE BREAST

Epithelial
— Duct papilloma.
— Pure adenoma (very rare).

Connective tissue
— Neurofibroma.
— Lipoma.

Mixed   Fibroadenoma.

Joseph Colt Bloodgood, 1867–1935. Surgeon, Johns Hopkins Hospital, Baltimore, Maryland, U.S.A.
David Howard Patey, 1899–1976. Surgeon, The Middlesex Hospital, London.

Duct Papilloma.—The majority of these tumours are single, but bilateral examples are not rare, and occasionally two or more ducts of the same breast are the seat of a papillary growth. The usual single papilloma often has a stalk, and is situated in one of the larger lactiferous ducts.

Clinical Features.—The condition is rare before the age of twenty-five, and usually occurs in women between thirty-five and fifty. In the majority of cases bright red blood or, less often, a dark blood-stained discharge from the nipple is the only symptom. On examination, a cystic swelling can sometimes be felt beneath the areola; pressure upon it will cause a discharge from the mouth of the affected duct on the nipple. The majority of patients are found to have a solitary papilloma which is benign but identical symptoms are associated with multiple papillomatosis which is undoubtedly premalignant and after months or years will transform into a duct carcinoma.

Treatment.—Amputation of the breast is unnecessary, the removal of the papilloma and the involved duct providing a cure. It is important not to express the blood before operation as it then may be difficult to identify the duct in the theatre.

Microdochectomy (after Hedley Atkins and Brigitte Wolff).—A lacrimal probe or length of stiff nylon suture is inserted into the duct from which the discharge is emerging and fixed to the skin of the nipple by fine silk stitches. The skin of the incision is infiltrated with adrenaline in saline (1 ml of adrenaline 1/1000 in 80 ml of isotonic saline). Using a pair of fine pointed scissors, a triangular area is cut 1 mm away from the point of entry of the probe. Skin flaps are then reflected and the probe together with the duct is excised to produce a mass of breast tissue about 2·5 cm in diameter. The lesion is nearly always situated within 4–5 cm of the nipple orifice. The whole specimen including the probe and triangular area of skin is removed intact.

Cone excision of the major ducts.—When the duct of origin of nipple bleeding is uncertain or when there is bleeding from multiple ducts, the entire major duct system can be excised for histological examination without sacrifice of the breast form. A circumareolar incision is made and a cone of tissue removed with its apex just deep to the surface of the nipple and its base on the pectoral fascia. The resulting defect is obliterated by a series of purse string sutures.

Fibroadenoma is the commonest tumour of the breast below the age of 35. Most form in the early post-pubertal years though they may not come to light until later. Fibroadenoma usually presents as a solitary, firm, well-defined, lobulated, extremely mobile lump, 1–3 cm in diameter. Two microscopical variants are seen, a pericanalicular where normal duct structures are surrounded by a concentric overgrowth of connective tissue stroma, and an intracanalicular where the stroma projects into the ducts to form elongated and distorted clefts. These two patterns are often seen in the same tumour and the distinction is unimportant. There is a well marked capsule. Malignant change (carcinoma or sarcoma) occurs extremely rarely. Treatment is by enucleation of the tumour through a cosmetically appropriate incision.

Massive Swellings of the Breast

These are:

1. *Diffuse hypertrophy*, which is usually bilateral (fig. 684).

2. *Giant Fibroadenoma* occurs occasionally, usually in teenage girls and clinically may mimic unilateral hypertrophy. It is locally excised through a submammary incision.

Sir Hedley John Barnard Atkins, 1905–1983. Past P.R.C.S., Emeritus Professor of Surgery, Guy's Hospital, London.
Brigitte Wolff, Contemporary. Formerly Clinical Assistant, Department of Surgery, Guy's Hospital, London.

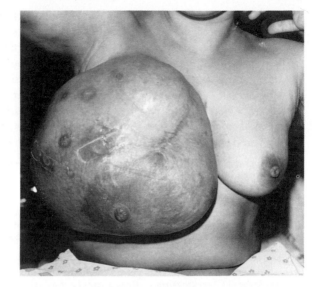

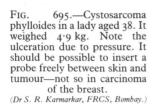

FIG. 695.—Cystosarcoma phylloides in a lady aged 38. It weighed 4·9 kg. Note the ulceration due to pressure. It should be possible to insert a probe freely between skin and tumour—not so in carcinoma of the breast.
(*Dr S. R. Karmarkar, FRCS, Bombay.*)

3. *Cystosarcoma Phylloides* (syn. Serocystic disease of Brodie)[1] usually occurs over the age of 40 but can appear in younger women (fig. 695). It presents as a large, sometimes massive tumour with an unevenly bosselated surface. It may undergo central softening and occasionally lead to ulceration of the overlying skin by pressure necrosis rather than infiltration. In spite of its size it remains mobile over the chest wall. Histologically there is a resemblance to intracanalicular fibroadenoma. Some tumours show malignant behaviour which can be predicted by the microscopic appearances of the stroma. These metastasise by the blood stream not by the lymphatics.

Treatment for the benign type is by wide local excision with a surrounding zone of normal breast tissue. Massive tumours may require simple mastectomy as does the malignant type.

When the Diagnosis of Carcinoma is in Doubt.—There will always be cases where the clinician cannot be sure whether a particular lump in the breast is an area of mammary dysplasia, a benign tumour or an early carcinoma. In doubtful cases it is essential to obtain a tissue diagnosis. This is often possible by needle biopsy (p. 713). In the event of a negative result, open biopsy of the mass is necessary. The diagnosis may be confirmed by frozen section histology which permits immediate procedure to definitive surgical management. In the absence of this facility it is wise to close the incision and await a formal histological report.

CARCINOMA OF THE BREAST

Breast cancer is the commonest malignant disease of women in England and Wales. It causes 12,000 deaths annually. It is estimated that one in 14 of all female children born will develop the disease during their lifetime. In spite of an immense amount of investigation there is still no known cause and its natural

---

[1] Phylloides—from the Greek φνλλωδησ = leaf-like. There are branching projections of the tumour tissue into the cystic cavities of this neoplasm.

Sir Benjamin Collins Brodie, 1783–1862. Surgeon, St. George's Hospital, London. Described this disease in 1840.

history is obscure. Women between forty-five and fifty-five are its most frequent victims, but many factors are known to influence its frequency.

While any portion of the breast may be attacked, the disease commences most frequently in the upper and outer quadrant (figs. 696 and 698). Unfortunately, so often the patient states that, although she noticed a lump in her breast while washing herself, she 'took no notice of it' because it was painless. Probably the average time between the patient finding the lump and reporting it is six weeks. Women should be urged to report to their doctors as soon as a lump in the breast is discovered.

(a) *Geographical.*—It occurs commonly in the Western World, England and Wales having a high incidence. It is a rare tumour in the East.

(b) *Genetic.*—It occurs more commonly in women with a family history of breast cancer than in the general population.

(c) *Endocrine.*—It appears to be commoner in nulliparous women than in women who have borne many children and have breast fed. It is also less common in women who have their first child at an early age especially if associated with late menarche and early menopause.

(d) *Milk Factor.*—Although an infective agent in the milk has been shown to transmit breast cancer in mice there is as yet no evidence to support this in the human.

Pathological Classification.—Breast cancer may arise from the epithelium of the duct system anywhere from the nipple end of major lactiferous ducts to the terminal duct unit which is in the breast lobule. The pathologist sometimes finds carcinoma which is entirely at the in situ stage either by chance in biopsies for a supposed benign condition, or following bleeding from the nipple, or in subclinical lesions detected by mammography. By the time of frank clinical presentation malignant cells have infiltrated the breast tissue—invasive breast carcinoma. The microscopical appearances vary from a well differentiated pattern with obvious transition from in situ carcinoma, usually ductal and only uncommonly lobular, to anaplastic where the breast is invaded by strands or clumps of anaplastic spheroidal or polygonal cells which often excite a considerable degree of stromal fibroblastic reaction (scirrhous carcinoma). Careful examination of multiple blocks from a given tumour usually shows a variety of histological appearances. Less common types include *colloid* carcinoma whose cells produce abundant mucin, and *medullary* carcinoma with solid sheets of large cells often associated with a marked lymphocytic reaction.

THE SPREAD OF MAMMARY CARCINOMA

(a) **Local Spread.**—The tumour increases in size and invades other portions of the breast. It tends to involve the skin and to penetrate the pectoral muscles, and even the chest wall.

(b) **Lymphatic spread** occurs in two ways; by *emboli*, composed of carcinoma cells, being swept along the lymphatic vessels, by the lymph stream; and *by permeation*, that is, actual growth of columns of cancer cells along the lumina of the lymphatic channels. The axillary lymph nodes and the internal mammary lymph nodes are involved comparatively early. Later, the supraclavicular lymph nodes, the opposite breast, and the mediastinum, are possible resting places for itinerant carcinoma cells. Finally, they may be found in lymph nodes even farther afield.

(c) **Spread by the Blood-stream.**—It is by this route that skeletal metastases occur (in order of frequency) in the lumbar vertebrae, femur, thoracic vertebrae, and the skull; they are generally osteolytic, pathological fractures occurring most often in a rib or a vertebra. In most instances it is by way of the blood-stream that metastases arrive in the liver, lung fields or brain from the breast, but secondary

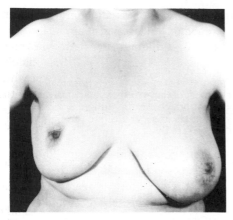

FIG. 696.—Scirrhous carcinoma of the right breast, upper outer quadrant and Stage III (below). Note shrinking and elevation of the breast with nipple retraction.

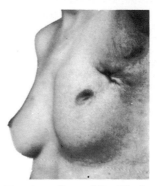

FIG. 697.—Stage IV. Nipple submerged, skin involved. Growth is adherent to chest wall.

deposits may also be carried to the liver via the lymphatics within the rectus sheath and the falciform ligament. The adrenal glands and the ovaries are also common sites for blood-borne metastases.

Clinical Types of Carcinoma of the Breast.—It is difficult to give any one growth a distinct classification, and clinical significance may be minimal. However, because the tumour may present in such a wide variety of ways, it is relevant to recognise certain clinical types:

Scirrhous carcinoma is the commonest form and is met with principally in middle aged or elderly women. Owing to an abundance of fibrous tissue the lump feels very hard, while its contour tends to be irregular. As the tumour advances it may cause indrawing of the nipple, the skin overlying (fig. 697) and tethering to the pectoral fascia deeply. The importance of recent retraction of the nipple has been alluded to already. In late cases there may be *peau d'orange* (fig. 699), ulceration of the skin and fixation to the chest wall.

If the breast containing a scirrhous carcinoma is cut with a knife so as to section the tumour, the following macroscopic characteristics will be noticed:

(1) The growth cuts with a grating sensation.

(2) The cut surfaces are concave.

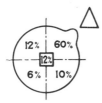

FIG. 698.—The relationship of carcinoma of the breast to the quadrants of the breast. (*Marshall and Higginbotham's statistics.*)

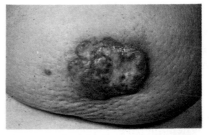

FIG. 699.—Paget's disease of the nipple. Note also the *peau d'orange* due to the underlying carcinoma.

Sir James Paget, 1814–1899. Surgeon, St. Bartholomew's Hospital, London.

(3) The colour of the cut surface is grey and may show small, granular, whitish streaks. Its appearance has been aptly likened to the interior of an unripe pear.

(4) There is no indication of a capsule, the tumour being fixed within the breast tissue.

Atrophic scirrhous carcinoma is an uncommon variant and is seen principally in aged, thin women with small breasts. The cellular element of the growth is comparatively sparse, its main constituent being the fibrous stroma. Although steadily progressive the disease runs a very chronic course, perhaps taking ten years or so to ulcerate through the skin, after which it is inclined to grow somewhat more rapidly.

Duct carcinoma may be impossible to distinguish from duct papilloma without the evidence of biopsy as both present with blood stained discharge from the nipple, though as a rule duct carcinoma is not seen below the age of 40.

Medullary carcinoma accounts for about 5% of all breast cancer and affects a somewhat earlier age group than the average. The primary tumour is soft and circumscribed, and may attain a large size. The prognosis is more favourable than for the commoner scirrhous type.

Inflammatory carcinoma (mastitis carcinomatosa) is a fortunately rare, highly aggressive cancer seen usually during pregnancy and lactation. The diseased breast is often painful—*a symptom occurring in some 10% of other breast cancers.* The reddened skin feels abnormally warm and cutaneous oedema, which indicates blockage of the subdermal lymphatics with carcinoma cells, usually extends over a considerable area, *i.e.* over one third or more of the breast. There may be retraction of the nipple. The important differential diagnosis is breast abscess and the clinical distinction may be difficult. Patients with mastitis carcinomatosa show no pyrexia or leucocytosis and oedema of the skin is usually more widespread than in abscess. The diagnosis is confirmed by biopsy.

Paget's disease of the nipple. (fig. 699) is a superficial manifestation of an underlying breast carcinoma. It presents as an eczema-like condition of the nipple and areola which persists in spite of local treatment. The nipple is eroded slowly and eventually disappears. If left an underlying carcinoma will sooner or later become clinically evident.

If eczema of the nipple or areola does not resolve after a few weeks appropriate medication, biopsy of the involved skin is essential. Microscopically Paget's disease is characterised by the presence of large, ovoid cells with abundant, clear, pale staining cytoplasm in the malpighian layer of the epidermis.

Treatment is by mastectomy and in the absence of a palpable lump in the breast the prognosis is good.

'Lipomatous' carcinoma.—True lipoma of the breast is extremely rare. However a scirrhous carcinoma may sometimes contract a covering of soft breast and subcutaneous tissue around itself to mimic a lipoma. It is therefore extremely dangerous to diagnose lipoma of the breast without histological proof.

CLINICAL STAGING OF CARCINOMA OF THE BREAST

When the patient is first examined, instead of categorising the growth in such vague terms as 'early', 'moderately advanced', or 'advanced', it is highly desirable to have some conventional method of expressing, in an explicit manner, the stage which has been reached. Not only does this provide a reasonably accurate indication of prognosis but it also provides a basis by which results of treatment can be compared. It is a prerequisite of any staging method that it must be accurate, and symptomless metastasis must be searched for by careful clinical examination and special investigations. The most valuable and least expensive screening tests are a standard chest x-ray and a serum alkaline phosphatase and gamma glutamine transaminase (gamma GT). Isotope scanning of the skeleton is often added (fig. 700); it is more sensitive than standard skeletal x-rays but less specific since inflammatory and degenerative conditions can produce an abnormal result. Abnormal liver function tests may be further elucidated by ultrasound or isotope scanning of the liver.

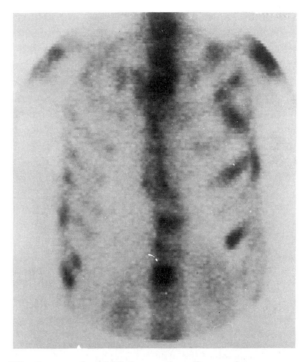

FIG. 700.—Skeletal isotope scan showing multiple 'hot spots' due to metastases.

T.N.M. Classification.—The International Union against Cancer has recommended a staging system known as T.N.M. (Tumour, Nodes, Metastases) (Chapter 8). Though this is receiving increasing acceptance, the Manchester system remains in wide use and is described here:

Stage I.—Growth confined to the breast. An area of adherence to, or ulceration of, the skin smaller than the periphery of the tumour does not affect staging. The tumour must not be adherent to the pectoral muscles or the chest wall.

Stage II.—Same as Stage I but there are affected *mobile* lymph nodes in the axilla of the same side. Clinical examination is notoriously inaccurate in assessing the significance of axillary lymph glands, for about one third of patients with no palpable glands have histological evidence of involvement and a similar proportion of patients with palpable glands have no evidence of tumour.

Stage III.—Skin involvement or *peau d'orange* larger than the tumour but still limited to the breast, tumour fixed to pectoral muscle but not to chest wall. Homolateral axillary lymph nodes matted together or fixed to chest wall, or homolateral supraclavicular nodes mobile or fixed, or oedema of the arm.

Stage IV.—Skin involvement wide of the breast and including 'cancer-encuirasse', complete fixation of tumour to chest wall, distant metastases either blood borne or lymph borne; this includes involvement of the opposite breast or axilla and deposits in bones and viscera such as lungs and liver.

PATHOLOGICAL STAGING AND PROGNOSIS OF OPERABLE BREAST CANCER

In patients with operable carcinoma of the breast (clinical stages I and II) the outlook for survival depends on a number of factors which include the size of the primary tumour and its hormone receptor status (receptor positive more favourable). The most accurate single prognostic factor however, is the *histological state of the axillary lymph nodes* as determined after surgical clearance or sampling of the axilla. Breast cancer often runs an indolent course and recurrence of metastasis may occasionally be seen as late as 20 or 30 years after treatment. For this reason it is better to consider 10-year survival data than the more usual 5-year figures for most other cancers. When the axillary nodes are free of tumour 75% of patients survive 10 years. With involvement of between 1 and 3 nodes this figure falls to 50% and when 4 or more nodes are involved only 25% are alive at 10 years. For *clinical stages* I and II the 10-year survival figures are respectively 54 and 25%. The relatively low figure for *clinical* stage I is due to the inclusion of patients whose axillary nodes are histologically positive and reflects the inaccuracy of clinical assessment of the axilla.

Prognosis in inoperable breast cancer (clinical stages III and IV).—The prospects of survival in these patients are extremely poor. Only 5% of women with stage III disease survive ten years. Survival for stage IV is close to zero.

PHENOMENA RESULTING FROM LYMPHATIC OBSTRUCTION IN LATE MAMMARY CARCINOMA

Peau d'orange is due to cutaneous lymphatic oedema. Where the infiltrated skin is tethered by the sweat ducts it cannot swell. The characteristic pitted appearance, so well likened to orange peel by French observers, has become a classical physical sign of advanced carcinoma of the breast. But it should be remembered that occasionally the same phenomenon is seen over an abscess, particularly a chronic abscess, of the breast.

Late oedema of the arm (*syn.* elephantiasis chirurgens) is a troublesome complication of surgery for breast cancer, especially when radical dissection of the axillary nodes is combined with radiotherapy to the axilla. The swelling appears at a time varying from several months to many years after operation, often without an obvious precipitating cause, though tumour recurrence must be excluded. The oedematous limb is susceptible to bacterial infections following quite minor trauma. These require vigorous and protracted antibiotic treatment since organisms tend to linger in the stagnant lymphatics. The treatment of late oedema is unsatisfactory. An elastic arm stocking is sometimes helpful, especially if the oedema can be reduced initially by elevation of the limb or the use of a pneumatic compression device. Diuretics are of little value.

Brawny arm can result from advanced neoplastic infiltration or unremoved or incompletely removed axillary or supraclavicular lymph nodes. The oedema, which is persistent and brawny (it does not pit), is due to lymphatic blockage, but in some cases venous obstruction is a contributory cause.

A forequarter amputation is merciful in selected cases, especially in order to relieve the intense pain caused by involvement of nerves in the axilla.

Cancer-en-Cuirasse.—Here, sometimes accompanied by a brawny arm, the chest wall is studded with carcinomatous nodules and the skin is so infiltrated that it has been likened to a coat of armour. Usually, though not necessarily, the condition appears in cases with local recurrence after mastectomy. Occasionally it is seen to follow the distribution of irradiation to the chest wall and axilla. The condition may respond to systemic treatment with hormones or cytotoxic agents. If these fail palliative measures to relieve pain and mental distress are prescribed; the prognosis for life is poor.

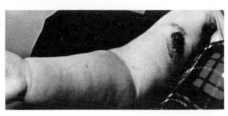

FIG. 701.—Lymphangiosarcoma developed 3 years after radical mastectomy. Patient well 6 years after forequarter amputation.
(R. P. Singh, FRCS, Karchana, India.)

Lymphangiosarcoma (fig. 701) is a rare complication of post-mastectomy lymph-oedema with an onset many years following the original surgery. It takes the form of multiple, subcutaneous nodules in the upper limb and must be distinguished from recurrent carcinoma of the breast. The prognosis is poor but some cases respond to cytotoxic therapy or irradiation. Interscapulo-thoracic (forequarter) amputation is sometimes indicated.

TREATMENT OF CANCER OF THE BREAST

The treatment of breast cancer is determined primarily by the stage of the disease. The factors affecting prognosis considered above indicate that the outlook is to a major extent influenced by the stage at which the patient first presents. In clinical stages I and II, where the surgeon plays a major role, eradication of local disease can be curative, especially when the axillary nodes are shown to be histologically free, and is therefore all important. At the other end of the spectrum in stage IV, cancer is manifestly widespread; systemic treatment must be considered though the value of locally directed therapy to control disease in the breast and regional nodes, and *e.g.* isolated bone metastases must not be overlooked. In stage III the local extent of disease usually rules out the possibility of curative surgery and although blood borne metastases are not yet detectable the low survival figures indicate that small subclinical deposits are almost always present.

Operable breast cancer (stages I and II)

Considerable argument and confusion exists regarding the management of disease at these potentially curable stages. Some authorities advocate surgical operations of varying magnitude, some irradiation and others a combination of surgery and irradiation. The continuing persistence of this controversy suggests that there is more than one 'correct' method of management. It is essential therefore to have a clear concept of the aims of treatment which are:

(1) To ensure long-term control of disease in the breast (local) and lymph node (regional) areas.

(2) As far as is consistent with 1 to conserve (or restore) local form and function.

(3) To prevent, *if possible*, the evolution of those occult metastases known to be present in a proportion of patients, no matter how thorough the staging.

The weapons available for loco-regional control are surgery and irradiation, alone or in combination. The basis of the surgical attack has for many years been radical mastectomy or one of its modifications; its aim is to remove the entire breast in continuity with radical dissection of the axillary contents. The classical radical mastectomy first described by Halsted[1] more than a hundred years ago is still widely used throughout the world and is therefore briefly described:

Radical mastectomy.—The breast and associated structures are dissected *en bloc*, and the excised mass is composed of:
1. The whole breast.
2. A large portion of skin, the centre of which overlies the tumour, but always includes the nipple. When there is much skin involvement more skin must be sacrificed.
3. The fat and fascia from the lower border of the clavicle to, and including, the upper quarter of the sheath of the rectus abdominis, and from the sternum to the anterior border of the latissimus dorsi.
4. The sternal portion of the pectoralis major and its fascial sheath.
5. The pectoralis minor and its fascial sheath.
6. The costocoracoid membrane.
7. All the fat, fascia, and lymph nodes of the axilla.
8. The fascia over, and a few of the superficial muscle fibres of, the anterior part of the external oblique, serratus anterior, the subscapularis, the exposed portion of the latissimus dorsi, and the upper part of the rectus abdominis (fig. 702).
During the operation every effort should be made to preserve:
1. The axillary vein.
2. The cephalic vein.
3. The long thoracic nerve of Bell (nerve to serratus anterior).
The middle or long subscapular nerve (nerve to latissimus dorsi) can be sacrificed without ill effect, and this should be done without hesitation if its division enables a more thorough dissection to be carried out.
At the completion of the operation, the wound is drained preferably using wide-bore suction tubes.
If a wide area of skin has been sacrificed, it may not be possible to approximate the skin edges completely. A deficiency is left which is treated by immediate or subsequent skin grafting.
After operation the arm is supported upon a pillow until the wound has healed, when early movement of the arm is encouraged. The movements of the arm after so extensive a loss of muscle are surprisingly good.
Patey operation. A popular modification of the Halsted operation is that devised by Patey in which total mastectomy is performed in continuity with radical axillary dissection but the pectoralis major muscle is conserved with resulting improvement in appearance and function.

While the results of radical mastectomy in terms of local control and survival have not been surpassed by any other method, the operation can be criticised on the following grounds:

(*a*) It ignores the internal mammary chain of lymph nodes which are involved especially when the primary tumour lies in the central area or medial quadrants of the breast. Extended radical mastectomy to include the internal mammary chain has been tried but does not improve survival.

(*b*) It overtreats the axilla when these nodes are uninvolved. The inaccuracy of clinical assessment of the axilla has already been referred to as have the complications of oedema of the upper limb and stiffness of the shoulder in some patients after radical axillary dissection. It must, however, be emphasised that axillary clearance is the only secure method of controlling metastatic nodes which are large enough to be clinically palpable.

---

[1] William Stewart Halsted, 1852–1922, Professor of Surgery, Johns Hopkins University, Baltimore, was responsible for evolving the radical amputation of the breast as performed today. The operation is often known as 'a complete Halsted'.

Sir Charles Bell, 1774–1842. Surgeon, Middlesex Hospital, London, and founder of its Medical School.
David Howard Patey, 1899–1976. Surgeon, The Middlesex Hospital, London.

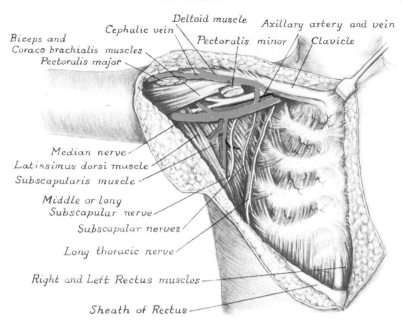

Biceps and
Coraco brachialis muscles
Pectoralis major
Cephalic vein
Deltoid muscle
Pectoralis minor
Axillary artery and vein
Clavicle

Median nerve
Latissimus dorsi muscle
Subscapularis muscle
Middle or long
Subscapular nerve
Subscapular nerves
Long thoracic nerve
Right and Left Rectus muscles
Sheath of Rectus

FIG. 702.—Radical mastectomy completed.

Simple mastectomy.—This means complete removal of the breast but the axilla is left undisturbed except for the region of the axillary tail which usually has attached to it a few nodes low in the anterior group. This operation controls the primary site and is adequate for regional control provided the axillary nodes contain no deposits. In view of the inaccuracy of clinical assessment of the axilla simple mastectomy should be combined with either:

(*a*) Scrupulous clinical follow-up; the axilla is dissected if nodes subsequently appear.
or:

(*b*) Post-operative irradiation to the axilla—which will unnecessarily treat a proportion of patients whose nodes are clear.
or:

(*c*) Surgical sampling of the lower axillary nodes as a guide to prognosis and to the need for additional radiotherapy if positive.

Can the breast be conserved?—Because of the mutilation of mastectomy which causes severe emotional upset in some women conservative surgery for patients with stage I carcinomas of small size (up to 2–3 cm), removing only the palpable tumour and a varying amount of apparently normal surrounding breast, has been under trial in many parts of the world. Such surgery alone is insufficient for local control because the primary lesion may have microscopic extensions beyond its visible margins and histological studies of mastectomy specimens show multi-focal cancers widespread throughout the breast in up to 40% of cases. Conservative surgery should therefore be followed by radiotherapy to the entire remaining breast. Axillary sampling at the time of excision of the primary will again guide prognosis and indicate the possible need for axillary irradiation. Such patients require very careful follow-up because a few develop late local recurrence within the breast which, if detected early, can still be controlled by mastectomy.

The results of this method of treatment, in terms both of local control of disease and survival, are equal to those of radical mastectomy. It must, however, be emphasised that breast conservation requires expert radiotherapy and suitable equipment. If these are not available, attempts at breast conservation are inadvisable.

The role of radiotherapy.—It can be seen that in the local/regional management of operable breast cancer radiotherapy and surgery are often complementary. Where conservative surgery is practised radiotherapy plays a major role treating those areas which are not included in the operative field, *i.e.* the remaining breast and regional nodes. After simple mastectomy radiotherapy to the axilla may be indicated as discussed above. After radical mastectomy the axilla does not require irradiation which is usually confined to those lymph node areas not included in the standard surgical field, *i.e.* the internal mammary and supraclavicular. The skin flaps are sometimes also irradiated if the primary tumour is large or tethered to the skin. Post-operative irradiation does not improve survival but it does reduce the incidence of local recurrence. Fears that radiotherapy might decrease survival by depressing the patient's immunity have not been confirmed.

Breast reconstruction.—Advances in the manufacture of breast prostheses and in the design of skin flaps have made it possible in highly selected cases to reconstruct the excised breast either at the time of mastectomy or at a later date should the patient not adjust to her deformity.

The problem of occult metastases.—The disappointing incidence of late blood borne metastases after successful local management of operable breast cancer, especially in the node-positive case, has led to trials of *adjuvant chemotherapy* in this latter high risk group. This is started immediately following completion of the primary treatment and continued for approximately one year. For pre-menopausal women, a combination of the cytotoxic drugs, cyclophosphamide, methotrexate and 5-fluorouracil has been used. For post-menopausal women the anti-oestrogen, tamoxifen has been given. A modest but definite prolongation of disease-free interval and of survival has now been established, though treatment is expensive and, in the case of the cytotoxic agents, toxic to the patient.

The present position in the management of operable breast cancer can be summarised as follows:

(1) *Radical mastectomy* (and the oncologically equivalent but less mutilating Patey modification) has stood the test of time as method of loco-regional control against which less extensive surgical procedures must be measured. Post-operative irradiation in selected cases improves local control but not survival.

(2) *Simple mastectomy and radiotherapy* offers equivalent control over prolonged periods of observation. Simple mastectomy with a watching policy for the axilla shows similar survival trends so far but has not been studied sufficiently long for universal acceptance.

(3) *Conservative surgery* is of established value in selected early cases. It demands highly skilled radiotherapy and scrupulous follow-up so that in the event of local failure salvage mastectomy can be performed without delay. Post mastectomy breast reconstruction, immediate or delayed, also calls for strict selection and special skills.

(4) There is a striking similarity in survival statistics whichever local method of treatment is used. The common factor in determining these figures is the stage

of disease at presentation. Prognosis is best predicted by the axillary node status as determined by axillary dissection or sampling. This allows the recognition of high risk patients for whom adjuvant systemic therapy can be given.

The Treatment of Locally Inoperable Carcinoma of the Breast.—In the presence of *peau d'orange*, matted or fixed axillary nodes (= transcapsular spread of tumour) or supraclavicular node involvement, even the most radical surgical operation will fail to encompass the disease and incision through the microscopically permeated tissues will often be followed by a condition worse than the original. For these patients the local treatment of choice is radiotherapy to the breast and lymph node areas. Sometimes the most advanced carcinomas will respond dramatically with disappearance of all palpable disease and healing of malignant ulceration. If the response to irradiation is substantial but incomplete selected patients may benefit from resection or residual disease, usually simple mastectomy. There is also a place for systemic treatment (see below) in some cases.

While most patients at this locally advanced stage will manifest metastases and die within a few years a small but unpredictable group will survive in good health for a considerable length of time.

Screening for Breast Cancer

Because the prognosis of breast cancer is closely related to stage at diagnosis, population screening programmes have been established in some centres in order to detect tumours before they come to the patient's notice. Women can be taught self-examination of the breasts but the most accurate screening method is the combination of careful clinical palpation by a trained observer, with mammography. Some palpable carcinomas are not visible on the mammogram and conversely mammography sometimes detects an impalpable carcinoma in its pre-clinical stage.

There is no doubt that a screened population yields patients with smaller primary tumours and a lesser degree of lymph node involvement as compared with an unscreened group. There has been uncertainty whether the resulting increase in survival from the time of *treatment* of these earlier stage patients represents a true benefit or whether such increase is simply equal to the period of clinical latency before diagnosis in the unscreened patient (so called lead time bias). The results of recent trials do suggest a survival advantage for screened women.

The disadvantages of population screening are expense and the possible hazard of repeated exposure of the breast to diagnostic x-rays; the latter danger is minimised by special low-dose equipment. Selective screening is specially indicated in high risk groups of women, *e.g.* those with a strong family history of breast cancer, and in the remaining breast following mastectomy where the cumulative incidence of a second carcinoma is approximately 1% per annum after the initial treatment.

The effects of pregnancy after radical mastectomy for carcinoma are unknown but most surgeons advise against having children within 3 years of operation. Similarly the use of small doses of oestrogens for menopausal symptoms or the contraceptive 'pill' may accelerate the growth of any remaining tumour tissue.

THE TREATMENT OF METASTATIC CARCINOMA OF THE BREAST

When the disease is widespread systemic treatment is indicated, though as has been mentioned local treatment is valuable for troublesome isolated deposits, *e.g.* excision of skin nodules, irradiation to painful bony deposits, internal fixation of pathological fractures *etc*.

Systemic therapy may be endocrine or cytotoxic:

Endocrine therapy

Some breast cancers respond to manipulation of their hormonal milieu by the administration of hormones or by ablation of endocrine glands. They are said to be hormone responsive (hormone dependent). Others unfortunately are autonomous (hormone independent).

1. **Hormone Responsive.**—About 30% of mammary carcinomas are hormone responsive; that is to say that their growth is controlled partly by one or more of the hormones involved in normal mammogenesis. When their hormonal milieu is altered to one that is disadvantageous to their continued growth they cease to proliferate or metastasise and many of their component cells perish. Unfortunately this regression following hormone manipulation is never permanent.

2. **Autonomous.**—The remaining 70% of carcinomas are composed of cells which require no hormonal stimulus to enable them to thrive, multiply and metastasise. Alteration of the hormonal status has an insignificant effect and usually no effect at all on tumour growth. Even if carcinomas belonging to group one are deprived of the hormone or hormones that stimulate them, after a varying number of months or years they, too, become autonomous.

Although the fact that some breast carcinomas are hormone responsive has been known for about seventy years, there is still no direct evidence as to which hormone or group of hormones is responsible. It has always been presumed that the term hormone responsive was synonymous with oestrogen responsive and that these cancers would cease to thrive if they were deprived of naturally occurring oestrogens. Indeed, most of the endocrine treatments for advanced cancer were aimed at those organs (*i.e.* the ovaries and adrenal glands) that are able to secrete oestrogens. During the past few years, however, since methods have become available for the accurate estimation of steroid hormones and their metabolites and of pituitary hormones it has become apparent that the problem is complex. Attempts to define hormone responsiveness in terms of the pattern of hormone levels in the blood or urine have so far been unhelpful. More recently methods of looking for oestrogen receptors in tumour cells or of examining the direct effect of various hormones on tumour cell cultures have been more hopeful in providing an answer. At the present state of our knowledge, however, treatment is still on an empirical basis, and although it has been found that certain combinations of sequences of drugs have a beneficial effect, we still do not know why this is so.

Major Endocrine Ablation.—After the synthesis of cortisone in the early 1950's it became possible to undertake the operation of bilateral total adrenalectomy. This removed an important source of extra ovarian oestrogen and was a valuable method of treatment for hormone dependent breast cancer in the post-menopausal patient or in premenopausal women following oöphorectomy. The adrenals were removed either via bilateral loin incisions or using the anterior route through a long vertical or transverse incision.

Removal of the pituitary gland (hypophysectomy) produced similar effects due to loss of trophic hormones controlling ovaries and adrenals and possibly also to loss of prolactin. The pituitary can be ablated either surgically or by the introduction of radioactive seeds into the pituitary fossa via a trocar and cannula inserted through the nose under radiographic control.

Bilateral adrenalectomy and hypophysectomy have been largely rendered obsolete by pharmacological advances in hormonal agents.

Oöphorectomy.—This was the first treatment designed to affect the endocrine status of patients with advanced carcinoma of the breast. It was first described in 1896 by Sir George Beatson, of the Western Infirmary in Glasgow, who published an account of two cases treated in this manner. Oöphorectomy or ovarian irradiation is still used extensively as a treatment of recurrent or advanced breast cancer and is beneficial in approximately 20–30% of cases. It is of value only before the menopause and the remission so produced can last up to two years or longer.

Androgens.—The administration of androgens probably accomplishes the same as an oöphorectomy although it could be argued that the former would also counteract the adrenal secretion of oestrogens. The remission rate and duration of remission are similar for the two forms of treatment. Administration is usually by injection, either in the form of testosterone propionate, 100 mg three times a week intramuscularly or one of the anabolic steroids, such as Durabolin 50 mg once a week intramuscularly. The great disadvantage of this form of treatment is the incidence of virilisation which, if severe, can be most distressing. With Durabolin, which has a more powerful anabolic and weaker androgenic effect, the incidence of side-effects is greatly diminished, and only a problem in 10 to 20% of cases. Androgens can be administered to all age groups, but are usually considered the treatment of choice for patients who are pre-menopausal or within five years of the menopause.

Oestrogens.—Although the prescription of oestrogens may seem contradictory to the theories of hormone responsiveness, it is an effective treatment. It should not be given unless the woman is more than five years postmenopausal. The response to the drug increases with age and may reach 60% in women over seventy. Overall the remission rate is approximately 40%. Side-effects do occur however; nausea and vomiting may be troublesome in the early stages and usually subside in time. Fluid retention and vaginal bleeding are a more persistent problem and if severe may mean that the treatment has to be stopped altogether or an alternative type of oestrogen used. Stilboestrol is the most commonly used agent, dose 1·0 mg t.d.s. There is no proof of increased benefit from higher doses sometimes recommended.

Antioestrogens.—Tamoxifen acts by competition at the cellular level and appears to be effective in both pre and post menopausal women. It has few significant side effects and is considered the agent of first choice. The usual dose is 20 mg daily. Since the introduction of Tamoxifen, androgens and oestrogens are much less often used; apart from the side effects mentioned they may also occasionally cause provocation of the disease, the most dangerous manifestation being acute hypercalcaemia.

Aminoglutethimide.—This drug produces a 'medical adrenalectomy' by blocking adrenal steroid systhesis through inhibition of the enzymatic conversion of cholesterol to pregnenolone; added glucocorticoid is required. The value of prolactin blocking drugs has so far been disappointing.

Progestogens.—Synthetic progestogens, *e.g.* medroxyprogesterone acetate, are also valuable in some hormone dependent breast cancers.

Cytotoxic Therapy

Fifty to 60% of patients with disseminated breast cancer respond to cytotoxic drugs though the duration of response is usually short. Combinations of drugs are more effective than single agents, among the most useful of which are cyclophosphamide, methotrexate, 5-fluorouracil, adriamycin and vincristine. The toxic side effects include nausea and vomiting, bone marrow depression and loss of hair.

Choice of systemic therapy.—Endocrine manipulation produces less unpleasant and dangerous side effects than cytotoxic agents, and the duration of response is usually longer. The likelihood of response to hormones is increased with increasing age; when the tempo of disease is slow (long free interval between treatment of primary and onset of metastases); when oestrogen receptors are present in significant amount; and when metastases are skeletal. For pre-menopausal women the first line of approach is ovarian ablation, surgical or radiotherapeutic. After the menopause Tamoxifen is the initial treatment of choice.

Cytotoxic therapy is more likely to be effective than endocrine in younger

Sir George Thomas Beatson, 1848–1933. Surgeon, Western Infirmary, Glasgow, Scotland.

patients; when the tempo of disease is fast; when oestrogen receptors are absent; and when there are visceral metastases.

THE 'FOLLOW-UP' OF CASES OF CARCINOMA OF THE BREAST

It is the duty of the surgeon to examine all his cases periodically for life, so that in event of recurrence he can inaugurate such treatment as is applicable without delay. The following indicates a routine suitable for this periodic examination:

History.—This includes an inquiry as to the physical energy, general health, and the presence of an unexplained cough. Symptoms that the patient usually ascribes to rheumatism, lumbago or sciatica (humerus, spine or femur) must be regarded with suspicion, for often skeletal metastases announce themselves in this way.

Examination.—The operation field is examined for nodules. The axillae, supraclavicular lymph nodes, and opposite breast[1] are palpated. The hand and arm are examined for oedema. The chest is percussed and auscultated and the abdomen examined for evidence of enlarged liver or ascites. If considered necessary, a rectal or vaginal examination is made in order to detect pelvic or ovarian metastases.

Radiography.—Regular annual mammography of the remaining breast and a routine radiographic examination of the chest are a valuable part of the follow-up. Further investigations, e.g. skeletal isotope scanning or x-rays, may be indicated according to the patient's symptoms.

THE MALE BREAST

Mastitis of puberty is discussed on p. 717.

Mastitis from local irritation is by no means rare in men; in civil life it usually occurs from wearing ill-fitting braces. It is not uncommon among soldiers carrying heavy equipment across their shoulders. The treatment is to remove the cause; substitution of a belt for braces is sound advice.

Gynaecomazia.—(*a*) *Idiopathic*.—Hypertrophy of the male breast may be unilateral or bilateral. The breasts enlarge at puberty, and sometimes present the characteristics of a well-developed female organ (fig. 703).

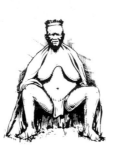

FIG. 703.—Chief Chengwayo, from a photograph by Schujelot.

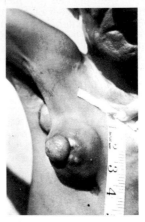

FIG. 704.—Carcinoma of the male breast.
(*Dr. Y. V. Shah, Vamnagar, India.*)

(*b*) *Hormonal*.—Enlargement of the breasts often accompanies stilboestrol therapy, *e.g.* for carcinoma of the prostate (Chapter 59); it may also occur as a result of a teratoma of the testis, in anorchism, and after castration. Rarely it may be a feature of ectopic hormonal production in a bronchial carcinoma and in adrenal or pituitary disease.

(*c*) *Associated with Leprosy*.—Gynaecomazia is very common in male persons suffering from leprosy. Possibly this is the result of bilateral testicular atrophy, which is a frequent accompaniment of leprosy (Bowesman).

---

[1] A few surgeons recommend early simple mastectomy on the contralateral breast because 7·5% of patients with carcinoma of the breast develop carcinoma in the contralateral breast.

Charles Bowesman, Contemporary. Formerly Surgical Specialist, lately Colonial Medical Service, Kumasi, Ghana.

(d) *Associated with Liver Failure.*—Gynaecomazia sometimes occurs in patients with cirrhosis due to failure of the liver to metabolise oestrogens.

(e) May occur in patients with *Klinefelter's syndrome* (a sexual anomaly giving a chromatin positive male and infertility). Certain drugs such as digitalis, spironolactone, cimetidine and isoniazid may also cause gynaecomazia.

Treatment.—Provided the patient is healthy and comparatively young, the treatment of idiopathic gynaecomazia is mastectomy with preservation of the nipple and areola, for their absence is subject to ridicule.

Mammary Dysplasia and Fibroadenoma are not unusual and present the same clinical features as in the female.

Carcinoma of the male breast (fig. 704) accounts for less than 1% of all cases of breast cancer. The known predisposing causes include gynaecomazia and disease associated with excess oestrogen (see (b), (c), (d) and (e) above). Presenting as a palpable lump in most cases in an age range from young to very old men it follows the same course as in the female. While it is expected that at presentation it is likely to be in the late stages (Manchester—above), because the breast is small and extramammary tissues are invaded early, this is not necessarily so and many patients are in stage I of the disease. The growth tends to be an infiltrating duct carcinoma.

Treatment.—Stage for stage the treatment is as for carcinoma in the female (see section above). Bilateral orchidectomy is the equivalent of oöphorectomy, but a higher proportion of men respond than women. Tamoxifen is proving to be the best hormonal agent and to be the treatment advised in the inoperable case, and always when orchidectomy is refused. The prognosis depends on the stage. The younger patient tends to come for help earlier than the older patient, to better effect. Because of the small size of the male breast, adequate local excision frequently results in a 'mastectomy'.

Other Tumours of the Breast

Lipoma.—A true lipoma is very rare (*cf.* lipomatous carcinoma p. 728).

Sarcoma of the breast is usually of the spindle-celled variety, and accounts for 0·5% of malignant tumours of the breast. Some of these growths arise in an intracanalicular fibroadenoma. It may be impossible to distinguish clinically a sarcoma of the breast from a medullary carcinoma, but areas of cystic degeneration suggest the probability of sarcoma. On incising the neoplasm its pale, friable consistency is characteristic. Sarcoma of the breast is met with most often in women between the ages of thirty and forty. Treatment is by simple mastectomy followed by radiotherapy. The prognosis depends on the stage and the histological type.

Metastases.—On rare occasions cancer elsewhere may present with a metastasis in the breast. The breast is also occasionally infiltrated by Hodgkin's disease (lymphoma) and other lymphomas.

Edmund William Klinefelter, Contemporary. Radiologist, Massachusetts General Hospital, Boston, Mass., U.S.A.

CHAPTER 40

THE THORAX

ANATOMY OF THE BRONCHIAL TREE

A thorough knowledge of the anatomy of the bronchial tree is essential, not only for the diagnosis of many chest conditions, but for the planning and execution of the majority of pulmonary operations.

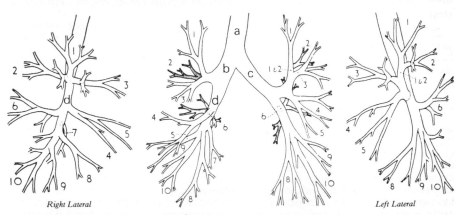

Right Lateral   Left Lateral

FIG. 705.—The bronchial tree with internationally adopted nomenclature.

RIGHT LUNG

1. Apical ⎫
2. Posterior ⎬ Upper Lobe.
3. Anterior ⎭
4. Lateral ⎫
5. Medial ⎬ Middle Lobe.
6. Apical ⎫
7. Medial (Cardiac):) ⎪
8. Anterior basal ⎬ Lower Lobe.
9. Lateral basal ⎪
10. Posterior basal ⎭

LEFT LUNG

1. Apical ⎫
2. Posterior ⎪
3. Anterior ⎬ Upper Lobe.
4. Superior lingular ⎪
5. Inferior lingular ⎭
6. Apical ⎫
8. Anterior basal ⎬ Lower Lobe.
9. Lateral basal ⎪
10. Posterior basal ⎭
(Segment 7 is absent in the left lung).

(a) Trachea, (b) R. main bronchus, (c) L. main bronchus, (d) Intermediate bronchus.

Fig. 705 illustrates the common pattern of the bronchial tree. Each bronchus is accompanied by a branch of the pulmonary artery and together they form a broncho-vascular pedicle supplying conical segments of lung tissue. The pulmonary veins lie between the segments with tributaries issuing from adjacent segments. Each segment is largely an independent unit which can be removed (segmental resection) without inter-fering with adjacent segments. The veins indicate the true position of the intersegmental plane, which must be followed accurately during the operation. Two or more bronchial arteries on each side enter the lung in the areolar tissue surrounding the bronchi. They arise from the descending thoracic aorta and supply the broncho-pulmonary tissues with arterialised blood. They develop links with the smaller pulmonary vessels which, in certain diseases, may enlarge considerably.

The trachea and main bronchi with their lobar and first segmental divisions can all be examined visually by bronchoscopy. This investigation will demonstrate abnormalities in size (stenosis, obstruction or dilatation), movement (immobility or spasm), shape or position. The examination may also reveal the presence of a tumour or an intrabronchial foreign body. Material for biopsy and secretions for cytological or bacteriological examination can be obtained. Only the proximal parts of the bronchial tree can be examined with the rigid bronchoscope even with the aid of a telescope. The flexible or fibreoptic bronchoscope can be introduced much farther into the bronchial tree and permits examination and biopsy of peripheral lesions. Biopsy under fluoroscopic control is useful.

A more detailed anatomical study can be made by bronchography, which consists of the introduction of radio-opaque material (iodised oil) into the bronchial tree. An attempt is made to fill all the branches of the bronchial tree on one side, and radiographs are taken in two or more planes. Bronchography provides information about the size and distribution of the bronchi, and will also demonstrate bronchial occlusion or narrowing.

Developmental Anomalies.—The trachea develops as a bud from the primitive foregut which soon divides into two main branches—the right and left main bronchus. Each bronchus continues to develop by branching so that all generations are present by the sixteenth week of intrauterine life. A fully developed segment has approximately 20 to 25 generations of branches. Failure of a main bronchus to develop results in *unilateral agenesis*, whilst failure of a lobar bronchus to develop produces *lobar agenesis*. Subsequent aberrations of development result in variations of the segmental pattern. Each developing bronchial bud becomes closely associated with the future pulmonary artery which covers its surface. Failure to link up with the pulmonary artery system occurs occasionally. In this case, ectopic bronchial buds develop anomalously, producing a mass of bronchial elements which often lose their connections with the parent bronchi. Vascular supply is derived direct from the descending aorta. In adult life the condition presents as a bizarre cystic mass, usually lying in the posterior aspect of the lower lobe with large systemic arteries the size of the radial artery or even larger entering the mass through the pulmonary ligament—*intralobar sequestration*. Infection of the cystic spaces is common and is the usual cause of symptoms. Removal of the lower lobe with the offending mass is recommended.

LUNG FUNCTION

The pulmonary alveoli allow the blood and inspired air almost to come into contact across the alveolar wall membrane. This enables the blood to take up oxygen from the air and discharge carbon dioxide into it, thus maintaining the normal levels of these gases in the lung. Any disturbance of this mechanism may, if severe enough, lead to changes in the blood gases.

Blood gas and pH determinations measure overall function. Measurement of the *mechanics of ventilation* (chest expansion, vital capacity, forced vital capacity) determine the patient's ability to ventilate. The movements of air in the tracheobronchial tree and of blood in the pulmonary vasculature can be determined by lung scanning with either inhaled (ventilation) or injected (perfusion) radioactive xenon. In this way the relationship between ventilation and perfusion (*ventilationperfusion ratio*) can be worked out. An outline of the pulmonary vascularity can be obtained with radio-opaque diatrizoate injected into the right ventricle (*pulmonary angiography*). Both lung scanning and pulmonary angiography are useful in the diagnosis of pulmonary embolism.

TECHNIQUE OF THORACOTOMY

The standard postero-lateral thoracotomy is through the bed of the 5th rib. The skin incision commences halfway between the midpoint of the vertebral border of the scapula

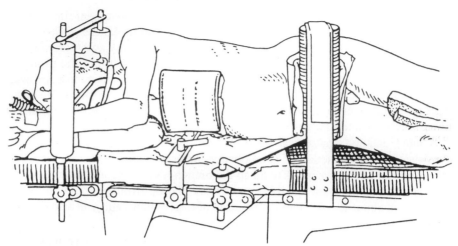

FIG. 706.—Anterior view of position for left posterolateral thoracotomy. Note position of chest and
pelvic supports.
(Reproduced from Hurt & Bates (1986) "Essentials of Thoracic Surgery", by permission of Butterworth & Co. Ltd.)

and the midline, extends forward 3–4 cm below the inferior angle of the scapula to the
anterior axillary line at the level of the 5th rib (figs 706 & 707). The superficial muscles
(latissimus dorsi and trapezius) are divided, deep to which are the serratus anterior anteriorly and the rhomboids posteriorly—parts of both these muscles are divided though the
serratus anterior may often be retracted and not divided. The periosteum is stripped from
the upper border of the rib and the rib bed and pleura are incised to allow a rib spreader
to be inserted. It is not necessary to resect a rib though if desired 3 cm of the posterior
end of a rib above or below the incision may be resected to improve the exposure, which
can also be facilitated by extending the incision further forward.

Before closing the chest one or two drains (apical for air and basal for fluid) are inserted
through separate stab incisions below the level of the thoracotomy incision and connected
to suction through an underwater seal (fig. 708). The ribs are brought together with an
approximator and the rib bed closed with a continuous 2/o nylon suture placed through
the intercostal muscles parallel to the rib above and below the incision, taking care not to
encircle the intercostal nerve as this would lead to persistent post-thoracotomy pain.
The muscles and skin are closed with continuous sutures of catgut and prolene or silk
respectively.

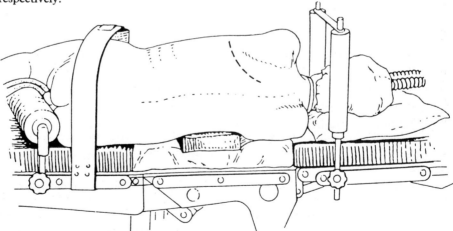

FIG. 707.—Posterior view of position for left posterolateral thoracotomy. Note position of pad under
patient's right chest.
(Reproduced from Hurt & Bates (1986) "Essentials of Thoracic Surgery", by permission of Butterworth & Co. Ltd.)

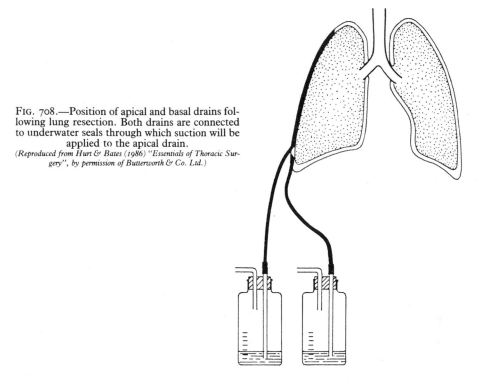

Fig. 708.—Position of apical and basal drains following lung resection. Both drains are connected to underwater seals through which suction will be applied to the apical drain.
(Reproduced from Hurt & Bates (1986) "Essentials of Thoracic Surgery", by permission of Butterworth & Co. Ltd.)

INJURIES TO THE CHEST

Apart from road accidents and stab-wounds chest injuries are not common in civil practice; in war, however, they constitute nearly 10% of all wounds, whilst of those killed in battle, 25% have chest injuries. They are often associated with injuries elsewhere, particularly the head and abdomen. Two main varieties are encountered—crush injuries and wounds—although in any particular patient both may be present.

Crush Injuries

These are common both in war and in civilian practice. The injury may be produced by a localised blow or a more extensive crushing force. Road accidents frequently result in severe crush injuries. Similar injuries can also be produced by concussion waves from explosions conveyed either through air or water (blast injuries).

The injuries may produce contusion of the chest wall, rib fractures, a stove-in chest, a flail chest, lung contusion or laceration, aortic rupture or myocardial damage.

Effects of a crush injury depend on its severity and the extent of involvement of chest wall, pleura and lung. The more severe forms interfere seriously with ventilation and coughing either from pain or from instability or deformity of the chest wall. The presence of blood or secretions in the bronchial tree makes ventilation still less effective. Respiration may, in addition, be depressed further by an associated head injury.

The serious interference with ventilation results in rapid and shallow respiration with cyanosis, tachycardia and hypotension. Respiration may be noisy from tracheo-bronchial secretions. Milder degrees of hypoxia produce cerebral confusion and restlessness, and this is followed by unconsciousness in severe cases.

Management in the early stages depends on a careful assessment of the damage. The chest wall is examined for paradoxical movement (multiple fractured ribs), depressions (stove-in chest) or sucking wounds. The posterior aspect of the chest should be examined as the patient is gently rolled on one side. The position of the mediastinum (trachea and apex beat) provides useful information concerning the presence of a pneumothorax, a haemothorax or massive collapse of the lung. An early chest x-ray is imperative for accurate diagnosis of the intrathoracic damage.

Early Treatment is directed at improving ventilation by the following means where indicated:

(1) Relief of pain with repeated small doses of morphine or other analgesics, or intercostal nerve block.

(2) Stabilisation of the chest wall: (*a*) strapping can be used in mild cases and temporarily in emergencies; (*b*) internal fixation of fractured ribs by wire or nails for more severe cases.

(3) Removal of pleural blood or air should they be large enough to compress the lung. Simple aspiration may be sufficient, but rapid reaccumulation may demand an indwelling tube or thoracotomy.

(4) Removal of tracheo-bronchial secretions may be effected by coughing after relief of pain. Bronchoscopic aspiration may be required but if secretions persist suction through an endotracheal tube or a tracheostomy is advisable.

(5) Repeated suction through an *endotracheal tube* or a *tracheostomy* (see also p. 639) is the most important measure in all serious cases. It permits effective and repeated aspiration of the tracheobronchial tree, eliminates the dead space of the oro-pharynx and reduces the work of respiration. If combined with intermittent positive pressure respiration (I.P.P.R.) it will eliminate paradoxical chest wall movements. Endotracheal suction will often transform the condition of a seriously ill patient. I.P.P.R. may be maintained for 10–14 days without the necessity for a tracheostomy. Repeated blood gas estimations are desirable to decide whether I.P.P.R. is required.

(6) Oxygen is usually necessary and is best administered by a mask.

(7) Blood transfusion, fluid replacement and vasopressor agents may be required to maintain the circulation.

Fractured Ribs.—(1) *Single rib fractures.* Single fractures of one or more ribs due to direct violence are a common complication of many varieties of chest trauma. The degree of pain depends on the number of ribs involved. Localised tenderness and crepitus are often elicited but the fractures may be difficult to demonstrate radiologically. Local support and analgesics are often all that are required for treatment (fig. 709). Intercostal nerve block may be required for persistent pain.

(2) *Double rib fractures.* A crushing injury of the chest will cause multiple fractures situated anteriorly and posteriorly ('stove-in' chest). This will often lead to loss of stability of the chest and paradoxical movement of the mobile portion

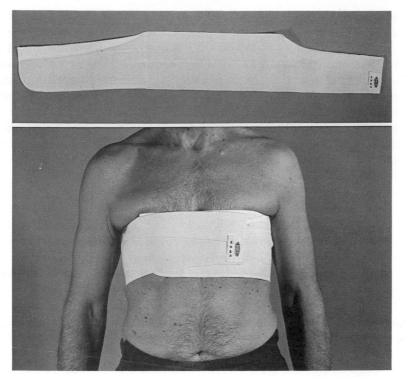

FIG. 709.—The elastic corset illustrated here is remarkably effective in reducing pain due to a fractured rib. It is frequently used in Europe and the author speaks from personal experience.

of chest wall, leading to respiratory difficulty, together with sputum and carbon dioxide retention.

(3) *Steering-wheel injury*. A particular type of injury (prevented by the wearing of seat belts) occurs in head-on car crashes, with a fracture/dislocation of the upper end of the sternum and bilateral fractures of the ribs at their anterior ends or costo-chondral junctions. This also will cause paradoxical respiration.

Treatment of 'stove-in' and flail chest.—Active treatment is essential in order to break the vicious circle of paradoxical chest wall movement leading to sputum retention, increased anoxia and increased respiratory movement and paradox.

Endotracheal intubation with positive pressure ventilation is indicated for the more severe injuries and will often control the situation. Ventilation may be required for several days until the chest wall stabilises. If ventilation is required for more than ten days a tracheostomy will be needed owing to the risks of laryngeal stenosis if an endotracheal tube is used for longer periods. Alternatively the fractured ribs may be secured with the use of stainless steel wire, intramedullary (Rush) nails or Judet clips (fig. 710) which are inserted at a formal thoracotomy in which any associated haemothorax or lung injury can also be treated. This should enable the period of artificial ventilation to be shortened or eliminated altogether.

Traumatic Pneumothorax.—Air in the pleural cavity appears commonly after many forms of trauma. In the majority it is associated with blood as well (*haemo-pneumothorax*). Air may reach the pleural cavity through a wound in the chest wall (*sucking wound*). More commonly air leaks from damaged lung; if the leak is valvular a considerable quantity of air will accumulate producing total collapse of the lung and displacement of the mediastinum towards the opposite side (*tension pneumothorax*). If the parietal pleura is damaged air may track into the subcutaneous tissues and cause *surgical emphysema*.

Sucking wounds should be sealed with an occlusive pad until definitive surgical repair can be arranged. A tension pneumothorax can be relieved in an emergency by plunging an unmounted aspirating needle into the chest which allows the air under tension to escape. Subsequently, a small soft catheter should be introduced through a cannula and connected to suction through a water seal.

Traumatic Haemothorax (see also p. 751).—Blood collects in the pleural cavity in the vast majority of chest injuries. The chest wall, lung or heart and great vessels (Chapter 41) may be the source of the bleeding. Bleeding is usually limited and should be dealt with by repeated daily aspirations after an initial interval of twenty-four hours to allow the bleeding vessel to seal. If the accumulation is large, earlier aspiration is necessary but, if progressive, a thoracotomy will be required to control the bleeding.

Pulmonary Contusion and Laceration.—The lung is injured in the majority of cases of moderate and severe trauma. Contusion results in areas of consolidation which will usually resolve spontaneously. Laceration permits the leakage of blood and air into the pleural cavity. Minor lacerations heal spontaneously, but more severe degrees produce persistent collapse of the lung and leakage of air and should be explored by thoracotomy. Secondary infection of the damaged lung is an important complication which can often be prevented by chemotherapy, bronchial aspirations and physiotherapy.

Fracture of Bronchus.—Severe crushing or deceleration injuries occasionally result in a transverse fracture of a bronchus which most commonly occurs at the origin of the more mobile left main bronchus. Total atelectasis and mediastinal surgical emphysema result. The condition can be confirmed at bronchoscopy. Early repair should result in a functioning lung, but delay will lead to irreversible infection and fibrosis.

Wounds of the Chest

These may be simple, or complicated by serious underlying visceral damage. In either case the wound may be penetrating or perforating (through and through wound). In all cases, however simple, it is necessary to exclude serious damage to either thoracic or abdominal viscera.

Simple wounds from stabs or bullets may give rise to little trouble—the external wound is small and usually clean. A haemothorax is usual and will require aspirations until the pleural cavity is dry.

Complicated wounds are common injuries with large missiles such as shell and bomb fragments and also modern high velocity bullets which produce extensive soft tissue damage (Chapter 2). This may be considerable and fragments of clothing, *etc.*, may be carried into the chest. Lung contusion and laceration is common and the mediastinal structures, the diaphragm and abdominal viscera may be involved.

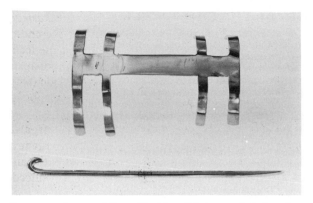
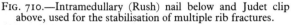

Fig. 710.—Intramedullary (Rush) nail below and Judet clip above, used for the stabilisation of multiple rib fractures.

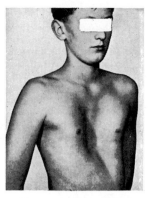

Fig. 711.—Funnel chest deformity.

Operative treatment will be required in the majority of cases, and should be carried out as soon as practicable after resuscitation. The only indication for emergency thoracotomy is uncontrollable internal or external bleeding.

Endotracheal anaesthesia is essential in order to ensure adequate ventilation and permit the removal of bronchial secretions during the operation. The chest wound is excised, rib fragments removed, and intercostal vessels ligated, if necessary. If the wound is conveniently situated, the pleural cavity can be explored through it, but if not, a separate thoracotomy is required. All blood, clot, and debris should be removed from the pleural cavity in addition to any retained foreign bodies. Lung lacerations should be sutured if small, or a formal resection carried out if more extensive. The pleural cavity should be drained through a separate stab incision. After operation it is essential that the lung should expand rapidly and completely; this is encouraged by suction drainage, breathing exercises and early ambulation.

Thoraco-abdominal Wounds.—These are always potentially serious owing to the involvement of both the abdomen and the chest; their importance depends on whether or not one of the hollow abdominal viscera is damaged. The predicted course of the missile should be considered in order to anticipate the visceral damage. Apart from serious involvement of the chest, as outlined above, the main indications for exploration are signs of persistent bleeding or evidence of involvement of a hollow viscus. The thoracic approach has the advantage of permitting correction of the thoracic injuries whilst giving adequate exposure of the upper abdomen through the diaphragm.

Shock Lung—Post-traumatic respiratory failure or shock lung may develop in 50% of patients after major trauma (Blaisdell). There is severe depression of gas exchange in the lungs due to pulmonary consolidation. Lung compliance is markedly decreased (stiff lung). Urgent treatment is required if a fatal outcome is to be avoided. Endotracheal intubation and positive pressure ventilation is instituted and large doses of steroids administered. Additionally, antibiotics and intravenous infusion are administered where indicated.

The condition is caused by micro-thrombo-embolism of small lung vessels following extensive intravascular coagulation produced by trauma. Similar changes are seen in septicaemia, after massive infusions of blood or clear fluids and following heart-lung bypass (pump lung).

F. William Blaisdell, Contemporary. Surgeon, San Francisco General Hospital.

DISEASES OF THE CHEST WALL

Kypho-scoliosis.—Deformities secondary to pleural and pulmonary disease are frequent unless preventive measures are taken; they can cause a considerable loss of pulmonary function, and may lead to repeated respiratory infections and cardiovascular disturbances. Vigorous breathing exercises can do much to prevent serious deformity provided they are initiated sufficiently early, but even in established cases some improvement can be expected. Primary kypho-scoliosis is considered in Chapter 21.

Tietze's disease is a not uncommon painful and non-suppurative swelling of the second or third costal cartilages. X-ray is negative. Reassurance and not exploration is required. Local heat will often relieve pain but injections of hydrocortisone into the perichondrium may be required to encourage resolution.

Funnel Chest (Pectus excavatum).—This deformity consists of a depression of the body of the sternum and the xiphoid process, combined with an inward curving of the costal cartilages and adjacent ribs. The deformity is usually minimal at birth, but becomes progressively more obvious during childhood. It predisposes to repeated respiratory infections and to cardiovascular disturbance, whilst the cosmetic appearances are frequently embarrassing (fig. 711).

Correction of the deformity is carried out through a transverse incision: the sternum and costal cartilages are exposed and the deformed costal cartilages are resected subperichondrially. The attachments of the diaphragm to the xiphoid process are detached and the sternum separated from the mediastinal tissues. A wedge osteotomy of the anterior table of the sternum is performed at the upper limit of the deformity, and the mobilised sternal body can then be easily elevated. The sternum should be maintained in an elevated position by a stainless steel strut which is placed beneath the sternum with the ends resting on the ribs laterally. The strut is removed after six months. The use of internal splinting has greatly improved the long-term cosmetic results.

Pigeon chest (Pectus carinatum) and other deformities may requires surgery for cosmetic reasons. The deformed ribs or cartilages should be resected.

Cold Abscess

The majority of cold abscesses of the chest wall are secondary to tuberculous intercostal lymphadenitis. A minority are associated with Pott's disease of the spine and tuberculosis of the ribs or sternum. The intercostal lymph nodes are situated posteriorly near the neck of the rib, or anteriorly in association with the internal mammary vessels. Tuberculous pus, forming in these sites, may track a considerable distance in the intercostal space before becoming subcutaneous. It usually reaches the superficial tissues by following the lateral or anterior branches of the intercostal vessels, and thus most commonly presents in the anterior axillary line or the parasternal region. The abscess has all the characteristics of a tuberculous cold abscess. Involvement of the skin and rupture is common in neglected cases, resulting in a persistent discharging sinus surrounded by typical tuberculous granulation tissue. A cold abscess must be distinguished from a lipoma or an empyema necessitatis; in the latter, the swelling is often tender and may exhibit an impulse on coughing, and is associated with the physical and radiological signs of an empyema.

The abscess should be treated by repeated aspirations through healthy skin with the instillation of streptomycin. If the abscess fails to respond to repeated aspirations, surgery will be required. The extent of the ramifications of the abscess should first be determined by the injection of iodised oil into the abscess. Ideally, the abscess and its ramifications should be completely excised, together with any underlying gland and secondarily involved bone; but if this is not practicable, the abscess should be evacuated, granulation tissue removed and the wound closed. Chronically discharging sinuses can sometimes be cured by regular

Alexander Tietze, 1864–1927. Surgeon, Breslau, Germany (now Wrocław, Poland).
Percivall Pott, 1714–1788. Surgeon, St. Bartholomew's Hospital, London.

instillations of streptomycin; alternatively, excision of the track is advisable. All patients should have a long course of chemotherapy.

Empyema Necessitatis

This is caused by an empyema perforating the chest wall and presenting with a subcutaneous collection of pus communicating, often by a tortuous channel, with the main pleural collection. The condition is seen either with a neglected or an undiagnosed empyema, or following aspirations of thin, highly infective pus from an empyema. In the latter case, the superficial tissues are infected by the seepage of pus through a needle track. The site of the subcutaneous abscess does not always correspond to the site of pleural perforation, as the abscess may track along the intercostal spaces before becoming superficial. The signs are those of a diffuse, fluctuant, tender swelling which may exhibit an impulse on coughing, and is associated with the clinical and radiological signs of an empyema. Treatment is primarily aimed at the empyema, which should be aspirated and drained. The superficial abscess may disappear as a result of aspirating the empyema, or may itself require separate aspirations or drainage.

Tumours of the Ribs

Rib tumours may be benign or malignant, and the latter either primary or secondary.

Benign tumours are frequently discovered by routine radiography. Many are symptomless and produce no external evidence of their presence. A few produce pain or an external swelling. The commonest is the chondroma (fig. 712(*a*) and (*b*)), whilst osteochondroma, multiple exostoses, fibrous dysplasia, lipoid granu-

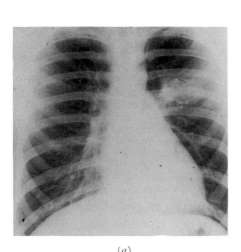 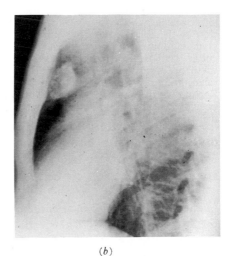

(*a*) (*b*)

FIG. 712.—(*a*) Calcifying chondroma of anterior portion of Left III rib. (*b*) Lateral view.

lomas and multiple myelomas are less common. Benign tumours usually produce expansion of the rib and are less dense radiologically than normal rib, whilst pathological fracture is rare. Malignant change can occur, especially in chondromas, and removal is advisable.

Primary malignant tumours are rare, the commonest being chondrosarcoma; they should be widely excised. Any sizeable deficiency of the thoracic cage which might result in paradoxical movement should be repaired with Marlex mesh or

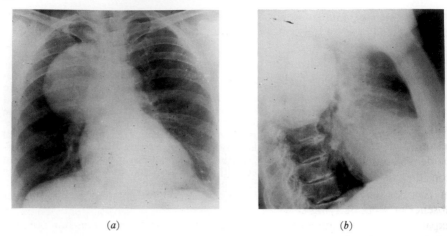

(a)   (b)

FIG. 713.—(a) Large neurofibroma of chest. (b) The lateral film shows the tumour lying posteriorly.

tantalum gauze. *Secondary deposits* in rib are particularly common in carcinoma of the lung and with breast cancer. The deposits are almost always painful and tender. They result in destruction of bone, and pathological fracture is common. X-ray therapy will usually relieve the pain.

Neurogenic Tumours

These are of two main types—*neurofibroma* (fig. 713 (a) and (b)) arising from the intercostal nerves and (2) *ganglioneuroma* from the sympathetic chain. The former appear close to the neck of the rib, whilst the latter lie slightly more medially applied to the vertebral bodies. They appear as a well-defined rounded shadow in the paravertebral gutter. They are usually symptomless, grow slowly and often cause widening of the upper rib spaces. A small percentage extend through the intervertebral foramen into the vertebral canal, where compression of the spinal cord may result in paraplegia (dumbbell tumour). Removal of the tumour is safe and simple and is recommended owing to the risks of malignant changes. Dumb-bell tumours, and particularly those with spinal-cord involvement, require urgent treatment. A small intraspinal extension can easily be removed from the chest, but extensive intraspinal tumours will require laminectomy for their removal; the latter can usually be carried out at the same time as the chest operation, but if very extensive, separate operations are advisable.

DISEASES OF THE PLEURA

Pneumothorax.—A pneumothorax is produced by the presence of air between the layers of the pleura. The air may be present alone or associated with serous fluid (*hydro-pneumothorax*), pus (*pyo-pneumothorax*), or blood (*haemo-pneumothorax*). Air may be deliberately introduced into the pleura (*diagnostic artificial pneumothorax*), be associated with trauma (*traumatic pneumothorax*), or may appear without any obvious exciting cause (*spontaneous pneumothorax*). The physical signs of a pneumothorax are a hyper-resonant percussion note with absent breath sounds. The trachea may be deviated. Radiographs reveal translucency on the affected side with absence of lung markings; the edge of the collapsed lung is usually visible.

Spontaneous Pneumothorax.—Causes:

(a) Tuberculous. (b) Non-tuberculous: (1) *Emphysematous bullae.* (2) *Solitary lung cysts.* (3) *Honeycomb or cystic lung.* (4) *Idiopathic.*

Tuberculous spontaneous pneumothorax is usually associated with obvious clinical or radiological signs of tuberculosis. The condition is produced by the rupture of a small subpleural tubercle or cavity, and is usually associated with infection or irritation of the pleura resulting in the appearance of fluid in the pleural cavity and a febrile reaction. Treatment depends on the underlying pulmonary lesion.

A non-tuberculous spontaneous pneumothorax by contrast is rarely associated with fluid formation or fever. In a minority an obvious underlying pulmonary lesion, such as an emphysematous bulla, a lung cyst, or a honeycomb lung, can be demonstrated. Absorption may occur spontaneously and rapidly, or may be considerably delayed (*chronic spontaneous pneumothorax*). Attacks may be single or repeated (*recurrent spontaneous pneumothorax*). With a first attack, in the absence of an underlying cause, air can be allowed to absorb spontaneously, or expansion can be encouraged by occasional aspirations. Should a tension pneumothorax occur an intercostal tube should be inserted, connected to an underwater seal and suction applied. This is preferable to a needle which may lacerate the lung as it expands or may become blocked.

Failure of absorption (*chronic spontaneous pneumothorax*), or repeated attacks (*recurrent spontaneous pneumothorax*), demand full investigations to determine the cause. The most useful investigations are tomography and thoracoscopy (inspection of the lung). These investigations may reveal:
(*a*) A localised lesion, such as a cyst.
(*b*) Generalised lesions, such as emphysema or honeycomb lung.
(*c*) Nothing abnormal.
A localised condition is best treated by thoracotomy and excision, but the latter two groups should be treated by artificial obliteration of the space (pleurodesis). This is achieved by the use of chemical or other irritants (5% silver nitrate, iodised talc, 0·5% camphor in oil) introduced either through a needle or applied to the lung surface at thoracoscopy. These irritants set up a diffuse pleuritis which will result in the fusion of the visceral to the parietal pleura if the two surfaces can be maintained in apposition. It is thus important to ensure that the lung expands rapidly and completely after pleurodesis by using catheter drainage with suction. Thoracotomy and an upper parietal pleurectomy is preferable for most cases as a recurrence so often occurs after a chemical pleurodesis. The lung leak is oversewn, cysts if present are excised and the parietal pleura at the apex is removed or abraded in order to ensure fusion of the lung to the chest wall and prevent recurrence.

Haemothorax.—Blood in the pleural cavity may occur in a variety of conditions and is often associated with air as well. The respiratory and cardiac movements defibrinate the blood as it reaches the pleural cavity so that the collection remains fluid. Massive clotting only occasionally occurs. Blood is a pleural irritant and its presence produces pain and shock in the early stages and later excites the formation of a considerable effusion. It is also an excellent culture medium and infection is relatively common.

Causes.—(1) Trauma (fig. 714).

(2) Post-operatively, following pulmonary, cardiac or oesophageal operations, cervical sympathectomy and occasionally after the introduction of a central venous pressure monitor line in the neck.

(3) Associated with new growths of lung, mediastinum or pleura.

(4) Leaking aneurysms.

(5) Spontaneous.

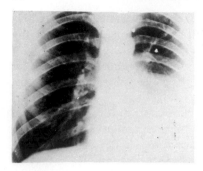

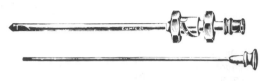

FIG. 714.—A left haemothorax with two retained metallic foreign bodies.

FIG. 715.—Abrams' Pleural Biopsy Punch.

The signs are those of a collection of fluid in the pleura, and the diagnosis is confirmed by exploration with a needle.

Treatment.—The initial treatment should be aimed at relieving pain, shock and blood loss. If signs of persistent bleeding are present, thoracotomy is advised. In all other cases the aim should be to remove the blood by aspiration as early and as completely as possible. Aspirations can be safely started twenty-four hours after the onset and should be repeated daily until no more fluid is obtained and the x-rays appear clear. Accidental or deliberate introduction of air must be avoided at all costs as it will lead to further collapse of the lung. Early and vigorous breathing exercises are advised.

A *clotted haemothorax* is diagnosed when the aspirating needle fails to remove a collection of blood. Liquefaction of the clot is often possible with streptokinase or trypsin ferments (Trypur®). An initial dose of 200,000 units of streptokinase or 1 ml of Trypur is injected into the clot and aspirations performed after twenty-four hours. Further doses can be given if the intial injection is not effective. In many instances however, the result is unsatisfactory, and thoracotomy with evacuation of clot and decortication of the lung is required.

An *infected haemothorax* should be treated initially with repeated aspirations and the instillation of suitable antibiotics. Early drainage or decortication will probably be required, owing to the difficulty of sterilising and aspirating the haemothorax if clotting has occurred.

Pleural Effusion.—The pleural cavity is constantly bathed in fluid which exudes from the visceral pleura and is absorbed by the parietal pleura. Any disturbance of the finely adjusted balance may result in the accumulation of fluid in the pleural cavity. Disturbances in osmotic or hydrostatic pressure produce a transudate (protein less than 3 g/100 ml); inflammatory lesions produce an exudate (protein more than 3 g/100 ml) and neoplasms produce variable changes and the fluid is often blood stained.

Pleural fluid when first formed gravitates to the most dependent part of the chest (usually posterior costo-phrenic angle), but later adhesions may lead to loculation.

Pleural fluid produces stony dullness with absent breath sounds and vocal fremitus with displacement of the mediastinum to the opposite side. Diagnosis can only be confirmed with the aspirating needle.

In all cases the aetiology must be determined by (*a*) bacteriological, biochemical and cytological analysis of fluid, (*b*), needle biopsy of pleura (Abrams) (fig.

Leon David Abrams, Contemporary. Thoracic Surgeon, United Birmingham Hospitals, England.

715), (c) thoracoscopic examination and biopsy of pleura, or (d) open thoracotomy.

In addition to these local measures a careful assessment of the lung and the heart is required and a search should be made for distant neoplasms (ovarian carcinoma, ovarian fibroma—Meigs' syndrome).

Pleural Tumours.—These may be benign or malignant and primary or secondary. A benign fibroma is rare, presents as a rounded shadow in the chest x-ray in an otherwise symptom-free patient. Finger clubbing is common. Malignant mesothelioma may affect the pleura diffusely, is often accompanied by pain and associated with a pleural effusion. These lesions are often associated with the inhalation of asbestos dust. Secondary pleural tumours are most often bronchial in origin, but the breast and ovary are also implicated. Secondary lesions are often associated with large, recurring blood-stained effusions.

Chylothorax.—Chyle may leak into the pleural cavity from the thoracic duct or its tributaries as a result of trauma (stab wounds, crush injuries, surgical injury) or obstruction by tumour. It is commonly mistaken for pus.

Chyle contains fat and the diagnosis depends on its demonstration by naked eye or microscope using Sudan III to stain the fat globules. Confirmation of the presence of chyle can be obtained by cholesterol and triglyceride estimations of the suspected fluid compared with fasting serum. Lipoprotein electrophoresis will reveal the presence of chylomicrons which are present in chyle.

Pseudochylous effusions have milky appearance not due to fat (cholesterol and calcium phosphate crystals, filarial parasites).

Chyliform effusions contain fat, but this has been derived from the breakdown of cells in encysted effusions. Distinction between chylous effusions and pseudo-chylous or chyliform effusions is possible using lipophilic dyes. A suitable dye is mixed with butter or oil and taken by mouth. Twelve to twenty-four hours later aspiration of the suspected fluid will be appropriately coloured if it be chylous. This technique can be used to aid identification of a leaking duct at thoracotomy.

Management will depend on the cause. The majority of surgically produced chylous effusions and some traumatic ones resolve with conservative measures (low fat diet and chest aspiration). If accumulation continues after a trial period of two weeks, thoracotomy is indicated to locate and suture or ligate the severed duct.

Empyema.—An empyema is a pleural abscess and consists of a collection of pus in the pleural cavity. The term is often wrongly used in a much wider sense to include all phases of pleural infection from an infected turbid effusion to a mature abscess containing thick pus. In the management of an empyema, it is just as important to consider the degree of localisation and pus formation as it is in other forms of septic cellulitis.

Aetiology.—An empyema is never primary. The majority are secondary to pulmonary infection, particularly pneumococcal pneumonia and broncho-pneumonia, but any infective process, such as tuberculosis, lung abscess and bronchiectasis may be complicated by an empyema. Any inflammatory condition in the vicinity of the pleura may give rise to an empyema, namely:

(a) Chest wall (wound, osteomyelitis of rib).

(b) Lung (pneumonia, abscess, bronchiectasis, tuberculosis, new growth).

(c) Post-operatively (thoracotomy).

(d) From the oesophagus (perforations, carcinoma).

(e) From below the diaphragm (subphrenic abscess).

Pathology.—In the common post-pneumonic empyema actual pleural infection is preceded by the development of a serous effusion. The pleura is subsequently invaded by organisms from the lung with associated inflammatory changes and further exudation of fluid. Fibrin is deposited on the surfaces of the pleura,

Joe Vincent Meigs, 1892–1963. Emeritus Professor of Clinical Gynaecology, Harvard University, Boston, U.S.A.

whilst intrapleural clotting is common in certain types which form a protein-rich exudate (pneumococcal empyema). The natural defences of the body are aimed at encircling the septic area by a barrier of fibrous tissue: this is initially achieved by the fusion of the lung to the chest wall at the periphery of the collection of fluid. Subsequently the fibrin deposits on the pleura are invaded by blood-vessels from the adjacent lung or chest wall with the formation of granulation tissue, and later of fibrous tissue. This process is progressive with an ever-increasing thickness of the wall of the empyema. Left to her own devices, nature will try to obliterate the empyema by converting it into a plaque of fibrous tissue. As the empyema becomes walled off by adhesions, the fluid thickens so that the presence of thick pus is a good indication that the empyema is localised and is unlikely to spread further. A mature empyema consists of visceral and parietal layers of fibrous tissue on the lung- and chest-wall surfaces respectively, with pus and debris between them. There is usually a good plane of cleavage between the wall of the empyema and the visceral pleura which is important in the operation of decortication. Secondary changes in the surrounding structures appear as the fibrous tissue contracts. The ribs are drawn together and lose their mobility. The diaphragm is elevated and fixed, and the mediastinum drawn towards the affected side. The lung is encased in a rigid covering of fibrous tissue and is immobile and functionless. The final picture of a neglected chronic empyema is a rigid contracted chest with relatively functionless lung underneath (frozen chest).

Clinical Features.—Empyemas, for convenience, can be divided into three groups: (1) Acute. (2) Subacute. (3) Chronic.

There are many potential causative organisms but many empyemas are sterile on the first aspiration owing to previous chemotherapy. The most frequently isolated organisms are therefore those resistant to the commoner antibiotics (*E. coli, Ps. pyocyaneus*, resistant staphylococci).

Acute Empyema.—The acute fulminating toxic empyema is now rare except when it follows perforation of the oesophagus or rupture of a lung abscess. There is profound toxaemia and shock with pleural pain and rapid, shallow respiration. The signs are those of pleural fluid, which should be confirmed by needle exploration. Early thoracotomy is required if the condition follows rupture or perforation of the oesophagus (see Chapter 43). Other cases should be treated by repeated aspirations with systemic and intrapleural antibiotics in an attempt to control the infection. If these measures fail to control the toxaemia, drainage should be carried out with an intercostal catheter inserted through a cannula and connected to an under-water seal, even though the pus is thin and the empyema not walled off. Subsequent management will be that of the subacute empyema.

Subacute Empyema.—The majority of empyemas present in a less severe form largely owing to the general use and efficiency of the antibiotics administered for the primary condition. As a result, an empyema may develop insidiously and its presence be completely overlooked. It should always be considered in cases of delayed resolution, slow convalescence or persistent fever following a pneumonic illness. Likewise, it should be suspected where the physical or radiological signs of resolution are inconclusive. Clinical signs are those of fluid with stony dullness, absent breath sounds, diminished chest movements, and displacement of viscera.

Chronic Empyema.—Many chronic empyemas are the result of mismanagement of the acute or subacute stages, some are due to failure to diagnose the original condition, and the remainder to some underlying pathology in the lung (bronchiectasis, lung abscess, tumour), pleura (foreign bodies, actinomycosis), or chest wall (rib sequestrum). Toxic absorption from the empyema is slight but symptoms of vague ill-health, febrile bouts, anaemia *etc.*, may occur. A chronic empyema may present in one of several ways, namely:

(1) A closed collection of pus completely walled off from its surroundings (*latent empyema*). If the pus is sterile, suspect tuberculosis.

(2) An empyema which is discharging either continuously or intermittently into a bronchus (*bronchopleural fistula*).

(3) An empyema which is discharging either continuously or intermittently through a sinus in the chest wall (*persistent empyema*).

Diagnosis.—An empyema is diagnosed by finding pus with an exploring needle. Failure to find pus may be due to:

(1) Use of too narrow a needle or the employment of an inefficient syringe.

(2) Selection of the wrong site for aspiration—usually too low.

(3) The presence of clot or fibrin tags which block the aspirating needle.

The commonest cause of failure is selection of the wrong site, but this should be avoided by a careful clinical and radiological examination beforehand. If pus is found, it is an advantage to keep two specimens—one for bacteriological studies, and the other for comparison with subsequent specimens.

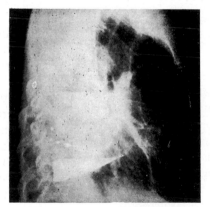 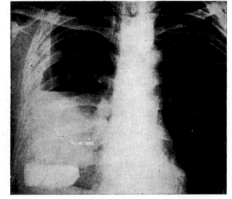

FIG. 716.—Lateral and postero-anterior radiograph of an empyema after injection of iodised oil to delineate the lower limits of the space prior to drainage. It is very important to order a radiograph with *extra* penetration to show the 12th rib and to be able to count the ribs from below.

Iodised oil should be injected into the empyema to show its lowest point and thus which rib to resect (fig. 716).

Having confirmed the diagnosis, it is important to determine if there is an underlying cause; whether the empyema is secondary to a carcinoma (always to be suspected over the age of 40 yrs, and excluded by bronchoscopy), underlying lung disease (lung abscess or bronchiectasis) or chronic infection (tuberculosis or actinomycosis).

Management.—The management depends on the stage in which the empyema is first diagnosed.

Stage I (Acute empyema). Initially all empyemas should be treated by aspiration repeated on alternate days, with the removal of as much pus as possible and the introduction of antibiotics. Only occasionally do aspirations fail to control infection, in which case drainage by intercostal tube should be carried out. If pus is still being produced after 14 days, this method of treatment should be abandoned as stage II has been reached. This method of treatment is especially valuable in children and the elderly.

Stage II (subacute empyema). Rib resection drainage is indicated if the pus is thick (more than one third sediment). Postoperative breathing exercises are *extremely* important.

The operation is carried out under local anaesthesia. The site selected for drainage lies immediately above the lowest limit of the empyema posteriorly. The lower posterior site is preferred because this is the most dependent part of the empyema with the patient sitting up in bed. An oblique incision through skin and muscles is made over the rib to be resected, as shown by previous lipoidal x-rays (fig. 716). The periosteum of a 5 cm segment of rib is elevated and the segment excised. A wide-bore aspirating needle should confirm that the correct rib has been removed and then the rib bed is incised, keeping towards its upper border to avoid damaging the intercostal vessels. The opening is enlarged to permit complete evacuation of the empyema and a thorough inspection and biopsy of the pleura. Drainage should at first be closed, using an under-water seal, but when the discharge is reduced to 60 ml daily open drainage should be instituted. Drainage must be maintained until the empyema cavity is completely obliterated, which may take as long as six to eight weeks. Premature removal of the tube is a frequent cause of chronicity. Control is effected by carrying out serial pleurograms with radio-opaque oil injected into the empyema cavity at intervals of three weeks. The tube should project 2·5 to 5 cm into the empyema cavity and will require little alteration until the final stages, when it should be adjusted to keep it 4 cm shorter than the empyema track.

Stage III (Chronic empyema). A decortication operation has become increasingly popular during the last 30 years. The operation aims at a complete removal of the empyema with its fibrous-tissue walls, leaving the lung and chest wall free to expand. It gives excellent functional results with minimal pleural thickening. Convalescence is rapid without the necessity for repeated dressings, and return to work is possible within a few weeks. The operation is, however, a major one requiring skilled anaesthesia and blood transfusion. It is indicated particularly for large and chronic empyemas, and for those secondary to bronchiectasis, lung abscess, or carcinoma where the underlying lung condition can be dealt with at the same time. It is contraindicated in the frail and elderly, or where complete resolution of a pneumonic process has not yet occurred.

Chronic empyema sinus. A chronic empyema sinus must always be examined radiologically following the instillation of radio-opaque iodised oil. It may be due to an underlying empyema, often surprisingly large. It may also be due to underlying lung disease, osteomyelitis of a rib or even a retained drainage tube. Most chronic empyema sinuses are due to improper treatment in the early stage—incorrect drainage site, premature tube removal, underlying lung disease or inadequate physiotherapy.

Tuberculous Empyema.—May be either a simple tuberculous infection or one complicated by secondary infection or a bronchopleural fistula. The majority are complications of an artificial pneumothorax or surgical treatment. They are much less common than they were, partly due to the widespread use of antituberculous drugs, but also to the decreased popularity of artificial pneumothorax. *Treatment* is basically the same as for any empyema, namely control of infection and obliteration of the pleural space, but is complicated by the presence or not of active tuberculosis of the lung or a bronchopleural fistula. Open drainage should be avoided as it will inevitably result in secondary infection of the space. Control of infection is often possible with regular aspiration and the use of systemic and intrapleural streptomycin, P.A.S., or I.N.A.H. The method adopted to obliterate the empyema depends on the condition of the underlying lung. If active pulmonary disease is present, either a thoracoplasty or a pleuropneumonectomy will be required after an adequate period of antituberculous chemotherapy. If the lung disease is controlled and inactive, obliteration may be possible by repeated aspirations over a prolonged period, or alternatively, by excision of the empyema. The operations of decortication and pleuropneumonectomy have dramatically altered the outlook in these cases.

Interlobar Empyema.—An interlobar empyema is a rarity, but one which is wrongly diagnosed with remarkable frequency. It can only occur when the interlobar space is completely shut off from the general pleural cavity. Occasionally a collection of pus remains localised in the fissure in cases of generalised pleural infection when the main collection has been adequately dealt with by aspiration. The diagnosis is largely a radiological one. The collection of fluid is oval or fusiform in shape with the long axis lying in the plane of one of the fissures. The appearances are easily confused with those of segmental atelectasis; if suspected, pus should be sought with an aspirating needle. Treatment consists of repeated aspirations with local intrapleural chemotherapy, or drainage if aspirations fail.

THE TRACHEA

Tracheal Stenosis.—Tracheal narrowing can be caused by extraluminal compression (carcinoma of thyroid, aortic aneurysms, aberrant aortic arch, enlarged lymph nodes, *etc*) or by fibrous strictures of the tracheal wall (tuberculous, post-tracheostomy) or by foreign bodies or intratracheal tumours (squamous cell carcinoma and cylindroma are the commonest tumours found).

The commonest type, at the present time, is stenosis following tracheostomy (Chapter 35). The stenosis most commonly occurs at the site of the inflatable cuff of a tracheostomy tube. It results from an ischaemic necrosis from an over-inflated cuff. It can be prevented by meticulous attention to tracheostomy drill and frequent deflation of the tracheostomy cuff. Less frequently, obstruction can occur at the level of the stoma and is usually the result of excessive resection of tracheal cartilage.

Resection of Trachea.—Up to six centimetres of the trachea or 5 cartilagenous rings can be resected and an end to end anastomosis carried out. The trachea is fully mobilised from the larynx to the carina to obtain relaxation. Lesions in the upper half of the trachea can be approached by a cervical collar incision but lower strictures may require a sternal splitting incision. The stricture or neoplasm is excised and an end to end anastomosis carried out with simple interrupted sutures. The patient should be nursed during the first week with the head fully flexed to avoid tension on the anastomosis. Replacement of a whole segment of the trachea by artificial prosthesis has not been entirely satisfactory. Best results have followed the use of pericardium reinforced with tantalum gauze or Marlex mesh.

DISEASES OF THE BRONCHI AND LUNG

Intrabronchial Foreign Bodies

Inhalation of foreign bodies is not a rare occurrence, particularly in children. In many instances the individual assumes that the foreign body has been expelled as the initial choking may soon pass. The commonest foreign bodies are teeth, mutton and rabbit bones, peanuts, pins, screws and nuts. The changes produced depend upon the size and nature of the foreign body. Small, smooth metallic

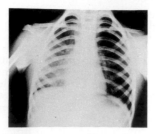

FIG. 717.— Obstructive emphysema of the left lung due to an inhaled peanut in the left main bronchus.

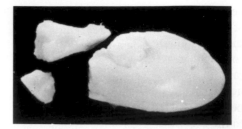

FIG. 718.—Peanut removed bronchoscopically from case illustrated in fig. 717.

foreign bodies produce little reaction, whilst larger foreign bodies may lead to partial or complete obstruction of one of the bronchi more commonly on the right side because of its more vertical position. Organic foreign bodies, particularly peanuts, produce marked inflammatory changes in the bronchial wall.

The clinical features may be:

(1) Wheezing, irritating cough and signs of unilateral obstructive emphysema (figs. 717 and 718).

(2) Symptoms due to atelectasis or pulmonary suppuration; cough, sputum, fever, *etc.*

(3) The patient may be symptomless.

Radiography is an essential investigation in every suspected case. If the foreign body is radio-opaque, it should be visible either in the postero-anterior or lateral film. In many instances the foreign body is either not opaque or is obscured by the heart shadow or secondary inflammatory changes.

Treatment.—Early bronchoscopy is essential in all suspected cases before oedema of the bronchial wall has occurred. An experienced anaesthetist is mandatory as the procedure may be difficult. A complete range of retrieval forceps should be available but if extraction proves to be impossible then a bronchotomy should be carried out through a postero-lateral thoracotomy. Rarely a lobectomy will be required if the foreign body has been present for a long time and has caused bronchiectasis.

Bronchiectasis

Bronchiectasis is a condition in which the bronchi are dilated and infected. There is usually some degree of collapse, so that on the bronchogram the bronchi appear to be closer together than normal. The lung parenchyma may also be affected and may be airless and fibrotic. On the other hand the lung itself may be relatively normal.

Aetiology. The two causes of bronchiectasis are external bronchial compression or internal bronchial occlusion.

1. *External bronchial compression* and consequent obstruction occur in childhood, due to glandular enlargement associated with measles, whooping cough or primary tuberculosis. The bronchial obstruction is followed by infection, which leads to mucosal ulceration, loss of bronchial cartilage and consequent weakening of the bronchial wall. The weakened bronchi later dilate due to the constant

negative pressure on the bronchial wall associated with respiration. Re-aeration of the collapsed lobe may occur later as the glandular compression subsides but the bronchi remain dilated and infected. The primary diseases are now much less common than 40 years ago and because of this bronchiectasis is now relatively rare. In addition the bronchial infection so often associated with these diseases is now treated much more promptly and efficiently with antibiotics and therefore permanent structural changes are much less likely to develop in the lung distal to the bronchial blockage.

2. *Internal bronchial occlusion* may occur from an unsuspected inhaled foreign body or an innocent bronchial tumour, leading to distal infection.

Pathology.—The bronchi appear thickened and irregular, whilst histologically there is marked destruction of all the normal elements and extensive infiltration of the remnants with inflammatory cells. The columnar epithelium is replaced by granulation tissue or by squamous or cuboidal epithelium. The lung supplied by the affected bronchi may be fibrotic and airless with loss of the alveolar pattern and infiltrated with inflammatory cells (bronchiectasis with an atelectatic lobe). In other cases the abnormal bronchi are surrounded by aerated lung tissue but the latter is usually emphysematous and relatively functionless. Bronchiectasis may be *cylindrical* or *saccular*. There is often an associated bronchitis.

Clinical Features.—In most cases the symptoms begin in childhood. Cough and purulent sputum which may be blood-stained, together with 'pneumonic' episodes of fever and increased sputum are the main features. A dry form of bronchiectasis sometimes occurs, in which infection is minimal, and repeated haemoptyses occur from the dilated bronchial arteries—so-called bronchiectasis haemorrhagia sicca. Clubbing of the fingers is common, and the patient usually has a 'wet' cough with moist sounds in the lungs.

Diagnosis. Except in advanced cases, the plain chest radiograph is frequently normal and the diagnosis is established by bronchogram, which must outline the whole of the bronchial tree on both sides. The lower lobes, right middle lobe and lingular segment of the left upper lobe are the areas most commonly affected. Bronchoscopy is advisable to exclude the presence of a foreign body or tumour.

Treatment.—In order to plan treatment it is essential to have good bronchograms of the whole of both lungs, so that the extent of the bronchiectasis can be accurately defined.

(*a*) *Prophylactic Treatment.*—Much can be done to prevent the development of bronchiectasis by treating the respiratory complications of measles and whooping cough with antibiotics and breathing exercises, and carrying out bronchoscopy at an early date should atelectasis occur.

(*b*) *Medical Treatment.*—If the bronchiectasis is not too severe it is possible for some patients to keep the disease under control by half hour periods of postural drainage night and morning, together with periods of prophylactic antibiotic therapy in the winter months and during exacerbations of infection. Postural drainage is carried out in a position designed to place the affected lobe above the draining bronchi, so that pus will drain by gravity from the lobe into the bronchus from whence it can be expectorated. Periods of half to one hour two or three times daily are advisable. Most patients will wish to have surgical treatment if this is possible.

(c) Surgical Treatment.—The aim of surgical treatment is to excise the affected segments or lobes and therefore it is essential that the disease be well localised and not scattered throughout both lungs. Removal of the affected area is by pneumonectomy, lobectomy or segmental resection (p. 740). If pneumonectomy is contemplated the contralateral lung must be normal. Bilateral lobectomy or segmental resection may also be undertaken but not more than 7–8 segments should be removed. Resection must be preceded by an adequate period of postural drainage and chemotherapy to reduce infection to a minimum. The results of resection for bronchiectasis are good and the patient's symptoms are greatly relieved, though if there is an associated chronic bronchitis, as is often the case, then the cough will not be abolished completely.

TUMOURS OF THE BRONCHI AND LUNG

With one or two rare exceptions[1], all pulmonary tumours arise from some part of the bronchial tree and are malignant in most cases (90–95 per cent of resected tumours).

Classification

Benign.—Carcinoid adenoma
        Hamartoma (fibroma, chondroma, lipoma, angioma)

Malignant

Primary.—Carcinoma (common).
  Alveolar-cell carcinoma (rare).
  Cylindroma (adenoid cystic carcinoma)
    (usually affects trachea) (rare)
  Sarcoma (rare).

Secondary.—Sarcoma.
  Teratoma of testis.
  Carcinoma (bowel, breast,
    thyroid, kidney).

Symptomatology.—The symptoms produced by a tumour may be due to the presence of an irritating lesion in the bronchial tree producing cough, sputum, wheezing and haemoptysis, or may be secondary (see Clinical Features).

Benign Tumours

Representing about 2% of all pulmonary tumours, they are slightly commoner in women and more frequent in the younger individual.

Pathology.—The tumours fall into two main anatomical groups, those arising from the larger bronchi and those situated in the periphery of the lung. The former are more common and are visible through the bronchoscope. The intra-bronchial portion of the tumour, however, may only represent a portion of the whole as there is often a large extra-bronchial portion (iceberg tumour). Peripheral tumours are not visible through a bronchoscope. Two main varieties are found: *carcinoid adenoma*, the commonest and most frequently found in the lobar or segmental bronchi; *hamartoma* most frequently occurs in the lung but is occasionally found in a large bronchus. Histologically the cells of the carcinoid tumour are regular, and well formed and consistent in appearance and tend to be arranged in solid acini. Mitoses are infrequent. The hamartoma is a composite tumour composed of two or more tissue elements. They represent an abnormal mixing or development of the normal components of the organ in which they occur. Thus, in the lung, cartilage, fat, glandular or vascular tissue and respiratory epithelium may be found. The hamartomas are usually described according to the preponderant tissue, *e.g.* chondromatous, haemangiomatous hamartoma, *etc.* (Chapter 8).

Clinical Features.—(1) Many are symptomless and found on routine radiography; this particularly applies to the peripheral types.

---

[1] Mesothelioma is another type of tumour but it originates from the pleural membrane. It is believed to occur more commonly in those who work with blue asbestos fibre.

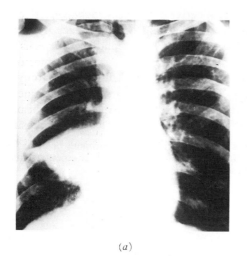
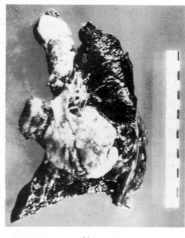

(a)   (b)

FIG. 719.—Adenocarcinoma right middle lobe. (a) Radiograph showing consolidation of right middle lobe and enlargement of mediastinal shadow. (b) Pneumonectomy specimen showing massive tumour in middle lobe and enlarged paratracheal nodes excised with the lung.

(2) Recurrent haemoptysis. The carcinoid adenoma is one of the causes of repeated large haemoptyses occurring over a period of years. There is frequently complete freedom from symptoms between attacks, though occasionally wheeziness and an irritating cough are present.

(3) Symptoms due to bronchial obstruction and lung infection. Simple uninfected atelectasis or pulmonary suppuration with abscess formation and bronchiectasis both occur commonly. In some cases of a lung abscess or an empyema, the underlying tumour is completely unsuspected until bronchoscopy is performed.

(4) Endocrine effects due to active secretion by the tumour cells, *e.g.* carcinoid syndrome.[1]

Diagnosis.—The diagnosis is often suggested by the history, but can only be confirmed by bronchoscopy. The carcinoid adenoma appears as a round, smooth or slightly lobulated raspberry-like tumour which is neither ulcerated nor necrotic. Tumours containing cartilage appear pale and hard and biopsy may be difficult. Bronchography may be necessary to determine the presence and extent of any secondary lung changes which will influence subsequent treatment.

Treatment.—Surgical resection is the treatment of choice. This can be planned conservatively as the risk of recurrence is negligible. Treatment by radon implantation, curettage or irradiation is ineffective and cannot be recommended. One or other of the following methods may be applicable to the individual case:

(1) *Bronchotomy.*—Local removal of the tumour with part of the bronchial wall if practicable for tumours of localised extent without extra-bronchial extension and without secondary lung damage.

(2) *Lung Resection.*—A lung resection as conservative as possible is required in those cases associated with permanent lung damage.

Carcinoma of the Bronchus

Aetiology.—The incidence of carcinoma of the bronchus has rapidly increased in the last 30 years and is now the commonest cancer in men, and the second commonest cancer in women (in the U.K.). It usually occurs over the age of 40 years but may appear earlier. Statistical surveys show that heavy cigarette smoking over many years predisposes to the development of lung cancer. The exposure

---

[1] Carcinoid tumours of bronchus are second in frequency only to those of the appendix; only a small minority produce systemic disturbances.

to other irritants, such as arsenic and radio-active substances (Schneeberg[1] cancer), exhaust fumes, sulphurous smoke and fog, and tarry particles from the roads may possibly be implicated. Workers in the chromate industry have a high incidence of lung cancer.

Pathology.—Three main macroscopic types are described:

(1) *Main Bronchus Tumours.*—The majority of tumours arise in the main bronchus or one of its primary or secondary divisions. They produce bronchial irritation and ulceration at an early stage and frequently give rise to bronchial obstruction. They are usually visible through the bronchoscope (fig. 719).

(2) *Peripheral Tumours.*—These are less common, arise from the smaller bronchi and may only be visible with the fibreoptic bronchoscope. They rarely produce secondary lung changes. Some are discovered at routine radiography (fig. 720).

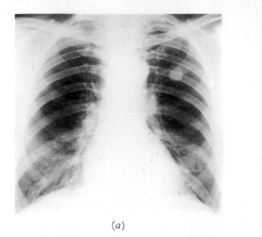 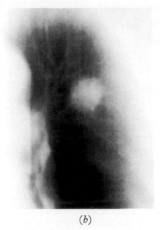

(a)   (b)

FIG. 720.—Peripheral lung carcinoma. (a) Typical 'coin lesion' in left upper lobe. (b) Tomogram shows spidery extensions into surrounding lung typical of carcinomatous invasion.

(3) *Pancoast 'Tumours'.*—These are essentially peripheral lung carcinomas arising at the apex of the lung. The tumour invades the brachial plexus, sympathetic chain, upper ribs and adjacent vertebrae producing the Pancoast syndrome (lower brachial plexus lesion, Horner's syndrome, an apical shadow, and rib erosion). The lesion is particularly distressing owing to the early production of intractable pain which is difficult to relieve, combined with a relatively slow growth.

Histology.—Three main histological types are recognised.[2]

(1) Squamous cell (epidermoid) carcinoma 50%.
(2) Anaplastic (a) Small cell (oat cell) 15%.
          (b) Large cell 5%.
(3) Adenocarcinoma 20%.

The anaplastic carcinomas are poorly differentiated tumours often exhibiting rapid growth with early metastases. They are more common in young individuals.

Spread of the growth.—(1) *By direct extension* into the mediastinum, pleura, chest wall or pericardium.

(2) *By the lymphatic system* to the hilar lymph nodes and thence to the subcarinal nodes or the paratracheal chain. The upper nodes of the chain are continuous with the inferior deep cervical group which may be detected by digital palpation

---

[1] The name of a district in Germany where these substances are mined.
[2] Based on WHO classification.

Henry Khumrath Pancoast, 1875–1939. Professor of Rontgenology, University of Pennsylvania, Philadelphia, U.S.A.
Johann Horner, 1831–1883. Professor of Ophthalmology, Zürich, described this syndrome in 1869.

deep to the insertion of the sternomastoid muscle. Other supraclavicular glands may be involved. Contralateral spread may occur from the left lower lobe to the right paratracheal nodes.

(3) *By the bloodstream* to the liver, brain, bones (ribs, vertebrae, pelvis and long bones), adrenal glands and skin.

Clinical Presentation.—Patients with carcinoma of the bronchus may present with symptoms due to the primary tumour, secondary deposits, one of the endocrine related syndromes, or a combination of any of these three manifestations:

Primary tumour.—The three most common symptoms are (1) cough with sputum lasting for more than 2–3 weeks or a *change in the character* of a chronic cough associated with chronic bronchitis, (2) haemoptysis, or (3) dyspnoea due to partial or complete bronchial obstruction. Chest pain and wheeze are less common symptoms. Any patient over the age of 40 years with these symptoms must be investigated to exclude a bronchial carcinoma, as also should any patient in whom there is an unduly slow radiological resolution of a pneumonitis or pneumonia.

The first symptoms may be due to invasion of the mediastinum causing (1) Pressure on superior vena cava causing SVC obstruction. (2) Pressure on recurrent laryngeal nerve causing hoarse voice. (3) Pressure on trachea or main bronchus causing stridor. (4) Pressure on oesophagus causing dysphagia.

Secondary deposits: (1) Brain (*a*) headaches and vomiting; (*b*) epileptiform fits; (*c*) weakness of a limb, leading to paralysis.

(2) Bone pain, especially in vertebrae, pelvis and long bones.

(3) Skin nodules.

Endocrine related symptoms. (1) Osteo-arthropathy – arthritic symptoms and finger clubbing.

(2) Carcinomatous neuropathy.

(3) Abnormal hormone secretion, causing hypokalaemia (muscle weakness), hyponatraemia (water retention), hypercalcaemia (confusion and drowsiness), gynaecomastia or Cushing's syndrome.

General symptoms.—Malaise, anorexia and loss of weight.

Investigations.—Investigations are necessary to establish the diagnosis and assess operability.

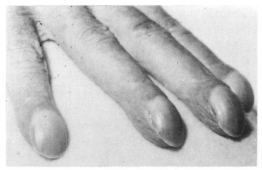

FIG. 721.—Gross finger clubbing in patient with lung cancer.

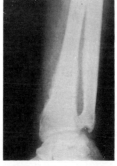

FIG. 722.—Periosteal changes seen in radius and ulna in patient with lung cancer and pulmonary osteo-arthropathy.

Harvey Cushing, 1869–1939. Professor of Surgery, Harvard University, Boston, U.S.A. (1912–1932). (See footnote p. 60.)

Chest X-Ray (which must include a lateral view) is abnormal in 98% of cases, There may be collapse/consolidation of a segment, lobe or lung, a well-defined shadow at the hilum or in the lung field, or a cavitated lesion, usually thick walled but sometimes thin walled.

Bronchoscopy by rigid or fibre-optic instrument is most important to obtain histology by biopsy or bronchial washings and also to assess operability – involvement of trachea, grossly widened carina between left and right main bronchus (due to involved carinal glands), rigidity of main bronchus near its origin, or visible tumour at the origin of a main bronchus will all signify inoperability. Peripheral tumours will not be visible.

Cytological examination of sputum will reveal malignant cells in about 60% of cases.

Needle biopsy of a peripheral lesion under radiographic control will often provide a histological diagnosis.

Barium Swallow.—This may provide evidence of mediastinal glandular involvement or less commonly actual involvement of oesophageal wall.

Tomography is useful in demonstrating enlarged mediastinal nodes.

Liver, brain and bone scanning is indicated if involvement of these organs is suspected.

CT whole body scanning is being increasingly employed for the detection of distant metastases, especially brain, liver and adrenal deposits.

Supraclavicular node biopsy is required if these nodes are enlarged.

Mediastinoscopy is a routine practice in some clinics to biopsy nodes from the paratracheal and inferior deep cervical groups. If contralateral nodes are involved resection of the lung tumour is contraindicated. If ipsilateral nodes are involved there is considerable controversy at the present time as to whether or not resection is indicated.

Diagnosis.—A positive histological diagnosis at bronchoscopy is available in about 70% of cases whilst malignant cells in the sputum or pleural fluid provide positive evidence in some of the remainder. In about 25% of cases, however, only a presumptive diagnosis can be made and these cases must have an exploratory thoracotomy if fit.

In the unproven case, a carcinoma is most likely to be confused with chronic suppurative pneumonia, a lung abscess, a solid tuberculous lesion or a benign tumour. Careful consideration of the history and response to antibiotics will often provide strong circumstantial evidence against a carcinoma, whilst tomography may be helpful in doubtful cases.

Treatment.—Surgical removal of the tumour offers the best prospects for cure. Radiotherapy is only very rarely curative and cytotoxic treatment is palliative only.

The aim of operative treatment must be the adequate removal of the primary tumour and the regional lymph nodes, but with the preservation of as much normal lung tissue as possible.

The extent of the lung resection will thus depend on the site of the tumour. Many patients will require a pneumonectomy (fig. 724) because of the position of the growth and the extent of lymph node involvement, but for growths confined to one lobe, a lobectomy is preferable as it is as effective in curing the

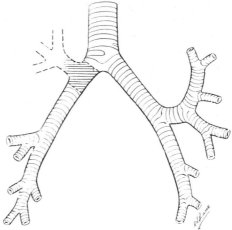

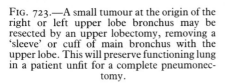

FIG. 723.—A small tumour at the origin of the right or left upper lobe bronchus may be resected by an upper lobectomy, removing a 'sleeve' or cuff of main bronchus with the upper lobe. This will preserve functioning lung in a patient unfit for a complete pneumonectomy.

patient as is pneumonectomy and furthermore carries a lower operative mortality. In some cases in which the growth is at the origin of an upper lobe bronchus and would be expected to require a pneumonectomy it is possible to remove the growth by the technique of upper lobectomy by 'sleeve' resection of a cuff of main bronchus (fig. 723), thus preserving some normal lung tissue. In all cases the paratracheal, subcarinal and para-aortic lymph nodes are removed. Limited resection of the chest wall, pericardium or diaphragm can be carried out should these structures be invaded. A localised peripheral tumour in an elderly patient with poor respiratory function may be treated by segmental resection.

In many thoracic surgical centres a pneumonectomy or lobectomy is carried out with equal frequency.

Lobectomy.—The operation is carried out through a postero-lateral thoracotomy. The relevant vein, artery and bronchus (in that order) are isolated by blunt dissection using

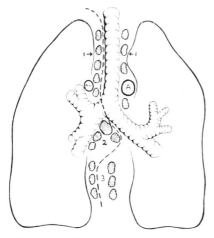

FIG. 724.—Right radical pneumonectomy. The dotted lines indicate the plane of dissection. A.V. = azygos vein. A. = aorta. I = paratracheal nodes. 2 = subcarinal nodes. 3 = para-aortic nodes.

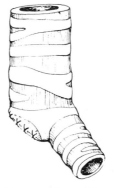

FIG. 725.—Sutured bronchus after right pneumonectomy. Note oblique division and absence of bronchial stump.

long curved artery forceps. The bronchus is divided between clamps and the vessels are securely ligated. The bronchus is closed by interrupted sutures of silk, thread, nylon or steel wire. Alternatively a stapler may be used. The lobe is then freed from its attachments to the parieties and mediastinum. Apical and basal pleural drainage tubes are inserted for the removal of air and blood respectively and to ensure the rapid and full expansion of the remaining lung.

Radical Pneumonectomy.—'One lung anaesthesia' is advisable. The feasibility of lung resection should be determined with as little lung disturbance as possible. At an early stage the pulmonary veins from the affected lobe should be tied to reduce the risks of tumour embolism. The remaining vessels are then isolated and divided after securing with double ligatures or a transfixed ligature. The bronchus is divided close to its origin after applying special bronchus clamps. The bronchus is closed with sutures of wire, nylon, or thread, using interrupted figure of eight stitches (figs. 724 and 725). Alternatively a stapler may be used.

The paratracheal and subcarinal and para-aortic lymph nodes should be removed with the lung. It may be necessary to open the pericardium in order to divide the pulmonary vessels.

Only 20% of lung cancers are considered suitable for exploration and of these one in ten is found to be too advanced for resection on exploration. The hospital mortality for pneumonectomy is 10% and for lobectomy is 5%, the deaths being due to respiratory infection, myocardial infarction or pulmonary embolus. Five-year survival (25–40%) is largely dependent on histological type and staging at the time of surgery as follows:

Stage I.—Growth confined to the lung.

Stage II.—Involvement of broncho-pulmonary lymph nodes at hilum.

Stage III.—Involvement of tracheo-bronchial (mediastinal) lymph nodes.

Stage IV.—Spread of growth outside the chest.

Squamous cell tumours have the best prognosis.

The following are contraindications to radical resection:
(1) A growth which involves the trachea or the origin of the main bronchus.
(2) Evidence of spread into the mediastinum with involvement of the oesophagus, recurrent laryngeal nerve or vena cava.
(3) Extensive invasion of the chest wall (fixed chest pain).
(4) Evidence of distant metastases.
(5) Patients over the age of seventy, unless fit for their years.
(6) Patients with poor respiratory reserve. (This can usually be assessed on clinical grounds with simple exercise tests.)
(7) Patients with serious ischaemic heart disease or generalised arterial disease.
(8) Patients with chronic bronchitis who have persistent signs in the normal lung. After operation they would be severely incapacitated (respiratory cripple).
(9) Involvement of phrenic nerve if growth is in upper lobe.

Palliative Resection.—At thoracotomy it is advisable to remove the lung with the primary tumour whenever possible even though the growth cannot be completely removed. Patients are better off without the primary tumour and die more peacefully from secondary deposits. Occasionally a deliberate palliative resection is justified in cases with repeated haemoptyses or with much pulmonary suppuration.

Radiotherapy.—The main use of radiotherapy is for the relief of the symptoms of superior vena caval obstruction, haemoptysis, and pain due to bone involvement. All of these respond dramatically, though survival is not appreciably lengthened. Radical treatment (4,000–5,000 cby) with the cobalt 'bomb' or the linear accelerator is given to some patients with some success, though the side effects of oesophagitis and radiation pneumonitis may be severe (fig. 726).

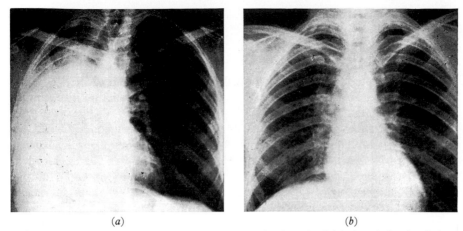

(a)   (b)

FIG. 726.—Main bronchus carcinoma, showing (a) total atelectasis of right lung before irradiation, and (b) aeration of the lung after treatment.

Pre-operative x-ray therapy has given disappointing results largely due to an increased incidence of broncho-pleural fistulas following resection.

Post-operative treatment is used occasionally where small areas of growth have not been removed (*e.g.* on the chest wall). Only fit patients should be treated if serious debilitating reactions are to be avoided.

Chemotherapy.—The use of cytotoxic drugs alone has been disappointing. Some benefit may follow their administration combined with surgery.

Secondary Lung Tumours.—Secondary deposits in the lungs from carcinomas and sarcomas occur frequently. The deposits are usually multiple but occasionally occur singly. In the absence of other evidence of malignant disease solitary lesions should be excised and many long-term cures have been obtained, especially in the case of hypernephroma or testicular teratoma.

Lung Abscess

A lung abscess is a localised area of lung infection, *with tissue necrosis,* due to an infection of such virulence that it is associated with thrombosis of the associated artery and vein. It is essentially the final stage in the development of a suppurative pneumonitis.

A large proportion of lung abscesses are secondary to chronic upper respiratory tract infection (sinusitis, tonsillitis or dental infection). They most commonly occur in the axillary subsegments of the upper lobe or the apical segment of the lower lobe and it is into these areas that infected material is inhaled whilst the patient is asleep and the cough reflex abolished.

Another important cause, especially in patients over the age of 40 years, is bronchial obstruction by carcinoma, leading to infection distal to the growth.

Classification.—Here based on aetiology

A. *Due to specific pneumonias*

1. Streptococcal—minimal sputum
2. Staphylococcal—loculated and resolve slowly
3. Pneumococcal—no specific features
4. Friedlander—elderly debilitated patients, sloughs often occur in abscess and associated with high mortality
5. Anaerobic—often from dental infection.

Carl Friedländer, 1847–1887. Pathologist, Friedrichshain Hospital, Berlin. Described this bacillus in 1882.

B. *Due to bronchial obstruction*
1. Carcinoma
2. Carcinoid or other benign tumour
3. Foreign body.

C. *Chronic upper respiratory tract infection*—sinusitis, tonsillitis or dental infection.

D. *Septicaemia*.

Pathology.—Infected material is inhaled into the bronchial tree and obstructs one of the smaller bronchi. The resulting atelectatic segment is invaded by pathogenic organisms producing pneumonic consolidation. The commonest organisms are *Haemophilus influenzae* and Pneumococci but invasion by mouth organisms (anaerobic streptococci and spirochaetes), coliform organisms and cross infection with drug-resistant staphylococci sometimes occur and may be detected by microscopy and culture of the sputum. Suppuration and necrosis develop in varying degrees within the involved segment, first with the production of a suppurative pneumonitis which later matures into an abscess. As pus accumulates, tension rises and eventually the abscess ruptures into the bronchus. This may be followed by complete expectoration of all sloughs and pus, and the inflammation may then subside. More commonly, however, a state of chronic infection with persistence of the abscess occurs. Progressive involvement of adjacent lung tissue or spread to other parts of the lung is possible.

Clinical Features.—The onset is often acute with influenza-like symptoms and variable toxaemia, but usually without any localising symptoms. After some days of ill-defined illness, pleural pain and a dry irritating cough will appear leading to the expectoration of considerable quantities of offensive blood-stained sputum. With successful treatment, resolution occurs slowly with reduction of toxicity and diminution of cough and sputum, but healing takes several weeks and can only be regarded as complete when cough and sputum have disappeared and radiographs are clear.

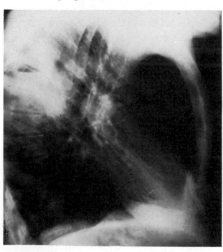 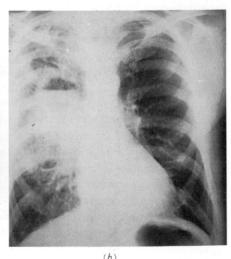

(a)   (b)

FIG. 727 (*a*) and (*b*).—Abscess in posterior segment of right upper lobe showing cavity with fluid level and surrounding zone of consolidation.

Complications.—(1) *Spread* of the disease to other parts of the lung by direct extension or by bronchial embolism: this is suggested by an exacerbation of symptoms and fresh radiograph changes.

(2) *Empyema.*—This is less common following the introduction of antibiotics. Persistent fever, pleural pain, and signs of a pleural effusion call for exploration of the pleura with a needle.

(3) *Cerebral Abscess.*—Pyaemic emboli reach the brain through the paravertebral system of veins (Collis). The resulting abscesses are usually multiple but occasionally single. The onset is usually accompanied by headaches and fever. A fit is occasionally the first symptom. The incidence of cerebral abscess has fallen markedly since the introduction of antibiotics.

(4) *Secondary Haemorrhage.*—Occasionally severe or fatal haemorrhage occurs.

Diagnosis.—The diagnosis is confirmed by the presence of a cavity on the chest x-ray (fig. 727), usually in the apex of the upper or lower lobe.

All cases must be investigated to determine the cause by:

(1) Bronchoscopy to exclude a foreign body or neoplasm.

(2) Complete bacteriological examination of the sputum including ?T.B.

(3) Examination of the teeth and upper respiratory tract.

Differential Diagnosis

The radiological appearance of a cavity in the lung may also be due to a breaking down carcinoma (seen on tomography to have thick irregular walls), tuberculosis, or numerous rare conditions such as mycoses, histoplasmosis, aspergillosis, hydatid cyst or congenital cyst. A small expectorated empyema may also cause confusion.

Treatment

1. *Medical.*—The majority (85%) of acute lung abscesses resolve satisfactorily on medical treatment. This consists of prolonged high dosage chemotherapy, together with postural drainage. The appropriate antibiotic is selected as soon as the bacteriology of the sputum is known. The dose of antibiotic must be two or three times the normal dose and the course must be prolonged—for at least 3 weeks and sometimes, as in the case of a staphylococcal abscess, as long as 6 weeks. The predominant organism in the sputum may change during the course of treatment and it may be necessary to change the antibiotic. The sputum bacteriology must therefore be checked periodically. Initially postural drainage should be carried out for 2-3 hours three times daily but as the abscess gradually resolves, so the periods of postural drainage may be reduced.

2. *Surgical.*—Surgical treatment is only required if medical treatment fails. This implies surgical resection (lobectomy—not segmentectomy) if the abscess becomes chronic and a cavity in the lung persists, as shown by tomography. The abscess may be chronic when first diagnosed, and resection may be indicated because a breaking down carcinoma cannot be excluded.

External drainage is no longer required now that most pulmonary infections can be satisfactory controlled with antibiotics. Twenty years ago it was sometimes necessary if copious sputum and toxicity persisted. A two stage rib resection drainage was carried out—the first stage to produce pleural adhesions and the second stage to open the cavity.

John Leigh Collis, Contemporary. Professor of Thoracic Surgery, United Birmingham Hospitals, England.

Lung Cysts

These may be divided into four groups:

(1) *Epithelial Cysts.*—These are developmental in origin and may be solitary and large or multiple and small. They are lined by respiratory epithelium and may have traces of cartilage, muscle or glands in their wall.

(2) *Emphysematous Cysts.*—These include a wide variety of conditions where the normal alveolar framework is destroyed or disrupted, resulting in large air spaces which may become further distended with air.

(3) *Parasitic cysts*, of which the commonest is the hydatid.

(4) *Pseudo-cysts.*—Certain inflammatory conditions of the lung result in cavity formation, and in many instances the cavities may closely resemble epithelial cysts. The cavities, when chronic, are often lined by squamous epithelium. These pseudo-cysts may occur in association with staphylococcal pneumonia, pulmonary tuberculosis, or following lung abscess. Their true nature is often suggested by their history, course, and radiological features, but the distinction is often difficult. They may develop a fungal infection (aspergilloma) leading to repeated life threatening haemoptyses.

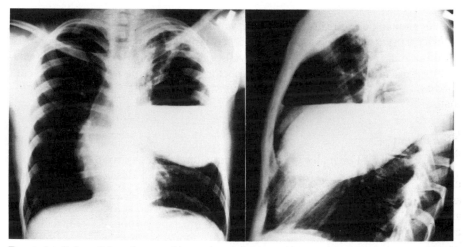

Fig. 728.—P.A. and lateral x-ray of large air and fluid containing congenital lung cyst occupying the greater part of the upper lobe. Removal by lobectomy.

Epithelial Cysts.—These are often associated with other congenital abnormalities (cervical rib, pulmonary stenosis, patent ductus) (fig. 728). They appear as spherical shadows in the x-ray with a thin, sharply defined wall. They may contain air, fluid, or both air and fluid. Symptoms may be produced by:

(1) The size of the cyst which compresses the lung and therefore causes dyspnoea and tightness in the chest. This is particularly so in infants and children where the thorax is small and the cyst often relatively large.

(2) Infection is common with the production of fever, cough and sputum. Radiography will demonstrate a fluid level in the cyst. Infection is usually readily controlled with antibiotics, but recurrence is frequent and removal indicated.

(3) Haemorrhage from cysts is usually associated with infection.

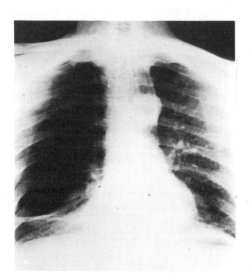

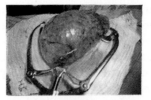

FIG. 730.—A giant emphyse-matous cyst which presented through the wound on opening the chest.

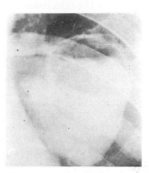

FIG. 729.—Giant emphysematous cyst of right upper lobe with compression of the lung and depression of the diaphragm.

FIG. 731.—Hydatid cyst. 'Water-lily' appearance.

Spontaneous pneumothorax is uncommon with epithelial cysts (cf. emphyse-matous cysts).

Treatment.—solitary cysts producing symptoms should be excised. Symptom-less cysts can be kept under observation. Infection of multiple cysts should be controlled by antibiotics if excision is not practicable.

Emphysematous Cysts.—Emphysematous cysts are due to degenerative changes in the lung, leading to rupture of the alveolar walls and abnormal disten-sion. Progressive coalescence of alveolar spaces combined with distension with air may result in the development of an enormous cyst (figs. 729 and 730). These cysts have no epithelial lining, and when large the remnants of the more resistant bronchi and blood vessels are seen stretching across the space. The changes may be limited to a small area of the lung, such as a segment or a lobe, or the condition may be generalised and bilateral.

Clincial Features.—The most important symptom is dyspnoea, which is due to a combination of compression of normal lung tissue by the cyst, increase in the dead space, and a poor gaseous exchange. Emphysematous cysts are frequently associated with chronic bronchitis. In such cases persistent coughing tends to distend the cysts still further, whilst the presence of bronchial secretions impairs respiratory function still more. The presence of bronchitis is a serious compli-cation which renders radical treatment more hazardous.

Spontaneous pneumothorax is a common and serious complication and may be the first presenting feature. Infection and haemorrhage are unusual (cf. epithelial cysts).

Treatment.—Emphysematous cysts which are not associated with generalised emphysematous changes should be excised, but if changes are widespread, excision is impracticable. Obliteration by plication with multiple sutures has given good results; it is applicable to multiple cysts and does not remove potentially functioning lung tissue. Removal of the pulmonary autonomic nerves can be combined with the above procedures; its chief value lies in the reduction of bronchial spasm. In cases complicated by a spontaneous pneumothorax, pleurodesis should be carried out to prevent further attacks of this serious complication.

Congenital obstructive emphysema.—This is a rare condition which occurs in infants, due to a congenital absence of bronchial cartilage. A 'ball valve' mechanism occurs in the bronchus of the affected lobe, usually the upper, which becomes increasingly distended. The treatment is lobectomy.

Hydatid disease of the lung has been largely eliminated from such countries as Australia and Iceland by control of dogs and the proper slaughtering of sheep. The disease remains endemic in Asia and parts of the Middle East but is now rare elsewhere.

Pulmonary hydatid cysts occur in about 15% of all cases; the cysts are usually solitary, but multiple or bilateral cysts are not uncommon. The disease is more common in children and young adults.

The cases may present in any of the following ways:

(1) On routine clinical or radiological examination and without symptoms.

(2) Dyspnoea, pain or tightness in chest due to the presence of a large cyst.

(3) Haemoptysis due to ulceration into the bronchus.

(4) Expectoration of watery fluid and 'grape skins' due to rupture into the bronchial tree. This event may produce severe distress with suffocating symptoms or even death if the leak is a large one. Anaphylactic shock and urticaria may occur.

(5) Symptoms due to secondary infection of the cyst, *viz*, cough, purulent sputum and fever.

Radiology is the most helpful investigation:

(1) An uncomplicated cyst appears as an almost spherical, sharply defined dense homogeneous opacity.

(2) Communication with the bronchial tree may result in a crescentic cap of air overlying the cyst (perivesicular pneumo-cyst).

(3) Rupture of the cyst permits air to enter the cyst and the laminated membrane collapses. This floats on any fluid which may be present, producing an irregular projection above the fluid level ('water-lily' appearance) (fig. 731).

(4) Infection results in disintegration of the laminated membrane with appearances simulating a lung abscess.

(5) Varying degrees of pneumonitis, atelectasis, or pleural effusion may accompany any of the above and modify the radiological appearance.

Diagnosis.—The most important point is to remember the condition. A history of residence in an endemic area may support the diagnosis. The intradermal test of Casoni will give a positive result in 75% of uncomplicated cysts provided fresh hydatid fluid is used. An eosinophilia of over 4% is suggestive of the condition.

Treatment.—Removal of the cyst is indicated in all cases owing to the considerable risk of serious or even fatal complications. The earlier operation of marsupialisation has been completely replaced by thoracotomy with enucleation of the cyst or lobectomy. Enucleation is employed for uncomplicated cysts without significant associated lung damage. Extreme care and utmost gentleness is required to remove the laminated membrane intact without spilling the contents with the risk of infecting the pleura or wound. The adventitia is carefully incised and the laminated membrane will usually slowly extrude itself. It should never be grasped with forceps as it is friable and is sure to tear. Extrusion can be expedited by gentle positive pressure by the anaesthetist. After removal, any bleeding-points or open bronchi are secured and the residual space can be obliterated by mattress sutures if desired. The pleura is drained as some leakage of air is inevitable.

Complicated cysts are best treated by a more formal resection (lobectomy), particularly if there is any surrounding lung damage.

Secondary Pleural Hydatid Disease.—This is an occasional but serious complication of rupture of a cyst into the pleura or of ill-executed surgery. Multiple cysts grow widely throughout the pleura and may invade the chest wall, diaphragm, or mediastinum. Radical pleuropneumonectomy offers the only hope of eradicating the disease.

Tomaso Casoni, 1880–1933. Physician, Ospedale Coloniale Vittorio Emanuele III, Tripoli, Libya.

Hepato-Bronchial Fistula is caused by the rupture of an infected hepatic cyst into the lung. The infected material traverses the subphrenic and pleural spaces (both being obliterated by adhesions) before discharging into the lung. It results in the production of bile stained sputum. Treatment demands a thoracotomy with resection of the affected lobe; the track through the diaphragm must be enlarged to expose the underlying residual cyst which is drained through an independent opening.

Pulmonary Oedema

Blood in the lung capillaries is separated from air in the alveolar spaces merely by the thin capillary wall and the alveolar membrane. Gaseous diffusion occurs readily across this membrane and any disturbance of the physico-chemical balance in the blood may permit the transudation of fluid from the capillaries into the alveolar spaces.

Initially, transudation occurs into the interstitial tissues of the lung, producing dyspnoea and cyanosis; later, when fluid reaches the alveoli, thin frothy blood-stained fluid is expectorated, often in considerable quantities. Coarse râles are audible throughout both lungs and radiographs show consolidated areas spreading from each hilum towards the periphery ('bat's wing' appearance).

Causes.—(1) Obstruction to the flow of blood through the left side of the heart as in left ventricular failure and mitral stenosis.

(2) Increased volume of blood reaching the lungs as may occur after excessive transfusion of blood or saline.

(3) Disturbances of osmotic pressure in the blood.

(4) Traumatic, such as follow the inhalation of certain noxious gases (phosgene, mustard gas), hot air, smoke or steam.

(5) Inflammatory, as in influenzal pneumonia.

(6) Associated with certain brain injuries and lesions of the brain stem.

(7) Fat embolism.

Treatment is urgently required along the following lines:

(1) Correction of the precipitating cause.

(2) Support of the heart and circulation with aminophylline (250 mg intravenously), digitalis (0·5 mg digoxin intramuscularly), pressor agents and oxygen.

(3) Morphine, which should be given intramuscularly, is particularly effective in left ventricular failure.

(4) Diuretics such as frusemide (Lasix®) 80 mg intravenously, repeated in one hour if necessary.

(5) Positive Pressure Ventilation is the most effective method of controlling pulmonary oedema and should not be delayed when the above measures are not immediately effective. Initially it can be employed with a cuffed plastic endotracheal tube, but tracheostomy will be necessary if ventilation is required for more than a week to ten days.

SURGICAL TREATMENT OF PULMONARY TUBERCULOSIS

In a book of this nature it is not possible to give more than an outline of the principles involved in the surgical treatment of pulmonary tuberculosis. Such treatment is usually an incident in the long-term management of the case, and as such can only be satisfactorily determined by consultation and discussion between physician and surgeon.

Principles of Treatment.—(1) *Rest.*—This is an essential part of treatment, though

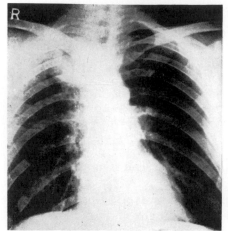

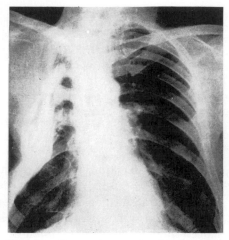

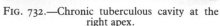

FIG. 732.—Chronic tuberculous cavity at the right apex.   FIG. 733.—Same case as in fig. 372 after thoracoplasty.

with the advent of antituberculous chemotherapy is now required for a very much shorter time.

(2) *Chemotherapy.*—The introduction of various anti-tuberculous drugs since 1950 has revolutionised the treatment of all forms of tuberculosis and has resulted in a world-wide reduction in the prevalence and importance of this disease. The drug regimen is discussed in Chapter 4.

(3) *Excision of Diseased Lung.*—Before the discovery of streptomycin in 1942, excision of tuberculous lungs usually met with disaster. Antibiotics used prior to, and as a cover for, operation have transformed the situation and resection has become the surgical therapy of choice. Resection has the advantage of removing the major foci of disease, leaving the body with the less formidable task of dealing with the residual disease.

(4) *Drainage of Pus.*—Apart from the drainage of a secondarily infected empyema this method has little application now, though in the past tuberculous lung cavities were treated by catheter drainage (Monaldi), or open external drainage (cavernostomy).

Management.—All cases should be treated with bed rest and chemotherapy for several months before any active measures are undertaken. In many instances prolonged treatment will result in complete arrest of the disease; in others a tuberculous cavity, a positive sputum, or bronchial damage requires more active treatment. Surgical measures are almost entirely employed for dealing with residual lesions which persist after adequate conservative treatment. Resection is the treatment of choice in nearly 90% of all cases requiring surgical aid. Thoracoplasty is employed only when the risks of resection are unduly high or the disease too widespread for safe removal.

Apart from the failures of medical treatment and the persistence of unstable foci, resection is indicated in patients with destroyed lobes, in tuberculous bronchiectasis and in large solid lesions (tuberculoma). Where there is an empyema as well, surgical treatment will probably be required.

Thoracoplasty.—This has been the standard method of treatment employing major collapse therapy. The operation is now performed infrequently owing to the greater efficiency and safety of lung resection. It is mainly used for cavities in the upper lobe associated with persistently positive sputum and resistant organisms (figs 732 and 733), especially where extensive disease makes resection too hazardous.

The aim of the operation is to relax the diseased area from all sides so that it will retract concentrically towards the hilum. Lateral relaxation is produced by removal of the upper ribs whilst apical relaxation is achieved by separating the lung from the apex and the mediastinum. The original operation was introduced by Sauerbruch and consisted of removal of ribs only (lateral thoracoplasty), but this operation has been replaced by Semb's modification which includes apicolysis in addition to rib removal.

Lung Resection.—Since the introduction of antibiotics, resection of tuberculous lesions has been widely practised and has given good results. The operation has the advantage of

Vincenzo Monaldi, Contemporary. Director, Tuberculosis Clinic, University of Naples, Italy.
Ernst Ferdinand Sauerbruch, 1875–1951. Successively Professor of Surgery at Zurich, Switzerland, and at Munich and Berlin, Germany.
Carl Boye Semb, 1895–1971. Professor of Surgery, University of Oslo.

removing the greater part of the diseased tissue, in leaving no external deformity, and disturbing respiratory function very little. But it cannot be safely employed in those with extensive disease. Before embarking on resection it is necessary to determine by tomography and bronchography whether the lung and bronchi to be left behind are free from disease. Pre-operative bronchoscopy is advisable, and if active tuberculous bronchitis is discovered, resection should be delayed until it is controlled by further chemotherapy. At operation it is advisable to remove all the obvious tuberculous disease, although small healed nodules may be safely left behind. In some cases the remaining lobes must be prevented from over-expanding either by temporary phrenic paralysis or by performing a small apical thoracoplasty. Over-distension of the lobe is likely to cause reactivation of dormant foci. It is unwise to carry out a resection if the organisms are resistant to all antibiotics.

Other Measures.—Minor collapse procedures, such as artificial pneumothorax, phrenic paralysis, and pneumoperitoneum and variations of the operation of thoracoplasty, such as extra-pleural pneumothorax and plombage, have been rendered obsolete by the continued efficiency of chemotherapeutic agents.

POST-OPERATIVE PULMONARY COMPLICATIONS

The pulmonary complications of general surgery are the cause of serious morbidity and an appreciable mortality, and yet they can be largely prevented by adequate pre-operative and post-operative care.

Predisposing Factors.—(1) *Type of Operation.*—Operations on the upper abdomen and on the upper respiratory tract are more commonly implicated than others, but no operation is exempt. Operations for septic conditions are more prone to be followed by complications.

(2) *Sex.*—Males are more commonly affected than females.

(3) *Age.*—Complications are particularly frequent in the very young and the elderly.

(4) *Chronic Bronchitis.*—Chronic bronchitis is an important predisposing condition.

(5) *Smoking.*—Due to chronic bronchitis, heavy smokers are more prone to complications than non-smokers. Morton records 60% of complications occurring in heavy smokers and less than 10% in non-smokers.

(6) *Anaesthetic.*—The anaesthetic plays some part though this is less than is usually thought. Trauma to the tracheo-bronchial tree should be avoided, and prolonged post-operative unconsciousness is undesirable.

(7) *Pain.*—Post-operative pain is an important factor as it restricts coughing and deep breathing.

(8) Lack of mobility in bed and dehydration predisposes to venous stasis and thrombosis.

(9) Abdominal distension due to paralytic ileus.

Excessive Bronchial Secretions

Abnormal bronchial secretions account for the majority of the chest complications of surgery. Many patients are a little 'chesty' following even the most trivial operation. This 'normal' post-operative bronchitis, however, may lead to very serious and perhaps fatal sequelae unless adequately controlled.

Preventative Measures.—Adequate time should be devoted to preparing patients for elective operations. This can usefully be done in a regular pre-operative clinic where breathing exercises and coughing instruction are given, dental sepsis is attended to and bronchitis treated by antibiotics. The latter may be continued into the post-operative period. A routine chest x-ray may reveal unsuspected tuberculous or other lesions. Smoking of cigarettes should be forbidden for several days before operation.

The following complications may be encountered, but it should be realised

Hugh John Vivian Morton, 1909–1981. Anaesthetist, Hillingdon Hospital, Uxbridge, Middlesex, England.

that one may merge into another, or neglect of one frequently leads to the production of more serious conditions.

(1) *Bronchitis*.—This is the commonest complication and is important in that it is often the precursor of more serious lesions. It may arise *de novo* or represent an exacerbation of a pre-existing bronchitis. The attack may vary considerably from a simple post-operative cough with mucopurulent sputum to severe suppurative bronchitis. Signs in the lungs are generalised, and there are no radiographic changes to be seen.

(2) *Bronchopneumonia*.—This is usually a sequel to the above. Patchy consolidation occurs with more profound systemic changes. The commonest organisms are *Haemophilus influenzae* and pneumococci but cross-infection with ward organisms such as drug-resistant staphylococci and *P. pyocyaneus* may occur. Their presence should be sought by microscopy and culture of the sputum. Signs are more localised and bronchial breathing may be heard. Radiographs will reveal patchy mottling.

(3) *Atelectasis*.—This is produced by occlusion of a bronchus by viscid bronchial secretions and is usually a sequel to bronchitis. The obstruction leads to absorption atelectasis of the involved lobe. Secondary invasion of the lobe by pathogenic organisms results in particularly serious changes. Depression of the cough reflex by oversedation and poor ventilation are important predisposing factors. Atelectasis usually occurs after the second post-operative night, when secretions accumulate during sleep, and by morning have blocked the bronchus. The patient does not feel so well and there may be slight fever, tachycardia and breathlessness. Cough and sputum may not be obvious as the latter cannot be expectorated. Signs consist of restricted movement of the affected side of the chest and diminished breath-sounds, impaired percussion note and bronchial breathing over the affected lobe. Radiography will reveal the dense opacity of the atelectatic lower lobe—seen as a straight line passing down from the hilum, which on the left side may be hidden behind the heart and only revealed by a penetrating radiograph (figs 734 & 735).

(4) *Lung Abscess*.—This usually follows bronchopneumonia or atelectasis in elderly patients and is the result of ineffective early treatment. It is a particularly serious complication which can lead to spreading suppuration throughout the lung by organisms which are by then often resistant to all drugs.

Treatment.—*Prophylactic*.—At the conclusion of an operation the tracheobronchial tree should be aspirated if any secretions are suspected. Early return of consciousness and the cough reflex are desirable. Subsequent physiotherapy with encouragement of expectoration are important. Pain should be controlled by repeated small doses of analgesics of which pethidine (50-100 mg) is the most useful, as it does not depress respiration.

The Established Case.—It is important to encourage the expectoration of sputum by all possible means. Much can be done by the physiotherapist and the nurse, whilst steam inhalations and mucolytic agents (Bisolvon) help to loosen the sputum. When the secretions cannot be adequately removed naturally, they must be removed by catheter suction. If the simpler measures are not soon effective *bronchoscopy* should be carried out. This can readily be performed in the ward with a rigid bronchoscope under minimal local anaesthesia so that the

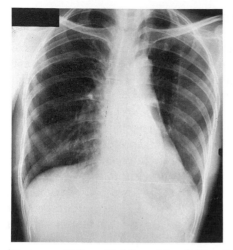

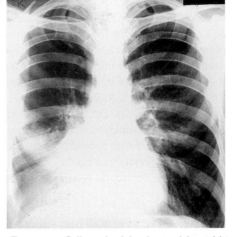

FIG. 734.—Collapsed left lower lobe, the line of which is just outside the heart shadow.

FIG. 735.—Collapsed right lower lobe with pneumonitis in adjacent right middle lobe.

cough reflex is preserved. A careful and unhurried clearance of the whole bronchial tree should be the aim. Bronchoscopy usually results in the aeration of an atelectatic lobe, but the condition may recur and further bronchoscopies be required. In such cases it is often preferable to perform a *tracheostomy*, particularly when secretions are profuse or the patient dyspnoeic. Tracheostomy by reducing the 'dead space' greatly improves the efficiency of respiration; it also provides easy access for repeated and atraumatic aspiration of the tracheobronchial tree.

A recent development is the use of a small plastic tube (Portex Ltd.) inserted under local anaesthesia through the cricothyroid membrane, through which secretions can be regularly aspirated with minimal disturbance to the patient (Matthews' Minitracheostomy).

Subphrenic Abscess (Chapter 49).

Broncho-pleural Fistula

This complication is one peculiar to thoracic operations involving resection of lung tissue. Several factors may be involved in its production.

(1) Poor surgical technique in closing the bronchus (sutures too tight, imperfectly placed or a long bronchial stump).

(2) State of the bronchial stump (malignant infiltration or tuberculous endobronchitis).

(3) Indifferent healing (elderly and debilitated patients, and after deep x-ray therapy).

Symptoms usually appear towards the end of the first week after operation; fever and blood-stained sputum are the first signs.

After a lobectomy air enters the pleural cavity producing a pneumothorax and collapse of the lung whilst pleural fluid enters the bronchial tree giving rise to a persistent cough with much thin blood-stained sputum.

Hugoe Matthews, Contemporary. Thoracic Surgeon, East Birmingham Hospital, England.

After a pneumonectomy serious flooding of the opposite bronchial tree may occur, leading to a fatal outcome unless promptly treated.

Treatment.—The first essential when a fistula is suspected is to anticipate and prevent flooding of the bronchial tree by early aspiration of fluid from the pleural cavity and by positioning the patient with the *affected side down.*

A small leak may be controlled by repeated aspirations or by temporary tube drainage until the fistula heals.

Larger fistulas should be treated at an early stage by re-opening the chest and resuturing the bronchus, after prelimary thoracoscopic aspiration of the pleural fluid. The suture line should be reinforced by a pedicled intercostal muscle graft. If the pleural cavity is already infected, however, it is better to drain the pleura and carry out bronchial repair at a later date.

Pulmonary Embolism (see Chapter 13).

Between 2 and 3% of all hospital deaths are due wholly, or in part, to pulmonary embolism. The condition is by no means limited to surgical wards. The clot most commonly originates in the veins of the calves, thighs or pelvis. Two types of venous lesions occur.

(1) *Thrombophlebitis.*—The thrombosis is secondary to infection or trauma. There is a marked inflammatory reaction and the resulting clot is firmly adherent to the vessel wall and is rarely dislodged.

(2) *Phlebothrombosis.*—Clotting is secondary to venous stasis and there is no inflammatory reaction in the veins. The clot is soft and insecurely attached to the vessel wall. Detachment of the clot is easy, particularly as the condition is often unsuspected and movements uninhibited (Chapter 13).

Clinical Features.—Pulmonary embolism is the most dangerous complication of phlebothrombosis. Much depends on the size of the embolus. *Small emboli* may be silent but the cumulative effect of many such episodes leads to a reduction in the pulmonary vascular bed resulting in pulmonary hypertension. Patients require permanent anticoagulants. *Medium emboli* lodge in branches of the pulmonary artery and result in pulmonary infarction without any haemo-dynamic disturbances. Classically the onset is abrupt with pain in the chest, dyspnoea, and haemoptysis. Chest radiographs reveal a triangular infarcted segment. Signs of venous thrombosis may or may not be present. Anticoagulants should be administered without delay and the patient immobilised for one week. Recurrent emboli are frequent. *Large emboli* lodge in the main pulmonary artery or one of its major branches. They produce serious haemodynamic disturbances which may be fatal (p. 779). Confusion with coronary thrombosis is easy but an E.C.G. is often of diagnostic value, showing right ventricular strain in pulmonary infarction. A massive pulmonary embolus may produce immediate death from ventricular fibrillation or complete obstruction of the circulation. Such cases often have an urgent desire for a bed-pan but are dead before one is produced. Those who survive complain of severe praecordial pain, tightness in the chest, and marked dyspnoea. Shock is great and the patient becomes grey and cold with a rapid, feeble pulse, low blood pressure, and raised venous pressure. Death may occur at any moment, but the longer the patient survives the better are his prospects of recovery.

Management of Massive Pulmonary Embolism.—Patients fall into one of two categories:

(*a*) Those who succumb within 2 hours of the embolism, and

(*b*) Those who survive this critical period.

In the former group cardiac arrest is frequent and closed cardiac massage will be required. This may serve to dislodge the clot and permit a limited pulmonary circulation. There is insufficient time to mount cardio-pulmonary bypass, and pulmonary embolectomy with temporary inflow occlusion should be attempted (see below).

In the second group a reasonable though precarious cardiac output is maintained and there is time to carry out essential investigations, to transfer the patient to a special centre or prepare cardio-pulmonary bypass. Confirmation of the diagnosis is essential by angio-cardiography before definitive treatment is started. The cardiac catheter is left in the pulmonary artery and 600,000 units of streptokinase is injected followed by 100,000 units hourly for 72 hours. Laboratory control of coagulation and lysis are essential. Improvement in cardiac output should occur within 6 hours. Thrombolytic therapy should be continued for 3–4 days in favourable cases. If deterioration sets in, pulmonary embolectomy should be performed. Heparin should not be used with fibrino-lysins.

Pulmonary Embolectomy without Bypass (Trendelenburg Type).—The pulmonary artery is exposed through a left fourth space thoractomy. Several stay sutures are placed on either side of the proposed incision in the pulmonary artery. A clamp is placed across the base of the pulmonary artery and aorta through the transverse sinus. The pulmonary artery is incised and clot removed with a sucker. Both branches of the pulmonary artery must be explored with the sucker end. After 90–120 seconds of occlusion the arteriotomy is controlled with a clamp and the occlusion clamp across aorta and pulmonary artery removed.

Pulmonary Embolectomy with Bypass.—Anaesthesia is not started until the pump is primed and the surgical staff scrubbed.

A mid sternal splitting incision gives quick access to the heart. A large venous tube is inserted into the right atrium and arterial return effected through a small incision in the ascending aorta. Bypass is then established and the pulmonary artery opened and clot removed with sponge forceps or a sucker. Careful exploration of the pulmonary arteries on both sides should be carried out and all fragments of clot removed.

Pulmonary Embolectomy with Inflow Occlusion.—This procedure is advised where bypass facilities are not available. The heart is exposed through a median sternotomy, the pericardium is opened longitudinally. Tapes are placed around both cavae. With the tape tightened, the right ventricle rapidly becomes empty and the pulmonary artery can be opened and clot removed with forceps and suction. Venous occlusion should only be maintained for about 60 seconds but can be reapplied several times to enable all clot to be removed.

Venous Thrombectomy.—Removal of residual clot by a Fogarty catheter is advocated by many surgeons to reduce the likelihood of further emboli and to help re-establish a normal circulation in the affected limb. Ligation or plication of the inferior vena cava is advocated by some to prevent further emboli reaching the lungs (Chapter 13).

LUNG TRANSPLANTATION

Transplantation of the lung has been successfully carried out on many occasions but to date the longest survivor died 10 months after the operation. Many technical problems such as ischaemia at the bronchial suture line and stenosis of the vascular anastomoses remain to be solved. In addition, the problems of rejection are not fully solved. At the present time, combined heart and lung transplantation appears to offer a better chance of survival for patients with primary lung disease than lung transplantation alone (Chapters 41, 62).

Friedrich Trendelenburg, 1844–1924 (see footnote, Chapter 5). Described pulmonary embolectomy in 1908. The operation was first performed successfully by Martin Kirscher (see footnote, p. 298) in 1924.
Thomas J. Fogarty, Contemporary. Assistant Professor of Surgery, Stanford University, San Francisco, California, U.S.A.

THE DIAPHRAGM

Herniation of an abdominal viscus through the diaphragm into the chest may occur through a congenital or acquired defect. *Congenital herniae* occur at certain well-recognised points (fig. 736) and are due to a failure of fusion of the various elements which make up the diaphragm. Such herniae usually have a well-defined sac and adhesions are uncommon. Other congenital malformations may be present.

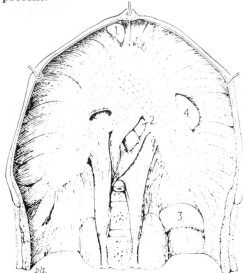

FIG. 736.—The usual sites of congenital diaphragmatic herniae. 1. Foramen of Morgagni. 2. Oesophageal hiatus. 3. Foramen of Bochdalek (pleuro-peritoneal hernia) (this may be situated more anteriorly). 4. Dome.

Acquired herniae may be due to trauma or may be through the oesophageal hiatus (see Chapter 43).

With the exception of acquired oesophageal hiatus hernia in adults, the symptoms in children will be due to acute respiratory embarrassment or incipient or actual intestinal obstruction, or in adults will be vague dyspeptic symptoms or definite subacute obstruction.

Surgical repair is advisable in all cases, usually through a low thoracotomy and with repair of the defect with a double row of non-absorbable sutures. In neonates a subcostal incision is advisable as there is frequently an associated malrotation of the bowel which must be corrected by dividing Ladd's band or repositioning the bowel.

(1) **Eventration.**—This condition is due to atrophy and loss of muscle of part or all of one leaf of the diaphragm, which becomes fibrous tissue covered with pleura and peritoneum. The thin, flaccid diaphragm is raised and immobile. Symptoms are uncommon and the condition is usually discovered on routine x-ray. If respiration is embarrassed plication is indicated.

(2) **Oesophageal Hiatus Hernia.**—This may occur as a congenital abnormality but more usually occurs as an acquired condition in the middle-aged or elderly. It is considered in Chapter 43.

(3) **Hernia through the Foramen of Morgagni.**—The defect lies between the sternal and costal attachments of the diaphragm and is therefore situated anteriorly and contains transverse colon. It is more common on the right (fig. 737). It

William Edwards Ladd, 1880–1967. Professor of Child Surgery, Harvard University, Boston, U.S.A.
Giovanni Battista Morgagni, 1682–1771. Professor of Anatomy, Padua, Italy for 56 years; from 1715 until his death in his 90th year.

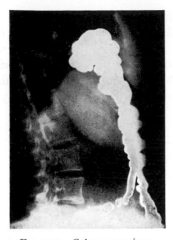

FIG. 737.—Colon occupying a
Morgagni hernia.
(*Dr. Oliver Smith, Birmingham.*)

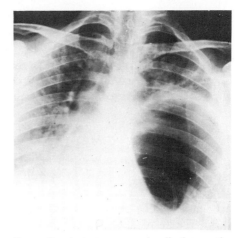

FIG. 738.—A large traumatic diaphragmatic
hernia with dilated stomach occupying much of
the chest.

FIG. 739.—Foramen of Bochdalek hernia on the
left side in an infant. The left pleural cavity is
occupied by intestine, the mediastinum is displaced to the right, and the right lung is very
little aerated.

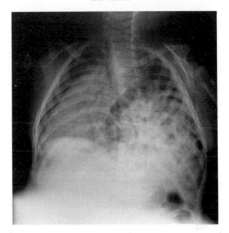

usually presents in adults and there may be symptoms of subacute obstruction
but more commonly the patient is symptom free.

(4) **Hernia through the Foramen of Bochdalek** (Pleuro-peritoneal Canal).—
This opening is in the dome of the diaphragm posteriorly and provides a free
communication between the abdominal and pleural cavities. The hernia, which
has no sac and is usually on the left side, presents in neonates or children, causing
respiratory difficulty or incipient or actual obstruction of the small or large intestine (fig. 739).

(5) **Traumatic Diaphragmatic Hernia.**—Rupture of the diaphragm
(fig. 738), unless due to a penetrating injury (sword thrust or bullet wound)
follows severe crush injury to the abdomen (*e.g.* a road traffic accident or a fall
from a height). Rupture can also occur from a crushing injury with the trunk
flexed (*e.g.* in mining accidents). It is a bursting injury and produces a long linear
tear in the dome of the diaphragm (usually on the left) and herniation of the
stomach and/or transverse colon. There is often delay in making the diagnosis
until distension of the stomach and respiratory embarrassment occur. The initial

Victor Alexander Bochdalek, 1801–1883. Professor of Anatomy, Prague, Czechoslovakia.

radiographic examination should reveal the diagnosis but the basal opacity may initially be confused with that of pleural fluid or basal consolidation. The condition may resemble a pneumothorax.

Clinical examination reveals that the breath sounds have been replaced by bowel sounds, unless intestinal ileus produces silence. Repair of the hernia should always be undertaken with the minimum delay.

MEDIASTINAL TUMOURS

Mediastinal tumours occur from infancy to old age in both sexes. About 50% are symptomless and are picked up on a routine chest radiograph. The size of the tumour bears no relation to possible symptoms—a small tumour may compress a bronchus leading to atelectasis of a lobe or lung and consequent dyspnoea, or a very large dermoid or neurofibroma may cause no symptoms at all.

The symptoms of a mediastinal tumour are due to pressure effects on (a) recurrent laryngeal nerve—hoarse voice; (b) trachea or bronchus–dyspnoea due to compression; (c) oesophagus—dysphagia; (d) superior vena cava—fullness of face; (e) sympathetic chain—small pupil, ptosis and unilateral sweating of the face (Horner's syndrome).

All mediastinal tumours gradually enlarge and sooner or later cause pressure symptoms. This may occur suddenly if there is a haemorrhage into the tumour. Phrenic or recurrent laryngeal nerve involvement almost always implies malignant change.

In practice, a thoracotomy is usually required both for diagnosis and treatment, as many of these tumours are potentially malignant and may suddenly increase in size if a haemorrhage occurs into them.

Mediastinal tumours are best classified according to their position on the chest x-ray. A lateral view is essential.

(1) **Anterior Mediastinal Tumours** (from above downwards)
   Retrosternal goitre.
   Thymic tumours and cysts.
   Teratoma and dermoid cyst.
   Pleuro-pericardial cyst.
(2) **Posterior Mediastinal Tumours**
   Neurogenic tumours (neurofibroma, ganglioneuroma).
(3) **Central Mediastinum**
   Lymphadenopathies (these are often multifocal and the lesions are characteristically lobulated). Secondary carcinoma, tuberculous adenitis, lymphomas, and sarcoid are the commonest varieties.
   Foregut duplication cysts (bronchogenic or gastrogenic).
   Lipoma.

Retrosternal Goitre (Chapter 37).—This produces an anterior mediastinal tumour of characteristic shape. It is frequently bilateral though usually larger on one side. The tumour has a broad base superiorly which merges and cannot be separated from the tissues of the neck on radiological examination. Calcification is not uncommon as the tumour has probably been present for many years. This is one of the few tumours which compress the trachea (scabbard trachea, fig. 740).

Removal through a cervical incision is usually possible, and only occasionally

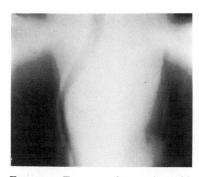

FIG. 740.—Tomogram from patient with retrosternal goitre showing displacement and compression of the trachea. Note line of thyroid shadow which passes directly upwards into the neck.

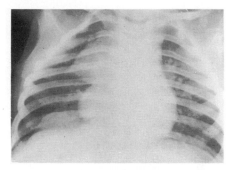

FIG. 741.—Typical sail-shaped upper mediastinal shadow due to enlarged thymus in an infant.

is a sternal-splitting approach required. It should be remembered that the blood vessels serving the thyroid are in the neck!

THE THYMUS

Anatomy.—The gland originates as a diverticulum of the third and sometimes the fourth pharyngeal pouch on each side. Epithelial in origin, it soon assumes a lymphoid character. The body of the thymus consists of two lobes closely applied to one another in the middle line, overlying the upper part of the pericardium and the great vessels, and extending upwards into the base of the neck. Each lobe is overlapped by pleura, and above this level has a slender pole passing to the isthmus of the thyroid. The blood supply of the gland is derived mainly from the internal mammary arteries. After puberty, the thymus commences to atrophy, and is replaced by fat, but even up to, and after, the age of fifty, the gland still contains a considerable amount of characteristic lymphoid tissue with epithelial elements, notably Hassall's corpuscles.

The Thymus and Immunity.—Most of our knowledge about the relationship of the thymus to immune processes is derived from observations made on thymectomised young mice and other mammals. Immunologically-active lymphocytes first appear in the thymus and are later seeded in other conglomerations of lymphoid tissue. Early thymectomy results in a depletion or absence of these cells in the body. In addition there may be depletion in immunoglobulin levels and some antibody responses are decreased or delayed. The thymectomised mice will accept homograft transplants with little or no evidence of rejection.

Hyperplasia of the thymus occurs in toxic goitre, acromegaly, in some cases of Addison's disease, after castration, after bilateral adrenalectomy, and in myasthenia gravis. In infancy the gland may be enlarged (fig. 741). In the past this condition was called '*status thymo-lymphaticus*' and thought to be an explanation of sudden death under anaesthesia in children. This theory is no longer acceptable. Enlargement of the gland in infants may compress the trachea causing stridor and wheeziness (thymic asthma). Symptoms usually subside spontaneously but if severe and persistent, treatment with radiotherapy or surgery may be required.

Tumours of the thymus are not uncommon. Classification is difficult, but Thompson and Thackray describe three main histological types: (1) Epithelial. (2) Lymphoid. (3) Teratomatous. The epithelial type is the commonest. Cyst formation, lobulation by fibrous tissue, necrosis, and calcification are sometimes seen. Between 10% and 20% of thymic tumours are associated with myasthenia. Conversely, about 15% of myasthenics are found to have a thymic tumour; half are invasive and malignant and associated with severe and intractable disease; the remainder are histologically indistinguishable from normal thymic tissue and are non-invasive and do not appear to influence the severity of the myasthenia nor its response to treatment. Thymic tumours occupy the anterior compartment of the superior mediastinum. The majority of tumours are discovered by routine radiography (fig. 742). Tumours visible on both sides of the normal mediastinal contour are likely to

Arthur Hill Hassall, 1817–1894. General Practitioner, Microscopist and Chemical Analyst, Kensington, London.
Robert Edward Mervyn Thompson, Contemporary. Reader in Bacteriology, Middlesex Hospital, London.
Alan Christopher Thackray, Contemporary. Professor of Morbid Histology, Middlesex Hospital, London.

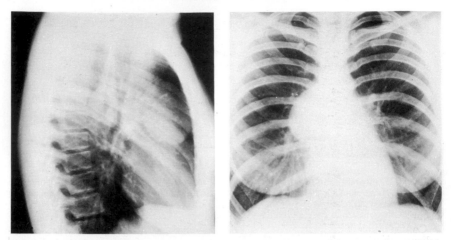

Fig. 742.—PA and lateral radiograph of thymic cyst. The mass occupies the anterior superior mediastinum.

be invasive and malignant (fig. 743). A few may produce signs of superior mediastinal
obstruction.

Removal of the tumours is advised in the majority of patients owing to the very real
risks of progressive growth and the development of invasive characteristics. The tumour
is approached by a sternal-splitting incision which gives excellent access and facilitates
complete removal. If the tumour is invading the surrounding structures widely a biopsy
only should be taken and excision not attempted. The correct treatment is radiotherapy.

Myasthenia Gravis.—In this disease the transmission of motor-nerve impulses at the
neuromuscular junctions is blocked by interference with the action of the transmitter—
acetylcholine—upon the muscle fibres.

Clinical Features.—The disease occurs in both sexes and commences, as a rule, in
early adult life. The essential symptoms are profound fatigue after modest exertion, and
transient paresis of voluntary muscles. Muscles supplied both by the cranial and spinal
nerves are affected, the extrinsic ocular muscles being involved most constantly. Usually
ptosis (fig. 745), a squint, and diplopia are the first symptoms. Later manifestations are
drooping of the mandible, with weakness of mastication and difficulty in swallowing. The
voice becomes weak, and in some cases death occurs within a few months from involvement of the muscles of respiration. Usually the disease runs a chronic progressive course,

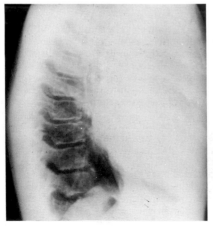
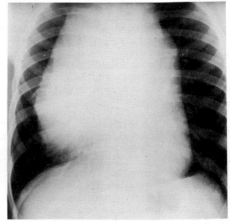

Fig. 743.—Lateral and PA radiograph of malignant thymoma. The tumour presents on both sides
of the mediastinum. In the lateral film it is seen to lie anteriorly.

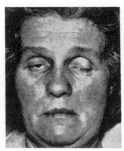

FIG. 744.—Myasthenia gravis. Before neostigmine.
(*Arthur Makey, FRCS, London.*)

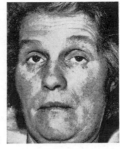

FIG. 745.—Myasthenia gravis. One hour after neostigmine.
(*Arthur Makey, FRCS, London.*)

but partial remissions occur. The reflexes remain normal, and there is no sensory loss. Occasionally myasthenia gravis complicates primary thyrotoxicosis. Should a patient with myasthenia gravis become pregnant, remission of symptoms during pregnancy often occurs.

Confirmatory Tests.—(1) Edrophonium chloride (Tensilon®), 10 mg intravenously relieves signs and symptoms of myasthenia in 1 minute though they usually return in 10 minutes. Tensilon is only used diagnostically in this way because it has such a short action. Alternatively 2 mg neostigmine and 0·65 mg atropine can be given but the response is delayed for ½-1 hour (figs. 744 and 745). (2) The affected muscles often show the myasthenic reaction—fatigue with faradic, but not with galvanic, stimulation.

Radiography, particularly a lateral radiograph, of the superior mediastinum should always be undertaken. In 15% of cases a thymic neoplasm is revealed. Apart from tumours, there is no x-ray evidence of thymic enlargements in myasthenic patients.

Treatment.—Medical.—Orally, from 4 to 15 tablets (15 mg each) of neostigmine can be given in the twenty-four hours. They should be so spaced as to enable meals to be taken without difficulty in mastication. Pyridostigmine (Mestinon®) is a related longer-acting compound which can be used in combination with, or instead of, neostigmine. It is particularly valuable for nocturnal administration. In critical cases neostigmine may be given in a slow drip infusion. Oral potassium salts given in large dosage (12 g per day) are often beneficial. Ephedrine and Guanidine may also be of benefit. Atropine should be administered if bowel activity is increased by the anti-cholinesterase drugs.

Surgical Treatment.—Thymectomy is advised for those patients who are not adequately controlled by medical measures and especially for the more severe cases. Best results are obtained in younger patients especially females with a short history and in these the indications are less strict. The operation, however, should not be denied the elderly male patient with a long history if medical management is proving difficult. The presence of a thymic tumour makes a good operative result less likely and some recommend pre-operative radiotherapy in such cases.

Thymectomy.[1]—Muscle relaxants are currently advised by many anaesthetists on the basis that 24 hours of artificial ventilation after operation has many advantages and permits the clinician to omit all drugs during this period.

The gland is best approached by a vertical full sternal splitting incision. The pleural cavities should be avoided if possible but if opened an intercostal drainage tube should be inserted at the end of the operation and connected to an under-water seal.

The gland is readily found as it is usually larger than normal. It is dissected carefully from its surroundings and removed in its entirety. The thymic vein passes directly backwards from the posterior aspect of the thymus to the left innominate vein and should be carefully displayed and divided after ligation. The mediastinum and the pleural cavity should all be drained for at least 24 hours.

After operation the patient is best managed in an intensive care unit, for respiratory problems are the main concern. An immediate post-operative chest radiograph is important to exclude a pneumothorax or a haemothorax. Artificial ventilation through an endotracheal tube for 24 hours is advisable. Thereafter the patient may be weaned from the ventilator, provided there is no respiratory infection and the patient's respiratory muscles are strong enough. Tracheal suction may be required. A nasogastric tube will allow the crushed anticholinesterase drugs to be given into the stomach, which is the most effective

---

[1] Alfred Blalock, 1899–1964. Professor of Surgery, Johns Hopkins University, Baltimore, was the first to perform thymectomy successfully for myasthenia gravis in 1939.

(a)

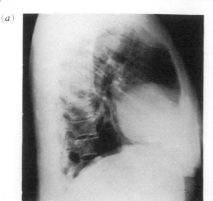

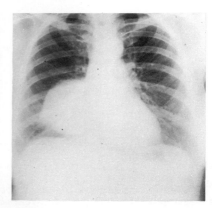

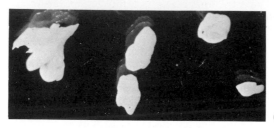

FIG. 746.—(a) Lateral and PA radiograph of patient with a mediastinal teratoma. The tumour lies anteriorly and
with a pedicle attached beneath the
aortic arch. (b) X-ray of excised tumour
showing formation of teeth.

(b)

route, but they should be withheld until their need is apparent so as to prevent the serious
complication of a cholinergic crisis.

Results of Treatment.—The operation mortality is approximately 5%. Complete
remission is obtained in nearly 50% of favourable cases (young females with a short history)
whilst many of the remainder are able to manage more satisfactorily on smaller doses of
drugs. In the older age group the results are less dramatic and are often delayed. In
patients with invasive thymic tumour the results may be disappointing even when the
tumour has been totally excised.

Pre-operative radiotherapy is only occasionally employed at the present time being
usually reserved for the acute case with a radiologically visible tumour.

Teratomas and Dermoid Cysts.—Teratomas and dermoid cysts contain tissue from the three embryological germinal layers (Chapter 8). They occur almost
always in the anterior mediastinum closely related to the anterior surface of the
pericardium and the great vessels (fig. 746). They may grow to a surprisingly
large size before they cause symptoms. These are due to pressure effects upon
the trachea, bronchus, great veins, oesophagus and phrenic or recurrent laryngeal
nerves. They are often slightly lobulated and may project into either side of the
chest. Irregular areas of calcification, bone or tooth formation are sometimes seen
and malignant change may occur.

Rapid increase in size without malignant change is sometimes associated with
pregnancy. Occasionally a positive Aschheim Zondek test is obtained in non-
pregnant patients. Removal is indicated in all cases, and is best carried out
through a wide lateral thoracotomy or a median sternotomy.

Mediastinal Cysts.—These are usually developmental in origin and may be associated
with the trachea, bronchi, or oesophagus (foregut cyst), pericardium (pleuro-pericardial
on 'spring-water' cyst) or lymph nodes (lymphogenous cysts).

Foregut cysts are likely to become infected and may rupture into the trachea, oesophagus, lung or bronchus. Removal is desirable.

Selmar Aschheim, Contemporary. Formerly Honorary Professor of Gynaecology, University of Berlin.
Bernhardt Zondek, 1891–1966. Professor of Obstetrics and Gynaecology, Hadassah Medical School, Hebrew University, Jerusalem, Israel.
Aschheim and Zondek described this text for pregnancy in a joint paper in 1928.

CHAPTER 41

THE HEART AND PERICARDIUM

SPECIAL METHODS OF INVESTIGATION

Modern cardiac surgery demands precise methods of investigation to provide accurate anatomical and physiological details of the various cardiac abnormalities. It is only when such information is available that a precise diagnosis can be made and surgical treatment planned. The most important available methods are:

(1) **Radiology** (standard techniques and fluoroscopy). Such examinations provide details of the contour and size of the cardiac chambers. Plain films also give a wealth of information on the pulmonary circulation. In departments of radiology fortunate enough to have a CT scanner further information on the pericardium and other thoracic structures can be obtained. This information can be increased by the use of reduction enhancement.

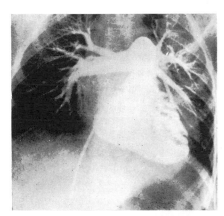 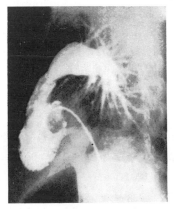

FIG. 747.—Normal angiocardiogram showing the right side of the heart and pulmonary arteries.

(2) **Angiocardiography** (figs 747 & 748).—The chambers of the heart and great vessels can be outlined by the injection of 30-80 ml of Niopam 370 under high pressure. Visual information can be recorded on either cine-film or cut films depending on whether static or dynamic information is required. Important anatomical information concerning the size and shape of the heart chambers, the presence of a shunt or of the function of a valve can be obtained. The pulmonary artery and its branches, and the aorta and the aortic root can also be visualised in detail. By manipulation of this data with computer technology refined images can be obtained, a technique called Digital Subtraction Angiography (DSA). Of great importance today is the delineation of the anatomy of the coronary arteries to allow accurate revascularisation for patients with angina. This is carried out routinely, again using Niopam 370 in a dose of 4-8 ml per artery selected.

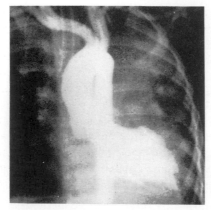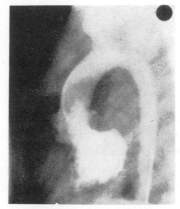

Fig. 748.—Normal angiocardiogram showing the left side of the heart and aorta.

(3) **Cardiac Catheterisation.**—A fine catheter is introduced through a vein or an artery into the heart where its passage can be followed by fluoroscopy and blood samples and pressure tracings recorded. This investigation supplies functional as well as anatomical data.

(4) **Measurement of Cardiac Output.**—Cardiac output is an important assessment of left ventricular function and peripheral vascular tone, which in turn may affect both the risks of operation and the subsequent relief of symptoms. Output can be estimated by the Fick principle after measurement of the oxygen consumption and the venous and arterial oxygen contents, by thermodilution techniques, or by the use of tracer dyes. The determination has been simplified by computerised techniques. (See also Swan Ganz P.C.W.P. measurement, p. 64.)

(5) **Echocardiography.**—Beams of high speed ultrasound waves are directed

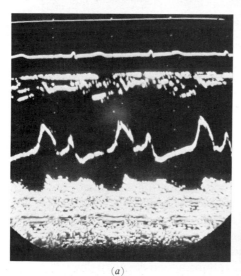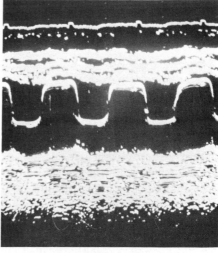

(a)   (b)

Fig. 749.—Movements of anterior leaflet of mitral valve as recorded by ultrasound, (a) normal cusp; (b) mitral stenois. The flat top of the tracing indicates reduced movement of valve leaflets during diastole.

(D. Gibson, London.)

Adolf Fick, 1829–1901. German Physiologist.

through the heart. Whenever the vibrations cross a boundary or interface, vibrations will be reflected back to the transmitting source provided the reflecting surface lies at right angles to the original beam. By accurate placing of the transmitter the movements of the aortic leaflet of the mitral valve, the anterior and posterior walls of the heart and the ventricular septum can all be recorded and important information obtained (fig. 749 (*a*) and (*b*)). Thickening, calcification and poor mobility of the anterior mitral cusp can be clearly demonstrated and indications for closed or open mitral valvotomy determined from this investigation alone, thus often avoiding the need for cardiac catheterisation and angiocardiography. Similarly pericardial effusions and atrial tumours can be diagnosed with certainty. Recent developments have included the investigation of all forms of congenital heart disease by two-dimensional (2-D) and pulsed Doppler echocardiography.

(6) **Radionuclear Studies** (fig. 750).—A major advance in the understanding of myocardial function in both health and disease has been the development of radionuclear imaging. Techniques are available using a gamma camera to assess both the way in which the ventricles are moving (MUGA Scans), and the blood supply to the heart (Thallium scans). By coupling radio-active material to specific antimyocardial monoclonal antibodies areas of the heart damaged during a heart attack or by other disease processes can be delineated.

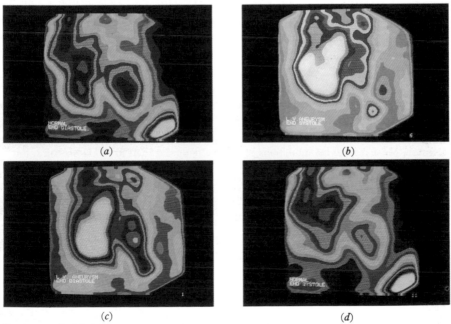

(*a*)   (*b*)

(*c*)   (*d*)

FIG. 750.—Gated radionuclide blood pool images (MUGA scans). The intensity of radioactivity is represented by the colours. Red represents a very 'hot' region whereas the various shades of green represent less radioactivity. The greater the volume of blood the greater will be the intensity of the radioactivity. (*a*) A normal left ventricle at the end of diastole. (*b*) The same ventricle at the end of systole. The decrease in volume of the left ventricle can be seen indicating that the ventricle is functioning well. (*c*) This scan is of a patient with a left ventricular aneurysm and the elongated appearance of the aneurysmal ventricle is well seen. (*d*) At the end of systole in the same ventricle a pool of blood can be seen remaining at the apex of the heart. This is within the aneurysmal sac.

Doppler, see p. 197.

(7) **Magnetic Resonance Imaging.**—It is becoming possible to create images of the working heart both in-vivo and in-vitro by the application of a very powerful magnetic field around the area of interest. The potential advantage of this technique is that information on the local biochemistry may be obtained in addition to a detailed visual image. This technology is highly expensive and is not widely available.

CARDIO-RESPIRATORY RESUSCITATION

In cardiothoracic emergencies the heart and lungs should be considered as one unit: where there is circulatory failure, both pulmonary and cardiac support will be required. Although in the early stages of a crisis only one element may be affected, its failure very rapidly implicates the other. Thus, respiratory failure rapidly leads to cardiac arrest and vice versa.

Circulatory failure is common in civil life—electrocution, drowning, asphyxia, and major trauma account for many cases. In addition, circulatory arrest may occur in any hospital department. It is more commonly associated with major surgical procedures especially those performed for cardiac conditions, but minor operations and diagnostic procedures are not immune. If lives are to be saved, it is essential that the mechanism of production and the methods of correction of circulatory arrest should be clearly understood. Not only should vulnerable departments be supplied with the necessary basic instruments for dealing with the emergency, but both medical and nursing personnel should be thoroughly familiar with the procedure of resuscitation.

Causes of Cardiac Arrest.—The following are the factors usually responsible for cardiac arrest:

(1) **Hypoxia.**—Myocardial hypoxia is probably the most frequent and important precipitating cause of arrest. It can be produced by a variety of means, such as respiratory obstruction, serious haemorrhage, a sudden severe fall in blood pressure or coronary air embolism. Haemorrhage from the heart is always more serious than that from the peripheral circulation owing to a marked decrease of cardiac output and rapid fall in blood pressure. Most cardiac manipulations produce a temporary fall in blood pressure, but if they are repeated or prolonged, severe and irreversible changes may develop.

(2) **Metabolic.**—The heart muscle is exceedingly sensitive to alterations in its biochemical environment. In particular it is very sensitive to alterations in the extra-cellular levels of potassium. Indeed the fact that the heart will arrest in diastole in the presence of hyperkalaemia is the basis of myocardial protection using cardioplegic solutions.

(3) **The State of the Myocardium.**—A healthy myocardium will stand moderate manipulation and hypoxia without ill effect, but a diseased myocardium (ischaemic, bacterial, viral) has less reserve, and relatively minor disturbances may cause failure.

(4) **Drug Induced.**—Many anaesthetic agents can induce dysrhythmias and hypotension, particularly if associated with hypoxia. Inotropic drugs such as isoprenaline, adrenaline and dopamine, if used inappropriately can also cause ventricular dysrhythmias leading to ventricular fibrillation. Beta-blockers, calcium antagonists, and other vasodilators, particularly if used in combination, can lead to profound hypotension and asystole.

Types of Cardiac Arrest.—Sudden acute cardiac failure may be produced by:

(1) **Circulatory Obstruction.**—By a massive pulmonary embolism, air embolism, or accidental occlusion of one of the main vessels.

(2) **Asystole.**—This is usually due to severe myocardial depression. The heart beat becomes slow and feeble and finally stops. The myocardium is flabby, dilated, and cyanosed.

(3) **Ventricular Fibrillation** is usually associated with an irritable heart as a result of manipulation, trauma or drugs. In such cases, the myocardium is less depressed and more likely to recover than in the former group.

Management of Cardiac Arrest.—Speedy recognition is essential if the circulation is to be restored before irreversible damage has been done to the brain. Diagnosis is based upon an absent cardiac impulse and carotid pulse. Respiratory arrest will very rapidly follow a cardiac arrest, even if it does not precede it. Within one or two minutes the pupils will begin to dilate signalling the onset of cerebral damage which will rapidly become irreversible. This usually occurs 3-5 minutes after cerebral perfusion has ceased. The heart may recover after slightly longer periods of absent circulation, but this is of no consolation if the patient is 'brain dead'. For this reason the rapid institution of cardiac massage is essential.

Vulnerable departments should prepare a simple chart outlining essential procedure for guidance to both medical and nursing staff.

Management is divided into two phases:

(*a*) **Emergency.**—These measures are carried out by the man on the spot and consist of *mouth to mouth ventilation* and *closed cardiac massage*. These can both be performed by one operator in the ratio of one breath to ten chest compressions, but are more efficiently carried out by two. (Full technical details are available in all first-aid manuals.) These two measures should be continued without interruption until a heart beat or spontaneous respirations return or until expert help arrives. If performed effectively, the vital organs can be kept alive for a few hours by these measures alone. Correction of metabolic acidosis as outlined in the next section should be started as soon as possible.

(*b*) **Subsequent Management.**—Further management depends on the arrival of expert help and appropriate equipment (endotracheal tubes, ventilating apparatus, cardiograph, electrical defibrillator and thoracotomy set).

1. *Ventilation:* At the earliest possible moment an endotracheal tube should be passed and positive pressure ventilation started.

2. *Cardiograph:* Electrocardiographic monitoring should be established as soon as possible in order to determine the type of cardiac arrest (asystole or ventricular fibrillation) and demonstrate any signs of recovery.

3. *Cardiac massage:* Closed massage should be continued until cardiography is available. Further action depends on the type of rhythm.

(*a*) If ventricular fibrillation is present, attempt external defibrillation. If this is unsuccessful, give an intravenous or intracardiac injection of 100 mg lignocaine or 250 mg of procaine amide, or 5 ml of 10% calcium chloride, and attempt defibrillation after an interval of two to three minutes with continued cardiac massage. As a last resort expose the heart and carry out open massage and drug administration.

(*b*) If asystole has developed, inject 10 ml of 1:10,000 adrenaline or 0·01 mg isoprenaline into the circulation. This should induce ventricular fibrillation in which case proceed as in 3(*a*) above. If there is no response, open the chest and carry out open massage with further injections of adrenaline or isoprenaline.

(*c*) **Open Cardiac Massage.**—The chest should be opened through the fifth intercostal space on the left side by an intercostal incision extending from the sternum to the axilla. The wound does not bleed as there is no circulation. The only instrument required to permit bi-manual massage is a rib-spreader, but should this not be immediately available massage is quite possible with one hand. Massage is most efficient with two hands with the pericardium widely opened. One hand should be placed above and the other below the ventricular mass, and massage should be carried out with the flat of the hand and fingers rather than with the finger-tips. The rate should be about 50 times per minute, though this is guided by the need for a sufficient pause to permit diastolic filling. Massage should always be carried out gently as damage to the myocardium is possible if excessive force is used. The object of cardiac massage is to improve the tone of the myocardium, to increase the coronary flow, and ensure a supply of oxygenated blood to the brain. The arrested heart is distended, flaccid, and cyanosed, but after massage it should become smaller, firmer, and pinker. When tone has returned, attempts should be made to obtain normal beating. Before closing the chest pacemaker wires should be attached to the left ventricle in case of further episodes of arrest.

In Cardiac Surgical Units it is often possible to establish cardio-pulmonary bypass as an emergency to allow the heart time to recover.

4. *Correction of Metabolic Acidosis:* All patients develop acidosis after cardiac arrest and its presence may prevent resuscitation. Sixty ml of an 8·4% solution of sodium bicarbonate (1 mmol per ml) should be given intravenously as soon as possible and further doses administered to restore the pH to normal levels (Chapter 6).

Later Management.—After the restoration of normal rhythm and a normal blood pressure, a careful watch should be maintained in case of recurrence. Adequate steps should be taken to correct any metabolic acidosis. The main late complications are related to cerebral and renal damage resulting from the period of circulatory arrest. If return of consciousness is delayed, cerebral dehydration as described in Chapter 26 should be carried out. Total body hypothermia with reduction of temperature to 32°C may help to limit cerebral damage (p. 793). If renal activity is impaired, the measures described under renal anuria (Chapter 58) should be instituted.

THE SCOPE OF CARDIAC SURGERY

Operative treatment of cardiac abnormalities is advancing steadily, particularly with the advent of new techniques for controlling the circulation. The procedures can be, for practical purposes, placed in one of three groups:

(1) **Extracardiac Operations.**—These are carried out on the main vessels outside the heart or on the pericardium. The ventricles or atria are not directly interfered with so that cardiac function is not unduly disturbed. Examples include ligation of a patent ductus, excision of coarctation, systemic-pulmonary anatomoses, pericardectomy and resection of some thoracic aortic aneurysms.

(2) **Closed Intracardiac Operations.**—These are blind intracardiac procedures performed by instrument or finger and controlled by touch. Access is obtained to the interior of the heart through either the ventricular or atrial walls or through the base of one of the great vessels. Cardiac action is interfered with to some extent so that irregularity of heart action is liable to be encountered. Mitral valvotomy is the only closed procedure still used regularly.

(3) **Open Cardiac Operation.**—The desire of every surgeon is to operate with safety under direct vision on the open and motionless heart. The following techniques have allowed this goal to be largely achieved.

(a) *Extra-corporeal Circulation.*—The heart-lung machine, many commercial models of which are now available, has been in regular daily clinical use now for more than twenty years. During this time there has been a steady improvement in the equipment available in terms of both refinement and patient safety. Basic-

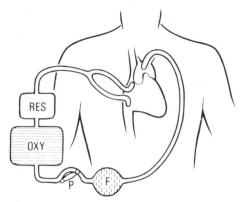
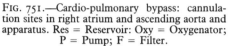

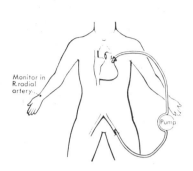

FIG. 751.—Cardio-pulmonary bypass: cannulation sites in right atrium and ascending aorta and apparatus. Res = Reservoir: Oxy = Oxygenator; P = Pump; F = Filter.

FIG. 752.—Left heart by-pass.

ally each consists of a pump and an oxygenator. Blood is withdrawn from the caval veins, passed through the oxygenator and returned to the arterial circulation through the ascending aorta or femoral artery (fig. 751). The blood is thus diverted from the heart and lungs but a good supply of well oxygenated blood is made available to the vital organs. Heart-lung machines provide the surgeon with periods of between two and three hours for intracardiac surgery with safety. By the use of an extracorporeal circulation many complicated congenital and acquired cardiac anomalies can be corrected.

Technique.—The majority of cardiac abnormalities are corrected through a median sternotomy incision. Immediately prior to cannulation the patient is heparinised with 3 mg/kg body weight. The ascending aorta is cannulated with a plastic tube through a purse string suture placed in the aortic adventitia and each cava is similarly cannulated through the right atrial wall. The cannulae are connected to the heart-lung machine after careful elimination of all bubbles of air. At the completion of the operation the cannulae are removed and the heparin is counteracted with protamine (6 mg/kg body weight). During heart-lung bypass the efficiency of the extracorporeal circulation is monitored by observing urinary output and by measurement of blood gases and determination of serum potassium.

(b) *Hypothermia.*—The metabolic needs of the body can be considerably reduced by cooling the tissues, thus enabling the latter to survive short periods of total deprivation of oxygen or longer periods of partial deprivation. Originally used as a sole technique, surface cooling of the body to 28–30°C gave a surgeon about 10 minutes of circulatory arrest before endangering the brain. This time permitted the performance of simple cardiac operations (closure of atrial defects and relief of pulmonary stenosis) but the technique has been almost entirely replaced by cardiopulmonary bypass. Greater safety with further reductions in body temperature can only be achieved with the use of cardiopulmonary bypass as ventricular fibrillation usually ensues at a temperature of about 25°C. With this technique, however, the body temperature can be reduced to 15–18°C and periods of up to 45 minutes or more of circulatory arrest can be tolerated. This technique is now widely used in the surgery of congenital heart disease in infants.

(c) *Left Heart Bypass.*—Left atrio-femoral or left heart bypass is a useful tech-

nique which facilitates operations on the thoracic aorta. The left atrium is cannulated and blood diverted with a pump into the femoral artery (fig. 752). The aorta
can now be cross-clamped and the left ventricle continues to supply the head and
upper extremities with blood whilst the bypass caters for the lower limbs and
abdominal viscera.

(d) *Femoro-femoral Bypass.*—The femoral artery and vein are each cannulated
and the blood is passed through an oxygenator before return to the body via the
femoral artery. Indications for its use are similar to left atrio-femoral bypass when
the left atrium is not readily accessible.

(e) *Vascular Shunts.*—Aortic anomalies such as aneurysms or coarctation can
be bypassed by shunting blood from the aortic arch or left subclavian to the
femoral artery. The use of a special heparinised tube for the creation of the shunt
eliminates the necessity for general body heparinisation.

Myocardial preservation.—For most operations on the heart today the surgeon
prefers a motionless relaxed heart for an appreciable length of time. This is
achieved with myocardial cooling and cardioplegic arrest. The infusion of a cold
solution containing an elevated concentration of potassium will cause the heart
to arrest in diastole. The vehicle for the potassium may be a crystalloid solution,
or the patient's own blood. It is usually infused at 4°C which also reduces myocardial temperature. Because the heart is not beating its consumption of oxygen is
dramatically reduced; this in conjunction with the effect of cooling conspires to
protect the myocardium for up to 2–4 hours with safety.

THE PERICARDIUM

Cardiac Tamponade.—An excessive accumulation of fluid in the pericardial
sac will compress the heart and prevent diastolic filling; this results in an increase
of the venous pressure and a reduction of the cardiac output. Occurring rapidly
(*e.g.* after injuries or cardiac surgery), it produces a shock-like state and if not
relieved may prove fatal. On clinical examination the area of cardiac dullness is
enlarged, the heart sounds are reduced, the jugular venous pulse is elevated, and
the pulse may be paradoxical (weaker on inspiration than on expiration). A chest
radiograph usually will reveal an enlarged cardiac silhouette. Immediate relief
can be obtained by aspiration but, if doubt remains, pericardial exploration is
indicated.

Aspiration of the Pericardium.—The pericardium should be explored with a
short-bevelled needle introduced alongside the xiphoid process in an upward and
backward direction with the needle at an angle of 45 degrees to the skin. This
site has the following advantages:

(a) It does not transgress the pleura.

(b) It is more likely to encounter fluid which frequently gravitates between
the diaphragm and the heart.

(c) It is less likely to damage the coronary vessels.

Acute Pericarditis.—Purulent pericarditis is now a rare complication of septicaemia,
pyaemia, pneumonia or empyema. Signs and symptoms may be vague, consisting of fever,
tachycardia or retrosternal pain. A friction rub may be heard and felt. X-rays may show
a large pear-shaped cardiac outline, whilst the electrocardiograph shows a characteristic
elevation of the S-T segment. The pericardium should be aspirated and suitable antibiotics

injected. Drainage of the pericardium is required if aspirations prove ineffective in controlling the infection. In certain circumstances it may be necessary formally to drain the pericardial effusion into the pleural space by means of an anterior thoracotomy. This is most common in cases of a malignant pleural effusion or certain connective tissue disorders. This is achieved by making an incision over the sixth intercostal space in the midclavicular line. This is carried through into the pleural space. A window of pericardium is excised approximately 3 cm square and sent for histological assessment. As a result any further collection of pericardial fluid will drain into the pleural space. This in turn can be drained by a pleural drainage tube.

Chronic Pericarditis (Constrictive Pericarditis; Pick's Disease).—In this condition there is marked thickening, fibrosis and calcification of the pericardium which confines the heart in a rigid inelastic casing preventing it from filling in diastole and emptying in systole. The majority of cases are a sequel to a tuberculous pericarditis, but occasional cases follow purulent pericarditis or a traumatic haemopericardium.

Haemodynamics.—Decreased diastolic filling leads to an accumulation of blood on the venous side. The jugular veins are engorged, pleural effusions may occur, the liver is enlarged, and ascites and oedema of the ankles may appear. On the arterial side, the blood pressure is low with a small pulse volume due to a reduced cardiac output. Fluoroscopy shows decreased or absent cardiac pulsation and pericardial calcification is commonly seen.

Treatment.—Surgical removal of the constricting pericardium is the only effective treatment; this will allow the heart to fill and empty normally.

The patient should be prepared by diuretics and aspirations of pleural or ascitic fluid. At operation (pericardectomy) it is essential to remove the thickened pericardium from the ventricles, and thickened or calcified plaques covering the atria or venae cavae should also be removed if possible.

CONGENITAL HEART DISEASE

Approximately six babies in every thousand live births have a congenital cardiac abnormality. Many are severe and complicated so that survival beyond a few weeks or months is unlikely. Of those who do survive infancy, the expectation of life is often markedly reduced so that surgical correction is desirable wherever possible.

The lesions are divided into those associated with a normal arterial oxygen saturation (acyanotic group) and those with reduced saturation (cyanotic group).

Acyanotic Congenital Heart Disease

1. PATENT DUCTUS ARTERIOSUS

This is one of the commonest abnormalities, accounting for 15% of all types. It may occur as an isolated condition (simple patent ductus) or as part of a more complex abnormality (complicated patent ductus). The mechanism of normal closure of the ductus and the causes of patency are not fully understood. However much evidence is accumulating to suggest that the local production of prostaglandins and the local oxygen tension are important. A rising pO_2 leads to constriction and prostaglandins to relaxation. The potency of both varies at various gestational ages. This information has led to the introduction of an infusion of PGE1 to maintain duct patency as a shunt in various congenital problems to allow time

Friedel Pick, 1876–1926. Professor of Laryngology, Prague, Czechoslovakia. Described this disease in 1896.

for carefully planned surgical correction to be carried out in the light of a full anatomical diagnosis.

Haemodynamics.—The ductus connects the left pulmonary artery with the aorta just distal to the origin of the left subclavian artery. As the pressure is higher in the aorta than in the pulmonary artery, blood will flow from the former into the latter vessel. As much as two to four times the normal cardiac output can flow through a patent ductus so that the amount of blood in the lungs is markedly increased and the pulmonary vessels are dilated (pulmonary plethora) and their pulsation increased (hilar dance). The additional circulation of blood through the lungs and the left side of the heart results in left ventricular hypertrophy.

Clinical Features.—Many cases are only discovered on routine examination in childhood, but a minority give rise to cardiac failure during the first year. The symptoms and signs of a Patent Ductus Arteriosus are consequent upon a left-to-right shunt. Therefore the severity of the problem is dictated by the size of the shunt. If the duct is large then the flow from aorta to pulmonary artery is dependent upon the pulmonary vascular resistance as the pressure will be equal in both vessels. As the pulmonary vascular resistance falls after birth with lung expansion there will be a rapid increase in pulmonary blood flow and the rapid development of congestive cardiac failure. On clinical examination the pulse will be collapsing in nature, there will be a thrusting left ventricular apical impulse and the praecordium will generally feel overactive. On auscultation there will be a systolic murmur maximal in the pulmonary area. As the difference in pressures develops the murmur takes on the well described 'machinery murmur' character-istics. With smaller patent ducts, the continuous murmur is audible earlier and the baby will not develop cardiac failure so rapidly. With the smallest types the baby may grow into adult life asymptomatically. All atypical cases should be investigated by cardiac catheterisation.

Complications.—(1) *Cardiac Failure.*—This is the most important compli-cation especially in infants and probably accounts for one-third of the deaths. Failure is preceded by progressive cardiac englargement.

(2) *Bacterial Endocarditis.*—Before the advent of antibiotics this was a frequent and fatal complication accounting for one-third of all deaths. Chemotherapy now permits control of the majority, but relapse is likely unless the ductus is ligated. Mycotic aneurysm formation is well documented following endocarditis but for-tunately is uncommon.

Prognosis.—The outlook for a simple patent ductus is difficult to determine because of the early introduction of surgical closure. A patent ductus never closes spontaneously, and it must be assumed that some patients die from cardiac failure later in adult life.

Treatment.—The results of surgical closure are so satisfactory and the operat-ive mortality so low that ligation can be recommended in all cases. Recanalisation is rare. Division and suture is practised by Gross and others in order to reduce the risks of recanalisation, but is probably only necessary for that short wide ductus which cannot be safely ligated.

The operation is carried out through a left-sided postero-lateral incision through the fourth space. The mediastinal pleura is incised over the aortic arch and the vagus nerve and its recurrent branch are retracted anteriorly. The areolar tissue is removed from the

Robert Edward Gross, Contemporary. Ladd Professor of Children's Surgery, Harvard University, Boston, Massachusetts, U.S.A.

surface of the ductus and the latter gently mobilised by blunt dissection. Occlusion is achieved by using two stout non-absorbable ligatures placed at either end of the ductus with a transfixion ligature between (Blalock). Occlusion by staples is also practised.

II. COARCTATION OF AORTA

Narrowing of the aorta may occur at any site, but, in the vast majority of cases, the stenosis lies immediately beyond the origin of the left subclavian artery in close relationship to the ductus or ligamentum arteriosum. The lesion accounts for 6% of all congenital cardiac anomalies.

Two main types are described according to the relationship of the ductus to the coarctation:

(1) **Post-ductal Type. Adult Coarctation.**—Sixty per cent of all cases are of this type. The ductus is patent in a minority and enters the aorta above the coarctation. The stenosis is abrupt with an internal lumen of 2 to 3 mm. Externally the aorta shows a characteristic indentation.

(2) **Pre-ductal Type. Infantile Coarctation.**—Here a patent ductus enters the aorta below the coarctation. Unoxygenated blood may pass from the pulmonary artery into the aorta and thence to the lower trunk and extremities. These areas are cyanosed, whilst the head, neck and upper extremities are pink (differential cyanosis). The stenosed aortic segment may be long and include one or more of the great vessels. Forty per cent of patients have other cardiac lesions. The mortality in the first year of life is considerable.

Clinical Features.—The obstruction results in hypertension above and hypotension below the constriction with collateral vessels linking the two areas. Symptoms can be divided into three groups:

(1) Those of proximal hypertension; headaches, irritability, excessive heart action, throbbing and pulsation in head and neck.

(2) Those due to peripheral hypotension; cold legs and intermittent claudication.

(3) Complications secondary to hypertension; left ventricular failure, intracranial haemorrhage, rupture of the aorta.

Characteristically there is marked pulsation of the carotid and subclavian arteries with evidence of left ventricular enlargement. Systolic murmurs are frequently audible over the praecordium and elsewhere over the thorax, due to the collateral vessels, although sometimes caused by associated aortic valve disease. Blood pressure in the arms is considerably elevated. Collateral vessels can be seen and felt over the thorax, particularly in the scapular region. Femoral, dorsalis pedis and posterior tibial pulses may be absent or weak. The femoral pulse, if present, is delayed when compared with the radial. X-rays show evidence of left ventricular enlargement, a prominent ascending aorta and an absent or abnormal aortic knuckle (fig. 753). Notching of the ribs due to large tortuous intercostal vessels is seen in adults but rarely in children under six.

Investigations.—Venous angiocardiography or retrograde aortography (fig. 754) are employed to demonstrate the site and type of the coarctation and the extent of collateral circulation.

Prognosis.—The condition is a serious one and it is estimated that very few patients survive beyond the age of forty-five years; the majority die from the effects of hypertension.

Treatment.—Both Crafoord and Gross independently in 1945 demonstrated that the stenosis could be excised and an end-to-end anastomosis safely per-

Alfred Blalock, 1899–1964. Professor of Surgery, Johns Hopkins University, Baltimore, Maryland, U.S.A.
Clarence Crafoord, Contemporary. Professor Emeritus of Thoracic Surgery, Karolinska Institut, Stockholm.

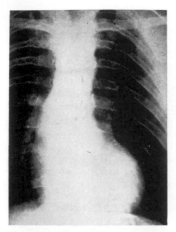

FIG. 753.—Coarctation of aorta showing a promiment ascending aorta, double aortic knuckle and rib notching.

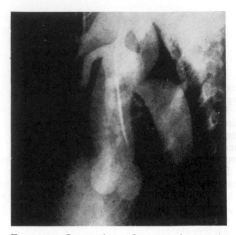

FIG. 754.—Coarctation of aorta. Aortogram showing the stenosis and the marked collateral vessels.

formed. Occasionally a graft is required to bridge a wide defect in cases with a long hypoplastic segment or with a post-stenotic aneurysm. Aortic homografts were originally employed but they calcify and narrow with age and have been superseded by grafts of crimped Teflon or Dacron (Chapter 14). All children and young adults should be operated upon.

The operation is carried out through a left postero-lateral incision through the fourth intercostal space. The large anastomotic vessels in the chest wall are ligated. The aorta is mobilised widely both above and below the constriction, great care being taken not to injure the large thin-walled intercostal and mediastinal vessels arising from the distal segment. The ligamentum arteriosum is divided: the aorta is clamped above and below the constriction and the latter excised (fig. 755). An end-to-end anastomosis is performed using a fine continuous suture. The clamps should be released slowly and any leak from the suture-line controlled by pressure.

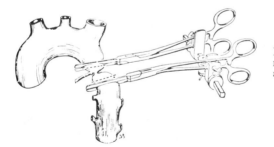

FIG. 755.—Coarctation of aorta. The mobilised aorta is clamped prior to excision and anastomosis. The clamps are held in position with the adjustable Brom's vice.

For patients with long coarctations a plastic reconstruction may be easier than an end-to-end anastomosis. The constricted zone is incised longitudinally and an oval patch of Dacron is inserted. An alternative approach developed by Hamilton, which is particularly suitable for infants, uses the left subclavian artery as an autologous onlay patch. All procedures in the young may need operative revision later in life.

Results of the Operation.—The over-all mortality rate is under 3%, but in children it is considerably lower. A normal blood pressure in both upper and lower limbs is usual in children; in adults some elevation in blood pressure may

Gerard Brom, Contemporary. Academisch Ziekenhuis, Leiden, Holland.
David Ian Hamilton, Contemporary. Cardiac Surgeon, Royal Liverpool Children's Hospital.

persist, but the femoral pulse is no longer delayed. Relief of symptoms is the rule.

III. CONGENITAL VALVAR ABNORMALITIES

Developmental abnormalities can occur with any of the valves, resulting in stenosis, regurgitation or combined lesions. Less frequently obstruction may occur in the subvalvar region.

Stenotic lesions in the pulmonary or aortic valves are commonest (all other varieties are rare). Classically the commissures are fused to form a dome-shaped valve with a small central orifice. Bicuspid valves and other complex varieties are not uncommon. The stenotic valve produces an ejection systolic murmur and thrill and evidence of Right (pulmonary stenosis) or Left (aortic stenosis) Ventricular Hypertrophy.

Both lesions can be corrected by open operation with heart-lung bypass with good results. The operation of closed pulmonary valvotomy (Brock) is rarely employed now.

IV. ATRIAL SEPTAL DEFECT

Defects of the septum between the atria account for 7% of congenital cardiac anomalies; they allow blood to flow from the left to the right atrium (L–R shunt) so that the right side of the heart and lungs are overfilled whilst the left side receives less blood than usual. Although the deformity may cause little disability during childhood and early adult life, it is a serious condition with troublesome symptoms appearing in middle life associated with the onset of atrial fibrillation.

The defects are of three main types depending on which part of the developing atrial septum is defective:

(*a*) *Secundum defect:* commonest and simplest; lies centrally in septum; caused by failure of septum secundum; direct suture closure often possible.

(*b*) *Primum defect:* caused by failure of septum primum; often associated with abnormal cleft of the mitral valve and mitral regurgitation; occurs low in the septum—there is no septal tissue separating mitral and tricuspid valves; always requires a patch for closure.

(*c*) *Sinus venosus defect:* due to failure of incorporation of sinus venosus into the atrium proper; occurs high in the septum and often associated with abnormal pulmonary venous drainage; usually requires a patch for closure.

Signs are due to over-filling and over-activity of the right side of the heart and lungs. The right ventricle is palpably enlarged and active. The pulmonary arteries are dilated and actively pulsatile (hilar dance) and increased flow produces a pulmonary systolic murmur. The second heart sound is widely split due to bundle branch block. The E.C.G. shows right bundle branch block and right ventricular hypertrophy (secundum defect).

Closure of the defect is readily performed by direct suture under vision with the aid of extracorporeal circulation.

The more complicated atrial defects (ostium primum: atrio-ventricular canal) can be corrected but the risks of operation are higher.

V. VENTRICULAR SEPTAL DEFECT

Isolated defects of the ventricular septum are one of the commonest congenital lesions (22%). In addition, they occur frequently as part of more complex anomalies (Fallot's tetralogy, transposition, *etc.*).

The defects may be single or multiple and vary from 1–3 cm in diameter. They

Russell Claude Brock (Lord Brock of Wimbledon), 1903–1980. Surgeon, Guy's Hospital and Brompton Hospital, London and President, Royal College of Surgeons of England.

are most often situated in the fibrous part of the septum close to the aortic and tricuspid valves.

Isolated ventricular septal defect allows the passage of blood from the left to the right ventricle resulting in over-filling of the right heart, with pulmonary plethora and hypertension.

The lesion is a serious one, over 50% of patients dying during the first few months of life.

The defect is repaired with the aid of an extracorporeal circulation using either direct sutures or inserting a patch of Dacron or pericardium. The operative approach is either through the anterior wall of the right ventricle or from the right atrium via the tricuspid valve.

The operative mortality is 5% and the most serious complications are due to the production of complete heart block or incomplete closure of the defect. In infants a stout ligature can be applied around the pulmonary artery (pulmonary banding) to restrict the flow of blood into the lungs. Closure of the defect and removal of the pulmonary artery band is carried out at a later date, although the results when compared with direct closure are not so good.

Cyanotic Congenital Heart Disease

The cyanotic heart lesions include a number of different abnormalities, the commonest of which is Fallot's tetralogy (fig. 756). The abnormalities are multiple and complex and often difficult to determine accurately, but all have central

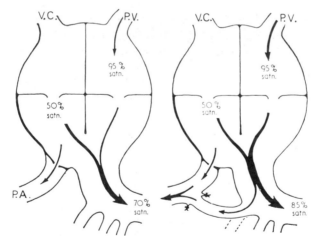

FIG. 756.—Haemodynamics of Fallot's tetralogy before and after Blalock's operation. Note the ventricular septal defect, the over-riding aorta, pulmonary stenosis and right ventricular hypertrophy which make up the tetralogy.

V.C. = Vena Cava
P.V. = Pulmonary Vein
P.A. = Pulmonary Artery

cyanosis due to an intracardiac shunt from the right to the left side. From the surgical point of view the state of the pulmonary circulation is by far the most important consideration. If this is deficient (pulmonary ischaemia), then surgical means can be taken to improve it and thereby increase exercise tolerance and decrease cyanosis. If, however, the lungs are overfilled (pulmonary plethora), or the pressure considerably raised (pulmonary hypertension) it may be difficult or impossible to carry out a corrective procedure with safety. The exact type of surgical procedure will depend on obtaining accurate haemodynamic and ana-

Etienne Louis Arthur Fallot, 1850–1911. Professor of Medicine, Marseilles, France.

tomical details of the abnormality by angiocardiography and cardiac catheterisation.

1. FALLOT'S TETRALOGY

This is the commonest of the cyanotic conditions and accounts for about 10% of all cases of congenital heart disease.

The tetrad originally described by Fallot in 1888 consists of (1) stenois of the pulmonary tract; (2) a ventricular septal defect; (3) an aorta which straddles the ventricular defect and over-rides both ventricles and (4) right ventricular hypertrophy.

The patient is usually undersized with considerable physical disability including central cyanosis and finger clubbing. The heart is small and quiet and there is a systolic murmur and thrill in the pulmonary area. All degrees of severity are encountered from those who are only cyanosed with exercise, to others who are deeply and permanently cyanosed in whom the arterial oxygen saturation rarely rises above 60%. The mortality in infancy in this latter group is considerable, but those of less severity may survive into adult life.

All patients require careful investigation with cardiac catheterisation, angiocardiography and dye studies to provide accurate anatomical details of the lesion and indicate the most favourable type of operation.

Fallot's Tetralogy is capable of complete surgical correction and this should be the aim in every case. However, in the very young and in those patients with hypoplastic right ventricular outflow tract some surgeons advise a palliative anastomotic operation designed to increase the pulmonary blood flow, to improve the patient's clinical condition and perhaps help the hypoplastic outflow tract to develop. Definitive total correction would then be carried out at a later date.

(i) **Anastomotic Procedures.**—These aim at increasing the blood flow to the lungs by creating a shunt between the aorta or one of its branches and the pulmonary artery. The Blalock operation is the most popular and consists of an anastomosis between the left subclavian artery and the left pulmonary artery.

A posterolateral left thoracotomy through the fourth space gives good access. The pulmonary artery is mobilised and doubly clamped as it lies in the lung hilum. The subclavian artery is fully mobilised and divided near the first rib, the proximal end of the subclavian is then anastomosed to the upper border of the pulmonary artery (fig. 757). A continuous thrill can be felt over the anastomosis on releasing the clamps.

Alternative anastomotic procedures are available where a Blalock operation cannot be done or in infants. Descending aorta—left pulmonary artery (Potts) ascending aorta—right pulmonary artery (Waterston-Cooley) or superior vena cava—right pulmonary artery (Glenn) are those most frequently employed.

(ii) **Complete Correction.**—This should be considered in every case but may be deferred in infants and the more severe examples where palliative anastomotic procedures are performed initially.

The operation is carried out under cardio-pulmonary bypass with additional hypothermia. The ventricular septal defect is closed with a Dacron patch. The pulmonary valvar and infundibular obstruction is relieved and an outflow tract patch of Dacron inserted to enlarge the track if necessary.

The operative mortality is about 10%. The results of total correction are dramatic and gratifying. Long term follow-up demonstrates continued good health.

Willis John Potts, 1895–1968. Surgeon, Children's Memorial Hospital, Chicago, Illinois, U.S.A.
David James Waterston, Contemporary. Formerly Surgeon, Hospital for Sick Children, Great Ormond Street.
Denton A. Cooley, Contemporary. Professor of Surgery, Baylor University, Houston, Texas, U.S.A.
William W. L. Glenn, Contemporary. Professor of Surgery, Yale Univerity, New Haven, Connecticut, U.S.A.

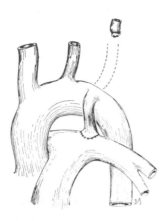

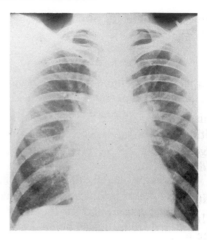

FIG. 757.— Subclavian-pulmonary anastomosis (Blalock) for Fallot's tetralogy.

FIG. 758.—Mitral stenosis showing enlargement of the 'pulmonary bay' and the pulmonary arteries.

II. TRANSPOSITION OF THE GREAT VESSELS

After Fallot's tetralogy this is the next most common cause of cyanotic congenital heart disease and frequently presents with severe symptoms in infancy. The aorta arises from the right ventricle and the pulmonary artery from the left ventricle. The greater and the lesser circulations are thus separated and life is only possible if there is a communication between the two through an atrial or a ventricular defect or a patent ductus arteriosus. Death in the neonatal period is common due to inadequate communications between the circuits.

The child is deeply cyanosed and severely incapacitated. The lungs may be plethoric or oligaemic depending on associated pulmonary stenosis. Diagnosis is confirmed by cardiac catheterisation and angiocardiography.

Management in infancy is aimed at improving the shunting between the circuits by creating or enlarging an atrial defect. This is effected in infants by rupturing the septum with a balloon catheter passed transvenously through the foramen ovale (Balloon Septostomy: Rashkind). Alternatively, portions of the septum can be excised by the technique of Blalock and Hanlon. If the child survives the first year with or without surgical aid a more radical correction can be contemplated.

The most popular surgical approach to this abnormality in many institutions has been the creation of a baffle within the atria to divert the returning blood to the appropriate ventricle to restore the normal circulation. Two principle operations have been described to bring this about. In one, a piece of material is cut to shape and sewn over the pulmonary veins to form a channel to divert the blood into the right atrium. The blood returning from the superior and inferior caval veins is diverted on the other side of the baffle into the left atrium. Various materials may be used. These include Dacron, PTFE, and pericardium. This operation is known as the Mustard procedure. An alternative procedure was developed by Senning in which the right atrial wall is tailored to make the baffle within the atria.

Both of these procedures have recently been superceded in other institutions by an operation in which the great arteries are 'switched' to their opposite ventricles. This is referred to as an anatomical correction because it results in the systemic ventricle being connected to the systemic great artery. This operation was first developed by Jatene and

William Jacobson Rashkind, Contemporary. Surgeon, Children's Hospital, Philadelphia, Pa., U.S.A.
Cyril Rollins Hanlon, Contemporary. Professor of Surgery, St. Louis University Hospitals, Missouri, U.S.A.
Ake Senning, Contemporary. Professor of Surgery, Zurich.
William T. Mustard, Contemporary. Associate Professor of Cardiovascular Surgery, Hospital for Sick Children, Toronto, Canada.
Jatene, Contemporary. Surgeon, Brazil.

colleagues in Brazil. A major contribution to its extended use has been by Yacoub and colleagues in the United Kingdom.

ACQUIRED HEART DISEASE

Inflammatory and degenerative changes are responsible for the majority of the acquired lesions of surgical interest although cardiac injuries and tumours constitute a small but important group. Rheumatism has a predilection for the mitral and aortic valves, syphilis for the aortic valve and aortic wall, whilst degenerative lesions are frequent in the aortic and mitral valves, coronary vessels and myocardium.

Mitral Valve Disease

Inflammation of the mitral valve is the commonest sequel of rheumatic carditis. The original attack of rheumatism may be so mild as to pass unnoticed. Only half the patients with mitral stenosis give a history of rheumatic fever or chorea. The condition affects women more frequently then men, and symptoms are commonest during the third and fourth decades.

Pathology.—The cardiac manifestations of rheumatism are widespread with involvement of all three layers, but it is mainly the mitral and aortic valve involvement which leads to later disturbances. The essential lesion is the Aschoff nodule. These produce swelling and roughening of the valve cusps and fibrin is deposited on the roughened

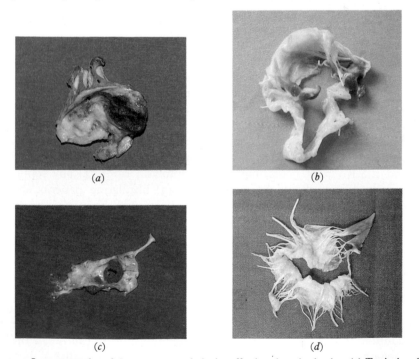

(a)

(b)

(c)

(d)

FIG. 759.—Some examples of the common pathologies affecting the mitral valve. (a) Typical end-stage rheumatic degeneration demonstrating the thickened, fused and shortened chordae tendinae, calcified and ulcerated leaflets and commissural fusion. (b) A 'floppy' valve with myxomatous degeneration. (c) Ulcerating bacterial endocarditis (d) A ruptured papillary muscle after myocardial infarction.

Magdi Yacoub, Contemporary, Surgeon, National Heart Hospital, London.
Karl Albert Ludwig Aschoff, 1866–1942. Professor of Pathology, Freiburg, Germany. Described the Aschoff nodule in 1904.

surfaces. Later organisation with fibrosis and calcification may occur. As a result the valve leaflets become fused, thickened, rigid and immobile. All grades are encountered from simple fusion of the commissures and mild fibrosis (but with preservation of mobility) to grossly calcified, fixed and functionless valves. The valve orifice is oval or slit-like with an average opening of 1 cm in its long axis in those patients submitted for operation.

The mitral valve mechanism may be affected by lesions other than rheumatism. Acute or subacute bacterial infection, ruptured chordae tendineae, papillary muscle dysfunction after myocardial infarction, and degenerative valve disease. Most of these conditions result in mitral regurgitation (fig. 759).

Haemodynamics.—Disease of the leaflets or subvalvar apparatus may result in obstruction to forward flow or the regurgitation of blood from the left ventricle to the left atrium. Often combinations of stenosis and regurgitation are present. In either case there is a reduction of forward flow from the left ventricle and a build up of blood in the lungs.

Clinical Features.—These can be considered briefly under four headings:

(1) Those due to a low cardiac output: tiredness, a small volume pulse and pale, cold extremities.

(2) Those due to disturbances of the pulmonary circulation: exertional dyspnoea, pulmonary oedema, nocturnal dyspnoea, haemoptysis and bronchitis.

(3) Those due to failure of the right ventricle: congestive heart failure with engorged veins, large liver, ascites and peripheral oedema.

(4) Systemic embolism by clot dislodged from the left atrial appendage.

Investigations.—These are required to determine the type and severity of the valve lesion and the presence or not of additional lesions such as other valve lesions or coronary artery disease which may complicate management.

Investigations may include radiology (fig. 758), echocardiography (fig. 749), cardiac catheterisation and angio-cardiography.

Indications for Operation.—Operation should be considered in any patient who has debilitating symptoms which cannot be controlled by medical means. Patients with little disability or few symptoms should be deferred.

Left ventricular function is one of the most important factors in determining risks, whilst in older patients the presence of significant coronary artery disease may affect the outcome.

There are few contraindications to operation in the symptomatic patient but certain factors may cause delay: (1) evidence of active rheumatism such as fever, raised E.S.R., joint pains, high anti-streptolysin titre; (2) any septic focus, especially dental, should be attended to; (3) fibrillating patients should be adequately controlled with digitalis; (4) patients with congestive heart failure should have optimum treatment before surgery; (5) pregnancy is no bar to mitral valve surgery if symptoms are demanding.

Mitral Valve Surgery

Closed mitral valvotomy was one of the earliest and most successful of cardiac operations. The operation has largely been superseded by open valvotomy though it is still practised in some centres. The advantage of an open procedure is that in addition to separation of the commissures the surgeon can repair the valve, can separate fused chordae tendineae and reduce the circumference of the annulus if this is stretched (annuloplasty).

Closed Valvotomy.—A good result from a closed valvotomy can be expected where the valve is mobile and neither thickened nor calcified. Regurgitation should be absent

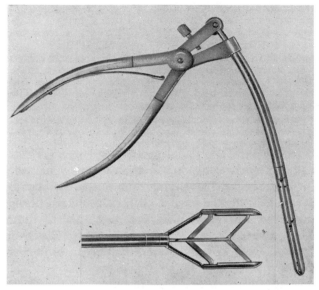

FIG. 760.—Transventricular adjustable mitral valve dilator.
(*Tubbs.*)

and the patient in sinus rhythm. The operation is carried out through a left antero-lateral thoracotomy. The valve is split with an expanding dilator (Tubbs, fig. 760) inserted through a stab wound in the apex of the left ventricle with the right index finger inserted into the left atrium through its appendage to control the split. The appendage is amputated at the end of the procedure to minimise risk of embolism.

Open Valve Repair (Open Valvotomy).—This is carried out with the aid of cardiopulmonary bypass through a sternal splitting incision. The valve is carefully inspected with the ventricle both relaxed and distended. Fused commissures can be carefully and accurately incised and fused chordae tendineae carefully separated. Any tears or irregularities of the leaflet mechanism can be repaired. If the annulus is dilated and producing regurgitation an annuloplasty of the posterio-medial commissure can be done. A somewhat better effect can be gained by the implantation of a flexible ring shaped to the normal contour of the mitral annulus. Examples of this have been developed by Carpentier and Duran.

Valve Replacement.—Replacement of the valve is indicated for a grossly diseased valve or where attempts at open valve repair have failed. The valve is excised and a suitable prosthesis sutured to the annulus with interrupted or continuous sutures. The surgeon has a choice of ball valve or valve mechanical prosthesis or a tissue valve (porcine heterograft) fig. 761).

Postoperative Care.—In the immediate postoperative period it is essential to maintain normal blood gases and normal electrolytes. Potassium is the most important after mitral valve surgery as total body potassium is likely to be low and a low serum potassium may provoke serious rhythm disorders.

Cardiac output is best monitored by observing skin temperature and urinary output in addition to blood pressure and pulse rate. A diminished cardiac output may be improved by reducing peripheral resistance with an infusion of sodium nitroprusside (50 mg in 100 ml), or by infusion of inotropic agents such as isoprenaline (2 mg in 500 ml), adrenalin (10 mg in 500 ml) or dopamine (800 mg in 500 ml).

Rhythm disorders are not infrequent. The patient should be adequately digitalised and the serum potassium must be within normal limits. If control is still not

Osward Sydney Tubbs, Contemporary. Formerly Cardiothoracic Surgeon, St. Bartholomew's Hospital, London.
Alain Carpentier, Contemporary. Cardiac Surgeon, Paris, France.
Carlos Duran, Contemporary. Cardiac Surgeon, Santander, Spain.

possible intravenous lignocaine, or verapamil (Cordilox) should be used but with caution.

Results of Treatment.—Closed mitral valvotomy gives good long term results in 75% of patients and with a mortality of approximately 5%. However, not all patients with dominant stenosis are suitable. Open valvotomy provides a better chance of a perfect operation but also a risk of failure demanding valve replacement. Operative risks are similar to those of closed valvotomy. Mitral valve replacement is employed for more severely diseased valves and carries a similar mortality.

Long Term Results—Restenosis can occur after both open and closed valvotomy in which case either a second valvotomy or a valve replacement will be required. All mechanical prostheses are potentially thrombogenic and need anticoagulation. This is effected with oral anticoagulants (Dindevan, Warfarin) in doses sufficient to maintain a prothrombin time of twice normal. If anticoagulants cannot be used or prove ineffective, drugs to prevent platelet adherence (aspirin, dipyridamole (Persantin)) can be used additionally. In spite of this, systemic embolism still occurs in a small number of patients.

All prostheses are foreign bodies in the circulation and are liable to become the focus of infection by bacteria, yeasts or fungi. The infection may seriously damage the prosthesis or its moorings leading to malfunction. Infection can sometimes be controlled with suitable antibiotics though often this can only be achieved by excising the prosthesis, sterilising the tissues and replacing with a new valve.

Valve Prosthesis.—The perfect artifical heart valve has yet to be designed. The surgeon today has the choice of three basic types—ball valve, disc or hinge valve and tissue valve.

The ball valve (fig. 761)(*a*) is simple in construction and with a simple mechanism unlikely to go wrong. It is thrombogenic as the poppet is partially obstructing the forward flow. The disc valves (fig. 761(*c*)) are less obstructive but the mechanism is more complicated and therefore more liable to develop malfunction. Damage to the red cells with haemolysis and anaemia can occur with both types of mechanical valve. Tissue valves (fig. 761(*b*)) have the best flow patterns and are least thrombogenic but their durability remains suspect. The present popular glutaraldehyde-treated porcine heterograft would appear to have a life of at least 7–10 years.

Aortic Valve Disease

The aortic valve may be affected by congenital, inflammatory or degenerative processes, resulting in stenosis, incompetence or combined lesions.

Aortic Stenosis.—The obstruction impedes the forward flow of blood from the left ventricle producing angina, syncope and effort dyspnoea. The left ventricle is hypertrophied and a coarse systolic murmur and thrill are discernible in the aortic area. The arterial pulse is slow-rising and sustained (anacrotic or plateau pulse) and the pulse pressure is small.

The lesion is serious; children are liable to sudden death and adults with symptoms have a life expectancy of only a few years.

Surgery, with the aid of extracorporeal circulation, plays an important role in the management of the condition. *Open valvotomy* with division of fused commissures is often possible in children. *Valve replacement* will be required for grossly destroyed or heavily calcified valves.

Aortic Regurgitation.—A leaking aortic valve produces considerable left ventricular dilation in addition to hypertrophy. Symptoms are similar to those of

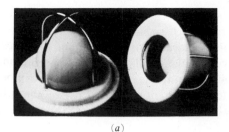

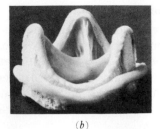

(a)   (b)

FIG. 761.—Cardiac valve prostheses: (a) Starr-Edwards silicone ball prostheses, model
6120. (b) Carpentier-Edwards
porcine aortic valve heterograft.
(c) Björk-Shiley tilting disc
valve.

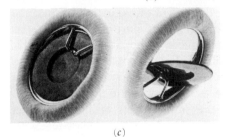

(c)

aortic stenosis. In addition to an aortic systolic murmur, a diastolic murmur is
audible along the left sternal edge. The pulse is characteristically quick rising
(Corrigan or water-hammer) with a high systolic and low diastolic pressure resulting in a large pulse pressure.

Isolated cases are capable of correction by suture (tears) or patching (perforations), but the majority are best treated by excision and replacement.

Aortic Valve Replacement.—This is carried out with the aid of heart lung
bypass through a sternal splitting incision. The valve is exposed with an incision
in the aortic root after cross-clamping the aorta. Cardioplegia and myocardial
cooling are used for protection of the myocardium during the ischaemic period.

The valve is carefully excised and calcium dissected from the valve ring. The
prosthesis is sutured to the valve ring with interrupted sutures. The surgeon has
a choice of the usual mechanical valves—a caged ball valve (fig. 761(a) and (c) a
mounted heterograft (fig. 761(b)) or a free homograft (Ross and Barratt-Boyes).

Results of Aortic Valve Replacement.—Early mortality is approximately 3%.
The later mortality and morbidity is determined by valve dysfunction, thrombo-
embolism, haemolysis or infection. Associated lesions, especially coronary artery
disease, are important causes of later mortality but generally the clinical results
are very satisfactory.

Cardiac Tumours

Tumours of the heart are relatively uncommon; they may occur in the ventricle or
atrium. The commonest is the myxoma of the atrium (80% of all tumours) and of these
the majority (75%) occur in the left atrium.

Left atrial myxomas simulate mitral stenosis; they obstruct the flow of blood through
the left atrium producing pulmonary venous engorgement and hypertension. Systemic
embolism and postural syncope are important symptoms.

The condition simulates mitral stenosis but is distinguished from it by a shorter and
more progressive history, evidence of toxicity (fever, raised E.S.R., anaemia) and disturbances of plasma proteins.

The lesion can be demonstrated by angiography and by ultra-sound (echocardiography,
p. 788) and can be completely removed with the aid of extracorporeal circulation.

Sir Dominic John Corrigan, 1802–1880. Physician, Jervis Street Hospital, Dublin. Described the water-hammer pulse of aortic incompetence
  in 1832.
Donald Nixon Ross, Comtemporary. Cardiac Surgeon, National Heart Hospital, London.
Sir Brian Barratt-Boyes, Contemporary. Cardiac Surgeon, Auckland, New Zealand.
Albert Starr, Contemporary. Professor of Surgery, University of Oregon, Portland, Oregon, U.S.A.
Alain Carpentier, Contemporary. Cardiac Surgeon, Hôpital Broussais, Paris.
Viking Olaf Björk, Contemporary. Formerly Cardiac Surgeon, Karolinska Sjukhuset, Stockholm, Sweden

Disorders of Rhythm

Heart block or complete atrio-ventricular dissociation may occur as a manifestation of congenital cardiac lesions, as a complication of ischaemic heart disease or the result of surgical treatment of ventricular or allied defects. The commonest cause remains degeneration of the conduction tissue in old age whereby the atrial impulse fails to stimulate the ventricle owing to interference with the conduction of the bundle of His. The ventricles beat independently at a rate of 25 to 50 per minute.

The dangers of this situation are that the slow rate impairs cardiac output and may lead to heart failure and also that a sudden slowing or cessation of the beat may produce syncope (Stokes-Adams attack), or death.

Artificial electrical pacemakers have been designed to stimulate the heart at appropriate rates and may be of either the *fixed rate* or *demand* types. The stimulating electrode is applied to the ventricle from the *endocardial* or *epicardial* aspect. With the introduction of lithium-powered generators, pacemaker systems (fig. 762) should now last at least seven years before requiring replacement.

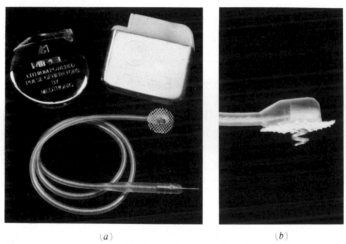

(a)   (b)

FIG. 762.—Implantable pacemakers: (*a*) Two varieties (Medtronic and Telectronic) of lithium-powered generators and pacemaker lead. These units should operate for at least 7 years. (*b*) Close-up view of the pacemaker electrode which is inserted into the myocardium.

Ischaemic Heart Disease

Atherosclerosis of the coronary arteries occurs with increasing frequency in Western civilisation. Between 1951 and 1975 the proportion of deaths in England and Wales due to ischaemic heart disease rose from 10·5% to 26·0% of the total.

Narrowing of the coronary arteries deprives the myocardium of oxygen. When severe enough, chest pain is produced (angina). Total occlusion results in death of myocardial tissue (infarction = necrosis). Angina thus indicates a serious deprivation of myocardial blood supply which may lead to infarction and death if allowed to progress.

Surgery has a role to play both in the relief of angina by revascularisation of the myocardium and in the management of the complications of infarction.

Wilhelm His (Junior), 1863–1934. Professor of Medicine, Berlin. Described the atrio-ventricular bundle in 1893.
William Stokes, 1804–1878. Regius Professor of Medicine, Dublin. Described this condition in 1846, and drew attention to the cases reported
*   by Adams in 1827.*
Robert Adams, 1791–1875. Regius Professor of Surgery, Dublin.

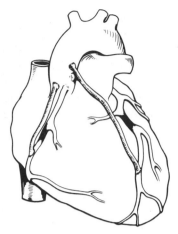

FIG. 763.—Diagrammatic representation of double coronary vein graft to obstructed right coronary artery and left anterior descending.

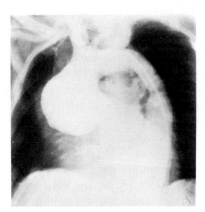

FIG. 764.—Saccular aneurysm of the ascending aorta.

The natural history of angina pectoris depends primarily on the extent of the coronary arterial disease and the functional state of the left ventricle. Full investigations including coronary arteriography and left ventriculography are therefore necessary before surgery can be considered. Patients with relatively mild arterial disease and angina that can be controlled by β blockers should be treated medically. The remainder should be considered for surgical treatment.

Coronary Artery Bypass Graft.—There are two principle ways of achieving this. By far the most commonly used technique until recently, is aorto-coronary bypass grafting using a segment of reversed long saphenous vein. Proximally it is attached to the ascending aorta and distally it is attached to the coronary artery beyond the occlusion (fig. 763). Several individual lengths of vein may be used, or a single length may be anastomosed in side to side fashion to several coronary artery branches as a sequential graft. It is argued that the greater run-off along such a graft leads to longer term patency. In either event the long term patency of saphenous vein is, although better than any synthetic material, still only 65–70% at 10 years in the best reported series. This fact has led to the search for a better long-term conduit.

The internal mammary artery is being used with increasing frequency and 10 year patency rates of greater than 90% are being reported. In this operation either or both internal mammary arteries are dissected from behind the anterior chest wall leaving their take-off from the Subclavian artery intact. The distal end is then anastomosed to the cornorary artery branch in question. It is possible to use sequential anastomoses with this vessel also. Generally speaking the right sided vessel will reach the right coronary artery proximal to the acute margin of the heart, and the left anterior descending branch of the left main coronary artery, and the left sided vessel will reach most of the branches of the left coronary artery.

The risks of these operations depend almost entirely upon left ventricular function. For routine patients the mortality should now be less than 1%.

Most patients gain complete relief from their angina and there is increasing evidence that the prognosis of patients with triple vessel disease is improved.

Left Ventricular Aneurysm.—Myocardial infarction results in death of muscle. Healing is by scar tissue and this scar may stretch and form an aneurysm. The presence of an aneurysm adversely effects the function of the heart and results in heart failure. Fibrin is deposited on the walls of the aneurysm and may be dislodged as an embolus. The aneurysm should be resected using cardiopulmonary bypass and the left ventricle reconstituted by suturing the edges of the aneurysm together.

The operative risks are approximately 10% and prospects of long term survival are quite good.

Other Complications of Infarction.—The interventricular septum or the papillary muscles supporting the tricuspid or mitral valves may be damaged after infarction. Rupture of the septum (acquired VSD) and papillary muscle dysfunction of the mitral valve may result. Either lesion seriously affects cardiac function but both can be corrected surgically.

Support of the circulation by means of intra-aortic balloon pump counterpulsation may be useful before and after the operation.

AORTIC ANEURYSMS

The surgery of the aorta has made considerable strides since the introduction of aortic grafts and the advent of hypothermia and methods of cardio-pulmonary bypass. It is now possible to occlude the aorta with safety for reasonable periods, and to bridge considerable defects, so that the two chief deterrents to reconstructive aortic surgery have largely disappeared.

Aortic aneurysms due to syphilis or degenerative changes may be fusiform, saccular (fig. 764) or dissecting. The diagnosis may be straightforward, but is often notoriously difficult. Although aortography has provided a useful diagnostic procedure, much better information may be gained with contrast CT scanning.

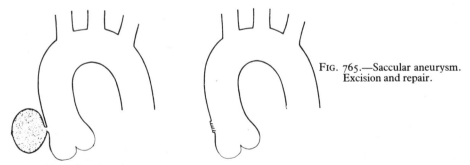

Fig. 765.—Saccular aneurysm. Excision and repair.

Treatment of Aneurysms.— (1) *Excision and Repair. Aneurysmorrhaphy (Matas).*—Applicable to smaller saccular aneurysms. Consists of excision of the sac with direct suture of the neck. Not applicable to fusiform aneurysm or saccular aneurysms with a wide neck (fig. 765 and also Chapter 14).

(2) *Excision and Grafting.*—This involves excision of the aneurysm and adjacent aorta and its replacement with a prosthesis (woven crimped Dacron) (fig.

Rudolph Matas, 1860–1957. Professor of Surgery, Tulane University, New Orleans, Louisiana, U.S.A.

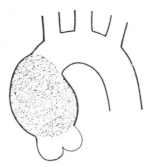
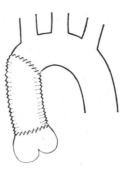

FIG. 766.—Fusiform aneurysm of the ascending aorta. Excision and grafting.

766). Heart-lung bypass is required for aneurysms of the ascending aorta or aortic arch, but the simpler left atrio-femoral bypass or heparinised vascular shunt (p. 794) is all that is required for aneurysms of the descending thoracic aorta.

(3) *Excision and Plastic Repair.*—The aneurysm is excised and the aortic defect is repaired by an insert of woven Dacron (fig. 767). This method is applicable to saccular aneurysms of the aortic arch and avoids the elaborate anastomoses required for replacement of the arch.

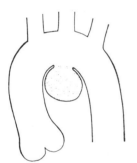
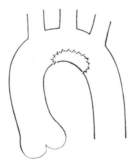

FIG. 767.—Aneurysm of the aortic arch. Localised excision and plastic repair.

Dissecting Aneurysms.—These are produced by a split in the intima and internal portion of the media, allowing blood to enter the media and extend both distally and proximally resulting in a double lumen aorta (fig. 768). The aneurysms may rupture externally or into the pericardium with fatal results, may

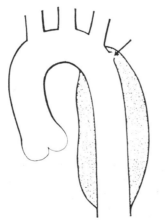
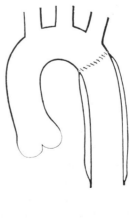

FIG. 768.—Dissecting aneurysm of the descending aorta. Excision of area of rupture and reconstitution of the aorta. The arrow indicates the site of the intimal tear.

undermine the attachments of the aortic valve, producing aortic incompetence or occlude vital branches of the aorta (coronary, carotid, renal, *etc.*) with serious consequences. Dissection may be related to systemic hypertension or defective aortic wall as in Marfan's disease.

The lesion is a serious one with a high mortality within a few days of onset, but a minority survive for some years. In the early stages dissection may be limited by the use of hypotensive drugs. Operative treatment with excision and anastomosis of the reconstituted ends offers hope of limiting further dissection for which some form of bypass circulation is necessary.

Vascular Rings (Dysphagia Lusoria[1]).—Abnormal development of the aortic arch and its branches (*e.g.* double aortic arch, right subclavian arising from descending aorta) may result in obstruction of the trachea and oesophagus by vessels which surround them both in front and behind. The anomaly may pass unnoticed, but occasionally in children severe dyspnoea, stridor and dysphagia may develop and require urgent treatment. Occasionally symptoms only occur later in life due to enlargement of the vessels.

A barium swallow reveals a posterior indentation of the oesophagus by the abnormal vessel. If symptoms are severe a left thoracotomy should be performed and the abnormal vessel divided or transposed.

CARDIOTHORACIC TRAUMA

Road accidents and other high-speed injuries may cause acute traumatic rupture of the aorta. This usually occurs between the left subclavian artery and the ligamentum arteriosum. Aortic rupture should always be suspected in deceleration injuries where there is widening of the mediastinum and unexplained hypotension. The diagnosis is confirmed by aortography. The natural history of traumatic rupture of the aorta is poor and emergency operation is indicated for either repair or replacement with a Dacron graft. These patients often have other extensive injuries and the recent introduction of heparinised vascular shunts (p. 794), thereby avoiding systemic heparinisation during the period of aortic clamping, has been an important advance.

Stab wounds of the chest may penetrate the lungs or heart. After initial clinical assessment a chest radiograph should be taken and the patient carefully observed. A pneumothorax or haemothorax should be treated by intercostal tube drainage. Most stab wounds of the heart present with signs of haemorrhage or cardiac tamponade. Providing the cardiovascular function remains stable it is sometimes reasonable to defer exploratory operation. However, frequent assessment by an experienced cardiac surgeon is important if this policy is followed, because late tamponade or continuing haemorrhage is possible.

CARDIAC TRANSPLANTATION (also see Chapter 62)

The first human heart transplant was performed by Christiaan Barnard in 1967. During the next decade considerable advances were made by Dr Shumway's group at Stanford University. In the last five years many more centres have

---

[1] Lusus = game, sport or jest. Condition originally described as 'Lusus naturae'—a jest or sport of nature. First noted by Bayford in 1761.

Bernard Jean Antonin Marfan, 1858–1942. (See footnote, Chapter 21).
David Bayford, 1739–90. Surgeon and Physician, Lewes, Sussex. He was born probably in the Hertfordshire village where Mr McNeill Love lived in his later years. He was granted the degree M.D. by the Archbishop of Canterbury, a rare means of obtaining a medical degree which still exists today.
Christiaan Barnard, Contemporary. Professor of Cardiac Surgery, Groote Schuur Hospital, Cape Town, South Africa.
Norman Shumway, Contemporary. Professor of Surgery, Stanford University, California, U.S.A.

started transplant programmes and most patients undergoing heart transplantation can now anticipate 75% and 50% chances of being alive after one and four years respectively.

The main reasons for this improved outlook include better selection of recipients, earlier detection and better management of acute rejection episodes, fewer postoperative infections, and a declining incidence of coronary atheroma in the transplanted heart.

Patients selected for transplantation should have terminal heart disease not amenable to further medical or conventional surgical treatment. They should preferably be less than 50 years of age, should have no active infection, and the pulmonary vascular resistance should not be unduly elevated. There should be ABO blood group compatability between donor and recipient and a negative lymphocyte crossmatch between donor cells and recipient serum. The degree of HLA tissue typing mismatch does not seem to affect the prognosis. Permanent immunosuppression with cyclosporin A, corticosteroids and azathioprine is necessary and most late complications are related to this. The advent of more effective and less toxic immunosuppressive agents will further expand the indications and reduce the cost of the procedure.

HEART AND LUNG TRANSPLANTATION

More recently combined heart and lung transplatation has been used successfully to treat patients with primary pulmonary hypertension or with pulmonary hypertension secondary to cardiac disease. Patients with primary lung disease may also benefit from this procedure in the future.

CHAPTER 42

ANASTOMOSES

Background

The experience of bowel surgery until the latter part of the 19th century was limited to dealing with protruding intestine following abdominal injury usually sustained during wars. If a laceration of the bowel was encountered attempts were made to repair it using the jaws of ants (described by Susruta & Albucasis), or by suturing (Celsus). Probably the first surgeon to describe a suture made from animal gut was Albucasis. In Salerno, Italy, between the 12th and 14th Centuries, it was advised that if a piece of bowel had to be repaired it should be done over a stent of elder wood or animal trachea. Alternatives for dealing with injured intestine was to suture it to the abdominal wall to create a fistula or do nothing and let nature take its course. The latter management was frequently considered safer.

For centuries, no attempt was made to define the process of healing of the gastrointestinal tract. However, in 1812, Travers reported that intestinal wounds healed as a result of 'adhesive inflammation' binding down the peritoneal ('serosal') coat. Fourteen years later Lembert described a suturing technique in which serosa to serosa apposition was obtained.

As a consequence of the adaption of the Listerian principles of wound care and antiseptic surgery (Chapter 1) (together with general anaesthesia) surgeons in the second half of the 19th Century began to embark upon laparotomies with the express purpose of resecting a piece of intestine and subsequently restoring continuity. Gastro-intestinal surgery expanded rapidly and with it various methods of suturing the bowel together. All were modifications of Lembert's basic principles and were reviewed by Senn in 1893. A year earlier Murphy introduced his button but adverse reports appeared in the surgical literature citing colo-colic anastomotic stricture which resulted in the patient's death.

In 1893 Senn advised two-layer interrupted anastomoses. His suture was of fine aseptic silk applied with ordinary sewing needles. Halsted favoured a one-layer anastomosis without penetration of the lumen. In contrast Connell in 1903 strongly recommended a single layer of interrupted sutures which passed through all coats of the bowel and with the knots ligated intraluminally. Kocher also suggested an all-coats suture technique in two layers using catgut and silk. In 1907 Kerr & Parker used a temporary suture to close the bowel whilst the permanent sutures were inserted; once the anastomosis was completed these preliminary sutures were removed. Schoemaker & Remkin (1928) performed end-to-end anastomoses over narrow crushing clamps.

In 1922 Halsted described a closed colorectal technique in which the bowel was crushed, ligated and divided at the resection margins. Next submucosal buttress sutures joined the two ends of the bowel and finally an instrument with a knife blade was passed per rectum through the anastomotic diaphragm to divide the two sutures which had closed the lumen: the forerunner of our contemporary stapling devices.

The closed method of anastomosis has been replaced by the open method for three major reasons: (a) the introduction of antibiotics, (b) improved pre-operative bowel cleansing, and (c) the use of atraumatic sutures.

Alexis Carrell was a recognised revolutionist in vascular surgery. In 1902 he described a suture technique he had developed that created a perfect end-to-end anastomosis of blood vessels. His method employed 3 retaining sutures which, when drawn taut, pulled the edges into an equilateral triangle which could then be easily sutured. This technique preserved the full patency of the lumen, and gave a smooth interior surface to reduce platelet and fibrin deposition.

Anastomotic healing is influenced by many factors and it is difficult to assess the influence of any single factor especially in the clinical situation. Healing depends on fibroblastic response and on the formation of plentiful collagen in the submucosa round the anastomosis. *The general, specific and local factors influencing anastomotic healing are listed in Table 1.*

TABLE 1

FACTORS INFLUENCING ANASTOMOTIC HEALING

General	Specific	Local
Age eg. *infancy & old age*	*Anaemia*	Site of Anastomosis
Circumstances	*Suture Line Disease*	(i) *Oesophagus*
(i) Elective surgery	*Irradiated tissue*	(ii) *Rectum*
(ii) *Emergency surgery*	*Infected Anastomosis*	(iii) *Extraperitoneal*
(iii) *Obstructed bowel*	*Antibiotics*	*Proximal faecal loading*
Malignancy		*Dilated proximal bowel*
Sepsis		Suture technique
Drugs		(i) Mucosal inversion
(i) *Corticosteroids*		(ii) One v. two layer
(ii) *Immunosuppressives*		Suture material
Malnutrition		(i) Absorbent v. non—
Anaemia		absorbent
Jaundice		Good blood supply
Uraemia		No tension
Irradiation		Drain
		Stimuli eg. feeding or drugs

Adverse factors in italics

The surgeon should be aware of good techniques relating to the main sites of anastomoses.

TABLE 2

SITES OF ANASTOMOSES

(a) Gastro-intestinal	*(b) Urological*	*(c) Vascular*
(i) Oesophagus	(i) ureter	(i) aorta
(ii) Stomach	(ii) bladder	(ii) peripheral artery e.g. femoral
(iii) Small intestine	(iii) urethra	(iii) vein e.g. portal
(iv) Biliary and pancreatic	(iv) vas deferens	(iv) lymphatic
(v) Large intestine		(v) coronary artery
		(vi) microvascular e.g. cerebral

TECHNIQUES FOR THE COMMONER ANASTOMOSES

(A) Gastro-intestinal Anastomoses

Certain important generalisations can be made: (a) *Exposure.*—Any anastomosis becomes difficult if the surgical access and exposure are poor. This may be caused by inadequate anaesthesia and muscle relaxation, poor assistance, a badly placed and/or too short incision, and less than perfect illumination. Poor access may also result from inadequate mobilisation of the viscera and this is more likely to occur in oesophageal, colonic and rectal anastomoses as these parts of the gastro-intestinal tract are anatomically fixed and deeply situated.

(b) *Blood Supply.*—The only absolute criterion of an adequate blood supply prior to anastomosis is free bleeding from the cut edges of the bowel. The blood supply can be compromised by undue tension on the suture line, devascularisation of the bowel during mobilisation, strangulation of the tissues by tightly knotted sutures, and the excessive use of diathermy.

(c) *Suture Technique.*—Experimental work and clinical trials have shown that inverted suture lines are superior to everted ones though this principle has been challenged by Ravitch. The vast majority of surgeons use an open method of intestinal anastomosis. One aspect which remains a controversy is the use of one or two layers. The latter was devised by Czerny and is probably the most popular technique still today. It is alleged that a single layer results in less ischaemia and tissue necrosis and less narrowing of the lumen. Studies in both experimental animals and man have shown no great difference between the two techniques. Anastomoses involving the extraperitoneal portion of the rectum and also the oesophagus are better performed using a single layer full thickness technique, as this preserves the blood supply and full lumen width better than a two-layer technique. Gastro-intestinal anastomoses can be performed end-to-end, end-to-side or side-to-side and can be either 'open' or 'closed'. Generally the method used in any one operation is standard. In the United Kingdom the majority of surgeons employ the 'open' method removing the clamps following the placement of the outer, posterior, serosal layer of sutures. The following methods are used for uniting parts of the gastro-intestinal tract:

(1) The Open End-to-end Two-layer Technique (fig. 769 a—d)

The divided ends of the bowel are held in crushing clamps and light occlusion clamps are applied across the bowel avoiding the mesentery. The outer posterior layer of sutures are placed usually in a continuous manner (fig. 769a) but interrupted sutures can also be used. The crushing clamps are then removed by amputation.

The inner layers of sutures are then inserted commencing at the antimesenteric border with the knot on the serosal surface. A continuous over and over technique is used, care being taken to include all coats of the bowel wall and avoiding grasping the mucosa with forceps.

The mesenteric corner of the anastomosis is securely invaginated by using a Connell suture (fig. 769b) and the anterior aspect closed using a continuous Connell technique (fig. 769c) or a simple over and over technique. The suture is then tied to its other end. The anastomosis is completed by an anterior row of serosal sutures either continuous from the posterior layer or interrupted (fig. 769d). The mesentery of the small intestine must be closed in every case and the anastomosis checked for patency (fig. 769d inset).

An alternative to the above procedure is to place the inner all-coats layer first

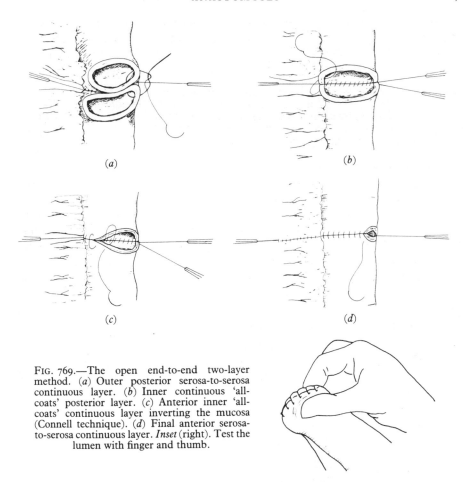

(a)

(b)

(c)

(d)

FIG. 769.—The open end-to-end two-layer method. (*a*) Outer posterior serosa-to-serosa continuous layer. (*b*) Inner continuous 'all-coats' posterior layer. (*c*) Anterior inner 'all-coats' continuous layer inverting the mucosa (Connell technique). (*d*) Final anterior serosa-to-serosa continuous layer. *Inset* (right). Test the lumen with finger and thumb.

and then the outer layer, rotating the anastomosis to complete the posterior aspect. This is not recommended when the mesentery is very fatty.

If there is disparity of the bowel ends, the smaller lumen orifice can be widened by cutting along its antimesenteric border (Cheatle's manoeuvre).

(2) **The Open End-to-end One-layer Technique** (fig. 770 *a* & *b*)

This method is increasingly favoured for end-to-end anastomoses in areas of the gastro-intestinal tract where the blood supply is poor, where there is no serosal coat or the lumen is small. In infants, a one-layer technique is the rule. Many surgeons favour the use of a one-layer open technique for the oesophagus and lower rectum.

After preliminary corner stitches are inserted to steady and approximate the posterior walls of the anastomosis (fig. 770*a*), a series of interrupted deep 'all-coat' sutures of un- or delayed-absorbable material (Dexon, Vicryl, Silk or Linen are all suitable) are inserted 5mm apart. After the corners have been reached, the suturing is continued along the anterior walls as interrupted Lembert stitches with a wide margin of muscle coat as shown (fig. 770*b*): some surgeons use

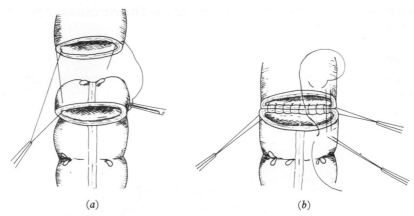

(a)   (b)

FIG. 770.—The open end-to-end one-layer technique. (a) Stay sutures at corners to approximate and steady the posterior walls. (b) After completing the posterior layer, the anterior layer is continued by interrupted Lembert sutures.

interrupted Connell sutures, but these are less haemostatic and turn in more tissue than the technique illustrated.

(3) The Closed End-to-end Single-layer Technique (fig. 771)

The single-layer inverting closed anastomosis with interrupted non-absorbable sutures was first advised by Halsted. The technique has been modified to incorporate the submucosa so that only the mucosa is excluded. It is commenced by inserting two angle stitches which are held untied. Posterior sutures are then placed longitudinally approximately 5mm apart (fig. 771). Once finished, the anterior layer is inserted in a similar fashion. Once in place the clamps are slipped out, the angle sutures tied and lastly the anterior ones. Patency must always be checked with finger and thumb (fig. 769d inset).

(4) End-to-side Anastomosis (fig. 772)

This technique is used particularly in surgery of the oesophagus, stomach and when there is significant disparity between two ends of intestine.

One end of the bowel must be closed and this is usually performed with a two-

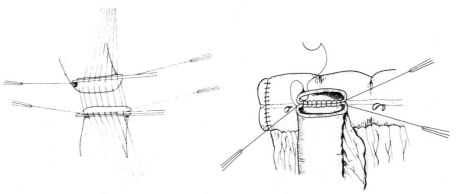

FIG. 771.—Closed technique.   FIG. 772.—End-to-side technique.

layer technique or alternatively by a row of staples. The anastomosis is performed as for an end-to-end one (fig. 769 *a—d*).

(5) Side-to-side Anastomosis

These are usually performed to by-pass an obstruction. Both ends are closed before the side-to-side anastomosis is carried out when the anastomosis is between two separate divided lengths of bowel.

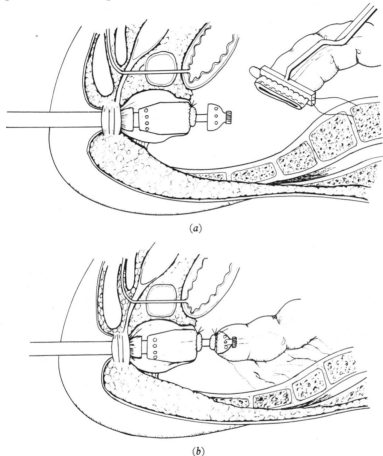

(*a*)

(*b*)

Fig. 773 *a* and *b*.—Circular stapling device being used for a low rectal anastomosis. The proximal end of colon has been divided between linear staples prior to using the Furness clamp to put in the purse-string suture.

(6) Stapling Techniques (figs 773 & 774)

(i) Preliminary closure of the bowel ends can be performed using linear staples (fig. 773) which can be cut away once the purse-string suture is in place.

(ii) End-to-end anastomosis is performed using circular stapling devices (E.E.A.—Autosuture and I.L.S.—Ethicon). Purse-string sutures must be carefully placed and for this the Furness clamp can be utilised (fig. 773*a*). Circular staples are very useful for oesophageal and rectal anastomoses. A rectal anastomosis is illustrated in fig. 773.

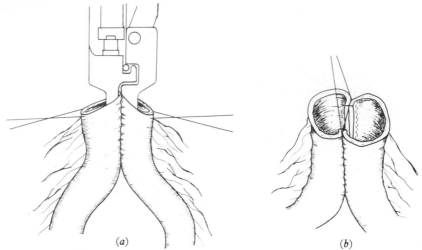

FIG. 774.—GIA linear stapling device (*a*) applying the staples, (*b*) the bowel ends must be closed over when the linear stapling device has been 'fired' and removed.

(iii) Side-to-side anastomoses can be performed using the G.I.A. stapler and this is useful for small bowel and ileo-colic anastomoses (fig. 774).

Special Sites

Oesophageal Anastomoses.—When suturing the oesophagus, horizontal mattress sutures should be used as they have less tendency to cut through the oesophageal muscle than vertical mattress sutures. The *cervical oesophagus* can be anastomosed to stomach, colon or jejunum. Providing there is no tension and the blood supply to the intestine brought up to the neck is adequate, these anastomoses heal well. The stomach is the simplest method of reconstruction but reflux can be a problem. The sutures are placed as horizontal mattress sutures in one layer (and the author now uses P.D.S.[1] for almost all intestinal anastomoses). The *thoracic oesophagus* is usually anastomosed to stomach (the Ivor Lewis operation) or jejunum. The technique used is the same though the circular stapling device can be used. The *abdominal oesophagus* is almost always anastomosed to jejunum either as a Roux-en-Y or to a loop and the circular stapling device is increasingly used in this situation following total gastrectomy. **Gastric Anastomoses.**—Following partial gastrectomy continuity is restored either to duodenum (Bilroth I partial gastrectomy) or to jejunum (Polya partial gastrectomy— fig. 775 *a* & *b*). The latter can be ante-colic or retro-colic and should be performed by joining lesser curve to afferent loop, the latter being kept as short as possible. Because of the excellent blood supply absorbable sutures can be used and placed in a continuous manner. If the operation has been for carcinoma, *e.g.* a radical subtotal gastrectomy, it is advisable to make the anastomoses ante-colic in case of recurrence and to use non-absorbable sutures or P.D.S. for the outer layer. Closure of the duodenum or stomach can be performed using linear stapling devices. **Small Intestinal Anastomoses.**—Jejuno-jejunal, jejuno-ileal, ileo-ileal, ileo-colic and ileo-rectal anastomoses are all performed following resections for

---

[1] P.D.S. = Polydioxanone suture.

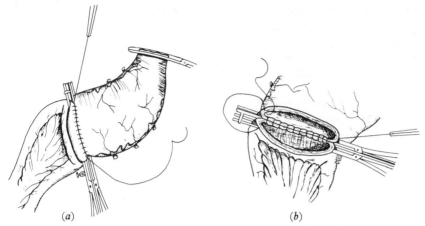

(a) (b)

FIG. 775.—Showing the gastro-jejunal anastomosis during a Polya-type gastrectomy. (a) The posterior continuous layer being inserted. The gastric area to be removed is being used as a tractor before being cut away, (b) the stomach has been cut away and the anterior layer is started.

different disease processes. Like the stomach, the small intestine has an excellent blood supply and therefore continuous sutures can be used though following right hemi-colectomy and total colectomy the ileo-colic and ileo-rectal anastomoses are best performed with an outer layer of interrupted sutures. It is always advisable to slant the clamps so that less antimesenteric border is left. The G.I.A. stapling device can be used for any of these anastomoses. **Colo-colic and Colo-Rectal Anastomoses.**—Because (1) the vascular supply is less good, (2) distension from gas occurs and (3) the contents are faecal, large intestinal anastomoses do not heal well. Two layers of interrupted sutures are ideal though many surgeons do use only one layer. It is the author's practice to use one layer only for extraperitoneal anastomoses following anterior resection but for very low rectal anastomoses the circular stapling device is usually used (fig. 773). No anastomosis should be performed if the colon has not been well prepared. If the colon is loaded a low rectal anastomosis will be placed in jeopardy. The advent of 'on table' lavage popularised at St Mary's Hospital, London (Dudley), is employed by the author which ensures an empty colon above the subsequent anastomosis. A self-retaining catheter is inserted into the caecum usually via the base of the appendix following appendicectomy or via the terminal ileum and scavenger tubing tied in place over the cut colon. Hartman's solution is then passed via the catheter until all faecal matter has been expelled from the colon via the scavenger tubing and the effluent is clear. The author retains the catheter as a tube caecostomy which acts as a gas vent. The terminal portion of the colon tied round the scavenger tubing is resected prior to anastomosis. The rectal stump is also lavaged from above and the effluent collected via a proctoscope in the anus. It is usual practice in cancer cases to employ a cytocidal fluid and mercuric perchloride[1] or noxythiolin is used. It should be stated that prior to resection tapes are placed round the bowel and tied to ensure no malignant cells are exfoliated and reimplanted.

---

1 Because mercuric perchloride is a poison, it should be used dilute (1:400) and the solution washed out immediately.

Hugh Dudley, Contemporary. Professor of Surgery, St Mary's Hospital, London.

Biliary and Pancreatic Anastomoses.—Either cholecyst-jejunostomy or choledocho-jejunostomy is used to bypass unresectable carcinoma of the head of the pancreas. Following cholecyst-jejunostomy a jejuno-jejunostomy distal to it is often performed. Also, if there is danger of duodenal occlusion gastro-jejunostomy is also performed.

For benign strictures of the common bile duct, excision and primary anastomosis may be possible. Otherwise a Roux loop is used as for malignant strictures. Most surgeons splint these anastomoses bringing the stent out well away from the anastomosis. Pancreatic duct anastomosis to jejunum is likewise splinted, performed in a single layer and for all these anastomoses P.D.S. is advocated. A non-absorbable suture in the biliary tree could lead to stone formation.

(B) Urological (fig. 776)

Most anastomoses are uretero-vesical but uretero-ureteric and uretero-ileal (fig. 776) are also performed. Uretero-colic anastomoses are performed less commonly as an ileal bladder is preferable. The ureter should always be spatulated to increase the size of the anastomosis and splinting is usual. Sutures are usually absorbable and placed either continuously or interrupted. As in the biliary tree non-absorbable material, especially if braided, could lead to stone formation. (See also Urinary Diversion in Chapter 58, fig. 1275.)

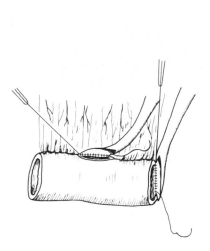
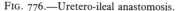

FIG. 776.—Uretero-ileal anastomosis.

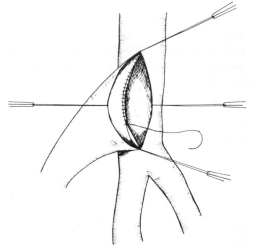

FIG. 777.—A typical end-to-side vascular anastomosis. In this case a vein is being anastomosed to the common femoral artery (to by-pass an obstruction to the superficial femoral artery in Hunter's canal).

(C) Vascular (fig. 777)

Except rarely, e.g. following trauma, when a severed vessel can be repaired primarily, most anastomoses are made to auto-grafts or to veins (fig. 777). The suture material used must be non-absorbable and continuous though occasionally with small vessels (e.g. fistula formation for haemodialysis) interrupted sutures are used. When placed end-to-end the graft or vein should be stretched to increase the orifice size. Micro-vascular anastomosis are always done with interrupted sutures. *If a vascular anastomosis is close to a joint, e.g. to the hip joint in the groin, excessive movement at that joint should be avoided until the anastomosis is healed.* (See also Chapter 14, figs. 179, 180 and 210.)

PROTECTING AN ANASTOMOSIS

All anastomoses should be made without tension in an area of good blood supply. Colonic anastomoses can be protected from the faecal stream by a proximal colostomy. Drains should lie *alongside* and *not on* the suture line. Gastrointestinal movement can be delayed or reduced by a policy of gastric suction, IV feeding and anti-spasmodic drugs (Buscopan). Oesophageal and rectal anastomoses can be checked by water-soluble contrast examinations before precautions against breakdown are discontinued. Drains can be a source of sepsis and should be removed immediately they have ceased to lead off significant quantities of fluid (or a track has formed—usually after 7 or 8 days).

If adverse healing factors are present (Table 1) precautions should be taken against breakdown, e.g. a diverting colostomy.

SUTURE MATERIALS

TABLE 3

SUTURE MATERIALS: PROPERTIES

ABSORBABLE	NON-ABSORBABLE
Catgut, collagen, homopolymer of glycolide, copolymers of glycolide and lactide, homopolymer of polydioxanone	Polyester, polyamide, polypropylene, polyethylene, steel, silk, cotton, linen
BIOLOGICAL	MAN-MADE
Catgut, collagen, silk, linen, cotton	Polyester, polyamide, polypropylene, polyglycolide, polylactide, polydioxanone, steel
MONOFILAMENT	MULTIFILAMENT
Polyamide, polypropylene, polyethylene, polydioxanone, catgut, steel	Polyester, polyamide, polyglycolide, polylactide, silk, cotton, linen, steel
BRAIDED	TWISTED
Polyester, polyamide, polyglycolide, polylactide, silk	Cotton, linen
COATED	UNCOATED
Polyester, polyglycolide, polylactide, cotton, linen	Polyamide, polypropylene, polyethylene, catgut, collagen, steel

A suture should be chosen with the following properties in mind:
 (i) strength
(ii) minimal reaction

(iii) easy handling characteristics

(iv) good knotting security.

The different properties of individual sutures are classified in Table 3.

(1) **Absorbable.**—Catgut is the oldest suture material known to man and is made from the submucosa of sheep intestines. It can be chromacised or plain and is still the most frequently used suture material in intestinal anastomoses.

Suture material is absorbed in one of two ways. The first applies to catgut and collagen where the absorption mechanism is by enzymatic digestion. The other method is one of preliminary hydrolysis which is the effect of water on the suture material and does not require the same cellular involvement as does catgut with its proteolytic digestive enzymes. Hydrolysis is increased with rise in temperature or pH changes. Fig. 778 demonstrates in general terms the comparative absorption times for catgut, Dexon (homopolymer of glycolide), Vicryl (copolymer of glycolide and lactide) and P.D.S. (polydioxanone). Once a suture has been broken up by hydrolysis, polymorphonuclear and other macrophages (e.g. giant cells) can digest even so-called unabsorbable material.

As the material absorbs it loses its tensile strength (fig. 778).

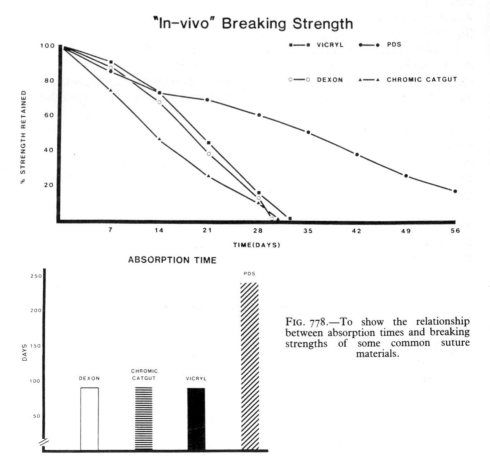

FIG. 778.—To show the relationship between absorption times and breaking strengths of some common suture materials.

(2) **Delayed or Non-absorbable.**—Very few sutures are truly completely unabsorbable.

Silk is derived from the cocoon of the silkworm larva. The suture is braided round a core and coated with wax to reduce capillary action. Tissue reaction is greater than to the synthetic non-absorbables because silk is a foreign protein. For those reasons the author will not use silk in anastomoses and prefers using a monofilament synthetic suture if a non-absorbable suture is deemed necessary. Wire sutures are ideal for qualities of inertness and permanence, but are difficult to work with. Vicryl is easy to use, has good qualities of minimal tissue reaction and absorption, but is expensive. Dexon has a prolonged absorption time and is cheaper, but its knotting qualities are less satisfactory.

(3) **Staples.**—Circular, linear and linear-cutting stapling devices are used to form anastomoses. The devices carrying these staples can be disposable or reusable. Until 1986 the staples were always non-absorbable being made of stainless steel. However, absorbable staples have now been developed and are on trial. The circular stapling device is used for oesophageal and rectal anastomoses. Their use is no 'short cut' to the joining of two pieces of intestine. The preparation of the bowel ends and the placement of the purse-string sutures must be carefully executed. They do, however, help in situations where the placement of sutures would be difficult, e.g. a low anterior resection in a patient with a narrow pelvis (fig. 773).

Linear stapling for anastomoses leaves awkward edges and ends (fig. 774) and is not favoured by the author. Linear-cutting staplers can save time if very long closures or multiple anastomoses are necessary but have no other benefit over hand-sutured anastomoses.

It is necessary to choose suture material which has the best characteristics for carrying out an anastomosis in a particular site. Vascular anastomoses require fine suture materials with minimal tissue reaction: strength is a secondary consideration: Vicryl is commonly used. Gut anastomoses require good handling qualities with secure knotting: pliancy is also important, as is strength when the intestine begins to contract: plain catgut is unsuitable for intestinal anastomoses, but chromic catgut can be used for gastric and small intestinal unions. Rectal and oesophageal anastomoses should employ an unabsorbable layer of stitches because these areas combine many adverse factors with the requirement to withstand powerful contractile activity.

COMPLICATIONS

There are four main complications:

(i) Haemorrhage
(ii) Leakage
(iii) Stenosis
(iv) Diverticular Formation (Aneurysmal at vascular anastomoses).

(i) **Haemorrhage.**—This can occur at the suture line or from the mesentery. The Connell suture is non-haemostatic and therefore should not be used if the cut intestine has an excellent blood supply, e.g. the stomach.

Haemorrhage can be immediate (reactionary) or later (secondary) though this is rare. If the bleeding causes systemic effects, a laparotomy must be performed and the anastomosis resected and refashioned.

(ii) **Leakage.**—Oesophageal and colonic anastomoses are most prone to leak. The outcome depends on the size of the leak and its anatomical site. As already stated, the healing of anastomoses depends on a good blood supply and no tension. With colonic anastomoses a clean bowel is also necessary.

(iii) **Stenosis.**—Can be caused by excessive inversion especially with two-layer anastomoses. An inadequate stoma in the first place or ischaemia can also lead to subsequent stenoses. Circular staples, especially double rows, are prone to cause narrowing due to the rigidity.

(iv) **Diverticular Formation.**—Caused by either a weakness of the wall or from a poor blood supply, a 'blow-out' occurs which is contained, i.e. perforation does not occur.

TABLE 4

PREVENTION OF COMPLICATIONS

AVOID	ENSURE
Excessive inversion of mucosa	Adequate blood supply
Compromised anti-mesenteric blood supply	No tension
	Adequate stoma
Ischaemic intestinal margins	'Clean' bowel
Haematoma at anastomosis	Gentle handling of tissues
Gap at mesenteric angle	Equality of ends
Exposed mucosa	
Unequal ends	

Although anastomoses depend on the many factors mentioned, a good technique is vitally important. Anastomoses should never be rushed or performed if the above conditions cannot be fulfilled. A few extra minutes spent pays handsome dividends.

CHAPTER 43

THE OESOPHAGUS

Surgical Anatomy.—The oesophagus is a fibromuscular tube 25 cm long occupying the posterior mediastinum and extending from the cricopharyngeal sphincter to the cardia of the stomach; 4 cm of this tube lies below the diaphragm. The musculature of the upper one-third is mainly striated, giving way to smooth muscle below. It is lined by squamous epithelium which is replaced by specialised epithelium at the level of the hiatus similar to gastric mucosa but without oxyntic and peptic cells. This specialised mucosa lines the lower 3 cm. The parasympathetic supply is mediated by the vagus through an extrinsic and intrinsic plexus. The intrinsic plexus has no Meissner's network which is present elsewhere through the alimentary canal, and Auerbach's plexus is present only in the lower two-thirds.

There are three physiological constrictions in this tube with distinct lesions at each level as shown in fig. 779. The figures 15, 25 and 40 are very important to the oesophagoscopist. They represent the situations of anatomical narrowing where difficulty may be experienced in the passage of instruments and where foreign bodies may be arrested. They are also the sites of election for innocent strictures and for carcinoma of the oesophagus.

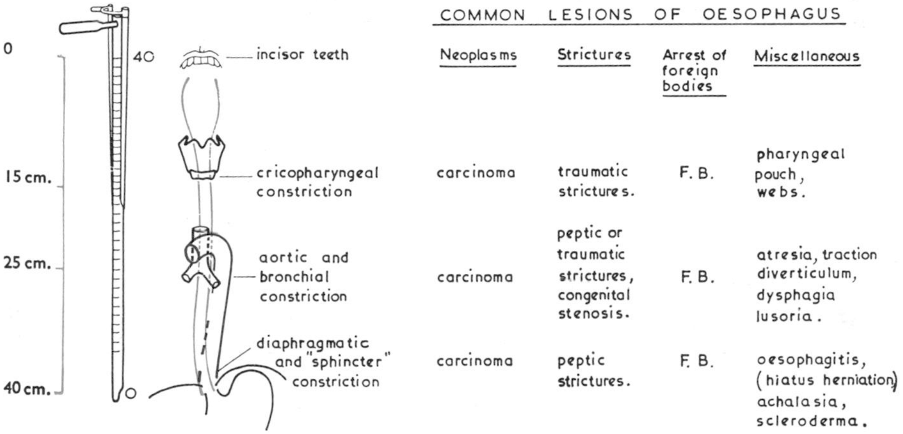

		COMMON	LESIONS	OF	OESOPHAGUS
	incisor teeth	Neoplasms	Strictures	Arrest of foreign bodies	Miscellaneous
15 cm.	cricopharyngeal constriction	carcinoma	traumatic strictures.	F. B.	pharyngeal pouch, webs.
25 cm.	aortic and bronchial constriction	carcinoma	peptic or traumatic strictures, congenital stenosis.	F. B.	atresia, traction diverticulum, dysphagia lusoria.
40 cm.	diaphragmatic and "sphincter" constriction	carcinoma	peptic strictures.	F. B.	oesophagitis, (hiatus herniation) achalasia, scleroderma.

FIG. 779.—Common lesions at various levels of the oesophagus. An oesophagoscope is drawn to the left of the diagram. Levels are less exact with a flexible endoscope.

(L. R. Celestin, FRCS, Bristol.)

Physiology.—The main function of the oesophagus is to form part of a coordinated mechanism transferring food from the mouth to the stomach. The initial movement of food through the oropharynx is induced voluntarily and involves sequential contraction of the oropharyngeal musculature together with simultaneous closure of the nasal and respiratory passages and opening of the upper oesophageal or cricopharyngeal sphincter. The body of the oesophagus then sweeps the food bolus by an involuntary peristaltic wave, through a relaxed gastro-oesophageal sphincter zone, into the stomach.

The cricopharyngeal sphincter is normally closed at rest and serves as a protective mechanism against regurgitation of oesophageal contents into the respiratory passages. Failure of it to relax on swallowing may pre-dispose to the development of a pharyngeal pouch (propulsion diverticulum, Chapter 34).

At the lower end of the oesophagus there is a physiological sphincter which together with other anatomical mechanisms (p. 836) prevent materials especially gastric acid or

Georg Meissner, 1829–1905. Professor of Physiology, Göttingen, Germany.
Leopold Auerbach, 1828–1897. Professor of Neuropathology, Breslau, Germany. (Now Wrocław, Poland.)

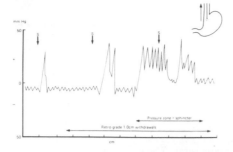

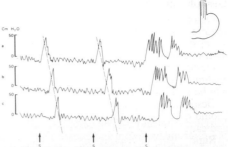

FIG. 780.—Small balloon (0·5 cm diam) pull-through study of normal human gastro-oeso-phageal junction. The small swings on the record represent respiratory movements: these are upward ('positive') below the diaphragm and downward ('negative') with inspiration above the diaphragm. This reversal of respiratory move-ment marks the hiatus. Note the responses to swallows (S) with a contractile response in the body of the oesophagus and a relaxation response in the sphincter zone.

FIG. 781.—Triple water-filled 'open-tip' tube study of normal lower oesophagus and gastro-oesophageal sphincter zone. Note the swallowing contractions in the body of the oesophagus are sequential, i.e. peristaltic. The tubes are record-ing at 1·0 cm intervals from each tip. The sphincter relaxes normally in sequence with each contraction arriving down the lower oesophagus.

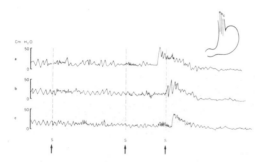

FIG. 782.—Triple 'open-tip' tube study of achalasia. Note that in contrast to the normal oesophagus: (i) there is no contractile response in the body of the oesophagus to a swallow; (ii) the sphincter zone retains a normal pressure, but does not relax with swallowing; (iii) the expected drop in press-ure when the units enter the oesophagus is absent (compare with fig. 781).

bile refluxing along the natural pressure gradient between the abdominal and thoracic cavities. The tone of the lower oesophageal sphincter is influenced by gastrointestinal hormones, anti-cholinergic drugs and smoking. The displaced sphincter loses tonus and permits reflux to occur, especially if the lower oesophagus also loses peristaltic activity (Earlam).

The presence and function of the physiological sphincter can be tested by manometric methods using small balloons and open-tip perfused tubes (Code). The normal gastro-oesophageal junction is 3-4 cm long and has a pressure of 30 cm H_2O (by open-tip tube) and higher (by balloon) (fig. 780). The oesophagus is a peristaltic organ, and the sphincter relaxes in advance of the peristaltic wave (fig. 781). Abnormal conditions e.g. achalasia (fig. 782) or scleroderma show changes in both oesophageal peristalsis and sphincter tonus and function.

Dysphagia is the term used to describe difficulty (not pain) in swallowing; there are two types—oropharyngeal and oesophageal. The type of dysphagia is important. It may be dysphagia for solids or fluids, intermittent or progressive, precise or vague in its appreci-ation. *Pain* may be present. Painful dysphagia is usually due to oesophagitis. *Regurgi-tation*—It is important to record the volume, contents, presence of blood or bile and the reaction to litmus. Loss of weight, anaemia, cachexia and change of voice are also import-ant symptoms.

Radiography is a most valuable investigation. A *straight film* will show an opaque foreign body and the site of its arrest (figs. 787, 788). A *barium swallow* is essential: screening will show the motility and films, taken as necessary, will delineate size, distortion or the presence of a space-occupying lesion. It is important to take a film with the patient in the prone head-down position to assess the degree of regurgitation.

Richard Earlam, Contemporary. Surgeon, The London Hospital.
C. F. Code, Contemporary. Emeritus Professor of Physiology: Mayo Clinic, Rochester, Minn., U.S.A.

Oesophagoscopy

Oesophagoscopy is necessary for the investigation of most oesophageal conditions. It is required to view the inside of the oesophagus and the oesophagogastric junction, to obtain a biopsy, for the removal of foreign bodies and to dilate strictures. There are two types of instrument available—the rigid and the flexible fibreoptic oesphagoscope.

Oesophagoscopy with a rigid oesophagoscope should never be carried out without a preliminary barium swallow—if this rule is broken, then sooner or later the oesophagus will be perforated during the examination.

Oesophagoscopy is a much more dangerous examination than a bronchoscopy and should never be undertaken lightly. Of all the foreign bodies which enter the oesophagus and cause a perforation, the oesophagoscope itself is without doubt the most frequent.

Rigid oesophagoscopy (fig. 783).—The teeth and lips must be protected during the examination. The Negus type of instrument is preferable, for it is elliptical in shape and has proximal illumination. Oesophagoscopy is carried out under general anaesthesia, with the head extended as in bronchoscopy but the head slightly flexed on the neck and the neck on the trunk. A slight foot-down tilt of the operating table will help to prevent gastric reflux. The well-lubricated instrument is passed into the mouth usually on the right side, and guided down with the fingers of the left hand to a position behind the epiglottis and the cricoid cartilage. This will view the cricopharyngeal inlet, through which the instrument must be passed. This is the most difficult part of the examination. If there is any difficulty a small bougie should be gently passed into the upper oesophagus as a guide and the oesophagoscope passed over it into the upper oesophagus. It may help if the anaesthetist grasps the whole larynx in his hand and draws it forwards. It may also help if at this stage the anaesthetist temporarily deflates the cuff on the endotracheal tube. The instrument should slide in without any force being required—if force is required, then either it is going in the wrong direction or a stricture is present, which should have been seen on the preliminary barium swallow. Alternatively, the patient is not adequately relaxed and the upper oesophageal sphincter is in spasm.

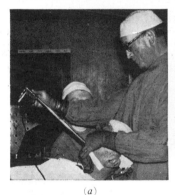
(a)

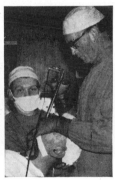
(b)

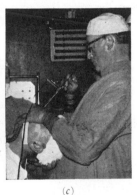
(c)

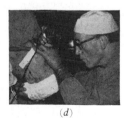
(d)

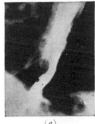
(e)

FIG. 783.—Oesophagoscopy. (a) With the patient's shoulders slightly raised and neck fully flexed, the oesophagoscope is guided by the endoscopist's left hand over the dorsum of the tongue to the posterior pharyngeal wall. (b) The head is slightly extended and the instrument has been passed under vision behind the endotracheal tube. The tip of the instrument is now behind the cricoid cartilage and on levering the larynx forwards the crico-pharyngeal fold is seen. (c) As the head and neck are gradually extended the instrument is advanced under vision. The mid-thoracic oesophagus is now being inspected. (d) The head and neck are now completely extended and the oesophagoscope has advanced until the 40 cm mark is opposite the upper incisor teeth. At this level the cardia normally comes into view but in this case the oesophageal carcinoma (e) is seen.

(Norman C. Tanner, FRCS, London.)

Sir Victor Ewings Negus, 1887–1974. Surgeon, Ear, Nose and Throat Department, King's College Hospital, London.

Once the cricopharyngeal sphincter has been passed, there is usually no difficulty in passing the instrument the full length of the oesophagus, unless a stricture is present or the patient is excessively kyphotic. If a stricture is present there may be a considerable amount of retained fluid and food debris in the dilated oesophagus proximal to the stricture and considerable time and several sucker tubes (which will have become blocked) may be required before an adequate view is obtained.

The oesophageal mucosa should be inspected and biopsied for evidence of reflux oeso-phagitis. If a stricture or growth is present a biopsy should be taken.

Fibre-optic Oesophagoscopy (see fig. 841, Chapter 44).—The flexible fibre-optic oeso-phagoscope has a number of advantages, but also a number of disadvantages. It may be passed under local anaesthesia and, because the patient is conscious, useful information concerning the oesophageal hiatus and possible reflux may be obtained. In addition, it may be passed on into the stomach. Being flexible it is less likely to damage the oesophagus. On the other hand, the biopsy obtained is small and its use is very difficult if there is a large amount of retained food, as in achalasia of the oesophagus or some cases of carcinoma. The removal of foreign bodies is not possible. It is ideally suited to exclude serious pathology.

pH Measurements

These are increasingly being carried out to estimate the presence or absence of reflux with change in posture and also to decide whether the pain of which the patient complains is indeed due to acid reflux into the oesophagus.

Therapeutic Procedures

Removal of foreign bodies.—Some objects are removed fairly easily and in these cases it is usually necessary to withdraw the oesophagoscope at the same time as the retrieving forceps which are holding the foreign body. If the foreign body is sharp or jagged and is likely to damage the oesophagus during its removal, it is preferable to open the oesophagus above the object through a right thoracotomy.

Dilation of stricture.—Benign and malignant strictures may require dilatation with boug-ies, which must be well-lubricated and introduced without too much force. It is remark-ably easy to perforate the oesophagus or to produce a false passage. The Maloney mercury-filled bougies are probably the safest type of bougie to use, although if these are not available, gum elastic bougies or Eder-Puestow metal olives threaded over a guide wire may be used.

CONGENITAL ABNORMALITIES

These may be:

1. Atresia with or without tracheo-oesophageal fistula.

2. Stenosis—rare.

3. 'Short' oesophagus with hiatus hernia—rare. Most cases of 'short' oesoph-agus are the *consequence* of a hiatus hernia.

4. Dysphagia lusoria (compression by an abnormal artery, Chapter 41).

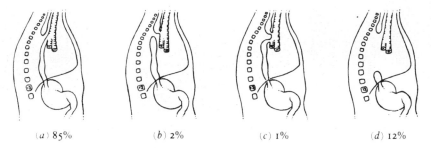

(a) 85%   (b) 2%   (c) 1%   (d) 12%

FIG. 784.—Congenital oesophageal atresia. (*a*) Lower segment opens into the trachea. (*b*) Upper segment opens into the trachea. (*c* Both segments open into the trachea. (*d*) Both segments end blindly and the mid-oesphagus is absent.

Congenital atresia of the oesophagus is usually associated with a tracheo-oesophageal fistula. Referring to fig. 784, it will be seen that in 85% of cases it is the *lower* segment that communicates with the trachea.

It is important to be aware of this abnormality, because its recognition within forty-eight hours of birth, and subsquent surgical correction, is the only hope of survival.

Clinical Features.—The new-bown babe regurgitates all its first, and every feed. Saliva pours, almost continuously, from its mouth. This is *the* sign of oesophageal atresia—it does not occur in any other condition. Attacks of coughing[1] and cyanosis occur on feeding. It should be suspected in all cases of hydramnios, a condition which is present in 50% of cases of atresia.

Clinical Confirmation of the Diagnosis.—A No. 10 soft rubber catheter is introduced into the oesophagus through the mouth. Should an obstruction be encountered about 10 cm from the lips, the diagnosis is practically certain.

Radiological Confirmation.—On no account should barium emulsion be given in these cases. Injection of 1 ml of dionosil down the catheter will demonstrate the obstruction. During this examination the supine position is advised, because in the rare event of the atresia belonging to categories (*b*) or (*c*), the medium is less likely to enter the trachea. In all cases the dionosil should be aspirated after the radiograph has been taken. Gas in the stomach will confirm that the lower end of the oesophagus reaches the trachea and that an anastomosis can be carried out (fig. 785).

Pre-operative Treatment.—Surgical intervention is urgent. Aspiration pneumonia is nearly always present and penicillin should be given. Dehydration should be corrected and naturally nothing should be given by mouth.

Operation.—The best approach is through a right-sided thoracotomy incision at the level of the fifth intercostal space (fig. 786). The azygos vein is divided between ligatures,

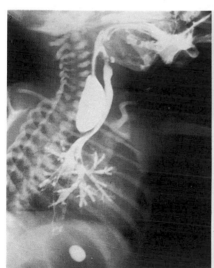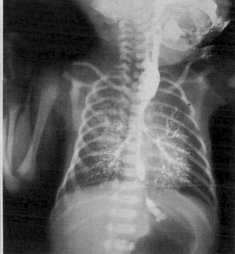

FIG. 785.—Tracheo-oesophageal fistula—radiographs in which excess dionosil was injected through the oesophageal catheter. Note the air and dionosil in the stomach, which indicates the presence of a lower oesophageal segment.
(Courtesy of Raymond Hurt.)

[1] In type (*a*) the patient coughs up frothy mucus, perhaps tinged with bile.

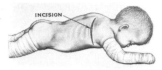

FIG. 786.—Thoracotomy for congenital oesophageal atresia.

the upper segment of the oesophagus is located by a catheter within it, and freed gently from the surrounding structure. The lower segment is divided at its entrance into the trachea, the opening in which is closed. An opening is made into the blind upper segment and anastomosis carried out between this opening and the lower segment.

Post-operative Care.—A special nurse skilled in aspirating the pharynx and an oxygen tent-incubator are highly desirable.

Prognosis.—The two post-operative complications are pneumonia and leakage of the anastomosis. With early diagnosis and skilled pre- and post-operative care, however, the mortality rate in a specialised paediatric unit should be under 10%.

Oesophageal Stenosis.—This a rare congenital organic narrowing of the lumen of the oesophagus and is a cause of dysphagia. It occurs anywhere in the oesophagus.

'Short' oesophagus with hiatus hernia.—In almost all cases the shortness is in reality secondary to a reflux oesophagitis due to a hiatus hernia and it is highly questionable whether an oesophagus is *ever* congenitally short (see p. 835).

Dysphagia Lusoria or **Oesophageal Compression by an Abnormal Artery** is discussed in Chapter 41.

FOREIGN BODIES IN THE OESOPHAGUS

All manner of swallowed foreign bodies have become arrested in the oesophagus: coins, pins, and dentures (figs 787, 788) head the list. All cases should have an urgent x-ray examination—including a dilute barium or water-soluble contrast medium (Gastrografin) swallow. Whenever possible the patient should be screened before oesophagoscopy is undertaken. Rigid oesophagoscopy is necessary in almost all cases.

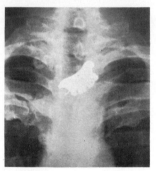

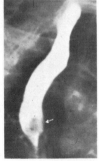

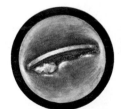

FIG. 787.—False teeth impacted in oesophagus.
(The late Dr. James F. Brailsford, Birmingham.)

FIG. 788.—Damson-stone outlined by barium, indicated by the arrow.

FIG. 789.—An 'old' penny in the oesophagus as seen through an oesophagoscope.

The foreign body is visualised (fig. 789), and, if necessary, manipulated into a favourable position so that it may be grasped with suitable forceps introduced through the oesophagoscope. The oesophagoscope, together with the forceps still grasping the foreign body, is then gently withdrawn.

INJURIES

Perforation of the oesophagus can result from the inexpert use of an oesophagoscope or a gastroscope; usually the beak of the instrument is thrust through the thin posterior wall of the pharynx just above the cricopharyngeal sphincter or the wall is crushed between the shaft of the instrument and a rigid, osteoarthritic cervical spine. Perforation just above an oesophageal stricture can occur from oesophagoscopy or bouginage. It also can result from removal of a piece of growth for biopsy, but probably the most frequent cause of perforation is a sharp foreign body plus instrumentation to remove it.

Often the perforation goes unrecognised by the oesophagoscopist until general distress and great pain on swallowing saliva or fluid, and dyspnoea, become apparent. In such circumstances the possibility of a tear should be considered at once. An x-ray is essential; this discloses the presence of air in the mediastinum, the pleural cavity, or in the neck which may be palpable (surgical emphysema). In doubtful cases the radiograph should be repeated after the patient has swallowed a small quantity of gastrografin. When the wall of the oesophagus has been perforated, urgent operation under antibiotic cover is indicated. When the cervical oesophagus has been ruptured, an incision along the anterior border of the sternomastoid (usually the left), with lateral retraction of the carotid sheath, gives access to the site of the perforation (fig. 790), which is closed in two layers, If the mid or lower oesophagus is involved, thoracotomy must be performed. In non-malignant cases timely suture is usually followed by recovery.

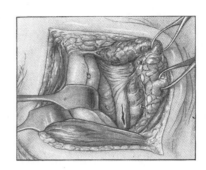

FIG. 790.—Exposure of a tear in the cervical oesophagus. In this case there was surgical emphysema on the right side of the neck.

When the symptoms are delayed, and radiography is negative, the perforation is in all probability a very small one. In this case massive antibiotic treatment with parenteral feeding is usually successful.

Corrosive fluid ingestion.—See page 847.

SPONTANEOUS RUPTURE OF THE OESOPHAGUS

Aetiology.—Instead of the cricopharyngeus relaxing, as is usual during vomiting, it contracts. The pressure within the oesophagus rises so steeply that the organ bursts at its weakest point. The condition is similar to the linear tears of the cardia in the Mallory-Weiss syndrome (Chapter 44).

Pathology.—The necropsy findings[1] are remarkably constant. There is a longitudinal tear 1 to 4 cm in length in the posterior wall of the extreme lower end of the oesophagus nearly always on the left side. Following perforation, the mediastinum becomes filled with air and gastric contents. Later the mediastinal pleura gives way, and air and gastric contents enter the pleural cavity. Less commonly a rupture may occur in the middle third of the oesophagus.

Clinical features are also remarkably constant. Following a meal, vomiting occurs. During vomiting, agonising pain is experienced in the thorax, and the patient soon becomes shocked. Board-like rigidity may occur and a misdiagnosis of coronary infarction, perforated peptic ulcer or acute pancreatitis may easily be made unless the chest is examined carefully and a chest x-ray taken in the erect position. Surgical emphysema may appear in the suprasternal notch. Hyper-resonance and absence of breath-sounds over one lung indicate a pneumothorax. The pain is so intense that even i.v. morphine fails to relieve it.

Radiography.—Mediastinal emphysema is soon seen; later, when the mediastinal pleura has ruptured, a hydro-pneumothorax will develop. This diagnosis should be confirmed by a gastrografin swallow.

---

[1] Spontaneous rupture of the oesophagus has been found at necropsy in cases of severe head injury and other cerebral lesions, doubtless due to vomiting and retching.

Treatment.—Recovery has followed immediate thoracotomy, opening widely the mediastinum, suture of the perforation, and closure of the thorax with drainage, providing this is carried out within 12 hours. If later than 12 hours the edges of the oesophageal tear will have become friable and suture (though it should be attempted) is unlikely to be successful. In these cases it is important to obtain early expansion of the lung by the insertion of two drainage tubes connected to an underwater drainage bottle and suction. In addition a feeding gastrostomy should be carried out.

OESOPHAGEAL DIVERTICULUM

Pulsion diverticulum is rare, and occurs where a blood vessel enters the oesophagus. The majority are associated with neuro-muscular incoordination which is the cause of occasional dysphagia (fig. 811). They are commonest at the lower end of the oesophagus.

PHARYNGEAL DIVERTICULUM (see Chapter 34)

OESOPHAGEAL VARICES (see Chapter 45)

PARALYSIS

The passage of food along the gullet is dependent entirely upon involuntary muscular peristalsis. When the neuromuscular mechanism of deglutition is paralysed, as occurs occasionally, notably as a complication of tetanus or diphtheria, or in motor neurone disease, ingested material is regurgitated. In established cases the difficulty must be overcome by feeding through a stomach tube.

OESOPHAGITIS

This may be *acute*—following burns or scalds, infective (spreading from the pharynx), or peptic, sometimes from the trauma of an indwelling stomach tube; or *chronic*—the most important cause is reflux of acid gastric juices due to a sliding hiatus hernia. Alkaline juices may also reflux following oesophago-duodeno-stomy or oesophago-jejunostomy without a Roux-en-Y loop. Reflux is common in pregnant women, but usually resolves after delivery.

Pathology.—The changes are maximal at the lower end of the oesophagus. Essentially there is loss of epithelium with replacement by bleeding granulation tissue. Although the symptoms are experienced by day, acid damage is done by night when the recumbent

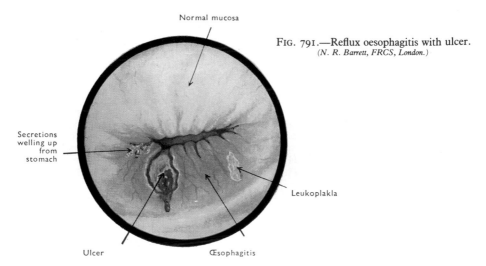

Normal mucosa

FIG. 791.—Reflux oesophagitis with ulcer.
(*N. R. Barrett, FRCS, London.*)

Secretions welling up from stomach

Leukoplakla

Ulcer   Œsophagitis

César Roux, 1857–1934. Professor of Surgery and Gynaecology, Lausanne, Switzerland. (See footnote Chapter 44.)

position allows the peptic juices to flow into the oesophagus. As soon as inflammation of the epithelium occurs, there is vagal hyperactivity so that the longitudinal muscle contracts and draws the cardia more and more up into the thorax and also hyperacidity is increased. Thus a vicious circle of oesophagitis—longitudinal muscle spasm—upward displacement of the cardia—increased acid regurgitation ensues. It is likely that the reflux oesophagitis so often encountered during pregnancy is due to a temporary sliding hiatus hernia resulting from increased intra-abdominal pressure; after delivery the hernia usually reduces itself, but it sometimes recurs apart from pregnancy later in life (fig. 791). Some hormones which are increased during pregnancy relax smooth muscle (progesterone) and can diminish the tone of the gastro-oesophageal sphincter.

Clinical Features.—Reflux oesophagitis is the commonest affection of the oesophagus, but its manifestations are not always clear-cut.

Pain.—In the majority, pain is the presenting symptom. At first, it is retrosternal and later may radiate between the shoulder blades, down either arm or up the side of the neck to the ear. This referred pain may simulate angina and is an expression of the sympathetic innervation. It tends to occur when the patient lies down to sleep and keeps him awake (in contradistinction to the pain of duodenal ulcer which wakes the patient from a sound sleep at about 2 a.m.). It is relieved by sitting upright and sometimes by taking alkalis.

Heartburn with regurgitation of bitter fluid is very common.

Dysphagia.—A complaint that food sticks in the region of the lower oesophagus is a fairly frequent symptom of oesophagitis. It occurs long before any stenosis has developed, and is probably an indication of oedema and spasm. Later, dysphagia is constant and becomes progressively worse as the stenosis develops.

Occult blood is present in the stools in a large percentage of cases.

Secondary anaemia is not uncommon. The oesophagitis may only be uncovered when a routine search is made for the cause of such anaemia.

Diagnosis.—A barium swallow x-ray of the oesophagus will reveal the causative sliding hernia and also a stenosis if this has developed. *Oesophagoscopy* will usually confirm the diagnosis. On examination, the mucous membrane of the lower end of the oesophagus is velvety, scarlet, and bleeds readily. Additional white areas of desquamating epithelium may also be seen in the inflamed area.

Treatment is that of the cause, notably that of hiatus hernia (p. 838). Recently the H_2 antagonists—ranitidine and cimetidine (Zantac®, Tagamet®) have proven a useful adjunct to treatment. They have still to be established as a safe long-term remedy (Chapter 44).

Barrett's ulcer is ulceration in the lower oesophagus due to acid secretion from ectopic gastric mucosa in the oesophagus *proximal* to the oesophago-gastric junction (fig. 792), although some specialists believe that gastric reflux is the real cause.

HIATUS HERNIA

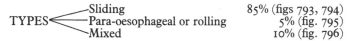

TYPES
Sliding   85% (figs 793, 794)
Para-oesophageal or rolling   5% (fig. 795)
Mixed   10% (fig. 796)

Ninety-eight per cent of diaphragmatic herniae (Chapter 40) occur through the oesophageal hiatus. Sir Astley Cooper was the first to insist that oesophageal hiatus hernia was acquired, and not congenital. While probably this is true in the majority of cases, the fact is that it may occur in early infancy, and rapidly proceed to stricture and oesophageal shortening, a condition erroneously described as 'congenital short oesophagus'. A true congenital short oesophagus is almost unknown.

Norman Rupert Barrett, 1903–1979. Surgeon, St. Thomas's Hospital, London.
Sir Astley Paston Cooper, 1768–1841. Surgeon, Guy's Hospital, London.

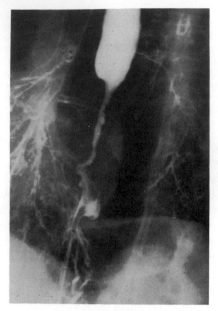

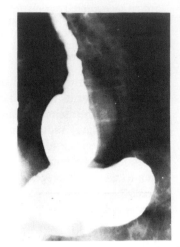

FIG. 792.—Oesophageal stenosis with
Barrett's ulcer.
(*Elizabeth M. Gordon, FRCS, London.*)

FIG. 793.—A large sliding hiatus
hernia.

1. Sliding Hiatus Hernia

Anatomy of Cardiac Sphincter.—There is undoubtedly a functional intrinsic physiological sphincter-like mechanism at the cardia although it cannot be demonstrated anatomically (see 'Physiology' p. 827). This is expressed as a zone of relatively high intra-luminal pressure which prevents regurgitation from the stomach. This important function is augmented by six factors: 1, the valvular effects of the oesophago-gastric angle (fig. 798); 2, the pinchcock action of the right crus (fig. 799); 3, the 'rosette-like' folds of the gastric mucous membrane at the cardia; 4, the presence of a length (about 4 cm) of intra-abdominal oesophagus (p. 838); 5, circular muscle fibres around lower end of the oesophagus; 6, a band of muscle which commences in the fundus of the stomach and passes around the oesophago-gastric junction (fig. 797).

Mechanism of Herniation.—The cardiac orifice and a portion of the stomach immediately adjacent pass into the posterior mediastinum, carrying with them a small peritoneal sac applied to the left side of the stomach. The right side of the hernia is derived from the 'bare area' of the stomach, and consequently is bereft of peritoneum (fig. 794). Branches of the left gastric artery supplying the prolapsed stomach also pass through the hiatus.

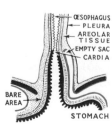

FIG. 794.—Sliding oeso-
phageal hiatus hernia.
(*After N. R. Barrett, FRCS,
London.*)

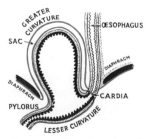

FIG. 795.—Para-oesophageal
hernia.

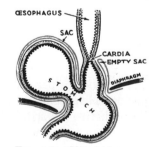

FIG. 796.—Mixed hiatus
hernia.

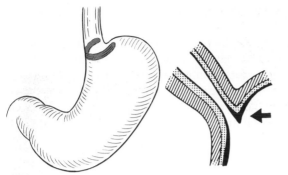

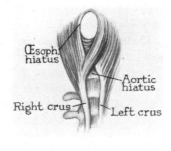

Fig. 797.—Band of muscle in stomach which passes around the oesophago-gastric junction.

Fig. 798.—The valvular mechanism of the cardia.

Fig. 799.—The right crus forms the entire musculotendinous diaphragmatic ring around the oesophagus.

Aetiology of Herniation.—There are several factors in the development of this hernia:

1. Muscular degeneration of increasing age.
2. Increased intra-abdominal pressure as in large ovarian cysts, pregnancy, increasing weight and the wearing of tight corsets.
3. Increase of fatty tissue in the hiatus with decreased elasticity of the crus as occurs in obese women.
4. Once regurgitation is established, oesophageal spasm and later even oesophageal fibrosis will pull more and more stomach into the chest.

Clinical Features.—These are similar to those of reflux oesophagitis (see p. 834). The majority of the patients are over forty years of age, and women are more often affected than men (female, fifty, fat, fertile: cf gallstones). A duodenal or gastric ulcer may be present as well. Gall stones, diverticulitis coli and hiatus hernia are not uncommonly associated (Saint's Triad, Chapter 47).

Complications of Hiatus Hernia.—The following complications of hiatus hernia occur, although there are no statistics to show in what proportion of patients these will develop. It has been said that 10% of patients with symptoms of oesophagitis will later develop a stricture (Flavell).

1. *Oesophagitis*—leading to anaemia and late stricture formation—common.

2. *Inhalation pneumonitis*—from recurring reflux—not very common.

3. *Obstruction or strangulation*—in large hernia, due to volvulus—uncommon.

Hiatus Hernia in Infants

Hiatus hernia with oesophagitis occurs in infants. The outstanding clinical feature is effortless vomiting of small amounts, often blood-tinged, starting soon after birth.

Radiography.—In order to demonstrate a sliding hiatus hernia radiologically, technique is important. During the course of a routine barium meal the patient is turned into a semi-prone position on the right side and the table tilted into a 20° Trendelenburg position. In the case of a true hiatus hernia, barium will regurgitate into the hernia without the aid of any additional pressure (fig. 793). If there is no regurgitation from the hernia into the oesophagus, there are usually no symptoms and no treatment is necessary.

Oesophagoscopy reveals varying degrees of inflammation of the lower end of the oesophagus (p. 835). The most valid sign of a hiatus hernia is reflux of gastric juice through the cardia, best seen during oesophagoscopy under surface

Geoffrey Flavell, Contemporary. Thoracic Surgeon, The London Hospital, England.
Friedrich Trendelenburg, 1844–1924. Professor of Surgery, Leipzig, Germany (see footnote Chapter 5).

anaesthesia. Furthermore the cardia will open on inspiration, whereas it normally closes and descends.

Differential Diagnosis.—Now that the prone head down position is routine in all barium meals, hiatus hernia and reflux are a not infrequent finding. Above the age of 60 years about 50% of all patients coming for a barium meal examination have a demonstrable hiatus hernia at some time or other (Airth). One must therefore be vigilant lest cholelithiasis, peptic ulcer, or diverticulitis be overlooked in a patient with an incidental hiatus hernia.

Treatment of Hiatus Hernia

The treatment of hiatus hernia may be medical or surgical. In all cases, however, weight reduction is most important, and many patient's symptoms will improve dramatically, or even disappear, if a significant amount of weight is lost.

An uncomplicated hernia which is causing no symptoms and is only discovered incidentally does not as a rule require treatment.

It is difficult at present to assess the role of ranitidine or cimetidine (Zantac®, Tagamet®), which undoubtedly relieve some of the symptoms of a hiatus hernia, though of course they do nothing to prevent the reflux and do not relieve the feeling of retrosternal discomfort and distension of which so many of these patients complain.

1. **Medical Treatment.**—The principles to be followed are:
1. The patient must sleep in a semi-recumbent position propped up with pillows and with the lower end of the bed raised on a chair. Five out of six patients benefit from lying on the left side at night.
2. The patient should avoid heavy work, lifting weights and excessive bending.
3. Six small, non-bulky meals should be taken daily, instead of three; food should be masticated thoroughly, and eaten slowly. The maintenance of the upright position after meals is sometimes of benefit.
4. Mucaine (a surface anaesthetic) and antacids such as Nulacin® may control symptoms.
5. If the patient is obese, reduction of weight is very important.
6. Correction of anaemia if present.
Especially when the patient is old or follows a sedentary occupation, these simple measures may bring about and maintain such a remarkable improvement that the question of operation can be postposed indefinitely. In other circumstances operation should be advised.

Medical Treatment in Infancy.—The baby should be nursed in an upright position and given a semi-solid diet as soon as possible. The most practical method of maintaining the sitting position is by an almost legless chair made of plaster of Paris, which can be used both in the cot and the perambulator. Some children lose all symptoms when they start to walk; some of the remainder will require surgery.

2. **Surgical Treatment.**—The aim of surgical repair is to: (*a*) Replace the oesophago-gastric junction below the diaphragm; (*b*) Reduce the size of the oesophageal hiatus; (*c*) Produce an anti-reflux mechanism. *It should be carried out in all patients who have a para-oesophageal hernia, providing they are fit.* In patients who have a sliding hernia the indications are more controversial. Surgical treatment should be advised if medical treatment proves to be unsatisfactory and is essential if significant oesophagitis is present at oesophagoscopy, which should be done in most cases.

Which approach—thoracic or abdominal?—There are two approaches in common use—abdominal or thoracic. The guiding principle of surgical repair is to ensure a length of at least 4 cm of intra-abdominal oesophagus and to prevent this segment from returning to the chest. The positive intra-abdominal pressure of inspiration closes this segment of gullet thus preventing the reflux of gastric juice into the thoracic oesophagus (Keen).

The anti-reflux operations devised independently in 1955 by Belsey and by Nissen are the most widely used operations in Europe and North America. The Belsey repair can

Graham Robertson Airth, Contemporary. Radiologist, Southmead Hospital, Bristol, England.
Gerald Keen, Contemporary. Thoracic Surgeon, Royal Infirmary, Bristol, England.
Rudolph Nissen, Contemporary. Formerly Professor of Surgery, Istanbul, Turkey, and Basle, Switzerland.
Ronald Belsey, Contemporary. Consultant Thoracic Surgeon, Frenchay Hospital, Bristol, England.

only be carried out through the chest whilst the Nissen fundoplication may be performed through the abdomen or the chest. Unfortunately the choice of operation and operative approach often depends mainly on the experience of the surgeon but there is now an increasing realisation by all surgeons that the thoracic approach provides a much better exposure and makes it much easier to carry out a satisfactory repair. However, the trans-thoracic approach limits the ability of the surgeon to diagnose and treat other conditions which may be present, e.g. gallstones.

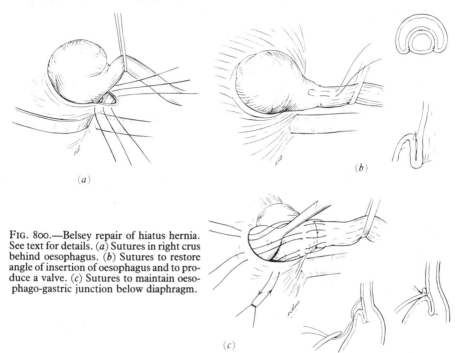

(a)

(b)

(c)

FIG. 800.—Belsey repair of hiatus hernia. See text for details. (a) Sutures in right crus behind oesophagus. (b) Sutures to restore angle of insertion of oesophagus and to produce a valve. (c) Sutures to maintain oesophago-gastric junction below diaphragm.

1. **Belsey Mark IV Operation.**—The Mark IV operation represents the fourth modification of the anti-reflux repair originated by Belsey. It is the repair most widely used in the United Kingdom. It not only reduces the size of the hiatal ring but it also produces a valve at the oesophago-gastric junction to prevent reflux. The results of the operation are good and the recurrence rate is small.

A postero-lateral thoracotomy is made through the 8th rib bed. The oesophagus and cardia are mobilised and fat from the anterior surface of the cardia is excised. The edges of the right crus are defined and 4 interrupted silk sutures are placed *behind* the oesophagus to be tied later. The angle of insertion of the oesophagus is restored by 4 interrupted silk mattress sutures placed between the anterior surface of the oesophagus and the adjacent fundus of the stomach, so as to wrap the stomach around the anterior two thirds of the oesophagus (fig. 800). A second row of interrupted silk mattress sutures is then placed between the oesophago-gastric junction and the under surface of the diaphragm to maintain this area below the diaphragm. Finally the previously placed crural sutures are tied, with care to be sure that the opening is not too small.

2. **Nissen Fundo-plication.**—This operation may be carried out through the chest or the abdomen. The fundus of the stomach is wrapped around the lower 5 cm of the oesophagus. There is, unfortunately, a very definite incidence of the 'gas-bloat' syndrome in which the patients complain of dysphagia and a considerable amount of abdominal gaseous distension due to an inability to bring up wind. A left upper abdominal incision is made in the line of the left margin of the rectus abdominis and the left lobe of the liver is mobilised to expose the cardia. A transverse incision at the hiatus is then made to expose the lower oesophagus and the crura. It is important to clear the abdominal oesophagus for 5 to 7·5 cm both behind the oesophagus and along the upper part of the lesser curve. The fundus of the stomach is freed, its anterior aspect is brought round behind the

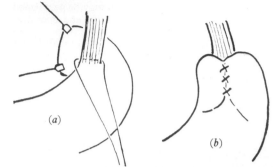

FIG. 801.—(a) Mobilisation of the gastric fundus with tissue forceps and a rubber catheter round the oesophagus. (b) Plication of the gastric fundus.

oesophagus and sutured anteriorly (fig. 801). Splenectomy may be required. Some believe that vagotomy with a drainage operation (Chapter 44) or more recently Highly Selective Vagotomy (Chapter 44) is advisable; this view is not widely shared. The operation is best carried out with a large bore stomach tube in position in order to prevent narrowing of the oesophagus. Lesions of the stomach, duodenum, gall bladder and colon may be dealt with at the same time. Late recurrence is reported to be uncommon.

The operation through the chest is carried out by an approach through the bed of the left 8th rib.

3. **Leigh Collis Gastroplasty.**—The Leigh Collis gastroplasty is performed through a thoraco-abdominal incision. It is of special value if the oesophagus is short due to previous oesophagitis. A tube of stomach is made which has the effect of extending the oesophagus into the abdomen (fig 802). The oesophageal hiatus is then reduced is size and around this tube.

4. **Angelchik prosthesis.**—In this new technique, after reduction of the hernia a plastic ring is placed around the oesophago-gastric junction. The large size of the prosthesis prevents herniation of the stomach into the chest. Late complications have occurred following this operation and it is too early to evaluate the long term value of this procedure:

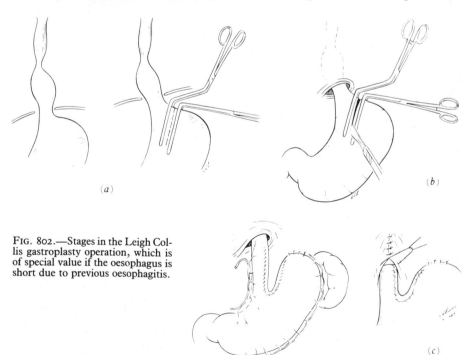

FIG. 802.—Stages in the Leigh Collis gastroplasty operation, which is of special value if the oesophagus is short due to previous oesophagitis.

John Leigh Collis, Contemporary. Emeritus Professor of Thoracic Surgery, Queen Elizabeth Hospital, Birmingham, England.

complications have included persistent dysphagia, stenosis, perforation and displacement of prosthesis. The procedure is also used for cases which have had dilation of a stricture above a hiatus hernia (see below).

Treatment of Stricture due to Reflux Oesophagitis.—It is often difficult to diagnose these strictures with certainty and their management frequently causes considerable problems, as many of these patients are old and frail. The differential diagnosis is clearly carcinoma but neither a negative biopsy nor the presence of a hiatus hernia excludes this condition—the biopsy may not have been deep enough to reach the carcinoma and a hiatus hernia may be present together with a carcinoma. It may only be possible to make the correct diagnosis at operation and even then only with difficulty for benign strictures are often extremely fibrotic.

The stricture should not merely be dilated, as this only leads to *increased* regurgitation and therefore increased stricture formation later. The very old may be excluded from this rule.

The following five procedures are available:

(1) *Occasional bouginage*, together with sleep in the semi-upright position and liberal antacids (magnesium trisilicate and ? cimetidine). Theoretically this is incorrect treatment but it may suffice in mild cases in elderly patients unfit for major surgery.

(2) *Dilatation of stricture and repair of hiatus hernia*. The repair of the hernia will abolish the reflux oesophagitis and the stricture will decrease once the oesophagitis is controlled. This is the ideal treatment.

(3) *Partial oesophago-gastrectomy*, with a high anastomosis. This will be necessary in some cases if the stricture cannot be dilated satisfactorily, providing the patient is fit. There is an appreciable risk of further oesophagitis and stricture formation, but this can be minimised by active antacid therapy.

(4) *Thal procedure*—in which the stricture is opened longitudinally and the oesophageal defect closed by suturing the adjacent fundus of stomach on to the edges of the oesophageal opening (fig. 803).

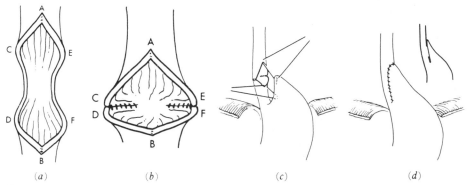

FIG. 803.—Thal's patch. (*a*) Longitudinal incision (A–B) through stricture. (*b*) Enlargement of lumen by approximating C to D, E to F. (*c*) Onlay patch of gastric fundus to oesophageal defect. (*d*) The completed patch. (Inset shows longitudinal section through patch.)
(*Reproduced by permission of the Royal College of Surgeons of Edinburgh.*)

(5) *Milstein procedure*—in which the stricture is opened longitudinally and closed transversely—as in a pyloroplasty. Reflux is prevented by a Nissen fundoplication.

(6) *Angelchik prosthesis*.—After reduction of the hiatus hernia, and dilation of the stricture, reflux is prevented by surrounding the oesophago-gastric junction with a plastic collar placed just above the cardia and held in place by tapes. Serious complications have been reported in a few cases (e.g. perforation) due to displacement of the prosthesis, and many patients experience dysphagia (see also above).

2. Para-oesophageal ('Rolling') Hernia

This is a true hernia into which the greater curvature of the stomach (figs. 804 and 805) or, very rarely, the whole stomach itself, ascends into a preformed sac lying in the mediastinum (fig 795). Acute dilatation or volvulus of the intrathoracic stomach may result in serious symptoms or death and such hernias are best repaired early.

Alan P. Thal, Contemporary. Surgeon, Kansas City, Kansas, U.S.A.
Ben Milstein, Contemporary. Consultant Thoracic Surgeon, Papworth Hospital, Cambridge, England.

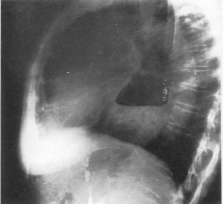

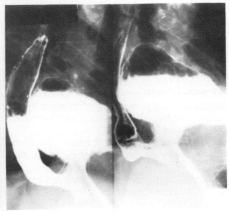

Fig. 804.—Para-oesophageal hernia. A fluid level is seen in the chest.

Fig. 805.—Barium study of this case.

A pure para-oesophageal hernia is extremely rare and in practice it is almost always combined with some degree of slide.

Clinical Features.—Regurgitant oesophagitis and peri-oesophagitis are *not* features of this condition since the cardia remains in its normal position (fig. 794). The gastro-oesophageal angle is not disturbed and the competence of the cardia is not impaired. Symptoms therefore rarely appear until the hernia is large (fig. 803), and they are variable: (*a*) intermittent dysphagia; (*b*) cardiac symptoms due to pressure on the heart; (*c*) occasionally bouts of hiccough from irritation of the phrenic nerve. These symptoms are most frequently due to a recurrent gastric volvulus (Chapter 44).

Operation.—The Belsey Mark IV repair should be carried out. Alternatively, the Hill repair (fig. 806) should be performed through the abdomen. The oesophago-gastric junction is anchored by sutures placed between it and the median arcuate ligament overlying the aorta and then the hiatus reduced in size by sutures placed to approximate the right crus, as in the Belsey repair.

3. Mixed Hiatus Hernia

The symptoms of a mixed hernia are variable, depending on the degree of reflux. It should be treated by the Belsey Mark IV repair or a Nissen fundoplication as already described.

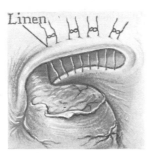

Fig. 806.—Hill repair of a para-oesophageal hernia. The sutures to approximate the crus should extend *behind* the oesophagus (not shown in this illustration).
(*After S. W. Harrington.*)

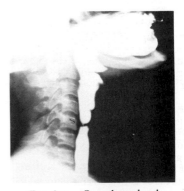

Fig. 807.—Oesophageal web.
(*H. Talib, FRCS, Baghdad.*)

Stuart William Harrington, Contemporary. Emeritus Professor of Surgery, Mayo Graduate School of Medicine, Rochester, Minnesota, U.S.A.
Lucius Hill, Contemporary. Surgeon, Mason Clinic, Seattle, Washington, U.S.A.

CHRONIC OESOPHAGEAL OBSTRUCTION

The causes of chronic oesophageal obstruction can be classified as follows:

Congenital

Acquired

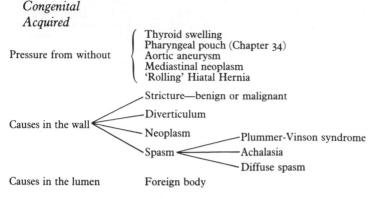

Pressure from without
- Thyroid swelling
- Pharyngeal pouch (Chapter 34)
- Aortic aneurysm
- Mediastinal neoplasm
- 'Rolling' Hiatal Hernia

Causes in the wall
- Stricture—benign or malignant
- Diverticulum
- Neoplasm
- Spasm
  - Plummer-Vinson syndrome
  - Achalasia
  - Diffuse spasm

Causes in the lumen — Foreign body

LOCALISED MUSCULAR SPASM

There are two important clinical entities associated with muscular conditions of the oesophagus. One effects the pharyngo-oesophageal junction and is known as the Plummer-Vinson syndrome. The other affects the extreme lower end of the oesophagus and is called cardiospasm, or achalasia.

THE PLUMMER-VINSON SYNDROME

This syndrome was first described by Paterson and Kelly in 1919. It is however commonly called after Plummer and Vinson (two Mayo Clinic physicians) who described it again in 1921. The patient is nearly always a middle-aged woman who complains of difficulty in swallowing. Severe retching spells occur and classically the patient fears choking. Provided the clinician is aware of the existence of the syndrome, thoughtful examination nearly always provides clues to the diagnosis, but not all the following are necessarily in evidence in a given case.

The tongue is usually devoid of papillae, smooth and pale, but rarely inflamed or sore.

The lips and corners of the mouth are often cracked, giving the mouth a pursed appearance.

The finger-nails are brittle, and tend to be spoon-shaped (koilonychia).

The spleen is enlarged in the same ratio as in other iron-deficiency anaemias.

The bone marrow is devoid of stainable iron stores.

The blood.—Hypochromic[1] anaemia is always present, the serum iron levels being particularly low. Usually dysphagia precedes the anaemia, which is due to lack of iron and other requirements of a balanced diet.

Achlorhydria is often present, as is usually the case in iron-deficient anaemia.

Dysphagia is due to spasm of the circular muscle fibres at the extreme upper portion of the oesophagus. This is associated with the formation of webs (fig. 807). The mucous membrane is hyperkeratotic in places, and desquamated in others; it is extremely friable and easily traumatised by the passage of an oesophagoscope. In long-standing cases the orifice looks like a mere pin-hole. This lesion is definitely a precarcinomatous condition. If a carcinoma is present it is usually very radio-sensitive.

Treatment.—The dysphagia yields readily to dilatation of the stricture through an oesophagoscope. As always, gentleness must be used; even so, in cases of some chronicity, bleeding will occur. The administration of tab. ferrous sulphate, 0·3 g t.d.s., together with vitamins, is indicated. Some patients require intramuscular or intravenous iron. Sometimes blood transfusion is necessary. Hyperalimentation with a liquid diet through a gastric aspiration tube helps to bring about regeneration of the desquamated epithelium of the mucous membrane of the oesophagus. Once the anaemia is under control and the patient can swallow an adequate diet, rapid improvement occurs and usually is maintained.

---

[1] Hypochromic anaemia is so-called because the red blood-corpuscles contain less haemoglobin than normal.

Henry Stanley Plummer, 1874–1957, Physician, Mayo Clinic, Rochester, Minnesota, U.S.A.
Porter Paisley Vinson, 1890–1959. Physician, Mayo Clinic, Rochester, Minnesota, U.S.A.
Donald Rose Paterson, 1862–1939. Surgeon, Ear, Nose and Throat Department, Royal Infirmary, Cardiff, Wales.
Adam Brown Kelly, 1865–1941. Surgeon, Ear, Nose and Throat Department, Victoria Infirmary, Glasgow, Scotland.

ACHALASIA OF THE OESOPHAGUS (*syn.* 'CARDIOSPASM')

Aetiology.—Achalasia is a disease of the oesophagus, the exact cause of which still remains unsolved.

It consists essentially of a failure of integration of the parasympathetic impulses so that oesophageal peristalsis is disorganised, and there is failure of relaxation of the cardia. These result in a *functional* obstruction. An epidemic variety has been described in Breslau and was associated with Vitamin B_1 deficiency on the one hand and trypanosomiasis on the other (Chagas' disease). Stress and emotional upsets are also associated with achalasia.

The oesophagus consists of a dilated tortuous sac above and a narrow neck below. The elements of Auerbach's plexus are defective though ganglia are present (cf. Hirschsprung's disease (Chapter 50) where they are completely absent). There is marked stasis and a retention oesophagitis due to the presence of a foul smelling liquid. Like stasis anywhere, it predisposes to diverticula and it is pre-cancerous.

Clinical Features.—Usually achalasia of the oesophagus occurs in women

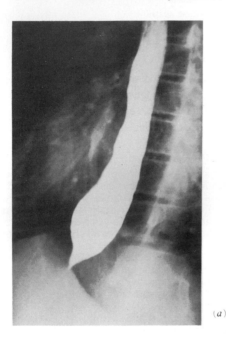

(*a*)

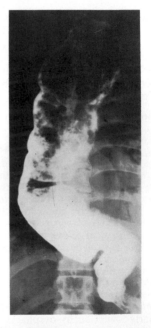

(*c*)

(*b*)

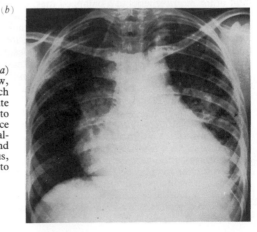

FIG. 808.—Achalasia of the oesophagus. (*a*) Typical appearance after barium swallow, showing smooth outline of the stricture, which narrows to a point at its lower end. (*b*) Late stage, showing grossly dilated oesophagus to right of mediastinum, together with evidence of an inhalation pneumonitis. (*c*) Barium swallow of same patient, showing tortuosity and sigmoid appearance of lower oesophagus, together with eccentric position of opening into stomach.

Carlos Chagas, 1879–1934. Professor of Tropical Medicine, Rio de Janeiro, Brazil.

20–40 years of age, but it can occur at any time of adult life and in both sexes. The history is one of progressive dysphagia; there are several special features.

The onset is insidious and, more often than not, the patient seeks relief only after the symptoms have been present for many years. Although the patient says she vomits, on closer interrogation it becomes apparent that there is *regurgitation* of food, often several hours after the meal. In advanced cases mucus and froth are brought up in considerable quantities. There may be retrosternal discomfort, foetid flatulence and aspiration pneumonitis. A toxic 'rheumatoid' arthritis may occur.

As a result of the obstruction the patient fails to obtain sufficient nourishment, and consequently remains in a state of continual ill-health, rendering normal activities impossible.

The *radiographic findings* are most important. Characteristic features are:
1. A smooth pencil-shaped narrowing of the lower segment (fig 808*a*).
2. Dilatation and later tortuosity and recumbency of the lower oesophagus (fig. 808*b*, *c*).
3. Lack of a gas bubble in the stomach.
4. Inco-ordinated peristalsis which is hypersensitive to acetyl-choline (when Carbachol 0·25 mg is injected intramuscularly abnormal peristaltic contractions occur).

Oesophagoscopy.—Once the instrument has passed the cricoid cartilage it appears to enter a gaping cave partially filled with dirty water, which laps to and fro with respiratory movement. When the fluid has been aspirated the cardiac orifice is located with difficulty, owing to its contracted state and often eccentric position.

Manometry.—If facilities are available pressure recordings from the oesophagus and sphincter zone will show an aperistaltic oesophagus with an unrelaxing (*but* not hypertonic) sphincter (fig. 782).

Treatment.—The essential is the disruption of the constricting fibres of the cardia either from without (by Heller's operation) or from within (by the Negus hydrostatic bag).

Operative treatment becomes necessary in the majority of cases.

Heller's Operation (*Oesophagocardiomyotomy*).—A *thoracic approach* should be used as otherwise it is not possible to make a sufficiently long myotomy. A left postero-lateral thoracotomy along the lower border of the 8th rib is made, the lower end of the oesophagus is mobilised and the cardiac end of the stomach gently drawn up through the hiatus. A single anteriorly placed incision is made through the longitudinal and circular muscle fibres of the oesophagus down to the mucosa, which will then pout through the divided muscle (fig. 809). Artery forceps should be used to separate the mucosa from the muscle, the incision in which should extend from 1 cm below the oesophago-gastric junction to 2 cm above the thickened muscle in the oesophagus, thus making an incision 8–10 cm long. Great care must be taken to divide all circular muscle and not to perforate the mucosa. If the mucosa is opened this will be obvious and it should be closed with interrupted 4/0 *silk* sutures on an arterial needle. Care must be taken to avoid the vagus.

Post-operatively fluids should be withheld for two days, then fluids only allowed for the next three days and semi-solids after a week.

Achalasia is sometimes associated with a hiatus hernia. If so the hernia should be repaired by the Belsey Mark IV technique.

The abdominal approach, through a high left paramedian incision, involves retraction of the left lobe of the liver to the right, retraction of the stomach downwards to display the abdominal portion of the oesophagus. After careful dissection encircling the oesophagus, and additional mobilisation, and retraction with a soft rubber sling, a longitudinal incision is made into the muscle and deepened to the mucosa (fig. 809), according to the technique described above.

Negus hydrostatic bag.—The stricture may be dilated by self-bouginage with a Hurst mercury loaded bougie or by forceful dilatation with a Negus hydrostatic bag passed at oesophagoscopy (fig. 810). The bougie may curl up inside the dilated oesophagus, or the

Ernst Heller, Surgeon, St. George's Hospital, Leipzig, Germany.
Sir Victor Negus, 1887–1974. Ear, Nose and Throat Surgeon, Kings College Hospital, London.

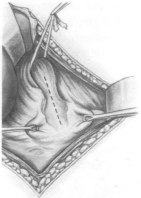

FIG. 809.—Heller's operation showing the length and position of the
incision dividing the muscular coats.
(After P. Thorek, Chicago, U.S.A.)

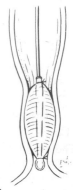

FIG. 810.—Negus hydrostatic bag.

identification of the oesophago-gastric opening at oesophagoscopy may be very difficult for it is often placed eccentrically (fig. 808). Moreover there is a 5% risk of perforation from hydrostatic dilatation. Neither of these procedures is therefore satisfactory or safe, though usually advised in the first instance in the United States and in some countries in Europe.

DIFFUSE SPASM (PRESBYOESOPHAGUS)

In this condition multiple areas of spasm (fig. 811) may be seen throughout the oesophagus ('corkscrew oesophagus'). Like scleroderma, however, it does not proceed to the massive dilatation seen in achalasia. 85% of cases are men over 60 (Flavell).

The condition presents as mild dysphagia with pain on swallowing felt mainly in the root of the neck but may be discovered accidentally during barium meal examination. The patient is usually of a nervous disposition. Treatment is by dilatation, although there is evidence that cholinergic antagonists and cholinesterase inhibitors may ultimately prove useful.

SCLERODERMA

Oesophageal manifestations of this distressing systemic disease are not uncommon, although the peripheral cutaneous, vascular and arthritic changes are more frequently seen.

The disease has a male: female ratio of 1:2 and is of the collagen variety.

Due to loss of muscle tonus at the gastro-oesophageal junction zone, reflux oesophagitis develops. A stricture then occurs with dysphagia. Anti-reflux measures—both medical [H₂ blockers] and surgical [Angelchik prosthesis]—may be used for treatment.

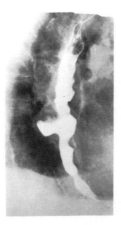

FIG. 811.—Diffuse spasm.
A diverticulum is present
in the mid-oesophagus.

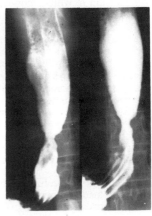

FIG. 812.—Scleroderma of
the oesophagus.

Geoffrey Flavell, Contemporary Retired. Surgeon, The London Hospital, England.

Widespread infiltration of the mucosa of the viscus with fibrous tissue leads to ineffectual contraction and eventually to a suspension of peristalsis and shortening particularly in its distal half (fig. 812). Areas of spasm may occur proximal to this. In its fully developed state surgical replacement of the lower oesophagus may be required.

BENIGN STRICTURES

A benign stricture at the lower end of the oesophagus (excluding cardiospasm) may be due to: 1. Corrosive fluid ingestion; 2. Reflux oesophagitis due to a hiatus hernia (see page 834).

1. Corrosive Fluid Ingestion

The ingestion of corrosive fluids, though now uncommon in the Western World, is relatively common in Asia and Africa where acetic acid is extensively used for the curing of rubber, and caustic soda for the manufacture of soap from palm oil. The lower oesophagus is the area most frequently affected. Reflex spasm at the lower end of the oesophagus following the swallowing of the corrosive leads to stasis and consequently severe and often a haemorrhagic oesophagitis. Necrosis of mucosa and even underlying muscle may occur, leading to severe stricture formation later.

A barium swallow in the erect position together with views in the Trendelenburg position with pressure on the abdomen will demonstrate the exact length and severity of the stricture.

Treatment. No attempt should be made during the first week to dilate the stricture, as there is a very high risk of oesophageal perforation due to the acute inflammatory state of the oesophagus. Steroids should be given for 6 weeks to minimise fibrosis, together with penicillin and metronidazole (Flagyl). Oral fluids should be withheld for one week. After the first week, when the acute stage has subsided, an attempt should be made to dilate the stricture at oesophagoscopy with a bougie (fig. 813) and this may be followed by self-bougienage. If there is difficulty in finding the opening, a thread may be swallowed to act

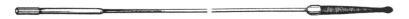

FIG. 813.—Chevalier Jackson's carrot-shaped oesophageal bougie.

as a guide and then a bougie with an eye at the end may be guided down over the thread. Retrograde dilation through a gastrostomy may be required if it is impossible to dilate from above. This is possible because the lower end of the stricture is always conical, as opposed to the proximal end where the opening is often placed eccentrically and may be difficult to identify.

A radical resection operation is ultimately required in about 40% of cases due to: complete stenosis; fistula formation; failure of bougienage to provide an adequate lumen; inability of patient to persevere with bougienage.

The possible operations are: 1. Local excision of stricture if it is short; 2. High oesophagogastrectomy—but risk of reflux oesophagitis later (Lewis type of operation—see page 852; 3. Cervical oesophago-gastrostomy (McKeown type of operation—see page 852); 4. Colon or jejunum interposition.

BENIGN TUMOURS

Benign tumours of the oesophagus are rare and comprise less than 1% of all oesophageal tumours. A leiomyoma is the commonest tumour but a papilloma, fibroma or lipoma may occur. They may develop anywhere in the oesophagus and cause a pedunculated swelling within the lumen, a tumour within the wall or remain outside the oesophagus. They only rarely cause symptoms because the oesophageal lumen is displaced around the tumour and therefore obstruction does not occur. They may cause haemorrhage from mucosal ulceration, a sense of fullness behind the sternum, bronchial compression, or only be found on a routine chest radiograph.

A barium swallow will show a smooth filling defect in the oesophagus and at oesophagoscopy this will be confirmed, often with intact mucosa over the tumour. Biopsy may cause full thickness perforation of the oesophageal wall with infection and therefore should not be performed.

Chevalier Jackson, 1865–1958. Professor of Bronchoscopy and Oesophagoscopy, Jefferson Medical College, Philadelphia, Pennsylvania, U.S.A.

Treatment is by thoracotomy with enucleation of the tumour (without opening the mucosa) or by local oesophageal resection.

CARCINOMA OF THE OESOPHAGUS

Carcinoma of the oesophagus occurs over the age of 45 years more commonly in men than in women, comprises about 5% of all carcinoma and causes about 3000 deaths each year in the United Kingdom. Probably no other carcinoma causes greater misery to the patient, due to the development of inability to swallow even fluids, and therefore in the terminal stages inhalation pulmonary symptoms. It occurs more commonly and at an earlier age in China, Japan and Russia, probably due to a more irritant diet.

Up to 24% 5 year survival after surgical resection has been obtained by Dark, Jackson and McKeown in reports from three different thoracic centres. But nonetheless the overall survival figures for oesophageal resection for carcinoma are very poor and only a few surgeons experienced in this type of surgery obtain such a high success rate.

Pathology.—The lesion may be a squamous cell carcinoma or an adenocarcinoma. The latter occurs essentially at the lower end from the lower 3 cm lined by columnar epithelium. Some adenocarcinomas of the lower oesophagus may really be gastric in origin. Squamous-cell carcinoma occurs usually at one of the three areas of constriction (fig. 779). The incidence is shown in fig. 814.

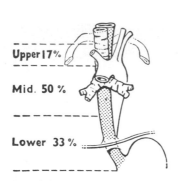

FIG. 814.—The relative frequency of squamous-celled carcinoma in various portions of the oesophagus.

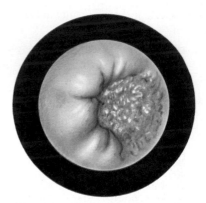

FIG. 815.—Carcinoma of the oesophagus as seen through an oesophagoscope.
(A. Lawrence Abel, FRCS, London.)

Macroscopically three types can be recognised:

1. An annular stenosing lesion usually found at the cardia.
2. An epitheliomatous ulcer with raised everted edges.
3. A fungating cauliflower-like friable mass.

Spread: (a) *Direct.*—This is the main method of spread and the most important to the surgeon. It is both transverse and longitudinal in direction and erodes the muscular wall to invade the important structures of the neck and posterior mediastinum, as well as the left main bronchus and trachea. It may perforate and lead to mediastinitis; rarely it causes massive fatal bleeding from the aorta. On the left side the recurrent laryngeal nerve may be involved ('hoarseness').

(b) *Lymphatic.*—Submucosal lymphatic permeation may lead to satellite nodules away

John Dark, Contemporary. Consultant Thoracic Surgeon, Wythenshaw Hospital, Manchester, England.
John Jackson, 1921–1985. Consultant Thoracic Surgeon, Harefield Hospital, England.
Kenneth Charles McKeown, Contemporary. Consultant Surgeon, Darlington Memorial Hospital, Darlington, England.

from the main tumour. Similarly, embolic spread to surrounding lymph nodes occurs. From the cervical oesophagus the spread is to the lymph nodes of the supraclavicular triangles. From the thoracic oesophagus metastases pass to the para-oesophageal and tracheo-bronchial lymph nodes, with downward extension to the subdiaphragmatic nodes. In the case of the abdominal oesophagus, spread is to the lymph nodes along the lesser curvature of the stomach, and thence to those around the coeliac axis. In the main, lymphatic metastases occur in a *downward* direction.

(c) *Bloodstream.*—Metastases to the liver are fairly common.

Clinical Features.—The disease usually, though not always, presents over the age of 45 years, more commonly in men than in women.

The leading symptom—indeed, often the only symptom—of this fell disease is dysphagia. Sometimes, owing to sloughing of a portion of the growth, for a time swallowing becomes easier, but as a rule the difficulty is steadily progressive. Only 40% of patients report within three months; too often the patient procrastinates and seeks advice when he can swallow liquids only, by which time considerable weight loss has occurred. Regurgitation (oesophageal pseudo-vomiting) is a fairly common symptom. The regurgitated material is alkaline, mixed with saliva, and possibly streaked with blood. In growths situated in the lower part of the oesophagus, anorexia is sometimes a feature. Pain, if it occurs, is usually a late manifestation, but it is not in itself a contraindication to an exploratory operation.

Radiography after barium emulsion has been swallowed should be carried out in every case of dysphagia (fig 816, 817).

Oesophagoscopy must always be performed but a positive biopsy is not always obtained. It will only be positive in 50% of cases and surgical exploration may be necessary to establish the diagnosis.

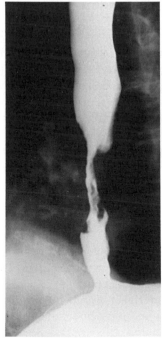

FIG. 816.—Carcinoma of the oesophagus: typical appearance.
(Courtesy of Raymond Hurt.)

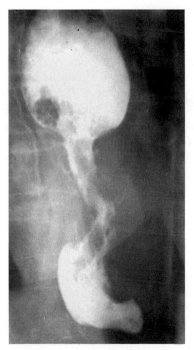

FIG. 817.—Bulky carcinoma of oesphagus.
(Courtesy of Raymond Hurt.)

Raymond Hurt, Contemporary. Surgeon, St Bartholomew's Hospital, London.

Bronchosocopy should be undertaken. In middle third growths the trachea or left main bronchus may be involved, often causing cough and sputum. A broncho-oesophageal fistula may develop later associated with greatly increased cough.

Exfoliative Cytology.—In China, lavage of the oesophagus and examination of the fluid for malignant cells have led to the discovery of an early carcinoma when radiology and oesophagoscopy have been negative.

Ultrasound.—In all cases secondary liver deposits should be excluded by ultrasound, which is probably more reliable than CT scanning.

Many of these patients have a long-standing nutritional deficiency and therefore haemoglobin, plasma proteins and blood chemistry must all be checked and corrected if necessary. Vitamin C (ascorbic acid) supplement will aid wound healing. Ten or more days pre-operative preparation will go far to minimise post-operative complications.

PRINCIPLES OF TREATMENT

A gastrostomy should *never* be carried out for oesophageal carcinoma. It is no longer required as a pre-operative measure to improve a patient's nutrition, for this can now be satisfactorily carried out by an indwelling 'Clinifeed' tube through the nose into the stomach, or by modern regimes for intravenous feeding. It should never be carried out merely to prolong the life of a patient who is unable to swallow, as the subsequent state of the patient when the inevitable inhalation lung complications occur due to inability to swallow saliva is most distressing.

The treatment should aim either at cure or, if this is impossible, at the relief of symptoms.

Curative Treatment

The operative problem is to remove the tumour and to restore continuity by the interposition of stomach, jejunum or colon. Curative treatment should be attempted providing: 1. The patient is fit enough on general appearance to withstand a very major surgical procedure. 2. There is no evidence of spread of the growth to the supraclavicular glands, tracheo-bronchial tree or liver.

1. *Post cricoid carcinoma*

Post cricoid carcinoma of the oesophagus should be treated by radiotherapy. The alternative surgical treatment of pharyngolaryngectomy with gastric transposition (Ong), colon transposition (Belsey) or plastic tube insertion (Stuart) is a very major undertaking associated with a high complication rate.

2. *Carcinoma of upper third of oesophagus*

Early diagnosis of carcinoma of the upper third of the oesophagus is rare and when dysphagia occurs there are often malignant glands in the neck or a recurrent laryngeal nerve paralysis, indicating inoperability. The only treatment that is then possible is radiotherapy. Only rarely is the growth operable, in which case a McKeown 3 stage oesophagectomy may be undertaken (for details see later) or the growth may be excised and continuity restored after by jejunal or colonic transposition.

3. *Carcinoma of middle third of oesophagus*

A growth of this site may become adherent to the aorta, vena azygos or left

Ronald Belsey, Contemporary. Consultant Thoracic Surgeon, Frenchay Hospital, Bristol, England.
G. B. Ong, Contemporary. Former Professor of Surgery, University of Hong Kong.
D. W. Stuart, Contemporary. Surgeon, North Staffordshire Royal Infirmary, Stoke-on-Trent.

main bronchus. There is an increasing tendency to treat carcinoma of the middle third of the oesophagus by radiotherapy rather than by surgery, for the surgical results are bad and the complication rate relatively high.

If surgery is undertaken, the operation is partial oesophago-gastrectomy with anastomosis above the level of the aortic arch. Only about one fifth of the stomach is removed. This is best carried out by a right thoracotomy (Ivor Lewis operation), though it may also be performed less easily through a left thoraco-abdominal approach.

Right thoracotomy (Ivor Lewis operation), through the 5th rib bed, preceded by a laparotomy to mobilise the stomach and to confirm the absence of extensive abdominal metastases. This approach is preferable as the access for the anastomosis, which is so vital a part of the operation, is not hampered by the aortic arch as it is through a left thoracotomy (fig. 818).

Left thoraco-abdominal approach, through a long skin and muscle incision, with entry into the chest through the 8th rib bed (extended onto the abdomen if necessary) and a radial incision in the diaphragm for the stomach mobilisation, together with entry through the 5th rib bed (through the same skin and muscle incision) for the anastomosis ('two rib' approach).

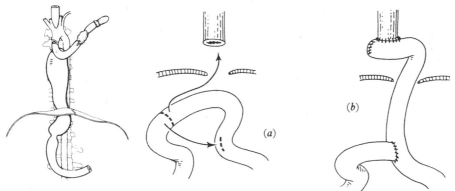

FIG. 818.—Resection of the oesophagus for a growth in its middle third, utilising the mobilised stomach for restoring the continuity of the alimentary tract (semi-diagrammatic).

FIG. 819.—Roux-en-Y anastomosis of the jejunum to the oesphagus to prevent reflux. (a) The jejunum is transected and (b) the proximal jejunum is anastomosed end-to-side to the distal end of the loop lower down.

(Reproduced from Hurt and Bates (1986) "Essentials of Thoracic Surgery", by permission of Butterworth & Co. Ltd.)

4. *Carcinoma of lower third of oesophagus*

A carcinoma of the lower third of the oesophagus may be resected by a partial oesophago-gastrectomy through a thoraco-abdominal incision through the 8th rib bed, extended onto the abdomen. A larger portion of the stomach is removed than in middle third growths—about three fifths, often together with the spleen.

If the patient has had a previous partial gastrectomy or duodenal ulceration with consequent fibrosis and contraction, it may be difficult to carry out the oesophago-gastric anastomosis without tension. Alternative procedures then available are:

a. Jejunal Roux-en-Y loop—this technique, which involves two anastomoses, is used to prevent bile and pancreatic juice from entering the lower oesophagus, where they would cause an oesophagitis and subsequent stricture (fig. 819).

Ivor Lewis, 1895–1982. Surgeon, North Middlesex Hospital, London, England.

b. Transverse colon interposition, with vascular supply maintained by middle colic artery.

5. *Squamous cell lesions*

Radiotherapy can be preferred as a first line treatment.

Detailed Technique of Partial Oesophago-Gastrectomy

1. **Through right thoracotomy** (preceded by laparotomy to mobilise stomach) (Ivor Lewis operation).

(*a*) *Paramedian incision.*—An opening is made in the gastro-colic omentum along the greater curve of the stomach, preserving the right gastro-epiploic arch. The short gastric and left gastro-epiploic arteries are divided. The gastro-hepatic omentum is next divided with preservation of the right gastric artery. The stomach is mobilised along the lesser curve and the left gastric artery divided close to the coeliac axis. Nodes are often involved in this area and should be removed. The blood supply to the mobilised stomach thus depends on the preservation of the right gastric artery and the right gastro-epiploic arcade. The oesophageal hiatus is defined and stretched if necessary. A pyloroplasty (or pyloromyotomy) is performed to prevent post-operative gastric distension, as both vagi have inevitably been divided.

(*b*) *Right thoracotomy* through 5th rib bed. The azygos vein is divided and the oesophagus and stomach are drawn up into the chest. The stomach is divided obliquely and closed in two layers. Alternatively the stapler may be used to close the stomach and the staples covered with a continuous inverting suture. The oesophagus is divided 4–6 cm above the growth—this distance is essential as the submucous spread of the carcinoma is always more extensive than anticipated. A two layer anastomosis is then made between the oesophagus and a separate opening in the fundus of the stomach. A naso-gastric tube should be passed into the stomach remnant for post-operative suction. The chest is drained by an apical tube and also a basal tube, the end of which is placed near the anastomosis, and finally the chest is closed in layers.

2. **Through left thoracotomy** (with a 'two rib' approach for middle third growths when the oesophago-gastric anastomosis will be high in the chest).

A long postero-lateral incision is made along the eighth rib and extended onto the abdomen towards the umbilicus. The rib bed is opened and a radial incision made in the diaphragm from the oesophageal hiatus laterally. This will give access for the stomach mobilisation as described above for the Ivor Lewis operation. The stomach is divided obliquely, turned upwards and the oesophageal carcinoma mobilised. The site of transection of the oesophagus should be 4–6 cm above the growth as submucous spread of the growth is always more than is anticipated. An oesophago-gastric anastomosis is made, as already described. If the growth is in the middle third of the oesophagus then a separate entry (through the same skin and muscle incision) should be made through the fifth rib bed to give adequate access for the anastomosis, which in middle third growths should be medial or lateral to the aortic arch. A nasogastric tube should be passed into the stomach remnant for post-operative suction. The chest is drained by an apical tube and also a basal tube, the end of which is placed near the anastomosis. Finally the chest is closed in layers.

Total Oesophagectomy

Total oesophagectomy, with anastomosis of the fundus of the stomach to the oesophagus in the neck (McKeown three stage operation) has recently been advised for growths in the upper half of the oesophagus. If an anastomotic leak occurs after this operation, it will not be of any serious consequence because pleural contamination will not occur. The leak will be in the neck, it will soon heal and the usually fatal outcome of this complication will be avoided.

The first two stages are those of the Lewis operation, with complete mobilisation of the stomach and thoracic oesophagus. The cervical oesophagus is then exposed through an incision along the anterior border of the right sternomastoid. The omohyoid muscle, middle thyroid vein and inferior thyroid artery are divided and the oesophagus and stomach drawn up into the wound. This exposure should *not* be done on the left side as the chyle duct may be damaged. The oesophagus and stomach are transected as described above and the anastomosis performed.

McKeown has reported 253 oesophageal resections, with a 12% operative mortality and a 24% 5 year survival rate.

Combination treatments.—Nakayama has produced excellent figures combining pre-operation irradiation (to 'sterilise' the area of the growth) followed by oesophageal resection with replacement by stomach.

Palliative Treatment

If the growth is inoperable because of the general condition of the patient, presence of metastases, or found to be unresectable at thoracotomy or laparotomy, then a palliative procedure should be carried out to enable the patient to swallow.

This may be by the insertion of a tube into the oesophagus through the growth or by a palliative short circuit operation. This may be combined with radiotherapy if thought advisable.

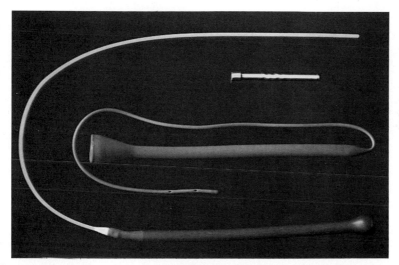

Fig. 820.—3 different types of tube for internal by-pass palliation of an oesophageal carcinoma. The Celestin tube (bottom) is commonly used. The Mousseau-Barbin tube (centre) is not recommended as there is a considerable risk of late necrosis/perforation of the oesophageal wall. The Souttar tube (top) can be inserted through an oesophagoscope and does not need a gastrotomy.

1. **Internal tube through growth.**—Several types of tube are available (fig. 820).

(a) *Souttar tube* (coiled German silver wire). The stricture is first dilated with gum elastic bougies to the size of the Souttar tube to be passed. A smaller size bougie is passed again through the stricture and then the Souttar tube passed over this bougie and *pushed* into the stricture. This technique reduces the risk of perforation, which nevertheless is still a definite hazard at the time of the initial dilatation. This tube, or any other type of tube, is not satisfactory for growths at the upper end of the oesophagus, where it will cause laryngeal irritation.

(b) *Celestin tube* (armoured rubber tube with a long tail). This tube has a tulip-shaped proximal end which effectively prevents its onward progress through the stricture. Its lumen is considerably larger than that of the Souttar tube. It may be introduced by passing the tail of the tube through the stricture into the stomach at oesophagoscopy and then making a small opening in the stomach at laparotomy and *pulling* the tube down until its upper end sits snugly above tumour (fig. 820).

Alternatively it is now possible to place a Celestin tube at oesophagoscopy with the use of a special introducer in satisfactory position through the stricture, without also performing a laparotomy.

K. Nakayama, Contemporary. Professor of Surgery, Institute of Gastroenterology, Women's Medical College, Tokyo, Japan.
Sir Henry Sessions Souttar, 1875–1964. Surgeon, The London Hospital.
Louis Roger Celestin, Contemporary. Surgeon, Frenchay Hospital, Bristol, England.

2. **Palliative short circuit operation.**—If the growth is found to be unresectable at operation a palliative oesophago-gastrostomy or oesophago-jejunostomy with a Roux loop (to prevent gastric reflux) may be carried out (fig. 819). There is, of course, the risk of an anastomotic leak, and because of this it is preferable to insert a Souttar or Celestin tube (fig. 820).

Terminal Complications.—Unresected, the growth causes death in one of the following ways:

1. Progressive cachexia and dehydration.
2. Pneumonia from perforation into some part of the bronchial tree.
3. Mediastinitis from perforation into the posterior mediastinum.
4. Erosion of the aorta (rare).

CHAPTER 44

THE STOMACH AND DUODENUM

SURGICAL ANATOMY

Blood Supply

Arterial Supply (fig. 821).—(*a*) The left gastric artery, the smallest branch of the coeliac axis, runs towards the cardiac orifice and thence along the lesser curvature, from left to right, to join (*b*) the right gastric artery, which arises from the hepatic artery and pursues a course from right to left along the lesser curvature. (*c*) The gastroduodenal artery is the largest branch of the hepatic artery. It passes behind the first part of the duodenum, where it bifurcates into the superior pancreatico-duodenal artery and (*d*) the right gastro-epiploic artery. (*e*) The left gastro-epiploic artery is the largest branch of the splenic artery. (*f*) Vasa brevia (short gastric arteries) are five to seven small vessels that spring from the splenic artery towards its termination, and are distributed to the fundus of the stomach. An important feature of the gastric circulation is the large number of arterio-venous shunts in the submucosa of the lesser curve. These are opened up by vagotomy.

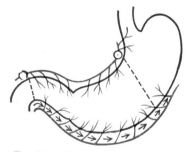

FIG. 821.—The main arteries of the stomach. Circles denote where the R. and L. gastric are divided. Arrows denote place of section of gastro-epiploic arteries. Dotted lines show where stomach is divided in partial gastrectomy.

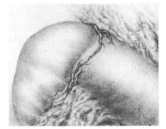

FIG. 822.—The pre-pyloric vein of Mayo.

Veins.—Those corresponding to the right and left gastric arteries terminate in the portal vein. Those corresponding to the left gastro-epiploic artery and vasa brevia join the splenic vein, while the right gastro-epiploic vein empties into the superior mesenteric vein. In the living, the veins of Mayo (fig. 822) are helpful landmarks in distinguishing the pyloric canal from the first part of the duodenum.

Lymphatics are described on p. 896 in connection with malignant neoplasms of the stomach with which they are so intimately concerned.

Innervation.—The vagus nerves are the motor and sensory nerves of the stomach. Fig. 823 shows the general disposition of the nerves, and their branches. Familiarity with the common distribution and main variations of the nerves is important owing to the swing from truncal to proximal gastric (syn. highly selective, parietal cell) vagotomy (Johnston, Amdrup) operations for duodenal ulcer (p. 877). The entire gastrointestinal tract has an extensive intrinsic innervation, grouped in two principal plexuses: the **myenteric plexus** of Auerbach and the **submucous plexus** of Meissner. The intrinsic nerves, which contain as many neurones as the spinal cord are important for all aspects of gastrointestinal function. After transection and anastomosis of the gut, the continuity of the intrinsic nerves is usually restored within a few weeks.

William James Mayo, 1861–1939. Surgeon, Mayo Clinic, Rochester, Minnesota, U.S.A. The pre-pyloric vein should be called the Vein of Latarjet as it was first described by André Latarjet (1876–1947), Professor of Anatomy, Lyons, France.
Leopold Auerbach, 1828–1897. Professor of Neuropathology, Breslau.
Georg Meissner, 1829–1905. German physiologist.
David Johnston, Contemporary. Professor of Surgery, Leeds, England.
Eric Amdrup, Contemporary. Professor of Surgery, Aarhus, Denmark.

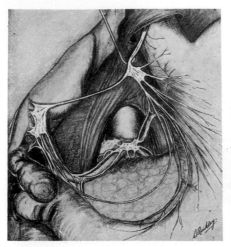 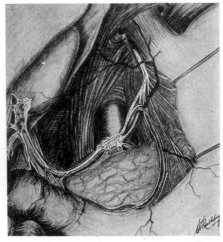

A   B

FIG. 823.—A, anterior and B, posterior vagus nerve. Showing distribution to stomach, coeliac, and subhepatic plexuses (*C. V. Ruckley, FRCS, Edinburgh*). The anterior and posterior nerves of Latarjet are seen crossing the pancreas on their way to supply the pylorus. The sympathetic innervation of the organ may carry a proportion of pain transmitting fibres.

Histology

Gastric Epithelial Cells lining the stomach are of the columnar type. They are filled with mucigenous granules and are responsible for the lubrication of contents. About a third of them regenerate daily by mitosis. They do not respond to acid secretagogues.

Parietal Cells.—These occur only in the body of the stomach and lie in the gastric crypts. Electron-microscopic studies show many inter-cellular canaliculi which communicate with the crypt lumen. They are responsible for the secretion of isotonic HCl to a pH of 0·9. In a normal adult male the parietal cell population is of the order of 1 billion whilst in about two-thirds of duodenal ulcer cases this may be nearly doubled. In the Zollinger-Ellison syndrome (Chapter 48) a four-fold increase has been reported. In gastric ulcer the count is low.

Chief Cells.—These lie mainly in the proximal part of the gastric crypts in the fundic mucosa and are responsible for the secretion of pepsinogen.

Endocrine Cells.—The mid-zone of the gastric mucosa contains G-cells, which synthesise gastrin. G-cells are found mainly in the gastric antrum, and their distribution differs from that of parietal cells on which gastrin acts. The number of G-cells may be increased in duodenal (but not gastric) ulcer patients, and is greatly increased in the condition known as G-cell hyperplasia (Polak). Other types of cells which secrete regulatory peptides occur in the gastric mucosa. These include D-cells, which contain somatostatin; it is probable that this peptide is involved in the negative feedback of gastric acid secretion, through its local action (paracrine) on adjacent exocrine cells.

PHYSIOLOGY OF THE STOMACH AND DUODENUM

The important physiological functions of the stomach and duodenum are secretory and motor. The stomach acts as a reservoir from which food, ingested over a period of minutes, is released over a period of hours after undergoing acid and peptic digestion into the duodenum. The most important action of the stomach, however, is not chemical but mechanical; lumps of solid food are broken down to small particles before being released by the antrum. In the duodenum, the mixed food and gastric secretions, now known as 'chyme', are brought to neutral pH by duodenal and pancreatic secretion of bicarbonate, and the osmolarity of the chyme is equilibrated with plasma. In addition, various nutrients stimulate the release from endocrine cells in the duodenal mucosa of polypeptides which modulate the secretory and motor activity of the digestive tract. The rate at which chyme is delivered from the stomach is dependent upon the osmolarity and the fat and caloric content of the chyme through receptors in the proximal duodenal mucosa (Hunt).

Julia M. Polak, Contemporary. Histopathologist, Hammersmith Hospital, London.
Jack Naylor Hunt, Contemporary. Professor of Physiology, Houston, Texas, U.S.A.

Secretion of Gastric Juice

The gastric juice consists mainly of pepsin, intrinsic factors, ions and other organic solutes in dilute hydrochloric acid. Conventionally, three phases of secretion of gastric juice are recognised.

1. **Cephalic.**—This is mediated by vagal activity, both from psychic arousal as demonstrated by Pavlov, and reflexly from antral stimulation (Uvnäs).

2. **Gastric.**—Gastrins are polypeptides differing in secretogenic potency and molecular size, but identical in action (Gregory), which are released from antral G-cells in response to mechanical distension of the antrum, and to meat proteins. After release from the G-cell, gastrin reaches the parietal cell *via* the systemic circulation. Secretion of acid is controlled by negative feedback; when intragastric pH falls below 3, due to acid secretion, the release of gastrin is inhibited. Because of the buffering capacity of a mixed meal, acid output is high for half an hour after eating, but falls thereafter. The role of histamine, long known as a potent stimulus of gastric acid secretion, has been a matter of controversy, but it now seems likely that gastrin acts on the parietal cell through the release of histamine in conjunction with cholecystokinin, acetyl choline and possibly noradrenaline.

3. **Intestinal.**—Prolongation of acid secretion for some hours after feeding was originally ascribed to 'intestinal factors'; but, since a mixed meal is not emptied from the stomach for several hours, it is probably due, for the most part, to prolonged gastrin release from mechanical stimulation of the antrum. The effect of chyme in the intestine on gastric secretion is largely inhibitory in order to preserve the neutral pH of the duodenum. Duodenal acidification provokes secretin and bulbogastrone release which inhibits gastric acid secretion (Grossman), and other intestinal polypeptides are probably implicated in this regulation; such polypeptides are termed 'gastrones'.

Pepsin Secretion

The secretion of pepsin is usually coupled to H+ secretion, but may be varied by cholinergic stimuli and by polypeptide hormones.

Gastric Mucus

The gastric mucosa is covered and lubricated by this viscid secretion, which is composed of mucopolysaccharides. As with pepsin, its secretion may be evoked by vagal stimulation on feeding. Its pH is alkaline, and it has considerable buffering capacity (up to 80 mmol/l, Hollander).

Gastric mucus forms a physiological barrier which protects the mucosa from mechanical damage and the effects of gastric acid. This protective function is strengthened by the secretion of small amounts of bicarbonate into the mucus layer, to produce a pH gradient. Davenport has suggested that this barrier is broken in cases of gastric ulcer, leading to back diffusion of H+ ion into mucosal cells; this would account in part for the apparently reduced secretion of acid in such patients, although the reduced number of parietal cells in such patients may produce hyposecretion. The barrier may be damaged by bile acids, refluxed through the pylorus and by drugs such as salicylates and alcohol. Irritation of the gastric mucosa may lead to excess mucus production.

Duodenal Exocrine Secretion

Although the duodenum is a relatively short tube, its surface area is extensive, due to the arrangement of the mucosa in transverse folds, the valvulae conniventes ('winking' valves). In the first and second part of the duodenum, an alkaline secretion is produced by Brunner's glands into the crypts of Lieberkühn: the volume of secretion is related to the amount of acid delivered through the pylorus. This alkaline secretion is largely responsible for correcting the pH of chyme to neutrality.

Gastric and Duodenal Endocrine Secretion

Both in variety and quantity of secreted polypeptides, the alimentary tract may be justly termed the largest endocrine organ in the body. Although a gastrointestinal hormone, secretin, was the first hormone to be described in physiological terms by Bayliss and Starling, the majority of gastrointestinal polypeptide hormones have been described in the last decade, following advances in immunoassay, cytochemistry and protein chemistry. While the physiology of these substances is still uncertain, there are some facts which are generally agreed.

Börje Karl Magnus Uvnäs, Contemporary. Professor of Physiology, University of Stockholm, Sweden.
Roderic Alfred Gregory, Contemporary. Holt Professor of Physiology, University of Liverpool.
Morton Grossman, 1919–1982. Director of the Center for Ulcer Research, Los Angeles, California, U.S.A.
Frederick G. Hollander, Contemporary. Surgeon, Mercy Hospital, San Diego, California, U.S.A.
Horace Davenport, Contemporary. Professor of Physiology, University of Michigan, Ann Arbor, Michigan, U.S.A.
Johann Conrad Brunner, 1653–1729. Anatomist, Basle, Switzerland.
Johann Nathanael Lieberkühn, 1711–1756. German Anatomist.
William Maddock Bayliss, 1860–1924. Physiologist, University College Hospital, London.
Ernest Henry Starling, 1866–1927. Physiologist, University College Hospital, London.

Structure of the Polypeptides

The majority of the polypeptides may be divided into two groups, on the basis of their structure. *Gastrin* and *cholecystokinin-pancreozymin* (CCK-PZ) have structural and functional affinities, with similar terminal amino-acid chains; both polypeptides occur in man in several variants of different peptide chain lengths. *Secretin, enteroglucagon* and *gastric inhibitory peptide* (GIP) have numerous structural affinities. Some polypeptides, such as *motilin*, appear to be unique in structure.

Localisation

The secretory cells of the polypeptide hormones are scattered among the epithelial cells of the gastrointestinal mucosa and are not aggregated in discrete glands. Gastrin is largely confined to the gastric antrum; most of the others are secreted in the small intestine, and principally in the duodenum. All secretory cells are adjacent to the lumen of the digestive tract, and luminal stimuli provoking polypeptide release (such as peptones releasing gastrin) have been identified in some cases. Polypeptides are also found in myenteric nerves, and the existence of 'peptidergic' nerves has been postulated (Polak). Most polypeptides normally found in the gut have also been identified within neurones in the central nervous system.

Function

Most of the polypeptides seem to be implicated in the control of digestive exocrine secretion, either exciting or inhibiting secretion. Gastrin provokes gastric acid secretion, secretin and CCK-PZ induce pancreatic secretion, while secretin inhibits gastric acid secretion.

A second role for the gastrointestinal polypeptides is in the control of gastrointestinal motor activity. CCK-PZ is the agent which mediates gall-bladder contraction, while gastrin stimulates gastric motor activity. Many other motor effects have been described, but, again, no clear picture has yet emerged.

The proximity of some endocrine cells to their exocrine target cells has led to the suggestion that *paracrine* effects (passage of polypeptide from secretory cell to target cell by local spread) may occur, but this is difficult to prove, and proof is as yet lacking. It is also likely that the function of polypeptides is as *neurotransmitters* or *neuromodulators* in the intrinsic nerve plexuses of the gut.

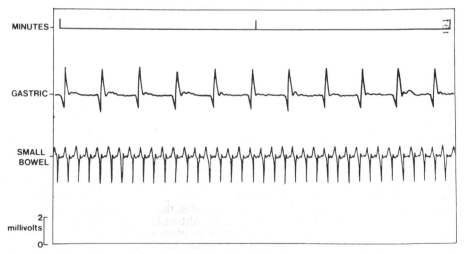

FIG. 824.—Pacemaking activity recorded at a single site in the canine stomach (upper trace) and duodenum (lower trace). In man, pacemaking activity is slower: 3/min in the stomach and 10–11/min in the duodenum.

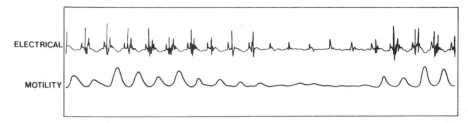

FIG. 825.—Simultaneous recording of myoelectric activity from a serosal electrode in the canine small intestine (upper trace) and intraluminal pressure adjacent to the site of the electrode. Regular pacemaking (small deflections) is visible, but pressure changes only occur when spike bursts (large deflections) follow the pacemaking wave.

Gastroduodenal Motor Activity

The complex sequence of digestive and absorptive processes acting on ingested nutrients requires the orderly propulsion of luminal content through different regions at different rates; this is accomplished by neurohumoral regulation of the contractile activity of the smooth muscle which completely invests the digestive tract.

The motor activity of the stomach and duodenum is rhythmic, and is controlled by waves of electrical depolarisation, known as *slow waves*. Slow waves are generated at proximal pacemaking sites in the stomach and duodenum, and spread aborally through the longitudinal smooth muscle fibres at speeds of several centimetres per second. The gastric pacemaker, in the gastric fundus, emits three slow waves per minute which descend to, but do not pass, the pylorus. Duodenal slow waves are generated by a pacemaker immediately distal to the pylorus (Hermon-Taylor) at a rate of ten per minute. These rhythmic slow waves, sometimes known as the *basic electrical rhythm*, resemble the electrocardiogram in nature and function: slow wave recording from the serosal surface of stomach and duodenum show rhythmic changes similar to, but slower than, the E.C.G. (fig. 824).

Since smooth muscle contraction at any site can occur only during the passage of a slow wave, pacemaker activity controls the *timing* of motor activity, and also the *direction*, as the slow waves travel caudally. But (unlike the E.C.G.) gastric and duodenal slow waves do *not* invariably initiate contraction during their passage. Simultaneous recording of duodenal electrical activity and intraluminal pressure change (fig. 825) shows regular slow wave activity, but pressure changes only occur with slow waves which show associated spike bursts (fig. 825). Intrinsic and extrinsic neural and humoral changes, as yet not fully explained, determine whether or not a slow wave will produce contraction; it is these factors, which integrate the motor activity of stomach and small intestine with the processes of digestion and absorption.

Gastric Emptying

The mixing and slow emptying of a mixed meal from the stomach is accomplished by means of the 'antral pump'. Gastrin release stimulates gastric motor activity by a slight increase in slow wave frequency, and a marked increase in the associated contractile activity. Caudal contraction waves propel contents into the gastric antrum (fig. 826): as the antrum fills, the pylorus, which has no resting tone, opens to allow the escape of some chyme. When the contraction wave reaches the pylorus, it closes, and the continuing antral contraction produces retropulsion of antral contents into the gastric corpus. Thus each contraction wave produces both the escape of a small quantity of chyme and the mixing of the remainder; in this way, the capacity of the duodenum to restore the pH of chyme to neutrality is not overcome. The volume lost through the pylorus with each contraction will depend upon the viscosity and the amount of solid in the gastric contents; fluids are emptied more rapidly.

Fasting *vs.* Feeding

There is a striking difference between the overall pattern of gastroduodenal motor activity during fasting, and following feeding. During fasting, a few minutes of active motor activity is followed by an hour or more of absent motor activity; this cycle of

John Hermon-Taylor, Contemporary. Professor of Surgery, St. George's Hospital, London.

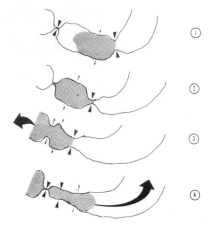

FIG. 826.—Sequential stages of gastric emptying. The pacemaker site and direction of slow wave propagation are shown at the right; the caudal propagation of contraction is shown in sequence from 1 to 4. Gastric contents are propelled into the antrum by the wave of contraction coupled to the slow wave (1, 2); as the antrum contracts, some content is expelled through the lax pylorus (3) as antral pressure rises. When the contraction wave reaches the pylorus (4), it closes, and antral pressure leads to retropulsion of gastric contents.

antral pump

alternating brief activity and prolonged inertia is repeated indefinitely in the absence of food. This pattern is not merely cyclical; it is also migratory. The brief phases of motor activity occur synchronously in stomach and proximal duodenum; as they decline, the activity 'front' passes caudally to the distal duodenum, and so on along the length of the small intestine (fig. 827). By contrast with the slow waves, the migration speed of these fronts is slow; passage from the stomach to the terminal ileum takes 1–2 hours, and the appearance of a new gastroduodenal front coincides approximately with arrival of the previous front at the terminal ileum. These migratory complexes were described in the first decade of the 20th century as 'hunger contractions'; more recently, the migrating complex has been termed the intestinal 'housekeeper' (Code) serving to propel fasting secretions and debris. Again in contrast to pacemaking activity, the 'clock' which controls the genesis of fasting front lies outside the smooth muscle, possibly in the myenteric plexus. The duodenum is important in the integration of this activity; there is evidence that one of the duodenal hormones, *motilin*, is implicated in this fasting control.

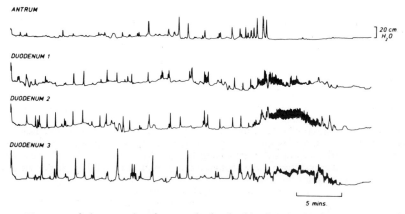

FIG. 827.—The onset of a human migrating complex in a healthy fasted subject registered by simultaneous recording from four pressure sensors equispaced between antrum and jejunum. At each site, pressure activity terminates in a burst of phasic contraction at 10/minute: this is the activity 'front' (see text).

Charles F. Code, Contemporary. Emeritus Professor of Physiology, Mayo Clinic, Rochester, U.S.A.

The transit of the 'housekeeping' front would be too fast to allow digestion and absorption of food to be complete; on feeding, the 'housekeeper' is immediately abolished, to be replaced at all levels of the intestine by intermittent contractile activity, permitting agitation and mixing of the chyme without rapid passage. When the stomach is empty, the fasting pattern resumes. The effects of feeding on the pattern of gastric motor activity can be partially simulated by the administration of gastrin (Code). It seems probable that other gastrointestinal polypeptide hormones will be shown to be implicated in the regulation of motor activity, and it may be that further study will lead to clarification of some of the common but ill-defined 'functional bowel syndromes' as disorders of neurohumoral regulation.

CURRENT TESTS OF GASTRIC SECRETION

(1) Peak Acid Output test (Pentagastrin)
(2) Insulin Test (Hollander)

TABLE I
Average H^+ response in mmol Acid

	Basal	Peak
Normal	5	27
Gastric Ulcer	2	15
Duodenal Ulcer	6	38
Zollinger-Ellison Syndrome	>60% of PAOp	

(1) **Peak Acid Output** (Pentagastrin).—Basal secretion is measured by aspiration of the fasting stomach for 1 control hour. Then the pentagastrin test is performed. Gastric acid secretion may be maximally stimulated using pentagastrin (Peptavlon I.C.I.). Side effects are negligible, $6\mu g/kg$ body weight is administered s.c., or i.m. and 15 minute samples are collected during the subsequent hour. (See Table I.) The two highest consecutive 15 minute aliquots of acid secretion, titrated to pH7, are taken; added; and multiplied by 2: the resulting figure being the peak acid output (PAOp) expressed in mmols H^+ (Baron). The mean values found in different conditions are shown in Table I.

Only limited reliance may be placed on such tests if they are not carried out by experienced investigators. It can be taken, however, that a patient cannot have *less* acid than is aspirated. He *may* have more. If the technique is faulty this will not be realised.

The tests are of value in the diagnosis of the Zollinger-Ellison syndrome (Chapter 48). In duodenal ulcer they may be a useful guide to which operation is more suited to the patient, *e.g.* where low, vagotomy and drainage—where high (45 mmol and above), vagotomy and antrectomy or partial gastrectomy.

Achlorhydria, by definition, occurs when a stomach cannot produce juice with a pH of less than 7·0 even after maximal stimulation. It occurs in 18% of patients with gastric carcinoma (Baron).

(2) **Insulin Test** (Hollander).—Since acid production following hypoglycaemia is attributed to direct vagal action on the parietal cell mass, insulin given to a patient who has had a vagotomy performed should result in no increase in acid production. This test is thus valuable post-operatively to verify the completeness of vagal section. To a fasting patient 2 units/10 kg soluble insulin are given intravenously, and serial quarter-hourly gastric aspirations performed for the next two hours. Blood-sugar levels are also measured at frequent intervals to ensure that the level falls below 35 mg/ (2 mmol/l) 100 ml—the level necessary to guarantee adequate vagal stimulation.

Early response.—A rise in concentration of 20 mmol per litre above the basal level in the first hour suggests incomplete vagotomy. If the basal samples were anacid, a concentration of 10 mmol per litre is regarded as positive.

Delayed response.—A rise in the concentration of acid secreted may occur between the first and second hours. This is thought to be due to vagal gastrin release. It is abolished by antrectomy. It suggests a less than complete vagotomy.

An early negative Hollander test may become positive some years later. The importance of this finding is not yet clear.

In addition, the glucose tolerance curve, an x-ray of the pituitary fossa, the serum calcium and phosphorus levels, and the urinary 17-ketosteroids may help to elucidate the difficult case with an endocrine background (multiple adenoma syndrome).

Jeremy Hugh Baron, Contemporary. Consulting Physician, St. Charles Hospital and Hammersmith Hospital, London.

Estimation of circulating gastrin.—Radio-immunoassay techniques are available. The principles of assay are:

A specific antigen is raised against gastrin. The biological sample competes with radioactive isotope-labelled hormone for combination with the antigen. The gastrin in the sample quantitatively inhibits the antigen binding with labelled hormone. The degree of inhibition gives a measure of gastrin in the sample. The findings have proved useful in diagnosis of the Zollinger-Ellison syndrome (Chapter 48).

Atrophy of Gastric Mucosa.—Atrophy may be due to duodenal regurgitation or it may be due to antibodies in the blood specific for the cytoplasm of the parietal cells. Such antibodies are found in pernicious anaemia in which there is also an antibody against intrinsic factor.

CURRENT TESTS OF DUODENAL SECRETION

No standard test of duodenal secretion exists, but monitoring of pH in the proximal duodenum may reveal an excessive fall in pH after a meal due to acid hypersecretion associated with duodenal ulcer.

CURRENT TESTS OF GASTRODUODENAL MOTOR ACTIVITY

Gastric emptying of a semi-solid meal can be monitored in a number of ways; the most reliable is the use of a gamma camera to follow the emptying of a meal of scrambled eggs labelled with Technetium. This may be of value in assessing the results of surgery on the gastric outlet.

HYPERTROPHIC PYLORIC STENOSIS OF INFANTS

Aetiology.—The cause of the condition, which occurs 3 or 4 times in every 1000 births, is unknown. Several theories have been propounded, the most acceptable being that the condition is due to an achalasia (primary failure of the pylorus to relax). In a small proportion (about 7%) of cases the abnormality appears in certain families with greater frequency than can be accounted for by coincidence. In these families, one parent bears the scar of an operation for hypertrophic stenosis in infancy, and in 50% of cases it is the mother, which, when the much higher incidence in the male is taken into consideration, is remarkable. In these families a brother is affected similarly in 10% and a sister in 2% of cases.

Pathology.—The musculature of the pyloric antrum is always hypertrophied. Proceeding distally, the hypertrophy increases, to reach its zenith in the circular fibres of the pylorus. Here the muscle layer is so thick that the mucosa is compressed, and often the lumen admits only a fine probe. As estimated at operation, the size of the pyloric 'lump' is proportional to the duration of the symptoms. The hypertrophy terminates abruptly, the duodenum being normal.

Clinical Features.—Characteristically first-born male infants are most commonly affected.

The peak incidence for the onset of symptoms is between the third and sixth weeks of life; however, the condition can commence before that time, and as late as the seventh week. The pillars upon which the diagnosis rests are:

Vomiting is the presenting symptom in all cases and within two or three days it becomes forcible and projectile. Bile is not present in the vomit. Immediately after vomiting the baby is often very hungry.

Visible Peristalsis.—After the child has been fed, peristaltic waves may be seen passing from left to right across the upper abdomen (fig. 829). A good light is essential for this; the abdomen should be watched throughout a feed until vomiting occurs.

The Presence of a Lump.—The palpation of the hypertrophied pylorus is the

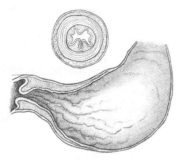

FIG. 828.—Pyloric stenosis of infants. Longitudinal and transverse sections of the stomach to show the enormous muscular hypertrophy. Note the abrupt termination.

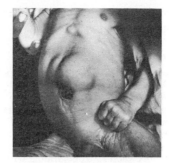

FIG. 829.—Visible peristalsis in hypertrophic pyloric stenosis: it is unusual for the waves to be so obvious.
(Alan Kark, FRCS, London.)

most essential step in reaching a diagnosis. The surgeon should palpate under the liver with a warm hand. It may be helpful to examine the child more than once. The lump is most easily felt when the child is given a feed.

Constipation is usually present, and when a stool is passed it is small and dry, resembling that of a rabbit. It is important to ask the mother about napkins; if the child is dehydrated, they are not wet and the case is correspondingly more urgent.

Loss of Weight.—One of the most striking signs of infants suffering from hypertrophic pyloric stenosis is loss of weight. Moreover, it is not long before the infant begins to look emaciated and dehydrated.

Often a change from one type of feeding to another brings about a remission. Consequently a series of changes in diet are sometimes made before the diagnosis is established, by which time the infant's condition may be pitiable.

In premature infants, in whom the condition is not uncommon, the symptomatology is often paradoxical. There is anorexia instead of a voracious appetite; the vomiting is regurgitant rather than projectile, and so frequently is peristalsis normally visible in these attenuated subjects that its significance is liable to be disregarded. None the less, amidst this sea of bewilderment one diagnostic rock remains—a hypertrophied pylorus can be felt through the poorly-developed abdominal wall with comparative ease.

Radiography.—The diagnosis should be made on a careful clinical examination and an x-ray is rarely necessary. To be diagnostic, a barium meal should show persistent narrowing and elongation of the pyloric canal.

Differential Diagnosis.—Conditions from which hypertrophic pyloric stenosis must be differentiated are (*a*) intracranial haemorrhage; (*b*) duodenal atresia; (*c*) high intestinal obstruction, *e.g.* volvulus neonatorum (Chapter 51). In (*b*) and (*c*) bile will be present in the vomitus.

Treatment.—The majority of paediatricians believe that surgery is the treatment of choice: the condition is immediately and completely corrected and the child is well within twenty-four hours. Babies who are admitted in a dehydrated condition should receive sufficient dextrose-saline solution, given intravenously, to restore the fluid and electrolyte balance. This results in a remarkable improvement in the general condition: the sunken eyes and cheeks and depressed fontanelle fill out; the dry skin and mucous membrane become moist, and the output of urine increases.

Medical Treatment

In cases complicated by infection, especially of the mouth, medical treatment is advisable because of the increased risk of post-operative gastro-enteritis, even if operation would otherwise be indicated.

In subacute cases the patient often reaches the age of two months before the symptoms become obvious and if, as a result of medical treatment, the gastric residue decreases in amount, a cure by non-operative means can be anticipated.

Eumydrin (atropine methylnitrate) 1:10,000 of water, freshly made, is given half an hour before each feed, beginning with 0·5 to 1 ml and increasing to 2·5 ml to control the symptoms. Toxic symptoms (erythema and hyperpyrexia), though less common than when atropine is employed, do occur with Eumydrin,[1] and are signs that the dose of the drug should be decreased or its use discontinued. Small, frequent feeds of milk (if possible the mother's milk), diluted with 5% dextrose, are given. Eumydrin must never be given until a firm diagnosis has been made.

Surgical Treatment.—After correction of dehydration, operation is performed without delay. The recovery rate approaches 100% in early cases.

Ramstedt's Operation.—*Preliminary Preparation.*—The stomach is washed out with saline several times; finally, one hour before operation. Immediately before operation gastric aspiration must be performed, and continued throughout the operation. The prevention of chilling is of great importance. To this end the temperature of the operating theatre should be high (27°C) and the infant's body is encased in wool, the upper abdomen alone being accessible.

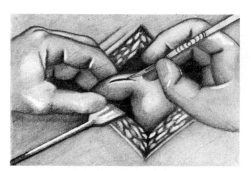

FIG. 830.—Ramstedt's operation.

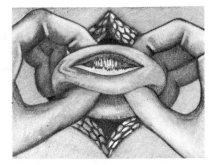

FIG. 831.—Showing the hypertrophied muscle divided and the mucous membrane bulging into the incision.

Operation.—Local anaesthesia is advisable only if the child is in good condition and the services of an anaesthetist skilled in anaesthesia of infants are not available. The abdomen is opened by a grid-iron[2] incision in the upper right quadrant of the abdomen. The hypertrophied pylorus is delivered and rotated so that its superior surface comes into view; thus the least vascular portion can be selected for the incision. In order to ascertain the distal limit of the hypertrophied pylorus the surgeon invaginates the duodenum with his index finger. The incision is made through the serosa only from this point along the whole length of the lump (fig. 830). Because the hypertrophied pylorus is the consistency of an unripe pear, splitting of muscle coats can be accomplished with a blunt dissector. On separating the edges with artery forceps the pyloric mucosa bulges into the cleft which has been made in the muscle (fig. 831). Great care is taken not to penetrate the mucosa,

---

[1] Eumydrin was introduced as a therapeutic improvement on atropine in the treatment of congenital pyloric stenosis by Svensgaard in 1935.
[2] Transverse through the skin and the anterior rectus sheath, and splitting the rectus muscle vertically.

Elisabeth Svensgaard, 1894–1952. Physician, Rigshospitalet, Copenhagen.
Wilhelm Conrad Ramstedt, 1867–1963. Surgeon, Rafael Clinic, Munster, Germany. Performed his first pyloromyotomy in 1911. He discovered in church records that his grandfather had misspelt the family name with two 'm's, so in 1920 he reverted to the original spelling.

an accident which is liable to occur while dividing the most distal part of the constricting fibres which are in the vicinity of the duodenal 'fornix' (fig. 828). In order to be sure that there is no perforation, some air is squeezed from the stomach into the duodenum. If a perforation has occurred, it is closed by a wisp of omentum held in place by three or four interrupted sutures of fine catgut. The free entry of air into the duodenum indicates adequate division of the muscle. Haemostasis must be meticulous. The abdominal incision is repaired. It is important to remove the wool from the infant's body as soon as the operation is over, or hyperthermia may occur.

After-treatment.—A small feed of not more than 5 ml should be given one hour after operation, and after that the feeds can be rapidly increased. The child should be feeding normally in forty-eight hours and if there is no vomiting at this time, it is the practice in many hospitals to send the child home early—no later than forty-eight hours. If the mucosa was accidentally opened at operation, it is wise not to feed the child orally for forty-eight hours.

Complications:

(*a*) *Post-operative pyrexia* is rather common and is not necessarily of serious consequence. If protracted, tepid sponging is advisable.

(*b*) *Gastro-enteritis* is minimised by absolute cleanliness of feeding utensils, segregation and sending the child home as soon as convenient.

(*c*) *Disruption of the wound* is also rare, and is more liable to occur in emaciated subjects. The use of the grid-iron incision in these cases has reduced the incidence of this complication.

Hypertrophic pyloric stenosis of adults is a definite entity and may be mistaken for carcinoma of the pylorus. When a diagnosis can be made with certainty, pyloroplasty or a gastro-jejunostomy (p. 878) gives excellent results; when doubt exists, a Billroth I gastrectomy is done. Microscopical examination of the specimen shows fibrosis of the myenteric plexus (contrary to the corresponding condition in the infant).

CONGENITAL ATRESIA OF THE DUODENUM

There is stenosis, usually complete, across the duodenum (fig. 832). This occurs at the point of fusion of the fore- and mid-gut, and consequently lies in the neighbourhood of the ampulla of Vater. It is frequently accompanied by other congenital defects. The infant vomits *from birth*, and daily rapidly loses weight. In contra-distinction to congenital pyloric

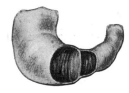

FIG. 832.—Congenital septum of duodenal obstruction at the commencement of the third part of the duodenum. The gut above is enormously dilated.
(After W. E. Ladd.)

stenosis *the vomit contains bile*. Laparotomy should be undertaken without delay. Duodeno-jejunostomy is the best procedure when, as is usually the case, the obstruction is in the second or third part of the duodenum (Ladd). In these cases the stoma is difficult to keep open and it is wise to introduce a fine plastic tube through a gastrostomy opening, through the stomach across the stoma and down into the jejunum for a few inches. This should be retained for several days for feeding purposes.

PEPTIC ULCERS

These occur in the presence of acid and pepsin. The two main types are gastric and duodenal, but they also occur at the stoma after gastro-jejunostomy, at the lower end of the oesophagus and in a Meckel's diverticulum in association with ectopic gastric mucosa. Therefore beware of the term 'peptic ulcer', it embraces five different types of condition.

Christian Albert Theodor Billroth, 1829–1894. Professor of Surgery, Vienna.
Abraham Vater, 1684–1751. Professor of Anatomy and Botany, Wittenberg, Germany.
William Edwards Ladd, 1880–1967. Professor of Child Surgery, Harvard University, Boston, Massachusetts, U.S.A.

ACUTE PEPTIC ULCERS

Aetiology.—Acute gastric ulcers are thought to be due to disruption of the gastric mucosal barrier. They appear as multiple erosions and at least half the patients give a history of ingestion of drugs, including aspirin, or one of the other members of the non-steroidal anti-inflammatory group. Classically they present with haemorrhage and this at present is seen in older patients with arthritis receiving one of the drugs mentioned above.

Pathology.—Acute peptic ulcers are frequently multiple—in 75% of cases more than three of these lesions are present. They can occur in any part of the stomach, but in the duodenum they are almost confined to the first part. These ulcers are oval or circular in shape and vary in size from 1 to 2 mm in diameter (when they are called erosions) to 1 cm or more in diameter. They are shallow, punched out, and seldom invade the muscular coats. When healing occurs acute peptic ulcers are unlikely to leave scars.

Clinical features.—Acute peptic ulcers probably occur with great frequency. They give rise to short-lived attacks of dyspepsia which are not diagnosed, and the ulcer heals. Usually they are recognised only when they cause haematemesis. Occasionally an acute ulcer, particularly when it is situated on the anterior wall of the duodenum, perforates. By gastroscopy, it has been ascertained that acute peptic ulcers can be the cause of haematemesis at all ages and in both sexes. Such lesions have been seen to progress to chronic ulceration (Tanner).

Treatment.—If possible the cause must be removed. Under medical treatment acute peptic ulcers tend to heal rapidly. Blood transfusions may be required for haematemesis. Dietetic irregularities must be corrected in order to prevent recurrence or chronicity.

Stress ulcers.—These constitute a special group of acute ulcers. They occur most frequently in patients in intensive therapy units. There is usually a history of hypotension from haemorrhage, endotoxic shock or cardiac infarction. Sometimes they are seen after cerebral trauma or neurosurgical operations (Cushing's Ulcer) but it has been held that these are not true stress ulcers. After major burns two types of ulcer occur (Curling's Ulcer). Within the first forty-eight hours multiple acute erosions may develop anywhere in the body and fundus of the stomach (14% of cases). The antrum and duodenum are unaffected. These are thought to be true stress ulcers. Later, during convalescence, acute duodenal ulcers may occur (9%) which sometimes become chronic. These are probably not stress ulcers.

As to aetiology, there may be mucosal ischaemia due to vascular shunting and associated disseminated intravascular coagulation as well as reflux of duodenal contents into the stomach. The output of gastric mucous substance is also increased and there is shedding of the surface epithelial cells, all of which predisposes to ulceration. Patients on steroids may develop similar lesions, sometimes referred to as Steroid Ulcers.

CHRONIC DUODENAL ULCER

Aetiology.—Most patients, although by no means all, have gastric hypersecretion of acid. Duodenal ulcer patients tend to have a larger than normal parietal cell mass.

Norman Cecil Tanner, 1906–1982. Surgeon, Charing Cross Hospital, London.
Harvey Cushing, 1869–1939. Professor of Surgery, Harvard University, Boston, Mass., U.S.A.
Thomas Blizard Curling, 1811–1888. Surgeon, The London Hospital. Described this ulcer in 1842.

(*a*) *Genetic and Blood Groups.*—There is definite evidence that chronic ulcers occur in families. Moreover, persons of blood group O are about three times more likely to develop a peptic ulcer than are persons of other blood groups. It seems possible that the ABO genes may modify the size of the parietal cell mass.

(*b*) *Neurogenic Theory.*—Stimulation of the vagus results in gastric hyper-secretion and hypermotility. Stress and anxiety may be a cause of duodenal ulcer and, if so, may exert their effect via the vagus.

(*c*) *Accessory Causes.*—Inadequate mastication, alcohol, irregular meals, excessive smoking and vitamin deficiency have, at one time or another, been blamed. It has been conclusively shown that smoking delays healing.

(*d*) *Endocrine.*—The effects of emotional, as well as physical stress are hormon-ally transmitted to the stomach via the pituitary adreno-cortical axis. There are specific endocrine disorders which may be associated with severe or intractable ulceration. These include (1) the Zollinger-Ellison syndrome, where a non-beta cell tumour secreting 'gastrin' occurs in the pancreas (Chapter 48); (2) the Mul-tiple Adenoma Syndrome, where adenomas occur in the pituitary, adrenal, pan-creatic and parathyroid glands (Chapter 38); (3) hyperparathyroidism (Chapter 38).

Incidence.—Duodenal ulcer, rare before the age of 16, becomes more frequent as middle age approaches and in England nearly 10% of men aged 45 to 54 years have been or are afflicted. However, since the mid-1950's the incidence has been falling, particularly in men, although now in the later 1980's it has plateaued with a male to female ratio of 2:1. Occupation has surprisingly little bearing on the condition; high incidences have been found among foremen, while significantly low incidences occur among agricultural workers (Doll). The popular belief that bus drivers are especially liable to this condition has not been substantiated. In many parts of the world, e.g. USA, Scandinavia, this disease is as common as it is in Great Britain. Conversely, the incidence among Africans and Asiatics living in their native land is comparatively low, except in the newly emerging nations where the local population are assuming increasing responsibility. Duodenal ulcer is found four times more commonly than gastric ulcer in patients under the age of 35 years but after 45 years of age it is only one or two times more common. In Scotland the ratio of duodenal to gastric ulcer is higher than in England, while in India the ratio of duodenal to gastric ulcers is 30:1.

Pathology.—Ulcers, whether gastric or duodenal, tend to occur in alkaline mucosa. The ulcer bearing area is shown (shaded) in fig. 833. A chronic duodenal ulcer invades the muscular coats, which it tends to penetrate. When a gastric or duodenal ulcer heals, the site is covered by a mucosal scar. Fibrosis, the result of recurrent ulceration, causes deformities, including pyloric stenosis and hourglass contracture of the stomach (see Chronic Complications).

In the duodenum the ulcer is nearly always situated in the first part and some-times two 'kissing' ulcers are present: one on the anterior surface and one on the posterior surface of the first 3 cm of the duodenum. An anterior ulcer may perforate, a posterior one carries the risk of haemorrhage by erosion of a large vessel.

Microscopical Examination.—There is nearly always greater destruction of the muscular coat than of the mucosa. The base of the ulcer is covered by a thin

Sir William Richard Shaboe Doll, Contemporary. Formerly Regius Professor of Medicine, Oxford, England.

layer of granulation tissue. The arteries in the neighbourhood show evidence of endarteritis obliterans. Often there are no nerves in the floor of the ulcer but always many in the edge. The terminations of these nerves are bulbous, akin to those in an amputation stump (Kinsella). At the margin of the ulcer there may be epithelial proliferation, and downgrowths of glandular tissue are apt to be found, which are sometimes misinterpreted as indicating a carcinomatus change (Newcomb).

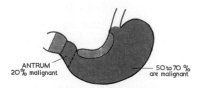

FIG. 833.—*Shaded Area.*—The common area for benign ulcers in stomach and duodenum. *Red Area.*—In this area ulcers carry a high risk of malignancy.

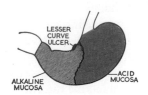

FIG. 834.—Area of gastritis (alkaline) in gastric ulcer. Red area = acid mucosa.

CHRONIC GASTRIC ULCER

Aetiology.—Chronic gastric ulcer is associated with either normal or hyposecretion, atrophic gastritis, and usually occurs in a later age group. The one constant association is with smoking, particularly of cigarettes, which may account for the fact that it is less common in social groups I and II.

Incidence.—Only 1–2% of the population suffer from this condition and the sex ratio is equal.

Pathology.—A chronic gastric ulcer is usually larger than a chronic duodenal ulcer. It varies in size, but in a well-established case it will admit the tip of a finger. The floor of a chronic gastric ulcer is situated in the muscular coats of the stomach, and as time goes on the ulcer occupying the posterior wall becomes adherent to and later invades (chronic perforation) the pancreas. In the same way, a chronic ulcer situated on the antero-superior aspect of the stomach can penetrate the liver, while a saddle-shaped ulcer situated on the lesser curve can, and often does, penetrate both the liver and the pancreas.

As with duodenal ulcer, gastric ulcers tend to occur in the nonacid secreting mucosa at the boundary with the body of the stomach (fig. 833), this area being much smaller than the area of chronic gastritis (fig. 834) which is the precursor of chronic gastric ulcer.

Microscopical Examination.—The microscopy of a chronic gastric ulcer is similar to that of a chronic duodenal ulcer and has been described above.

Do Peptic Ulcers become malignant?—A chronic duodenal ulcer never becomes carcinomatous. On the other hand, a chronic gastric ulcer may become malignant, but how frequently this change takes place is a matter of great difference of opinion (see above). It would seem probable that it does not exceed 0·5%. Even **giant ulcers** (those with a crater of more than 2·5 cm in diameter) are seldom carcinomatous.

Appearance of chronic gastric or duodenal ulcer at operation.—A chronic peptic ulcer may present as a white scar under the peritoneal coat. Delicate vascular adhesions,

Victor John Kinsella, Contemporary. Consulting Surgeon, St. Vincent's Hospital, Sydney, Australia.
Wilfrid Davidson Newcomb, 1889–1971. Professor of Pathology, St. Mary's Hospital, London.

salmon pink and fluffy in appearance, can often be observed in the immediate neighbour-hood of the peritoneal aspect of the ulcer. At other times the ulcer must be sought for by palpation; induration, frequently extensive in the case of a gastric ulcer, is centred over the mucosal lesion. When the ulcer is situated in the duodenum, the surrounding induration is not so evident, but if the ulcer is situated on the posterior wall it may be possible to feel the crater with the tip of the finger. A useful method of confirming the presence of a peptic ulcer, particularly one situated on the anterior wall of the duodenum, is to rub the peritoneal surface gently with a swab; the peritoneum overlying the ulcer becomes speckled, as though sprinkled with cayenne pepper (fig. 835), a characteristic phenomenon due to minute petechial haemorrhages.

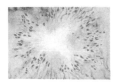

Fig. 835.—Petechial haemorrhages around the peritoneal aspect of a chronic peptic ulcer. These become more obvious after gently rubbing the surface with gauze.

If there is any doubt about the presence of an ulcer, a longitudinal gastrotomy incision should be made and the mucosal area inspected. Ulcers in the pyloric channel (p. 885), and around the cardia, may be missed if this is not done.

THE CLINICAL FEATURES OF GASTRIC AND DUODENAL ULCERS CONTRASTED

It is useful to record the patient's history under seven headings.

Chronic Gastric Ulcer.—The patient is usually beyond middle age, and by reason of a restricted diet is often thin. In many instances the patient appears anaemic, and this is often confirmed by a haemoglobin estimation. On careful enquiry certain features of the dyspepsia become manifest. Typically there is:

1. *Periodicity.*—The attacks last for several weeks, and are followed by inter-vals of freedom from two to six months. The attacks are more in evidence in the spring and autumn and should be recorded.

2. *Pain* is epigastric, and may occur immediately, or any time up to two hours, after food. Pain may radiate through the back, is relieved by lying down flat and practically never occurs at night.

3. *Vomiting.*—In over 50% of cases vomiting is a notable symptom. It relieves the pain, and may be self-induced.

In the 'pyloric channel' ulcer vomiting may be the predominant or only symptom and the barium meal may be negative. Endoscopy is essential in order to make the diagnosis. Pyloric channel deformity may be the precursor of a lesser curve gastric ulcer.

4. *Haematemesis and Melaena.*—At some time or other 30% of patients with gastric ulcers suffer from bleeding from the ulcer. The ratio of haematemesis to melaena is about 60:40.

5. *Appetite* is good, but the sufferer is afraid to eat.

6. *Diet.*—The patient learns to avoid fried foods, stews, curries, and twice cooked meat. Milk, eggs, and fish are the staple diet.

7. *Weight.*—Usually by the time the surgeon is consulted there has been some loss of weight.

On examination there is frequently deep tenderness in the mid-line of the epigastrium a few inches above the umbilicus.

Chronic duodenal ulcer can occur at any time during adult life, but is commonest between the ages of twenty-five and fifty. It is more common in men, who appear otherwise healthy.

1. *Periodicity* is usually well marked, and classically the attacks come on in the spring and in the autumn and are precipitated by 'work, worry, or weather'. These attacks usually last from two to six weeks, with decreasing intervals of freedom from one to six months.

2. *Pain* is severe, and may double up the patient. It usually occurs one to two and a half hours after food. As it is often relieved by food, the pain is known as 'hunger pain', and, classically, the patient carries biscuits, which he eats at frequent intervals to prevent this gastric torment. The pain, which is also relieved by alkalis, often awakens the patient round about 2 a.m. but is usually absent at the normal hour of rising.

3. *Vomiting* is rare in duodenal ulceration unless it is self-induced or stenosis has occurred. Regurgitation of burning fluid into the mouth ('water-brash') together with pain deep to the sternum ('heart-burn') due to reflux oesophagitis are common complaints (1:10).

4. *Haematemesis and melaena*, which occur in the ratio of 40:60, but sometimes together, are rather more frequent than in the case of gastric ulcer.

5. *Appetite* is exceptionally good, but the patient sometimes refrains from eating solid food during the attacks.

6. *Diet.*—In contradistinction to patients with a chronic gastric ulcer, those suffering from duodenal ulcer who have not been ordered a special diet seldom display much dietetic discrimination, although some of the more intelligent find it advisable to avoid fried food.

7. *Weight.*—Usually there is no loss of weight; indeed, the patient often becomes plump (partly because of the ingestion of milk to relieve pain).

On examination it is not unusual to find localised deep tenderness in the right hypochondrium.

Overall, in men, there is a 5% risk of perforation and this risk is increased in those who have perforated previously. Likewise, about 10% of patients will have a significant bleed. But, if they present with haemorrhage, the probability of re-bleeding within 10 years rises to 75%.

Summary

	Gastric Ulcer	Duodenal Ulcer
Periodicity	Present	Well marked
Pain	Soon after eating, but not when lying down	Two hours after food Night pain
Vomiting	Considerable vomiting	No vomiting
Hæmorrhage	Hæmatemesis is more frequent than melæna	Melæna more frequent than hæmatemesis
Appetite	Afraid to eat	Good
Diet	Lives on milk and fish	Eats almost anything
Weight	Loses weight	No loss in weight

SPECIAL METHODS OF INVESTIGATION

Barium Meal.—The radiological findings are often conclusive. In a lesser curve *gastric ulcer* a niche will be seen projecting from the usually smooth outline (fig. 836). The

Berkeley George Andrew Moynihan (Lord Moynihan of Leeds), 1865–1936. Professor of Clinical Surgery, Leeds, England, was the first to describe 'hunger pain'.

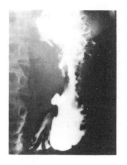

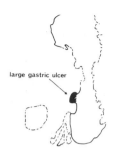

FIG. 836.—Typical gastric ulcer on the lesser curve.

FIG. 837.—Antral ulcer.

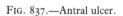

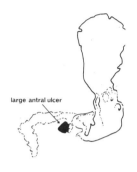

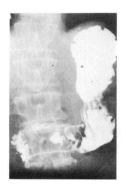

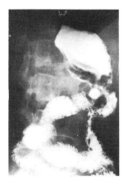

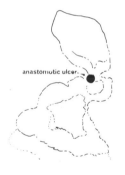

FIG. 838.—Anastomotic ulcer.

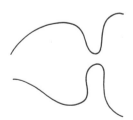

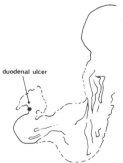

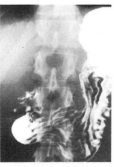

FIG. 839.—Normal duodenal cap filled with barium.

FIG. 840.—Duodenal ulcer.

stomach is often hypotonic and J-shaped and hangs low in the pelvis. In *antral ulcer* the appearance of the niche is similar (fig. 837). *Anastomotic ulcers* can also be shown (fig. 838) although only about 30% can be demonstrated. In *duodenal ulcers* diagnosis depends on demonstrating an ulcer crater filled with barium—this is positive evidence of an 'active' ulcer (fig. 840). In longstanding ulcers so much scar tissue is present that it is often impossible to show an ulcer crater with a persistent flake of barium. Where, however, deformity is *constant* the inference is that there has been a chronic cicatrical process due to an ulcer. In such a case the folds of scar tissue converge on the ulcer site, and if this '*rugal convergence*' can be shown, there is a very strong suspicion that an ulcer is present. It is important to recognise the shape of the normal duodenal cap when distended with barium (fig. 839). The appearances of pyloric stenosis (fig. 858) and hour-glass deformity (fig. 859) are characteristic.

Blood Studies.—A haemoglobin estimation may show evidence of chronic blood loss.

Studies of Gastric Function.—These are described in the section on gastric physiology on p. 856.

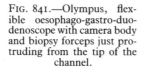

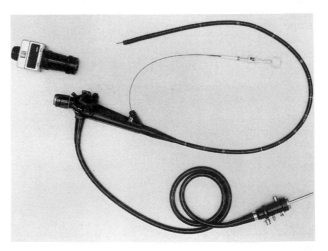

FIG. 841.—Olympus, flexible oesophago-gastro-duodenoscope with camera body and biopsy forceps just protruding from the tip of the channel.

Gastroduodenoscopy requires special training and considerable experience but affords valuable information. By its employment the whole of the interior of the stomach as well as the oesophagus, the first part and the proximal section of the second part of the duodenum and both efferent and afferent limbs of a gastrojejunostomy if present (Hirschowitz) can be adequately scrutinised (fig. 841).

The fibrescope is an instrument in which glass fibre provides the image transmission system and is therefore flexible.

Following the development of the gastrocamera in Japan there is now a wide range of endoscopes which allow biopsies to be taken under direct vision. Photographs may be taken by still or cinecamera and television methods.

Indications.—Gastroduodenoscopy is valuable in the diagnosis of shallow gastric ulcers that do not show on radiography, in checking the results of medical treatment in cases of chronic gastric ulcer, in the differential diagnosis between a chronic peptic ulcer (figs. 842

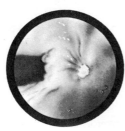

FIG. 842.—Gastroscopic view of the lesser curvature showing a gastric ulcer above the entrance to the antrum.
(*W. W. Davey, FRCS*)

FIG. 843.—Gastroscopy—early carcinomatous change in a chronic gastric ulcer in a patient undergoing medical treatment.
(*Hermon Taylor, FRCS, London.*)

Basil I. Hirschowitz, Contemporary. Professor of Medicine, University of Alabama, Birmingham, U.S.A.

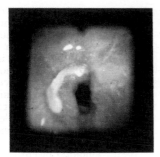

FIG. 844.—Benign prepyloric
ulcer.

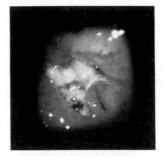

FIG. 845.—Neoplastic ulcer
involving the pylorus.

and 844) and a carcinoma (figs. 843 and 845), in the diagnosis of a small gastric neoplasm, in the detection of certain forms of gastritis, in the examination of the stoma in cases of suspected gastro-jejunal ulcer, and in the diagnosis of duodenal ulcer.

TREATMENT OF CHRONIC UNCOMPLICATED GASTRIC AND DUODENAL ULCER

CONSERVATIVE MANAGEMENT

All are agreed that in the absence of complications threatening life, the treatment of a proven chronic gastric or duodenal ulcer should in the first instance be conservative (medical). There is no doubt that the patient benefits from close and continuing collaboration between surgeon and physician, and that this collaboration is improved when each has a clear understanding of both conservative and surgical therapy. The management of the two conditions is similar in some respects, but there are important differences.

Aims of Conservative Treatment

The aim of treatment is the *relief of symptoms*; this is often, but not always, synonymous with healing; typical symptoms may persist in the absence of a detectable lesion, while a frank ulcer (10%) may be virtually asymptomatic. Since gastric acid is the main provocative factor the control of acid secretion is the essential therapy. The introduction of drugs which selectively and specifically block acid secretion has increased the effectiveness of conservative therapy without, so far as can be ascertained, altering the natural history of the chronic disorder.

Chronic Gastric Ulcer.—Prior to the institution of treatment, accurate diagnosis is essential. Endoscopic inspection and biopsy of the ulcer must be performed; in general, the size of the lesion is best assessed radiologically. Once the lesion has been confirmed as benign, symptomatic treatment is instituted. Although secretion of acid may be subnormal, H_2 receptor blockade with either cimetidine or ranitidine will secure healing in more than half the patients in a period of 6 weeks. Provocative agents should be avoided, including chemical irritants such as aspirin, corticosteroids, non-steroidal anti-inflammatory agents, and alcohol. Cigarette smoking should be stopped as it is known to delay gastric healing. There is no specific ulcer diet, but foods which provoke symptoms should be avoided.

Six weeks after the institution of treatment, objective evidence of healing must be obtained. Endoscopy is the simplest test, and gives a good estimate of partial healing even when resolution is incomplete. If there is no clear evidence of healing, four-quadrant endoscopic biopsy is essential, and if the ulcer persists, a Billroth I gastectomy is indicated.

Chronic Duodenal Ulcer.—Even though the aetiology of duodenal ulcer in relation to acid secretion remains a matter of controversy, there is no doubt that (1) active duodenal ulcer disease is often associated with increased gastric acid secretion and (2) that the pain of duodenal ulcer arises from the contact of acid with the lesion (Dragstedt). Thus, for duodenal ulcer, the control of gastric acid secretion is logical treatment. It has to be remembered that spontaneous healing of duodenal ulcers within 6 weeks is common, and the aim of treatment is the abolition of pain during the healing phase as well as avoiding

Lester Reynold Dragstedt, 1893–1975. Research Professor of Surgery, University of Florida, Gainsville, U.S.A.

possible perpetuation of the ulcer by acid. Traditional doses of antacid are helpful in the immediate relief of symptoms, but fall far short of the doses required to buffer secreted acid. Large doses of antacid (such as 120 ml daily of an aluminium and magnesium hydroxide mixture) will significantly neutralise gastric acid but are not very acceptable, partly because of a high incidence of diarrhoea on this regime.

H2-Receptor Antagonists.—At the parietal cell level, acid secretion is mediated partly by histamine acting on H2 histamine receptors. Recently, drugs have been developed which specifically block these receptors, without other significant effects. The first such drug to be introduced was cimetidine (Black), and its effect is virtual abolition of resting (or basal) acid secretion and, in normal therapeutic dosage, reduction by half of meal or gastrin stimulated acid secretion. Ranitidine, a later drug, has a similar spectrum of activity to cimetidine. The timing of doses is related to the timing of maximum risk to the lesion. Acid secretion is stimulated by a meal, but the meal itself will buffer the acid for about one hour after food. After that time, continuing secretion induces a fall in gastric pH, and it is then that the pH in the duodenal bulb falls. Although the fall in pH will cut off acid secretion by negative feedback, duodenal ulcer patients in particular tend to have defective autoregulation, with prolongation of the acid secretion after the buffer capacity of the meal is exhausted (Malagelada). In practice, however, it is night time secretion that is reduced and one 800 mg dose of cimetidine at bedtime has become the accepted way of using this drug. Ranitidine, equally effective, is given as 150 mg twice daily.

Aspects of Management

General and Specific.—The diagnosis is made on the basis of x-ray findings (of which deformity of the duodenal bulb is the most characteristic) and the presence of symptoms. Endoscopic confirmation of an ulcer crater is not indicated unless the diagnosis remains in doubt. The same general lines of treatment follow as for gastric ulcer in terms of dietary modification and avoidance of irritants. There is no evidence that smoking delays healing of duodenal ulcer, but reduction or cessation of cigarette smoking often alleviates persistent symptoms and reduces the likelihood of recurrence.

Relapses.—Most relapses in case of chronic duodenal ulcer disease will respond to the standard regime. As there is no evidence that H2-receptor antagonists alter the natural history of the disease, relapses may occur as expected, and two or three courses of treatment per year ('interval therapy') may be necessary. Prolonged treatment ('maintenance therapy') with a nocturnal dose only will keep symptoms at bay, and apparently prevent relapse. Since there is evidence that prolonged treatment may mask the symptoms of recurrent ulceration, complications of ulcer can occur on such a regime.

Prolonged Therapy.—In the present state of knowledge, there must be doubts about the wisdom of prolonged maintenance therapy; apart from the possibility of unwanted side-effects,[1] it is not always acceptable to patients, and it is also expensive. Where symptoms can only be controlled by such measures, assessment of the patient for elective surgery is advocated.

Warning.—Since duodenal ulcer disease may be lifelong, physicians must beware diagnostic complacency. Gallstone disease presents with similar symptoms, and 'ulcer' symptoms which do not respond to antacids or H2-receptor antagonists in a chronic duodenal ulcer patient should always raise the suspicion that there is other pathology, and lead to appropriate investigations. In uncomplicated cases, where symptoms rapidly respond to treatment, repeated radiology and endoscopy is neither helpful nor necessary.

SURGICAL TREATMENT

Indications for Operation.—Where healing has not progressed under medical treatment or where there is any doubt about the histology, operation is indicated. Less frequently, the ulcer may be in the antrum or in the prepyloric region. Antral ulcers have a 10% and prepyloric ulcers a 20% chance of being malignant when they are first diagnosed radiologically. These ulcers therefore must be regarded with considerable suspicion, and endoscopy with four quadrant biopsy

---

[1] Gynaecomastia has been reported in association with high doses of cimetidine.

Sir James Black, Contemporary. Pharmacologist, Wellcome Laboratories, Kent.
J. R. Malagelada, Contemporary. Gastroenterologist, Mayo Clinic.

is mandatory. Biopsy, however, is often difficult to achieve from ulcers in this region and requires the services of a highly skilled endoscopist. Where such a person is not available, it is wise to submit these patients to operation, because of the high risk of malignancy. Medical treatment unless covered by biopsy evidence, is unjustified in such cases.

It is wise to let the duodenal ulcer patient 'earn' his operation. If surgery is done early in the disease before he has had much pain or a complication, he will be likely to resent some of the sequelae of surgery. In general, the following facts suggest the need for surgery:

(a) Intractable pain, or recurrence of pain with frequent loss of work, failure to respond to adequate medical treatment.

(b) Complications, e.g. pyloric stenosis, hour-glass deformity, perforation, or bleeding.

(c) In general, ulcers which have been present for five years are unlikely to heal (Watkinson). It has been suggested that the risks of operation approximate to the risks of having a peptic ulcer for five years.

Assessment for operation.—Since the advisability of operation, the type of operation, and additional operative procedures may be affected by the results of assessing the patient, it is important to note:

1. The age, sex and general condition of the patient, including the cardiovascular, respiratory and renal systems.

2. The presence of pyloric stenosis, bleeding, combined gastric and duodenal ulcers, hiatus hernia, gallstones and other gastrointestinal disorders.

Aims of operations.—Surgical treatment for peptic ulcers aims to cure the ulcers with the maximum effectiveness, the minimum danger and side effects. The variety of operations performed testifies to the lack of agreement among surgeons. Because duodenal and gastric ulcers are considered to be *different disease entities*, the aims of operation differ for each type of ulcer.

Gastric ulcer.—Gastric ulcer is not associated with high levels of gastric acid secretion.

1. Orthodox surgical treatment aims at excision of the ulcer-bearing area and the stomach distal to the ulcer.

2. Improving the emptying of the stomach.

3. Prevention of complications.

4. To ensure that malignant ulcers are removed and avoid the risk of such a change in benign lesions.

Duodenal ulcer.—1. Operation aims to reduce the acid contact with the ulcer by diverting acid through a stoma as in gastroenterostomy, by removing part of the parietal cell mass as in gastrectomy, or by reducing stimuli to acid secretion by vagotomy and by antrectomy.

2. Correction of ill effects of the ulcer, such as pyloric stenosis, or haemorrhage.

3. Prevention of complications.

Mortality.—The average national mortality for gastrectomy is 2%, but this figure is greater in the elderly. The mortality after vagotomy with a simple drainage procedure is 0·75%. Gastrectomy is a more difficult operation and usually takes longer.

Geoffrey Watkinson, Contemporary. Physician, Western Infirmary, Glasgow, Scotland.

The sequelae of gastrectomy, and truncal vagotomy and gastric drainage, both immediate and remote, are now well established (p. 889).

Operations

For gastric surgery, the upper abdomen may be opened by a right paramedian incision. Having verified the diagnosis and ensured the absence of other pathology, the subsequent procedure differs according to the operation to be carried out.

Operations for Gastric Ulcer

The classical operation is the Billroth I partial gastrectomy.

The stomach is mobilised by division of the main arteries as shown in fig. 821. The distal part, including the ulcer, is resected. The cut edge of the remnant is partially closed, leaving a stoma at the lower end which matches the lumen of the duodenum. The duodenum may be mobilised by Kocher's method, with division of the peritoneum around its convex border, allowing union of the stomach and duodenum without tension (fig. 846). The stoma should be as large as possible.

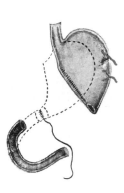

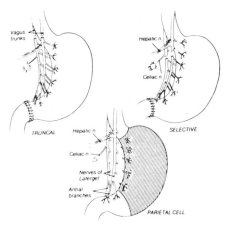

Fig. 846.—Billroth I operation. Dotted lines show rotation of the stomach, mobilisation of the duodenum, and the anastomosis in progress.

Fig. 847.—Diagrammatic representation of the three types of vagotomy. 1. Truncal vagotomy. 2. Selective vagotomy. 3. Proximal gastric (parietal cell or highly selective) vagotomy.
(Dr Paul H. Jordan, Houston, Texas.)

Selection of operation for gastric ulcer

1. Billroth I partial gastrectomy is followed by recurrent ulcer in less than 1%. The resected ulcer is available for histological examination to confirm that it is benign.

2. Billroth II gastrectomy with resection of the stomach below a high benign gastric ulcer invariably results in healing of the ulcer. The operative difficulty, and consequent risk, is reduced. The post-operative nutritional state of the patient is better following a conservative resection.

3. Vagotomy and pyloroplasty has been advocated as a conservative operation for benign gastric ulcer. Biopsy of the ulcer, with frozen section histology, is essential to confirm the benign nature of the ulcer. The theoretical basis for employing this operation is hotly discussed. In both 2 and 3 an ulcer cancer may be missed.

Theodor Kocher, 1841–1917. Professor of Surgery, Berne, Switzerland.

4. Proximal gastric vagotomy with excision of the ulcer has also been described, This has the advantage of disturbing the gastric physiology least and securing biopsy evidence of the benign nature of the ulcer. This method however is not fully evaluated and therefore not accepted by all surgeons.

Operations for Duodenal Ulcer

1. **Vagotomy (Vagus Nerve Section) with Gastric Drainage.**—Truncal vagotomy has the twofold effect of reducing hypermotility and hypersecretion of the stomach. Unfortunately it also causes gastric retention. It is therefore essential to perform some sort of 'drainage procedure' such as pyloroplasty or gastro-jejunostomy to correct this. Truncal vagotomy moreover may be followed by severe episodic attacks of diarrhoea.

The main varieties of vagotomy are as follows:

(*a*) *Truncal Vagotomy* (fig. 847).—The abdomen is opened by a right upper paramedian incision, the diagnosis is confirmed, and the other abdominal organs are examined. The left lobe of the liver is mobilised by dividing the left triangular ligament close to its hepatic attachment. The peritoneum to the left of the oesophagus is incised and the right index finger encircles the oesophagus in order (*a*) to pass the soft rubber tube which is used for traction purposes, and (*b*) to identify the position of the posterior vagus trunk, which is thicker than the anterior nerve trunks, and lies almost entirely free from the oesophagus. With the oesophagus taut it is possible to make a thorough search for and divide all the anterior vagal fibres. Two centimetres of the posterior vagus are resected.

(*b*) *Selective Vagotomy* (fig. 847).—The operation is not widely used.

Both of the above operations are associated with gastric stasis and pylorospasm following the vagal denervation and hence a gastric drainage procedure must be carried out (see below).

(*c*) *Proximal gastric vagotomy* (*highly selective vagotomy* or *parietal cell vagotomy*) (fig. 847) preserves the innervation of the pylorus and hence a drainage procedure is unnecessary. In this the anterior and posterior nerves of Latarjet are identified (fig. 823). Their terminal fibres reach the antral wall about 5–7 cm above the pylorus. They are preserved and with them the innervation of the pylorus. The stomach is now pulled to the left and its lesser curve laid bare from just above this point of entry of these nerves right up to the cardia. The main vagal trunks are now identified, drawn aside and the lower 5–7 cm of oesophagus are cleared circumferentially of the nerve fibrils and vessels. The operation has been widely adopted because of the minimal disturbance of gastric physiology consistent with adequate acid and pepsin reduction and healing of the ulcer.

(*d*) *Lesser Curve Seromyotomy* (Taylor, 1979). This procedure of either the anterior lesser curve with posterior truncal vagotomy or of both the anterior and posterior aspects of the lesser curve results in a similar type of gastric denervation to proximal gastric vagotomy. It has not become universally accepted.

2. Billroth II Gastrectomy

The lesser sac is opened through the gastro-hepatic omentum and the left hand introduced behind the stomach. Holding the stomach in this manner, the blood vessels and omentum along the greater curvature are divided and ligated. It is safer to do this between the gastro-epiploic artery and the greater curve. It is important at this stage to see that damage is not done to the spleen itself. The dissection is carried on to the first part of the duodenum below, and up to include the lower short gastric vessels above. The right gastric artery is divided. The duodenum is then divided and closed by at least two layers of inverting sutures. Great care is needed to avoid damage to the common bile duct. With the stomach held up, the left gastric artery is now divided. The stomach is turned over to the left and a clamp is applied to permit removal of about 60% of the stomach. End-to-side gastro-jejunal anastomosis is now made, so that the afferent loop is as short as possible.

Thomas Taylor, Contemporary. Manchester Royal Infirmary, England.

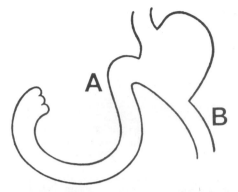

FIG. 848.—Polya type of gastrectomy. The duodenum is closed, and the first piece of jejunum is joined to the stomach remnant. A = afferent 'loop', B = efferent 'loop'.

If this is achieved by a retrocolic anastomosis at the duodeno-jejunal flexure it becomes the Polya variety of the Billroth II gastrectomy and the closure of the mesocolic leaf around the anastomosis is of paramount importance (fig. 848). There are still many surgeons who advocate an antecolic anastomosis. The addition of 'valves' offers no increased benefit. If the surgeon is not absolutely satisfied with the duodenal closure, a soft drainage tube should be put down to, but not touching, the duodenal stump (see p. 887).

Historical

In January 1881, Billroth of Vienna performed the first successful gastrectomy, and in September of the same year Wolfler introduced the operation of gastro-enterostomy. The original Billroth operations consisted of gastric resection followed by gastro-duodenal anastomosis (Billroth I technique).

In 1885, the Billroth II operation was introduced as a two-stage procedure, more by accident than design. A preliminary gastro-enterostomy was done on a gravely ill patient with a pyloric carcinoma. Contrary to expectations, the patient improved, and the stomach was resected, distal to the anastomosis. It soon became evident that the use of a gastro-jejunal anastomosis after gastric resection could be safer and easier than the Billroth I procedure. Now there are some forty modifications in technique of the Billroth II procedure—the main variations involving the use of an antecolic or retrocolic anastomosis, the direction of peristalsis in the jejunal loop, and the use of a full-width stoma or a restricted stoma with a 'valve'.

GASTRIC DRAINAGE PROCEDURES

There are three main types:

(1) **Gastro-jejunostomy.**—The essential feature of this procedure is to establish an anastomosis at the most dependent part of the stomach, which is the greater curve on the posterior wall. A short-loop posterior operation with a vertical stoma extending to the greater curvature (fig. 849) is the type of operation that gives the best results. In this

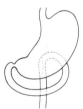

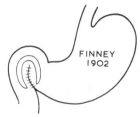

FINNEY 1902

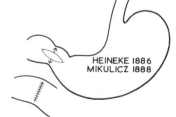

HEINEKE 1886 MIKULICZ 1888

FIG. 849.—The posterior, vertical, short-loop retrocolic gastro-jejunostomy of Mayo.

FIG. 850.—Finney pyloroplasty. The adjacent antrum and duodenum is approximated and an inverted U incision is sutured to give a wide gastro-duodenal anastomosis.

FIG. 851.—Heineke-Mikulicz pyloroplasty. A longitudinal incision of 6 cm is closed transversely by a layer of interrupted silk sutures, reinforced by a large omental patch.

Eugen Alexander Polya, 1876–1944. Surgeon, St. Stephen's Hospital, Budapest, Hungary.
Anton Wolfler, 1850–1917. Professor of Surgery, Prague, Czechoslovakia.
Walther Hermann Heineke, 1834–1901. Surgeon, Erlangen, Germany.
Johann von Mikulicz-Radecki, 1850–1905. Professor of Surgery, Breslau, Germany (now Wroclaw, Poland).
John Miller Turpin Finney, 1863–1942. Surgeon, Johns Hopkins Hospital, Baltimore, Maryland, U.S.A.

operation the stoma should be larger than in gastrectomy. Dragstedt and Tanner advocate an anterior anastomosis made in the pre-pyloric area. The risk of recurrent ulcer is less, and if it does occur, it is easier to deal with.

(2) **Pyloroplasty.**—The aim here is to produce free drainage by division of the pyloric ring. This can be done by two methods, that of Heineke-Mikulicz or that of Finney (figs. 850 and 851).

(3) **Antrectomy.**—In addition to acting as a drainage procedure, antrectomy also abolishes the hormonal phase of gastric secretion. A gastrojejunal anastomosis is made.

The operation is combined with truncal vagotomy. Care must be taken that all of the antral mucosa is removed; hence in practice, a hemigastrectomy is done.

SELECTING OPERATIONS FOR DUODENAL ULCER

The mortality rates and recurrent ulcer rates following different operations for duodenal ulcer are set out in fig. 852. Simple operations carry a low mortality, but a high rate of recurrence. More complicated operations carry a higher risk to life but are more effective in curing peptic ulceration. The operative risks are increased in elderly patients, in patients with concomitant disease, in those operated upon in emergency conditions because of bleeding. In contrast, all elective operations carry low risks in young, fit patients.

	Mortality	Recurrence
Gastrojejunostomy	Les than 1%	40%
Vagotomy + Gastrojejunostomy } Vagotomy + Pyloroplasty }	Less than 1%	5%
Highly Selective Vagotomy	Less than 1%	10%
2/3 Gastrectomy	2%	1–4–%
Vagotomy + Antrectomy (hemigastrectomy)	2%	1%

FIG. 852.—Mortality and recurrent ulcer rates following operations for duodenal ulcer.

Truncal Vagotomy plus a drainage operation is at present the most widely used procedure, but here the problem of postvagotomy diarrhoea, which is significant in up to 8% of patients and may be present in a lesser form in up to 30%, is a serious drawback (p. 891) and cannot be cured.

Selective Vagotomy.—Used very infrequently.

Proximal Gastric Vagotomy.—Data on the long-term results are not yet available. After it, the Hollander test for incompleteness of vagotomy becomes positive within a year in over half. It must not be carried out if the pylorus is narrowed by scarring. Although tedious to do, the patients seem to tolerate the operation easily and nothing is resected. The important point about this procedure is that it is not followed by diarrhoea, dumping or bilious vomiting (all complications that defy effective treatment). The recurrent ulceration rate is variously reported and may well be between 8 and 11%—but a recurrent ulcer can be treated either with drugs or by further surgery and does not represent a disaster for the patient.

Gastrectomy.—Must be recognised to be an ablative procedure and is not much practised nowadays for chronic duodenal ulcer, the long-term sequelae being regarded as too heavy a price to pay for a relatively benign condition.

Vagotomy and Antrectomy.—Is regarded by some as a reasonable alternative and less mutilating then gastrectomy itself, but the mortality rate for this procedure (fig. 749) is the same although the long-term sequelae are less than for gastrectomy.

Gastro-jejunostomy.—It would be remiss not to mention the great value of this operation as the *sole* procedure for the treatment of duodenal ulcer. It has been practised for the whole of this century and has given great benefits to hosts of patients. Its mortality is low, but unfortunately the ulcer-recurrence rate following this steadily increases with time, *e.g.* it may be as much as 40% within twenty-five years after operation. It still has a value, however, in the elderly (especially women) with pyloric stenosis in whom the gastric acidity remains low after ten days thorough gastric lavage. Women do not do well after gastrectomy of the Billroth II type and rarely, if ever, should a woman be submitted to this operation for simple duodenal ulceration.

LOCAL COMPLICATIONS OF CHRONIC PEPTIC ULCER

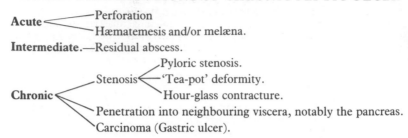

Acute — Perforation

Hæmatemesis and/or melæna.

Intermediate.—Residual abscess.

Chronic —

Stenosis — Pyloric stenosis.

'Tea-pot' deformity.

Hour-glass contracture.

Penetration into neighbouring viscera, notably the pancreas.

Carcinoma (Gastric ulcer).

PERFORATED PEPTIC ULCER

Sex.—The ratio is 8 men to 1 woman.

Age.—The highest incidence is between forty-five and fifty-five years.

Most often a peptic ulcer that perforates is situated on the anterior surface of the duodenum; much less frequently it is situated on the anterior surface of the stomach, usually near the lesser curvature or the pyloric antrum. Rarely an ulcer on the posterior wall of the stomach perforates into the lesser sac. In 80% of cases there is a history—often a long history—of peptic ulceration. In 20% there is no such history; it is a 'silent' chronic ulcer that perforates, especially in those patients who are being treated with cortisone. Usually the symptoms of perforation occur with dramatic suddenness.

The gastric or duodenal contents escape through the perforation into the general peritoneal cavity, resulting in peritoneal irritation (peritonism). At that moment the victim cries out in agony, and, at any rate if the perforation is a large one and the stomach is full, he is riveted temporarily to the spot where the perforation felled him. The peritoneum reacts to this chemical irritation by secreting peritoneal fluid copiously and this gives relief of pain for a short time. This *stage of reaction* lasts from three to six hours, and is followed by diffuse bacterial peritonitis.

Clinical Features

1. *Massive perforation.*—In the early stage of peritoneal irritation, the patient is pale, anxious, and loath to move. The temperature may be subnormal but the pulse is raised to 80–90. The abdomen is held still, moving little or not at all with respiration (fig. 853). The whole abdomen is tender with board-like rigidity. It is dull to percussion. Sufficient gas may have escaped to reduce liver dullness in the mid-axillary line. Pelvic tenderness may be elicited on rectal examination.

After three to six hours, the pain, tenderness, and rigidity may lessen. The temperature rises to normal or higher. However, the pulse remains high, the bowel sounds are absent. This temporary improvement has rightly been called the 'period of illusion'.

After six hours, the stage of diffuse peritonitis develops, accompanied by

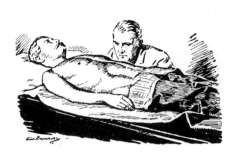

FIG. 853.—A sketch of Mr. Hamilton Bailey watching for abdominal movement on respiration. In cases of perforated peptic ulcer abdominal movement is restricted or absent.

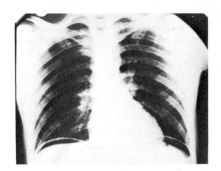

FIG. 854.—Plain x-ray of a perforated duodenal ulcer showing gas beneath the diaphragm.
(Dr. R. Vecht, Bristol.)

silent abdominal distention. Enough free fluid may have collected to be clinically detectable. The rising pulse rate marks the progressive deterioration in the patient's condition with each hour that passes without operative treatment.

2. *Subacute perforation.*—The pain may be less severe, less generalised with definite tenderness but equivocal guarding and rigidity when the perforation is small, and occurs in a robust, phlegmatic patient. Bowel sounds frequently persist. A small amount of fluid may track down the paracolic gutter, producing pain and tenderness in the right iliac fossa, simulating appendicitis. It is important to establish the site of onset of the pain.

Diagnostic aids.—A plain x-ray of the abdomen with the patient erect reveals a translucent area beneath the right cupola of the diaphragm in 70% of cases (fig. 854). Bile-stained fluid may be aspirated from the peritoneal cavity; it is alkaline to litmus.

Treatment.—Morphine should not be given until written permission for operation has been obtained. Operation, as soon as the general condition permits, is usually the best course. Laparotomy is performed and the typical oedema with a curious punched-out ulcer of the anterior wall of the juxtapyloric region is found. The perforation is closed with interrupted sutures reinforced with an omental patch. In the case of a gastric ulcer a biopsy *must* be taken as there is a risk of malignancy. In large perforations it is advisable to reinforce the suture line with a patch of omentum. *Thorough peritoneal toilet is essential.* With a mechanical sucker fluid and food debris are removed from the peritoneal cavity. Drainage of the peritoneal cavity is employed.

The immediate after-treatment consists of continuous gastric aspiration supplemented by intravenous fluid. Antibiotic therapy and breathing exercises are important in the elderly, and in cases where operation is more than six hours after perforation.

Pyloroplasty with vagotomy may be carried out only if the patient would merit elective surgery for the ulcer before the perforation occurred, if the perforation is recent, if the patient is fit, if the surgeon is experienced and backed by a fully trained supporting team (Kirk).

Follow-up of Patients after Perforation.—As might be expected, there is a transient remission of symptoms due to the rest in bed and the careful dietetic supervision during convalescence. Elderly patients and those of any age with a short dyspeptic history are likely to remain symptom-free after successful treatment of a perforation (Illingworth).

Sir Charles Frederic William Illingworth, Contemporary. Emeritus Regius Professor of Surgery, Glasgow, Scotland.
Hamilton Bailey, 1894–1961. Surgeon, Royal Northern Hospital, London.
Raymond Maurice Kirk, Contemporary. Surgeon, Royal Free Hospital, London.

Nevertheless, within one year 40% of patients relapse, and within five years 70%. On this account, those who survive perforation should be followed up as outpatients, so that if symptoms suggesting renewed activity of the ulcer occur, timely treatment can be instituted.

Residual Abscess.—This may occur after perforation in any of the subphrenic spaces (Chapter 49) or in the pelvis.

HAEMATEMESIS AND MELAENA

Aetiology.—

Chronic peptic ulcer	65% of cases.
Acute peptic ulcer Multiple erosions	} 30% of cases.
Oesophageal varices (Chapter 45) Carcinoma of the stomach Mallory-Weiss syndrome Peptic ulcer in a Meckel's diverticulum (Chapter 50) Purpura (Chapter 46) Haemophilia Pernicious and other anaemias Ehlers Danlos Syndrome	} 5% of cases.

(Compiled mainly from statistics by Sir Francis Avery Jones, London.)

Special Types.—Chronic Peptic Ulcer.—Slight bleeding due to trauma from solid food occurs frequently from all chronic peptic ulcers; such bleeding is demonstrated by finding traces of blood during gastric analysis and occult blood in the stools. With advancing age and the associated arteriosclerosis there is an increasing risk of severe haemorrhage due to the erosion of an artery in the base of the ulcer. Occasionally the artery is of considerable size, viz. the splenic or gastro-duodenal artery; more usually it is a branch of one of these vessels. Once a sclerotic artery has been eroded, even if it is sealed by clot, it is liable to bleed again (fig. 855). Even when a large vessels is eroded, death seldom results from the initial haemorrhage. Far more frequently a large haemorrhage is heralded by two or three smaller ones on consecutive days, as in other cases of secondary haemorrhage.

Acute Peptic Ulcer (p. 866).—This may be solitary or present as multiple erosions

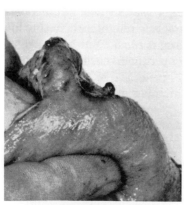

Fig. 855.—A gastric ulcer with an eroded and aneurysmal artery temporarily sealed by clot.
(Norman C. Tanner, FRCS, London.)

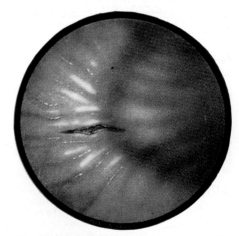

Fig. 856.—A healing mucosal tear extending across the oesophagogastric junction.
(Prof. Michael Atkinson, Nottingham, and the Editor and Publishers of 'Gut'.)

Sir Francis Avery Jones, Contemporary. Physician, Central Middlesex Hospital, London.
George Kenneth Mallory, Contemporary. Professor of Pathology, Boston University, Boston, Mass., U.S.A.
Soma Weiss, 1899–1942. Hersey Professor of Physic, Harvard University, Boston, Mass., U.S.A.

all over the stomach. The diagnosis is established by gastroscopy. It should be treated conservatively and all drugs withdrawn. Cimetidine (300 mg i.v. 2–4 times daily if renal function is satisfactory) may control the bleeding. It is particularly useful in stress ulcers.

Mallory-Weiss Syndrome.—This condition has specific features—the patient, usually a man over fifty, has a prolonged vomiting bout, often after imbibing alcohol. Having vomited gastric contents, he suddenly starts to vomit blood profusely and persistently, and becomes exsanguinated. As a result of the straining and retching a longitudinal tear of the mucosa just below the cardia occurs and gives rise to the sudden onset of haematemesis (fig. 856). The violent vomiting is sometimes due to migraine or vertigo. The diagnosis can be made on the history and is easily confirmed by gastroscopy.

In over 90% of cases the condition responds to sedation, blood transfusion and if necessary, pitressin. In the remainder, laparotomy is done and the linear tear exposed through a gastrotomy incision. It can then be sutured.

Clinical Features in General.—Initial features are usually faintness, sweating, and pallor; occasionally the patient collapses. Soon afterwards there is haematemesis, which is effortless, vomiting of coffee-ground material or bright-red blood. Later, black tarry stools (melaena) or red clotted blood may be passed per rectum.

Treatment.—*On admission* the collapsed patient is laid flat, with one pillow under the head, and the foot of the bed is raised. He is accorded the usual number of blankets for the time of year, and not heated artificially in any way. If restlessness is in evidence, morphine 15 mg is given intravenously and repeated in four hours if necessary. A plasma expander such as Haemaccel is given and if the situation is desperate due to hypovolaemia from acute loss of blood, type specific *uncrossmatched* blood must be given to avoid delay. The evils of the 'Shock Syndrome' will only be prevented if the blood volume and thus cardiac output and peripheral perfusion are rapidly restored. A pulse chart, if necessary half-hourly, is compiled, and a careful watch is kept on the blood pressure, central venous pressure, urinary output and peripheral perfusion.

Very soon after a severe haemorrhage the haemoglobin concentration is often unchanged, and therefore no reliance should be placed upon it at this critical time. After three hours, estimations, repeated at frequent intervals, provide helpful information.

Signs that bleeding has very seriously depleted the blood volume and is probably continuing are a cold nose, increasing pallor, increasing pulse-rate, beads of sweat on the forehead, and clammy palms of the hands (Chapter 5).

Management:

Conservative (Medical) or Surgical Regimen?—This decision should be made by joint consultation and co-operation between the physician and surgeon. They will take into consideration the following factors:

Response to Treatment.—Above all, if there is recurrent or profuse bleeding while the patient is under adequate conservative treatment, the call for surgery is compelling.

Age.—Seventy per cent of cases of bleeding are over the age of forty-five. After this age operation is increasingly necessary.

Chronicity of Ulcer.—The patient with a short history is more likely to respond to conservative treatment than one whose history suggests a deep penetrating ulcer. Sometimes, on account of cerebral anoxia, the patient's history is unreliable, when it will be necessary to obtain all possible information from the relatives. If he has been treated at another hospital, no time should be lost in contacting that hospital because all-important x-ray evidence may be forth-coming.

Ingestion of Drugs.—The patient must be closely questioned about the ingestion of aspirin, other non-steroidal anti-inflammatory drugs, or cortisone. If so, with-drawal of these drugs may suffice.

Condition of Arterial Tree.—The presence of arterio-sclerosis as evidenced by the history, the radial artery, fundal and electrocardiographic changes suggest the likelihood of recurrent bleeding.

Ancillary Aids.—As far as possible the exact cause of the bleeding should be made before operation:

Oesophagogastroscopy using the fibreoptic type of endoscope is the ideal means of doing this. The patient's pharynx is sprayed with local anaesthetic and sedation is achieved with Valium or other appropriate drugs. The instrument is then passed and the oesophagus examined. It is usually possible to exclude bleeding from varices in this way. If these are not seen, the instrument is passed into the stomach and the blood aspirated through its lumen. Should multiple clots be present the instrument is manipulated around them and often the site of bleeding can be located. Acute ulceration, erosions or the Mallory-Weiss syndrome (p. 883) may be seen. If blood is seen coming back through the pylorus, it is highly likely that a duodenal ulcer is the cause of the bleeding.

Conservative Treatment.—In addition to absolute rest, the essentials are:

Blood Transfusion.—When the estimated blood loss has been replenished, a drip trans-fusion is continued at the rate of 30 drops a minute for as long as is deemed necessary. The aim always is to render and maintain the cardiac output and peripheral perfusion. In addition, frequent pulse-rate, C.V.P. and blood-pressure readings are continued for a minimum three days after the apparent cessation of haemorrhage (Chapter 5).

Morphine.—Sufficient intravenous morphine is prescribed to allay anxiety.

H$_2$-Receptor Antagonists (p. 874).—These should be given intravenously.

Diet.—As soon as it is established that surgery is unlikely to be required a light diet is allowed. It is essential that an accurate fluid balance-sheet be kept. The patient is given the routine treatment for peptic ulcer (p. 874).

Prevention of Pulmonary Complications.—These patients are prone to develop respirat-ory infection, and not a few of them have bronchitis, with or without emphysema. Regular chest physiotherapy and prophylactic antibiotics are essential.

Operative Treatment.—A decision should be made within 48 hours of the commencement of bleeding, particularly if the patient rebleeds. Experience has shown that when operation is delayed beyond that time the mortality rises steeply.

Before the patient is anaesthetised it is essential to ascertain that the blood transfusion is capable of rapid acceleration. In this connection, sometimes it is advisable, in order to provide a stream of blood equivalent to that of the splenic or the gastro-duodenal artery, to set up a second transfusion into a second vein. The aim of the operation is to stop the bleeding. If a gastric ulcer is the source of the bleeding, gastrotomy and underrunning of the offending vessel is all that is required; the point being to limit the scale of the operation in an already sick patient. Rarely, gastrectomy will be required. Alternatively, vagotomy and a wide pyloroplasty may be carried out together with direct suture of the bleeding vessel in the ulcer base if it is duodenal.

When no ulcer is found on external examination of the stomach, a gastrotomy, extended to gastroduodenotomy, should be made to expose occult ulcers, erosions, vascular 'raspberry' malformations (Gius), and cardiac tears (p. 883). Whenever possible, bleeding should be controlled by suture, diathermy and local excision-biopsy with suture. A 'blind' gastrectomy should be avoided but, if deemed necessary, the Billroth II type is favoured.

John Armes Gius, Contemporary. Professor of Surgery, University of Iowa, Iowa City, Iowa, U.S.A.

Should no cause be found, examination of the rest of the gastrointestinal tract, and of structures which may bleed into the gut, must be meticulously performed.

CHRONIC COMPLICATIONS

1. **Pyloric stenosis** is usually the result of cicatrisation from a duodenal or juxta-pyloric ulcer. Not infrequently it is due to a carcinoma situated at or near the pylorus. Classically, pyloric stenosis occurs in women with a slow silent onset, but when there is a long standing history of ulcer the following modifications are evident:

History.—*Periodicity* is lost.

Pain and *fullness* become more pronounced towards evening. The patients can usually eat breakfast, a very small lunch, and nothing thereafter because they feel full.

Vomiting.—Very large foul and frothy vomits are characteristic. They usually occur once a day, commonly in the evening. Classically, the patient recognises currants or other undigested particulate matter eaten one or more days previously. Vomiting usually gives considerable relief.

On Examination.—In thin subjects the outline of the enlarged stomach can sometimes be observed. Visible peristaltic waves passing from left to right (fig. 857) are characteristic. A succussion splash is heard. These patients may be mentally confused as a result of alkalosis.

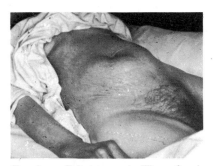

FIG. 857.—Pyloric stenosis. Wave of peristalsis passing from left to right. Note that outline of stomach extends well below umbilicus.

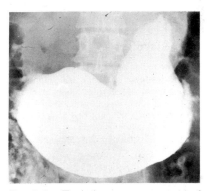

FIG. 858.—Typical x-ray appearance of pyloric stenosis.

Barium Meal.—The stomach is large and low (fig. 858), it is never empty, and the barium is mixed with food residue. There is much delay in its evacuation.

Treatment.—Operation in this condition carries a high mortality unless the patient is carefully prepared. Preliminary treatment by gastric lavage with saline through a wide-bore tube for 4–5 days, a high-protein fluid diet, and correction of electrolytes and vitamin deficiencies is necessary. Potassium and chlorides are usually deficient. A normal output of urine indicates adequate hydration (Chapter 6). Where chronic duodenal ulcer is the cause, truncal vagotomy and gastrojejunostomy is preferred because regardless of the degree of duodenal disease it is always feasible. Some have advocated Billroth II gastrectomy but the mortality is higher.

2. **Hour-glass stomach** occurs almost exclusively in women, is usually silent, and is due to cicatricial contracture around a saddle-shaped lesser-curve ulcer. In extreme cases the stomach is divided into two compartments, united by a channel which barely admits a pencil (fig. 859). The condition is sometimes associated with pyloric stenosis.

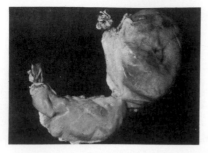

FIG. 859.—Hour-glass stomach.

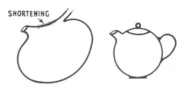

FIG. 860.—'Tea-pot' stomach.

History.—*Periodicity* is lost. The symptoms have become practically constant.
Vomiting is more frequent, and gives no relief to the discomfort.
The *appetite* becomes poor.
Weight.—Loss may be so great that carcinoma is suspected.
Barium meal is often characteristic. We have known of cases of hour-glass stomach being reported as pyloric stenosis, owing to failure of the second pouch to fill. True hour-glass stomach must be distinguished from gastric spasm of the hour-glass type, which is sometimes associated with an uncomplicated ulcer on the lesser curvature.
Gastroscopy.—The gastroscope enters the upper compartment of the stomach, and the narrow, scarred channel leading to the lower compartment is usually seen.
Treatment.—Billroth I gastrectomy, with removal of the second pouch and the isthmus, is the best treatment.

3. **Penetration of pancreas** may occur with posteriorly disposed gastric and duodenal ulcers.

History.—The main change is that pain is referred to the back and may be aggravated by stooping or exercise and *relieved by lying down*. The back pain may be so prominent that the patient is referred in the first instance to an orthopaedic surgeon.
Treatment.—Recognition of this feature of the ulcer is an indication for surgery, not only for relief of pain but also because of the possibility of torrential haemorrhage.

4. **Malignant Change.**—This only occurs in gastric ulcers and is rare in lesser curve ulcers proximal to the angulus (p. 868). Endoscopy and biopsy are essential if it is decided to offer medical treatment for an *apparently* benign ulcer.

History and Barium Meal.—This often gives no guide to the seriousness of the condition. The important point is a constant awareness of the possibility of malignancy *de novo* at all times. Over 20% of all antral ulcers seen on x-ray examination for the first time are malignant, or have been malignant, from the start. It should be remembered that even malignant ulcers may initially appear to respond to cimetidine.

5. **'Tea-pot' Stomach.**—Cicatrisation around a long-standing gastric ulcer often causes shortening of the lesser curvature, thus producing the 'tea-pot' deformity of the stomach (fig. 860).

'Tea-pot' or 'handbag' stomach is not uncommon. Unless the deformity is known to the radiologist it is likely to be diagnosed as a congenital abnormality or as the result of a carcinoma. These patients may present with symptoms and signs of pyloric stenosis.

COMPLICATIONS AFTER GASTRIC OPERATIONS

(1) Complications following any operation (*e.g.* pulmonary, cardiac, thrombotic).

(2) *Specific* complications of gastric operations.

A. **Early**	B. **Remote**
1. Haemorrhage from anastomotic line.	6. Recurrent ulcer.
2. Paralytic ileus.	7. Gastro-jejuno-colic fistula.
3. Stomal obstruction.	8. Post-gastrectomy syndromes.
4. Duodenal fistula.	9. Intestinal obstruction.
5. Acute post-operative pancreatitis.	10. Pulmonary tuberculosis.
	11. Anaemia.
	12. Decalcifying bone disease.
	13. Carcinoma in remnant.
	14. Gallstones.

1. **Haemorrhage from Anastomotic Line.**—If it does occur, morphia should be given together with a slow blood transfusion. If the haemorrhage is *severe* and *persistent*, the abdomen should be re-opened, continuous gastric lavage started and the anastomosis oversewn with continuous through-and-through catgut. The stomach is not opened. With control of the haemorrhage, the washouts become clear. If this measure fails, the stomach must be opened and the cause of the bleeding found.

2. **Paralytic Ileus.**—Is treated by 'drip and suction' (Chapter 51).

3. **Stomal Obstruction.**—This includes five different conditions: (*a*) Due to oedema of the actual stoma or of adjacent small bowel. This occurs more frquently after a gastro-duodenal anastomosis—hence the need for a large stoma in this operation. It is important to persevere with gastric aspiration and intravenous therapy maintaining correct electrolyte balance, especially of potassium. After a Billroth II gastrectomy, the stoma should function and the patient be absorbing fluids within 3 days. The Billroth I operation stoma often takes 5 days to open up.

(*b*) Due to the occurrence of *retrograde jejuno-gastric intussusception*. This, of course, only occurs after a gastro-jejunal anastomosis and may appear immediately or after many weeks or months. The stomach completely fails to empty and a filling defect can be clearly seen on x-ray with a small amount of barium. The intussusception may reduce following the barium or gastric saline lavage or the adoption of the sitting or standing position. If it does not respond to these measures (and it usually does in a few hours), an operation must be done to reduce the intussusception by gentle downward traction. An attempt may be made to anchor the loop by stitching or enteroanastomosis.

(*c*) Due to ball-valve obstruction of the duodenum by hypertrophied and oedematous mucosa of the antrum in a Billroth I anastomosis. Excision of the excess mucosa is all that is required.

(*d*) Due to technical factors—for example hitching of the efferent loop in Billroth II gastrectomy with resultant narrowing of the outflow tract of the stomach.

(*e*) *Apparent stomal obstruction* due to an atonic stomach. Endoscopy in this case will demonstrate a widely patent stoma.

4. **Duodenal fistula ('Blow-out')** is an infrequent, but very serious, complication of Billroth II gastrectomy with a maximal incidence about the fourth day.

Prevention.—There are two important points in technique.

(*a*) Construction of the stoma in such a way that afferent loop contents have free egress. A drain down to the duodenal stump, or even into the duodenum (formal fistula) are worthwhile safeguards if trouble is anticipated. When a blow-out occurs the duodenal sutures give way and, if drainage was not provided at the time of the operation, there is intense thoraco-abdominal pain, which is not infrequently mistaken for acute basal pneumonia with pleurisy. Unless prompt action is taken, diffuse peritonitis ensues.

(*b*) Avoid operating on a hot duodenum, *i.e.* where the ulcer is active and inflamed. Choose another operation, *e.g.* vagotomy and gastrojejunostomy.

Treatment consists in providing free drainage down to the duodenum with peritoneal toilet by suction. When drainage of the periduodenal tissues was not provided at the time of the gastrectomy, a small subcostal incision is made down to the duodenum. In either event, sump suction drainage is instituted until, and even after, the track of an external duodenal fistula has become defined. All oral fluids are stopped and the patient is maintained on total parenteral nutrition. Providing there is *no* distal obstruction the duodenal-cutaneous fistula will always close; it may however take some time and one of our patients took 43 days.

5. **Acute post-operative pancreatitis** is rare. The condition carries a high mortality rate. Treatment is along the usual lines (Chapter 48).

6. **Recurrent Ulcer.**—This includes the true anastomotic ulcer (gastro-jejunal, gastro-duodenal or jejunal ulcer) or a gastric ulcer in the remnant. True anastomotic ulceration has an incidence of 3% after a Billroth II gastrectomy, 5 to 7% after vagotomy and gastro-enterostomy, and up to 40% following gastro-enterostomy (fig. 861). The symptoms which appear usually within two years after operation consist of severe persistent pain, 'boring' in type, which is worse within a few minutes of taking food. The pain passes down the left side of the abdomen, sometimes into the perineum, but may be felt in the lower left chest especially following an ante-colic anastomosis. It is not relieved by antacids or milk. Bleeding manifest as haematemesis, melaena, occult blood, or secondary anaemia is common and perforation may occur. Gastroscopy is the most accurate way of making the diagnosis.

Management.—Conservative treatment with H_2 receptor blockers is nearly always effective but relapse occurs directly they are withdrawn. Other causes of abdominal pain must be excluded. A considerable number of patients with symptoms after gastric surgery fit into the 'functional' category and no relevant pathology can be demonstrated. They tend to be over investigated, under diagnosed and re-operation may be disastrous.

In patients with true recurrence, hypergastrinaemia and hypercalcaemia must be looked for. If present the appropriate further investigations and then treatment of the primary condition will result in healing of the ulcer.

(a) **Following Billroth II gastrectomy.**—An anastomotic ulcer may be obvious or require the opening of the anterior suture line. If the stoma is adequate and acid hypersecretion is present, vagotomy will cure the patient. If low acid secretion is found, revision gastrectomy with a fresh anastomosis to correct stasis is advisable.

(b) **Following Billroth I gastrectomy.**—Anastomotic ulcers should be treated by vagotomy. Recurrent gastric ulcer should be treated by higher gastrectomy, including the ulcer in the resected specimen. A Polya type operation is preferred.

(c) **Following gastro-enterostomy.**—Provided the stoma has not been narrowed by the scarring, vagotomy will effect a cure.

(d) **Following Vagotomy and a drainage operation.**—The Hollander Test (p. 857) should reveal incomplete nerve section. A search must be made for an intact vagal trunk in order to divide it. The drainage operation should not be changed but it must be functioning adequately. If an intact vagus nerve cannot be found, the operation should be converted to an antrectomy, preferably with Billroth I type anastomosis. If, however, a gastric ulcer is present, Billroth I conversion should be carried out, resecting the ulcer with the specimen.

7. **Gastro-jejuno-colic fistula**—is a complication of gastro-jejunal ulcer, and more often follows simple gastro-enterostomy than partial gastrectomy. The ulcer penetrates and erodes the transverse colon. Usually the symptoms of anastomotic ulcer disappear soon after the fistula develops, but in their place the unfortunate patient is troubled with severe diarrhoea after every meal, and eructates foul gas. Exceptionally the patient vomits fragments of formed faeces. Loss of weight and strength, dehydration, and anaemia complete the picture. It is important to stress that this final picture may be of extremely rapid onset so that the patient becomes desperately ill within two to three weeks. Severe malabsorption is shown by the presence of cachexia, hypoproteinaemic oedema, and steatorrhoea. The chief factor producing the rapid deterioration of the patient is the bacterial contamination of the jejunum by colonic contents with resulting disturbance of the absorptive mechanisms. It is *not* that the gastric contents pass directly into the colon. The diagnosis is established by a barium enema; in more than half the patients a barium meal may fail to reveal a fistula (fig. 862). *The sudden onset of severe diarrhoea in a patient who has a gastro-enterostomy must always raise the serious possibility of this condition.*

Treatment.—This consists of a resection of the fistula with repair of the colon and

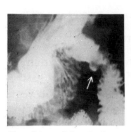

FIG. 861.—Jejunal ulcer
following   gastro-jejun-
ostomy.
(The late Dr. K. J. Yeo, London.)

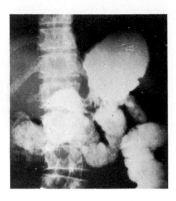

FIG. 862.—Gastrocolic fistula.
(Courtesy Dr Vachhani.)

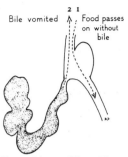

FIG.   863.— The afferent
loop syndrome. The food (1)
passes out of the gastric remnant before the bile (2) is
ejected.
(After Charles Wells, FRCS.)

jejunum, together with either vagotomy or a high partial gastrectomy. This can be one of the most difficult procedures that any surgeon may be called upon to do.

Some of these patients are extremely ill, and may require resuscitative measures, oral antibiotics and intravenous feeding before operation is attempted.

8. Post-gastrectomy Syndromes

Gastrectomy may cause reduced secretion of HCl, pepsin, intrinsic factor and pancreatic enzymes, inadequate mixing of food with enzymes and bile, reduced absorption of protein, fat, calcium, vitamin D and iron, rapid absorption of glucose, increased intestinal motility, and creation of a blind loop (*i.e.* the afferent loop, fig. 863).

The effects of some of those changes may appear a few weeks after operation, especially the post-cibal syndromes. It may be several years, however, before the absorption defects produce apparent nutritional disturbances.

The various **Post-gastrectomy Syndromes** therefore may be classified as follows:

A. Post-cibal Syndromes

(i) Early post-cibal syndrome (*syn.* early dumping).
(ii) Late post-cibal syndrome (*syn.* hypoglycaemia or late dumping).
(iii) Bilious vomiting.

B. Nutritional Syndromes

(i)	Weight loss.	(v)	Megaloblastic anaemia
(ii)	Steatorrhoea.	(vi)	Vitamin B deficiency.
(iii)	Diarrhoea.	(vii)	Calcium deficiency.
(iv)	Iron-deficiency anaemia.	(viii)	Gross malabsorption states.

By and large the higher the resection, the greater the risk of post gastrectomy troubles. In addition, these syndromes are best prevented if the normal duodenal pathway is maintained— and not by-passed.

Post-cibal Syndromes—Early and Late

In general, these occur more frequently in women than in men, and are seen following the Billroth II operation rather than the Billroth I. Time relation to meals permits classification into early and late varieties; the main features of these are summarised in the table on page 890.

The Early Post-cibal Syndrome.—This syndrome, consisting of abdominal and vasomotor symptoms, is seen in the majority of patients during convalescence, and persists in 5–12%. A variety of causes may be involved—rapid emptying of the stomach with increased small bowel activity, distension of the afferent loop, and a fall of blood volume (of the order of 13%), especially in patients susceptible to such changes. According to Le Quesne, there is a primary disorder of carbohydrate metabolism. Following the ingestion of glucose, there is initial transient hyperglycaemia. This suppresses further absorption

Leslie Philip Le Quesne, C.B.E. Contemporary. Formerly Professor of Surgery, Middlesex Hospital, London.

	Early	*Late*
1. Incidence	5–12%	5%
2. Relation to meals	Immediately afterwards	During second hour afterwards
3. Duration of attack	Thirty to forty minutes	Thirty to forty minutes
4. Long-term	Severe cases indefinitely	Two to five years
5. Relief by	Lying down	More food, glucose
6. Aggravated by	More food	Exercise
7. Precipitating factor	Bulk of food, especially if wet	Carbohydrates
8. Chief symptoms	Epigastric fullness Sweating Sensation of warmth Tachycardia Occasionally colic, diarrhœa	Tremor Faintness Epigastric emptiness Nausea
9. Occurrence	Commonest after Polya	After any type of gastrectomy

of glucose, which is retained in the intestine, resulting in fluid shift from the blood to the lumen of the intestine. Both increased intestinal activity and fall of blood volume may occur.

Treatment.—Time must be allowed to elapse for the syndrome to subside naturally. Meals should be small in bulk and dry. Milk and carbohydrate meals should be avoided. Belladonna or codeine may reduce intestinal activity. It is important to maintain the haemoglobin level as near 100% as practicable. When the syndrome persists, especially when associated with nutritional defects, conversion of a Billroth II anastomosis to a Billroth I is the operation of choice. Alternatively various conventional operations have been described all of which are designed to slow the rate of gastric emptying. For example, the interposition of a 10 cm antiperistaltic jejunal loop between stomach and duodenum described by Henley.

Late Post-cibal Syndrome.—This is not a common or a serious cause of symptoms. It is almost certainly due to a low blood sugar, occurs two hours after meals, and may be seen in some 5% of patients. After the initial hyperglycaemia there is a rapid fall of blood sugar to 50 mg (2·8 mmol/l)/100 ml or so. This rapid fall is probably due to increased insulin sensitivity.

Bilious Vomiting.—This symptom is usually an isolated feature but may be associated with dumping. It occurs in 10 to 15% of patients and consists of vomiting of bile unmixed with food. The vomiting is intermittent rather than after every meal. In the Billroth II operation the cause is probably transient obstruction of the afferent loop. This symptom can be eliminated almost entirely by a retrocolic anastomosis with the shortest possible afferent loop, *i.e.* into the duodeno-jejunal junction.

Nutritional Disturbances

Weight Loss.—This is a well recognised feature, occurring in some 50% of patients. It is the rule after total gastrectomy, common after the Billroth II operation, and infrequent after the Billroth I. It is due to reduced intake of food, and diminished absorption, and is particularly liable to occur in patients with postcibal symptoms. It is not necessarily serious, and indeed may have a beneficial effect. There is a reduced incidence of coronary disease following gastrectomy.

It is essential in these patients to exclude reactivation of previous tuberculous disease.

Steatorrhoea.—This has a similar incidence to weight loss, and is due to poor mixing of food and enzymes, reduced pancreatic output, and inactivation of pancreatic enzymes in the afferent loop. If it appears slowly after operation, the cause may be latent intestinal disease such as jejunal atrophy or the development of a cul-de-sac phenomenon (*i.e.* blind loop, fig. 1022) in the afferent loop.

Diarrhoea.—Most patients say that their bowel habits are much improved after gastrectomy, but some 5% have diarrhoea, either episodic or persistent. It may be related to intestinal hurry or to steatorrhoea. Diphenoxylate or loperamide may be helpful in managing this problem.

Iron-deficiency Anaemia.—This is a progressive condition after gastrectomy, and may be seen in some 40% of patients, particularly when the duodenum is by-passed. If occult blood loss is excluded, daily supplements of iron are essential.

Megaloblastic Anaemia.—Although invariable several years after total gastrectomy, it is rare following partial gastrectomy. It may occur as an isolated lesion due to gastric mucosal atrophy, or as part of a gross malabsorption defect (*vide infra*). There is evidence of reduced serum vitamin B_{12} levels in some 25 to 50% of patients five to ten years after partial gastrectomy. Intramuscular vitamin B_{12} (Cyanocobalamin) 100 µg weekly is given until the blood is normal; thereafter a maintenance dose each month is necessary.

Vitamin B Deficiency.—This occurs in roughly 10% of patients, and is manifest by angular stomatitis, glossitis, or peripheral neuritis. A regular supplement is the best method of prevention.

Calcium Deficiency.—Reduced acidity in the proximal intestine may interfere with calcium absorption, and some 40% of patients may become deficient. Bone changes may occur in some 5% and although such changes are usually seen associated with steatorrhoea, they may occur independently.

Gross Malabsorption States.—In less than 1% of patients, a severe malabsorption syndrome may develop. Conversion to a Billroth I is usually effective.

Post-vagotomy Syndromes

Effects of Vagotomy.—In addition to its gastric secretory effects, truncal vagotomy may produce undesirable side effects. The loss of gastric motility produces gastric distension, with delayed emptying, resulting in a persistent gastric splash, nausea, loss of appetite, foul eructations, vomiting and abdominal pain. Gastric ulceration may occur. The effect of vagotomy on the rest of the bowel is variable. About 30% of patients have an increase in bowel habits; of these a very small number suffer from variable diarrhoea which at its worst is urgent, episodic, uncontrollable and watery.

Vagotomy and inadequate drainage operation.—When no drainage operation accompanies vagotomy, gastric emptying may be inadequate, partly resulting from duodenal ulcer scarring, partly resulting from the reduced gastric motility following vagotomy. It is not possible to estimate the size of the pyloroduodenal canal by inspection from outside; moreover the site of narrowing is inconstant. Pyloroplasty in which the duodenotomy does not extend beyond any narrowing is similarly inadequate. A small, badly sited gastroenterostomy stoma may not allow the stomach to empty. Symptoms of gastric retention follow, and can be relieved by performing an adequate drainage operation.

Vagotomy and adequate drainage operation.—In spite of apparently adequate complementary surgery following vagotomy, some patients have symptoms of gastric retention after operation. Failure of gastric emptying may continue for up to 3 weeks, even though the stoma is patent and bile can be aspirated from the stomach. This functional disability slowly resolves. However, post-prandial fullness, regurgitation of bitter fluid into the mouth, and abdominal colic are experienced by some patients for longer periods.

The post-operative effects may be linked not to the vagotomy but to the complementary operation. As a result, the merits of each operation are hotly debated.

Because the symptoms tend to improve, conservative treatment usually suffices. The patient is advised to take small dry meals, with fluids taken between meals. Foods which are found to produce symptoms are temporarily discontinued.

Metoclopramide and more recently bethanecol 5 mg four times daily before meals (Catchpole) have been used with success.

Diarrhoea may be controlled by codeine phosphate or similar drug.

Recurrent ulcer after vagotomy.—The insulin test of gastric secretion confirms that vagotomy is incomplete. If the symptoms do not respond to medical treatment, re-operation is performed. If a vagal trunk is found and divided, provided that the existing drainage procedure is adequate, nothing more should be done. If no residual intact vagal fibres are found, gastric resection is necessary. If a gastric ulcer is found, gastrectomy should be performed. The possibility that the Zollinger-Ellison syndrome may be present should be borne in mind.

Intestinal Obstruction

(*a*) **Herniation Obstruction.**—In cases of a Billroth II gastrectomy with an antecolic

Bernard Newman Catchpole, Contemporary. Professor of Surgery, Perth, Western Australia.

anastomosis, small intestine herniates through a gap between the anastomosis and the transverse mesocolon, either from right to left or from left to right. It is easily prevented by a few stitches between the anastomosis and the transverse mesocolon at the time of gastrectomy (Stammers).

Clinical Features.—Usually symptoms of high intestinal obstruction commence between the third and eighteenth post-operative days, but often these symptoms soon become atypical because gastric aspiration is instituted after the first or second vomit. For the same reason colicky pains, so typical of intestinal obstruction, are often lacking; in most cases the pain is continuous, and increases in severity.

Treatment.—Even if the condition is only suspected, the abdomen should be reopened. The hernia is usually reducible, but gangrene has occurred from long delay. The gap should be closed as detailed above and gangrenous bowel resected if necessary.

(*b*) Bolus Obstruction.—The commonest cause of this is a piece of unmasticated orange pith which, in the absence of the pylorus, is able to pass into the small intestine and lodges about two feet from the ileo-caecal valve. Clinically, it is not unlike gallstone obturation (Chapter 51) but occurs in a younger age group. *Every patient who has had the pylorus excised or by-passed must be told to masticate thoroughly and not to swallow orange pith or dried fruits.*

Pulmonary Tuberculosis

Patients after both gastrectomy and truncal vagotomy with drainage show slight but definite increased susceptibility to pulmonary tuberculosis, probably due to reactivation of a latent focus owing to diminished nutrition.

Carcinoma

Following gastrectomy, especially for a gastric ulcer, the gastric remnant is slightly more prone to develop a carcinoma than is a normal stomach. This may appear after a latent period of fifteen to twenty years or more. It is because of such a complication following gastrectomy that the recent results of vagotomy plus a drainage procedure must be accepted with some reserve as carcinoma may follow this operation also.

Gallstones

There is no good evidence that the incidence increases after gastric surgery.

GASTRIC NEOPLASMS

Benign Tumours.—Although they constitute 3% of all gastric neoplasms benign tumours of the stomach are so over-shadowed by the frequency and gravity of gastric carcinoma that they tend to be forgotten.

Leiomyoma is the most common benign neoplasm of the stomach. Sometimes it grows mainly towards the serosal coat, in which case it is symptomless, and attracts notice only when it is large enough to constitute a painless, smooth lump in the epigastrium. It may cause a low-grade fever. More usually a leiomyoma protrudes towards the lumen of the stomach, and gives rise to melaena, mild indigestion, and epigastric pain, in that order. Haematemesis is, however, the most common symptom, and results from deep central ulceration of the tumour. Radiography after a barium meal reveals a space-filling lesion (fig. 864). Necrobiosis of the tumour has led to perforation of the serosal surface with intraperitoneal bleeding, and even to perforation of the stomach. Local excision is curative.

Neurofibroma and Neurilemmoma.—A tumour arising from a nerve sheath gives rise to exactly the same symptoms as a leiomyoma.

Adenomatous polypus, sometimes single, but more often multiple, is, as a rule, situated in the distal half of the stomach. Usually the symptoms are bleeding and abdominal pain. Achlorhydria is present in nearly all cases. Rarely a pedunculated adenomatous polypus of the pyloric antrum is carried into the pyloric canal, there to cause pyloric obstruction. The diagnosis rests on gastroscopy and/or x-ray. It is wise to regard multiple polypi as premalignant, and accordingly perform partial gastrectomy so as to include all the polypi; a single polypus can be excised locally.

Adenomatous Polypi and Pernicious Anaemia.—In pernicious anaemia there is severe

Francis Alan Roland Stammers, 1898–1982. Emeritus Professor of Surgery, Birmingham, England.

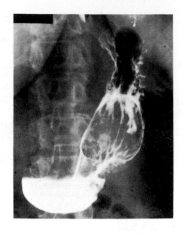

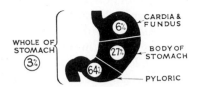

FIG. 865.—Incidence of carcinoma in various positions of the stomach.

FIG. 864.—Leiomyoma of stomach. A round space filling defect in the mid-stomach with small ulcer cavity at 3 o'clock.

atrophy of that portion of the gastric mucosa containing the fundal glands, and this provides a fertile bed for precarcinomatous adenomatous polypi to flourish. In about one in five cases of pernicious anaemia gastroscopy reveals adenomatous polypi. It is for this reason that patients suffering from pernicious anaemia are recommended to undergo annual gastroscopy and a barium meal.

An aberrant pancreas has been found arising in the wall of the stomach from time to time. Usually partial gastrectomy has been performed by a surgeon mistaking it for a carcinoma.

Menetrier's Disease.—A condition in which there is giant hypertrophy of the mucosa of the gastric fundus with cystic changes in the crypts, the antrum being spared. There is inconclusive evidence that the condition may predispose to carcinoma. It is associated with protein loss and may require surgical treatment, partial gastrectomy being the usual operation used. It should be distinguished from the hyperrugosity of the gastric mucosa, which may be associated with the Zollinger-Ellison syndrome (Chapter 48), but here there is no evidence of protein loss and there is acid hypersecretion.

CARCINOMA OF THE STOMACH

Carcinoma of the stomach is one of the 'captains of the men of death'. In 1959, 14,076 persons died from this cause in England and Wales but, fortunately, it now appears to be decreasing and the Registrar General's Mortality Statistics for 1984 indicate that 6,177 men and 4,183 women died of the disease that year. While from early adult life to senility no age is exempt, the highest incidence is between forty and sixty years of age. Three times as many males as females fall victims to this disease.

Aetiology.—There are a few definite pre-malignant conditions and risk factors. These are a gastric polypus, pernicious anaemia, the post-gastrectomy and post-truncal vagotomy stomach, autoimmune and environmental gastritis, gastric mucosal dysplasia, cigarette smoking, patients with long standing dyspepsia, genetic make-up and possibly, but only rarely, a gastric ulcer (p. 868). Ingested carcinogens seem to be important. Furthermore, substances that cause an irritative gastritis, such as neat spirits as drunk in Scandinavia, Holland, and Czechoslovakia, may increase the incidence of carcinoma. The geographical distribution of this disease is important and may prove a most profitable avenue in the study of aetiology. An interesting example of this is the differing incidence in the North and South of Iceland. Crude smoked salmon was the staple diet of the Northerners who have a much higher incidence than those in the South. Aird found a higher incidence of gastric carcinoma in people with blood group A.

Pathology.—*Macroscopically* five types can be recognised:

Pierre Menetrier, 1859–1935. French Physician.
Ian Aird, 1905–1962. Professor of Surgery, Royal Postgraduate Medical School, London.

Type 1.—A cauliflower-like growth with sharply defined edges. Its surface is indurated. Later it ulcerates.

Type 2.—An ulcer with an irregular indurated edge. Sometimes small superficial ulcers are present in the immediate vicinity.

Type 3.—Colloid carcinoma.

Type 4.—Scirrhous localised or diffuse (leather-bottle, fig. 868).

Type 5.—Carcinoma secondary to a chronic gastric ulcer (p. 868).

Early gastric cancer is classified into Type I: protruded; type II: superficial; type III: excavated.

Microscopically.—Since 1950 early gastric cancer has come to be recognised at first in Japan and later in all other parts of the world. These lesions are limited to the submucosa irrespective of lymph node metastases. The growth is usually columnar-celled, but cubical, and even squamous-celled neoplasms arise near the oesophageal orifice. The last type probably arises within the oesophagus.

Site: The most common site for the neoplasm is in the prepyloric region (fig. 865); when carcinoma follows pernicious anaemia, however, it is more likely to be fundal and polypoid.

The Spread of Carcinoma of the Stomach.—No better example of the various modes by which carcinoma spreads can be taken than the case of the stomach.

1. *Direct Spread.*—As the growth enlarges, it tends to invade neighbouring structures. The pancreas, transverse colon, mesocolon, oesophagus, or liver may be involved.

2. *Lymphatic Spread* (fig. 870): both by emboli and permeation.

3. *Spread by the Blood-stream.*

4. *Transperitoneal Implantation.*—Carcinoma cells sometimes pass from the stomach into the peritoneal cavity. They gravitate to the pelvis, where secondary tumours palpable on rectal examination may develop. On occasions, in the female, they alight upon the ovaries, giving rise to **Krukenberg's tumours**, which are liable to cause diagnostic confusion. These tumours are premenopausal, because after the climacteric the ovaries atrophy and thus are unlikely to give sustenance to tumour cells. In some cases Krukenberg's tumours are not the result of transcoelomic implantation, but are due to retrograde lymphatic permeation, especially from a carcinoma of the colon.

Clinical Features.—This is a very difficult disease to diagnose early, not only because of the diversity of its presentation but also because of the time-lag between the commencement of the growth and the appearance of symptoms:

1. Gastric distension: inability to take a normal meal, vomiting.

2. Anorexia leading to loss of weight.

3. Anaemia, tiredness, weakness, pallor.

4. Persistent pain; no response to treatment—no periodicity.

Clinical groups.—i. The '*new dyspepsia*' *after forty*—vague but *persistent* indigestion occurring in a patient who has never previously had 'stomach trouble'.

ii. *Insidious Onset.*—Especially in a man: he feels tired and weak, and the three A's may be in evidence—Anaemia, Anorexia, and Asthenia. Although the majority have an iron-deficiency anaemia, a few may present with a macrocytic anaemia.

iii. The *obstructive* types—carcinoma of the cardia presents with dysphagia; carcinoma of the pylorus with fullness, belching, and then vomiting.

iv. *Lump.*—The incidental discovery of a lump in the epigastrium, no other symptoms being present, is sometimes the cause of the patient seeking advice. In about 30% of cases a lump can be palpated.

Friedrich Ernst Krukenberg, 1870–1946. Ophthalmologist, Halle, Germany, wrote a classic paper on malignant tumours of the ovary in 1896.

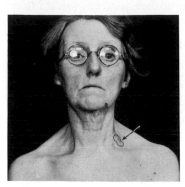

FIG. 866.—Troisier's sign found in the course of a routine examination for vague dyspepsia of recent origin. In this case there was a visible as well as a palpable mass of lymph nodes in the left supraclavicular fossa.

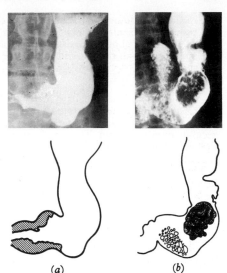

(a)   (b)

FIG. 867.—Barium-meal x-ray in carcinoma of (a) the antrum and (b) the body of the stomach.

v. *Silent.*—Carcinoma of the body of the stomach may be silent but give rise to features in other organs, such as obstructive jaundice due to secondary deposits in the liver, ascites from carcinomatosis of the peritoneum (Chapter 49), Krukenberg's tumours (see above), Trousseau's sign (phlebo-thrombosis of superficial veins of leg), or Troisier's sign (fig. 866).

INVESTIGATIONS IN A SUSPECTED CASE

If the diagnosis of this dread condition is to be made earlier, it is essential that attention is paid to the following investigations in *all* cases of indigestion.

Haemoglobin—anaemia is present in 45% of cases.

Occult blood is present in the stools in 80% of cases.

Where necessary, repeated tests should be done. It is important to remember that a negative test does *not* exclude a neoplasm.

Radiology.—While a skilled radiologist attains a high degree of accuracy in the interpretation of a double contrast barium meal, small lesions are liable to escape notice, particularly if too much barium is given initially. Irregularities of the cardia or fundus are inclined to be overlooked unless the technique includes an examination in the inverted position. Flat growths may remain undetected in the early stages. Radio-diagnosis is accurate in 90% for pyloric growths, 75% for the cardia, and 60% for neoplasm of the body, but in only 47% of patients with conclusive radiological findings (filling defects) (fig. 867) is the neoplasm found to be potentially curable by resection.

Gastric Secretory Studies.—The majority have either achlorhydria (p. 861) or hypochlorhydria.

Gastroscopy.—If the tumour can be visualised, its characteristics are obvious. Its nodularity, the presence of several irregular superficial ulcers, the multicoloured base, the immotility of the adjacent mucosa, all point to the nature of the lesion. Multiple biopsies are essential.

Armand Trousseau, 1801–1867. Physician, Hôtel-Dieu, Paris. It was this sign which first caused him to suspect his own gastric carcinoma.
Charles Émile Troisier, 1844–1919. Professor of Pathology, Paris.

Exfoliative Cytology.—Examination of cells found in the washings after gastric lavage has proved sufficiently reliable to confirm a diagnosis of carcinoma of the stomach in doubtful cases in about 70% of cases. Negative results are ignored.

Laparotomy.—If there is still reasonable doubt after all these tests, it is wise to explore the abdomen.

COLLOID CARCINOMA

The stomach appears infiltrated in all its layers by a kind of areolar tissue, the interspaces of which contain a transparent gelatinous substance. Groups of cancer cells often line the accumulations of colloid. The tubular glands are extremely distended with this substance. Colloid carcinoma represents about 6% of the total cases of gastric carcinoma. It is this type of carcinoma which classically gives rise to the Krukenberg phenomenon (p. 894).

The treatment is the same as that for leather-bottle stomach and the prognosis is almost equally gloomy.

LEATHER-BOTTLE STOMACH (*syn.* LINITIS PLASTICA)

There is a generalised and a localised form of leather-bottle stomach.

When localised, it is the pyloric antrum that is mainly involved. The stomach wall is enormously thickened (fig. 868), and feels, as its name implies, like leather.

The enormous proliferation of fibrous tissue involves especially the submucosa, which often appears as a dense layer, mother-of-pearl in appearance. Astonishingly, the whole of the mucous membrane looks and feels quite normal. It is often difficult or impossible to find any evidence of carcinoma, even in serial sections, but metastases are usually found in the regional lymph nodes. When distant metastases occur they are usually found in the liver or the ovary; on rare occasions bones are involved.

The symptoms are those of pyloric obstruction, but the small capacity of the stomach as revealed radiologically by a barium meal (fig. 869) makes the diagnosis tolerably certain.

Boeck's sarcoid of the stomach occurs occasionally (Chapter 9), and gives symptoms and x-ray findings identical with those of leather-bottle stomach.

Crohn's Disease (Chapter 50) may affect the stomach and mimic linitis plastica.

Carcinoma of the pancreas invading the posterior wall may be misleading.

TREATMENT OF CARCINOMA OF THE STOMACH

In the localised variety, partial gastrectomy, and in the diffuse, total gastrectomy, offer hope of prolonging life, but the results, especially in the more common generalised variety, are among the worst, if not *the* worst, of all varieties of carcinoma of the stomach.

No description of the treatment of carcinoma of the stomach is comprehensible without a knowledge of its lymphatic drainage (fig. 870).

The lymphatic vessels of the stomach arise in its submucous and subperitoneal layers, and divide into four main sets that accompany corresponding blood-vessels. Each set drains both the anterior and the posterior surfaces of the stomach, and although they intercommunicate, their valves direct the lymph flow as follows:

The lymphatics of the proximal half of the stomach drain primarily into the left gastric and the splenic lymph nodes, and thence into the left, middle, and right superior pancreatic lymph nodes.

The lymphatics of the antrum drain into the right gastric lymph nodes superiorly and the right gastroepiploic and subpyloric lymph nodes inferiorly.

The lymphatics of the pylorus drain into the right gastric (suprapyloric) superiorly and the subpyloric lymph nodes, situated around the gastro-duodenal artery, inferiorly.

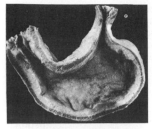

FIG. 868. — Leather-bottle stomach, showing the enormous thickening of the stomach wall.

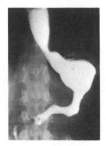

FIG. 869.—X-ray of a case of leather-bottle stomach.

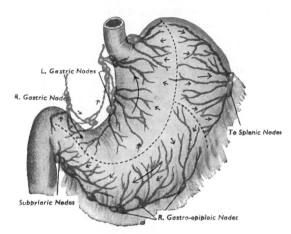

FIG. 870.—The lymphatic drainage of the stomach.
(*After Jamieson and Dobson.*)

The efferent lymphatics from the suprapyloric lymph nodes converge un the para-aortic lymph nodes around the coeliac axis, while the efferent lymphatics from the sub-pyloric lymph nodes pass to the main superior mesenteric lymph nodes situated around the origin of the superior mesenteric artery. The lymphatic vessels related to the cardiac orifice of the stomach communicate freely with those of the oesophagus.

Whether or not there is histological evidence of regional lymph node involvement makes a tremendous difference in the prognosis of *completely operable* cases of carcinoma of the stomach. It must be remembered that retrograde (or downward) spread may occur if the upper lymphatics are blocked.

Forty per cent of patients without regional lymph node involvement survive five years or more, whereas less than 10% with regional lymph node involvement survive this length of time.

Prognosis.—The most significant feature is the stage of the cancer. In Japan 90%, and in Birmingham (U.K.) 70·4% survived 5 years (age adjusted) following resection for early gastric cancer. These figures are to be compared with an overall 5 year survival rate following resection for more advanced cancers of 33% at best and 4·7% at worst.

There can be no doubt that radical resection of cancers of the distal stomach is well worthwhile and if the nodes are free of metastases the 5 year survival is approximately 50%. In fact, surgery is all that can be offered to these patients and therefore, virtually always, should be carried out.

Operative Treatment:

Nomenclature.—A 'curative' resection consists of removing a block of tissue, including the growth, a margin of at least 4 cm beyond its palpable limits with the stomach unstretched, and the related lymph nodes. The term radical gastrectomy should be reserved for a monoblock dissection fulfilling these requirements, thus bringing the term 'radical' into line with operations for carcinoma in other situations, *e.g.* the breast. Radical operations upon the stomach are of three varieties—(1) radical total gastrectomy, (2) radical upper gastrectomy, and (3) radical lower gastrectomy.

Incision.—Where possible an abdominal approach is to be preferred to an abdomino-thoracic. The latter carries an increased risk. The deciding factor for the use of an abdomino-thoracic incision is involvement of the gastro-oesophageal junction.

Operability.—As soon as the abdomen is opened, a firm plan, based on the extent of the growth, must be made. The decision is of profound importance and calls for considerable clinical judgement. There are three possibilities—radical surgery, palliative surgery, or the lesion may be inoperable.

Signs of Inoperability.—In general, these depend on the extent of the growth which include (1) fixation to the pancreas or posterior abdominal wall or involvement of the mesentery especially the origin of the superior mesenteric vessels, (2) gross local involvements of lymph nodes leading to fixity and evidence of retrograde spread downwards in the pre-aortic lymph nodes, (3) the presence of secondaries in the liver—an exception may be made in the case of a solitary resectable nodule, (4) peritoneal seedlings either locally or in the pelvis. A Krukenberg tumour does not of itself make the case inoperable.

Radical Operations

1. **Total gastrectomy.**—Indicated for growth involving the upper or middle two-thirds of the stomach. An upper left paramedian incision is made. The spleen with its hilar lymph nodes, the stomach, the splenic vessels, the tail and body of the pancreas are mobilised from left to right *en bloc*, the operation being essentially retroperitoneal. The left gastric artery and the splenic vessels are ligated retroperitoneally. The lymph nodes around the coeliac axis and cardiac orifice are freed, and the lesser omentum is detached as far from the stomach as possible. Similarly, the subpyloric lymph nodes are mobilised and the greater omentum is detached from the transverse colon. The cut edge of the pancreas is closed with sutures and a soft rubber drain is passed down to this site, to be brought out through a separate stab incision. The stomach having been excised, the continuity of the alimentary canal can be restored in the manner shown in fig. 871; this procedure is valuable because it prevents regurgitation of bile and pancreatic juice into the oesophagus, which is so vulnerable to these digestive ferments. An oesophago-duodenostomy should not be done as an *alkaline* oesophagitis so frequently follows. If a thoraco-abdominal incision has been necessary, the diaphragm must be carefully repaired with non-absorbable sutures. Waterseal drainage of the pleural cavity is instituted.

Post-operative Care of Total Gastrectomy.—Here nutritional disorders, *e.g.* weight loss, steatorrhoea, and macrocytic anaemia are the rule. The first two appear early but the anaemia takes five or six years to develop. These patients need frequent small meals of high protein, high calorie content, and regular vitamin B_{12} supplements (100 to 200µg monthly).

2. **Partial Gastrectomy.**—This operation for carcinoma of the pyloric end of the stomach involves separation of the greater omentum from the colon in its entirety, separation of the lesser omentum from the liver, freeing the subpyloric lymph nodes, and removal of the spleen and body and tail of the pancreas. The left gastric vessels and the right gastro-epiploic vessels are divided at their origin, stripping all fatty and lymphatic tissue around them towards the stomach. The operation is then completed by a Billroth II anastomosis.

Palliative Operations

1. *Partial Gastrectomy.*—Offers the best palliation, whatever the extent of the lesion or the involvement of adjacent structures. It is feasible in 70% of cases. A Billroth II type is preferred.

2. *Gastro-jejunostomy.*—For irremovable pyloric carcinoma gastro-jejunostomy should be performed some distance from the tumour, so that the advancing growth will not invade the stoma, at any rate for some time.

3. For *obstruction of the cardia* considerable relief can be obtained by the introduction of a *plastic tube* (Chapter 43). This is the most valuable manoeuvre in those patients whose days are numbered. It is preferable to a palliative oesophago-jejunostomy which carries a high operative mortality in these debilitated patients.

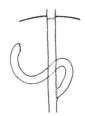

FIG. 871.— Total gastrectomy with oesophago jejunostomy-en-Y (Roux's method).

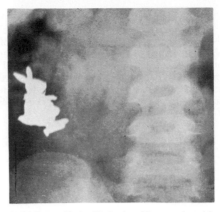

FIG. 872.—Embedded in Normacol, this foreign body was passed naturally in three days.

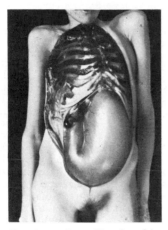

FIG. 873.—Acute dilatation of the stomach seen at necropsy.

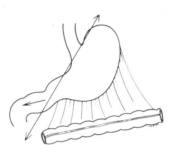

FIG. 874.—Volvulus of stomach—common axis of rotation.

SARCOMA OF THE STOMACH

Sarcoma of the stomach accounts for about 1% of gastric neoplasms.

Lymphosarcoma is the most common variety. In contradistinction to lymphosarcoma of the small bowel which is multiple, this tumour is usually solitary. In all inoperable cases a piece of the growth should be removed for histological examination. Although radio-sensitive, the best treatment, if circumscribed, is gastrectomy. Chemotherapy may be useful.

Leiomyosarcoma.—The first symptom may be a massive haematemesis and/or melaena. The presence of a barium-filled sinus extending into the tumour visualised by x-rays is extremely characteristic of leiomyosarcoma. Unlike a carcinoma of similar dimensions, the gastric acidity is unchanged. Usually these tumours metastasise late, and, when they do, secondary growths are often found in the liver. The treatment is partial gastrectomy. The tumour is more vascular than a carcinoma. It is stressed particularly that leiomyosarcomas should be attacked with vigour, regardless of the magnitude of the procedure, as the results are so much more gratifying than those of carcinoma of the stomach. At least 50% of the patients are alive five years after the operation.

Neurofibrosarcoma behaves precisely as a leiomyosarcoma, from which it is distinguished only by histological examination.

Fibrosarcoma, derived from the subserosa, is the rarest variety and the least malignant; it sometimes gives rise to a tumour of immense size, and in the female such a tumour is liable to be mistaken for an ovarian cyst.

César Roux, 1857–1934. Professor of Surgery and Gynaecology, Lausanne, Switzerland. Described this method of forming a jejunal conduit, which has so many uses in modern gastro-intestinal surgery, in 1908.

DUODENAL NEOPLASMS

Neoplasms of the duodenum are very rare. Adenomas have been reported as causes of severe melaena. Carcinoma of the first part of the duodenum is so rare that many of great experience have never seen a case. There is an apparent bar to spread of carcinoma of the pyloric end of the stomach into the duodenal mucosa, but there is no such obstacle to the spread in the subserous layer which, indeed, occurs with some frequency—hence the necessity for excising 2·5 cm of the duodenum when performing radical lower partial gastrectomy. Carcinoma of the second and third parts occurs. It may occlude the ampulla of Vater.

MISCELLANEOUS CONDITIONS OF THE STOMACH AND DUODENUM

Foreign Bodies in the Stomach

A variety of ingested foreign bodies reach the stomach. Fortunately, for the most part they are opaque to x-rays (fig. 872). Sharply pointed or long objects are best removed promptly by gastrotomy because they have difficulty in negotiating the curves of the duodenum. Rounded, smaller foreign bodies may be left to pass along the natural passages. Suitable doses of Normacol form a gelatinous pabulum, in which the article becomes embedded during its transit along the alimentary tract. X-ray examinations should be undertaken sparingly.

Hair-ball of the Stomach (Trichobezoar).—An example of this rare condition is usually to be found on the shelves of pathological museums. Trichobezoars occur almost exclusively in females, and in 80% of cases the patient is a psychiatric case. Trichobezoars can give rise to gastro-duodenal ulceration leading to haematemesis, perforation, peritonitis, or obstruction. A trichobezoar shows well on radiography. The treatment is removal by gastrotomy.

Acute Dilatation of the Stomach (fig. 873)

Unfortunately this term has been allowed to slip into surgical teaching as though it was some mysterious condition. It frequently represents poor post-operative care in which an undiagnosed or inadequately treated paralytic ileus results in gastric retention. Fluid, often in large volumes, is sequestered in the stomach and upper intestine and if the patient is at the same time dehydrated then hypovolaemic reduction in cardiac output results. The way to avoid this sequence of events is to maintain drip and suck and a proper fluid and electrolyte balance. The volume of fluid vomited by the patient can be so large that spill-over into the lungs can occur, causing an acute shock-like state (Mendelsohn reaction). The condition is not limited to operations on the stomach.

Volvulus of the Stomach

Rotation of the stomach usually occurs around the axis made by its two fixed points, *i.e.* the cardia and the pylorus (fig. 874). Although the rotation can occur in a horizontal or vertical direction, in its common form the greater curve with the colon moves upwards to lie under the cupola of the left diaphragm (fig. 875). An important predisposing cause of this event is eventration of the diaphragm from whatever cause. It is probable that the colon moves up first and takes the stomach with it. The condition is usually intermittent, but it may present in an acute form. The patient takes a small amount of food and he feels

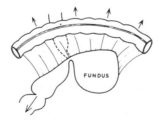

FIG. 875.—Volvulus of stomach—colon passes upwards and greater curve of stomach is inverted.

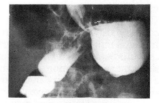

FIG. 876.—Volvulus of stomach—barium meal findings.

full; there is slight epigastric pain and retching. He has to wait a while, and he may find that if he lies flat he can then eat some more. The diagnosis is established by a barium meal (fig. 876). It is often impossible to pass a stomach tube.

Treatment.—Operation is the only satisfactory form of treatment. The greater curvature of the stomach must be completely freed from the colon by division of the gastrocolic omentum. It is probable that this of itself is adequate. A further safeguard, however, consists of fixing the greater curve to the duodeno-jejunal flexure (or better, the fourth part of the duodenum), as in a posterior gastro-enterostomy but without a stoma.

Where the rotation occurs as the result of and into a large hiatal defect, the essential treatment consists of closure of the hiatus around the oesophagus.

Gastric Tetany

Tetany due to alkalosis may occur where there is a long-continued vomiting, gastric aspiration, or excessive ingestion of alkali. The extracellular alkalosis is always accompanied by cellular acidosis, potassium depletion, and a fall in the blood calcium (parathyroid tetany). Clinically there are muscle spasms in the extremities, shallow respiration, and cyanosis. The stomach must be kept empty by a tube and the blood electrolytes estimated so that the specific deficiencies may be rapidly corrected. Whilst these are being done, continuous intravenous dextrose saline with calcium gluconate should be given. Even when the chloride deficit is corrected, the alkalosis may persist and this is indicative of the need for potassium.

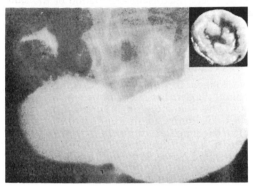

Fig. 877.—Prolapsing gastric mucosa. Inset.—The prolapse viewed from the duodenal aspect of the pylorus.
(L. H. Appleby, FRCS, Vancouver.)

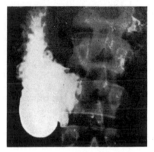

Fig. 878.—Duodenal ileus. Note the abrupt obstruction to the third part of the duodenum.

Prolapsing Gastric Mucosa.—This is an x-ray finding. Hypertrophied gastric mucosa prolapses through the pylorus (fig. 877 (inset)). Pyloric obstruction has been attributed to this phenomenon.

Giant rugal hypertrophy of the stomach is a descriptive name given to a condition which may manifest itself clinically as a protein-losing gastro-enteropathy. Recognition of this feature may necessitate gastrectomy. The thick folds can be demonstrated radiologically, seen at gastroscopy, and palpated at laparotomy. There is not the slightest evidence that this condition is premalignant, nor is it inflammatory.

Duodenal Diverticulum

There are two varieties:

1. **Primary diverticulum** of the second and third parts of the duodenum. They occur on the concave border, are usually single but may be multiple, and commonly arise at the portal of entry of the blood-vessels into the duodenal wall. In 90% of cases they are an incidental finding during the course of a barium meal. It is wise not to incriminate them as a cause of symptoms but to make a thorough search for pathology elsewhere. Rarely, a large diverticulum near the ampulla of Vater may cause jaundice. In addition, if a diverticulum is persistently tender when visualised during screening or if it retains barium

for days, then it may be justifiable to operate. The duodenum is mobilised, turned medially, and the diverticulum dissected free. The duodenum is then opened opposite the diverticulum which is seized, inverted into the lumen, and is ligated. The duodenum is then closed and the fascia over the site of the diverticulum oversewn. The duodenum is deficient of peritoneum in this area and the operation may be complicated by a fistula.

2. **Secondary Diverticula.**—These occur in the first part of the duodenum and are the result of scarring following duodenal ulceration. They are responsible for the trifoliate duodenum seen on x-ray.

Chronic duodenal ileus is a rare condition which may mimic pyloric stenosis. The duodenum is dilated up to the superior mesenteric vessels. The dilated segment has a characteristically smooth outline (fig. 878). It is a radiological diagnosis rather than a clinical one. Some advocate duodeno-jejunostomy for this condition, but the results are disappointing.

Duodenal Fistula

The most usual causes are as follows:
1. As a complication of gastrectomy.
2. An abscess connected with a perforated duodenal ulcer.
3. Traumatic rupture of the duodenum (see below).
4. As a complication of transduodenal sphincterotomy, right nephrectomy, or right colectomy.

The fistula discharges bile and pancreatic juice which cause excoriation of the skin. Excessive discharge may quickly lead to dehydration, electrolyte imbalance, and hypoproteinaemia. The management consists essentially of three procedures:
1. Protection of the skin with a barrier cream.
2. Continuous and efficient suction drainage of the fistula which may be facilitated by gravity—the patient lying prone.
3. Stopping all oral intake.
4. Total parenteral nutrition for however long it takes the fistula to close.

Note that it is essential to exclude any distal duodenal or intestinal obstruction.

Traumatic Rupture of the Duodenum.—This is an increasingly common problem in hospitals near a fast main road (see seat belt syndrome, Chapter 49). If the rupture is extraperitoneal the initial symptoms are often slight and the condition is overlooked until an abscess forms. When the abscess is opened a fistula develops. With intraperitoneal rupture the clinical features resemble a perforated duodenal ulcer. Laparotomy is performed and the tear can usually be sutured.

Traumatic fistulae of the first part usually close spontaneously—those of the second and third part are formidable indeed. They present such a grave problem that it is worth considering a duodeno-jejunal anastomosis to overlie the defect if this cannot be closed easily at the primary operation.

CHAPTER 45

THE LIVER

Surgical Anatomy and Physiology.—The dual afferent blood supply, consisting of the hepatic artery and the portal vein, singles out the liver from all other organs. That the portal vein has no valves is basic to the understanding of portal hypertension. Both the portal and the hepatic veins have well-defined coats of unstriated muscle which together with the hepatic artery control the blood flow through the liver.

The blood in the sinusoids is derived from two sources:

1. The portal system conveys between 60 and 80% of the afferent blood to the liver, together with the products of digestion from the alimentary canal and the endocrine secretions, from the stomach, pancreas and small intestine. No less than one-fifth of the portal blood comes from the spleen.

2. The hepatic artery which supplies 25% of the 1500 ml blood that enters the liver each minute provides oxygen for the liver, and, by a delicate pressure arrangement with the portal venules determines the blood flow through the liver lobules. The pressure relationships of the hepatic artery (100–150 mmHg), the portal vein (8–12 mmHg) and the hepatic veins (1–4 mmHg) testify further as to the unique nature of the circulation through the liver. During exercise the blood flow through the liver, normally about 40% of the cardiac output, falls sharply in favour of the heart, brain and muscles.

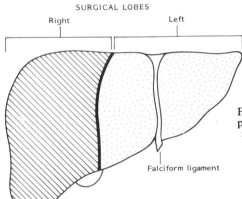

SURGICAL LOBES

Right   Left

Falciform ligament

FIG. 879.—The 'surgical' lobes of the liver compared with the usual anatomical division into right and left lobes by the falciform ligament.

Surgical Lobes of the Liver (fig. 879)

The right and left branches of the hepatic artery do not supply the two main anatomical lobes as such. Their territory has a boundary running along the gall-bladder bed and thence upwards over the anterior surface to the inferior vena cava, down this vessel to return to the porta hepatis. The biliary ducts and branches of the portal vein follow the hepatic arterial branches. In this way the liver is divided into two surgical lobes, right and left, by a major avascular fissure. The blood from the liver is drained by three major hepatic veins, the middle one of which is located in the major fissure. Knowledge of the anatomy of the surgical lobes is particularly important in planning hepatic resections for injury or tumours.

Functions of the Liver:

1. The formation of bile and the metabolism of bilirubin and of bile salts.
2. The synthesis of albumin, fibrinogen, and prothrombin.

3. Storage and metabolism of carbohydrates, including the conversion of monosacchar-ides (*e.g.* dextrose) into glycogen, and vice versa.

4. Formation of phospholipids and cholesterol, synthesis of fatty acids from carbo-hydrate, and other steps in fat metabolism.

5. Deamination of amino-acids with formation of urea. Removal of ammonia from portal blood.

6. Heat production. Intermediate metabolism, both anabolic and catabolic, in the liver requires a large amount of energy derived from the conversion of adenosine triphosphate (ATP) to adenosine diphosphate (ADP) as well as aerobic oxygenation via the Krebs cycle. A byproduct of these activities is the production of an excessive amount of energy in the form of heat.

7. Reticulo-endothelial activities.

8. Storage of vitamin B12 (cyanocobalamin) and vitamin A.

9. Iron and copper storage.

10. Destruction of bacteria. Bacteria, especially Gram-positive cocci, have been found repeatedly in samples of portal blood taken at laparotomy for non-infected conditions. It is therefore believed that the liver destroys many bacteria that gain entrance to the body through the portal tributaries.

11. Detoxication of drugs and hormones, *e.g.* benzodiazopines; oestrogens.

Regeneration.—Unlike other organs, the liver possesses a remarkable ability to replace lost tissue rapidly and completely by compensatory cellular hypertrophy and hyperplasia. This permits wide resection for a localised hepatic neoplasm, and removal of large portions of doubtfully viable liver tissue in cases of severe trauma.

HEPATOCELLULAR FAILURE

Hepatocellular failure can complicate almost all forms of liver disease and may be precipitated by intercurrent infection, a surgical operation, administration of a general anaesthetic, bleeding or even narcotics.

Clinical Features.—The most marked features are weakness and general fail-ure in health. Jaundice is usually present. The hyperdynamic circulation is mani-fested by flushed extremities and bounding pulse. The patient may be cyanosed. Fever is common and septicaemia is found terminally. Foetor hepaticus, a sweet-ish, musty odour, is frequently noticeable. Spider angiomas are found in the vascular territory of the superior vena cava. Appearance of fresh crops of spider naevi suggest progressive liver disease and their disappearance accompanies improving hepatic function. Palmar erythema (liver palms) affects mainly the thenar and hypothenar eminencies.

Other changes include loss of axillary and pubic hair, and white nails. In the male, gynaecomastia and testicular atrophy may be found in chronic hepatic failure of the cirrhotic.

On occasion, as the result of massive death of liver cells, usually in acute viral hepatitis, there may be sudden, severe impairment of hepatic function—*fulminant hepatic failure.* Acute liver failure has also been observed following exposure to drugs, such as carbon tetrachloride, multiple exposures to halothane and after cytotoxic drugs. Personality changes occur, proceeding to delirium, nightmares and uncooperative behaviour, in addition to those features described above. There is usually an accompanying failure of the kidneys.

Treatment.—Precipitating factors must be looked for and treated. Gastro-intestinal haemorrhage may require blood transfusion; an acute infection may be dealt with by antibiotics. Electrolyte abnormalities, especially hypokalaemia, should be corrected.

If the patient can eat, a high carbohydrate diet should be given. Nutrition and

Hans Christian Joachim Gram, 1853–1938. Professor of Medicine, Copenhagen.

fluid intake have to be maintained in the unconscious patient by the use of a nasogastric tube or intravenous infusion. Diuretics, morphine and paraldehyde should be avoided because they may precipitate or potentiate coma.

In acute failure with coma, very skilled and intensive treatment is required. Hypoglycaemia and electrolyte abnormalities will require particular attention. For renal failure with hyperkalaemia, peritoneal or haemodialysis should be performed. Bleeding due to abnormalities in clotting mechanisms and infection will require skilled haematological and bacteriological treatment. The overall mortality of fulminant hepatic failure is high, between 70–90% in comatose patients, but spontaneous recovery has been noted in 10–20% of patients.

For patients whose condition is not responding, but who are thought to have potentially reversible failure, temporary hepatic support should be considered. These measures include exchange blood transfusion, cross circulation between donor and patient, extracorporeal perfusion of the patient's blood through a pig's liver and, recently, perfusion of the patient's blood through columns of activated charcoal. The results of these various treatments are uncontrolled and their long-term benefit remains doubtful.

PORTA-SYSTEMIC ENCEPHALOPATHY

This chronic fluctuating neuropsychiatric disorder occurs when much blood is bypassing the liver (either because of cirrhosis or via a surgically-created porta-systemic shunt) and when there is a degree of hepatic insufficiency. Toxic products of bacterial degradation of nitrogenous material within the bowel are normally absorbed and are removed by the liver. In chronic liver disease—and also because of direct access to the systemic circulation via collateral vessels, surgical shunts or intra-hepatic communications—these toxic products may reach the brain where they exert a deleterious effect. Ammonia is probably one of the toxic products responsible for hepatic encephalopathy, but amino-butyric acid, mercaptan, methionine and short chain fatty acids have also been incriminated. These products are normally metabolised in the liver, and the syndrome rarely occurs unless the liver function is impaired. It thus tends to be precipitated by a large protein meal or an upper gastro-intestinal haemorrhage. Other precipitating factors include potassium depletion, frequently accompanying drug-induced diuresis, uraemia and narcotics. In individual patients it is often difficult to determine to what extent the symptoms are due to this cause or to liver-cell damage. In patients who have had symptoms for some years, organic changes have been found in the cerebral cortex or in the spinal cord.

Clinical Features.—It is characterised by disorientation and a flapping tremor of the outstretched hands. Cogwheel rigidity of the limbs and ankle clonus may be elicited, and the patient may pass rapidly into deep coma. Intellectual deterioration and changes in personality, slurring of speech, can be observed frequently. On the electroencephalogram there is marked slowing of the frequency down to the delta range. Sometimes the brain may recover equally rapidly when the source of the toxic products is removed from the alimentary canal.

Treatment.—Measures to reduce the amount of nitrogenous material in the bowel, its breakdown by bacteria and its absorbtion are effective, viz:

1. Restriction of dietary protein (less than 20 g daily).

2. Removal of blood from bowel by purgation (Mag. Sulph. 5–15 g), enemas.

3. Administration of antibiotics orally or rectally, especially non-absorbed antibiotics such as neomycin (1 g 4 times daily).

4. Oral lactulose (a disaccharide), whose mode of action is still unclear, may be of value (30–50 ml, 3–4 times daily).

Other measures include the avoidance of sedatives and the correction of vitamin and electrolyte deficiencies.

SPECIAL METHODS OF INVESTIGATING THE LIVER

A. Liver Function Tests.—Owing to its many and varied functions, there is no single test by which the liver can be stated to be functioning normally. Therefore several tests are usually undertaken in each patient, and in some instances the individual test must be repeated. No less than 80% of the liver can be out of action without affecting individual tests, and in patients with cirrhosis they may all be within normal limits. Among a large number of tests available the following are the most useful:

1. **Serum Bilirubin Estimation.**—A value of conjugated bilirubin exceeding 7 μmol/l (0·4 mg/ 100 ml) is one of the most valuable indices of either stasis within the biliary tree or hepato-cellular damage, but it is of no value in distinguishing the one from the other.

2. **Serum alkaline phosphatase.**—Normal value 3 to 13 King–Armstrong (K–A) or 1·5–4 Bodansky units. A high alkaline phosphatase (>100 iu) with low transaminase levels favours obstructive jaundice but the alkaline phosphatase can be high in cholestatic jaundice and hepatitis.

3. **Estimation of serum albumin** is a good general test of hepatic function, as the liver is the only site of its production. A level below 25 g/l (2·5 g/100 ml) indicates that liver function is greatly impaired (in the absence of an obvious source of excessive loss) and, if an operation is essential, only the minimum should be done. Above 30 g/l (3·0 g/100 ml) is satisfactory.

4. **Serum Transaminases (aminotransferases).**—These are enzymes present in liver cells and heart muscle. Increased values (over 100 units) are found in hepatocellular disease but only in prolonged obstructive jaundice when liver damage occurs.

5. **Plasma prothrombin index**, if *low* is an indication for pre-operative vitamin K therapy. Where there is little or no response to vitamin K, extensive hepatocellular damage is almost certain. Owing to large reserves a satisfactory reponse does not exclude considerable liver damage.

6. **5-nucleotidase and γ-glutamyl transferase.**—The concentration of these enzymes in the blood is not affected by osteoblastic activity and they are therefore of value in determining the origin of a rise in alkaline phosphatase, which may be influenced by bony and intestinal, as well as hepatic, activity. γ-glutamyl transferase is raised particularly in alcoholic liver disease.

7. **Alphafetoprotein.**—Very high levels of this abnormal protein are almost diagnostic of hepatoma.

8. **Specific Tests** for particular forms of liver disease include:
(*a*) For haemochromatosis—serum iron, total iron-binding capacity, serum ferritin
(*b*) Wilson's disease—serum copper, urinary copper, serum caesuloplasmin
(*c*) α-l-antitrypsin deficiency- α-l-antitrypsin

9. **Immunological tests** in liver disease:
(*a*) Antimitochondrial antibody ⎫
(*b*) Antinuclear antibody ⎪ Primary biliary cirrhosis
(*c*) Anti-smooth muscle antibody ⎬ and
(*d*) Liver membrane antibody ⎭ Chronic active hepatitis

B. Liver biopsy is a common procedure of considerable diagnostic value. It should never be attempted until the presence or absence of a bleeding tendency on the part of the patient has been ascertained by all accepted tests, and if present, remedied. The

Earl Judson King, 1901–1962. Professor of Chemical Pathology, University of London (Royal Post-Graduate Medical School).
Arthur Riley Armstrong, Contemporary. Director of Department of Laboratories, Hamilton Health Association, Hamilton, Ontario, Canada.
Aaron Bodansky, 1887–1961. Biochemist, Hospital for Joint Diseases, New York City, U.S.A.

procedure is hazardous in the presence of ascites, hepatic adenoma, and hydatid disease of the liver must be excluded as accidental puncture can spread the disease throughout the peritoneal cavity or give rise to anaphylactic shock. The puncture is carried out on the right side or in the epigastrium. The Menghini needle or a Tru-cut needle are the best. Sections are cut from the cylindrical specimen obtained. Haemorrhage or biliary peritonitis are complications. Liver biopsy is of particular value in generalised liver disease, *e.g.* cirrhosis, reticulosis and hepatitis. Local disease such as tumours, focal granulomas, *etc.* may be missed. A combination of peritoneoscopy with needle liver biopsy enables a tissue sample to be taken directly from a focal abnormality and the needle can be guided by ultrasound or a CT scan (see below).

C. Imaging techniques.

1. **Non-invasive methods.**—(*a*) *A plain x-ray* of the abdomen is only of limited diagnostic value, but may show calcification, *e.g.* in a hydatid cyst (fig. 880).

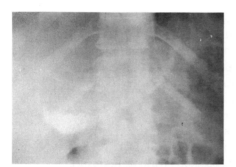

FIG. 880.—Calcification in the wall of a hydatid cyst.

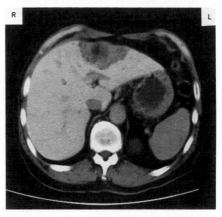

FIG. 881.—CT scan of the liver showing an obvious tumour on its anterior surface. The tumour is a primary hepatoma.

(*b*) *Grey-scale Ultrasound.*—This is a safe, simple and non-invasive method which is of particular value in demonstrating dilation of bile ducts and stones in the gall-bladder (Chapter 47) as well as primary and secondary liver tumours and cysts.

(*c*) *Computed axial tomography.*—Although a promising technique, its primary disadvantage is its expense and limited availability. Is of considerable value in showing the nature and relations of tumours and cysts in the liver (fig. 881). As it is expensive it is used to find out more about a tumour that has been first diagnosed on ultrasound.

(*d*) *Radio-active scanning.*—A gamma emitting isotope such as [198]colloidal gold and [69]Technetium is taken up by the reticulo-endothelial system and can be useful in focal lesions in the liver. Rose-bengal labelled with ^{131}I is taken up by the liver parenchyma but unfortunately its concentration in the gallbladder interferes with delineation of the liver edge.

The normal liver presents an even distribution of activity and lesions which do not take up isotopes, *e.g.* abscesses, cysts and tumours, appear as defects in the scan. Also extrinsic lesions such as subphrenic abscesses can be detected. Lesions greater than 2 cm can be detected readily, but false positive scans are a problem.

Generalised decrease in uptake suggests a diffuse hepatocellular disorder such as cirrhosis. Radioactive scanning is being used less, now that ultrasound is widely available.

2. **Invasive methods.**—(*a*) **Angiography** by means of coeliac axis or superior mesenteric arteriograms is occasionally valuable in detecting changes in the vascularity of the liver, either due to vascular obstruction or to an avascular lesion such as a cyst or abscess, or to a vascular tumour. In cases of portal hypertension films in the venous phase of superior mesenteric angiography are useful. Splenic puncture is more hazardous but if a fine needle is used, it is an acceptable alternative.

(*b*) Percutaneous transhepatic cholangiography (Chapter 47).
(*c*) Endoscopic retrograde cholangiopancreatography (ERCP), Chapter 47.

Georgio Menghini, Contemporary. Physician, Perugia, Italy.

INJURIES

Rupture of the liver, is an extremely grave accident, and in a considerable proportion of cases it is associated with other serious injuries. Consequently the mortality is high (up to 20%, rising to 50% if four or more organs are injured). The violence that produces this injury is usually of a crushing type or from the steering wheel of a car in collision. Rupture of the right lobe is much more common than of the left, because it is larger and less mobile; usually the tear is on the anterior or the superior surface of the organ. Often a rib, or ribs, on the right side are fractured. Less commonly, wounds are of the penetrating type, due to knife or missile.

Most of the problems of injury of the liver are caused by haemorrhage, leakage of bile and devitalisation of liver tissue. Haemorrhage may be free into the peritoneal cavity and the patient presents with the clinical picture of massive intra-abdominal haemorrhage, perhaps indistinguishable from rupture of the spleen but suggested by localising signs of pain, tenderness and rigidity in the right upper quadrant of the abdomen. Bleeding within the liver may form a large haematoma, which may later become infected to form an abscess, or it can rupture into the bile duct giving rise to haemobilia. Biliary leakage can lead to biliary peritonitis with subsequent abscess or cyst formation. Infarction of liver tissue due to occlusion of blood supply can be complicated by an abscess within the liver or immediately above or below that organ.

Diagnosis.—Liver damage must be suspected in any patient with upper abdominal or lower chest injuries. But when there is doubt, especially if peritoneal signs are difficult to elicit, as in an unconscious patient, peritoneal lavage to detect haemoperitoneum may be helpful.

Treatment.—A blood transfusion is of cardinal importance, and in all cases laparotomy must be undertaken.

Operation.—The abdomen is opened either through a right paramedian incision, with extension into the right thorax or by median sternotomy, if required for major hepatic lobectomy, or through a midline incision which can be extended into the chest as a median sternotomy. Bleeding vessels in the wall and depths of fissures and tears should be ligated, but it is important that all pulped liver and portions of doubtful viability should be removed. In presence of rapid bleeding packing and pressure allows the anaesthetist to restore the blood pressure by transfusion, and temporary occlusion of the hepatic artery and portal vein in the free edge of the lesser omentum may permit accurate ligation of vessels in the wound. Failure to debride non-viable liver tissue favours infection and secondary haemorrhage.

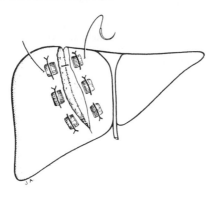

Fig. 882.—Repair of liver tear. Mattress sutures are first inserted parallel to the tear and then under-run with coapting stitches. Ox fibrin 'buffers' may also be used to prevent sutures tearing out.

Simple tears may be opposed by sutures (fig. 882). Soft drains placed in the vicinity of the injury should be brought out through a separate incision.

Packing should be avoided except as a temporary measure or may be used by the less experienced surgeon to allow the patient to be transported to a centre where resection can be performed. Hepatic artery *or* portal vein ligation may also be used as a last resort, if temporary clamping of one or the other has been found to control the bleeding. With extensive haematoma formation and rupture of liver tissue, a major hepatic resection occasionally may be required, frequently a right hepatic lobectomy, *i.e.* removal of the right anatomical lobe and medial segment of left lobe, along with quadrate and caudate lobes. Following such major operations the abdominal cavity must be drained because leakage of bile occurs from torn ducts. It is still a matter of discussion whether the bile ducts should be drained after resection. Following major hepatic resections, complications such as abscess formation, haemobilia, hypoalbuminaemia and coagulation defects may occur. The mortality for hepatic injury is about 10%.

Penetrating Wounds of the liver occur as a result of gunshot injuries and stab wounds. When, as is commonly the case, the wound of entrance is in the right lower thorax, the thoraco-abdominal approach, excising the wound of entrance, is advisable. In some cases the wound of the liver is comparatively small, and no serious bleeding occurs; but in all cases, laparotomy must be performed to exclude damage to other organs. If the wound is a large one, the principles of arresting haemorrhage given above are employed. High velocity bullets can produce extensive intrahepatic damage with little damage on the surface. Injuries of the inferior vena cava or rupture of the hepatic veins are nearly always fatal but occasionally can be repaired by gaining control above as well as below the rupture via a lower median sternotomy.

ENLARGEMENTS OF THE LIVER

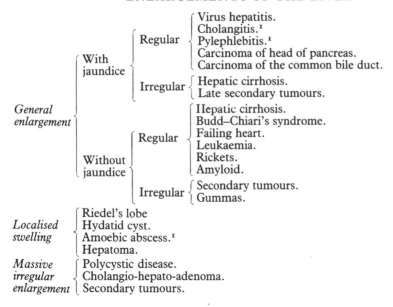

General enlargement

With jaundice

Regular
- Virus hepatitis.
- Cholangitis.[1]
- Pylephlebitis.[1]
- Carcinoma of head of pancreas.
- Carcinoma of the common bile duct.

Irregular
- Hepatic cirrhosis.
- Late secondary tumours.

Without jaundice

Regular
- Hepatic cirrhosis.
- Budd–Chiari's syndrome.
- Failing heart.
- Leukaemia.
- Rickets.
- Amyloid.

Irregular
- Secondary tumours.
- Gummas.

Localised swelling
- Riedel's lobe
- Hydatid cyst.
- Amoebic abscess.[1]
- Hepatoma.

Massive irregular enlargement
- Polycystic disease.
- Cholangio-hepato-adenoma.
- Secondary tumours.

VIRUS HEPATITIS

Hepatitis can be caused by a number of viruses. The term Hepatis A Virus (HAV) is used for short-incubation disease, formerly called 'Infective Hepatitis'; Hepatitis B Virus

---

[1] Intermittent pyrexia, sometimes rigors, occur.

Bernhard Riedel, 1846–1916. Professor of Surgery, Jena, Germany.

(HBV) is used for long-incubation disease, hitherto called 'Serum Hepatitis'. Our knowledge of the latter type of disease has been advanced by the discovery of hepatitis B (Australia) antigen.[1]

Hepatitis A Virus occurs in sporadic and epidemic forms. The virus (type A) is excreted in the faeces and this is probably the method of spread. It is the commonest form of jaundice in children and young adults, and there is no evidence that one attack confers immunity. The incubation period is from three to five weeks.

The condition commences with anorexia, nausea and perhaps vomiting, with malaise and fever, and jaundice appears after about three days. The liver may be palpable and tender, and occasionally there is transient ascites. The fever subsides shortly after the jaundice appears. Usually the jaundice disappears after two or three weeks, but it may persist very much longer. In such cases, the diagnosis from extrahepatic biliary obstruction may be difficult, and liver function tests may not give a clear distinction.

Following infective hepatitis, forms of chronic liver disease, and hepatocellular disease, do not occur. Most patients recover completely. However, a few develop acute or subacute hepatic necrosis which accounts for the mortality of 3%.

Gammaglobulin is effective in preventing or modifying Type A virus hepatitis and is usually given to household contacts who have not already had the disease. Antibiotics are of no value. Steroids may be given to those with prolonged cholestasis to lower the serum bilirubin. It is regarded as important that the patient should avoid alcohol or strenuous exercise for some months after all symptoms and signs have subsided. A small proportion of patients have recurrent attacks of mild symptoms persisting for a year or more.

Hepatitis B Virus.—See Chapter 4.

CHOLANGITIS (syn. INTERMITTENT HEPATIC FEVER OF CHARCOT)

By cholangitis is meant a state of inflammation of the bile ducts, but it is the radicles of the biliary tree within the liver that are the main site of the infection. Cholangitis can occur as the result of obstruction of the common bile duct by a gallstone (Chapter 47) or a stricture, or in mucoviscidosis (Chapter 47). Suppurative cholangitis (Chapter 47), like pylephlebitis, may be followed by the formation of multiple liver abscesses. The symptoms of cholangitis are biliary colic, jaundice, chills and fever. There is usually a marked leucocytosis. There is often septicaemia with a positive blood culture for *E. coli* and other intestinal organisms. Gram-negative shock may develop. Although the treatment of cholangitis is ultimately the removal of the cause, most cases of cholangitis can be brought under control by an intravenous antibiotic, *e.g.* a cephalosporin or aminoglycoside. The bile duct must be decompressed by the establishment of drainage by non-operative or operative means. In some patients the picture of septic shock predominates and the hepatobiliary origin of the infection may not be evident on superficial examination.

PYLEPHLEBITIS (syn. PORTAL PYAEMIA)

Pathology.—Pylephlebitis can follow a suppurative disease in any part drained by the portal system, but usually arises as a complication of apprendicitis or diverticulitis. The process commences as a thrombophlebitis of a small vein draining the infected lesion. The thrombus spreads to a larger collecting vessel, and pieces of infected thrombus break off and are swept into the liver, where they lodge and form abscesses. Cultures show a mixed infection in which *Esch. coli* is prominently represented.

Clinical Features.—Pylephlebitis is characterised by a hectic temperature and the occurrence of repeated rigors. Moderate ascites is sometimes present. The patient soon becomes slightly jaundiced, the liver is somewhat enlarged and tender and the serum bilirubin is raised.

Blood culture is positive in 50% of cases if blood is withdrawn during or immediately after a rigor.

Prophylaxis.—The most important means of preventing pylephlebitis is to administer a broad spectrum antibiotic in cases of fulminating appendicitis or diverticulitis.

Treatment.—As the organisms responsible are mixed, initial chemotherapy should include broad-spectrum antibiotics such as amoxycillin and gentamicin administered parenterally. If bacteroides are identified, metronidazole should be given. Cloxacillin should be administered if staphylococci are identified. Blood transfusion is often required.

---

[1] So-called, because it was discovered in an Australian Aboriginal.

Jean-Martin Charcot, 1825–1893. Physician La Salpêtrière, Paris.

Prognosis.—When pylephlebitis is fully established the outlook was formerly almost hopeless, but with the use of antibiotics many cases recover. Extrahepatic portal venous obstruction is likely to develop later.

IDIOPATHIC PYOGENIC LIVER ABSCESS

Acute abscesses are usually multiple and may be associated with biliary or abdominal disease, but often, especially in elderly patients suffering from malnutrition, no cause can be found. The clinical features and treatment are similar to those described for pylephlebitis (see above).

Chronic abscesses are usually single and occur mainly in the elderly. The onset is often insidious, or even silent (cryptogenic abscess). A cause for the infection may be found in the biliary passage or intestinal tract, but in half the cases no source can be discovered. The patient presents with pyrexia, abdominal discomfort, an enlarged liver, and, in advanced cases, hepatic coma. Leucocytosis may be absent, but the serum albumin level rapidly falls, and anaemia develops. Hepatic scintiscanning, ultrasonic scanning and CT scanning have proved most helpful not only in permitting earlier diagnosis of fluid-filled hepatic masses but also in aiding the localisation of the abscess before exploration and drainage.

Treatment

The essential basis of treatment is the administration of an appropriate antibiotic, *e.g.* aminoglycoside, clindamycin, or metronidazole. Fine needle aspiration under ultrasound or CT scan guidance will enable a specimen to be obtained for staining and culture so that the appropriate antibiotic can be given. Where there are solitary abscesses or a large multiple abscess, drainage may be carried out percutaneously under ultrasonographic or CT control. When the abscess is secondary to intra-abdominal disease, laparotomy is required to treat the primary condition and to search for other abscesses in the liver, which should be drained by tube drainage. The drain is left in position until drainage ceases.

In most instances the cause of a liver abscess is apparent, or can be ascertained, infection reaching the liver in one of several ways, *viz:*

CAUSES OF ABSCESSES OF THE LIVER

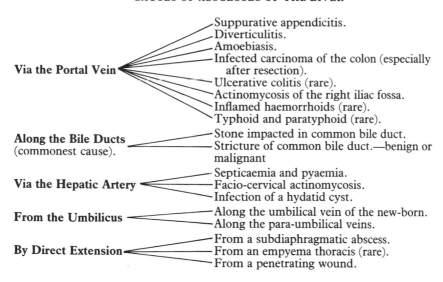

Via the Portal Vein
- Suppurative appendicitis.
- Diverticulitis.
- Amoebiasis.
- Infected carcinoma of the colon (especially after resection).
- Ulcerative colitis (rare).
- Actinomycosis of the right iliac fossa.
- Inflamed haemorrhoids (rare).
- Typhoid and paratyphoid (rare).

Along the Bile Ducts (commonest cause).
- Stone impacted in common bile duct.
- Stricture of common bile duct.—benign or malignant

Via the Hepatic Artery
- Septicaemia and pyaemia.
- Facio-cervical actinomycosis.
- Infection of a hydatid cyst.

From the Umbilicus
- Along the umbilical vein of the new-born.
- Along the para-umbilical veins.

By Direct Extension
- From a subdiaphragmatic abscess.
- From an empyema thoracis (rare).
- From a penetrating wound.

AMOEBIC LIVER ABSCESS (*syn.* TROPICAL ABSCESS, DYSENTERIC ABSCESS)

Amoebic abscess of the liver is one of the terminations of amoebic hepatitis, which in turn is a complication of amoebic dysentery—not so very uncommon. It is estimated that 10% of the world's population is infected.

Pathology.—*Entamoebae histolyticae* (fig. 883) pass from a focal lesion in the colonic wall into a radicle of the inferior mesenteric vein and via the portal vein they enter the liver to take up residence there, usually in the upper and posterior portion of the right lobe. In the liver the entamoebae colonise and live at the expense of the liver cells, causing localised liquefaction necrosis. The amount of liver destruction is proportional to the size of the colony, the resistance of the host and the extent of secondary infection. In 70% of cases, the abscess is solitary; in 30% more than one abscess is present. Characteristic pus from an amoebic liver abscess is chocolate-coloured, or like anchovy sauce, and consists of broken-down liver cells, leucocytes, and red blood cells; nevertheless, in an appreciable number of instances the pus is green, from being admixed with bile. In about half the cases the pus contains staphylococci, streptococci, and *Esch. coli*, as well as *E. histolytica*. In the remainder the pus is sterile, but except in long-standing cases, motile entamoebae can be demonstrated in the last few drops of pus to be withdrawn, or from a scraping of the abscess wall at operation. Commonly perihepatitis causes the liver to become fixed to the diaphragm or the abdominal wall.

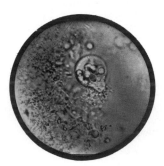

FIG. 883.—Entamoeba histolytica.

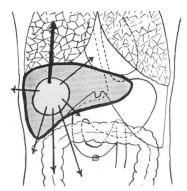

FIG. 884.—Directions in which a tropical liver abscess may burst.
(After Sir Zachary Cope, FRCS)

Course.—An amoebic abscess of the liver runs a variable course:

1. In early stages of amoebic hepatitis with abscess threatening, resolution may occur under emetine or metronidazole treatment, but some authorities doubt whether there is really a stage of hepatitis without abscess formation; it is more probable that treatment results in cure of a small abscess or abscesses (Milroy Paul).

2. When an abscess forms the liver enlarges, most often in an upward direction. It is at this stage that surgical intervention is called for.

3. It may become encapsulated and remain dormant for long periods.

4. Unrecognised and untreated, it may burst into (*a*) the right lung, (*b*) the peritoneal cavity, (*c*) the right pleural cavity, in that order, or, more rarely, into a hollow viscus (fig. 884). Exceptionally the abscess points subcutaneously. Erosion into the lung and the expectoration of a quantity of chocolate-coloured sputum sometimes results in a natural cure.

Milroy Paul, Contemporary. Formerly Professor of Surgery, University of Ceylon.

Bacterial infection is a rather frequent and serious complication of amoebic abscess. While a solitary amoebic abscess is usually amenable to combined specific drug and surgical treatment, the prognosis in cases of multiple amoebic liver abscesses is extremely poor.

Clinical Features.—As a rule, the condition develops soon after an attack of amoebic dysentery while the patient is resident in a tropical or sub-tropical country. Less frequently its appearance is delayed, sometimes for many months; exceptionally it has occurred more than thirty years after returning home from the tropics. Occasionally an amoebic abscess develops in a carrier who has not had overt dysentery; indeed, it sometimes appears in persons who have had mild diarrhoea not diagnosed as dysentery, and consequently have not had treatment for that condition. There is a striking predominance in young males.

Early Symptoms.—Anaemia, loss of weight, and an earthy complexion are often the first symptoms.

Pyrexia rising to 38°C or more, at night, with profuse sweating, is usually present. Rigors occur, especially in the early stages.

Pain is constantly present in the liver area, and is occasionally referred to the right shoulder. Jarring increases the pain so that the patient learns to try to support his enlarged liver with his hands when he walks.

Tenderness and *rigidity* in acute cases are comparable to that of acute cholecystitis. In chronic cases tenderness may be absent.

Enlargement of the liver may be demonstrated (fig. 885) but it is not unusual for an abscess to be present in a liver which is fixed by perihepatitis, and therefore the liver cannot enlarge in a downward direction.

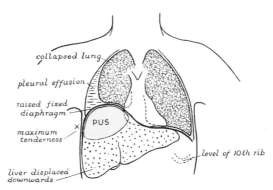

Fig. 885.—The physical signs of a tropical liver abscess (commonest site). *(After A. T. Andreasen.)*

Isotope scanning of the liver, using *ultra-sound* techniques and CT scanning, may help to localise the abscess.

Basal lung signs on the corresponding side.

Leucocytosis is present in nearly all cases. Polymorphonuclear cells constitute, at the most, only 75% of the total count. Anaemia, if present at all, is not marked.

Examination of several stools for amoebae and cysts should be undertaken, but their absence does not exclude the diagnosis.

Sigmoidoscopy sometimes reveals the characteristic ulcers (Chapter 50) and the parasites may be seen on a mucosal biopsy.

Radiography (antero-posterior and lateral positions) often reveals an elevation and fixation of the right cupola of the diaphragm.

Often an absolute diagnosis is possible only on finding typical pus by exploratory aspiration.

Occasionally an amoebic liver abscess does not give rise to symptoms; healed lesions have been found at necropsy and calcified lesions (that may have been abscesses) have been revealed radiologically.

Liver function tests are often unhelpful and liver biopsy is not recommended because of the risk of contamination of the pleural cavity. Aspiration of the abscess will not necessarily confirm the diagnosis, because often amoebae are not seen.

Serological Tests.—The indirect haemagglutination test, which is sensitive and reliable, is positive in most affected patients. The gel diffusion precipitive test is simple and inexpensive, and is positive in 95% liver abscesses.

Treatment.—The treatment of choice is metronidazole (Flagyl) 800 mg three times daily for 7–10 days. Failures are few and side affects much less than with the more toxic emetine and chloroquine.

Aspiration.—Small abscesses respond without aspiration. Needle aspiration should be used if there is a lack of response to five days of metronidazole treatment, if the abscess is very large and the patient very toxic. A secondarily infected abscess should be treated similarly in the first instance; indeed, such infection can be discovered only by bacteriological examination of the pus.

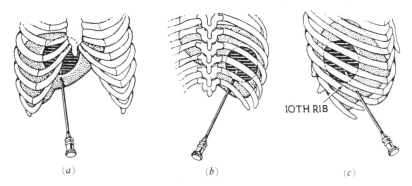

FIG. 886.—Aspiration of an amoebic hepatic abscess; (*a*) in the anterior part of the liver; (*b*) in the posterior part of the liver; (*c*) located near the dome of the diaphragm.

Technique.—Aspiration must be conducted in the operating theatre. A long needle is necessary, and its bore should be wide (1–2 mm), as the pus is usually thick in consistency. The important technique of percutaneous introduction of the hollow needle (under local anaesthesia) into the abscess cavity in various locations is shown in fig. 886. In some cases the abscess eludes the aspirating needle, in which event laparotomy must be performed, thus allowing the liver to be explored by the aspirating needle more thoroughly. At the same time laparotomy permits the exclusion of a primary carcinoma of the liver which, in coloured races, sometimes closely resembles an amoebic liver abscess in its onset and physical signs, and at times is even accompanied by a low pyrexia. When the abdomen is open, packs, impregnated with a solution of erythromycin 1:1000, are so arranged as to isolate the liver. On aspiration the abscess is thoroughly emptied by syringe suction. The incision is closed completely *and on no account should a drainage tube be employed*. Its use leads to invasion of its track by amoebae and in some cases a fatal spreading infection of the abdominal wall (Amoebiasis cutis).

After Treatment.—A full course of specific drug therapy should be given after aspiration.

ACTINOMYCOSIS OF THE LIVER

Actinomycosis (Chapter 4) produces the well-known 'honeycomb' liver. Actinomyces reach the organ: 1. Via the portal vein from actinomycosis of the right iliac fossa (60%). 2. Via the hepatic artery from a more distant primary focus, *e.g.* facio-cervical actinomycosis—about 30%. 3. From contiguous viscera, *e.g.* a penetrating peptic ulcer invading the liver—rare.

The disease is slow to develop. Gradually the liver tissue is destroyed and replaced by multiple abscesses.

Treatment.—Exploration is essential, and in every case of liver abscess of doubtful origin the pus should be examined for actinomyces. Long-acting penicillin in large doses, or other more suitable antibiotic therapy must be continued for some months.

TUBERCULOSIS OF THE LIVER

In 50% of necropsies upon patients who have died from tuberculosis, miliary tubercles are present in the liver. Local tuberculosis of the liver is usually diagnosed at necropsy, but occasionally at laparotomy. There is a large mass containing necrotic material. This lesion may be seen in children, and in negroes with little immunity. Less uncommon is a tuberculous abscess. The symptoms are identical with those of an amoebic abscess. The diagnosis is established by liver biopsy, and antituberculous drugs (Chapter 4) are highly effective.

HEPATIC SYPHILIS

Syphilis, always an accomplished actor, can, and does, deceive the clinician. Gummas give rise to rounded masses in the liver. These swellings may simulate a liver abscess. Syphilis of the liver is now a rarity.

HYDATID DISEASE OF THE LIVER

Although the larval stage of the parasite *Echinococcus Granulosus* can thrive in many parts of the body, in 80% of cases it does so in the liver; after ingestion it enters this organ through a radicle of the portal vein, and usually the right lobe is affected.

Source of Infection.—Dogs are the chief mediators of hydatid disease to human beings by direct contact. Humans may also eat salads on which the ova

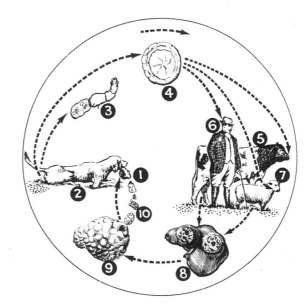

FIG. 887.—The life-cycle of the *Echinococcus Granulosus.* (1) Offal infected with hydatid cysts is eaten by a dog (2). The *Echinococcus Granulosus* (3) develops in the dog's intestine. This parasite is about 1 cm long and is made up of a head and three segments, the last of which contains about 500 ova (4). The ova are expelled from the dog's intestine on to grass, vegetables, etc. Cattle (5), human beings (6), or sheep (7) ingest the eggs. The liver (8) is the organ most frequently infected with hydatid cysts, a larval form of *Echinococcus Granulosus*. Such cysts (9) harbour thousands of heads of the parasite (scolices) (10).
(After V. P. Fontana, Montevideo.)

have been deposited. Animals, particularly sheep, are infected by eating contaminated grass (fig. 887). Once in the stomach, the ova burrow through the stomach wall to enter the portal system and the liver. Dogs become infected by feeding on offal of infested sheep and, to a lesser extent, cattle. As would be expected, the disease is relatively common in the sheep-rearing districts of Australasia and South America, Greece, Turkey, Iran and Iraq, while, for the same reason, in the British Isles, Wales shows the highest incidence.

In other parts of the world where the disease is common the life-cycle can be completed in other animals; thus pigs (not in styes) and occasionally horses can take the place of sheep and cattle, while in the frozen North (the disease is common among Red Indians and Eskimo) the wolf→moose→wolf often maintain the cycle.

Pathology.—A hydatid cyst consists of three layers.

1. *The adventitia (pseudocyst)*, consisting of fibrous tissue, the result of reaction of the liver to the parasite, is grey in colour and blended intimately with the liver, from which it is inseparable.

2. *The laminated membrane (ectocyst)* formed of the parasite itself is whitish and elastic, and contains the hydatid fluid. Indeed, this membrane closely resembles a child's uncoloured balloon filled with water, and unless bacterial infection has occurred it peels readily from the adventitia.

Hydatid fluid is crystal-clear; it registers a specific gravity of 1·005–1·009, contains no albumin, and when not too old, hooklets and scolices. The cyst grows very slowly.

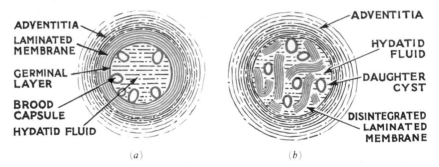

FIG. 888.—(*a*) Typical hydatid cyst. (*b*) Development of daughter cysts (not common).

3. The only living part of a hydatid cyst is a single layer of cells (germinal epithelium) lining the cyst (*endocyst*). This secretes: (*a*) internally: the hydatid fluid; (*b*) externally: the laminated membrane (fig. 888(*a*)). Brood capsules within the cyst develop from the germinal epithelium and are attached by pedicles to its innermost wall. Within the brood capsules, scolices (heads of future worms) develop. Should the laminated membrane become damaged, it disintegrates (Dew), and the brood capsules, becoming free, grow into daughter cysts (fig. 888(*b*)). In this event the mother cyst ceases to exist as such, the hydatid fluid and its content being confined by the adventitia only.

Clinical Features.—For a long time, perhaps for some years after the original infestation (which often occurs in childhood), a hydatid cyst remains symptomless (fig. 889). In the course of time a visible and palpable swelling in the upper

Sir Harold Dew, 1891–1962. Professor of Surgery, Sydney, Australia.

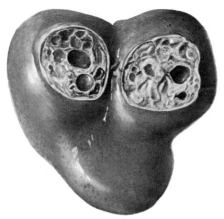

FIG. 889.—Multiple hydatid cysts in the liver. The patient, who had never left England, died after a street accident.

abdomen is discovered. The size which a hydatid may attain without causing serious disturbance to health would seem to be limited only by the capacity of the peritoneal cavity.

Naturally, when a patient hails from a locality where hydatid disease is rife, the diagnosis is simplified. An unruptured cyst presents as a rounded calcified shadow in the liver (fig. 890). Ultrasound and CT scanning (fig. 891) can localise the cyst and ERCP can show whether the cyst communicates with bile duct.

The intradermal test (Casoni's test) is positive in 75% of cases, but gives up to 40% false positives.

Recent serological tests, although more complicated, are of greater accuracy, *e.g.* indirect haemagglutination reaction.

A blood-count often, but not invariably, shows an eosinophilia (6% or more).

Course of the Disease.—1. Occasionally the parasite dies. The fluid is absorbed, and all that remains is an encapsuled, laminated, bile-stained membrane. In cases of long standing the walls of the cyst may calcify (fig. 890).

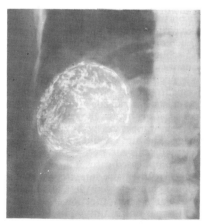

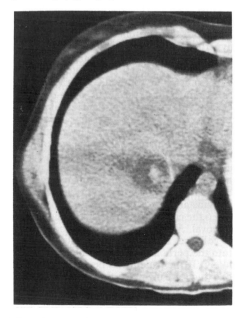

FIG. 890.—Calcification of hydatid cyst of the liver.
(H. Talib, FRCS, Baghdad.)

FIG. 891.—Liver CT scan (viewed from the feet of the patient). Calcifying hydatid cyst in posterior (paravertebral) part of right lobe.

Tommaso Casoni, 1880–1933. Physician, Ospedale Coloniale, Vittorio Emanuele III, Tripoli.

2. *Virus Hepatitis.*—The exact percentage of cases in which cirrhosis is an aftermath of virus hepatitis is debatable, and it varies in different localities.

3. *Chronic (Surgical) Biliary Obstruction,* leading to Secondary Biliary Cirrhosis.—This is to be distinguished from Primary Biliary Cirrhosis (Hanôt) an autoimmune disease of middle-aged women. In the latter the mitochondrial immunofluorescence test is positive in 98% (Sherlock).

4. *Infestation of the liver by schistosomiasis* undoubtedly is a principal cause of the condition in districts where schistosomiasis is rife.

5. *Nutritional Deficiency.*—In the tropics this appears to be a major factor. Its mode of action is as follows: some toxic agents and mild infections, harmless to the well-nourished, are liable to have a deleterious effect on the liver of protein-deficient individuals. Therefore protein deficiency is indirectly responsible for the cirrhosis.

6. *Haemochromatosis* (Bronzed Diabetes).

7. *Hepato-lenticular degeneration.*

8. *Chemical poisons:* carbon tetrachloride, arsenic, chloroform.

9. *Unknown.*—In many instances the cause is obscure. These account for half the cases seen in Great Britain (Sherlock).

Morphological Types

Three anatomical types are recognised:

(*a*) *micronodular* is characterised by irregular thick bands of fibrous tissue and by small regenerating nodules uniformly less than 3 mm diameter. It is often associated with alcoholism.

(*b*) *macronodular* is characterised by bands of fibrous tissue of varying thickness and nodules the majority of which are greater than 3 mm diameter. This type is also called postnecrotic.

(*c*) *mixed*—liver shows both micro- and macronodular features.

Pathology.—As a result of widespread parenchymal destruction and overgrowth of fibrous tissue, the tiny radicles of the portal and hepatic veins become compressed and distorted. In some cases there may be spasm of the portal veins. Arterioles resist this compression for a longer time than veins. As a consequence the cirrhotic liver becomes dependent upon the hepatic artery for the major portion of its blood supply, and in the desperate effort to maintain the circulation through the liver in these adverse circumstances, extensive intrahepatic communications develop between branches of the hepatic artery and the portal vein, and between the tributaries of the portal and hepatic veins.

Nature's intrahepatic shunts, combined with the opening up of the better-known extrahepatic porta-systemic communications, divert a large portion of the portal blood past the hepatic parenchyma into the systemic venous system. Thus the remaining hepatic cells are deprived of their fair share of portal blood.

Usually there is a fine fibrosis producing slight nodularity (Laënnec's cirrhosis[1] or hob-nail liver), but coarse lobulation may result from larger regeneration nodules (fig. 893)

Clinical Features:

The early stages of cirrhosis may be quiet and long. The liver hypertrophies. In some cases there are repeated attacks of slight jaundice with epigastric pain and vomiting. At each attack areas of the liver are destroyed and replaced by fibrous tissue, while the remainder hypertrophies.

Cirrhosis results in three major events—hepatocellular failure, portal hyper-

---

[1] Laënnec introduced the term from the Greek κιρρός = tawny, as the nodules are orange-yellow in colour.

Victor Charles Hanôt, 1844–1896. Physician, Hôpital Saint Antoine, Paris.
Dame Sheila Patricia Violet Sherlock, Contemporary, Professor of Medicine, Royal Free Hospital, London.
René Théophile Hyacinthe Laënnec, 1781–1826. Professor of Medicine, College de France, invented the stethoscope in 1819.

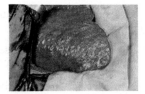

FIG. 892.—Portal cirrhosis.

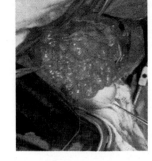

FIG. 894.—Spider naevus.

FIG. 893.—Portal cirrhosis with large regeneration nodules.

(Prof. R. Milnes Walker, FRCS, Bristol.)

tension and fluid retention. Later the liver commences to shrink. The spleen becomes enlarged, and usually increases in size with the raised portal blood pressure of which hepatic cirrhosis is the principal cause in adults. Functioning liver tissue is gradually destroyed and hepatocellular failure develops. About this time, especially in alcoholic subjects, two classical signs may appear: *Spider naevi*,[1] which are usually located around the face, neck, shoulders and the upper arms. Histologically they prove to be an overgrown end-artery with branching arterioles (fig. 894). *Palmar erythema*—the hands are warm, and the palms are bright red.

Bleeding from oesophageal varices occurs in about 40% of cases, and may be the first evidence of the disease. Not infrequently the superficial veins radiating from the umbilicus enlarge, forming a Caput Medusae (fig. 895). Progressive ascites occurs (fig. 896). Testicular atrophy and gynaecomasia are common in cirrhosis, no doubt due to increase of oestrogens in the blood. The failing liver is unable to neutralise these substances. In women there is a tendency to masculinisation. Dupuytren's contractures may develop (p. 419).

Once hepatic decompensation has occurred (if the patient escapes death from torrential haemorrhage from oesophageal varices), liver failure, like a sword of Damocles, sooner or later falls upon the sufferer from this disease.

Clinical Pathological Associations.—Cirrhosis, whatever its type, has certain clinical and pathological associations including splenomegaly, pancreatitis (especially in the alcoholic), gastrointestinal bleeding from varices, peptic ulcer or gastric erosions, primary liver cancer and liability to infections.

Liver Function Tests.—In compensated cirrhosis, tests may be normal, the most frequent abnormality being impairment of B.S.P. clearance. In decompensated disease, urobilinogen is usually present in the urine in excess and the plasma albumin is depressed.

Liver biopsy is usually necessary only for the diagnosis of a well-compensated case in order to confirm the diagnosis and assess prognosis.

---

[1] An older Miss Muffet
Decided to rough it
And lived upon whisky and gin.

Red hands and a spider
Developed outside her—
Such are the wages of sin.
(W. B. Bean.)

William Bennett Bean, Contemporary. Professor of Internal Medicine, University Hospitals, Iowa City, U.S.A.
Medusa, one of three Gorgons whose fine hair was turned into snakes (Greek mythology).
Damocles, a Greek who was feasted with a sword suspended above his head by a single hair (Greek mythology).

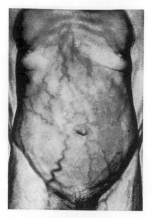

FIG. 895.—Enlargement of the veins of the abdominal wall in a case of portal hypertension. Infra-red photograph.
(The late A. H. Hunt FRCS, London.)

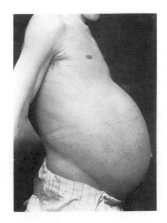

FIG. 896.—Hepatic cirrhosis with ascites.

Treatment.—There is no specific remedy for established cirrhosis, but the following measures may be helpful: (*a*) increased glucose intake; (*b*) alcohol forbidden; (*c*) high protein diet if there is no evidence of liver failure; (*d*) steroids should only be given in active chronic hepatitis.

Hepato-lenticular degeneration (*syn*. Wilson's disease) is an uncommon condition that is confined to children and young adults due to an hereditary error in copper metabolism. In infants the symptoms are those of cirrhosis. In adolescents a coarse tremor is commonly an initial symptom. As the disease progresses, muscular rigidity and dysarthria dominate the picture. Kayser-Fleischer rings in the eyes due to peripheral corneal opacity are present. Liver function tests give varying results. Liver biopsy shows cirrhosis. Serum caeruloplasmin and serum copper are decreased, and urinary copper increased. Increased liver copper can be demonstrated. Treatment is by penicillamine, which may have to be given for several years.

TREATMENT OF ASCITES

The cause.—The mechanisms of ascites in liver disease are complex. They are related partly to (i) increased formation of hepatic lymph, (ii) reduction in plasma albumin, (iii) retention of salt and water by the kidneys.

Diagnosis.—Clinically ascites is diagnosed by the presence of abdominal distension with dullness in the flank, eversion of the umbilicus and shifting dullness.

It is essential to exclude other causes of ascites, *e.g.* cardiac and renal disease, malnutrition, intra-abdominal malignancy. For this reason, before treatment is started, a small sample of ascitic fluid should be withdrawn by abdominal paracentesis. A sample should be examined for white cells and organisms to exclude bacterial peritonitis which may be clinically silent; malignant cells may be seen on cytological examination of the ascitic fluid. High concentration of amylase in the ascitic fluid suggests pancreatic disease. Discovery of milky fluid on paracentesis suggests a chylous ascites, which may be caused by malignant disease or, rarely, injury.

Treatment.—Conventional treatment consists of the prescription of a salt-free diet (with a sodium intake less than 20 mmol daily). Fluid intake need not be

Samuel Alexander Kinnier Wilson, 1878–1937. Neurologist, King's College Hospital, London.
Bernhard Kayser, 1869–1937. Germany Ophthalmologist.
Richard Fleischer, 1848–1909. German Physician.

restricted and potassium supplements may have to be given to treat the potassium depletion. Diuretics are usually given, usually in the form of spironolactone 200 mg per day and if necessary frusemide may have to be added. Potassium supplements are usually required when diuretics are given. Diuresis may be initiated by administering salt-poor albumin intravenously. While most forms of ascites respond to intensive medical treatment, operation may occasionally be required. Portasystemic shunts have no place in the treatment of ascites alone, but refractory ascites may be treated by a peritoneal-jugular shunt, in which a silastic tube transfers blood from the peritoneal cavity into the jugular vein in the neck. Various types of peritoneal-jugular shunt have been described (le Veen shunt and Denver shunt). Shunts are occasionally used in cirrhotic patients with ascites but may also be used in patients with malignant ascites. Complications include disseminated intravascular coagulation and infection. The commonest problem is thrombosis of the valve of the shunt, which would require its replacement.

PORTAL HYPERTENSION

Aetiology.—Increase of the portal venous blood pressure is due to an obstruction which can be (1) Pre-hepatic; (2) Intra-hepatic; (3) Post-hepatic.

1. **Pre-hepatic.**—About 20% of patients belong to this group. The patient with pre-hepatic portal obstruction is nearly always young, and often a child. The most usual cause for advice being sought is either a sudden haemorrhage or listlessness due to anaemia. On examination the liver is impalpable, but the spleen is obviously enlarged. The anaemia is usually due to oozing from oesophageal varices, but sometimes hypersplenism is a factor. As the liver is normal, or nearly so, liver function tests remain normal as the disease advances. Ascites does not occur unless there is active phlebitis in the portal vein. The obstruction arises in one of two ways:

(a) *There is congenital absence or abnormality of the portal vein.*

(b) *Thrombosis of the portal vein* due to extension of the normal obliterative process of the umbilical vein and ductus venosus (fig. 897) sometimes associated with omphalitis of the new-born.

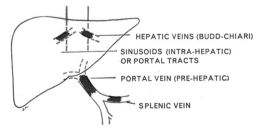

FIG. 897.—Sites of obstruction. The blocks in the veins represent possible sites of thrombus formation.
(After Sir James Learmonth, Edinburgh.)

HEPATIC VEINS (BUDD-CHIARI)

SINUSOIDS (INTRA-HEPATIC) OR PORTAL TRACTS

PORTAL VEIN (PRE-HEPATIC)

SPLENIC VEIN

(c) *Obstruction of the portal vein* in adults may be due to chronic pancreatitis and carcinoma of the pancreas, or thrombosis of the vein may follow acute pancreatitis.

The vein becomes replaced by a mass of collateral channels which have been described as a 'cavernoma'.

2. **Intra-hepatic** accounts for nearly 80% of all cases. The causes are cirrhosis

Harry le Veen, Contemporary. Professor of Surgery, University of S. Carolina, U.S.A.

(frequently alcoholic in origin) and schistosomiasis in which the blood-flow through the liver is obstructed. Enlarged porta-systemic venous communications are present long before serious oesophageal haemorrhage occurs. Oesophageal varices can be demonstrated radiologically or seen through an oesophagoscope. Enlargement of veins of the abdominal wall radiating from the umbilicus may be present (fig. 895). As long as hypertrophy of liver tissue is sufficient to compensate for the cellular destruction by cirrhosis, the liver function tests remain within normal limits.

3. **Post-hepatic** is rare. It may be caused by a constrictive pericarditis and tricuspid valvular incompetence, and it is also a component of the Budd-Chiari syndrome.

BUDD-CHIARI'S SYNDROME

This syndrome results from obstruction to the hepatic veins. Spontaneous thrombosis of the hepatic veins or neoplastic encroachment from other organs account for the majority of cases. The syndrome is also associated with clotting diseases, especially polycythaemia and the use of hormones for contraception and infertility. Some cases, presumably congenital, are caused by an obstruction of the suprahepatic portion of the inferior vena cava with a membraneous web. The importance lies in its potential curability by operation.

An acute form of the disease is seen in Jamaica and may be caused by plant extracts such as Senecio and Crotalaria used in herbal tea.

Clinical Features.—*In acute cases*, nausea, vomiting and severe pain, due to rapid enlargement of the liver as a result of congestion, are often followed by death from hypotensive shock.

A less sudden onset is characterised by rapidly accumulating ascites and signs of portal hypertension with a developing collateral circulation. Signs of hepatic insufficiency are unusually pronounced, and early death and hepatic coma are the rule. The simultaneous development of oedema of the legs testifies to involvement of the inferior vena cava in the occlusive process.

Chronic cases closely resemble hepatic cirrhosis which, indeed, may develop. Liver function tests indicate severe hepatic parenchymal damage, and rarely does the patient survive more than a few months. A few patients who do not die from hepatic coma succumb to haemorrhage from oesophageal varices, mesenteric infarction, or intercurrent infection. In short, the Budd-Chiari syndrome, when the occlusion is, or becomes, complete, must be looked upon as a harbinger of death.

Treatment.—In patients with membranous obstruction of the inferior vena cava, a transatrial meatotomy may be considered. In those in whom the portal vein and inferior vena cava are patent, a portacaval or mesocaval shunt should be tried for the relief of portal hypertension (but *not* an end-to-side shunt, fig. 904). In patients with a blocked inferior vena cava a meso-atrial shunt may be attempted.

Collateral Circulation.—When there is obstruction of blood flow to or from the liver, Nature endeavours to relieve the obstruction by opening up normally insignificant anastomotic channels.

When the obstruction is pre-hepatic, collaterals between the portal vein distal to the obstruction and the portal vein proximal to the obstruction enlarge. Thus insignificant venae comitantes of the hepatic artery and of the portal vein widely dilate. Depending upon the site of the obstruction, some of the collaterals between the portal and systemic venous systems, notably the oesophageal plexus, also become dilated.

When the obstruction is intra-hepatic, anastomotic channels outside the liver between the portal and systemic systems become engorged, dilate, and so an increasing proportion of the obstructed portal venous blood by-passes the liver.

George Budd, 1808–1882. Professor of Medicine, King's College Hospital, London. He was probably the first to describe the Budd-Chiari syndrome.
Hans Chiari, 1851–1916. Professor of Pathological Anatomy, Prague.

ANASTOMOSES BETWEEN THE PORTAL AND SYSTEMIC VENOUS SYSTEMS

	Site of Anastomosis	Portal Vessels	Systemic Vessels	Signs and Symptoms
1	Plexus around lower end of oesophagus.	Oesophageal branches of left gastric vein and short gastric veins.	Lower systemic oesophageal veins.	Haematemesis or melaena.
2	Around umbilicus.	Para-umbilical veins (accompany the round ligament of the liver).	Superficial veins of the anterior abdominal wall.	Caput Medusae.
3	Plexuses around lower third of rectum and anal canal.	Superior haemorrhoidal vein.	Middle and inferior haemorrhoidal veins.	Rectal varices (heavy bright red bleeding)—rare.
4	Extraperitoneal surfaces of abdominal organs.	Tributaries of superior and inferior mesenteric veins.	Subdiaphragmatic and retroperitoneal veins.	Silent.

The only ones which are dangerous to life are those in the submucosa of the oesophagus and upper end of the stomach. In patients with portal hypertension, haemorrhoids, if present, are usually of the idiopathic type but rectal varices can occur and can lead to severe haemorrhage (fig. 898).

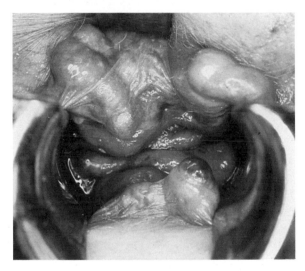

FIG. 898.—Large rectal varices in a case of portal hypertension (seen through an anal speculum). A very unusual type of haemorrhage.

Oesophageal Varices.—*Although called 'oesophageal' it is important to realise that these varices extend well into the stomach.* Oesophageal varices (fig. 899) are dilations of the normal submucosal oesophageal veins and are the most important collaterals of the portal circulation. Sometimes, as intra-abdominal pressure rises, *e.g.* when straining at stool or during heavy lifting, they rupture; in other cases the overlying mucosa becomes abraded by a rough bolus or excoriated by regurgitated gastric juice. Bleeding which is nearly always from the lower 5 cm of the oesophagus may be a slow ooze or sudden and severe. The presence of oesophageal varices can be demonstrated by:

(*a*) *Fibre-optic or rigid oesophagoscopy* will demonstrate them in all cases, and should be carried out along with gastroscopy to confirm the presence of varices and determine if they are the source of bleeding. The risks are not great in skilled hands, but if the lower oesophagus is full of fresh blood it may be impossible to see variceal bleeding. In such cases the diagnosis may be made by excluding duodenal and gastric lesions, or, if the patient's condition permits, by re-endo-scoping an hour or two later. If bleeding is very heavy and endoscopy is imposs-ible, tamponade (see below) may occasionally have to be started on the assumption that the bleeding is from oesophageal varices. If the bleeding is not immediately controlled, the diagnosis must again be questioned.

(b) *Radiology* after a barium swallow (fig. 899). In the great majority of cases oesophageal varices can be revealed by this method as filling defects. They may extend from below the gastroesophageal junction for 10–15 cm up the oesoph-agus. Perforating veins through the oesophageal wall connect them to the peri-oesophageal plexus. The presence of varices and the cause of the portal hyperten-sion, *e.g.* portal thrombosis or cirrhosis, can be demonstrated by *angiography*. The venous phase of a coeliac axis angiogram is now preferred to direct puncture of the spleen particularly as subtraction films give excellent definition.

Clinical Features.—If the patient is known to have hepatic cirrhosis, it should be assumed that the haemorrhage is coming from oesophageal varicose veins, although patients with cirrhosis of the liver are particularly likely to suffer also from a gastric or duodenal ulcer. In nearly all cases the spleen is palpably enlarged. Liver function tests, if abnormal, greatly favour hepatic cirrhosis as the cause of the haemorrhage. They are of value in deciding whether operation should be carried out because in those with a low serum albumin (below 25 g/l) and a high serum bilirubin the results of operation are poor.

Bleeding occurs in about 40% of all patients with cirrhosis and the initial episode of variceal haemorrhage is fatal in 50–60%. Usually two-thirds of those who survive will bleed again.

Treatment of Massive Haemorrhage from Oesophageal Varices

Rest, sedation, and replacement of blood will carry a few of the patients who are actively bleeding past the emergency period. For transfusion, fresh blood is particularly desirable. Careful monitoring of the blood pressure and central venous pressure is necessary.

By the time patients reach hospital about one third will have stopped bleeding, one third will be oozing and one third still bleeding heavily. There are four stages in management:

1. Resuscitation of the Patient

Ensuring a clear airway and rapid replacement of blood volume are the priorit-ies. Fluids containing sodium should be avoided because patients with liver disease retain sodium excessively, and great care must be taken with sedation as opiates and tranquillizers are normally metabolised in the liver.

2. Arrest of Haemorrhage

(a) *Tamponade.*—In patients who are still bleeding, the site of haemorrhage must be identified if possible (see above). Tamponade is the most direct and reliable method of arresting haemorrhage if carried out carefully by an experi-enced team. A Sengstaken type of tube with gastric and oesophageal balloons is

Robert William Sengstaken, Contemporary. Surgeon, Garden City, New York.

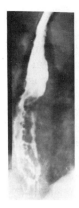

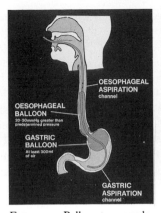

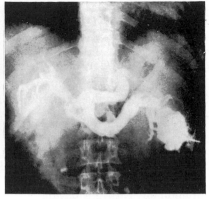

FIG.899.—Barium swallow showing filling defects due to oesophageal varices.

FIG. 900.—Balloon tamponade. Shows how the 4-channel tube is used to temporarily arrest active haemorrhage from gastro-oeso-phageal varices. The gastric channel can be used to wash out the stomach with ice-cold water to remove clots and decrease the gastric circulation.
(Courtesy of British Journal of Hospital Medicine.)

FIG. 901.—Splenoportograph in a case of intra-hepatic portal hypertension showing dilated splenic and portal veins.
(Professor R. Milnes Walker, FRCS, Bristol.)

the most commonly used (fig. 900) although a Linton tube with a single gastric balloon, drawn against the cardia by traction, is an alternative. Whichever is used there must be some method of aspirating saliva from the oesophagus to prevent inhalation pneumonia. The Sengstaken has now been modified with a fourth lumen, or a separate aspiration catheter can be attached to the older tubes. The gastric balloon should be inflated with 300–400 ml of air to ensure that the tube does not fall out and to compress the varices round the upper part of the stomach. (The pressure of the gastric balloon inside the stomach will be nearly the same as it was when inflated before insertion.) Once the gastric balloon is inflated in the right position, the oesophageal balloon is inflated to a volume which was found before insertion to produce an even distension. (The pressure should be 20–30 mmHg above that recorded before insertion, but if the pressure change is much higher than this, a little air should be let out of the balloon.) The tube is secured to the forehead to prevent it advancing into the stomach but strong traction is unnecessary; and the pressure in the balloon is measured at the beginning and checked at regular intervals to detect leaks. The tube is kept in position until the bleeding point is treated. This should not be more than 24 hours, preferably 12 hours. There is no point in deflating the balloons and then deciding what to do next as the rebleeding rate without further treatment is very high.

(b) *Drugs.*—Vasopressin (20 iu in 200 ml iv over 20 min and then 0·4 u/min for up to 24 hours) may be used to lower portal venous pressure and so reduce bleeding. Side effects include abdominal griping and coronary artery vasoconstriction so it must be used with caution in the elderly. Analogues of vasopressin (*e.g.* glypressin) are being evaluated and somatostatin has been used in some centres but is very expensive. Beta blocking drugs, although possibly of some use in special situations, have no place in acute variceal bleeding. *Morphine is contra-indicated.*

3. Treatment of Source of Bleeding

(a) *Endoscopic sclerotherapy* is now the simplest and safest way of treating haemorrhage from oesophageal varices and stops the bleeding in over 90% of cases. In the small number of patients in whom the bleeding continues, an operation must be considered (see below). If a Sengstaken tube is in position it should not be deflated until preparations are ready for immediate sclerotherapy.

Technique.—A rigid oesophagoscope may be used under general anaesthetic or a fibreoptic flexible oesophagoscope under sedation with pharyngeal analgesia. In addition, with the flexible endoscope, a sheath or balloon may be used to compress the remaining varices while one is being injected. In the *intravariceal* method 5–6 ml of ethanolamine oleate is injected into each varix at or just above the gastroesophageal junction to produce thrombosis. In the *paravasal* technique, *very small quantities* (0·5 ml) of sclerosant are injected in many different sites alongside each varix to produce perivascular fibrosis. If bleeding follows injection, balloon compression may be used for a short time afterwards. Sclerotherapy may be repeated the following day. Any anaesthetic must be given by an anaesthetist experienced in looking after patients with liver disease and even intravenous sedation must be used with caution in these patients. A general anaesthetic is best for very restless patients and those with large varices and heavy bleeding.

(b) *Operations.*—Emergency operations are avoided, if possible, in patients who are actually bleeding because of the high mortality, but if bleeding persists after sclerotherapy there is no alternative. There are two approaches: devascularisation and transection, or porta-systemic shunting (see below).

(i) *Devascularisation and transection operations.*—Over the years a number of operations have been devised, all incorporating a direct approach to the veins in the lower oesophagus. The Milnes-Walker and Borema-Crile procedures were transthoracic and involved direct ligation of the veins in the oesophagus, and Tanner's porta-azygos disconnection used an abdominal approach with transection of the upper stomach. These concepts have now been amalgamated into combined devascularisation transection operations, where the upper half of the stomach and lower part of the oesophagus are devascularised and then the gastro-oesophageal junction transected and reanastomosed, thereby interrupting the intramural and submucosal veins. The names of Siguira (Japan), Hassab (Egypt) are given to variations on this theme. If the vagal trunks are damaged during the procedure, a pyloroplasty must be added; the stapling gun makes the transection and reanastomosis relatively easy. The devascularisation must be continued well up the oesophagus when an abdominal incision is used (fig. 902).

The decision to operate must be made once it is clear that sclerotherapy is not likely to control the bleeding, before a series of injections has made the lower oesophagus oedematous and friable. The operation is not easy.

(ii) *Shunt operations.*—These are discussed below. They are best avoided in the presence of gastric bleeding except by very experienced surgeons. Before a shunt is contemplated, the site of portal block must be defined by angiography.

Robert Milnes Walker, 1903–1985. Professor of Surgery, Bristol, England.
George Crile, Jnr., Contemporary. Head of the Department of General Surgery, The Cleveland Clinic, Cleveland, Ohio, U.S.A.
Norman Cecil Tanner, 1906–1982. Consulting Surgeon, Charing Cross Hospital, London.

It is particularly important to diagnose a prehepatic portal block (which makes a portacaval shunt impossible).

4. General Management of Patient

Stopping the bleeding is the first priority but the general state of the patient must not be forgotten.

1. *Encephalopathy.*—Absorption of protein metabolites from the alimentary tract leads to encephalopathy. The bowel should be cleared of blood by enemas, purgatives (*e.g.* mag. sulphate) down the Sengstaken tube. In addition, lactulose and/or neomycin are given by mouth or tube to alter and reduce the proteolytic bacteria in the gut.

2. *Ascites.*—Spironolactone is the drug of choice. Fluid may be recycled into a vein using a special apparatus, but should *not* be drained by paracentesis.

3. *Correction of clotting problems.*—Vitamin K is given to correct the abnormal prothrombin time.

Prevention of rebleeding.—Usually the patient's bleeding is controlled temporarily by sclerotherapy. The decision must then be made about long term treatment. The alternatives are:

1. Repeated sclerotherapy with regular check endoscopies at two weeks, one month, three months and then six monthly, to diagnose and sclerose non-thrombosed varices or new varices that develop with time.

2. Devascularisation and oesophageal transection.

3. Porta-systemic shunts.

It is not yet clear which is the best long term management for patients with Grade A and Grade B liver function. In those with Grade C function, sclerotherapy is preferable to the considerable risks of operation (see fig. 903).

Prophylactic Treatment of Oesophageal Varices

There is no evidence yet that treatment of varices before they bleed prolongs survival. Controlled trials of prophylactic shunt operations showed no significant

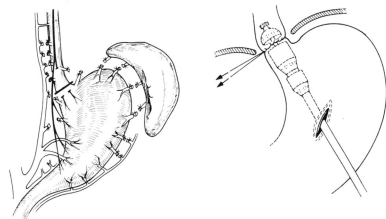

FIG. 902.—On the left, the vessels that need to be divided to interrupt the major feeders of bleeding varices are shown. On the right, the use of the stapling device to re-join the transected gastro-oesophageal junction is illustrated.

difference because of the mortality and complications of the operation. Whether prophylactic sclerotherapy, with its lower complication rate, will be successful remains to be seen.

Treatment of gastric varices.—It is rarely possible to inject gastric varices unless they are just around the cardia. Instead the treatment must be gastric devascularisation or shunt, together with direct ligation of the bleeding vein from inside the stomach.

Treatment of rectal varices (fig. 898).—The best treatment is direct ligation under anaesthetic using a continuous suture for about 5–6 cm along each varix. One of the newer, synthetic, slowly absorbed sutures is ideal. This relatively minor operation can be repeated if further varices develop.

Portal Hypertension

Splenoportography (Chapter 46) will usually display the site of the block, but if the portal vein does not fill, the cause may lie in a reversed flow in the splenic vein. If, therefore, there is suspicion that the portal vein may be obstructed, a venogram may also be done by injection into a mesenteric vein at laparotomy.

Measuring the Portal Blood Pressure.—One method is to record the intrasplenic pressure, and this can be done at the same time as transplenic portavenography. In cases of intra-hepatic obstruction an alternative method is to measure the wedged hepatic vein pressure. The technique is not especially difficult, and can be undertaken in any centre equipped for cardiac catheterisation. Following local anaesthesia and opening an antecubital vein as for cannulation, a cardiac catheter with only a terminal opening is passed into the vein. The catheter is advanced through the right auricle and inferior vena cava under radiological control. The tip is then insinuated into a hepatic vein until a peripheral radicle is occluded. It is important that the tip of the catheter should be in a peripheral position, so as to obviate obstruction by a bifurcation of the vein, and thus falsify results. Pressure recordings are then taken. The normal portal pressure is 8 to 12 mmHg (1·06–1·6 kPa). In cases of established cirrhosis it may rise to 30·0 mmHg (4 kPa) or more. The portal pressure is always high in cirrhotic patients who have oesophageal varices. The ascites of cirrhosis does not bear a direct relationship to elevated portal blood pressure, as was formerly believed. In specialised centres the patency of the portal vein can be confirmed and its pressure directly determined by passing a catheter, percutaneously inserted, into the liver and thence into the portal vein, and injecting contrast medium.

Treatment of Oesophageal Varices

At present, the preferred initial treatment for oesophageal varices is endoscopic injection sclerotherapy, because of its simplicity, lower mortality and repeatability. The technique has been described earlier (p. 928).

Indication for a Porta-systemic Shunting Operation

If bleeding cannot be controlled, emergency operation is required but is followed by high mortality and morbidity rates. If the patient has had several episodes of bleeding in the past, the operation may be performed electively after the patient's condition has been stabilised and provided that hepatic function is not severely impaired (see fig. 903).

Contraindications:

1. If the patient's serum albumin[1] is less than 30 g/l (3 g/100 ml).
2. If the patient is jaundiced significantly.
3. Massive ascites. Evacuation of this by suction at operation may lead to death on the table.
4. Operation should not be performed in a patient who has not bled from varices. Prophylactic operations do not prolong life and may reduce it.

---

[1] Normal level 3·6 to 4·5 g/100 ml (36–45 g/l).

Observations	Very suitable. A	Marginal. B	Unsuitable. C
Serum bilirubin (mg %)	Below 2·0	2·0–3·0	Over 3·0
Serum albumin (mg %)	Over 3·5	3·0–3·5	Below 3·0
Ascites	None	Easily controlled	Poorly controlled
Neurological disorder	None	Minimal	Coma
Nutritional status	Excellent	Good	Poor

FIG. 903.—Child's table indicating suitability of a patient with portal hypertension for shunt surgery.

Pre-operative treatment is directed mainly to correcting the accompanying hypochromic anaemia; blood transfusion is often required. Control of a bleeding tendency (secondary to impaired production of prothrombin) is essential and for this purpose vitamin K is given parenterally. If there is no immediate danger of renewed haemorrhage, those in whom a porta-systemic shunting operation is indicated are often benefitted greatly by a course of preoperative medical treatment. If ascites is present, a low sodium diet, in conjunction with diuretics, often causes absorption of ascitic fluid. If possible, paracentesis should be avoided. *Anaesthesia.*—In patients with liver disease great care must be taken with any sedation as most drugs are metabolised in the liver. Diazepam or another benzodiazepine (iv) is suitable for endoscopy if the dose is carefully titrated for each patient. For open operations or injection of varices in a confused or aggressive patient, an inhalant general anaesthetic is safer. Thiopentone induction followed by oxygen and nitrous oxide with suxamethonium as a relaxant does not rely on drugs whose metabolism is greatly affected by liver function (Ward).

OPERATIONS FOR PORTAL HYPERTENSION (fig. 904)

Preliminary investigations should have determined the cause of the venous block and its site. If doubt exists then an 'on-table' portal angiogram should be done, injecting contrast material into a suitable vein in the gastro-hepatic or superior mesenteric system.

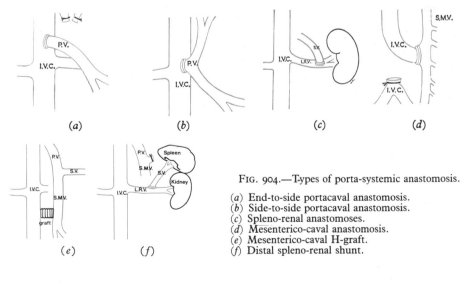

FIG. 904.—Types of porta-systemic anastomosis.

(a) End-to-side portacaval anastomosis.
(b) Side-to-side portacaval anastomosis.
(c) Spleno-renal anastomoses.
(d) Mesenterico-caval anastomosis.
(e) Mesenterico-caval H-graft.
(f) Distal spleno-renal shunt.

C.G. Child, Contemporary. Professor and Chairman, Dept. of Surgery, Michigan, U.S.A.
Michael Elliott Ward, Contemporary. Anaesthetist, Nuffield Department of Anaesthetics, Radcliffe Infirmary, Oxford.

1. **Portacaval Anastomosis.**—The traditional operation to decompress the splanchnic circulation is end-to-side portacaval shunt (fig. 904(a) provided that liver function is adequate and the portal vein is patent. The serum albumin level should be at least 30 g/l, and the serum bilirubin not more than 17 mmol/l.

The best approach is a subcostal one. The peritoneum is divided along the lower border of the right lobe of the liver and the lateral border of the duodenum. The portal vein is exposed by an incision through the peritoneum forming the anterior wall of the epiploic foramen, and a length of about 3 cm freed. An incision in the peritoneum over the vena cava exposes its anterior surface. The portal vein, or its two main branches, is now ligated at the hilum of the liver, a Blalock clamp placed on its lower end, and the vein divided.

After placing a side clamp on the vena cava, an incision is made in its anterior wall, and an end-to-side anastomosis made using everting fine silk sutures. The wound is closed with drainage.

With careful selection of cases the mortality of an elective porta-caval operation is about 6%, and recurrent bleeding from varices after this operation is most unusual.

Up to 30% of patients may have post-shunt encephalopathy because of venous deprivation of the liver and slow deterioration of liver function. Some surgeons believe that a side-to-side porta-caval anastomosis (fig. 904(b)) has a lower incidence of encephalopathy.

2. **Spleno-renal Anastomosis.** (fig. 904(c)—This may be performed if there is thrombosis of the portal vein, but it is contraindicated if the splenic vein is less than 1 cm in diameter as shown by venography. This operation is less effective than a portacaval anastomosis in preventing further haemorrhage, but carries a lower risk of encephalopathy. Owing to the small size of the splenic vein, this operation is rarely of value in cases of extrahepatic obstruction in children.

The operation is performed through a left thoraco-abdominal incision. The spleen is removed but during the dissection of the hilum as great a length as possible of the vein is carefully preserved. Enough vein is separated from the pancreas to allow its apposition to the renal vein, and it is temporarily occluded with a bull-dog clamp. The renal vein is dissected out and occluded by clamps or threads and the splenic vein anastomosed by everting sutures to an opening in its upper surface. To prevent engorgement of the kidney a temporary clamp may be put on the renal artery, but it should be released after fifteen minutes to allow a fresh flow of blood to the kidney.

3. **Superior Mesenterico-caval Anastomosis.** (fig. 904 (d) & (e)—When the portal vein is thrombosed this alternative may be possible. The inferior vena cava is divided just above its lower end, and ligated below. The proximal end is joined to the side of the superior mesenteric vein in the root of the mesentery. This operation is particularly indicated in children, who can tolerate complete division of the inferior vena cava without developing oedema of the lower limbs. Alternatively a shunt of synthetic material (Dacron) or of endogenous vein can be interposed between the superior mesenteric vein and the inferior vena cava. This mesentericocaval shunt (H-graft, 'jump' graft) is generally simpler to perform than the other operations, an advantage in emergency circumstances. It also can be carried out when the portal vein is occluded by thrombus. There is a high risk of late thrombosis in the graft. This operation does not reduce the risk of post-operative hepatoportal encephalopathy.

4. **Distal Splenorenal Shunt.** (fig. 904 (f)—Distal splenic vein is joined to the renal vein without splenectomy. The extrinsic gastric and lower oesophageal veins are ligated except the short gastric veins draining the stomach into the splenic bed. The objective is to decompress the critical area of the lower end of the oesophagus, yet preserving a venous blood supply to the liver. The incidence of encephalopathy is said to be low. The operation presents technical difficulties in the obese patient and those with splenomegaly.

Other shunt operations are being evaluated, including left gastric venocaval shunt, umbilicocaval shunt and arterialisation of the portal vein with portacaval shunt.

5. **Splenectomy.**—This has no place in the treatment of portal hypertension except in the very rare cases of thrombosis confined to the splenic vein, or in combination with some other operation.

6. **Other.**—When conditions are not ideal for time-consuming or sophisticated investigations, or when the patient's liver function is inadequate for a porta-systemic shunt or there is no suitable patent vein, it is desirable to make an effort to interrupt the communications between the left gastric (portal system) and oesophageal veins (azygos system)—porto-azygos disconnection—so cutting off the flow of portal blood to the varices by direct and simple methods.

(a) **Oesophageal Transection** (Milnes Walker).—The aim of this operation is to cut

Alfred Blalock, 1899–1964. Surgeon-in-Chief, Johns Hopkins Hospital, Baltimore, U.S.A.

off the flow of portal blood to the varices. Through a left trans-thoracic approach the lower end of the oesophagus is mobilised and the vagus nerves separated from it. The oesophagus is transected at the level of the hiatus in the diaphragm, and resutured with continuous sutures in the mucosa and submucosa which obliterate the vessels.

(*b*) **Suture of the Varices** after opening the lower part of the oesophagus longitudinally (Crile), just above the diaphragm. The varices, extending through the cardia are underrun with continuous chromic catgut.

(*c*) **Gastric Transection** (Tanner).—The aim is similar to that of oesophageal transection. Through a left thoraco-abdominal approach, the upper part of the stomach is transected and reanastomosed with continuous sutures to obliterate the blood vessels.

(*d*) **Oesophageal Stapling** (Johnston).—A simple way of interrupting dilated varices within the oesophageal wall is to pass a stapling instrument into the lower oesophagus through a small hole in the anterior wall of the stomach. When operated, the instrument simultaneously divides the oesophagus and joins it together again with staples which occlude the vessels. The results of this operation are reasonably effective and it has the merit of simplicity.

All of these operations may be helpful in emergency circumstances or when the splanchnic vessels are thrombosed, thus averting a shunt operation, but rebleeding is common.

NEOPLASMS OF THE LIVER

Benign:

Haemangioma occurs more commonly in the liver than in any other internal organ, and usually the neoplasm is of the cavernous type. As a rule, a haemangioma of the liver is solitary, and is found either at necropsy or incidentally at operation. Exceptionally, it becomes large enough to cause symptoms, in which event laparotomy is required to establish the diagnosis. The compressibility of the tumour makes the diagnosis unmistakable, and on no account should biopsy be performed, for the resulting haemorrhage is terrific. Radiotherapy is often useful in reducing the size of the tumour. Excision of tumour confined to a lobe necessitates hemi-hepatectomy.

Hepato-adenomas are composed of hepatic cells. Frequently multiple and small, they are distinguished with difficulty from the nodular hyperplasia of cirrhosis. There is no evidence that they become malignant. These tumours occur almost exclusively in women and are becoming more common because of the use of oral contraceptives. Their removal is unnecessary.

Cholangio-adenomas originate from the bile-ducts and form small subcapsular masses. They are found at operation or necropsy, and can simulate closely metastatic deposits, which should not be assumed without biopsy. They are harmless.

Malignant:

Primary carcinoma of the liver is uncommon in European races, but is by no means rare in Africans, Malayans, Chinese, and Japanese. The highest recorded incidence is in Mozambique where it is a thousand times as common as in most of Europe. In the majority of these patients it arises as a complication of cirrhosis. A similar ratio is not found among the coloured and white North American peoples. Two pathological varieties are described:

1. **Hepatocarcinoma** arises in the liver cells and constitutes about 80% of primary malignancies of the liver. There are great variations in the malignancy of this tumour, which may be multicentric in origin, particularly when it occurs in a cirrhotic liver. At one end of the scale is a relatively benign, firm, slowly growing tumour, and at the other a rapidly growing, soft neoplasm prone to undergo necrosis, which soon metastasies within the liver, or to the lymph nodes in the hilum of the liver, mediastinum or neck. The alphafetoprotein level is raised.

2. **Cholangiocarcinoma.**—(Chapter 47).

Clinical Features of Primary Carcinoma of the Liver.—These tumours occur

George Johnston, Contemporary. Surgeon, Royal Victoria Hospital, Belfast.

in children and in older people, but are rare between the ages of 20 and 40 except in those countries where the incidence is high and then this is the age group most affected. The usual train of events is anorexia, rapid loss of weight, and asthenia. On examination an enlarged liver is found and often a localised mass. Less frequently the patient presents on account of a swelling he has discovered in the upper abdomen: the swelling may, or may not, be tender, depending on the rate of growth. Neoplastic proliferation is sometimes so rapid as to cause a low pyrexia, in which event, in tropical countries, an amoebic abscess will be considered as a possible diagnosis. Every effort is made to seek a possible primary growth, bearing in mind that, at any rate in Caucasians, secondary carcinoma of the liver is immeasurably more common than primary carcinoma. In patients with primary liver cancer, α-1-fetoprotein (AFP) may be present in the plasma long before clinical features appear. AFP is a normal component of the plasma protein of the human fetus older than six weeks and disappears a few weeks after birth. It is a valuable screening method for patients with primary liver carcinoma with cirrhosis. Radio-scanning (p. 907) may be helpful and needle biopsy of the liver may establish the diagnosis. Additional diagnostic techniques include ultrasonic scanning, coeliac axis angiography and CT scanning (fig. 881).

Ascites is present in about 40% of patients at the time of the first examination; diagnostic aspiration often reveals blood-stained ascitic fluid. Such ascites resists therapy, and re-accumulates rapidly after paracentesis.

SECONDARY NEOPLASMS OF THE LIVER

Secondary Carcinoma.—As is well known, the liver is a favourite site for carcinomatous metastases. Characteristically, secondary growths in the liver, owing to degeneration of cells in the centre, are umbilicated. As a rule, carcinomatous deposits in the liver are multiple (figs. 905 and 906). Occasionally at lapar-

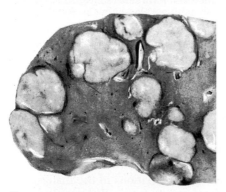

FIG. 905.—Secondary carcinoma of the liver.

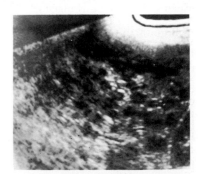

FIG. 906.—Multiple 'echo-free' or 'transonic' metastases in the liver from carcinoma of the breast.
(Dr. J. McIvor, FRCR, London.)

otomy a secondary growth in the liver is found to be apparently solitary and accessible (fig. 908). In such circumstances, provided that the primary growth can be or has been resected, excision of that part of the liver containing the neoplasm sometimes results in a long-lasting survival.

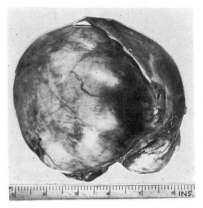

FIG. 907.—Hepatoma resected from the liver successfully.

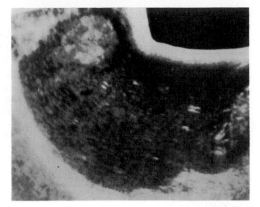

FIG. 908.—Solitary 'echogenic' metastasis in the liver arising from carcinoma of the colon, possibly suitable for lobectomy or hemi-hepatectomy.
(*Dr. J. McIvor, FRCR, London.*)

Secondary melanoma occurs particularly when the primary growth is in the eye. Fifteen years or more have elapsed between the removal of the primary growth and the appearance of secondary deposits.

Secondary carcinoid (argentaffin) tumours (Chapter 50) are rare; where they occur they often grow to a large size. There are always many hepatic metastases when malignant carcinoid of the small intestine or bronchus is associated with vasomotor abnormalities and pulmonary stenosis. The increased urinary excretion of 5-hydroxy-indole-acetic acid is helpful in making a diagnosis.

Secondary Sarcoma.—The liver is not an uncommon site for secondary deposits in cases of sarcoma, but the lungs show a much higher incidence.

Treatment of Neoplasms of the Liver

Secondary tumours of the liver are most resistant to treatment. Ligation of the hepatic artery to deprive the tumours of blood-supply and infusion of chemotherapeutic agents are not very effective. Occasionally where a solitary secondary nodule is located in one lobe of the liver, hepatic lobectomy may be carried out. This procedure is curative in some cases but may prolong life in others: if the nodule is superficial local resection can be an alternative to lobectomy.

The management of *primary hepatic tumours* is depressing because untreated patients survive only 3–5 months after diagnosis. Radiotherapy and chemotherapy have been disappointing. Attempts have been made to improve results by ligating the hepatic artery, considered to be the major feeding vessel for such tumours, but there is no evidence that the results are improved. Hepatic transplantation has been carried out for liver tumour but the results in terms of long-term survival are disappointing and it is only considered if there is no evidence of extrahepatic spread. Where primary hepatoma is located to one or other lobe of the liver, and provided that the rest of the liver itself is normal and not cirrhotic, the affected lobe of the liver may be excised (fig. 907). It is occasionally possible to resect a peripheral lesion in a cirrhotic liver leaving enough functioning tissue for the survival of the patient.

Resection of a Benign Tumour of the Liver.—In order to conserve blood, the hepatic artery and portal vein can be clamped lightly at the porta hepatis, and released every five minutes. Another very important point is that branches of the hepatic artery and the portal vein ramify through the liver in the portal canals: each of these canals is surrounded by a prolongation of Glisson's capsule which, when encountered with a blunt instrument, gives a sense of resistance. Thus, if liver tissue is dissected with the finger, it is possible to divide liver tissue, but spare the vessels, which can be clamped and ligated, or coagulated with diathermy, before division. The resection completed, the resulting raw surfaces of the cut liver are dealt with in the same manner as described for rupture of the liver.

Francis Glisson, 1598–1677. Regius Professor of Physic, Cambridge, England.

Hemi-hepatectomy.—A number of cases of successful removal of the surgical right lobe of the liver for primary and secondary tumours or for carcinoma of the gall-bladder have been reported. Removal of the surgical left lobe is less frequently necessary and left (anatomical) lobectomy usually suffices (Rodney Smith).

Right Hemi-hepatectomy.—After operability has been determined through a right paramedian incision, extension into a right thoraco-abdominal is achieved through the eighth interspace. The liver is mobilised and rotated forwards and upwards into the chest to expose the porta hepatis. Working from below upwards, the cystic artery and duct, the right hepatic duct, right hepatic artery, and right branch of the portal vein are successively divided between ligatures. The inferior vena cava is then exposed by mobilising the duodenum and head of pancreas and drawing them over to the left (Kocher's manoeuvre). It is then possible to expose, ligate, and divide the inconstant minor hepatic veins running from the right lobe into the cava, up as high as the site of entry of the right hepatic vein; great care must be taken not to obstruct the venous return in the vena cava. The liver is then divided from in front and above between the surgical lobes by diathermy or the 'finger fracture' technique. The right hepatic vein is then exposed and divided and also the right-sided branches of the middle hepatic vein as they are encountered. The raw surface of the left lobe is covered with the falciform ligament and it is wise to drain the entire area. Some surgeons advocate draining the common bile duct.

Liver Transplantation is dealt with in Chapter 62.

Rodney Smith (Lord Smith of Marlow), Contemporary. Formerly Surgeon, St. George's Hospital, London.
Theodor Kocher, 1841–1917. Professor of Clinical Surgery, University of Berne, Switzerland.

CHAPTER 46

THE SPLEEN

Anatomy.—The normal spleen weighs about 150 g and is situated posteriorly between the fundus of the stomach and the diaphragm in the line of the 10th rib. The tail of the pancreas is adjacent to the splenic hilum and in children the spleen rests on the left adrenal gland.

The cut surface of the spleen consists of areas of 'red pulp' within which can be seen pale, ovoid nodules (about 1mm diameter) of 'white pulp' (Malpighian bodies). The splenic artery divides at the hilus into branches which run along the trabeculae. These trabecular arteries pass into the white pulp (fig. 909) where they give off branches which are almost perpendicular to the central trunk. This produces a skimming effect by which plasma tends to pass down the branches to the white pulp and most of the red cells pass in the trabecular artery to the red pulp. The white pulp has an immune function whereas the red pulp filters abnormal red cells from the circulation. Phagocytosis of blood borne particles occurs in both areas.

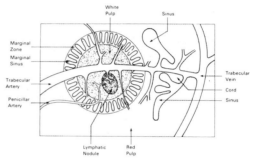

FIG. 909.—A central trabecular artery passing through the white pulp into the surrounding red pulp. A blood flow skimming effect results in most of the plasma passing down branches of the artery while the cells pass in the central trabecular artery directly to the red pulp.

The white pulp consists of a central trabecular artery surrounded by lymphatic nodules with germinal centres and periarterial lymphatic sheaths which provide a framework filled with lymphocytes and macrophages. At the edge of the white pulp is the marginal zone into which pass arteries from both the central artery and from peripheral 'penicillar' arteries. Plasma-rich blood which has passed through the central lymphatic nodules is filtered as it passes through the sinuses within the marginal zone, and particles are phagocytosed. Immunoglobulins produced in the lymphatic nodules enter the circulation through the sinuses in the marginal zone. Beyond the marginal zone is the red pulp which consists of cords and sinuses. Cell-concentrated blood passes in the trabecular artery through the centre of the white pulp to the red pulp cords. In order to pass from the cords to the sinuses, the red cell must elongate and become thinner. This filters abnormally shaped or rigid cells out of the circulation.

90% of the blood passing through the spleen moves through an 'open' circulation in which blood flows from arteries to cords and thence to sinuses. The remaining 10% bypasses the cords and sinuses by direct arteriovenous connections. The overall flow rate through the spleen is about 300 ml/min.

Functions of the Spleen.—The spleen is not essential to life and the effects of its removal are not obvious from clinical examination. The role of the spleen in health and disease has not been fully elucidated.[1] However, the spleen is known to have the following functions:

1. *Response to antigenic challenge.*.—There is a proliferation of T-lymphocytes within the lymphatic sheaths, and antibody-forming B-lymphocytes within the lymphatic nodules. This results in increased production of humoral immune factors of both B and T-

---

[1] Organum plenum mysterium (*Latin*) = Organ full of mystery (*Galen*).

Marcello Malpighi, 1628–1694. Pioneer Italian Microscopist, Pisa.
Galen, 130–200. First experimental physiologist and personal physician to the Roman emperors Marcus Aurelius Commodus and Septimus Severus.

cell origin: *antibody* (especially IgM), *tuftsin* (a peptide which stimulates phagocytosis by neutrophils), *opsonins*[1] (antibodies and other proteins which react with bacteria and fungi to make them more susceptible to phagocytosis), *properdin* (an immunoglobulin, found in unchallenged animals which have not formed antibody, that fixes complement to bacterial and fungal surface polysaccharides prior to phagocytosis), and *interferon* (a glycoprotein which exerts an antiviral effect by stimulating killer-cell/macrophage activity). Splenectomised patients develop decreased levels of all these factors, and this reduces resistance—in particular to encapsulated bacteria. 24 hours after production in the spleen, 75% of neutrophils either pass to other tissues or are destroyed. Neutropenia in hypersplenism occurs either because of granulocyte sequestration in the spleen, *e.g.* in hypersplenism, or because of splenic destruction of altered granulocytes as in autoimmune neutropenias.

2. *Destruction of abnormally shaped or rigid red cells* by 'culling' and 'pitting' which take place in the red pulp. Culling refers to the filtering and phagocytosis of old red blood cells which have either been damaged or contain inclusions such as nuclei, nuclear remnants (Howell-Jolly bodies), target cells, siderocytes and spherocytes. Pitting is the removal of certain inclusions *e.g.* red blood cell nuclei or malarial parasites from red blood cells without destroying the cells. The normal red cell life span of approximately 120 days is not prolonged after splenectomy because there are other sites of red cell destruction.

3. *Phagocytosis of foreign substances* by reticuloendothelial macrophages in the spleen. This is exemplified by the uptake of radio-opaque thorium into the spleen following administration of the contrast agent thorotrast which was once used in arteriography and cerebral ventriculography. Thorium can be seen in the spleen on plain x-ray 20 years after administration of the thorotrast. Radioactive decay of the thorium over this period can produce splenic fibrosis and hyposplenism. Particulate matter, and bacteria, fungi and protozoa are also removed from the circulation by these macrophages. A similar process of phagocytosis of abnormal lipoids is the cause of splenic enlargement in the lipoid dystrophies.

4. *Platelet reservoir.*—The spleen normally sequesters 30–40% of blood platelets. The lifespan of platelets in the circulation is about 10 days. In splenomegaly, up to 80% of the platelet pool can be sequestered in the spleen and this, together with accelerated platelet destruction, can result in thrombocytopenia. Platelet phagocytosis is a normal function of the spleen but in conditions such as idiopathic thrombocytopenic purpura it is accelerated. In some animals, but not in man, the spleen also contains a reserve of red cells which can be released into the circulation following a hypoxic stimulus.

5. *Erythrocyte production.*—Red blood cells are normally produced in the fetal spleen from the fourth month of development until birth. Erythropoesis does not take place in the spleen after birth unless marrow production of red cells is defective *e.g.* in myelofibrosis.

Investigation of the spleen

Conditions which cause splenomegaly can often be diagnosed by history, and physical and laboratory examination. For example a haemolytic anaemia is detectable by full blood count, reticulocyte count and tests for haemolysis. Similarly, splenomegaly associated with portal hypertension caused by hepatic cirrhosis is diagnosed by the physical signs of liver dysfunction, abnormal liver function tests and evidence of oesophageal varices. Many conditions which cause splenomegaly also cause lymphadenopathy. The cause of the splenomegaly should then be determined from investigations for diseases known to cause splenomegaly and lymphadenopathy—possibly including a lymph node biopsy. There are also more direct methods of investigating the spleen:

1. **Plain x-ray.**—The spleen may be visible as a soft tissue shadow in plain films of the upper abdomen. This finding, repeated at intervals, is evidence that the spleen is not ruptured. Calcification in the spleen may suggest an old infarct or a hydatid cyst. Multiple areas of calcification suggest splenic tuberculosis.

2. **Scanning.**—There are various techniques for scanning the spleen:

(*a*) *Ultrasound examination* of the spleen (fig. 910) can usually provide information about its size and consistency *e.g.* the presence of cysts. Ultrasound is the investigation of choice when there is difficulty in diagnosing a ruptured spleen or a subcapsular haematoma.

(*b*) In cases where ultrasound is not able to visualise the spleen *e.g.* where there is

---

[1] Opsonein (Gk) = to prepare food for.

William Henry Howell, 1960–1945. Professor of Physiology, Johns Hopkins University, Baltimore, U.S.A.
Justin Marie Jules Jolly, 1870–1953. Professor of Histophysiology, College de France, Paris.

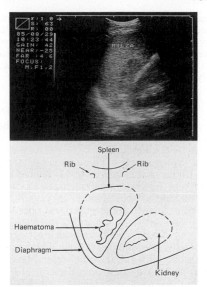

FIG. 910.—Ultrasound image obtained with a probe situated over the anterior aspect of the left lower ribs showing the spleen containing a haematoma. The left kidney is situated behind the spleen and the posterior diaphragm can be seen as it dips down posteriorly behind the left kidney. (*Courtesy of Dr L. Solbiati, Ospidale Busto Arsizio, Milan.*) The subcapsular splenic haematoma is shown near the hilar surface of the spleen, as the drawing below it illustrates.

surrounding bowel gas, *CT scanning* may be useful in diagnosing splenomegaly, a splenic infarct or haematoma. CT scanning is particularly useful in conditions where splenomegaly is associated with lymphadenopathy because the size of the para-aortic lymph nodes can be determined at the same examination (fig. 911).

(*c*) *Radioisotope scans* using ⁹⁹Tc-labelled colloid can also provide information about the position and size of the spleen. The ability of the spleen to remove damaged red cells from the circulation can be assessed by administering heat-damaged red cells, labelled with ⁵¹Cr, which are removed from the circulation in the splenic red pulp. Administration of platelets labelled with ¹¹¹In provides similar information about the sequestration of platelets in the spleen.

3. **Portal and splenic venogram.**—Occasionally visualisation of the splenic and portal

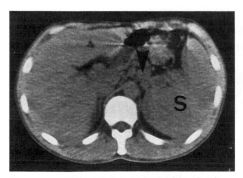

FIG. 911.—CT scan[1] showing an enlarged spleen (S) with enlarged para-aortic lymph nodes (arrowhead) in a case of leukaemia.
(*Dr Maurice Turner, The London Hospital.*)

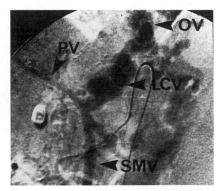

FIG. 912.—Venous phase of a selective mesenteric angiogram. The superior mesenteric vein (SMV) and portal vein (PV) are filled with contrast. Due to portal hypertension abnormal retrograde flow has occurred with flow from the portal vein via the coronary vein (LCV) adjacent to the stomach into oesophageal varices (OV) running up the lower part of the oesophagus.
(*Courtesy Dr. H. Nunnerley, King's College Hospital, London.*)

[1] Note that CT scans are viewed from the feet of the patient.

vein (fig. 912) can be helpful in the identification of a site of portal vein occlusion or in deciding whether the direction of flow along the portal vein is reversed. This can be done by taking films during the venous filling phase after coeliac and mesenteric angiography. Reversed flow along variceal collateral vessels can be seen better with computerised digital subtraction. Direct splenoportography via a needle puncture of the spleen is rarely necessary.

CONGENITAL ABNORMALITIES OF THE SPLEEN

1. **Absence of the spleen** is rare and when it occurs it is often associated with congenital heart disease. Patients without a spleen are occasionally subject to fatal infection (see Functions above).

2. **Splenunculi.**—These are single or multiple accessory spleens which are found near the hilum of the spleen (50%), related to the splenic vessels and behind the tail of the pancreas (30%) or in the splenic ligaments and mesocolon. They are important because if left behind at splenectomy, they undergo hyperplasia and lead to a recurrence of the disorder for which the spleen was removed.

3. **Hamartomas.**—Rarely, these are found in the spleen—usually incidentally at autopsy. They vary in size from less than a centimetre in diameter to masses large enough to produce abdominal swelling. There are two varieties: one mainly lymphoid resembling the white pulp and the other resembling the red pulp.

4. **Splenic cysts.**—Non-parasitic cysts are rare. They consist of true cysts formed from embryonal rests and include dermoids and mesenchymal inclusion cysts, or false cysts resulting from trauma which contain serous or haemorrhagic fluid.

RUPTURE OF THE SPLEEN

Splenic rupture can result from a blow to the abdomen, for example in a road traffic accident or a punch to the upper abdomen. The shock impact of a fall can also rupture the spleen, and in children splenic rupture can be produced by a fall from a bicycle—particularly if the handlebars strike the abdomen—or a swing. A splenic injury should be suspected if there are fractures of the overlying ribs. Less frequently the spleen may be lacerated by a knife or bullet. The spleen ruptures more easily when it is enlarged e.g. in infectious mononucleosis or malaria. Advantage was once taken of this in countries where malaria is endemic in the Far East. Murderers could achieve their purpose by digging a victim beneath the left ribs with a weapon known as a larang; the enlarged malarial spleen would rupture easily.

Cases of ruptured spleen may be divided into three groups:

1. **The Patient Succumbs Rapidly, Never Rallying from the Initial Shock.**— This type is comparatively rare in temperate climates; tearing of the splenic vessels and complete avulsion of the spleen from its pedicle[1] give rise to rapid shock which can be fatal within minutes.

2. **Initial shock; recovery from shock; signs of a ruptured spleen** is the usual type seen in surgical practice. After the initial shock has passed off, there are signs which point to intra-abdominal bleeding.

General signs of internal haemorrhage are variable. Perhaps the most helpful are increasing pallor, a rising pulse-rate, sighing respiration, and restlessness.

Local Signs.—(a) Abdominal rigidity is present in more than 50% of cases; it is most pronounced in the left upper quadrant.

(b) Local bruising and tenderness in the left upper abdominal quadrant.

---

[1] Favoured by adhesion of the spleen to the diaphragm.

(*c*) Abdominal distension commences about three hours after the accident, and is due to the irritative effect of the intraperitoneal blood which produces peritonism and ileus.

(*d*) Kehr's sign is pain referred to the left shoulder. There may be hyperaesthesia in this area. This sign can often be demonstrated a quarter of an hour after elevation of the foot of the bed. It is due to blood in contact with the under-surface of the diaphragm, the pain being mediated through afferent fibres in the phrenic nerve.

(*e*) Shifting dullness in the flanks is often present.

Ballance's sign is positive in about 25% of cases. There is a dull note in both flanks, but on the right side it can be made to shift, whereas on the left it is constant. The interpretation is that there is blood in the peritoneal cavity, but the blood in the neighbourhood of the lacerated spleen has coagulated.

(*f*) Rectal examination frequently reveals tenderness and sometimes a soft swelling, due to blood or clot in the rectovesical pouch.

3. **The Delayed Type of Case.**—After the initial shock has passed off, the symptoms of a *serious* intra-abdominal catastrophe are postponed for a variable period up to fifteen days, or even more. As a rule it is only a matter of minutes to an hour or so, during which time the patient often appears to have recovered from the blow. Thus a Rugby footballer may continue to play after a short rest, only to collapse later from internal haemorrhage.

Delay of serious intraperitoneal bleeding is explained in one of the following ways:
(*a*) The greater omentum, shuts off that portion of the general peritoneal cavity in the immediate vicinity of the bleeding (fig. 1011(*c*), Chapter 49).
(*b*) A subcapsular haematoma forms and later bursts.
(*c*) Blood-clot temporarily sealing the rent becomes digested by escaping ferments from the lacerated tail of the pancreas. What may happen is that a patient with a suspected rupture of the spleen is taken into hospital; the symptoms abate, and in due course he is allowed up and then he suddenly collapses. At other times fresh haemorrhage is heralded by a rising pulse-rate, increasing pallor, advancing to air-hunger and collapse. Such disasters can, and should, be prevented by careful re-examination and radiography.

Investigation.—Ultrasound examination of the spleen is the investigation of choice where there is difficulty in making a diagnosis of splenic rupture. The spleen can usually be visualised and a surrounding haematoma may suggest rupture (fig. 909). Serial examinations, by showing a change in splenic size, can identify an enlarging subcapsular haematoma.

A normal well-outlined spleen on plain x-ray of the upper abdomen, is a reliable sign of an intact spleen. The radiological signs of splenic rupture are: (1) Obliteration of the splenic outline. (2) Obliteration of the psoas shadow. (3) Indentation of the left side of the gastric air bubble. (4) Fracture of one of more lower ribs on the left side (present in 27% of cases). (5) Elevation of the left side of the diaphragm. (6) Free fluid between gas filled intestinal coils.

Treatment of Rupture of the Spleen.—Immediate laparotomy and splenectomy is the only reliable course. Blood is evacuated and, after injury to other viscera has been excluded, the abdomen is closed. When the organ is damaged by a stab wound or missile penetrating the left pleural cavity, access to the spleen is best obtained by excising the thoracic and diaphragmatic wounds, and enlarging the opening in the diaphragm. Blood transfused should be as required.

Recently in children splenorrhaphy is advised and several techniques of repairing the torn spleen are described, but this should *not* be attempted unless the surgeon has experience with the technique.

Hans Kehr, 1862–1916. Surgeon, Halberstädt, later Berlin. He died of septicaemia contracted during this work.
Sir Charles Alfred Ballance, 1856–1936. Surgeon, St. Thomas's Hospital, London.

Rupture of a Malarial Spleen.—As has been mentioned, in tropical countries this is a frequent catastrophe. The delayed type of rupture (following a trivial injury) is also very common, and the patient is admitted with a perisplenic haematoma. If splenectomy can be performed before the haematoma bursts into the general peritoneal cavity, the prognosis is less grave.

The operation is considerably more difficult than in the case of a ruptured normal spleen. Surgeons with tropical experience have surmounted these difficulties by ligating the splenic vessels as they run along the superior border of the body of the pancreas (fig. 913), before disturbing the haematoma (Andreasen) (and see p. 951).

ANEURYSM AND INFARCTION

Aneurysm of the splenic artery.—This is an uncommon condition; estimates of its incidence at autopsy vary between 0·04% and 1%. Whereas aneurysms of other arteries are more common in men, in the splenic artery they are about twice as common in women. They are usually single and situated on the main trunk of the splenic artery (fig. 913), but more than one is found in a quarter of cases.

The aneurysm is usually symptomless unless it ruptures. Occasionally it is palpable in the epigastrium or associated with a bruit over the left hypochondrium. It may be discovered accidentally, on plain x-ray of the upper abdomen, as a calcified ring situated to the left of the first lumbar vertebra. Rupture of the aneurysm is unsuspected in about half of all cases; it bursts into the peritoneal cavity and the symptoms resemble those of splenic rupture. Nearly half of all cases of rupture occur in patients less than 45 years of age, and a quarter of all cases are in pregnant women (usually in the last trimester of pregnancy or actually in labour).

The treatment of choice is splenectomy and removal of the length of artery bearing the aneurysm. If the aneurysm has eroded into the pancreas or is close to the origin of the splenic artery, then proximal and distal ligation of the sac is usually followed by thrombosis in the aneurysm. In younger patients, particularly women, with asymptomatic splenic artery anerysm, surgical treatment is indicated after the diagnosis has been confirmed by selective coeliac arteriography. The maternal mortality of surgery at the time of rupture, in late pregnancy, is over 70%. In elderly patients, particularly men, where an asymptomatic calcified aneurysm is detected on plain x-ray, there is less risk of rupture and surgery is not indicated.

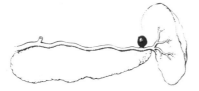

FIG. 913.—Usual position of a splenic aneurysm.
(After O. E. Owen, Caernarvon, Wales.)

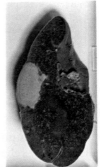

FIG. 914.—Infarct of the spleen.

Infarction of the spleen (fig. 914).—This occurs in patients with massive spleens resulting from a myeloproliferative syndrome, or with vascular occlusion produced by sickle cell disease or an embolus from an infected heart valve in bacterial endocarditis. The infarct may be asymptomatic or may cause left upper quadrant abdominal pain radiating to the left shoulder with splinting of the left hemidiaphragm, guarding and, at time, a friction rub heard over the splenic area. Sedation and bed rest are sufficient, except rarely when a septic infarct causes an abscess necessitating splenectomy.

Anthony Turner Andreasen, Contemporary. Surgeon, Kampala, Uganda.

ENLARGEMENT OF THE SPLEEN

The spleen is a meeting-place of medicine and surgery. The following is a useful table of the many causes of enlargement of the organ:

1. Infective

- *Bacterial—*
  - Typhoid and Paratyphoid.
  - Typhus.
  - Anthrax.
  - Tuberculosis.†
  - Septicaemia.
  - Abscess of the spleen.‡
- *Spirochaetal—*
  - Weil's disease.
  - Syphilis.
- *Viral—*
  - Infectious mononucleosis
  - Psittacosis.
- *Protozoal— & Parasitic—*
  - Malaria.
  - Schistosomiasis (Egyptian splenomegaly)†
  - Trypanosomiasis
  - Kala-azar.
  - Hydatid cyst.*
  - Tropical splenomegaly.†

2. Blood diseases

- Myelofibrosis.‡
- Acute leukaemia.
- Chronic leukaemia (lymphocytic or granulocytic).‡
- Pernicious anaemia.
- Polycythaemia vera.
- Erythroblastosis foetalis.
- Hereditary spherocytosis.*
- Autoimmune haemolytic anaemia.†
- Idiopathic Thrombocytopenic purpura.*
- Mediterranean anaemia (thalassaemia).‡
- Sickle cell disease‡

3. Metabolic

- Rickets.
- Amyloid.
- Porphyria.
- Gaucher's disease‡ (Chapter 45).

4. Circulatory

- *Infarct—*
  - Infective endocarditis.‡
  - Mitral stenosis.
- *Occlusion of the portal vein—*
  - Portal hypertension (Chapter 45).‡
  - Thrombophlebitis.†
  - Neoplastic, *e.g.* carcinoma of tail of pancreas.‡

5. Collagen Diseases

- Still's disease (Chapter 19).
- Felty's syndrome.† (Chapter 46).

6. Non-parasitic cysts

- Congenital.*
- Acquired.*

7. Neoplastic

- Angioma.*
- Primary fibrosarcoma.*
- Hodgkin's lymphoma.‡ (Chapter 9).
- Other lymphomas.‡

* Benefited by splenectomy.   † Often benefited by splenectomy.
‡ Splenectomy sometimes indicated.

In connection with the above Table, the following points should be noted. In idiopathic thrombocytopenic purpura the spleen, although somewhat enlarged, is seldom palpable. In psittacosis the enlarged spleen can be palpated regularly after the first few days of the illness; this enlargement is helpful to differentiating the condition from other varieties of

Adolph Weil, 1848–1916. Physician, Dorpat (Tartu), Estonia.

pneumonia. In portal hypertension the spleen is enlarged secondary to hepatic cirrhosis or portal vein thrombosis (Chapter 45).

Hereditary Spherocytosis.—The essential lesion is an increase in permeability of the red cell membrane to sodium. As the sodium leaks into the red cell its osmotic pressure rises, it swells and becomes more spherical and in consequence more fragile. The mechanism by which the cell rids itself of sodium—the sodium pump—has to work harder. This has two consequences (a) there is greater loss of membrane phospholipid and so a weakening of the membrane which thus becomes more fragile and (b) the energy and the oxygen requirements increase. These requirements are particularly difficult to satisfy in the spleen where there is a deficiency of both glucose and oxygen. Thus a large number of red cells are destroyed in the spleen, and splenectomy reduces this cell destruction. Splenectomy does not, of course, cure the congenital red cell membrane defect but it lessens the anaemia and makes the red cell survival time normal. The defect is transmitted by either parent as a Mendelian autosomal dominant.[1] Males and females are equally affected.

The circulating bilirubin is not conjugated with glycuronic acid. It is attached to albumin and is not excreted in the urine (alcholuric jaundice).[2]

Clinical Features.—Once the disease manifests itself, spontaneous remissions are almost unknown. As a rule the patient is pale and has jaundice, which at its height is of a pale daffodil hue. In established cases lassitude and undue fatigue are usually present, but they vary with the amount of haemolysis.

Sometimes the patient is born jaundiced, or becomes so early in life. In certain families the disease is characterised by severe crises of red-blood-cell destruction; thus, with the onset of a crisis, an erythrocyte count may fall from 4½ millions to 1½ millions in less than a week. Such crises are characterised by the sudden onset of pyrexia, abdominal pain, nausea, vomiting, and extreme pallor, followed by increased jaundice. These crises may be precipitated by acute infection, and can be so severe as to cause death in infancy or childhood. More usually the jaundice, although variable, is very mild, and may not appear until adolescent or even adult life. In adult cases there is often a history of attacks of gall-stone colic; indeed, 68% of untreated patients over the age of ten years have pigment stones in the gall-bladder. Every child with gall-stones should be investigated for evidence of hereditary spherocytosis and enquiry should be made amongst relatives of patients with spherocytosis for evidence of similar disease.

On examination the spleen is large, and in thin subjects it can be palpated easily. Sometimes the liver is also palpable. Chronic ulcers of the legs can occur in adults with the disease.

Haematological Investigations

The Fragility Test.—Increased fragility of erythrocytes characterises this disease. Normally, erthrocytes begin to haemolyse in 0·47% saline solution. In this condition haemolysis occurs in 0·6% or even in stronger solutions.

---

[1] In 1886 Mendel described 'dominant' and 'recessive' traits in hybrids. His work passed unnoticed for thirty-five years.

[2] Although there is excessive breakdown of red cells with transformation of liberated haemoglobin to bilirubin, the bilrubin compound so produced is excreted by the liver and not by the kidneys, thus favouring the formation of pigment gall-stones.

Gregor Johann Mendel, 1822–1884. Augustinian Monk and Naturalist, who later became Abbot of Brunn, Austria, (now Brno, Czechoslovakia). His work on inheritance was published in 1866 but passed almost unnoticed during his lifetime.

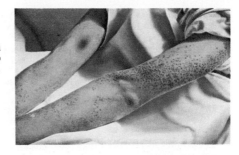

FIG. 915.—Purpura. The patient presented with symptoms of acute intestinal obstruction due to submucosal haemorrhage of the small intestine.

The Reticulocyte Count.—To compensate for the loss of erythrocytes by haemolysis, the bone marrow discharges into the circulation immature red cells, which differ from the adult cells by possessing a reticulum. This cannot be seen in the usual blood films, but can be demonstrated readily by vital stains. Crises are associated with reticulocytopenia, and hypoplasia of the erythroid element of the bone marrow. After a crisis the reticulocyte count is greatly increased.

Faecal urobilinogen is increased, as most of the urobilinogen is excreted by this route.

Use of Radioactive Chromium.[1]—Labelling of the patient's own red cells with ^{51}Cr will demonstrate the severity of red cell destruction and if this is accompanied by daily scanning over the spleen it will show the degree of red cell sequestration by the spleen. If splenic radioactivity is high, splenectomy will be of value.

Treatment.—All patients who have hereditary spherocytosis should be treated by splenectomy. Not, of course, that the spleen is at fault. The trouble lies with the red cells, but it is the spleen which will not let them survive sufficiently long to be of much service. After splenectomy, the spheroidal cells have a normal life span though they are still fragile.

In the great majority of cases splenectomy can be undertaken as an elective operation during a remission. In juvenile cases the age at which operation is recommended has been decreasing. If it is not imperative before, the optimum time seems to be about 7 years, *i.e.* before gall-stones have had time to form, but subsequent vulnerability to infection is reduced.

At operation (splenectomy) the gall-bladder should be palpated for gall-stones, and if they are present cholecystectomy can be undertaken then or at a later date, depending on the patient's fitness.

Following splenectomy, the patient soon recovers from the anaemia, which does not return. The jaundice disappears, but the tendency to haemolysis persist; it has been demonstrated twenty-five years after removal of the spleen. Ulcers of the leg due to this disease heal rapidly. In short (ruptured spleen excepted), in no other condition is splenectomy more successful. Owing to the absence of adhesions, the operation can be undertaken easily and expeditiously, which in part accounts for the very low operative mortality.

When a patient is anaemic, transfusion with whole blood or packed cells is of benefit, since red cell antibodies are not normally present.

Acquired autoimmune haemolytic anaemia

This may be due to a drug reaction, e.g. to alpha methyl dopa, to another disease, *e.g.* systemic lupus erythematosis, or its cause may be unknown. Red cell survival is reduced

---

[1] A solution of radioactive chromium salt is mixed with the patient's own blood and becomes attached to the red cells. When these are re-injected into the circulation the concentration of red cells in such organs as the spleen and liver can be counted by an external counter.

because of an immune reaction triggered by immunoglogulins or complement on the red cell surface. The red cell surface is damaged as a result of the binding of the Fc portion of the red cell antibody to a macrophage Fc receptor in the spleen. The red cell is thus rendered vulnerable to 'culling' within the splenic red pulp.

Clinical Features.—Autoimmune haemolytic anaemias are more common after the age of fifty, and in females. The spleen is enlarged in 50%, and pigment gallstones are present in 20%, of cases.

Investigations.—Anaemia is invariably present and may be associated with spherocytosis because of red cell membrane damage. The Coombs' test is usually but not invariably positive.

Treatment.—Usually the disease has an acute, self-limiting course and no treatment is necessary. Splenectomy should be considered if: (1) Corticosteroids are not effective. (2) The patient is developing complications from long-term steroid treatment. (3) Corticosteroids are contraindicated e.g. because of a history of peptic ulcer. 80% of patients respond to splenectomy.

Idiopathic Thrombocytopenic[1] Purpura (ITP)

Purpura[2].—Not all cases of purpura benefit from splenectomy. Purpura is defined as a focal haemorrhage into the skin. A history of purpura and evidence of it on examination should be sought before any surgical procedure is undertaken (fig. 915). Purpura may result from:

(1) Increased capillary fragility, as in steroid-induced or Henoch-Schönlein purpura.

(2) Defective platelets (thrombocytopathies), for example after taking aspirin which inhibits thromboxane and prostaglandin and reduces their property of making the platelet adhesive.

(3) A reduced number of normal platelets (thrombocytopenia). This can be a consequence of:

(a) Decreased platelet production by marrow megakaryocytes, for example because of marrow supression by cytotoxic chemotherapy, or in aplastic anaemia.

(b) Increased platelet consumption, as in seen in disseminated intravascular coagulation where the clotting cascade is triggered by septicaemia and platelets adhere to vascular endothelium, or in a large haemangioma in which platelets adhere to the abnormal endothelium.

(c) Increased platelet destruction by the spleen. This may be associated with autoimmune disease e.g. systemic lupus erythematosis; with drug reactions e.g. to quinine; and with certain infections e.g. mononucleosis. Alternatively, as in idiopathic thrombocytopenic purpura, the platelet destruction may not be associated with any other condition.

(d) Increased splenic sequestration of platelets. This can be associated with any condition which produces gross splenic enlargement, e.g. portal hypertension.

Splenectomy may sometimes be helpful in purpura associated with splenic destruction or sequestration (3c, 3d above). It is most reliably of use in idiopathic thrombocytopenic purpura.

Aetiology of ITP.—In most cases the low platelet count in ITP is due to the development of antibodies which damage the patient's own platelets.[3] Transfused platelets have a short survival time after transfusion into patients with ITP, and the children born to mothers with ITP may have a temporary, maternal antibody-induced, thrombocytopenia after birth.

Clinical Features.—Purpuric patches (ecchymoses) in the skin and mucous membranes (fig. 915) which tend to be more prominent in dependant areas because of a higher, gravity added, intravascular pressure. A tendency to spontaneous bleeding from mucous membranes e.g. epistaxis and in women to menorrhagia, and prolonged bleeding from minor wounds. Urinary and gastrointestinal

---

[1] Thrombocytopenia = poverty of thrombocytes (blood-platelets).
[2] Purpura = Porphyra (Gr) = purple.
[3] The normal blood-platelet count is 250,000 to 400,000 per mm³ (250 to 400×10⁹/l).

Robert Royston Amos Coombs, Contemporary. Quick Professor of Biology, Cambridge, England.
Eduard Heinrich Henoch, 1820–1910. Physician, Berlin.
Johannes Lucas Schönlein, 1793–1864. Physician, Berlin.

haemorrhage, and haemarthrosis are rare. Intracranial haemorrhage is also rare, but is the most frequent cause of death. Cutaneous ecchymoses may be found on examination and the tourniquet test is positive. The spleen is palpable in only 25% of cases, and gross splenic enlargement suggests that the diagnosis is not ITP.

Investigations.—The bleeding time is increased but the clotting and prothrombin times are normal. The platelet count in the peripheral blood film is reduced (usually less than $60 \times 10^9/1$). Examination of a bone marrow biopsy reveals a plentiful supply of platelet producing megakaryocytes.[1]

Treatment.—The behaviour of the disease is different in children and adults. In children, the disease regresses spontaneously in 75% of cases after one attack. Short courses of corticosteroids or occasionally azathioprine, are usually followed by recovery. Splenectomy is reserved for severe cases who have relapsed or girls approaching menarche. In adults, the initial attack is less severe than in children, but the disease relapses and becomes more severe. Splenectomy is indicated where the ITP has persisted for more than 6-9 months.

60% of patients can be regarded as cured, 20% will be improved and 15% or more will derive no benefit from the splenectomy. It is often, though not invariable, that a response to steroids predicts a good response to splenectomy. If severe bleeding has not been controlled by steroids, fresh blood transfusion or transfusion with platelet concentrates prior to operation is necessary. Splenectomy is contraindicated during the acute phase of ITP; the disease should first be controlled by medical treatment. Occasionally, in resistant cases, the anti-platelet immune response can temporarily be blocked by IgG transfusion to saturate the splenic Fc binding sites and reduce platelet destruction to allow the platelet count to rise at the time of surgery.

Splenectomy for other causes of thrombocytopenic purpura. Occasionally splenectomy is of benefit in thrombocytopenia due to systemic lupus erythematosis and in hypersplenism; also in purpura associated with 3(c) and (d)—p. 946.

Schistosomiasis

This is prevalent in Africa (particularly around the Nile delta), Asia and South America. It is caused by infection with *Schistosoma mansoni* in 75% of cases and by *Schistosoma haematobium* in 25% of cases. Splenic enlargement is produced by hyperplasia which is induced by phagocytosis of disintegrated worms, ova and toxins, and by portal hypertension which is the result of hepatic fibrosis (fig. 916).

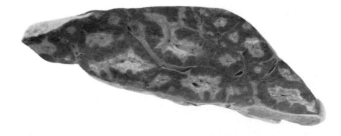

FIG. 916.— Periportal fibrosis of the liver in Egyptian splenomegaly.
(*Dr. Halawani, Cairo.*)

---

[1] Megakaryocytes, the giant cells of bone marrow, give origin to blood-platelets.

Sir Patrick Manson, 1844–1922. Practised in Formosa and Hong Kong. Later Physician, Dreadnought Hospital, Greenwich, London. He is regarded as the 'Father of Tropical Medicine'.

Clinical features.—Splenomegaly resulting from schistosomiasis can occur at any age and is more prevalent in males. The degree of splenic enlargement reflects the extent of hepatic fibrosis and may be massive.

Investigations

The urine and the faeces are examined for ova.

Liver function tests reveal a varying degree of hepatic impairment. A hypochromic anaemia is always present.

Treatment.—Successful treatment of established cases does not result in regression of the splenomegaly. Removal of the painful and bulky spleen is indicated where there is no evidence of hepatic or renal insufficiency. If ascites is present, portasystemic shunt should be combined with splenectomy.

Tropical Splenomegaly

Massive enlargement of the spleen occurs frequently in the tropics *e.g.* in malaria (especially in children), kala azar, and schistosomiasis (see above). In parts of Africa and New Guinea splenomegaly cannot be fully attributed to these diseases, because tropical splenomegaly is restricted to only a few adults in areas where malaria is endemic. The most likely explanation is an abnormal immune response to malaria or to unusual species of plasmodia. Malnutrition may also be a factor (there is a high incidence in lactating women).

The spleen is grossly enlarged (2000–4000 g). This is associated with anaemia (due to shortened red cell life) and thrombocytopenia (due to splenic sequestration of platelets) which respond to splenectomy. Splenectomy is indicated for those disabled by anaemia or by the weight of an enormous spleen. Splenectomy reduces immunity to malaria and therefore anti-malarial chemotherapy, *e.g.* 100 mg proguanil daily, should follow splenectomy in malaria endemic areas for life.

Hypersplenism due to Portal Hypertension

Splenomegaly invariably accompanies portal hypertension. This splenic enlargement results in thrombocytopenia (due to splenic sequestration of platelets) and granulopenia. These are permanently relieved when splenectomy accompanies the operation for relief of the portal hypertension. Shunt surgery alone does not have a similar effect.

Felty's Syndrome

A moderate number of patients with chronic rheumatoid arthritis develop mild leucopenia; in a few of these, neutropenia becomes extreme and usually is associated with enlargement of the spleen. This combination is referred to as Felty's syndrome. A remarkable characteristic of this syndrome is that the leucopenia and splenic enlargement are apparently unrelated to the severity of the arthritic changes; indeed, in some instances the arthritis has commenced to improve or has become quiescent by the time the low white-cell count and the splenomegaly become unmistakable. In those cases in which the arthritis is slight but the splenic enlargement and the blood changes are much in evidence, a diagnosis of primary splenic neutropenia is sometimes made.

Clinical Features.—Sufferers from Felty's syndrome are very prone to pyogenic infections of all varieties, infected ulcers around the ankles being particularly frequent. They are fatigued easily, lean, and unable to gain weight. It is impossible to say whether these symptoms should be attributed to the arthritic process or to the leucopaenia and spleno-

Augustus Roi Felty, 1895–1964. Physician, Hartford Hospital, Hartford, Connecticut, U.S.A.

megaly. As a rule the degree of splenic enlargement is not great. Enlargement of lymph nodes and generalised brown pigmentation of the skin are sometimes present.

Blood Examination.—The white-cell count shows persistent leucopenia varying between 1000 and 2000 per mm³ ($1\cdot0$–$2\cdot0\times10^9$/) with less than 20% of neutrophils. The greatest reduction is in the granulocytes. Neutrophils range from slightly below normal to virtually absent. There is almost always an associated anaemia of moderate severity.

Sternal Puncture.—The bone marrow shows increased cellularity with, in some cases, a deficiency of mature granulocytes.

Treatment.—The results of splenectomy are variable. Usually there is an improvement in the blood picture with increased neutrophils, but this improvement is not maintained. However, the liability to infections seems to be decreased in many cases and rheumatoid arthritis that has become resistant to steroid therapy may react favourably to steroid therapy once more.

Tuberculosis of the Spleen

Tuberculosis of the spleen is not so uncommon as is sometimes believed. It occurs chiefly in adults between twenty and forty years of age. When a patient has splenomegaly with asthenia, loss of weight and an evening temperature, it is well to bear in mind the possibility of the enlargement of the spleen being due to tuberculosis. Too often these signs lead to the erroneous diagnosis of leukaemia or some other disorder for which splenectomy is not indicated. Occasionally tuberculosis of the spleen produces portal hypertension. Another form is cold abscess, which is very rare. Splenic puncture, followed by culture, or guinea-pig inoculation, will yield positive results. A therapeutic test with antituberculous drugs (Chapter 4) brings about some improvement, and there is less danger of dissemination of tubercle bacilli if splenectomy is undertaken. The operation, which usually is rendered difficult because of adhesions, is contraindicated only if other active tuberculous lesions are present. Otherwise the results of splenectomy in tuberculosis of the spleen are excellent (Patel).

Neoplasms

The commonest benign tumour of the spleen is the haemangioma which may occasionally develop into a haemangiosarcoma. Splenectomy may be necessary. The commonest cause of neoplastic enlargement of the spleen is lymphoma. Splenectomy plays a part in the management of these conditions (Chapter 9).

Thalassaemia[1] (*syn.* **Cooley's anaemia; Mediterranean anaemia**)

Thalassaemia is the result of a defect in haemoglobin peptide chain synthesis which is transmitted as a dominant trait. The disease is really a group of related diseases—alpha, beta and gamma—depending on the haemoglobin peptide chain whose rate of synthesis is reduced. Most patients suffer from beta-thalassaemia in which a reduction in the rate of beta chain synthesis results in a decrease in haemoglobin A. In addition to a decrease in haemoglobin, intracellular precipitates (Heinz bodies) contribute to premature red cells destruction. The disease is no longer thought to be confined to the descendants of those living around the Mediterranean.

Clinical Features.—Gradations of disease range from heterozygous thalassaemia minor to homozygous thalassaemia major which is associated with chronic anaemia, jaundice and splenomegaly. Patients with homozygous thalassaemia major frequently develop clinical signs within the first year of life: retarded growth, enlarged head with slanting eyes and depressed nose, leg ulcers, jaundice and abdominal distension (due to splenomegaly).

Investigations.—Red cells are small, thin and misshapen, and have a characteristic resistance to osmotic lysis. In the more severe forms, nucleated red cells and other immature blood cells are seen. The final diagnosis is by haemoglobin electrophoresis.

Treatment.—Blood transfusion may be necessary to correct profound anaemia. Splenectomy is occasionally of benefit in patients who require frequent blood transfusion—particularly if they have developed haemolytic antibodies from repeated transfusion—and where the bulky spleen is uncomfortable or painful.

---

[1] Thalassaemia = Greek, Thalassa—Sea. (Because it was originally thought to be restricted to people of Mediterranean origin.)

Jean Patel, Contemporary. Professor of Clinical Surgery, Paris, France.
Thomas Benton Cooley, 1871–1945. Professor of Paediatrics, Wayne University, Detroit, U.S.A.

Sickle cell disease

Sick cell disease is a hereditary haemolytic anaemia, occurring mainly among those of African origin, in which the normal haemoglobin A is replaced by haemoglobin S (HbS). The HbS molecule crystallises when the blood oxygen tension is reduced and this distorts and elongates the red cell. This increases blood viscosity and obstructs the flow of blood through both the 'open' and 'closed' circulations in the spleen, and through other blood vessels. Splenic microinfarcts, splenomegaly and, later, autosplenectomy develop. This is associated with reduced antibody production and a reduced ability to filter bacteria— especially *Streptococcus pneumoniae*—in the spleen.

Clinical features.—The sickle cell trait can be detected in 9% of those of African origin but most are asymptomatic; sickle cell disease occurs in about 1% of Africans. Depending on the vessels affected by the vascular occlusion, patients may have bone or joint pain, priapism, neurological abnormalities, skin ulcers, or abdominal pain due to visceral blood stasis.

Investigations.—Characteristic sickle shaped cells can be seen in a blood film, but this has now been replaced by haemoglobin electrophoresis.

Treatment.—Hypoxia, which provokes a sickling crisis should be avoided, and particular care should be taken in patients with sickle cell anaemia undergoing anaesthesia. Adequate hydration and partial exchange transfusion may help in a crisis. Splenectomy is of benefit in a few patients where excessive splenic sequestration of red cells aggravates the anaemia. This hypersplenism may be chronic, which usually occurs in late childhood or adolescence, or acute which occurs in the first five years of life and may be precipitated by *Streptococcus pneumoniae* infection. Acute attacks of hypersplenism can usually be treated with packed red cell transfusion, but occasionally splenectomy is of benefit.

Porphyria

Porphyria is an hereditary error of catabolism of haemoglobin in which porphyrinuria occurs. The abdominal crises, which are characterised by violent intestinal colic with constipation, are liable to be precipitated by the administration of barbiturates, to which these patients have an idiosyncrasy. The patient is anaemic, frequently suffers from photo-sensitivity, and in advanced stages of the disease neurological or mental symptoms (from damage to the brain) are often present.[1] On examination the spleen will be found to be enlarged. On a number of occasions the splenic enlargement, which is usually well marked, has been overlooked and *the abdomen has been opened on the diagnosis of intestinal or appendicular colic*, with negative findings. Another manifestation of acute porphyria is spasmodic abdominal pain followed by jaundice.

Two methods of establishing the diagnosis are available:

The urine is sometimes normal in colour. Usually it is orange (which is often dismissed as 'concentrated'). If the specimen is left exposed to daylight for a few hours it develops a port-wine colour, particularly near the surface, where it is exposed to the air. There are several conclusive laboratory tests for porphyrinuria.

Radiography of the abdomen. Serial x-ray films show areas of intestinal spasm causing short segments of gaseous dilatation of the small and large intestine, especially of the caecum.

Treatment.—Often there is a striking decrease in the serum sodium level and the patient is improved considerably by infusion of normal saline solution with careful control of electrolytic balance. To relieve the abdominal pain methadone is the best drug. If a sedative is required, one of the phenothiazines (*e.g.* chlorpromazine) should be given. Splenectomy is not of value except in the uncommon erythropoietic type with splenomegaly.

Gaucher's Disease

As mentioned, the spleen may take an active part in the storage of abnormal lipoids, as does the remainder of the reticulo-endothelial system. In the case of Gaucher's disease the lipoid in question is glucocerebroside. Gaucher's disease, which is rare, is characterised by enormous enlargement of the spleen, which may weigh 8 or 9 lb (3·6 or 4·1 kg). In the majority of cases the splenic enlargement begins in early childhood, often before the

---

[1] King George III is believed to have suffered from this malady (a Royal malady).

Philippe Charles Ernest Gaucher, 1854–1918. Physician, Hospital St. Louis, Paris.

age of twelve, although the patient rarely seeks advice before adult life. Until the splenic enlargement becomes massive the symptoms are few. There is anaemia, a yellowish-brown discoloration of the skin of the hands and face, and a curious conjunctival thickening (pinguecula) that helps to clinch the clinical diagnosis. Slavonic and Jewish races appear to be more prone to the disease than the rest of humanity. The diagnosis is confirmed by finding Gaucher's cells in the bone marrow.

Treatment.—Splenectomy rids the patient of a large abdominal swelling, but the operation is difficult because of perisplenitis and friability of the splenic pulp. It does not greatly influence the course of the disease but because it reduces the hypersplenism (anaemia, leucopenia and thrombopenia) and makes the patient more comfortable it is worth doing.

Leukaemia

Leukaemia is one of the conditions to be considered in the differential diagnosis of splenomegaly. The diagnosis can be made by examination of a blood or marrow film. The main treatment is chemotherapy or radiotherapy; occasionally marrow transplantation is necessary. Splenectomy during the chronic phase of chronic granulocytic leukaemia will not reduce the incidence of blastic transformation or improve survival. The procedure should be reserved for hypersplenism occurring during the chronic phase, or for when bone marrow transplantation might be necessary. In rare instances the removal of a symptomatic enlarged spleen during the blastic phase produces relief but the period of relief is brief and the operation is hazardous.

Splenectomy is occasionally indicated for palliation of a painful bulky spleen in chronic lymphocytic leukaemia.

Abscess of the Spleen

If a splenic embolus is infected, and the primary condition does not prove fatal, a splenic abscess may be expected to follow. Other sources of metastatic abscesses of the spleen are typhoid and paratyphoid fever, osteomyelitis, otitis media and puerperal sepsis. An abscess in the upper pole of the spleen may rupture and form a left subdiaphragmatic abscess. If the abscess is in the lower pole, rupture results in diffuse peritonitis.

Treatment.—As a rule, owing to dense adhesions, drainage of the abscess is the only course. Very rarely, splenectomy may be possible with the abscess *in situ*.

SPLENECTOMY

The usual indications for splenectomy in the U.K. are:

1. Trauma—either following an accident or during a surgical operation *e.g.* when mobilising the splenic flexure of the colon.
2. Removal 'en bloc' with the stomach as part of radical gastrectomy.
3. Removal as part of the staging laparotomy undertaken before treatment of Hodgkin's lymphoma.
4. To reduce the anaemia or thrombocytopenia in spherocytosis, idiopathic thrombocytopenic purpura or hypersplenism.
5. In association with shunt or variceal surgery for portal hypertension.

Other indications for splenectomy are tabulated on p. 943.

Technique of Splenectomy.—Most surgeons use a left paramedian or left subcostal incision. For large spleens adherent to the diaphragm a thoraco-abdominal incision may be necessary. Before operation, the passage of a naso-gastric tube enables the stomach to be emptied. This eases the identification of the abdominal oesophagus and decompresses the stomach if acute gastric dilatation or paralytic ileus develop.

If the operation is for *traumatic rupture*, a quick mobilisation is necessary. The hand is passed round the outer surface of the spleen, the posterior layer of lieno-renal ligament (fig. 917) divided largely by blunt dissection, and the spleen rotated medially into the incision. A large pack is inserted and the short gastric vessels and those in the pedicle are ligated and divided. It is important to separate the tail of the pancreas from the vessels in the hilum before ligation (see below and Malarial Spleen p. 942).

For *other conditions* requiring splenectomy.—The first step is to open the gastro-splenic ligament and divide the short gastric vessels (fig. 917). The splenic vessels at the superior

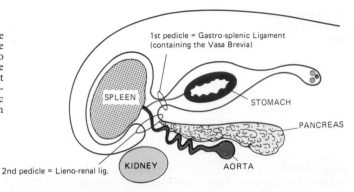

FIG. 917.—From the
surgical standpoint the
spleen may be said to
have two pedicles—the
gastrosplenic ligament
and the lieno-renal liga-
ment. The splenic
artery and vein lie in
the latter.

border of the pancreas are under-run with silk and ligated. The posterior surface of the
spleen is exposed, the posterior leaf of the lieno-renal ligament divided by long curved
scissors, and the spleen rotated medially, together with the tail and body of the pancreas.
The pancreas is separated from the hilum and the vessels dissected out, ligated, and
divided. Careful search must be made for accessory spleens. It is wise to drain the wound
in case damage to the pancreatic tail has occurred.

Post-operative complications.
1. Haemorrhage, if a ligature slips off the splenic artery.
2. Gastric dilatation following partial mobilisation of the stomach when ligating the short
   gastric veins. This can be controlled by nasogastric drainage for 24 hours post-operatively.
3. Haematemesis may rarely occur—possibly due to mucosal damage to the stomach
   when ligating the short gastric veins.
4. Left basal atelectasis, sometimes with a pleural effusion is common. This may be due
   to damage to or irritation of the left hemi-diaphragm or subphrenic abscess, and may
   be accompanied by persistent hiccough.
5. Damage to the tail of the pancreas during mobilisation of the splenic pedicle. This may
   produce a localised abscess, or if the area has been well drained, a pancreatic fistula.
   This may be associated with a left pleural effusion, a peritoneal effusion or abdominal
   wound dehiscence.
6. Splenectomy is frequently followed by a rise in the white cell and platelet count a few
   days after the operation. There may be a risk of thrombosis in the splenic or pancreatic
   veins if the platelet count rises to above 1000 × 10⁹/l and it is justifiable to anticoagulate
   the patient in this circumstance.
7. Gastric fistula due to damage of the greater curvature when ligating the short gastric
   vessels.
8. **Post splenectomy septicaemia.**—The spleen phagocytoses bacteria, particularly
encapsulated bacteria. Splenectomised patients show reduced antibody production when
challenged with particulate antigens, are deficient in tuftsin and may have reduced IgM
and properdin levels (see Functions, above). Splenectomised patients are at increased
risk of septicaemia due to *Streptococcus pneumoniae*, *Neisseria meningitidis*, *Haemophilus
influenzae*, and *Babesia microti*. The risk becomes ever bigger in splenectomised patients
treated with cytotoxic chemotherapy or radiation, and in patients who have undergone
splenectomy for thalassaemia, sickle cell disease and autoimmune anaemia or thrombocytopenia.
   Children who have undergone splenectomy should receive pneumococcal anti-toxin
(pneumovax) and antibiotic (erythromycin) cover until 18 years of age. Pneumococcal
vaccine should also be administered to adults, particularly those undergoing splenectomy
prior to chemotherapy or radiation. Splenectomised patients who live in malaria endemic
areas should receive anti-malarial prophylaxis.

CHAPTER 47

THE GALLBLADDER AND BILE DUCTS

SURGICAL ANATOMY AND PHYSIOLOGY

The gallbladder is pear shaped, 7·5 to 12·5 cm long, with a normal capacity of about 50 ml, but capable of considerable distension in certain pathological conditions. The anatomical subdivisions are a fundus, a body, and a neck which terminates in the narrow infundibulum. The muscle fibres in the wall of the gallbladder are arranged in a criss-cross manner, being particularly well developed in the neck. The mucous membrane contains indentations of the mucosa that sink into the muscle coat; these are the crypts of Luschka.

The cystic duct is about 2·5 cm in length. It contains the spiral value of Heister.

The common hepatic duct is usually less than 2·5 cm long, and is formed by the union of the right and left hepatic ducts.

The common bile duct, about 7·5 cm long, is formed by the junction of the cystic and common hepatic ducts. It is divided into four parts: 1. *The supraduodenal portion,* about 2·5 cm long, runs in the free edge of the lesser omentum. 2. *The retroduodenal portion.* 3. *The infraduodenal portion* lies in a groove, but at times in a tunnel in the posterior surface of the pancreas. 4. *The intraduodenal portion* passes obliquely through the wall of the second part of the duodenum where it is surrounded by the sphincter of Oddi. It terminates by opening on the summit of the papilla of Vater. Its various relationships to the pancreatic ducts are depicted in fig. 918.

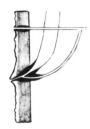 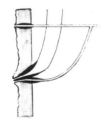 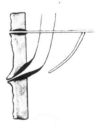

85% Common Channel   13% Separate openings   2% Atretic duct of Wirsung

FIG. 918.—Relationship between termination of common bile duct and pancreatic ducts.

The Arterial Supply of the Gallbladder.—The cystic artery, a branch of the right hepatic artery is usually given off *behind* the common hepatic duct (fig. 919(*a*)). Occasionally an accessory cystic artery arises from the gastroduodenal artery. In 15% of cases the right hepatic artery and/or the cystic artery cross in front of the common hepatic duct and the cystic duct (fig. 919(*b*)). The most dangerous anomalies are when the hepatic artery takes a tortuous course in front of the origin of the cystic duct or the right hepatic artery is tortuous, and the cystic artery is short. The tortuosity is known as the 'caterpillar turn' or Moynihan's 'hump' (fig. 919(*c*)). There is a possibility of liver infarction in accidental ligation of the hepatic artery.

Lymphatics.—The lymph vessels of the gallbladder (subserosal and submucous) drain into the *cystic lymph node of Lund* (the sentinel lymph node), which lies in the fork created by the junction of the cystic and common hepatic ducts. Efferent vessels from this lymph node go to the hilum of the liver, and to the coeliac lymph nodes. The subserosal lymphatic vessels of the gallbladder also connect with the subcapsular lymph channels of the liver, and this accounts for the frequent spread of carcinoma of the gallbladder to the liver.
Embryology (see Congenital Abnormalities).

Hubert Luschka, 1820–1875. Professor of Anatomy, Tübingen, Germany.
Lorenz Heister, 1683–1758. Professor of Surgery and Botany, Helmstädt, Germany.
Ruggero Oddi, 1845–1906. Physiologist, Perugia, Italy.
Abraham Vater, 1684–1751. Professor of Anatomy and Botany, Wittenberg, Germany.
Johann Georg Wirsung, d. 1643. Professor of Anatomy, Padua, Italy. Murdered when entering his house at night.
Berkeley George Andrew Moynihan (Lord Moynihan), 1865–1936. Professor of Clinical Surgery, Leeds, England.
Fred Bates Lund, 1865–1950. Surgeon, Boston City Hospital, Boston, Mass., U.S.A.

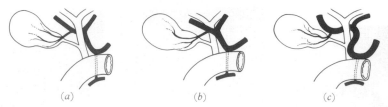

(a) (b) (c)

FIG. 919.—Arrangements of the arterial supply to the gallbladder.

Surgical Physiology

Bile, as it leaves the liver, is composed of 97% water, 1 to 2% bile salts and 1% pigments, cholesterol and fatty acids. The liver excretes bile at a rate estimated at 40 ml per hour.

The healthy gallbladder has several functions:

1. **Reservoir for Bile.**—During fasting, resistance to flow through the sphincter is high, and bile excreted by the liver is diverted to the gallbladder. After feeding, the resistance to flow through the spincter of Oddi is reduced, the gallbladder contracts and bile enters the duodenum. These motor responses of the biliary tract are in part effected by the hormone cholecystokinin, released by the upper intestinal mucosa in response to food, particularly fats.

2. **Concentration of Bile.**—By the active absorption of water, sodium, chloride, and bicarbonate by the mucous membrane of the gallbladder, the hepatic bile which enters the gallbladder becomes concentrated 5 to 10 times, with a corresponding increase in the proportion of bile salts, bile pigments, cholesterol, and calcium it contains.

3. **Secretion of Mucin.**—About 20 ml is secreted each twenty-four hours.

INVESTIGATIONS OF THE BILIARY TRACT IN RELATION TO DIAGNOSIS AND MANAGEMENT

Plain x-ray will show radio-opaque gallstones in 10% of cases (fig. 920). It will also show the rare cases of calcification of the gallbladder (porcelain gallbladder, fig. 921), and limey (lime water) bile (fig. 923). It will also show up air or gas in the duct system.

Oral cholecystography (Graham-Cole test) (figs. 922 and 924(a) and (b)):

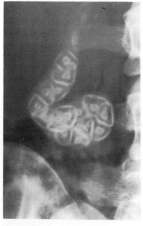

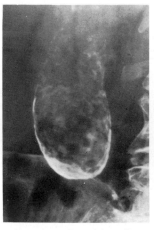

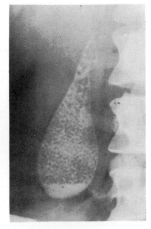

FIG. 920.—Plain radiograph showing radiopaque stones in the gallbladder; radiopaque stones are rare [10%]

FIG. 921.—Porcelain gall-bladder.

FIG. 922.—Non-opaque stones rendered visible by oral cholecy-stography.

Evarts Ambrose Graham, 1883–1957. Bixby Professor of Surgery, Washington University, St. Louis, Missouri, U.S.A.
Warren Henry Cole, Contemporary. Emeritus Professor of Surgery, University of Illinois, Chicago, U.S.A.

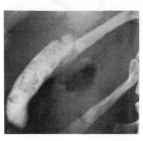

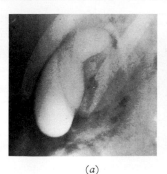

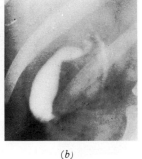

FIG. 923.—*Plain radiograph* showing a gallbladder filled with limey bile. Gallstones are present also.

(a)

(b)

FIG. 924.—(a) A normal cholecystogram. (b) Same after a fatty meal.

FIG. 925.—Simultaneous oral and intravenous cholecystography and cholangiography revealing a dilated gallbladder, a distended common bile duct, and a 'cut off' at the lower end of the duct due to a stone.

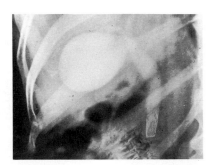

Telepaque[1] (Bayer Products Ltd.) is the contrast medium employed most commonly in the British Commonwealth and North America. A control x-ray is taken and then at about 18.00 hrs on the day before the next x-ray the patient has a meal, preferably containing some fat in order to empty the gallbladder. The medium is given by mouth, with water, at 21.00 hrs. Nothing to eat or drink is taken thereafter. Oblique films of the right upper abdomen are taken in the erect and supine position at 09.00 hrs the next day. A fatty meal or drink is then given to stimulate gallbladder contraction and another x-ray is taken (fig. 924(b)). Nonvisualisation of the gallbladder ('non-functioning gallbladder') may be due to failure of the patient to take the Telepaque tablets, vomiting, malabsorption, impaired liver function, a blocked cystic duct or severe gallbladder disease rendering it incapable of concentrating the contrast.

Intravenous cholangiography (Biligram[2]) permits radiological visualisation of the bile ducts (fig. 925). It is used in conjunction with oral cholecystography. Tomography[3] is helpful in delineating stones in the ducts; but compared with those methods in which contrast media are injected directly into the ducts (see below), the ducts are not well demonstrated. Indications for this investigation are becoming few.

Safety Precautions and Contraindications.—Substances containing iodine such as Biligram can give rise to severe anaphylactic reactions. Impaired renal function, macroglobulinaemia, multiple myelomatosis and thyrotoxicosis are contraindications.

This and oral cholecystography are not used if the patient is jaundiced with a plasma bilirubin level of over 50 μmol/l (3 mg/100 ml), because poorly functioning hepatocytes do not excrete the medium in sufficient concentration to be shown up by x-ray. Also acute cholecystitis precludes their use.

Ultrasonography (figs. 926–931) is non-invasive and is used as the initial imaging technique for the investigation of the patient suspected of having gallstones and of the jaundiced patient. It will demonstrate biliary calculi, dilatation of the biliary tree, and maybe a carcinoma of the pancreas occluding the common bile duct (Chapter 48). It may

---

[1] Iopanoic acid. B.P.
[2] Meglumine ioglycamate.
[3] Tomography = a method of placing one given plane into sharp focus while blurring others.

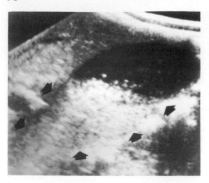

FIG. 926.—Multiple small gallstones filling part of the body and infundibulum of a large gallbladder.

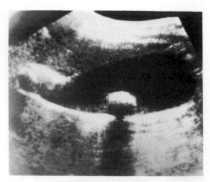

FIG. 927.—Single large gallstone casting an 'acoustic shadow'.

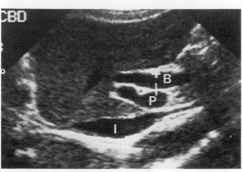

FIG. 928.—Longitudinal scan through the hilum of the liver showing the dilated common bile duct (B). P = portal vein; I = IVC.
(Dr J. E. Boultbee, Charing Cross Hospital.)

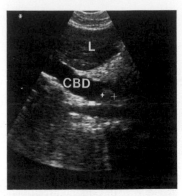

FIG. 929.—Longitudinal scan. Large stone with obstruction of the common bile duct which is dilated.
(Dr J. E. Boultbee, Charing Cross Hospital.)

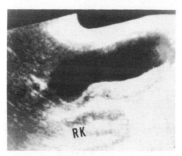

FIG. 930.—Mucocele of gallbladder which is now larger than the right kidney (RK).

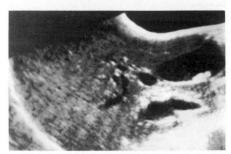

FIG. 931.—Dilatation of the intrahepatic and common bile ducts due to a calculus impacted at the sphincter of Oddi. There are calculi visible in the gallbladder.

(Figs 926, 927, 930 and 931 couresy of James McIvor, FDS, FRCR, London.)

also show stones in a non-functioning gallbladder. If it shows dilatation of part of the biliary tree, the patient may be advised to undergo endoscopic retrograde cholangiography (ERCP) and/or transhepatic cholangiography (PTC) (see below) in order to ascertain the nature and extent of blockage of the ducts. If no dilated ducts are shown, then it is likely that the jaundice stems from intrahepatic cholestasis (viral hepatitis, primary biliary cirrhosis, drugs etc.), and provided it is safe (no coagulopathy) a liver biopsy is the next appropriate investigation.

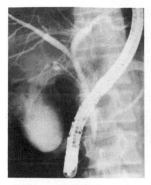

FIG. 932.—E.R.C.P.: Normal cholangiogram.

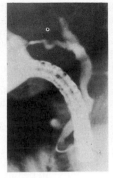

FIG. 933.—E.R.C.P.: Complete occlusion of common hepatic duct due to cholangio-carcinoma.

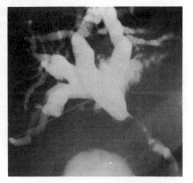

FIG. 934.—Percutaneous transhepatic cholangiogram in the same patient as fig. 933. Demonstrates the upper extent of the malignant stricture.

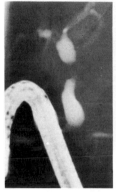

FIG. 935.—E.R.C.P.: Partial occlusion of bile duct by malignant stricture.

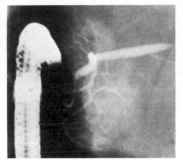

FIG. 936.—E.R.C.P.: Same patient as fig. 935. Complete block to main pancreatic duct indicates a pancreatic carcinoma.

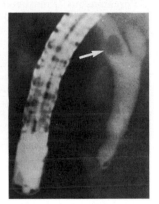

FIG. 937.—E.R.C.P.: Small solitary gallstone in bile duct following cholecystectomy.

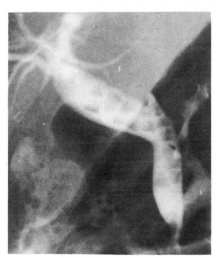

FIG. 938.—E.R.C.P.: Small multiple stones in a dilated common bile duct following cholecystectomy.

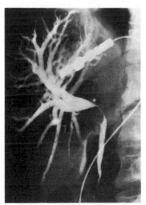

FIG. 939.—Transhepatic cholangiography showing a stricture of the common hepatic duct.

(Miss Phyllis George, FRCS, London.)

Radioisotope Scanning.—[131]I Rose Bengal and [99]Tc[m] labelled derivatives of imino-diacetic acid (HIDA, PIPIDA) are excreted in the bile and are used to visualise the biliary tree. In acute cholecystitis, the gallbladder is not seen. It is superior to ultrasonography in the diagnosis of this condition as it will aid the diagnosis of acute acalculous cholecystitis as well as the more common acute calculous cholecystitis. The technique can be used in the diagnosis of congenital biliary atresia and in the assessment of the patency of biliary-enteric anastomoses by noting whether the isotope fails to enter the intestine.

Computed Tomography (CT scan) provides similar information as ultrasonography. It is useful for those patients in whom ultrasonography is difficult, *e.g.* obese patients, or those with excessive bowel gas.

Endoscopic Retrograde Cholangio-Pancreatography (ERCP) (figs 932, 933, 934, 935, 936, 937 and 938).—The ampulla of Vater can be cannulated with the aid of a fibre-optic duodenoscope. The bile ducts are visualised after injecting water soluble contrast, thus differentiating surgical from medical causes of jaundice. Bile can be sent for cytological and microbiological examination, and brushings can be taken from strictures for cytolog-ical studies. Acute cholangitis may follow ERCP when a dilated and obstructed duct is filled. Antibiotics and expeditious surgery are then required. Refinements of the technique include endoscopic papillotomy to extract stones, passing catheters through strictures to provide external biliary drainage, and the placing of stents through strictures.

Percutaneous Transhepatic Cholangiography (PTC) (figs. 934 and 939).—This investigation should not be undertaken if the patient has a bleeding tendency. A history of cholangitis warrants the use of antibiotics. Under fluoroscopic control, a needle (the Chiba or Okuda needle) 15 cm long and 0·7 mm diameter is advanced into the liver through the eighth intercostal space in the mid-axillary line to a point about 2 cm short of the right margin of the vertebral column. The stylet is then removed, and whilst injecting Conray 280,[1] the needle is slowly withdrawn until contrast is seen to enter a biliary radicle. This technique has now been extended in order to place a catheter in the bile ducts to provide external biliary drainage in patients with biliary strictures. Also stents can be passed through strictures to provide antegrade drainage into the duodenum.

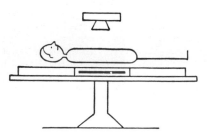

FIG. 940.—Per-operative cholangiogra-phy using a radiolucent table-top.

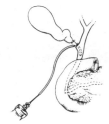

FIG. 941.—Per-oper-ative cholangiography. Method of introducing the medium.

Per-operative Cholangiography (figs 940, 941 and 942).—A cassette tunnel is placed beneath the patient at a level that will include the entire biliary tract. The cystic duct is opened and a fine polythene catheter is passed through it into the common bile duct for 3 cm. A ligature tied round the cystic duct and catheter prevents leakage. The catheter is filled with normal saline prior to insertion, so that there are no air bubbles present which would have a similar x-ray appearance to a radiolucent gallstone. Instruments and packs which might obscure the x-ray are removed, and the table is tilted 10° to the right side so that the spine and ducts are not superimposed. Three injections (3, 4 and 10 ml) are given of 25% Hypaque (sodium diatrizoate). An x-ray exposure follows each injection; respiration being interrupted to obviate any movement which would blur the picture. An x-ray image intensifier with T.V. display is a great asset as the operator can dispense with the blind exposures, and is able to take the x-ray picture when he knows he has given a satisfactory injection. A normal cholangiogram is sufficient evidence that exploration of

---

[1] Conray 280—Meglumine iothalamate 60% w/v.

Kunio Okuda, Contemporary. Professor of Medicine, Chiba University, Japan.

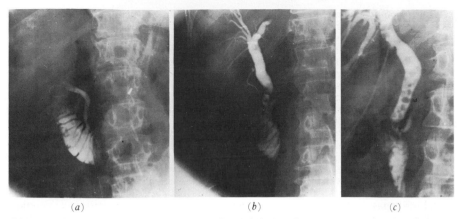

(a)   (b)   (c)

FIG. 942.—Per-operative cholangiography. (*a*) Gentle infusion of contrast, passing without hindrance into the duodenum. A normal duct with no problems. (*b*) The duct is dilated and there is a slight hold-up of contrast. No stones and no real indication to operate on the sphincter of Oddi (see Sphincterotomy). (*c*) All the ducts are dilated and contain many stones. There is narrowing of the lower end of the duct with reflux of contrast into the pancreatic duct. Sphincterotomy was performed.

the common bile duct is unnecessary. Failure of contrast to enter the duodenum may be due to sphincter spasm rather than an organic lesion. This possibility can be excluded by giving succinylcholine and repeating the x-rays. If the contrast still fails to enter the duodenum, or if the ducts contain stones, duct exploration should be carried out. *Note:* In about 20% of cases the medium flows along the duct of Wirsung. This is not necessarily pathological.

Operative Biliary Endoscopy (Choledochoscopy).—At operation a rigid (Storz) or flexible fibre-optic (Olympus) endoscope can be passed into the biliary tree. Stones can be identified and removed under direct vision, and strictures inspected and biopsied.

Per-operative Post-exploratory Cholangiography.—A cholangiogram via a catheter or the T-drainage tube may be performed, after choledochotomy, to make sure that all stones have been removed, and that there is no obstruction to the flow of bile into the duodenum.

Post-operative Cholangiography is performed 10–14 days after choledochotomy via the T-tube used for drainage of the common bile duct. The absence of stones and a normal flow of bile into the duodenum indicates that the T-tube can be removed.

CONGENITAL ABNORMALITIES OF THE GALLBLADDER AND BILE DUCTS

Embryology.—The hepatic diverticulum arises from the ventral wall of the foregut and elongates into a stalk to form the choledochus. A lateral bud is given off, which is destined to become the gallbladder and cystic duct. The embryonic hepatic duct sends out many branches which join up with the canaliculi between the liver cells. As is usual with embryonic tubular structures, hyperplasia obliterates the lumina of this ductal system, but normally

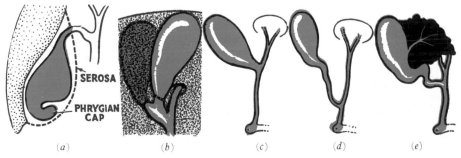

(a)   (b)   (c)   (d)   (e)

FIG. 943.—Some anatomical anomalies of the gallbladder and bile passages.

recanalisation occurs subsequently and bile begins to flow. During early foetal life the gallbladder is entirely intrahepatic.

A congenital anomaly of the biliary tract is found in 10% of necropsies.

Absence of the Gallbladder.—Occasionally the gallbladder is absent in man.

The Phrygian cap[1] (fig. 943(*a*)) is present in 2 to 6% of cholecystographies, and may be mistaken for a pathological deformity of the organ.

Floating Gallbladder.—The organ hangs on a mesentery which makes it liable to undergo torsion (p. 962).

Double Gallbladder.—Rarely (fig. 943(*b*)), the gallbladder is twinned. One of the twins may be intrahepatic. Cholecystography often fails to be diagnostic, because the shadows of the two gallbladders are superimposed. Double cholecystectomy should be performed.

Absence of the Cystic Duct (fig. 943(*c*)).—Injury of the common duct is liable to occur when cholecystectomy is performed in a patient with this abnormality. Meticulous dissection is required and the neck of the gallbladder is closed with a continuous fine suture.

Low Insertion of Cystic Duct (fig. 943(*d*)).—The cystic duct opens into the common duct near the ampulla. This common anomaly must be sought for particularly when considering a bypass operation for jaundice due to carcinoma of the duct or the pancreas.

An Accessory Cholecystohepatic Duct (fig. 943(*e*)) may open into the gallbladder and cause leakage after cholecystectomy. In the very rare anomaly where the right hepatic duct terminates in the gallbladder, cholecystostomy or partial cholecystectomy should be performed.

BILIARY ATRESIA (FIG. 944).

Aetiology and Pathology. Atresia is present in 1 per 10,000 live births. The aetiology is unknown. It may be the result of an inflammatory process, possibly viral in origin, rather than a failure of embryogenesis. Variable lengths of biliary tree are occluded. If a patent portion of the extrahepatic duct communicates with the intrahepatic ducts it is called a 'correctable' lesion (fig. 944 (*a*) and (*b*)). If no such communication exists the term 'noncorrectable' (fig. 944(*c*)), (*d*) and (*e*)) is applied. Ten per cent are 'correctable', 90% 'noncorrectable'.

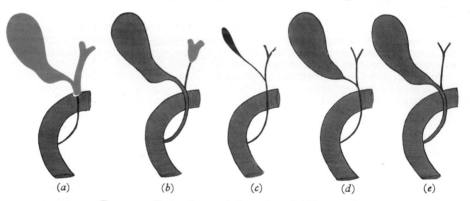

(*a*)   (*b*)   (*c*)   (*d*)   (*e*)

FIG. 944.—Types of congenital extrahepatic biliary atresia.

Clinical Features.—About one third of cases are jaundiced at birth. In all, however, jaundice is present by the end of the first week and deepens progressively. The meconium may be a little bile-stained but later the stools are pale and the urine dark. Prolonged steatorrhoea gives rise to osteomalacia (biliary rickets). Pruritis is severe. Clubbing and skin xanthomas, probably related to a raised serum cholesterol, may be present.

Differential Diagnosis.—This includes any form of jaundice in a neonate giving a cholestatic picture. Examples are α[1]anti trypsin deficiency, cholestasis associated with intravenous feeding, choledochal cyst and the inspissated bile syndrome. Neonatal hepatitis is the most difficult to differentiate. Both extrahepatic biliary atresia and neonatal hepatitis are associated with giant cell transformation of the hepatocytes. This makes liver biopsy of limited value in discriminating between the two conditions.

---

[1] The Phrygian cap refers to hats worn by peoples of Phrygia, an ancient country of Asia Minor. The cap was rather like a liberté cap of the French Revolution.

Diagnosis.—Liver function tests show a biochemical picture consistent with obstructive jaundice. Radiosotope scanning may reveal non-visualisation of the biliary tree and failure of the isotope to reach the intestine. A laparotomy is needed to confirm the diagnosis. A small subcostal incision is made and a cholangiogram performed, usually by injecting contrast into the gallbladder. If this is not possible a patent segment of the extrahepatic biliary tree is sought. A liver biopsy is taken. This may provide an alternative diagnosis if the biliary tree is patent.

Treatment.—In the 'correctable' case, a Roux-en-Y jejunal loop is anastomosed to the patent portion of the extrahepatic biliary tree communicating with the intrahepatic ducts. Kasai, after observing the presence of minute channels at the porta hepatis which communicate with the intrahepatic ducts devised the operation of hepatic portojejunostomy for the so-called noncorrectable cases. Fibrous tissue where the hepatic ducts should leave the liver at the porta hepatis is dissected free and divided flush with the liver capsule. To this area a loop of jejunum is anastomosed.

Prognosis.—Even though long term survival has been reported in both types of case, the overall results are not good in either category. Cholangitis, cirrhosis and portal hypertension are major complications, and is why hepatic transplantation is being tried as an alternative (Chapter 62).

Congenital Dilatation of the Intrahepatic Ducts (Caroli).—This rare congenital, non-familial condition is characterised by multiple, irregular, saccular dilatations of the intrahepatic ducts separated by segments of normal or stenotic ducts. Biliary stasis leads to stone formation and cholangitis. The patients present in childhood or in early adult life. Associated conditions include congenital hepatic fibrosis, medullary sponge kidney, and, rarely, cholangiocarcinoma. The mainstays of treatment are antibiotics for the cholangitis, and the removal of calculi. As the condition can be limited to one lobe of the liver, lobectomy may be indicated (Longmire).

CHOLEDOCHAL CYST

Congenital Choledochal cyst is due to a specific weakness in a part, or the whole, of the wall of the common bile duct. The commonest type is a fusiform dilatation of the common bile duct (figs. 945 and 946). This is a rare condition affecting females four times as commonly as males, Japanese being more prone to the condition than other races. The symptoms and signs seldom become manifest before the age of six months (only half the cases present before the age of twenty). The cyst may contain as much as 1 to 2 litres.

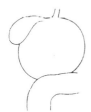

FIG. 945.—Choledochal cyst. Fusiform dilatation of the common bile duct. The gallbladder is not distended, and distension rarely occurs in the cystic or hepatic ducts.

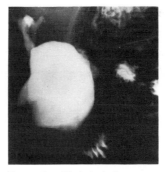

FIG. 946.—Choledochal cyst outlined by operative cholangiography.

Clinical Features.—There are attacks of jaundice of the obstructive type, which are usually accompanied by upper abdominal pain and pyrexia due to infection. In most cases a swelling is detected in the upper abdomen. Ultrasound will demonstrate its cystic nature. Untreated, the condition ultimately proves fatal, due to ascending cholangitis, biliary cirrhosis, or diffuse peritonitis following rupture of the cyst. Carcinoma may develop in a cyst.

Treatment.—If technically feasible the cyst should be excised, if not a choledocho-cystojejunostomy is performed.

César Roux, 1857–1934. Professor of Surgery and Gynaecology, Lausanne, Switzerland.
Morio Kasai, Contemporary. Professor of Surgery, Tokyo University, Japan.
Jacques Caroli, Professor of Medicine, Paris, France.
William Polk Longmire, Jr., Contemporary. Surgeon UCLA Medical Centre, Los Angeles, U.S.A.

INJURIES

1. **Trauma in the gallbladder and extrahepatic biliary tree** is rare and may be due to either a penetrating or crush injury. The physical signs are identical with those of rupture of the small intestine, with one notable addition—unmistakable jaundice, which appears within two or three hours of the accident in 65% of cases. When the abdomen is opened, bile is found within the peritoneal cavity.

Treatment of the various lesions is depicted in fig. 947, but when there is a small hole in the gallbladder (such as can occur from a penetrating wound), suture of the rent with drainage of the peritoneal cavity is indicated.

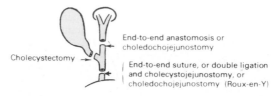

FIG. 947.—Methods of treating early complete tears of the biliary tract.

2. **Injuries of the Bile Ducts incurred during Operation** are discussed on p. 979.

TORSION OF THE GALLBLADDER

Torsion can occur in those rare instances where the gallbladder has a comparatively long mesentery—the so-called 'floating' gallbladder. There is a sudden agonising pain, with vomiting and shock. If the gallbladder becomes gangrenous or ruptures, the pain passes off instantaneously, but signs of diffuse peritonitis soon follow. Cholecystectomy is the treatment.

GALLSTONES (Cholelithiasis) (fig. 948)

Gallstones are the commonest biliary pathology. They are classified according to their chemical composition into cholesterol stones, mixed stones, and pigment stones. *Cholesterol stones*, comprising 6%, consist almost entirely of cholesterol and are often solitary (cholesterol solitaire). *Mixed stones* account for 90% of gallstones seen in the western hemisphere. Cholesterol is the major component. Other components include calcium bilirubinate, calcium phosphate, calcium carbonate, calcium palmitate and proteins. Usually they are multiple, and often they are faceted. *Pigment stones* are more common in the Far East than in the West. Composed almost entirely of calcium bilirubinate, they are mostly small, black and multiple. Some are hard and coral-like, others are soft and really concretions of sludge rather than stones.

Gas in Gallstones.—Rarely, the centre of a stone may contain radiolucent gas in a tri-radiate or bi-radiate fissure and this gives rise to characteristic dark shapes on x-ray—the *Mercedes Benz* or *Seagull* signs.

Limey bile

'Lime-water' bile is revealed in a plain radiograph (fig. 923) more clearly than if the gallbladder has been visualised by cholecystography. The opacity is the result of the gallbladder becoming filled with a mixture of calcium carbonate and calcium phosphate, usually the consistency of toothpaste. The condition tends to occur when there is a gradual obstruction of the cystic or common bile duct (*e.g.* chronic pancreatitis or carcinoma of the pancreas). Organisms are rarely grown from the emulsion.

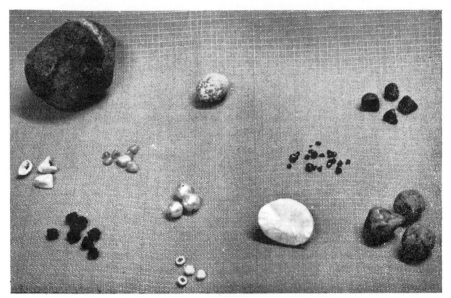

FIG. 948.—Gallstones (see text). Note, however, the three pearls, usually formed of calcium carbonate in the oyster around a parasite or a grain of sand.

Incidence of Gallstones.—A Fat, Fertile, Flatulent Female of Fifty is the classical sufferer from symptomatic gallstones.[1] Useful as is this clinical memorandum, it should be tempered with the knowledge that cholelithiasis occurs in both sexes, quite often at a much earlier age —even in childhood—and is more common in old age. In Europe 30% of females over 60 years of age have gallstones; however, two thirds are asymptomatic. Stones are rarer in Africa and in the Indian subcontinent.

Causal Factors in Gallstone Formation

The aetiology of gallstones is probably multifactorial. Factors implicated are 1. Metabolic, 2. Infective, 3. Bile stasis.

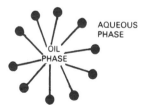

FIG. 949.—Diagram representing a spherical micelle formed by aggregation of bile-acid molecules. The rounded end of each molecule is water-loving (hydrophilic), whilst the stick-end is the hydrophobic part to which the water-insoluble cholesterol is adsorbed.

Cholesterol and Mixed stones.—*1. Metabolic.* Cholesterol, insoluble in water, is held in solution by the detergent action of bile acids and phospholipids with which it forms micelles (fig. 949). Bile containing cholesterol stones has an excess of cholesterol relative to bile salts and phospholipids thus allowing cholesterol crystals to form. Such bile is termed 'supersaturated' or 'lithogenic'. Bile cholesterol increases with age and is raised in women, particularly those taking the contraceptive pill[1], in obesity, and by clofibrate—a drug used in the treat-

---

[1] It is a sign of the times, and a signpost to causation that gallstones are being seen increasingly in Postpartum Primipara who were Prepregnancy 'Pill' takers (contraceptive pill).

ment of certain hyperlipoproteinaemias. The concentration of bile salts in bile is reduced by oestrogens, and also by factors which interrupt the enterohepatic circulation of the bile salts, *e.g.* ileal disease, resection or bypass and cholestyramine therapy. These conditions are all associated with an increased incidence of stones. But there are still some people with cholesterol supersaturation who remain free, suggesting that there are other factors which are important.

2. *Infection.*—The role of infection in causing stones is unclear. Often bile from patients with gallstones is sterile, but organisms have been cultured from the centres of gallstones: the radiolucent centre of many gallstones may represent mucus plugs originally formed around bacteria.[1]

3. *Bile stasis.*—Gallbladder contractility is reduced by oestrogens, in pregnancy and after truncal vagotomy, situations in which the incidence of gallstones is increased. Patients on long-term parenteral nutrition have a high incidence of stones. Lack of good oral intake precludes the release of cholecystokinin, the hormonal stimulant of gallbladder contraction released from the small bowel mucosa.

Pigment Stones are seen in patients with haemolysis, in which bilirubin production is increased. Examples are hereditary spherocytosis, sickle cell anaemia, thalassaemia, malaria, and mechanical destruction of red cells by prosthetic heart valves. Pigment stones are found in the ducts of patients with benign and malignant strictures. Also they are common in cirrhosis. Pigment stones in oriental countries are associated with infestations of the biliary tree by Clonorchis sinensis and Ascaris lumbricoides. E. Coli is often found in the bile of these patients. This bacterium produces the enzyme β glucuronidase which converts the bilirubin into its unconjugated, insoluble form. These stones are often present throughout the biliary tree including the intrahepatic ducts.

Gallstones in Relation to Other Disorders

Saint's Triad.—(i) Gallstones, (ii) Diverticulosis of the colon, and (iii) Hiatus hernia frequently coexist. It is important to find out which lesion is the cause of the patient's dyspeptic symptoms.

THE EFFECTS AND COMPLICATIONS OF GALLSTONES

Gallstones are usually found in the gallbladder, but may also be present in the bile ducts. The effects and complications of gallstones can be summarised as follows:

1. **In the gallbladder**   —Silent stones
   —Chronic Cholecystitis

   —Acute Cholecystitis $\left\{ \begin{array}{l} \text{gangrene} \\ \text{perforation} \\ \text{empyema} \end{array} \right.$

   —Mucocele
   —Carcinoma

2. **In the bile ducts**   —Obstructive jaundice
   —Cholangitis
   —Acute or acute relapsing pancreatitis

3. **In the intestine**   —Acute intestinal obstruction

Silent Gallstones.—It is possible for a calculus or calculi to be present in the gallbladder and to give rise to no symptoms during a long lifetime. As 10% of gallstones are radiopaque, they may be discovered accidentally on x-ray for another condition, *e.g.* on an intravenous urogram.

Most such patients should undergo cholecystectomy. If the patient is young and fit to withstand the operation, it is especially advisable, particularly in those patients with a non-functioning gallbladder, or those with diabetes mellitus, as they are more likely to encounter complications.

---

[1] Moynihan's aphorism = 'A gallstone is a tombstone erected to the memory of the organism within it'.

Charles Frederick Morris Saint, 1886–1973. Emeritus Professor of Surgery, Cape Town, South Africa.

CHRONIC CALCULOUS CHOLECYSTITIS

The gallbladder which contains stones may have a thickened fibrotic wall. Bacteria can be cultured from the bile in less than 30% of cases, and from the gallbladder wall slightly more. Failure to detect organisms in all cases has led to the suggestion that in some cases the inflammatory changes are a response to chemical irritants in the bile. A chronically inflamed gallbladder may be an incidental finding at laparotomy or autopsy with no symptoms referrable to it, or it may give rise to symptoms of varying severity. The symptoms are supposed to be due to either inflammation of the gallbladder wall or to obstruction of the outlet of the gallbladder by a stone impacted in Hartmann's pouch.[1]

Symptoms. 1. *Right hypochondrial pain*. Patients with chronic cholecystitis may experience episodes of right hypochondrial pain of varying severity. In some it is merely a discomfort, in others it is excruciating. The latter has been called gallstone colic, but it is rarely colicky in nature. Radiation to between the shoulder blades is frequent and it may be associated with nausea and vomiting. Fatty foods often precipitate it. It can last for several hours, but if an attack lasts for more than 12 hours, the diagnosis of acute cholecystitis should be considered. During an attack, tenderness in the hypochondrium is present. Murphy's sign may be positive.[2] This is elicited by asking the patient to breathe in whilst gently palpating the gallbladder area. The patient will experience pain and 'catch her breath' just before the zenith of inspiration. If the temperature and the white blood count are elevated, the diagnosis of acute cholecystitis should be considered.

2. *Flatulent Dyspepsia*. This term is used to describe a feeling of fullness after food associated with belching and heartburn. It is brought on by a large or a fatty meal. Some of these patients have gallstones and a proportion of these are relieved by cholecystectomy. However, other explanations should be sought before undertaking this, *e.g.* hiatus hernia, chronic pancreatitis, peptic ulcer.

Diagnosis.—Ultrasonography is usually the only investigation needed to show gallstones. In most cases they can also be seen by oral cholecystography. The biliary tree should be visualised radiologically in all cases of gallstones to detect duct stones. A per-operative cholangiogram is the usual technique. At least 10% of patients undergoing routine cholecystectomy have unsuspected duct stones.

Treatment.—(a) *Of biliary pain. Analgesics may be required. Severe pain* will require the administration of opiates even though these drugs are known to cause spasm of the sphincter of Oddi. This can be countered by the simultaneous administration of hyoscine butylbromide. Antiemetics may be needed. The patient should be put on a low fat diet until cholecystectomy.

(b) *Subsequent treatment*. Once a diagnosis has been made the gallbladder should be removed providing the patient is fit. A cholecystostomy is rarely indicated.

(c) *Dissolution of gallstones*. The bile acids, chenodeoxycholic and ursodeoxycholic acid taken orally will dissolve gallstones as long as they are radiolucent and the gallbladder is not 'non-functioning'. However, the treatment causes diarrhoea in half the patients and has to be continued for at least six months. Not all stones

---

[1] Hartmann's pouch is a dilatation of the neck of the gallbladder due to a stone. It is not found in the normal gallbladder.
[2] This sign is also named after Bernard Naunyn, 1839–1925, Professor of Medicine, Strasbourg, who described it in 1890, thirteen years before Murphy.

Robert Hartmann, 1831–1893. Professor of Anatomy, Berlin.
John Benjamin Murphy, 1857–1916. Professor of Surgery, North-western University, Chicago, U.S.A.

disappear and after cessation of treatment many recur. This treatment should only be considered in patients unfit for cholecystectomy, or for small retained stones of the biliary tree.

ACUTE CALCULOUS CHOLECYSTITIS

The gallbladder, often already affected by chronic cholecystitis, is acutely inflamed (fig. 950). In 95% of cases a gallstone is found impacted in Hartmann's pouch or obstructing the cystic duct. In most cases bacteria can be cultured from

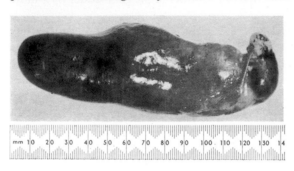

FIG. 950.—Acute obstructive cholecystitis in a Professor. A stone has impacted in Hartmann's pouch. Gangrene is occurring.

the bile or the gallbladder wall. The common organisms are E. Coli, Klebsiella Sp and Streptococcus faecalis (Keighley). Strict anaerobes, *e.g.* Bacteroides, are very uncommon. Gas forming organisms, *e.g.* Clostridia, may rarely infect the gallbladder. Gas is then seen in the gallbladder (fig. 951). Typhoidal infection is another serious infection, which may cause perforation. The sequelae to an attack of acute cholecystitis are:

1. When a certain degree of distension of the gallbladder has been reached, the mucous membrane tends to be lifted away from the sides of the stone and as a consequence the stone may slip back into the body of the gallbladder, and any mucoid (from a mucocele—see below) or muco-purulent contents of the gallbladder escape by way of the cystic duct.

2. Less frequently the impaction persists and an empyema (pyocele) of the gallbladder results.

3. On rare occasions the distended, inflamed gallbladder perforates. Doubtless the infrequency of perforation is due to the thickened walls of an organ that has long been the seat of chronic cholecystitis.

Perforation of the Gallbladder.—The site of perforation is either at the fundus, which is farthest away from the blood-supply, or, less commonly, at the neck from pressure necrosis of an impacted calculus. The sequelae are:

(*a*) **Local Abscess.**—On account of the present, and probably past, attacks of cholecystitis, there are adhesions between the gallbladder, the greater omentum, and the parietal peritoneum. Consequently, when an infected, obstructed gallbladder perforates the usual outcome is a local abscess.

(*b*) **Perforation into the general peritoneal cavity** occurs in only 0·5% of cases undergoing conservative treatment for acute cholecystitis, and the patient is usually a man. If the bile is infected diffuse peritonitis supervenes readily and rapidly, and the mortality is about 50% (Ellis).

Clinical Features of Acute Cholecystitis.—The onset is sudden, and pain is located mainly in the right hypochondrium. Severe nausea and vomiting are

Michael Robert Burch Keighley, Contemporary Professor of Surgery, University of Birmingham.
Harold Ellis, Contemporary. Professor of Surgery, Westminster Hospital, London.

features in the early stages. Pyrexia, sometimes to 38°C or more, is usual. A neutrophilia is present.

On examination tenderness and rigidity are found in the right hypochondrium. If the patient can be persuaded to relax, a mass consisting of the inflamed gallbladder with adherent greater omentum attached may be felt.

Boas's sign, if positive, is sometimes most helpful in distinguishing acute cholecystitis from other conditions. There is an area of hyperaesthesia between the ninth and the eleventh ribs posteriorly on the right side.

Diagnosis.—A chest and plain abdominal x-rays help to exclude other causes of the patient's symptoms and signs, and in a few cases will show radiopaque stones. Oral cholecystography is unreliable during an acute attack and is postponed until the patient has recovered. If a policy of early operation (see below) is adopted then ultrasonography, or HIDA scan may be useful to confirm the diagnosis.

Differential Diagnosis.—Conditions commonly presenting similarly to acute cholecystitis are appendicitis, perforated peptic ulcer and acute pancreatitis. Occasionally, acute pyelonephritis of the right kidney, myocardial infarction and right lower lobe pneumonia lead to confusion.

Treatment:

(*a*) **Conservative Treatment followed by Cholecystectomy.**—Experience shows that in more than 90% of cases the symptoms of acute cholecystitis subside with conservative measures. Non-operative treatment is based upon four principles:

1. *Nasogastric aspiration and intravenous fluids.*

2. *Analgesics.*

3. *Antibiotics.* As the cystic duct is blocked in most cases, the concentration of antibiotic in serum is more important than its concentration in bile. A broad spectrum antibiotic effective against Gram-negative aerobes is most appropriate, *e.g.* cephazolin, cefuroxime, or gentamicin. The new penicillins, such as mecillinam, mezlocillin, and ticarcillin may also be used.

4. *Subsequent Management.*—When the temperature, pulse, and other physical signs show that the inflammation is subsiding (usually by the third day) the naso-gastric tube is removed, and fluids followed by a fat free diet are given. Ultrasonography can be performed at any time to confirm the diagnosis. Cholecystectomy is performed during a subsequent admission after the acute attack has completely resolved, usually at least three weeks later.

Conservative treatment is not advised when there is uncertainty about the diagnosis, *e.g.* when high retrocaecal appendicitis or a perforated duodenal ulcer cannot be excluded.

Conservative treatment must be abandoned: If the pain and tenderness spreads across the abdomen and the pulse-rate rises. Cholecystectomy should be undertaken forthwith. In the very ill and the elderly patient it may be advisable to limit the operation to *cholecystostomy*[1]—usually a dependable, safe operative procedure, *but the gallbladder must be emptied of stones.*

(*b*) **Routine Early Operation.**—Some surgeons advocate urgent operation as a routine measure in cases of acute cholecystitis. Provided the operation is undertaken within forty-

---

[1] Elective cholecystectomy is still indicated in due course, in suitable patients. Cholecystostomy may relieve all symptoms, but some patients continue to suffer, and they may have an intermittent mucopurulent discharge from the drainage wound.

Ismar Isador Boas, 1858–1938. Gastroenterologist, Augusta Hospital, Berlin.

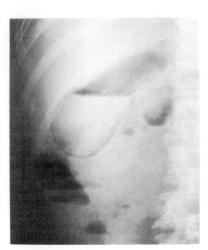

FIG. 951.—Gas in gallbladder and gallbladder wall (*Cl. welchii*). Emergency surgery is indicated.

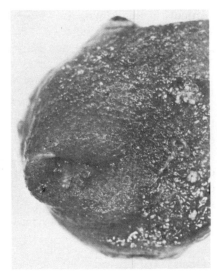

FIG. 952.—The interior of a strawberry gallbladder.

eight hours of the onset of the attack, the surgeon is experienced and excellent operating facilities are available, good results are claimed.

It is not proposed here to enter into a controversy on the merits and demerits of early and delayed operation for acute cholecystitis, but to state categorically that the most dangerous period for operation is between the seventh and fourteenth days of the attack. Should operation become imperative during this period, when the ducts are often obscured by oedema and immature fibrous tissue and the liver function is at a low ebb, it may be prudent to perform a simple cholecystostomy rather than a difficult cholecystectomy (see footnote[1] p. 973.)

Mucocele of the gallbladder.—This occurs when the neck of the gallbladder becomes obstructed by a stone but the contents remain sterile. The bile is absorbed and replaced by mucus secreted by the gallbladder epithelium. The gallbladder may be palpable. Enormous sizes and shapes (ramshorn) may be encountered. A mucocele also occurs in those cases of malignancy which occlude the cystic duct.

Empyema of the gallbladder.—The gallbladder appears to be filled with pus, but surprisingly in over half the cases bacteria cannot be cultured from the 'pus'. It may be a sequel of acute cholecystitis or the result of a mucocele becoming infected. The treatment is cholecystectomy.

ACALCULOUS CHOLECYSTITIS

Acute and chronic inflammation of the gallbladder can occur in the absence of stones and give rise to clinical pictures similar to calculous cholecystitis. Some patients have nonspecific inflammation of the gallbladder wall, whilst others have one of the cholecystoses. Oral cholecystography is more useful than ultrasound in the diagnosis in those patients presenting with chronic symptoms and radioisotope scanning in those presenting acutely. The identification of cholesterol crystals in a duodenal aspirate may also help. Acute acalculous cholecystitis is particularly seen in patients recovering from major surgery, trauma and burns. In these patients the diagnosis is often missed and the mortality is 20%.

The Cholecystoses

(Cholesterosis, Polyposis, Adenomyomatosis, Cholecystitis Glandularis Proliferans)

This is a not uncommon group of conditions affecting the gallbladder in which there are chronic inflammatory changes with hyperplasia of all the tissue elements.

Cholesterosis (*syn.* **Strawberry Gallbladder**).—In the fresh state the interior of the gallbladder looks something like a strawberry; the yellow specks (submucous aggregations of cholesterol crystals and cholesterol esters) correspond to the seeds (fig. 952). It may be associated with cholesterol stones.

FIG. 953.—Cholesterol polyposis.
(*D. J. Oakland, FRCS, Hereford.*)

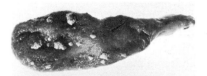

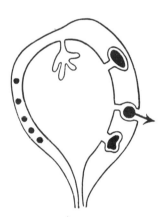

FIG. 954.—Types of cholecystitis glandularis proliferans (polypus, intramural or diverticular stones, and fistula).

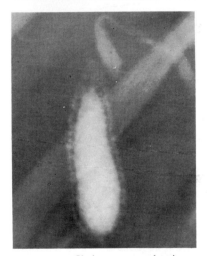

FIG. 955.—Cholecystogram showing cholecystitis glandularis proliferans.

Cholesterol Polyposis of the Gallbladder (fig. 953).—Cholecystography shows negative shadows in a functioning gallbladder. The shadows, which are adjacent to the wall of the gallbladder, remain constant in position and in relation to one another in all films of the series. Histologically, cholesterol polyposis is similar to the cholesterol-laden projections of the strawberry gallbladder, but the lesions are much less numerous and are relatively gigantic. The treatment is cholecystectomy.

Cholecystitis glandularis proliferans (polyp, adenomyomatosis, and intramural diverticulosis). Fig. 954 summarises the varieties of this condition. A polyp of the mucous membrane is fleshy and granulomatous. All layers of the gall-bladder wall may be thickened, but sometimes an incomplete septum forms which separates the hyperplastic from the normal. Intraparietal 'mixed' calculi may be present. These can be complicated by an intramural and, later, an extramural abscess. *Diverticulosis of the gallbladder* is usually manifest as black pigment stones impacted in the out-pouchings of the lacunae of Luschka.

Diverticulosis of the gallbladder may be demonstrated by cholecystography, especially when the gallbladder contracts after a fatty meal: there are small dots of contrast medium just outside the gallbladder (fig. 955). A septum may also be present (to be distinguished from the Phrygian cap—fig. 943). The treatment is cholecystectomy.

Typhoid gallbladder.—Salmonella typhi[1] or occasionally Salmonella typhimurium can infect the gallbladder. Acute cholecystitis can occur. More frequently, chronic cholecystitis occurs, the patient being a typhoid carrier excreting the bacteria in the bile. Gallstones may be present.[2] It is debatable whether the stones are secondary to the salmonella cholecystitis or whether pre-existing stones predispose the gallbladder to chronic infection. Howbeit, salmonella can frequently be cultured from these stones. Ampicillin and cholecystectomy are indicated.

Welchii infection.—See fig. 951.

CHOLECYSTECTOMY AND CHOLECYSTOSTOMY

1. **Preparation for Operation.**—The use of prophylactic antibiotics, usually a second generation cephalosporin, will reduce the incidence of wound infection. They should be given with the premedication. Provision is made for per-operative cholangiography by placing the patient on an appropriate operating table. Routine cholangiography is preferable to haphazard periodic attempts

2. **Laparotomy.**—A right paramedian or right subcostal incision is used. All the abdominal organs as well as the gallbladder must be examined.

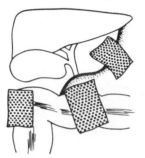

FIG. 956.—Cholecystectomy. Positions of the packs after identifying the colon, the duodenum and the stomach.

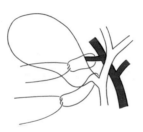

FIG. 957.—Ligatures are passed and tied round the cystic artery and cystic duct.

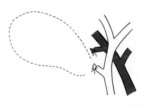

FIG. 958.—The gallbladder has been removed.

3. **Cholecystectomy.**—The area is now isolated with packs (fig. 956). If the gallbladder is greatly distended, it is aspirated through the fundus by means of a trocar and cannula attached to a suction apparatus. The neck of the gallbladder is grasped with spongeholding forceps. Then the very important dissection to display the junction of the cystic, the common hepatic, and the common bile ducts is commenced.[3] During the course of this dissection the cystic artery is found, and its relation to the common hepatic artery verified. The artery is then divided between ligatures at least 5 mm away from the hepatic duct (fig. 957). Cholangiography is performed at this stage both to confirm that the anatomy of the biliary tree has been correctly identified, as well as to check for stones in the main ducts: the 'dye' should enter the duodenum without undue delay. Only when anatomical and radiological tests are *both* satisfactory should any duct be divided. The cystic duct is then ligated. Forceps are applied to the gallbladder side and the cystic duct is divided. From below, upwards, the gallbladder is dissected from its bed, dividing the peritoneum

---

[1] 'Typhoid Mary', a cook-general who passed *Salmonella typhi* in her faeces and urine, was responsible for nearly a score of epidemics of typhoid in and around New York City.

[2] Surgeons should not give patients their stones after operation if there is any suspicion of typhoid!

[3] 'It is the left hand of my assistant that does all the work' (Moynihan). By splaying the fingers to depress the stomach and duodenum, he displays the biliary ducts, aided also by retraction of the quadrate lobe of the liver.

Daniel Elmer Salmon, 1850–1914. Veterinary Pathologist, Chief of the Bureau of Animal Industry, Washington, D.C., U.S.A.

on the gallbladder (fig. 958). The gallbladder having been removed and haemostasis assured, the abdominal wall is closed with drainage of the operation site, either using a suction drain or a corrugated drain.

Some Golden Rules in case of difficulty:

(1) Clear identification of the colon, the pylorus and duodenum is a prerequisite for a proper approach to the ductal and arterial system.

(2) A common duct hidden in fibrous tissue may be located by means of an aspirating syringe and fine needle.

(3) With severe inflammation in Calot's triangle[1] it may be wise to open the gallbladder, extract all the stones and bile, and excise as much of the wall of the gallbladder as possible. The cystic duct opening is closed by a catgut suture from 'within'. Any mucous membrane remaining on the hepatic side may be diathermied. An alternative is cholecystostomy.

(4) A clear indication of the position of the common and right hepatic duct in the danger area can be given by inserting a sound upwards through a choledochotomy.

A cholecystohepatic duct (fig. 943(e)), is present in about 0·5% of cases, and is usually the size and colour of a oo suture. Its possible presence must be remembered when separating the gallbladder from its bed, and, if recognised in time, it can be ligated. If avulsed from the liver, a persistent ooze of bile occurs from the ruptured end, which should be oversewn.

Cholecystostomy.—Two stay sutures are inserted on either side of the fundus, in order to steady the organ, the fluid contents of which are aspirated. The fundus is opened and stones are removed from the interior by Desjardins' forceps, aided, always, by a finger milking up a stone or stones from Hartmann's pouch. Minute calculi are often dislodged by strips of dry gauze passed into the interior. A large Foley catheter is placed in the gallbladder and the balloon inflated. The opening in the gallbladder is closed about the tube. The tube is brought through a portion of greater omentum, which is anchored to the gallbladder by the original stay sutures. The catheter is then brought to the surface through a separate stab incision. The abdominal incision is closed, and the catheter connected to a sterile bag. Seven to ten days later Hypaque injected down the catheter may be seen on x-ray to flow easily into common bile duct and duodenum. If no obstruction exists, removal of the catheter will be followed by closure of the biliary fistula within a week.

Indications for Choledochotomy at Cholecystectomy

In an environment where the modern diagnostic armamentarium described at the beginning of this chapter is not available and neither is peroperative cholangiography, it is as well to rehearse the traditional indications for choledochotomy, which are: (1) Stones can be felt in the ducts. (2) There is jaundice or a history of jaundice, or rigors. (3) A dilated common bile duct (10 mm diameter or more) is present. (4) The liver function tests are abnormal, in particular a raised alkaline phosphatase. Choledochotomy is described on p. 973.

Choledochotomy is described on p. 973.

SYMPTOMS PERSISTING AFTER CHOLECYSTECTOMY

In 15% of all cases, cholecystectomy fails to relieve the symptoms for which the operation was performed. Such patients have been described as having the 'post cholecystectomy syndrome', however it is a diagnosis which should only be made with caution. The symptoms are most commonly due to disease of organs other than the biliary tract, such as hiatus hernia, duodenal ulcer, pancreatitis, diverticulitis or the irritable bowel syndrome. If these can be eliminated, one of the following lesions of the biliary tract must be considered:

1. A stone in the common bile duct escaped detection at the original operation.
2. When a comparatively long stump of a cystic duct has been left behind as frequently

---

[1] Calot's triangle is bounded above by the liver, medially by the common hepatic duct and below by the cystic duct.

Jean François Calot, 1861–1944. Surgeon, Paris.
Abel Desjardins. Surgeon, Dispensaire Henri de Rothschild, Paris.

happens where the cystic duct joins the common bile duct lower than usual (fig. 943(*d*)), calculi may form in the remnant.

3. Operative damage to the common bile duct occurred, resulting in stricture of that duct.

Management.—Intravenous cholangiography and ERCP are valuable in determining the cause which is treated appropriately.

STONES IN THE BILE DUCTS

In addition to those in the gallbladder, stones may be present in the intra- and extrahepatic bile ducts. Usually they originate in the gallbladder and pass down the cystic duct. Sometimes they form in the ducts and are then called primary duct stones. Such stones are commonly encountered in the tropics where they may be secondary to infestation of the biliary tree by Ascaris lumbricoides and Clonorchis sinesis. They also occur in any condition causing prolonged biliary obstruction.

The consequences of duct stones are either obstruction to bile flow or infection—cholangitis. Stones in the bile ducts are more often associated with infected bile (80% of cases) than are stones in the gallbladder.

Symptoms.—The patient may be asymptomatic. Usually one or more of the symptoms, pain, jaundice and fever are present.

Pain is similar to the pain of cholecystitis. *Jaundice* may be intermittent or persistent. It is obstructive in type and therefore the urine is dark, the stools are pale and the skin itches (pruritis). *Fever* and rigors[1] indicate acute cholangitis. Rigors are uncommon in cholecystitis.

Charcot's Triad. The three symptoms occurring together constitute this triad and indicate acute cholangitis.

Signs.—Tenderness may be elicited in the epigastrium and right hypochrondrium. As a rule the gallbladder is impalpable. In the jaundiced patient it is useful to remember *Courvoisier's 'law'*[2]: 'In obstruction of the common bile duct due to stone, distension of the gallbladder seldom occurs; the organ usually is already shrivelled. In obstruction from other causes distension is common by comparison. Atrophy occurs only in 1 in 12 cases.' So, most patients with jaundice due to stone have a fibrotic non-distensible gallbladder, whilst those with malignant obstruction have a distensible gallbladder. Another factor is that malignant obstruction is often complete whereas stone obstruction may not be so complete as to cause distension.

Differential Diagnosis.—Calculous biliary obstruction is a very frequent cause of jaundice encountered in surgical practice (fig. 959). It is particularly important to distinguish between large duct obstruction and intrahepatic cholestasis resulting from obstruction of the bile canaliculi or the cholangioles within the portal tracts. Conditions causing the former include stones and pancreatic carcinoma and require operation. Conditions causing the latter include viral hepa-

---

[1] In Britain the two common causes for rigors are urinary and biliary obstruction with infection. In equatorial regions, malaria is the commonest cause.

[2] Of 187 cases, a shrivelled gallbladder was found in 70/87 with stones, and distension in 92/100 from other causes: 'Bei Steinobstruction des Choledochus ist Ectasie der Gallenblase selten; das Organ ist vorher schön gewöhnlich geschrumpft. Bei, Obstruction andrer Art ist dagegen Ectasie das Gewöhnliche; Atrophie besteht nur in 1/12 dieser Fälle.'

Jean Martin Charcot, 1825–1893. Physician, Hôpital Salpêtrière, Paris.
Ludwig Courvoisier, 1843–1918. Professor of Surgery, Basel, Switzerland.

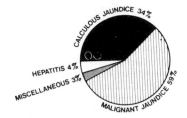

Fig. 959.—Incidence of jaundice in surgical practice (The London Hospital Surgical Unit, 1964–1973, 197 cases).

titis, drug induced jaundice and primary biliary cirrhosis, diseases not amenable to surgical treatment.

Diagnosis.—Liver function tests alone (Chapter 45) will not distinguish with certainty between intrahepatic cholestasis and large duct obstruction. Ultrasound, ERCP and PTC are the most useful investigations.

Complications.—1. Prolonged obstruction causes impairment of liver function which in some cases may progress to biliary cirrhosis. 'White bile' may be seen in the bile ducts at operation. 2. Suppurative Cholangitis. The bile ducts can become filled with pus. Liver abscesses and septicaemia result.

'White Bile'.—This phenomenon follows obstruction of a large duct. It is mostly mucus derived from the glands lining the ducts.

MANAGEMENT OF BILIARY OBSTRUCTION DUE TO STONE

Liver failure is treated if present. A high intake of glucose is instituted to build up the store of liver glycogen. Clotting abnormalities are usually due to failure to absorb Vitamin K. (This fat soluble vitamin requires bile salts for its absorption and these are lacking from the gut in obstructive jaundice. Vitamin K1 10 mg is given i.m. or i.v.) Blood cultures are taken and broad spectrum antibiotics administered if there is any evidence of cholangitis (fever, raised wbc.). Patients with obstructive jaundice, particularly if submitted to operation are prone to renal failure. Dehydration must be avoided and mannitol i.v. should be given prior to surgery to promote a diuresis.

Endoscopic papillotomy.—This technique can be used in patients unfit for operation, or who have previously had a cholecystectomy. An ERCP is performed and a specially designed diathermy wire is passed down the endoscope and used to divide the papilla of Vater. A Dormia basket (Chapter 57), or balloon catheter is then passed into the bile duct and the stones extracted.

Percutaneous removal of stones.—If stones are detected on a postoperative T-tube cholangiogram it may be possible to extract them through the T-tube track. Six weeks postoperatively, when a mature track has been allowed to form, the T-tube is removed and a steerable catheter and stone basket is passed down into the bile duct. The stone is grasped and extracted.

Percutaneous biliary drainage is an extension of the use of PTC. It was thought that its preoperative use by reducing jaundice and improving liver function would reduce operative mortality. However this has not been demonstrated.

Choledochotomy.—If a stone (or stones) is present in the common bile duct, its removal should have priority over cholecystectomy. Should the patient be unfit for cholecystectomy, or even cholecystostomy, the gallbladder should be removed on a future occasion.[1] In particular this may be the case in suppurative cholangitis.

---

[1] A living problem is better than a dead 'cert'. (Grey Turner.)

George Grey Turner, 1877–1951. Professor of Surgery, Postgraduate Medical School, London.

Supraduodenal Choledochotomy.—Most stones in the common bile duct can be removed by this route. If, as is often the case, a stone can be felt, an attempt is made to manoeuvre it into a position midway between the entrance of the cystic duct and the superior border of the duodenum. The stone is steadied between the finger and thumb. The duct is opened longitudinally directly on to the stone, enabling it to be removed by a malleable scoop or Desjardins' gallstone forceps. The interior of the duct is then explored upwards and downwards with the scoop for further stones.

When the stone cannot be felt, or cannot be manipulated into the optimum position just described, after incising the peritoneum overlying the common bile duct, a length of the underlying structure is displayed. As soon as about 2 cm of the common bile duct has been exposed, two stay sutures are placed in the duct and a longitudinal incision into the duct is made between them. Escaping bile is mopped up or removed by suction. Through this opening it may be possible to identify the stones and remove them with a scoop or forceps (fig. 960). A balloon catheter, similar to that used for embolectomy, and irrigation of the ducts with saline are useful additional methods. Choledochoscopy may be employed to confirm that all calculi have been removed. Usually drainage of the common bile duct is carried out by means of a T-tube (fig. 961).[1] The transverse limb, shortened if necessary to about 5 cm long, is inserted in the duct which is closed snugly about the vertical limb, using fine catgut on an atraumatic needle. The long limb is brought out through a separate stab wound and securely anchored to the skin. The bile draining from the tube is collected in a plastic bag by the side of the bed, its amount and character being noted. After 10 days the tube may be clamped for increasing periods, and the absence of pain and jaundice and the presence of bile in the stools indicate satisfactory flow into the duodenum. Hypaque is injected down the tube to obtain a cholangiogram, and if there are not filling defects in a well-outlined duct, and the 'contrast' enters the duodenum freely, the T-tube can be removed. Subsequent bile drainage is minimal and does not usually persist for more than a day.

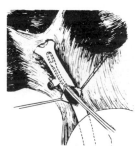

FIG. 960.—Choledochotomy. The stone is seized with Desjardins' forceps.

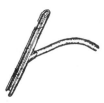

FIG. 961.— T-tube for draining the common bile duct.

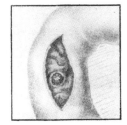

FIG. 962.—The trans-duodenal approach to a stone impacted in the ampulla of Vater.

Closure of the Common Duct without a T-tube.—If this procedure is attempted, it is most necessary to provide drainage placed in apposition to the common duct.

Transduodenal Sphincterotomy is indicated when a stone is found to be impacted near the ampulla of Vater (fig. 962) and it cannot be retrieved from above. Other indications are when the common bile duct is dilated and contains multiple stones and biliary sludge, and when the papilla is fibrosed and stenosed secondary to the passage of stones through it. Some surgeons prefer the method to supraduodenal choledochotomy to remove all duct stones.

The duodenum is opened in its second part between stay sutures, and the region of the ampulla brought into the opening by traction using tissue forceps. Removal of the stone or stones requires division of the duodenal papilla and the sphincter. A grooved director is passed through the papillary opening and up into the bile duct where it *must be palpated*.

---

[1] T-tubes should be of latex or rubber and only used once. Plastic tubes are 'hardened' by the bile and are difficult to remove. Latex (and rubber) stimulate the fibrinous adhesion of omentum to liver and colon to form a safe track. There is very little reaction to a plastic tube and therefore the risk of biliary peritonitis is greater.

The papilla and part or all of the sphincter is now divided at 10 o'clock. If the bile duct mucosa is sutured to that of the duodenum, the procedure is called a sphincteroplasty.

Choledochoduodenostomy is an alternative to transduodenal sphincterotomy when the common bile duct is dilated and contains multiple stones and sludge, particularly in the elderly (fig. 963).

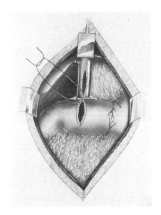

FIG. 963.—Choledochoduodenostomy. The stoma must be 2–3 cm long. The stoma is fashioned to extend as low as possible in order to reduce the collection of sludge in the 'sump' necessarily left in the retroduodenal portion of the duct. It must permit free entry and egress of fluid, for if it is large enough, regurgitant cholangitis does not occur and liver function is not impaired. The two openings are approximated with catgut, with several reinforcing fine silk sutures. A drain is inserted.

The operation is contraindicated if the common duct is not 1·5 cm or more in diameter or it is impossible to make a stoma of 2–3 cm. The convalescence is usually surprisingly placid. It is indeed a procedure which has commanded much support.

STRICTURE OF THE COMMON BILE DUCT $\Big\langle$ BENIGN $\Big\langle$ Post-operative 80% / Inflammatory 20% / MALIGNANT

Post-operative stricture concerns either the common bile duct or the common hepatic duct. In a few cases only the right hepatic duct is implicated. The stricture is the result of a preventable error in technique, during the performance of cholecystectomy:

1. Blind plunge application of a haemostat to a bleeding cystic or accessory cystic artery, or to the right hepatic artery, is likely to damage the common hepatic duct (fig. 964).

The prevention of this tragic happening is standardised. All unexpected haemorrhage in this region should be controlled initially by inserting an index finger into the foramen of Winslow, and pinching the free edge of the gastro-hepatic omentum between the finger and thumb. Temporary compression of the hepatic artery in this way allows the bleeding-point to be visualised and ligated accurately (Hogarth Pringle's manoeuvre).

2. Should cholecystectomy be performed by dissecting from the fundus (the fundus-first operation) too much traction applied to the freed gallbladder may so tent the common bile duct that any forceps intended for the cystic grasp the angulated main channel[1] (fig. 965).

3. Ignorance of the anatomical anomalies of the bile ducts.

4. Laceration of the common bile duct while exploring it for stones.

5. In 3% of cases of stricture of the common bile duct, injury occurs during partial gastrectomy for a penetrating duodenal ulcer.

---

[1] Forceps should not in fact ever be used for grasping the cystic duct prior to ligature (fig. 957).

Jacob Benignus Winslow, 1669–1760. Professor of Anatomy, Physic and Surgery, Paris.
James Hogarth Pringle, 1863–1941. Surgeon, Royal Infirmary, Glasgow, Scotland.

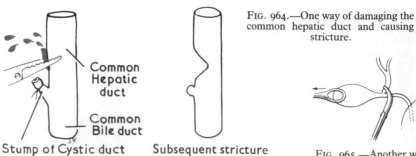

Stump of Cystic duct   Subsequent stricture

Common
Hepatic
duct

Common
Bile duct

FIG. 964.—One way of damaging the common hepatic duct and causing stricture.

FIG. 965.—Another way of damaging the ducts!

About 15% of injuries to the bile ducts are recognised at the time of the operation. In 85% of cases the injury declares itself post-operatively by: (*a*) a profuse and persistent discharge of bile if drainage has been provided, or bile peritonitis if such drainage has not been provided; (*b*) by deepening obstructive jaundice. When the obstruction is incomplete, jaundice is delayed until subsequent fibrosis renders the lumen of the duct inadequate.

Radiological Investigation of Biliary Strictures

(1) Cholangiography *via* a T-tube if present.
(2) ERCP
(3) Transhepatic cholangiography (figs 934 and 939).
(4) Ultrasound.

Treatment. In the debilitated patient, temporary external biliary drainage may be achieved by passing a catheter percutaneously into an intrahepatic duct. Also catheters may be passed through strictures at the time of ERCP and left to drain through the mouth. When the general condition of the patient has improved, definitive surgery can be undertaken. However, both these methods may be complicated by cholangitis and are not recommended for all cases.

Operations.—Occasionally a malignant stricture (carcinoma of the bile duct or head of the pancreas) may be resectable. Benign strictures and unresectable malignant strictures require bypass or stenting. Various procedures are available.

1. *Cholecystjejunostomy.* If the gallbladder is present and the cystic duct is assuredly patient, and the stricture well distal to the confluence of the cystic and common hepatic ducts, a loop of jejunum can be anastomosed to the gallbladder to provide drainage.

2. *Choledochojejunostomy..* Usually the upper end of the duct is anastomosed to the side of a Roux-en-Y limb of jejunum. This may have to be performed in the porta hepatis to the common hepatic duct.

3. *Choledochoduodenostomy* (see above). Best reserved for the localised obstruction in the distal bile duct.

4. *Insertion of a stent.* If bypass is impossible a stent may be positioned in a stricture, either at open operation or via PTC, or ERCP (fig. 968).

Sclerosing Cholangitis.—This term is used to describe fibrous thickening of the bile duct walls often associated with multiple strictures. The intra and extrahepatic ducts may be involved. It may occur secondary to duct stones, congenital lesions or operative trauma to the bile ducts. In a small number of cases, no such predisposing cause is found and the condition is called primary sclerosing cholangitis. About one third of the cases are associated with ulcerative colitis (Chapter 50). Multiple strictures separated by segments of duct of normal or increased diameter give a beaded appearance on radiological examination

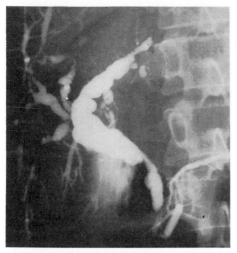

FIG. 966.—Sclerosing cholangitis in patient with ulcerative colitis visualised by ERCP.

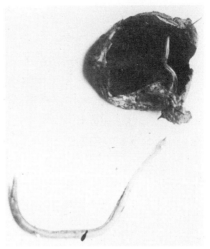

FIG. 967.—Ascaris projecting into the gallbladder.

(fig. 966). Prognosis is extremely variable. Some patients die from liver failure within months of diagnosis whilst others may live relatively symptom-free for many years.

The appropriate treatment is controversial. If a major stricture of the extrahepatic duct exists, benefit may be achieved from a by-pass procedure. Other cases have been treated successfully by T-tube drainage of the common bile duct, and by stenting of strictures. Often a short course of high dose steroids can be effective in relieving the fibrous strictures, either pre-operatively or beginning 10 days after surgery.

PARASITIC INFESTATION OF THE BILIARY TRACT

Biliary Ascariasis.—The round worm, Ascaris lumbricoides, commonly infests the intestine of inhabitants of Asia, Africa and Central America. It may enter the biliary tree through the ampulla of Vater and cause biliary pain. Complications include strictures, suppurative cholangitis, liver abscesses and empyema of the gallbladder. In the uncomplicated case antispasmodics can be given to relax the sphincter of Oddi and the worm will return to the small intestine to be dealt with by antihelmintic drugs. Operation may be required to remove the worm or the complications (fig. 967). Worms can also be extracted through the ampulla of Vater by ERCP.

Clonorchiasis (Asiatic cholangiohepatitis).—The disease is endemic in the Far East. The fluke, up to 25 mm long and 5 mm wide inhabits the bile ducts, including the intrahepatic ducts. Fibrous thickening of the duct walls occurs. Many cases are asymptomatic. Complications include biliary pain, stones, cholangitis, cirrhosis and bile duct carcinoma. Choledochotomy and T-tube drainage and in some cases choledocho-duodenostomy are required. Because a process of recurrent stone formation is set up, a choledochojejunostomy, with the loop affixed to the abdominal parietes, is made in some eastern centres to allow easy subsequent access to the duct system.

Hydatid Disease.—A large hydatid cyst may obstruct the hepatic ducts. Sometimes a cyst will rupture into the biliary tree and its contents cause obstructive jaundice or cholangitis, requiring the appropriate surgery (see Chapter 45).

CARCINOMA OF THE GALLBLADDER

Carcinoma of the gallbladder is rare in Western countries but commoner in India and Mexico. It is found in less than 1% of gallbladder operations. In over 90% of instances gallstones are present. The patients are mostly in the seventies (female: male ratio of 5:1). The usual type is a scirrhous carcinoma, but squamous cell and mixed squamous-adenocarcinomas are found. Spread is by direct

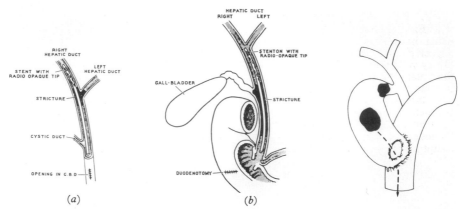

FIG. 968.—Insertion of a stent for (*a*) a high lesion and (*b*) a low
lesion (*after Ritchie and Maclean*).
(*From Annals of the Royal College of Surgeons.*)

FIG. 969.—Fistulation
of gallstone into duo-
denum.

invasion of the liver and portahepatis, by lymphatics to hilar lymph nodes, and by veins to the liver. Distant metastases are uncommon.

Clinical Features.—A small tumour may be found at cholecystectomy. Indeed all gallbladders should be opened at the time of removal and the mucosa inspected, and all resected gallbladders should be sectioned. When the tumour obstructs the cystic duct the patient may present with acute cholecystitis or a mucocele. Over half the cases present with obstructive jaundice and a palpable mass in the right hypochondrium.

Treatment and Prognosis.—On diagnosis at cholecystectomy, it may be considered advisable to resect part of the underlying liver (Smith), otherwise palliation only is possible. Jaundice may be relieved by a stent (fig. 968). The 5 year survival is 2–5%, but where the tumour is confined to the mucosa the figures improve to over 50%.

BILE DUCT CARCINOMA—CHOLANGIOCARCINOMA

Carcinoma of the bile ducts is even less common than gallbladder carcinoma. Stones are present in less than 30% of cases and males are slightly more affected than females. Patients with ulcerative colitis, primary sclerosing cholangitis, Clonorchiasis, choledochal cyst, and Caroli's disease have an increased risk of developing the condition. It is usually an adenocarcinoma of the scirrhous or papillary type.

Clinical Features.—Over 90% present with obstructive jaundice, less commonly with biliary pain and cholangitis.

Treatment.—The choledochoscope is very useful for obtaining histological proof at laparotomy. About half the lesions are situated in the hilar region. Rarely are they resectable. Intubation of the lesion with a transhepatic tube (passed through the lesion, liver and out through the skin) followed by radiotherapy offers palliation and some hope of prolonged survival (Terblanche). Tumours of the lower end of the common bile duct are often resectable by Whipple's operation (Chapter 48), and a 5 year survival of 30% may be expected (Tompkins).

Alexander David Willard Maclean, Contemporary. Surgeon, The London Hospital.
Lord Smith of Marlow, Contemporary. Past President, Royal College of Surgeons.
John Terblanche, Contemporary. Professor of Surgery, Cape Town, S.A.
Allen Oldfather Whipple, 1881–1963. Professor of Surgery, Columbia University, New York, U.S.A.
Ronald K. Tompkins, Contemporary. Professor of Surgery, UCLA Medical Centre, Los Angeles, U.S.A.

BILIARY FISTULAS

1. **External Fistulas.** Nearly all follow operations on the biliary tract, resulting from either damage to the main ducts or a leaking biliary anastomosis. They persist if there is a block preventing flow into the bowel (see principles, Chapter 8). The continuity of the biliary system in these cases must be restored. Radiography is very helpful in assessing the situation (*e.g.* sinograms, ERCP). Spontaneous restoration of normal flow may occur in some cases.

2. **Internal Fistulas.** A gallstone may ulcerate through the gallbladder wall into the stomach, duodenum or colon (fig. 969). Air is seen in the biliary tree on plain x-ray. If large enough the stone will obstruct the small intestine (gallstone ileus, Chapter 51). Stones entering the colon have been known to obstruct and so bring to light an otherwise symptomless carcinoma of the colon.

CHAPTER 48

THE PANCREAS

Surgical Anatomy.—The name pancreas is derived from the Greek 'pan' (all) and 'kreas' (flesh). It was originally thought to act as a cushion for the stomach. The gland weighs approximately 80g and is situated retroperitoneally. It is divided into a head and neck (comprising 46% of the whole organ), and a body and tail. The head lies within the curve of the duodenum. It overlies the body of the second lumbar vertebra and the aorta, but during respiration it moves up and down by 3–4 cm and forwards and backwards with the aortic pulse. The neck is that part of the pancreas which has the superior mesenteric vessels as a posterior relation (fig. 970). Coming off the side of the pancreatic head and passing to the left and behind the superior mesenteric vein, is the uncinate process. Short veins, which must be ligated in the pancreatectomy operation, pass from the uncinate process to the superior mesenteric vein. Behind the pancreas, at its upper border, the superior mesenteric vein joins the splenic vein to form the portal vein.

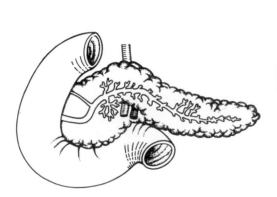 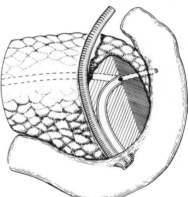

FIG. 970.—Anterior view of the pancreas. The head lies within the duodenal loop. The superior mesenteric vessels pass over the uncinate process and behind the neck of the pancreas. The superior mesenteric vein joins the splenic vein at the superior border of the pancreas to form the portal vein. The superior mesenteric artery lies to the left of the vein and joins the aorta behind the pancreas.

FIG. 971.—Posterior view of the head of the pancreas. The accessory duct (dorsal bud duct) passes superiorly and anteriorly to enter the second part of the duodenum. The main duct (ventral bud duct) passes posteriorly and inferiorly within the head of the pancreas to lie adjacent to and eventually fuse with the bile duct at the ampulla.

(Courtesy Annals Royal College of Surgeons of England.)

The pancreas develops as two buds (ventral and dorsal) from the primitive duodenum. The accessory pancreatic duct (Santorini) is the duct of the dorsal bud. It persists as the main duct of the body and tail of the pancreas and passes anteriorly through the head of the pancreas to enter the second part of the duodenum at the accessory papilla (fig. 971). The ventral bud duct, which forms the main pancreatic duct in the head of the pancreas, fuses with the dorsal duct in the pancreatic head and then runs posteriorly and inferiorly to lie next to and eventually join with the bile duct at the ampulla of Vater. Occasionally the main duct in the head (ventral bud duct) does not fuse with the accessory duct (dorsal bud duct). This gives rise to the condition of unfused ventral pancreas in which the body and tail of the pancreas drain exclusively through the accessory duodenal papilla and are vulnerable to accessory papillary stenosis.

Giovanni Domenico Santorini, 1681–1737. Professor of Anatomy and Medicine, Venice, Italy.
Abraham Vater, 1684–1751. Professor of Anatomy and Botany, Wittenberg, Germany.

Pancreatic acinar tissue is organised into lobules. The main duct ramifies into interlobular and intralobular ducts, ductules and finally acini. Acinar cells are clumped around a central lumen to form an acinus which communicates with the duct system. The pancreas thus consists of a network of fine ducts lined by secretory cells. Acinar tissue comprises about 84% of the pancreas, duct cells and blood vessels 4%, and endocrine cells (the islets of Langerhans) about 2%. The rest is connective tissues, blood vessels and fat.

The islets of Langerhans are more densely distributed in the tail of the pancreas. Islets consist of differing cell types: 75% are B cells (producing insulin), 20% A cells (glucagon), 5% D cells (somatostatin) and a small number of pancreatic polypeptide secreting cells. Within an islet, the B cells form an inner core surrounded by the other cells. Capillaries draining the islet cells drain into the portal vein, forming a pancreatic portal system.

Surgical Physiology.—In response to a meal, the pancreas secretes digestive enzymes in an alkaline (pH 8·4), bicarbonate rich fluid. Acinar cells synthesise and secrete digestive enzymes while the duct cells secrete bicarbonate. The daily secretion is about 1 litre, containing 5–8 g of protein in the form of enzymes. This secretion is under both neural and hormonal control. Stimulation of parasympathetic nerves in the vagus results in secretion of bicarbonate and enzymes, whereas stimulation of splanchnic sympathetic nerves inhibits secretion. The rate of secretion and the bicarbonate content of the pancreatic juice is increased by the hormone *secretin* which is released from the duodenal mucosa by luminal acid stimulation. Pancreatic enzyme secretion is potently stimulated by *pancreozymin* which is released from the duodenal mucosa by luminal fat and peptides. Pancreatic secretion can also be stimulated by hormones produced within the pancreas and small bowel, vasoactive intestinal peptide (VIP) and gastrin; and inhibited by the pancreatic hormones somatostatin, pancreatic polypeptide and glucagon.

Pancreatic secretion consists of a cephalic phase, initiated by the thought of food, a gastric phase produced by food in the stomach, and an intestinal phase mediated by secretin and pancreozymin release from the duodenum and jejunum. About 20 digestive enzymes are produced: *proteolytic enzymes, e.g.* trypsin; *lipolytic enzymes, e.g.* lipase; *starch splitting enzymes, e.g.* amylase, and *nucleic acid splitting enzymes, e.g.* ribonuclease.

Investigation of the pancreas.—It is possible to obtain information about: (a) pancreatic damage by measuring levels of pancreatic enzymes in body fluids; (b) pancreatic function, by measuring bicarbonate and enzymes produced in the pancreatic juice; and (c) morphological abnormality of the parenchyma and duct system by ultrasound and CT scan, and E.R.C.P.

(a) *Estimation of pancreatic enzymes in body fluids.*—When the pancreas is damaged, enzymes such as amylase, lipase, trypsin and chymotrypsin are released into the serum. Measurement of the serum amylase is the most widely used test of pancreatic damage. Amylases are hydrolytic enzymes which digest starch. They are found in pancreas, salivary gland, the lactating breast, fallopian tubes, and the liver and bile duct, but despite this variety of sources, a significant rise, in clinical practice, is most likely to arise from the pancreas. Amylase activity is often measured by the Somogyi unit which is defined as equivalent to 1 mg of glucose released by amylase from starch during 30 minutes incubation under the conditions of Somogyi's saccharogenic method. More recently an international unit has been introduced (1 Somogyi unit = 1·8 iu/l). The serum amylase rises within a few hours of pancreatic damage and declines again after about 48 hours, returning to normal within 4–8 days. Because of their sources of small amounts of amylase in the serum, a serum level of greater than 1,000 Somogyi units is generally required to support the diagnosis of pancreatic injury. The organ of origin of the amylase in the serum can be identified by isoenzyme analysis, but this is not routinely necessary. Measurement of urinary amylase can provide evidence of pancreatic damage for up to a week after the serum amylase has begun to fall. The normal rate of urinary amylase excretion is 4–75 iu/hr; considerably higher levels than this, with a wide fluctuation from hour to hour, are found in pancreatitis. Use of the amylase-creatinine clearance ratio has been advocated to overcome urinary collection difficulties. However, the test depends on four chemical estimations (including that for serum creatinine which is not very accurate by the colourimetric method) and is inaccurate where there is renal failure. Thus it probably provides no additional information and may be inaccurate.

(b) *Pancreatic function tests.*—Pancreatic secretion in response to a standardised stimulus can provide an assessment of the functional capacity of the gland. The tests can be divided into those where the stimulus to secretion is indirect—produced by the ingestion of a test meal; and those where it is directly produced by the injection of a hormone. The most widely used indirect method was introduced by Lundh in 1962. The duodenum is

Paul Langerhans, 1847–1888. Professor of Pathological Anatomy, Freiburg, Germany.
Michael Somogyi, 1883–1971. Biochemist, Jewish Hospital, St. Louis, Missouri, U.S.A.
Göran Lundh, Contemporary. Department of Surgery, University of Lund, Lund, Sweden.

intubated and a standard meal is ingested. The contents of the duodenum (pancreatic juice, bile and duodenal secretions) are collected and analysed for one of the pancreatic enzymes, usually trypsin. The test is limited because it does not measure the peak secretory capacity of the pancreas since secretion may be diminished by impaired neurohumoral stimulation of the pancreas rather than intrinsic pancreatic disease.

This objection is overcome by the secretin-pancreozymin test. A triple lumen tube is passed such that one aspiration channel is in the stomach and another in the duodenum while the third channel is used for perfusion of the duodenum with a non-absorbable marker such as polyethylene glycol. Aspiration via the stomach portal prevents gastric acid from neutralising duodenal bicarbonate. Secretin is given first and the duodenal contents collected. After 30 minutes pancreozymin is given and the duodenal collection continued for another 30 minutes. The completeness of duodenal recovery can be estimated from the recovery of non-absorbable marker. The test can also be performed more directly by endoscopic cannulation of the pancreatic duct. A permanently diminished maximal bicarbonate concentration and post-secretin bicarbonate output, and a reduced post-pancreozymin enzyme output are characteristic of relapsing chronic pancreatitis. In ductal obstruction arising either from a stricture or a calculus in chronic pancreatitis, or from pancreatic cancer, there is a reduced volume of secretion.

In addition to reduced exocrine function, abnormalities of endocrine function can also be identified. The mild diabetes mellitus of chronic pancreatitis is associated with a reduction in plasma insulin levels, in contrast to the raised levels found in maturity onset diabetes. Once carbohydrate intolerance occurs, insulin reserve and glucose tolerance is diminished. Transient glycosuria and hyperglycaemia may occur during the course of acute pancreatitis, but impairment in glucose tolerance is usually mild and does not persist. Measurement of circulating insulin and glucagon levels have not proved to be clinically useful in the management of pancreatic disease.

(c) *Detection of morphological abnormalities of the parenchyma and ducts.*—In cases where the changes are difficult to distinguish from pancreatitis, cytological examination of pancreatic juice obtained directly from the cannulated pancreas can confirm the radiological diagnosis (fig. 986).

The investigation is not free of side effects; cholangitis, amylasaemia and acute pancreatitis have occasionally been encountered.

(d) *Ultrasonography.*—In scanning the pancreas, the adjacent vessels, particularly the aorta, superior mesenteric artery and portal vein, are identified in longitudinal sections and then the pancreas is examined with axial or oblique sections 2–5 mm apart. The normal pancreas is moderately reflective. The best images are produced in thin subjects, but the images are poor in the obese with well developed surrounding fat planes.

Carcinoma of the pancreas in the head and body can be identified in most patients when they present clinically (fig. 972) but tumours less than 2 cm in diameter are not usually detected. Pseudocysts are easily recognised and pancreatic calcification produces highly reflective echoes with acoustic shadowing beyond. With real expertise a dilated pancreatic duct is recognisable. Jaundice is one of the major indications for ultrasonography. Obstructive jaundice is shown by the dilated intrahepatic ducts produced and the actual

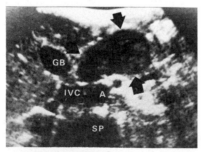

FIG. 972.—Carcinoma of the pancreas on a transverse ultrasound image of the upper abdomen (seen from the foot of the patient). GB Gallbladder; IVC Inferior vena cava; A Aorta; SP Spine.
(*J. McIvor, FRCR, London.*)

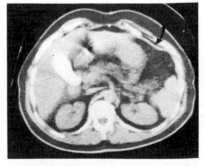

FIG. 973.—Chronic pancreatitis causing peritoneal thickening (curved arrow).

site of obstruction can often be identified particularly if a tumour is in the head of the pancreas.

(*e*) *Computed tomography* (CT scan).—(Figs 973–978.)

Pancreatic carcinoma larger than 3 cm is usually demonstrable whether in the head (fig.

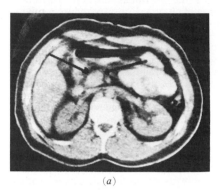

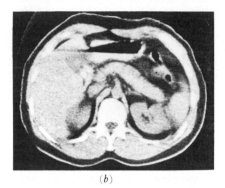

(*a*)

(*b*)

FIG. 974.—Normal pancreas on computed tomography. (All CT scans are viewed from the foot of the patient.) (*a*) The head of the pancreas (arrows) lies adjacent to the superior mesenteric artery and anterior to the inferior vena cava at the entry of the left renal vein which curves over the aorta. (*b*) The body and tail of the pancreas curves over the superior mesenteric artery with the tail of the pancreas lying in the angle between the left kidney and the spleen.

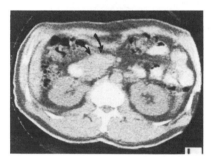

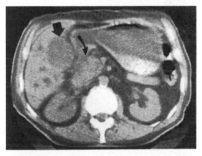

FIG. 975.—Carcinoma of the head of the pancreas (curved arrows) causing enlargement and lobulated margin.

FIG. 976.—Carcinoma of the head of the pancreas (curved arrow) with an enlarged gallbladder (broad arrow) and dilated ducts in the liver.

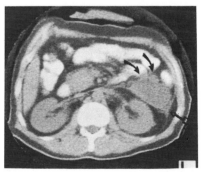

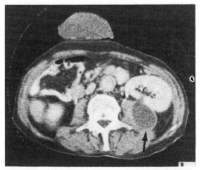

FIG. 977.—Pseudocyst in the region of the tail of the pancreas (curved arrows) associated with thickening of the transversalis fascia and anterior and posterior pararenal fascia (open arrow.)

FIG. 978.—Retroperitoneal pseudocyst displacing the kidney. A dense rim has appeared after intravenous contrast enhancement.

975), body or tail, but the adjacent duodenum and jejunum must be clearly labelled with an oral contrast agent, otherwise they may be mistaken for a tumour. Pseudocysts (figs. 977 and 978) are easily identified as well as pancreatic calcifications, gallstones, dilated intrahepatic ducts, and a distended gallbladder. In acute pancreatitis the surrounding inflammatory changes are frequently visible as well as the late thickening of the peritoneal reflections, particularly the anterior peri-renal fascia of Gerota. Contrary to ultrasonography, the best results are obtained with patients who have well developed fat planes. Abscesses and pseudocysts of the pancreas have similar appearances unless gas shadows can be identified indicating an abscess. In most cases the clinical findings are sufficiently distinctive allowing correct interpretation of the scanning images. The scope of diagnostic imaging is still limited. Endocrine tumours such as insulinomas and gastrinomas are not visualised when small, and are best demonstrated by selective arteriography. E.R.C.P. (fig. 985) is more effective in diagnosing tumours which obstruct or narrow the pancreatic duct even when small. However, the clear 3-dimensional view obtained with ultrasonography and computed tomography allows accurate placements of needles and catheters. Percutaneous drainage of pseudocysts and abscesses can save an otherwise inevitable laporatomy.

In the future other medical imaging systems will almost certainly be available. *Magnetic resonance imaging* (MRI) (Chapter 26, fig. 426) is non-ionizing and apparently harmless. Imaging in any plane is possible and blood vessels show particularly well.

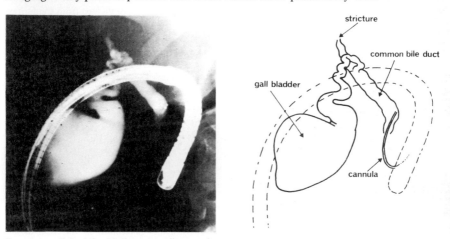

FIG. 979.—E.R.C.P. Malignant stricture of common hepatic duct. No contrast passes upwards beyond it.
(Dr. P. Cotton, London and The Lancet, 1972.)

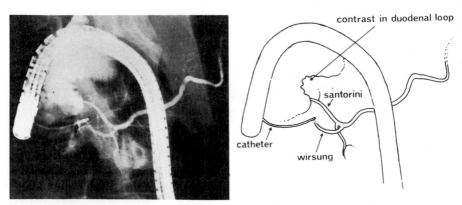

FIG. 980.—E.R.C.P.: Normal pancreatic duct with filling of duct of Santorini from the duct of Wirsung.
(Dr. P. Cotton, London.)

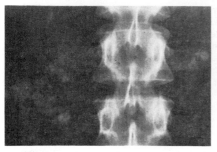

FIG. 981.—Plain abdominal x-ray: Chronic pancreatitis. Multiple opacities in the region of head and tail of pancreas.

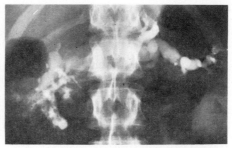

FIG. 982.—E.R.C.P.: Same patient as in fig. 981. Most of opacities lie within the duct system and are stones. Gross dilatation of ducts in body and tail due to obstruction by stones in head of pancreas.

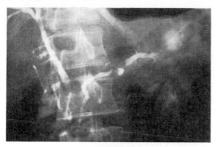

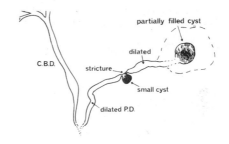

FIG. 983.—E.R.C.P.: Relapsing acute pancreatitis. Normal biliary tree. Pancreatogram shows stricture of main duct in the body with distal dilatation and cyst formation.
(Dr. P. Cotton, London, and Gut, 1972.)

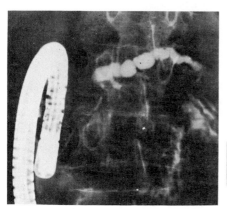

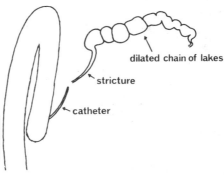

FIG. 984.—E.R.C.P.: Chronic pancreatitis. Long stricture of pancreatic duct in the head; distal pancreatic duct shows sacculation with intervening short strictures, 'chain of lakes'.
(Dr. P. Cotton, London.)

(f) *Endoscopic Retrograde Cholangio-Pancreatography*.—(E.R.C.P.).—The ampulla of Vater can now be cannulated using a side-viewing fibre-optic duodenoscope and the biliary and pancreatic ducts outlined with 65% Angiografin. This technique can be of value in confirming the presence or absence of a surgical cause of jaundice (fig. 979).

The retrograde pancreatogram will demonstrate the morphology of the pancreatic ducts. The normal anatomy is shown in fig. 980. Changes seen in chronic pancreatitis include strictures, dilated main ducts with stones (figs. 981 and 982) and first order branches and pancreatic cysts (fig. 983). The 'chain of lakes' appearance due to alternating strictures and duct sacculation is seen in fig. 984. The technique is of great value in both the diagnosis of chronic pancreatitis and in determining whether surgical intervention is indicated and which therapeutic procedure should be used.

In pancreatic carcinoma the main pancreatic duct is narrowed or completely obstructed at the site of the tumour with dilatation upstream of the obstruction but with a normal duct system downstream of the obstruction (fig. 985).

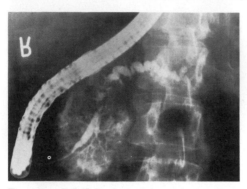

FIG. 985.—E.R.C.P.: Pancreatic carcinoma. Irregular stricture of main pancreatic duct with dilatation upstream of obstruction.

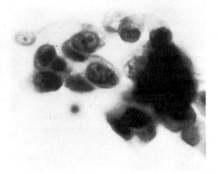

FIG. 986.—Group of adenocarcinoma cells from the pancreatic juice, collected at the time of E.R.C.P. of the patient illustrated in fig. 985.

CONGENITAL ABNORMALITIES

Cystic fibrosis.—This is inherited as an autosomal recessive. It most frequently occurs among Caucasians in whom it is the most commonly occurring inherited disorder (incidence 1 in 1,800 live births). Heterozygous carriers of the gene are asymptomatic, but recently it has proved possible to identify them by DNA analysis.

The disorder is due to a generalised dysfunction of exocrine glands whose aetiology is unknown. Glandular secretions have abnormal physicochemical properties resulting in: malabsorption due to pancreatic insufficiency, chronic pulmonary disease arising from blockage of bronchi and bronchioles, and elevated sodium and chloride ion concentrations in sweat. It is the commonest cause of chronic lung disease among children in developed countries.

Secretions precipitate in the lumen of pancreatic ducts causing blockage resulting in duct ectasia and fatty replacement of exocrine acinar tissue. The islets of Langerhans usually appear normal, but diabetes mellitus can occur in older patients. Steatorrhoea is usually present from birth resulting in stools which are bulky, oily and offensive. At birth the meconium may set in a sticky mass and produce intestinal obstruction—meconium ileus. Although about 15% of patients do not develop clinical steatorrhoea, most show complete exocrine insufficiency with the secretin-pancreozymin test.

The earliest clinical signs of cystic fibrosis are: poor growth and appetite, rancid greasy stools, abdominal distension, a persistent cough, emphysematous chest and finger clubbing. Later the liver may become cirrhotic due to bile duct plugging and the signs of portal hypertension may appear; cor pulmonale may develop; and the appearance of secondary sexual characteristics may be delayed. The mother may have noticed that the child is salty when kissed, and levels of sodium and chloride ions in the sweat above 90 mmol/l confirm the diagnosis.

Treatment is aimed at control of the secondary consequences of the disease. Malabsorption is treated by administration of pancreatic enzyme preparations, and pulmonary function preserved with physiotherapy and antibiotics. A suitable diet is low in fat but contains added salt to replace the high losses in sweat. With optimal treatment 80% of patients diagnosed early should survive to beyond their 19th year.

Congenital pancreatic hypoplasia.—This is usually associated with depressed bone marrow function, and occasionally with a variety of other abnormalities: metaphyseal dysostosis, thoracic dystrophy or hepatic dysfunction. There is gross pancreatic insufficiency associated with acinar fatty replacement, but endocrine function is not impaired. Neutropenia which can be cyclical over a period of about three weeks, results in an increased susceptibility to infection. Treatment is directed at the secondary consequences of repeated infection and malabsorption. The prognosis is better than that of cystic fibrosis, from which it can be differentiated by a normal sweat concentration of sodium and chloride.

Isolated pancreatic enzyme deficiencies.—Isolated deficiencies of lipase, amylase, trypsin, and intestinal enterokinase can occur: patients develop varying degrees of growth retardation and steatorrhoea. The diagnosis can be confirmed by the Lundh or secretin-pancreozymin tests.

Annular pancreas.—This is due to a failure of complete rotation of the ventral pancreatic bud during development (p. 980), so that a ring of pancreatic tissue surrounds the second or third part of the duodenum. It is more prevalent in the Down's syndrome child and in infants with other congenital gut abnormalities. It is one of the causes of obstructive vomiting in the neonate. The vomiting can be bile stained if the duodenal obstruction is below the ampulla of Vater. Peristaltic waves and upper abdominal distension may be seen, and plain abdominal x-ray shows the 'double-bubble' sign of the interrupted gastro-duodenal shadow produced by the rigid ring of pancreatic tissue. The usual treatment is bypass—duodenojejunostomy or duodenoduodenostomy. Attempts at resection of the band may result in a pancreatic fistula.

Ectopic pancreas.—This is found in the submucosa of some part of the stomach, duodenum, or small intestine (including Meckel's diverticulum), the gallbladder, adjoining the pancreas (*e.g.* in the hilum of the spleen) or (in 2% of carefully conducted necropsies) within the liver. Ectopic pancreas in the wall of the intestine is apt to be the starting-point of an intussusception. Ectopic pancreas in the wall of the stomach is liable to undergo cystic degeneration.

Congenital cystic disease of the pancreas.—This sometimes accompanies congenital disease of the kidneys and liver.

INJURIES TO THE PANCREAS

External Injury

The pancreas may be injured by direct blunt trauma or by a penetrating injury. Blunt trauma may come from a blow during an automobile or bicycle accident, or an unexpected punch into the relaxed abdomen. The commonest site of pancreatic injury is to the left of the neck of the pancreas, where it is most vulnerable as it overlies the aorta and lumbar spine. Occasionally a blow on the right side of the abdomen can lacerate the duodenum and pancreatic head. Penetrating injuries involving the pancreas frequently include injuries to the stomach, duodenum, colon, liver or spleen.

Presentation and management.—The most frequent presentation of blunt pancreatic trauma is epigastric pain. The serum amylase should be measured, as a rise is associated with 90% of cases of pancreatic injury. Ultrasound will demonstrate pancreatic oedema, haematoma or a pseudocyst (fig. 990). Persisting abdominal pain, prolonged elevation of the serum amylase or progression of physical signs will determine if laparotomy is necessary. At operation, the extent of injury is frequently underestimated because of a large surrounding haematoma. The whole pancreas should be visualised by entering the lesser sac and mobilising the duodenum and head of the pancreas. Injuries to the body or tail of the pancreas are best treated by distal resection to the point of injury. 80–90% of the normal gland can be removed without symptoms of insufficiency. Injuries to the pancreatic head and duodenum require partial pancreatoduodenectomy (Whipple procedure, see p. 999). There is a high incidence of duodenal breakdown following attempts at repair. Similarly, attempts at duct repair over a stent, anastomosing

Johann Friedrich Meckel (The Younger), 1781–1833. Professor of Anatomy and Surgery, Halle, Germany.
Allen Oldfather Whipple, 1881–1963. Professor of Surgery, Columbia University, New York, U.S.A.

both lacerated ends into a Roux-en-Y loop, and sphincterotomy to reduce resistance to flow of pancreatic juice and prevent a fistula, have not been successful. If a pancreatic pseudocyst develops, a cystogastrostomy should be carried out (fig. 991). Occasionally the consequences of pancreatic duct injury are not apparent until late, when pancreatitis due to traumatic pancreatic duct stenosis develops.

Prognosis.—The commonest cause of death is bleeding from the site of pancreatic rupture. The mortality of blunt pancreatic injury varies from 16 to 28% depending on the presence of associated injury—particularly to the duodenum. The mortality of penetrating injury to the pancreas with associated injuries to surrounding viscera approaches 50%.

Iatrogenic injury.—This can occur in four ways:

(1) Injury to the tail of the pancreas during splenectomy resulting in a pancreatic fistula.

(2) Injury to the accessory pancreatic duct (Santorini) during Bilroth II partial gastrectomy. This duct is the main duct in 10% of patients. A pancreatogram, done by cannulating the duct at the time of discovery, will demonstrate whether it is safe to ligate and divide the duct. If no alternative drainage duct can be demonstrated then the duct should be reanastomosed to the duodenum.

(3) Attempts at enucleation of islet cell tumours of the pancreas can result in fistulas. Enucleation should be avoided in favour of formal pancreatic resection.

(4) Duodenal or ampullary bleeding following sphincterotomy. This may require duodenotomy to control the bleeding.

Pancreatic fistula.—This usually follows operative trauma to the gland which in most cases was not suspected at the time.

Treatment.—The problems in the management of these fistulas are:

(1) *Fluid and Electrolyte Loss.*—In the presence of these fistulas the pancreas tends to hypersecrete and up to 2 litres may be lost in twenty-four hours. Such a loss of fluid and electrolytes may constitute a menace to life; they must therefore be replaced either by mouth or intravenously. In large losses, daily fluid and electrolyte balance must be maintained. If there is much loss, pancreatic extract should be given by mouth. Pancreatic secretion can be partially suppressed by diamox and atropine. The diet should consist of high protein and low carbohydrate. Total parenteral nutrition is frequently necessary.

(2) *Autodigestion of the Parietes.*—The skin should be protected by an ointment composed of 1% HCl in zinc oxide cream. A 'pure' pancreatic juice fistula is much less corrosive to the skin than a mixture of duodenal and pancreatic juice, because in the former the enzymes are not activated by the duodenal contents.

(3) *'Pooling' of the discharge* deeply in the wound. If possible, completely *dependent* drainage must be instituted; if necessary, the patient must lie prone. If this is not possible, continuous motor suction sump drainage must be carried out. In any case, the daily loss must be measured. Spontaneous closure occurs in 90% of cases, though this may take several months. Failure is usually due to inadequate dependent drainage.

If in spite of all these measures the fistula fails to close, it should be dissected to its source in the pancreas and drained into the stomach or into a Roux-en-Y jejunal loop.

PANCREATITIS

Classification.—The classification of pancreatitis has always been a problem. Two useful classifications are as follows:

A. **Classification by clinical presentation** (Marseilles[1]):

1. **Acute Pancreatitis** } *These return to normal when the primary cause is*
2. **Relapsing Acute Pancreatitis** } *removed*
3. **Chronic Pancreatitis** } *In these, even if the cause is removed, functional or*
4. **Relapsing Chronic Pancreatitis** } *structural damage still remains.*

B. **Classification according to aetiology[2]:**

1. **Biliary Tract Disease**   55% } *Aetiology is very*
2. **Alcoholism**   2% } *important in relating*
3. **Post-operative**   5% } *the natural history*
4. **Traumatic**   1% } *of the disease to*
5. **Rare causes** (e.g. mumps, hyperpara-   } *prognosis, long term*
   thyroidism, vascular disease)   2% } *treatment, and*
6. **Idiopathic**   35% } *prophylaxis.*

The latest consensus is that a division of pancreatitis into 'acute' and 'chronic' is most useful.

'Acute pancreatitis' is defined as an acute condition presenting with abdominal pain and usually associated with raised pancreatic enzymes in blood or urine due to inflammatory disease of the pancreas. Acute pancreatitis may recur.

'Chronic pancreatitis' is defined as a continuing inflammatory disease of the pancreas characterised by irreversible morphological change and typically causing pain and/or permanent loss of function. Many patients with chronic pancreatitis may have exacerbations, but the condition may be completely painless.

Acute Pancreatitis

Acute pancreatitis has an incidence of about 5 per 100,000 per year in the UK. The incidence among men is about the same as in women, but in men the peak age of incidence is about 30–40 years whereas in women it is 50–60 years. The condition is characterised by varying degrees of oedema, haemorrhage and necrosis of the pancreas and surrounding fat (fig. 987).

Aetiology.—There are two major causes of acute pancreatitis in the UK: biliary calculi (about 50% of all cases) and alcoholism (about 25% of all cases). The remaining 25% of cases is composed of a wide variety of conditions:

(a) After biliary or gastric surgery—especially after Bilroth II partial gastrectomy if the pancreatic duct is injured or if the afferent duodenal loop is obstructed producing a high duodenal pressure.

(b) After trauma, such as a blow, to the pancreas.

(c) Where there is distortion of the ampulla of Vater due to peptic ulcer or ampullary carcinoma.

(d) As a result of generalised disorders, such as hypercalcaemia, hyperlipaemia, diabetes mellitus and porphyria.

(e) In reaction to some drugs e.g. corticosteroids.

(f) Viral infiltration of the pancreas e.g. mumps virus.

(g) In some autoimmune diseases *e.g.* polyarteritis nodosa.

(h) After impaired pancreatic blood flow *e.g.* after cardiopulmonary bypass and following hypothermia.

---

[1] The Marseilles classification was adopted in 1963 in order to standardise analysis of this condition.
[2] Based on an analysis of 520 cases (Trapnell). Note the size of the group with no known cause (idiopathic). Recent studies suggest alcohol as the cause in 92% of acute necrotising pancreatitis, and even higher in chronic pancreatitis (Seligson).

John Eliot Trapnell, Contemporary. Surgeon, Royal Victoria Hospital, Bournemouth, England.
Ulf Seligson, Contemporary. Surgeon, Stockholm.

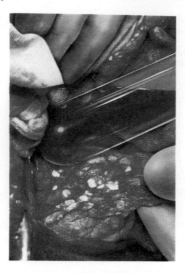

FIG. 987.—Widespread fat necroses of omentum. A test-tube has been filled with the blood-stained peritoneal fluid. This specimen was rich in amylase *Fat necroses* are dull, opaque, yellow-white areas suggestive of drops of wax. They are most abundant in the vicinity of the pancreas, but are widespread in the greater omentum and the mesentery. At necropsy they can sometimes be demonstrated beneath the pleura and pericardium, and even in the subsynovial fat of the knee joint. Fat necroses consist of small islands of saponification caused by the liberation of lipase, which splits fat into glycerol and fatty acids. Free fatty acids combine with calcium to form soaps= fat necrosis.
(*G. D. Adhia, FRCS, Bombay.*)

The mechanism of damage in pancreatitis is autodigestion of the gland by its own enzymes. Ligation of the pancreatic duct does not result in pancreatitis because proteolytic enzymes are not activated until they reach the duodenum. In pancreatitis produced by gallstones, it is thought that the passage of a calculus through the ampulla of Vater distends or splints the sphincter. When the duodenal pressure rises with spasm or contraction, duodenal contents reflux into the pancreas triggering the proteolytic enzymes and the inflammation.

High levels of alcohol ingestion have been shown to alter metabolism in acinar cells. It is thought that this metabolic disturbance, together with alterations in the composition of pancreatic juice forming protein plugs within pancreatic ducts, may be the cause of alcoholic pancreatitis.

Clinical features.—The main symptom is epigastric pain which is frequently severe and radiates to the left and right, and through to the back. This may be associated with anorexia, nausea and vomiting. On examination there may be abdominal guarding and bowel sounds may be reduced or absent. About 60% of patients are febrile and 50% are tachypnoeic while jaundice may be seen in about 10%. In less than 5% of cases, retroperitoneal haemorrhage can produce a bluish ecchymotic discoloration of the flanks (Grey-Turner's sign) and periumbilical area (Cullen's sign).

Investigations.—The serum amylase is elevated to above 1,000 Somogyi Units. Plain abdominal x-ray may show: (a) an air—containing slightly dilated loop of small bowel over the left upper quadrant, called a 'sentinel loop' and produced by the local involvement of small bowel adjacent to the pancreas. (b) Moderate distension of the duodenum with an air fluid level. (c) Mild distension of the transverse colon with collapse of the descending colon—the colon 'cut off' sign. Pancreatic ultrasound can confirm the pancreatic oedema, and may demonstrate whether calculi in the gall bladder or bile duct are present.

Treatment.—The course of pancreatitis varies from mild to fulminant and it is important, in management, to decide how serious the disease is. Criteria which identify high risk patients have been identified by Ransom, they are: old age;

George Grey Turner, 1877–1951. Professor of Surgery, Postgraduate Medical School, London. Formerly Professor of Surgery, University of Durham.
Thomas Stephen Cullen, 1868–1953. Professor of Gynaecology, Johns Hopkins University, Baltimore, U.S.A.

extent of rise in blood sugar, white cell count, liver function tests, blood urea and base deficit; extent of fall in serum calcium, haematocrit, and arterial oxygen tension; and the volume of fluid accummulated in extravascular spaces—'third space' collection.

The mainstays of treatment are bed rest, intravenous fluids, nasogastric decompression, and pain control with opiates—preferably pethidine with an antispasmodic which has less tendency to produce ampullary sphincter spasm. Attempts to reduce pancreatic secretion with anticholinergics, glucagon, calcitonin, somatostatin, vasopressin, acetazolamide and isoprenaline have been shown to be of no value. Similarly, anti-enzyme preparations such as aprotinin, epsilon-aminocaproic acid, snake anti-venom, and chlorophyll-a have shown no benefit. While trials of peritoneal lavage have shown no overall significant advantage, occasional patients with severe disease do seem to be improved.

It has been proposed that operation, at the time of an attack, with exploration of the ampulla of Vater will improve a significant proportion of patients with gallstone pancreatitis in whom a bile duct stone is arrested at the ampulla producing duodenopancreatic reflux. Removal of the stone might then relieve the attack. Exploration of the ampulla at this stage carries a high risk of morbidity and mortality, and it has not yet been shown that the benefits outweigh the deficits. If undertaken, surgical exploration of the ampulla should only be carried out by an experienced biliary surgeon. Endoscopic sphincterotomy and extraction of biliary stones may be a less traumatic way of removing troublesome calculi during an attack of acute pancreatitis. Occasionally, following a severe attack of necrotising pancreatitis, pancreatectomy of the necrotic sequestrum may be of value. All pancreatic tissue distal to the necrotic tissue should be removed, otherwise a pancreatic fistula may develop.

Complications

Shock.—Volume deficits resulting from gastrointestinal fluid loss, and 'third space' collections in peritoneal and pleural cavities, and the extravascular space produce hypovolaemic shock. This may be associated with a fall in haematocrit, due to retroperitoneal haemorrhage, and electrolyte disturbance. The central venous pressure should be monitored and fluid replacement, in the form of whole blood, plasma expanders, or albumin should be administered. Later reabsorbtion of fluid from 'third space' may lead to pulmonary oedema.

Pulmonary insufficiency.—Minimal degrees of hypoxia are common, and occasionally marked hypoxia can occur. This is due to a combination of factors: retroperitoneal oedema, elevation of the diaphragm, reduced ventilation due to pain, right to left arterial shunting of blood in the lungs, intravascular coagulation of platelets in the lungs, activation of phospholipase A with loss of pulmonary surfactant, and increased affinity of oxyhaemoglobin for oxygen. Early provision of supplementary oxygen, especially to high risk older patients reduces the mortality. Occasionally, positive pressure ventilation is of benefit.

Infection.—Secondary infection of necrotic tissue in the pancreatic bed produces an abscess one or two weeks after the initial attack has subsided in 1·3–4·5% of all cases of acute pancreatitis. This carries a high mortality, and operative debridement of the area, with resection of distal pancreatic tissue offers the best chance of recovery.

Hypercalcaemia—occurs in 3–30% of cases. The mechanism is not fully understood. It was originally thought to be due to binding of calcium in calcium soaps within areas of fat necrosis, but this does not account for the amounts of calcium involved. Raised plasma levels of glucagon and calcitonin, and deficiencies in parathormone may be additional causes. A serum calcium level below 2·0 mmol/l is associated with a poor prognosis. Tetany due to hypercalcaemia can be treated with intravenous calcium gluconate. In some

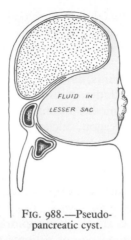

FIG. 988.—Pseudo-
pancreatic cyst.

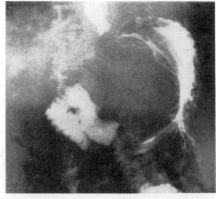

FIG. 989.—Barium meal—Pseudo-pancreatic
cyst displacing stomach.
(Lord Smith, London, in Trans. med. Soc. Lond.)

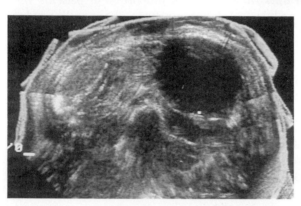

FIG. 990.—Ultrasound of pancreatic pseudocyst (tail). A large
fluid-filled area is seen in the tail
of the pancreas.
(Dr. J. Boultbee, Charing Cross Hospital.)

cases the tetany may be resistent to massive doses of calcium and this carries a very poor prognosis.

Colonic stricture—results from scarring of the transverse mesocolon and colon at the point where it overlies the pancreas. This is not as rare as was once thought and can be mistaken for a colon carcinoma.

Pseudocyst.—Ultrasound in cases of acute pancreatitis suggests that about half of all cases are complicated by the formation of pseudocysts, but 20–40% of these resolve spontaneously. A pancreatic pseudocyst is a collection of fluid in the lesser sac (fig. 988) which accumulates after damage to the pancreas. In order of frequency, the pseudocyst projects (a) between the stomach and the transverse colon; (b) between the stomach and liver; (c) behind or below the transverse colon. An epigastric swelling appears during the conservative treatment of pancreatitis, or in traumatic cases during or after convalescence for an injury that did not merit laparotomy. Exceptionally the patient is admitted with a pseudocyst of the pancreas and gives a history of an attack of severe abdominal pain that occurred a week or more previously.

On examination there is a swelling, sometimes as large as a melon, placed centrally above the umbilicus: the swelling is fixed, and in many instances it is so tense that fluctuation cannot be elicited. As a rule, transmitted pulsation from the abdominal aorta is very noticeable and the diagnosis of an aneurysm may be considered, although in the latter case the pulsation is expansile and, in the knee-elbow position the pulsation is much diminished. Moreover, in the case of a pancreatic cyst, a bruit is absent and the swelling, which is the presenting feature, is much broader. A Ryle's tube passed into the stomach may be palpable over the swelling if the patient is thin (Baid). Mesenteric cysts are rare and very mobile. A barium meal shows projection of the cyst into hollow viscera, especially the stomach (fig. 989). Every case of acute pancreatitis must be observed for the develop-

J. C. Baid, M.S., Contemporary. Surgeon, Jodhpur, India.

ment of a pseudocyst. Ultrasound and CT scanning[1] are valuable investigations. The earlier a pseudocyst appears the worse the prognosis.

Treatment.—It is necessary to distinguish between acute and chronic pseudocyst formation. Acute pseudocysts commonly arise after severe attacks of pancreatitis. About 20–40% of these will resolve without treatment and so no action should be taken during the first weeks after they have been recognised unless there is clinical evidence that the cyst has become infected. Serial ultrasonic measurements will give a good indication of how the cyst is progressing and should show spontaneous resolution if this is occurring. Where, however, infection has supervened or when the cyst has been present for 2–3 months or is over 6 cm in diameter, operative treatment is recommended because of the risk to life from spontaneous rupture. The treatment is cysto-gastrostomy. The stomach is opened through its anterior wall and an incision of at least 6 cm made through the posterior wall into the cyst. Haemostasis is secured with a circumferential running suture and the anterior wall of the stomach is closed (fig. 991). The contents of the cyst then drain into the stomach. Convalescence is shortened thereby and the complications referred to are obviated. Curiously, food does not enter the sac, as might be expected. The opening must be large enough to allow for subsequent contraction. Bleeding from the incised edge may follow and this is the major post-operative hazard. Cysto-jejunostomy is equally effective.

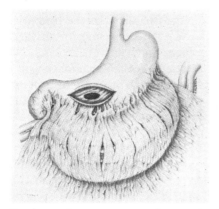

FIG. 991.—Cysto-gastrostomy for pseudo-pancreatic cyst.

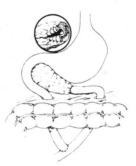

FIG. 992.—Retrograde pancreatojejunostomy.
(*After M. K. Du Val, Jnr.*)

Prognosis of acute pancreatitis.—The mortality varies according to the severity of disease, varying from 3–10% for oedematous pancreatitis, 40–50% for necrotising pancreatitis to nearly 100% for patients in whom the gland is completely necrosed.

Patients who have recovered from pancreatitis produced by gallstones should undergo cholecystectomy, and either operative or endoscopic removal of any bile duct stones. This should be done within a couple of months of the attack, before another attack develops. Some advocate that cholecystectomy should be carried out before the patient is discharged from hospital after recovery from an attack of acute pancreatitis, while others feel that an early operation may be attended by more complications *e.g.* pseudocyst formation. Other causes of pancreatitis should be sought, and where identified, they should be treated *e.g.* hyperparathyroidism. Some alcoholics will be warned off further drinking by the fear of another attack.

20–50% of all patients with acute pancreatitis suffer a further attack.

---

[1] Originated in 1968 in the EMI Central Research Laboratories.

Chronic Pancreatitis

Chronic pancreatitis is characterised by the persistence of pancreatic damage even if the primary cause of the pancreatitis is eradicated. The prevalence of chronic pancreatitic change found at autopsy is about 300 per 100,000, but the prevalence of clinically significant disease during life is much less than this. It occurs more frequently in men (M:F, 4:1) and the mean age of onset is about 40 years of age.

Pathology and aetiology.—At the onset of the disease, when symptoms have developed, the pancreas may appear normal. Later, the pancreas enlarges and becomes hard due to sclerosis while the ducts become distorted and dilated with areas of ectasia. Calcified stones, weighing from a few milligrams to as much as 200 g may form within the ducts. The ducts become occluded with gelatinous protein-rich fluid and debris to form cysts. Histologically the lesions affect a particular lobule producing ductular metaplasia and atrophy of acini, hyperplasia of duct epithelium, and interlobular fibrosis. In cases where there is significant clinical abnormality, the changes affect a large part or all of the pancreas, and the pancreas may be surrounded by sclerosis which can narrow the arteries, lymphatics, portal and splenic veins, bile ducts, and transverse colon.

The most frequent cause of chronic pancreatitis is high alcohol consumption accompanied by a diet which is high in protein and fat. The mechanism of damage is not understood, but alcohol appears to change the amount and content of pancreatic juice, resulting in the formation of protein plugs which occlude the pancreatic ducts. Other causes are: pancreatic duct obstruction due to stricture *e.g.* after trauma or acute pancreatitis, or to occlusion by pancreatic cancer; hyperparathyroidism; cystic fibrosis; hereditary pancreatitis; infantile malnutrition; and a large unexplained 'idiopathic' group. Occasionally stenosis of the ampulla of Vater can result in chronic pancreatitis, and where the ventral and dorsal pancreatic buds have remained unfused (p. 980) stenosis of the accessory papilla may produce pancreatitis changes which spare the ventral pancreatic bud in the head of the pancreas.

Clinical features.—Epigastric pain (93% of cases) which is referred to the left (29%) and right (44%) hypochondrium, and through to the back (56%). Sometimes the pain is exacerbated by taking alcohol. Weight loss resulting from loss of appetite produced by pain and malabsorbtion. Gross malabsorbtion or diabetes mellitus are late features. Examination is usually unhelpful but jaundice may be seen in about 3% of cases due to narrowing of the retropancreatic bile duct. A tender hard epigastric mass may indicate the formation of a cyst or may even be a cancer.

Investigation.—In the early stages, when there is little parenchymal damage, a transient rise in serum amylase after a painful crisis may be the only detectable abnormality. An evocative test in which a rise in serum amylase occurs after stimulation with secretin-pancreozymin may confirm the diagnosis at this stage. Later, when chronic changes have developed, the Lundh or secretin-pancreozymin tests. (p 982) become abnormal. A high lactoferrin level in pancreatic juice obtained at E.R.C.P. is a specific test for calcifying chronic pancreatitis. Steatorrhoea is found in about 30% of cases, and only develops when the pancreatic insufficiency has become severe.

A plain abdominal x-ray (fig. 981) demonstrates calcification in 65% of cases of chronic pancreatitis. Ultrasound of the pancreas shows enlargement of the pancreas with cysts and dilated ducts. CT scan may be useful in the exclusion of other retroperitoneal sources of pain e.g. lymphadenopathy or a retroperitoneal sarcoma. E.R.C.P. can demonstrate a ductal or papillary stricture acting as a trigger lesion for pancreatitis, duct anomalies e.g. ventral unfused pancreas, and the extent of disease as assessed by the degree of duct distortion. E.R.C.P. is also used to establish whether surgical treatment is likely to be of benefit, and if so, the type of operation.

Treatment.—A diet containing about 100 g protein and 100 g fat per day and absolute abstention from alcohol. Pancreatic enzyme supplement (Pancrex), even in the absence of steatorrhoea, may reduce the frequency of painful crises. Medium chain triglyceride and vitamin D supplements may also be required for malabsorbtion. Pain can be very troublesome and should be controlled by the use of suitably strong analgesia. Occasionally splanchnic nerve block may provide relief. The pain often remits if the patient abstains from alcohol. If diabetes mellitus occurs it can usually be controlled initially with oral agents, but later, insulin may be required.

Medical management is often able to ensure a reasonable life for the patient, but surgery is occasionally indicated when the disease is not controlled despite abstention from alcohol. 45% of the pancreas i.e. the body and tail or most of the pancreas (95%) leaving only a thin rim within the duodenum can be excised. Where there is reduced drainage through the head of the pancreas with a dilated proximal pancreatic duct (fig. 984), retrograde pancreatico-jejunostomy can be of benefit (fig. 992). Where there are multiple duct strictures, the duct can be laid open on the anterior surface and a side-to-side pancreatico-jejunal anastomosis (Puestow) over a length of at least 10 cm can be carried out. Sphincterotomy, either at laparotomy or done endoscopically, is valuable where stenosis of the main or accessory duct sphincter can be demonstrated.

Prognosis.—Drainage or excision procedures provide relief from pain in two-thirds of the patients selected for surgery, but patients undergoing extensive resection eventually become malnourished due to the poor quality of residual pancreas. The life expectancy of patients who abstain from alcohol and undergo surgery for chronic pancreatitis, is the same as for the normal population.

CARCINOMA OF THE PANCREAS

Carcinoma of the Exocrine Pancreas

Pancreatic carcinoma is one of the five most commonly occurring cancers in the UK (incidence 12 per 100,000 population per year). The incidence reported has doubled in the last twenty years. This is partly as a result of more accurate diagnosis—previously the source of many pancreatic cancers was not identified—and partly because the condition has become more common. It afflicts males and females to the same degree (M:F, 1.03:1), and occurs more frequently in older people—about half of all patients are aged over 70 years at the time of onset.

Charles B. Puestow, Contemporary. Professor of Surgery Emeritus, The Abraham Lincoln School of Medicine, University of Illinois, U.S.A.

Pathology and aetiology.—More than 75% of all cases are adenocarcinomas which morphologically resemble the duct cell. This does not mean that the tumour always arises from the duct cell which comprises less than 4% of the pancreas, see p. 981. It is likely that the majority arise from primitive stem cells which normally differentiate into both acinar and duct cells. A considerable desmoblastic response is often seen; in some areas there are only a few isolated clusters of tumour cells widely separated by bands of collagen. Carcinoma-in-situ in ducts adjacent to the cancer occurs in about 19% of cases, suggesting that some cases may be multicentric in origin. There is a slight preponderance of tumours arising in the head and neck of the pancreas compared to the body and tail (head and neck: e.g. body and tail, 1·8:1). In cases where the tumour is situated towards the head, pancreatitic changes may develop in the body of the pancreas proximal to the tumour.

About 1% of pancreatic cancers are cystadenocarcinomas. These are large cystic tumours which are more slow growing than other pancreatic cancers.

Epidemiological studies have suggested an association with tobacco smoking which is less strong and takes longer to develop than the association between smoking and bronchial carcinoma. A western diet, high in protein and fat may also promote pancreatic carcinoma. There is no evidence that the disease is more prevalent among alcoholics, but there may be a slightly increased incidence in patients with chronic pancreatitis.

Clinical features.—The most frequent symptoms are non-specific: weight loss, pain and anorexia. The prevalence of these and of jaundice vary with the position in the pancreas where the tumour is situated:

Symptom	Ampulla (%)	Head/neck (%)	Body/tail (%)
Weight loss	62	83	71
Pain	38	48	90
Jaundice	77	65	0
Painless jaundice	46	27	0
Anorexia	69	44	52
Thrombophlebitis	8	8	9·5

Jaundice is only present in two thirds of cases with tumours in the pancreatic head. Painless jaundice which is widely believed to be synonymous with ampullary carcinoma, in fact is only found in a minority of cases. Thus in many cases the diagnosis of pancreatic cancer is made from non-specific symptoms. The site of the pain depends on the situation of the tumour. In tumours of the head of the pancreas the pain is to the right of the epigastrium, whereas in tumours affecting the body the pain is to the left of the epigastrium. Back pain is due to involvement of retropancreatic nerves and to pancreatic duct obstruction and stasis within the pancreas.

On examination there is generalised wasting and the liver is palpable in about 50% of cases. This does not denote inoperability since it may be due to biliary obstruction and not to hepatic metastases. Although the gall bladder is frequently distended at laparotomy, it can be palpated on clinical examination in about 30% of tumours in the head of the pancreas and 50% of ampullary tumours. Courvoisier first drew attention to this association in 1890 when he suggested of the gall bladder that 'when the common duct is obstructed by a stone, dilatation is rare;

Ludwig Courvoisier, 1843–1918. Professor of Surgery, Basle, Switzerland.

when the duct is obstructed in some other way, dilatation is common!' This was because biliary calculi tended to create a non-distensible gall bladder as a result of cholecystitis[1]. If the growth is situated in the body of the pancreas, it may occasionally be palpable and may transmit the aortic pulsation. Splenic vein thrombosis may occur in about 10% of cases and this may result in splenomegaly.

Investigation.—There is no single test which is unequivocally abnormal in all patients. With the exception of ampullary cancers which can produce jaundice when they are small, the diagnosis is usually made late. A high index of suspicion is required in the investigation of patients complaining of weight loss or upper abdominal and back pain. The serum alkaline phosphatase may be elevated, even in the absence of jaundice. Obstruction of the main pancreatic duct leads to a reduction in the volume of pancreatic secretions after stimulation with secretin-pancreozymin. Reduction in flow can be identified in 95% of patients with tumours in the head of the pancreas and 59% of those with tumours in the body. Cytological examination of pancreatic juice may reveal tumour cells.

Enlargement of the pancreas due to a tumour in the head of the pancreas can be identified by hypotonic duodenogram in which the duodenal loop is widened and there may be duodenal mucosal irregularity due to tumour invasion (figs 993–996). Pancreatic ultrasound may show a mass (fig. 972), together with a dilated pancreatic duct or common bile duct if occluded. CT scan may show an enlarged pancreas and can also show whether regional para-aortic lymphatics are involved (figs 975, 976). Both CT and ultrasound may show whether hepatic metastases are present.

Probably the most sensitive investigation, which is able to demonstrate lesions as small as 1 cm in diameter is selective coeliac and superior mesenteric angiography. This can reveal irregular narrowing of vessels, distortion of their usual course, tumour circulation, and compression of the splenic, superior mesenteric or portal veins.

Duodenoscopy can reveal ampullary cancers which can be biopsied at the same time. A pancreatogram taken at E.R.C.P. may demonstrate a typical sharp duct occlusion, but by the time this has occurred the tumour size usually exceeds 2 cm in diameter. Pancreatic juice can be collected at E.R.C.P. for cytological examination (fig. 986).

Management.—At the time of presentation, the disease is beyond surgical resection in over 80% of cases. This is either because of local spread into the superior mesenteric vein, para-aortic or mesenteric lymphadenopathy, or hepatic metastases. In view of this, and the advanced age of presentation in a high proportion of cases, about 95% of all cases of pancreatic carcinoma are treated palliatively. Pain is controlled with strong analgesics, if necessary opiates. Pancreatic supplements may help to reduce weight loss. Jaundice produced by biliary obstruction is associated with unpleasant pruritus, and this can be corrected by biliary bypass. Biliary bypass is necessary in about 30% of all patients with pancreatic cancer. Probably the best method of bypass is the roux-en-Y choledochojejunostomy, but the simpler cholecystjejunostomy is more frequently performed (fig. 997). The disadvantage of the latter is that bile must drain through

[1] See footnote, p. 972.

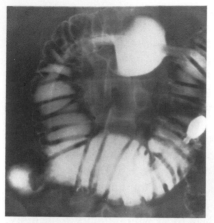

FIG. 993.—Normal hypotonic duodenogram.

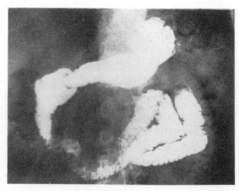

FIG. 994.—Barium meal showing widened duodenal loop and the reversed 3 sign.
(*Lord Smith, P.P.R.C.S., London*, Trans. med. Soc. Lond.)

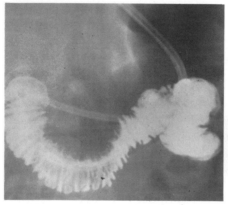

FIG. 995.—Carcinoma of head of pancreas. 'Rose thorning' of medial wall of duodenum.

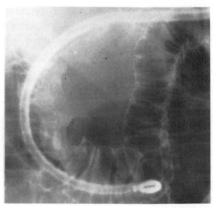

FIG. 996.—Carcinoma of ampulla. Filling defect in region of ampulla.

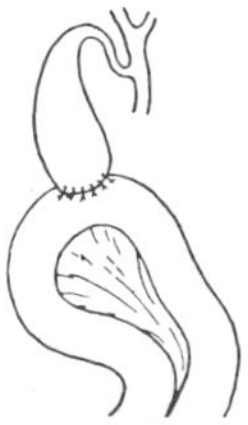

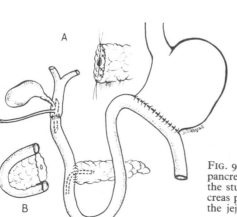

FIG. 997.—Cholecystjejunostomy. Some surgeons also perform an entero-enterostomy lower down so that intestinal contents are diverted from the biliary tree.

FIG. 998.—Reconstruction after pancreatoduodenectomy. Inset A, the stump of the body of the pancreas prepared for anatomosis with the jejunum. Inset B, the portion removed.
(*After H. A. Zintel.*)

the cystic duct which is narrow, and if inserted low into the bile duct is vulnerable to occlusion by tumour growth. About 20% of patients with tumours producing obstructive jaundice may also develop duodenal obstruction. Some surgeons routinely perform a prophylactic gastroenterostomy at the time of biliary bypass. This prolongs the operation, increases the morbidity, and if there is no obstruction at the time of operation may not remain patent. As the procedure carries disadvantages, and is not necessary in the majority of patients, it probably should not be carried out as a routine. Anastomosis of the dilated pancreatic duct side to side to the back of the stomach has also been advocated as a means of relieving the pain of pancreatic obstruction. However this has not been widely adopted. Transduodenal Truecut biopsy of the pancreas, at the time of laparotomy, may produce an abscess or a haematoma and, if negative, does not exclude the diagnosis because the malignant area may not have been sampled. As it may be hazardous, and does not contribute vital information to the patient's management Truecut biopsy should be avoided. Recently, endoscopic stenting through the occluded bile duct at E.R.C.P. has provided a non-surgical alternative to biliary bypass. This approach has two main disadvantages: (a) cholangitis is more likely because of the presence of a foreign body in the bile duct and a greater degree of biliary stasis, (b) the tumour is not accurately staged at laparotomy, and therefore a potentially resectable tumour may be treated by a biliary stent. Thus this technique should be reserved for elderly or frail patients in whom a laparotomy would be hazardous.

Surgical resection.—Tumours less then 3 cm in diameter are usually resectable whereas those greater than 8 cm are unresectable. Resectable tumours are most frequently situated near the ampulla and tumours in the body of the pancreas are almost always unresectable. Thus when resection is possible, the area resected is the head and neck of the pancreas together with the duodenum (Whipple's procedure). Overall, only about 5% of all cases of pancreatic cancer in the UK undergo resection. Attempts at percutaneous ultrasound guided needle biopsy of the tumour preoperatively should be avoided since it has been shown that this can disseminate malignant cells along the needle track. It may not be possible to make a tissue diagnosis prior to removal of a suspicious pancreatic mass, and the surgeon should be prepared to resect without a tissue diagnosis where there is sufficient clinical suspicion.

Pancreatoduodenectomy.—Pre-operative management.—Jaundiced patients undergoing major surgery are at risk of developing acute renal failure—the 'hepato-renal syndrome'. This is not fully understood, but it appears to have a septicaemic basis which may be provoked by reduced reticuloendothelial function and increased absorbtion of bacterial toxins from the gut. Jaundiced patients undergoing surgery should receive perioperative antibiotic cover, and Mannitol 10 g before and during surgery together with adequate fluid replacement to ensure a good diuresis. Clotting may be disordered because of Vitamin K malabsorbtion from the gut and Vitamin K supplement (10 mg, intramuscular for one or two days pre-op) should be given and continued until the jaundice has receded. Transcutaneous drainage of the hepatic ducts to reduce the jaundice prior to surgery does not reduce morbidity because of a high risk of infecting the obstructed biliary system.

A long right paramedian incision is made. Explore the abdomen and the area thoroughly. Involved lymph nodes, fixity of the tumour, and liver secondaries rule out radical surgery. Expose the duodenum by separating the right half of the transverse colon and the hepatic flexure from their peritoneal attachments and dissect out the common bile duct above the duodenum. Mobilise the duodenum by dividing the peritoneum along its right border so that it can be lifted off the inferior vena cava. Clear the superior mesenteric vessles and make sure that these and the portal vein are not involved in growth.

If the growth is operable the operation may proceed. Divide the common bile duct above the duodenum, mobilise the duodenum and pyloric antrum and ligate and divide the right gastric, right gastro-epiploic, and gastro-duodenal vessels. The duodenojejunal flexure is exposed and divided and the inferior pancreaticoduodenal vessels are ligated. The superior mesenteric vessels in the region of the uncinate process must be carefully exposed. The pancreatic venous radicles there are very short and tenuous, and may be torn easily. Reconstruction is now carried out as in fig. 998. Alternatively, the pancreas may be anastomosed end-to-end with the jejunum and the bile duct end-to-side.

The abdomen is now closed, but the areas of the biliary and pancreatic anastomoses must be drained. A fine pancreatic duct stent can be very useful in preventing a pancreatic fistula.

Regional Pancreatectomy.—Fortner has shown that involvement of the superior mesenteric vein adjacent to the uncinate process is not a contraindication to resection. The superior mesenteric vein segment can be excised and an end to end anastomosis to the portal vein performed. This operation, together with a wider lymphatic clearance is called regional pancreatectomy. It has increased the resectability rate, but improvement in survival has not been demonstrated. Occasionally, total pancreatectomy is performed where it seems that the growth may be multicentric. Because of the associated partial gastrectomy, duodenectomy and the loss of glucagon as well as insulin secreting cells this results in an unstable diabetes mellitus in which hypoglycaemia can readily occur. Long term survival is unusual.

Attempts at treatment by radioactive implantation with ^{125}I seeds, external beam irradiation and cytotoxic chemotherapy have not produced significant improvements in survival.

Prognosis.—Overall the median survival is about 9 months from the time of diagnosis with less than 5% of all patients surviving for 5 years. However patients with ampullary tumours undergoing resection have a 5-year survival of about 30%. Thus patients with ampullary tumours should always undergo resection if feasible. There is no evidence that surgical resection, which has an operative mortality of about 15% can achieve a cure for resectable tumours of the head or body of the pancreas. However, it is likely that, even if cure cannot be achieved by resection, survival is prolonged and the symptoms produced by the local expansion of the primary growth are avoided. Thus resection should be carried out, where technically feasible, in suitably fit patients

ENDOCRINE TUMOURS OF THE PANCREAS

The islets of Langerhans contain three types of cells: alpha, beta, and gamma, and of these the beta-cell is most common. Tumours of these endocrine cells comprise 1% of all pancreatic tumours.

Pathology.—The actual islet-cell lesion may be one of the following:

(1) Generalised hyperplasia; (2) discrete adenoma; (3) generalised adenomatosis; (4) carcinomas. Two-thirds of islet lesions occur in the body or tail of the pancreas. Approximately in one-third of cases they are multiple and in one-third they are malignant.

Such lesions may be associated with similar states in other endocrine glands, especially the anterior pituitary, the parathyroids, and the adrenal cortex (multiple endocrine adenomatosis).

The condition is usually familial. Such cells are now believed to comprise an APUD cell system (Amine Precursor Uptake and Decarboxylation). An apudoma is a tumour derived from these cells. It is neuroectodermal in type and secretes its normal peptide hormone, or variants, and sometimes others as well. Gastrinoma, Vipoma, Glucagonoma, Insulinoma, Nesidioblastoma, Somatostatinoma, and Pancreatic Polypepidoma are described. All have similar morphologic characteristics but can be distinguished by radioimmunoassay.

J. G. Fortner, Contemporary. Attending Surgeon, Memorial Sloan-Kettering Cancer Center, New York, U.S.A.
Paul Langerhans, 1847–1888. Professor of Pathological Anatomy, Freiburg, Germany.

Clinically, in overt cases, there may be: (1) Hyperinsulinism. (2) Features of other endocrine lesions, *e.g.* enlarged sella turcica, altered phosphorus and calcium blood levels, and increased keto-steroids in the urine. (3) Peptic ulceration. (4) Zollinger-Ellison syndrome (p. 1002).

Of these it is only possible here to discuss (1) and (4).

HYPERINSULINISM (BETA-CELL TUMOUR). INSULINOMA

Clinical features are not stereotyped, and unless the attending clinician is alive to the bizarre symptoms to which it gives rise, insulinoma of the pancreas, still somewhat of an enigma, will often continue to be displayed only at that final Court of Appeal—the post-mortem room, for so often the patient is diagnosed as psycho-neurotic, epileptic, a malingerer, or a sufferer from organic nervous disease.

The attacks, due to hypoglycaemia, come at irregular intervals and often with progressively increasing frequency and severity. Four stages are recognised, and in the beginning the attacks do not necessarily progress beyond the first or second stages.

Stage 1.—Often the symptoms simulate duodenal ulcer, awakening the patient in the early hours of the morning with vague abdominal discomfort, relieved by carbohydrates. At other times nervous symptoms predominate. There is a vague feeling of being unwell, a disinclination for exertion, and possibly some disorientation.

Stage 2.—Trembling, sweating, dizziness, blurring of vision, and great hunger.

Stage 3.—Sluggish mind, inarticulate speech, inco-ordinated movements, diplopia, sometimes hallucinations.

Stage 4.—Fits indistinguishable from epilepsy[1] passing into semi-consciousness or coma, with dilated pupils and extreme spasticity. In course of time intellectual deterioration is liable to follow.

Usually the patient is an adult under forty years of age, but a few cases have occurred in children. Because eating relieves the symptoms, over-weight not infrequently results. Pain is not a feature of benign insulinoma, but is present in most cases where a malignant change has occurred.

In a few instances the tumour contains sufficient calcium to show in a radiograph.

Diagnosis.—The three criteria (Whipple's triad), which, if present, suggest the diagnosis are:

1. An attack, as described above, occurs in the fasting state (*i.e.* in the morning) or with exercise.

2. During the height of the attack there is a hypoglycaemia below 45 mg per 100 ml (2·5 mmol/l) of blood.

3. The symptoms are relieved by glucose.

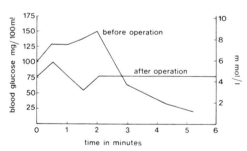

FIG. 999.—The hypoglycaemia caused by the islet-cell tumour is cured by operation.

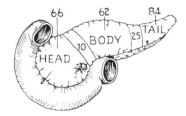

FIG. 1000.—Site of the insulin-secreting adenoma in 254 cases. Seven were situated in an ectopic pancreas. Twenty were overlooked at operation.
(*J. M. Howard et al., Philadelphia.*)

Confirmation depends on the identification of fasting hypoglycaemia (fig 999), associated with elevated human insulin levels as measured by radioimmunoassay. Further confirmation may be sought by more elaborate insulin stimulation and suppression tests.

Treatment.—The only curative treatment is extirpation of the tumour or tumours. An intravenous drip infusion of isotonic dextrose solution is started, laparotomy is performed

---

[1] The brain cannot store dextrose, which it requires in large amounts. Deprivation of this essential brings about a burst of nervous energy; the higher centres are affected first.

Allen Oldfather Whipple, 1881–1963. Valentine Mott Professor of Surgery, Columbia University College of Physicians and Surgeons, New York, U.S.A.

The Bacteroides.—Only recently has the frequency and importance of the presence of bacteroides in the causation of peritonitis been realised. These Gram-negative, non-sporing organisms though predominant in the lower intestine often escape detection because they are strictly anaerobic, and slow to grow on culture media unless there is an adequate carbon-dioxide tension in the anaerobic apparatus (Gillespie), In many laboratories, the culture is discarded if there is no growth in forty-eight hours. These organisms are resistant to penicillin and streptomycin but sensitive to metronidazole, clindamycin and lincomycin and the new cephalosporin compounds. Since the widespread use of metronidazole ('Flagyl') bacteroides infections have diminished greatly.

Bacteria NOT *from the Alimentary Canal.*—Examples are peritonitis due to the gonococcus, beta-haemolytic streptococcus, pneumococcus, and the *M. tuberculosis*. Since the advent of antibiotics haemolytic streptococcal peritonitis has lost many of its dreaded lethal properties. In young girls and women, pelvic infection via the Fallopian tubes is responsible for a high proportion of 'non-alimentary' infections (*e.g.* gonococcus and streptococcus) but bacteroides is also found normally in the female genital tract.

PATHS OF BACTERIAL INVASION

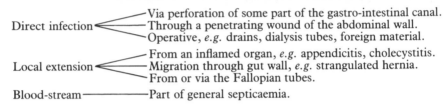

Direct infection —— Via perforation of some part of the gastro-intestinal canal.
Through a penetrating wound of the abdominal wall.
Operative, *e.g.* drains, dialysis tubes, foreign material.

Local extension —— From an inflamed organ, *e.g.* appendicitis, cholecystitis.
Migration through gut wall, *e.g.* strangulated hernia.
From or via the Fallopian tubes.

Blood-stream ————— Part of general septicaemia.

Even in non-bacterial peritonitis (*e.g.* intraperitoneal rupture of the bladder or a haemoperitoneum) the peritoneum soon becomes infected by transmigration of organisms from the bowel, and it is not long (often a matter of hours) before chemical peritonitis becomes a peritonitis in the cusual meaning of the term.

Natural Factors which favour Localisation of Peritonitis. These factors are anatomical, pathological and surgical.

Anatomical.—Excluding the subphrenic spaces, the greater sac of the peritoneum is divided into (*a*) the pelvis, and (*b*) the peritoneal cavity proper. The latter is re-divided into a supracolic and an infracolic compartment by the transverse colon and transverse mesocolon, which deter the spread of infection from one to the other. When the supracolic compartment overflows, as is often the case when a gastric ulcer perforates, it does so over the colon into the infracolic compartment, or, by way of the right paracolic gutter to the right iliac fossa, and thence to the pelvis. Posture can assist in directing collections into the pelvis, as in the 'Sherren' regime for perforated appendicitis.

Pathological.—The clinical course is largely governed by the manner in which adhesions form around the affected organ. Inflamed peritoneum loses its glistening appearance and becomes reddened and velvety. Flakes of fibrin appear and cause coils of intestine to become adherent to one another and to the parieties. There is an outpouring of serous fluid rich in leucocytes and antibodies that soon become turbid; if localisation occurs, the turbid fluid becomes frank pus. Peristalsis is retarded in affected coils, and this helps in preventing distribution of the infection to other coils. The greater omentum, by enveloping and becoming adherent to inflamed structures, often forms a substantial barrier to the spread of infection.

Surgical.—Drains are frequently used post-operatively to assist localisation (and exit) of intra-abdominal collections: their value is disputed.

William Alexander Gillespie, Contemporary. Formerly Professor of Clinical Bacteriology, University of Bristol.
Gabriele Fallopio (Fallopius), 1523–1563. Professor of Anatomy, Surgery and Botany, Padua, Italy.

Natural Factors which tend to cause Diffusion of Peritonitis

(*a*) A prime factor in the spread of peritonitis is whether it develops rapidly or slowly. If an inflamed appendix (fig. 1001) or other hollow viscus perforates before localisation has taken place, there is a gush of intestinal contents into the peritoneal cavity which spreads over a large area almost instantaneously.

(*b*) The ingestion of food, or even water, by stimulating peristaltic action, hinders localisation. Violent peristalsis occasioned by the administration of a purgative or an enema, causes a widespread distribution of an infection that would otherwise have remained localised.

(*c*) When the virulence of the infecting organism is so great as to render the localisation of the infection difficult or impossible.

(*d*) In children the omentum is small, and natural immunity underdeveloped.

(*e*) Injudicious and rough handling of localised collections, *e.g.* appendix mass or pericolic abscess.

(*f*) Deficient natural resistance ('immune deficiency'): this can result from drugs (*e.g.* steroids), disease (*e.g.* AIDS*) or old age.

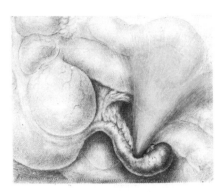

FIG. 1001.—Sudden perforation, especially if engendered by purgation, often results in an immediate widespread bacterial peritonitis.

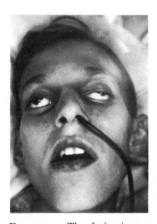

FIG. 1002.—The facies in terminal diffuse peritonitis.

CLINICAL FEATURES

Localised peritonitis is bound up intimately with the causative lesion, and the initial symptoms and signs are those of that lesion. When the peritoneum becomes inflamed the temperature, and especially the pulse-rate, rise. The pain increases and usually there is associated vomiting. The most important sign is guarding and rigidity of the abdominal wall over the area of the abdomen which is involved, with a positive 'release' sign. If inflammation arises under the diaphragm, shoulder tip ('phrenic') pain may be felt. In cases of pelvic peritonitis arising from an inflamed appendix in the pelvic position or from salpingitis, the abdominal signs are often slight, deep tenderness of one or both lower quadrants alone being present, but a rectal or vaginal examination reveals tenderness, often

*AIDS = acquired immune deficiency syndrome (Chapter 4).

exquisite, of the pelvic peritoneum. With appropriate treatment localised peritonitis usually resolves. In about 20% of cases an abscess follows. Infrequently, localised peritonitis becomes diffuse. Conversely, in favourable circumstances diffuse peritonitis can become localised, most frequently in the pelvis.

Diffuse (*syn.* **Generalised**) **Peritonitis.**—1. *Onset.*—Pain, which is severe and is made worse by moving or breathing. It is first experienced at the site of the original lesion, and spreads outwards from this point. Vomiting may occur. The patient usually lies still. Tenderness and rigidity on palpation are typically found when the peritonitis affects the anterior abdominal wall. Abdominal tenderness, and rigidity are diminished or absent if the anterior wall is unaffected, as in pelvic peritonitis or, rarely, peritonitis in the lesser sac. Patients with pelvic peritonitis may complain of urinary symptoms; they are tender on rectal or vaginal examination. Infrequent bowel sounds may still be heard for a few hours but they cease with the onset of paralytic ileus. The pulse rises progressively, but if the peritoneum is deluged with irritant fluid, there is a sudden rise. The temperature changes are variable.

2. *Intermediate.*—Peritonitis may resolve, so that the pulse slows, the pain and tenderness diminish, leaving a silent, soft, abdomen. (These are features that can easily mislead the observer.) The condition may localise, producing one or more abscesses, with overlying swelling and tenderness.

3. *Terminal.*—If resolution or localisation have not occurred, the abdomen remains silent, and increasingly distends. Circulatory failure ensues, with cold, clammy extremities, sunken eyes, dry tongue, thready (irregular) pulse, drawn and anxious face (Hippocratic facies—fig. 1002). The patient finally lapses into unconsciousness. With adequate treatment, this condition is rarely seen in hospitals.

Diagnostic aids.—Investigations will not save the need for careful confirmation of the history and physical signs, which are tenderness, guarding and rigidity with a distending silent abdomen. It is unwise to rely slavishly on any single symptom or sign; not one is incontrovertible.

A battery of investigations *may* elucidate a doubtful diagnosis. More often, they only confuse it. Peritonitis usually, but not always, produces leucocytosis. *Peritoneal diagnostic aspiration* may be helpful but is usually unnecessary. After infiltrating the skin of the abdomen with local anaesthetic, the peritoneum is entered in each quadrant with a sterile needle attached to a syringe, into which is sucked any free fluid. Bile-stained fluid indicates perforated peptic ulcer, the presence of pus indicates bacterial peritonitis; blood is aspirated in a high proportion of patients with intraperitoneal bleeding. When aspiration fails, the introduction of a small quantity of sterile physiological saline, followed after a few minutes by peritoneal aspiration may produce fluid of diagnostic value.

An x-ray film of the abdomen (fig. 1003) may reveal free air, or confirm the presence of dilated gas-filled loops of bowel with multiple fluid levels. If the patient is too ill for an 'erect' film to demonstrate free air collecting under the diaphragm, a lateral decubitus film is just as useful.

Serum amylase estimation may uphold the diagnosis of pancreatitis, provided it is remembered that raised values are frequently found following other abdominal catastrophes, and operations, e.g. perforated duodenal ulcer.

Treatment

The essential principles in the treatment of peritonitis are: (1) Correction of circulating volume and any electrolyte imbalance. (2) Decompression. (3) Antibiotics. (4) Appropriate surgical treatment.

Hippocrates, by common consent the Father of Medicine, was born on the Greek Island of Cos, off Turkey, about 460 B.C. and died in 375 B.C.

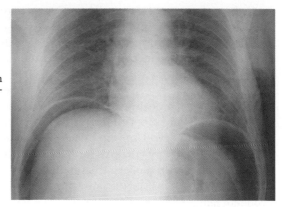

FIG. 1003.—Gas under the diaphragm in a case of free perforation with peritonitis.
(*Dr. C. P. Reynolds, London Hospital.*)

1. *Intravenous Fluids.*—These patients are frequently hypovolaemic with electrolyte disturbances. The plasma volume must be restored and the plasma electrolyte concentrations corrected. Plasma protein depletion may need correction—inflamed peritoneum leaks protein calamitously and continuously. If the patient's recovery is delayed for more than 7 to 10 days, intravenous feeding ('hyperalimentation') is required.

2. *A nasograstric tube* is passed into the stomach, which is aspirated. Intermittent aspiration is maintained until the paralytic ileus resulting from peritonitis has recovered. After operation, measured volumes of water are allowed by mouth, when only small amounts are being aspirated. If the abdomen is soft and not tender, and bowel sounds return, oral feeding may be progressively introduced. It is important not to prolong the ileus by missing this stage.

3. *Antibiotics.*—Administration of antibiotics prevents the multiplication of bacteria, and the release of endotoxins. As the infection is usually a mixed one, initially parenteral ampicillin, gentamicin and metronidazole may be given.

4. *Surgical correction of the underlying cause* must not be delayed in appropriate cases, once the patient is fit for operation. At the same time the results of peritonitis are corrected—necrotic material and pus are removed from the peritoneal cavity (see Peritoneal Toilet, below).

Ancillary Care

5. *A fluid balance chart* must be started at once so that daily output by gastric aspiration and urine are known, losses from the lungs, skin, and in faeces are estimated, so that the intake requirements can be calculated and seen to have been administered.

Throughout recovery, the haematocrit values, blood electrolytes, and urea must be checked.

6. *Intravenous fluids* are continued after operation until the patient can be fully maintained by oral feeding. If recovery is delayed, high caloric, vitamin-rich supplements must be added to the balanced electrolyte solutions.

7. The patient, nursed in the sitting-up position, must be relieved of pain before and after operation. Once the diagnosis has been made morphine may be given, and small doses continued for 48 hours. Freedom from pain allows early mobilisation and adequate physiotherapy in the post-operative period, to prevent basal collapse, deep-vein thrombosis and pulmonary embolism.

Treatment of the Cause.—If the condition is amenable to surgery, such as in perforated appendicitis, gangrenous cholecystitis, diverticulitis, peptic ulcer or rarely in perforation of the small bowel, operation must be carried out as soon as the patient is fit for anaesthesia. This is usually within a few hours. In peritonitis due to pancreatitis, salpingitis, or in cases of primary peritonitis of streptococcal or pneumococcal origin, conservative treatment is the procedure of choice (if the diagnosis can be made with certainty).

Peritoneal Toilet.—In surgery for general peritonitis it is essential that after the cause has been dealt with, the whole peritoneal cavity should be explored with the sucker and mopped dry, if necessary until all sero-purulent exudate is removed. The use of a large volume of antibiotic saturated saline (1–2 litres) has been shown to be very effective for 'cleaning' the peritoneum (Matheson).

Prognosis.—With modern treatment diffuse peritonitis carries a mortality of about 10%. The lethal factors are (*a*) bacterial toxaemia, (*b*) paralytic ileus, (*c*) bronchopneumonia, (*d*) electrolyte-imbalance, (*e*) renal failure, (*f*) undrained collections, (*g*) bone-marrow suppression, (*h*) 'multi-system breakdown'.

COMPLICATIONS OF PERITONITIS

All the complications of a severe bacterial infection are possible, but the special complications of peritonitis are as follows:

(1) *Acute intestinal obstruction due to peritoneal adhesions*. This usually gives central colicky abdominal pain with evidence of gas and fluid levels confined to the upper portion of the small intestine on x-ray. It is more common with localised peritonitis. It is essential to distinguish this from:

(2) *Paralytic ileus* where there is usually little pain and gas-filled loops with fluid levels are seen distributed throughout the small and large intestines on the x-ray film. In intestinal obstruction, bowel sounds are increased. In paralytic ileus bowel sounds are reduced or absent.

(3) *Residual abscesses.*—Abscess formation following local or diffuse peritonitis usually occupies one of the situations shown in fig. 1004. When palpable, an intraperitoneal abscess should be monitored by marking out its limitations on the abdominal wall, and meticulous daily examination. In the majority of cases, with the aid of antibiotic treatment, the mass becomes smaller and smaller, and finally is impalpable. In others, the abscess fails to resolve, or becomes larger, in which event it must be opened. In many situations, by waiting a few days the abscess becomes adherent to the abdominal wall, so that it can be drained without opening the general peritoneal cavity.

In the case of a laterally-placed abscess, the incision is made on the lateral side of the swelling. The layers of the abdominal wall are divided until the peritoneum is reached. With the finger, the extra peritoneal tissues are separated from the peritoneum until the abscess is opened. A drainage tube is inserted; if the path is tortuous, a Penrose drain (a thin tube of latex rubber containing a wick of gauze) is valuable.

PELVIC ABSCESS

The pelvis is the commonest site of an intraperitoneal abscess, because the vermiform appendix is often pelvic in position and also the Fallopian tubes are frequent foci of infection. A pelvic abscess can also occur as a sequel to any case of diffuse peritonitis. Pus can accumulate in this area without serious constitutional disturbance, and unless the patient is examined carefully from day to day, such abscesses may attain considerable proportions before being recognised. The most characteristic symptoms of a pelvic abscess are diarrhoea and the passage of mucus in the stools. It is no exaggeration to say that the

N. A. Matheson, Contemporary. Surgeon, Aberdeen Royal Infirmary.
Charles Bingham Penrose, 1862–1925. Professor of Gynaecology, University of Pennsylvania, Philadelphia, U.S.A.

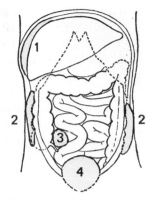

FIG. 1004.—Common situations for residual abscesses. 1. Subphrenic. 2. Paracolic. 3. Appendix. 4. Pelvic.

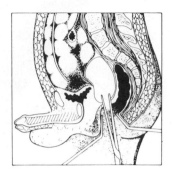

FIG. 1005.—Opening a pelvic abscess into the rectum.

passage of mucus, occurring for the first time in a patient who has, or is recovering from, peritonitis, is pathognomonic of pelvic abscess. Rectal examination reveals a bulging of the anterior rectal wall which, when the abscess is ripe, becomes softly cystic. Left to Nature, a proportion of these abscesses burst into the rectum, after which the patient nearly always recovers rapidly. If this possible happy termination does not readily occur, the abscess should be drained deliberately. In women vaginal drainage through the posterior fornix is often chosen. In other cases, where the abscess is definitely pointing into the rectum, rectal drainage (fig. 1005) is employed. If any uncertainty exists as to the presence of pus, an aspirating needle introduced through the rectal wall into the bulging swelling will settle the question. Occasionally, in the case of a large abscess which can be palpated above the pubes, after the bladder has been emptied by catheterisation, lower laparotomy should be undertaken in order to be quite certain of the diagnosis. Provided the abscess is shut off from the general peritoneal cavity, a point which can be ascertained undeniably when the abdomen has been opened, rectal drainage of a pelvic abscess is far preferable to suprapubic drainage, which breaks down Nature's barriers and exposes the general peritoneal cavity to the dangers of spreading infection. Occasionally, drainage tubes can be inserted blindly from the surface under radiological (ultrasonic) guidance.

SUBPHRENIC ABSCESS

Anatomy.—The complicated arrangement of the peritoneum results in the formation of four intraperitoneal and three extraperitoneal spaces in which pus may collect. Three of these spaces are on either side of the body, and one approximately in the mid line (fig. 1006).

Left Anterior intraperitoneal, bounded above by the diaphragm, behind by the left triangular ligament and left lobe of the liver, the gastro-hepatic omentum and anterior surface of the stomach. To the right is the falciform ligament, and to the left the spleen, gastrosplenic omentum, and diaphragm. The common cause of an abscess here is following operations on the stomach, the tail of the pancreas, the spleen or the splenic flexure of the colon or in diverticulitis.

Left Posterior intraperitoneal is another name for the 'lesser' sac. The commonest type of suppuration here is the pancreatic pseudo-cyst. In practice perforated gastric ulcer rarely causes a collection here, because the potential space is obliterated by adhesions.

Right Anterior intraperitoneal, which lies between the right lobe of the liver and the diaphragm. It is limited posteriorly by the anterior layer of the coronary and the right triangular ligaments, and to the left by the falciform ligament. Common causes here are perforating cholecystitis, a perforated duodenal ulcer, a duodenal cap 'blow out' and appendicitis.

Right Posterior intraperitoneal (*syn.* Rutherford Morison's kidney pouch) lies transversely beneath the right lobe of the liver. It is bounded on the right by the right lobe of the liver and the diaphragm. To the left is situated the foramen of Winslow, and below

James Rutherford Morison, 1853–1939. Professor of Surgery, Durham, England.
Jacob Benignus Winslow, 1669–1760. Professor of Anatomy, Physic and Surgery, Paris.

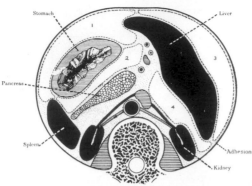

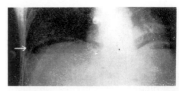

FIG. 1007.—Radiograph in erect position showing subphrenic abscess containing gas.

FIG. 1006.—Transverse section through the lesser sac. Intra-peritoneal subphrenic abscesses may occupy. 1. left anterior space. 2. left posterior space (lesser sac). 3. right anterior space which becomes shut off by adhesions from 4, right posterior space.

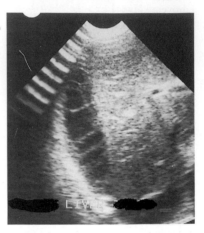

FIG. 1008.—Subphrenic abscess. Ultrasonogram shows loculated dark area under diaphragm (left) in a girl aged 18 yrs who had perforated her appendix 3 weeks earlier.
(Dr. C. P. Reynolds, London Hospital.)

this lies the duodenum. In front are the liver and gallbladder, and behind, the upper part of the right kidney and diaphragm. The space is bounded above by the liver, and below by the transverse colon and hepatic flexure. It is the deepest space of the four and the commonest site of a subphrenic abscess which usually arises from appendicitis, cholecystitis, a perforated duodenal ulcer or following upper abdominal surgery.

Extraperitoneal.—There are three of these:

Right and Left extraperitoneal which are terms given to perinephric abscesses (Chapter 57).

Midline extraperitoneal which is another name for the 'bare' area of the liver which may develop an abscess in amoebic hepatitis (the commonest cause) or it may be a pyogenic liver abscess (Chapter 45).

Clinical Features.—The symptoms and signs of subphrenic infection are frequently unspecific, and it is well to remember the aphorism, 'Pus somewhere, pus nowhere else, pus under diaphragm'.

Symptoms.—A common history is that when some infective focus in the abdominal cavity has been dealt with, the condition of the patient improves temporarily, but after an interval of a few days or weeks, symptoms of toxaemia reappear. The condition of the patient steadily, and often rapidly, deteriorates. Sweating, wasting, and anorexia are present. There is sometimes epigastric fullness and pain, or pain in the shoulder on the affected side, owing to irritation of sensory fibres in the phrenic nerve, referred along the descending branches of the cervical plexus. Persistent hiccup may be a presenting symptom.

Signs.—A swinging pyrexia is usually present, unless antibiotics or drugs (steroids) have interfered. If the abscess is anterior, abdominal examination will reveal some tenderness, rigidity, or even a palpable swelling. Sometimes the liver is displaced downwards, but more often it is fixed by adhesions. Examination of the chest is important, and in the majority of cases collapse of the lung or evidence of basal effusion or empyema is to be found.

Accessory Investigations.—(i) *Blood Count.*—A relative and absolute leucocytosis is usual.

(ii) *X-ray.*—A plain radiograph sometimes demonstrates the presence of gas (fig. 1007) or a pleural effusion. On screening, the diaphragm is often seen to be elevated (so-called 'tented' diaphragm) and its movements impaired.

(iii) Ultrasound and scanning have proved contributory (fig. 1008).

Differential Diagnosis.—Pylephlebitis, tropical abscess, pulmonary collapse, and empyema give rise to most of the diagnostic difficulties.

Treatment.—The clinical course of suspected cases is watched, and blood and radiological examinations are made at suitable intervals. If suppuration seems probable, surgical intervention is indicated, but if skilled help is available it is sometimes possible to insert a fine percutaneous drainage tube 'blindly' under combined ultrasonic and fluoroscopic control. The same tube can be used to instil antibiotic solutions into the abscess cavity. To pass an aspirating needle at the bedside through the pleura and diaphragm invites catastrophic spread of the infection into the pleural cavity.

If a swelling can be detected in the subcostal region or in the loin, an incision is made over the site of maximum tenderness, or over any area where oedema or redness is discovered. The parietes usually form part of the abscess wall, so that contamination of the general peritoneal cavity is unlikely.

If no swelling is apparent, the subphrenic spaces should be explored either by an anterior sub-costal approach or from behind after removal of the *outer part* of the twelfth rib according to the position of abscess if indicated on a lateral x-ray film (see above). With the posterior approach the pleura must *not* be opened, and after the fibres of the diaphragm have been separated a finger is inserted beneath the diaphragm so as to explore the adjacent area.

Thus both approaches must be extra-serous to avoid dissemination of pus into the peritoneal or pleural cavities.

When the cavity is reached, all the fibrinous loculi must be broken down with the finger and one or two drains or drainage tubes must be fully inserted. These drains are withdrawn gradually during the next ten days and the closure of the cavity checked by x-ray sinograms.

The appropriate antibiotics are given in support.

Post-operative Peritonitis.—The patient is ill, with raised pulse and peripheral circulatory failure. Following post-operative leakage from a suture line, the general condition of a patient is far more grave than if the patient had suffered leakage from a perforated peptic ulcer with no preceding operation. Local symptoms and signs are less definite.[1] Abdominal pain may not be prominent, tenderness may be masked by the presence of a recent wound. The patient's deterioration may be wrongly attributed to pulmonary collapse which is usually concomitant.

Peritonitis follows abdominal operations more frequently than is realised. The principles of treatment do not differ from those of peritonitis of other origin. Antibiotic therapy alone is inadequate; no antibiotic can stay the onslaught of

---

[1]Particularly if steroids are being given.

bacterial peritonitis due to leakage from a suture line, which must be dealt with appropriately.

Peritonitis in Patients under Treatment with Steroids.—Pain is frequently slight or absent. Physical signs are similarly vague and misleading.

Peritonitis in Children.—The diagnosis is in some ways more difficult, in other ways more easy, than in adults. If a history can be taken it is plain and unembroidered. Any physical signs elicited by a gentle, patient, and sympathetic examiner are meaningful.

Peritonitis in Senile Patients.—These can be as fractious as children and unable to give a reliable history. Abdominal tenderness is usually well localised, but guarding and rigidity are less marked because the abdominal muscles are thin and weak.

Bile Peritonitis.—Unless there is reason to suspect that a bile duct was damaged at an operation in which drainage was not provided, it is improbable that bile as a cause of peritonitis will be thought of until the abdomen has been opened and bile is seen therein. The common causes of bile peritonitis are: (1) following biliary surgery—damage to the common bile duct, slipping of a ligature on the cystic duct, leakage from a divided accessory bile duct in the gallbladder bed or dislodgement of a T-tube drain in the early post-operative phase; (2) following perforation or gangrene of the gallbladder or leakage from a choledochus cyst; and (3) following gastro-duodenal surgery, e.g. duodenal cap 'blow out' or leakage from a suture line.

Unless the bile has extravasated slowly, and the collection becomes shut off from the general peritoneal cavity there are signs of diffuse peritonitis with a degree of shock. After a few hours a tinge of jaundice is not unusual. Local drainage, and when necessary suprapubic peritoneal drainage, is imperative, and if performed early enough, these measures will often save the patient' slife. When bile is seen issuing from a perforation of some part of the biliary tree, a drainage tube should be passed through the opening and secured there. Infected bile is more lethal than sterile bile. The gallbladder, if present, should be drained. A ruptured duodenum must be drained; it is too oedematous to repair.

Meconium Peritonitis. Meconium is a sterile mixture of epithelial cells, mucin, salts, fats, and bile, and is formed when the fetus commences to swallow amniotic fluid. By the third month of intra-uterine life the upper third of the small intestine has become filled with meconium; by the fourth month the accumulation has reached the ileo-caecal valve; during the remainder of intra-uterine life the colon becomes increasingly filled.

Meconium peritonitis is an aseptic peritonitis which develops late in intra-uterine life or during, or just after, delivery. Meconium enters the peritoneal cavity through an intestinal perforation, and in over 50% of cases the perforation is the result of some form of neonatal intestinal obstruction; in the remainder no cause for the perforation is discernible. When meconium, which is sterile, enters the peritoneal cavity an exudate is secreted that organises rapidly; matting of intestinal loops occurs, and in many cases in a matter of weeks the extruded meconium becomes calcified.

Meconium remains sterile until about three hours after birth; thereafter, unless the perforation has become sealed, sterile meconium peritonitis gives place to acute bacterial peritonitis which, unless treated promptly, is rapidly fatal.

Clinical Features.—Meconium peritonitis should always be considered when a baby is born with a tense abdomen. There is vomiting, and failure to discharge meconium. The differential diagnosis between neonatal intestinal obstruction and peritonitis is, in many cases, virtually impossible; indeed, in half the cases both are present. Free fluid in the peritoneal cavity is often sufficient to give a fluid thrill. In many cases there are exocrine secretary deficiencies elsewhere, *e.g.* lungs, pancreas, salivary glands (*Syn.* 'muco-viscidosis'). Bronchial obstruction by mucus plugs can be an immediate cause of fatal pneumonia.

Radiography (fig. 1009).—Free air in the peritoneal cavity, an abundant quantity of abdominal fluid, fluid levels, calcification (often most distinct on the surface of the liver or the spleen, and most readily seen in a lateral view) are characteristic findings, all of which are unlikely to be present in every case. Meconium peritonitis has been diagnosed by radiography of the foetus *in utero* two days before birth.

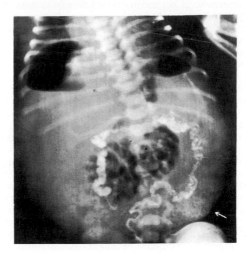

FIG. 1009.—Meconium peritonitis. Note: Free air and fluid in the peritoneal cavity; intra-abdominal calcification [↖] and on the spleen; air in the small intestine; micro-colon shown by a barium enema.

(*Dr. Jack Lester, Copenhagen.*)

Treatment.—The prognosis is bad, but recovery has followed prompt operation in some cases. The greatest chance of survival is in those patients who have an intestinal perforation but no intestinal obstruction, in which case closing the perforation and draining the peritoneal cavity is all-sufficient, and can be performed expeditiously. Intestinal lavage can prevent reformation of meconium bolus' obstruction and supplements of pancreatic exocrine enzymes may be necessary until adult life. If there is an associated pulmonary problem, the condition requires special treatment (*e.g.* O_2, bronchial lavage, nebulisers and long-term use of antibiotics).

Pneumococcal Peritonitis.—There are two forms of this disease:
1. Primary.
2. Secondary to pneumonia.

Primary pneumococcal peritonitis is much the more common. The patient is often an under-nourished girl between three and six years of age, and it is probable that the infection sometimes occurs via the vagina and Fallopian tubes, for pneumococci have been cultured from patients' vaginas. At other times, and always in males, doubtless the infection is blood-borne from the upper respiratory tract or the middle ear. After the age of ten years pneumococcal peritonitis is most unusual. Children with nephritis are more liable to this condition than others. During the past thirty years the incidence of pneumococcal peritonitis has declined greatly and the condition is now rare, Perhaps this is on account of the greater cleanliness and higher standard of living of what were the poorer classes, as well as early use of antibiotics to treat infections.

Clinical Features.—The onset is sudden, and the earliest symptom is pain localised to the lower half of the abdomen. The temperature is raised to 39.8°C or more, and there is usually frequent vomiting. After twenty-four to forty-eight hours profuse diarrhoea, occasionally blood-stained, is characteristic. There is usually increased frequency of micturition. The last two symptoms are due to severe pelvic peritonitis. Herpes on the lip or nostril is often present. In acute forms of the disease, even in cases where there is no involvement of a lung, there is a tinge of cyanosis of the lips and cheeks, and movement of the alae nasi is often discernible. On examination rigidity is usually bilateral, but is less than in most cases of acute appendicitis with peritonitis.

Differential Diagnosis.—A leucocytosis of 30,000/mm³ ($30 \times 10^9/1$) or more with approximately 90% polymorphs speaks more for pneumococcal peritonitis than appendicitis. Even so, it is often impossible, especially in males, to exclude perforated appendicitis. The other condition which is extremely difficult to differentiate from primary peritonitis in its early stage is pneumonia. An unduly high respiratory rate and the absence of abdominal rigidity are the most important signs supporting the diagnosis of pneumonia, which is usually clarified by a radiograph of the thorax.

Treatment.—*Early operation* is always required. After correcting dehydration and electrolyte imbalance, a short paramedian incision is made over the right rectus abdominis. The peritoneum is incised. Should the exudate be odourless and sticky, the diagnosis of pneumococcal peritonitis is practically certain, but it is desirable to perform a routine laparotomy to exclude other lesions. Assuming that no other cause for the peritonitis is discovered, some of the exudate is removed with a syringe, and sent to the laboratory for culture and sensitivity tests. Thorough peritoneal toilet is carried out and the incision closed. The patient is returned to bed and antibiotic and fluid replacement therapy continued. Gastrointestinal suction drainage is essential.

Primary streptococcal peritonitis of infants and children is rather more frequent than the foregoing but still uncommon. When a streptococcus is the infecting organism, the peritoneal exudate is thin, slightly cloudy, and contains flecks of fibrin. From the standpoints of clinical aspects and treatment, streptococcal peritonitis in infants and children does not differ from those detailed in the account of pneumococcal peritonitis (*vide supra*), but the mortality is higher. An intravaginal foreign body should always be looked for in female patients, *e.g.* a toy.

Idiopathic streptococcal and staphylococcal peritonitis in adults is fortunately rare, for prior to the antibiotic era it was nearly always fatal, and the mortality is still very high. Rightly, in early cases the abdomen is opened, usually on a diagnosis of acute appendicitis. In streptococcal peritonitis the peritoneal exudate is odourless, thin, contains small flecks of fibrin, and may be blood-stained. In these circumstances pus is removed by suction, the abdomen closed with suprapubic drainage, and the measures detailed in the conservative treatment of peritonitis carried out. Recently the use of intravaginal tampons has led to an increased incidence of *Staph. aureus* infections: these can be associated with 'toxic shock syndrome'.

Peritonitis following Abortion/Parturition.—The abortionist has usually pushed an instrument through the uterine vault and streptococcal peritonitis follows. When peritonitis follows puerperal infection, it is a notifiable disease. It is more common after first deliveries. Rigidity is seldom much in evidence; this, at any rate in part, is due to the stretched condition of the abdominal musculature. The lochia may be offensive but not necessarily so. Diarrhoea is common.

Treatment.—Provided the infection is limited strictly to the pelvis, the correct treatment is rest for the alimentary canal, intravenous fluids, the required antibiotic, and attention to electrolyte balance. Posterior colpotomy may be necessary if a pelvic abscess forms. If the peritonitis is generalised, the patient is usually extremely ill and drainage is advisable. This is best carried out by making a small suprapubic incision under local anaesthesia and inserting a drain. This can be done with the patient in bed, if necessary.

In the pre-antibiotic era the mortality of general peritonitis following parturition or abortion was at least 50%; with antibiotic therapy and timely operation, the mortality has fallen to less than 10% (Brews).

Periodic peritonitis is characterised by abdominal pain and tenderness, mild pyrexia, polymorphonuclear leucocytosis, and occasionally pain in the thorax and joints. The duration of an attack is twenty-four to seventy-two hours, when it is followed by complete remission, but exacerbations recur at regular intervals. Most of the patients have undergone appendicectomy in childhood. The disease, often familial, is limited principally to Arabs, Armenians, and Jews; other peoples occasionally are affected. At laparotomy, which may be necessary to exclude other causes, the peritoneum—particularly in the vicinity of the spleen and the gallbladder—is inflamed. There is no evidence that the interior of these organs is abnormal.

Differential Diagnosis.—Patients with abdominal epilepsy do not have positive physical signs of pyrexia, and their attacks are usually controlled by anti-convulsive medication.

The aetiology of periodic peritonitis is unknown, and no form of treatment has been found to be of the slightest avail.

Usually children are affected, but it is not rare for the disease to make its first appearance in early adult life, when females outnumber males by two to one. Exceptionally the disease becomes manifest in patients over forty years of age.

Richard Alan Brews, 1902–1965. Obstetric and Gynaecological Surgeon, The London Hospital.

TUBERCULOUS PERITONITIS

Acute Tuberculous Peritonitis.—Tuberculous peritonitis sometimes has an onset that resembles so closely acute peritonitis that the abdomen is opened. Straw-coloured fluid escapes, and tubercles[1] are seen scattered over the peritoneum and greater omentum. Tubercles occasionally simulate fat necroses or the nodules of peritoneal carcinomatosis. On opening the abdomen and finding tuberculous peritonitis, the fluid is evacuated, some being retained for bacteriological study. A portion of the diseased omentum is removed for histological confirmation of the diagnosis, and the wound closed without drainage.

At other times, although acute abdominal symptoms arise, the presence of ascites makes the diagnosis of acute tuberculous peritonitis reasonably evident.

Chronic Tuberculous Peritonitis.—Although the incidence of turberculous peritonitis has declined in Britain, in many parts of the world where measures for eradicating tuberculosis (especially the disease in cows) are enforced less strictly, the condition still occurs.

Presentation.—Abdominal pain is present in 90%, fever in 60%, loss of weight 60%, ascites 60%, night sweats 37%, abdominal mass 26%.

Origin of the infection:

1. From tuberculous mesenteric lymph nodes.
2. From tuberculosis of the ileo-caecal region.
3. From a tuberculous pyosalpinx.
4. Blood-borne infection from pulmonary tuberculosis, usually the 'miliary' but occasionally the 'cavitating' form.

There are four varieties of tuberculous peritonitis:

1. **Ascitic Form.**—The peritoneum is studded with tubercles, and the peritoneal cavity becomes filled with pale, straw-coloured fluid. The onset is insidious. There is loss of energy, facial pallor, and some loss of weight. The patient is usually brought for advice because of enlargement of the abdomen. Pain is often completely absent; in other cases there is considerable abdominal discomfort which may be associated with constipation or diarrhoea. On inspection dilated veins can be seen coursing beneath the skin of the abdominal wall. Shifting dullness can be elicited readily. In the male child congenital hydroceles sometimes appear, due to the patent processi vaginales becoming filled with ascitic fluid from the peritoneal cavity. Because of the increased intra-abdominal pressure, an umbilical hernia commonly occurs. On abdominal palpation a transverse solid mass can often be detected. This is rolled-up greater omentum infiltrated with tubercles.

The diagnosis is seldom difficult, except when it occurs in an acute form or when it first appears in an adult, in which case it has to be differentiated from other forms of ascites, especially from malignant secondary deposits. A positive Mantoux test in a child with ascites strongly suggests, and a negative test is good evidence against, tuberculosis. In adults this test is of negligible value. The diagnosis of tuberculous peritonitis having been made, it is always important to look for tuberculous disease elsewhere, and in this respect the possibility of tuberculous salpingitis in females should be remembered. A chest x-ray should always be taken before a laparotomy is performed.

The fluid is pale yellow, usually clear, and rich in lymphocytes. The specific gravity is comparatively high, often 1·020 or over. Even after centrifugation, rarely can the *Mycobact. tuberculosis* be found, but its presence can be demonstrated by culture or by guinea-pig inoculation.

Treatment.—See guidelines, Chapter 4. If the general condition is good, the patient can return home and, if an adult, to light work, before the course of chemotherapy has been completed.

2. **Encysted** (*Syn.* **Loculated**) **form** is similar to the above, but one part of the abdominal cavity alone is involved. Thus is producted a localised intra-abdominal swelling which gives rise to difficulty in diagnosis. In a female above the age of puberty, when the swelling is in the pelvis, an ovarian cyst will probably be diagnosed. In the case of a child it is sometimes difficult to distinguish the swelling from a mesenteric cyst. For these reasons laparotomy is often performed, and if an encapsulated collection of fluid is found, it is evacuated and the abdomen is closed. The general treatment already detailed is required, but the response to this treatment is more rapid. Late intestinal obstruction is a possible complication.

---

[1]Early tubercles are greyish and translucent. They soon undergo caseation, and appear white or yellow, and are then less difficult to distinguish from carcinoma.

Charles Mantoux, 1877–1947. Physician, Le Cannet, Alpes Maritimes, France.

3. **Fibrous** (*syn.* **plastic**) **form** is characterised by the production of widespread adhesions, which cause coils of intestine, especially the ileum, to become matted together and distended. These distended coils act as a 'blind loop' and give rise to steatorrhoea, wasting and attacks of abdominal pain. On examination the adherent intestine with omentum attached, together with the thickened mesentery, may give rise to a palpable swelling or swellings. The first intimation of the disease may be subacute or acute intestinal obstruction. Sometimes the cause of the obstruction can be remedied easily by the division of bands. Lateral anastomosis between an obviously dilated loop and a collapsed loop of small intestine should not be done or the 'blind loop' syndrome is a certain outcome. If the adhesions are accompanied by fibrous strictures of the ileum as well, it is best to excise the affected bowel, provided not too much of the small intestine needs to be sacrificed. If adhesions only are present a plication may be performed (Chapter 51). This is a dangerous condition and the surgeon must adhere to strict physiological principles in its treatment. Fortunately, chemotherapy after adequate surgery will rapidly bring it under control.

4. **Purulent form** is rare. When it occurs, usually it is secondary to tuberculous salpingitis. Amidst a mass of adherent intestine and omentum, tuberculous pus is present. Sizeable cold abscesses are wont to form, and point on the surface, commonly near the umbilicus, or burst into the bowel. In addition to prolonged general treatment, operative treatment may be necessary for the evacuation of cold abscesses and possibly for intestinal obstruction. If the patient survives long enough to overcome the infection, it may be possible to close a faecal fistula, which otherwise usually persists because of obstruction distal to it. Closure must therefore be combined with some form of anastomosis between the segment of intestine above the fistula and an unobstructed area below. The prognosis of this variety of turberculous peritonitis is relatively poor.

SCLEROSING PERITONITIS

Practolol, a β-adrenergic blocking agent used in the treatment of cardiovascular disorders, has been found to be associated with the late development of a sclerosing condition in the peritoneum which may cause intestinal obstruction. At laparotomy the condition resembles plastic tuberculous peritonitis. It may be confused with mesothelioma or carcinoid syndrome. Lysis of the adhesions is indicated. The condition may cause recurrent obstruction.

PERITONEAL BANDS AND ADHESIONS

Congenital bands and membranes occur in the peritoneum as described in textbooks of anatomy. None of them causes intestinal obstruction except an obliterated vitello-intestinal duct.

Peritoneal adhesions are discussed in Chapter 51.

Talc Granuloma.—Talc (silicate of magnesium) should never be used as a lubricant for rubber gloves for it is a cause of peritoneal adhesions and granulomas in the Fallopian tubes. Potassium bitartrate, which is completely soluble, is free from these serious objections. *Starch peritonitis* (see below).

ASCITES

Ascites, an excess of serous fluid within the peritoneal cavity, can be recognised clinically only when the amount of fluid present exceeds 1500 ml; in the obese a greater quantity than this is necessary before there is clear evidence of the presence of intraperitoneal fluid.

Mechanism of Ascites.—The balanced effects of plasma and peritoneal colloid osmotic pressures and hydrostatic pressures determine the exchange of fluid between the capillaries and the peritoneal fluid. Normal intraperitoneal pressure and normal peritoneal fluid colloid osmotic pressure cannot be measured. Protein-rich fluid enters the peritoneal cavity when capillary permeability to protein is increased, as in peritonitis and carcinomatosis peritonei. Capillary pressure may be increased because of generalised water retention, cardiac failure, constrictive pericarditis, or vena caval obstruction. Capillary pressure is raised selectively in the portal venous system in the Budd-Chiari syndrome (Chapter 45), portal cirrhosis, or extrahepatic venous obstruction.

Plasma colloid osmotic pressure may be lowered in patients with reduced intake, diminished absorption, abnormal losses, or defective protein synthesis as occurs in cirrhosis.

Clinical Features.—The abdomen is distended evenly, with fullness of the flanks, which are dull to percussion. Usually shifting dullness is present, but when there is a very large accumulation of fluid, this sign is absent. In such cases, on flicking the abdominal wall, a characteristic fluid thrill is transmitted from one side to the other. In the female, ascites must be differentiated from an enormous ovarian cyst.

Type 1. Due to Congestive Heart Failure.—This, the commonest cause of ascites, is due to chronic venous stasis in the thoracic segment of the inferior vena cava, and consequent obstruction to the venous outflow from the liver. There is stasis also in the superior vena cava, as evinced by engorgement of the veins of the neck—a striking sign in this condition. The ascitic fluid is light yellow serum of low specific gravity, about 1·010.

Type 2. Due to Hepatic or Biliary disease (Chapter 45).—In cirrhosis there is obstruction to the venous outflow of the liver due to obliterative fibrosis of the intrahepatic venous bed. Lymph flow may be increased. In the Budd-Chiari syndrome (Chapter 45), thrombosis or obstruction of the hepatic veins is responsible for the back-pressure.

Type 3. Due to Tuberculous Peritonitis.

Type 4. Secondary Carcinoma of the Peritoneum.—Again the ascites is due to excessive outpouring, due to lymphatic blockage. The fluid is dark yellow and frequently blood-stained. The specific gravity is high—1·020 or over. Microscopical examination often reveals cancer cells, especially if large quantities of fluid are 'spun-down' to produce a concentrated deposit for sampling.

Type 5. Chronic Constrictive Pericarditis (syn. *Pick's Disease*).—In addition to the peritoneal effusion, effusions occur into the pleural cavity. These effusions are due to engorgement of the venae cavae consequent upon diminished capacity of the right side of the heart.

Type 6. Due to depletion of blood protein consequent upon albuminuria or starvation. The ascites in this instance is due to alterations in the osmotic pressure of the capillary blood.

Type 7. Meigs' Syndrome.—This is ascites and pleural effusion associated with solid fibroma of the ovary. The effusions disappear when the tumour is excised.

Treatment.—Ascites may be tapped (paracentesis abdominis) but unless other measures are taken, the fluid soon re-accumulates and repeated tappings remove valuable protein. Dietary sodium restriction to 200 mg per day is frequently successful. Diuretics may be effective in selected patients.

If portal venous pressure is raised, it may be possible to lower it by treatment of the primary condition. (See Chapter 45.)

Paracentesis Abdominis.—The bladder having been emptied by a catheter, under local anaesthesia puncture of the peritoneum is carried out with a moderate-sized trocar and cannula at one of the points shown in fig. 1010. In cases where the effusion is due to cardiac failure the fluid must be evacuated slowly. In other circumstances this precaution is unnecessary. If the cannula becomes blocked with fibrin, it is cleared with a stylet. After the fluid has been evacuated the puncture is sealed, and a tight binder is applied to the abdomen. Some surgeons prefer to perform the 'tap' over the liver beneath the costal margin, or in the midline beneath the xiphisternum.

Friedel Pick, 1876–1926. Professor of Laryngology, Prague, Czechoslovakia. (See footnote, p. 795)
Joe Vincent Meigs, 1892–1964. Gynaecological Surgeon, Massachusetts General Hospital, Boston, Mass., U.S.A.

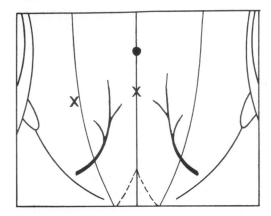

FIG. 1010..—Usual points of puncture for tapping ascites. The bladder must be emptied by a catheter before the puncture is made. Note the relationship of the sites of the puncture to the inferior epigastric artery.

(Drs. V. C. and V. V. Shah, Jamnagar, India.)

Permanent Drainage of Ascitic Fluid.—In rare cases where ascites accumulates rapidly after paracentesis, and the patient is otherwise fit, permanent drainage of the ascitic fluid renders the patient more comfortable. A number of procedures have been described of which *Peritoneo-Venous Shunts* are becoming popular. Similar in concept to shunts for hydrocephalus (Chapter 26), a catheter (*e.g.* of silicone) is constructed with a valve so as to allow one way flow from the peritoneum to a central vein (*e.g.* internal jugular). A chamber, placed subcutaneously over the chest wall may be included for manual compression. Insertion is relatively simple. The complications include overloading the venous system, cardiac failure, and disseminated intravascular coagulopathy (D.I.C., Chapter 5) from fibrin degradation products (FDP) entering the circulation. The procedure may also be used for patients with terminal malignant ascites, giving improved quality of life, at the expense of dissemination of malignant cells (Le Veen Shunt).

STARCH PERITONITIS

Like talc, starch powder has found disfavour as a surgical glove lubricant. In a few starch-sensitive patients it causes a painful ascites, fortunately of limited duration. Should laparotomy be performed, any small granulomas in, say, the omentum, will be found to contain birefringent starch particles.

PERITONEAL LOOSE BODIES (Peritoneal mice)

Peritoneal loose bodies almost never cause symptoms. One or more may be found in a hernial sac or in the pouch of Douglas. The loose body may come from an appendix epiploica that has undergone axial rotation, followed by necrosis of its pedicle, and detachment, but they are also found in those who suffer from subacute attacks of pancreatitis. These hyaline bodies attain the size of a pea or bean, and contain saponified fat surrounded by fibrin.

NEOPLASMS OF THE PERITONEUM

Carcinoma peritonei is a common terminal event in many cases of carcinoma of the stomach, colon, ovary, or other abdominal organs and also of the breast and bronchus. The peritoneum, both parietal and visceral, is studded with secondary growths, and the peritoneal cavity becomes filled with clear, straw-coloured, or blood-stained ascitic fluid.

The main forms of peritoneal metastases are:

   1. Discrete nodules. This is by far the most common variety.

   2. Plaques varying in size and colour.

   3. Diffuse adhesions. This form occurs at a late stage of the disease, and gives rise, sometimes, to a 'frozen pelvis'.

Harry le Veen, Contemporary. Professor of Surgery, University of S. Carolina, U.S.A.
James Douglas, 1675–1742. Anatomist and Obstetrician, London.

Gravity probably determines the distribution of free malignant cells within the peritoneal cavity. Cells not caught in peritoneal folds along the attachments of mesenteries gravitate into the pelvic pouches or into a hernial sac, enlargement of which is occasionally the first indication of the condition. Implantation occurs also on the greater omentum, the appendices epiploicae, and the inferior surface of the diaphragm.

Differential Diagnosis.—Early discrete tubercles common in tuberculous peritonitis are greyish and translucent, and closely resemble the discrete nodules of peritoneal carcinomatosis, but the latter feel hard when rolled between the finger and the thumb, making the differential diagnosis tolerably simple. Fat necroses usually can be distinguished from carcinomatous nodules by their opacity. Peritoneal hydatids can also simulate malignant disease after rupture of a hydatid cyst.

It is remarkable how often patients riddled with intraperitoneal carcinoma preserve their nutrition, and look and feel comparatively well until the terminal stage.

Treatment.—Ascites due to carcinomatosis of the peritoneum can be considerable ameliorated by instillations of radio-active gold and chemo-cytotoxic agents, *e.g.* methotrexate. Tamoxifen[1] can dramatically ameliorate ascites due to breast cancers which are oestrogen dependent.

Radio-active gold (^{198}Au) has a half-life of two and a half days, and is supplied as a purple colloidal solution. One hundred millicuries or more of the solution are introduced into the peritoneal cavity after paracentesis. To improve distribution the foot of the bed is raised; then the patient lies on one side and then on the other, and finally prone, each for fifteen minutes. There follows a period of nausea, but approximately half the patients so treated are benefited for a time. The treatment is of no avail if, after paracentesis, the secondary deposits can be palpated, as the isotope can penetrate only to a depth of 1 millimetre.

Radio-active chromic phosphate (^{32}P) ia also supplied as a colloidal solution, and is as effective as gold. Not only is it less expensive, but this solution requires none of the troublesome precautions connected with the protection of personnel. It emanates pure beta radiation, and has a longer half-life, viz 14·3 days. In its administration rubber gloves are the only protection needed.

Pseudomyxoma Peritonei.—This rare condition occurs more frequently in females. The abdomen is filled with a yellow jelly, large quantities of which are often more or less encysted. The condition arises in one of two ways: more often from rupture of a pseudomucinous cyst of the ovary, less often from rupture of a mucocele of the appendix. It is painless, and there is no impairment of general health for a long time. When the condition arises from the appendix the mass is often more localised, but in cases of ovarian origin the whole peritoneal cavity is involved. Although an abdomen distended with what seems to be fluid that cannot be made to shift should suggest the possibility, it is highly improbable that a correct pre-operative diagnosis will be made. At laparotomy masses of jelly are scooped out, and the primary focus, if it can be found, is removed. Unfortunately, recurrence is usual. When pseudomyxoma peritonei arises from a mucocele of the appendix, repeated recurrence is less common. Pseudomyxoma peritonei is locally malignant but does not give rise to metastases. Occasionally the condition responds to radio-active isotopes, which certainly should be employed in recurrent cases. Interferon has also been used in the treatment of this condition.

Mesothelioma.—As in the pleural cavity this is a highly malignant tumour. Asbestos is a recognised cause. It has a predilection for the pelvic peritoneum and may mimic puboprostatic carcinoma, clinically. It is not radio-sensitive. Alkylating agents have given remissions. Benign forms are reported. Recent multiple regimes of chemo-cytotoxic agents have been reported as curative for *early* forms of malignant mesothelioma.

---

[1] Tamoxifen = oestrogen receptor-site competitor.

PERITONEOSCOPY (LAPAROSCOPY)

The peritoneoscope resembles a cystoscope. Preferably under general anaesthesia, a midline incision 6 mm long is made close to the umbilicus. A trocar and cannula are pushed into the peritoneal cavity and the requisite amount of CO_2 (1 to 1½ litres) is introduced. The patient is tilted so that the gas will rise into the upper abdomen or the pelvis, as required. The telescope is inserted via a special cannula and the organs inspected. Biopsy of a particular area of the liver is possible, but haemorrhage from it is not infrequent. Air embolism is another possible danger.

THE GREATER OMENTUM

Rutherford Morison called the greater omentum 'the abdominal policeman'.[1] Relatively larger and structurally more substantial in the adult than in the child, the discharge of its life-saving constabulary duties becomes more effective after puberty, and remains unabated throughout life. The greater omentum attempts, often successfully, to limit intraperitoneal infective and other noxious processes (fig. 1011). For instance, an acutely inflamed appendix is often found wrapped

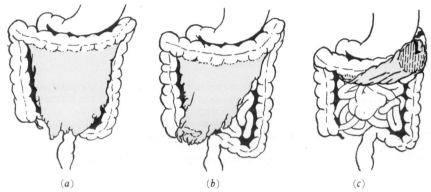

(a) (b) (c)

FIG. 1011.—The greater omentum. (a) Normal. (b) In appendicitis.
(c) In a (comparatively small) laceration of the spleen.

in omentum, and this saves many a patient from developing diffuse peritonitis. Some sufferers from herniae are also greatly indebted to this structure, for it often plugs the neck of a hernial sac and prevents a coil of intestine from becoming strangulated.

Apart from a small portion of it becoming gangrenous while performing the last-mentioned duty (strangulated omentocele), this good Samaritan[2] of the peritoneal cavity seldom itself becomes diseased; when it does become overwhelmed, as in tuberculous peritonitis and carcinomatosis peritonei, it becomes rolled like a scroll.

Torsion of the Omentum.—Torsion of the omentum is a rare emergency, and consequently is seldom diagnosed correctly. It is usually mistaken for appendicitis with somewhat abnormal signs. It may be primary or secondary to an adhesion of the omentum, to an old focus of infection, or to a hernia. Successive herniations of a portion of the omentum into a hernial sac of irregular bore are credited with giving the necessary stimulus to omental torsion.

---

[1] But it has not any feet, *i.e.* it does not move across the abdomen of its own volition, but passively due to peristalsis, and it may be pushed by the movements of the abdominal wall into an area of immobility (rigidity) where there is local peritoneal irritation.

[2] Samaritan, an inhabitant of Samaria, Jordan. The parable of the Good Samaritan is told in the Bible, *Luke x*, 30–37.

The patient is most frequently a middle-aged, obese male. A tender lump may be present in the abdomen. The blood supply having been jeopardised, the twisted mass sometimes becomes gangrenous, in which case bacterial peritonitis soon follows.

Treatment.—The abdomen having been opened, the pedicle above the twist is ligated securely and the mass removed.

Omental Cyst (see below).

THE MESENTERY

A wound of the mesentery can follow a severe abdominal contusion,[1] and is a cause of haemoperitoneum. In about 60% of cases the mesenteric laceration is associated with a rupture of the intestine. If the tear is a large one, and especially if it is transverse (fig. 1012), the blood supply to the neighbouring intestine is cut off, and a limited resection of gut is imperative. Small wounds and wounds in the long axis (fig. 1013) should be sutured. If extensive damage to the mesenteric arcade of vessels is associated with damage to contiguous intestine, exteriorisation of the damaged segment is preferable to excision and suture.

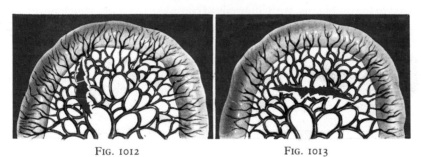

FIG. 1012   FIG. 1013

Laceration of the mesentery, a common injury in car accidents. A transverse tear (fig. 1012) often imperils the blood supply of a segment of intestine, making resection necessary. A longitudinal tear (fig. 1013) can be closed by suture.

Torsion of the Mesentery (see Volvulus Neonatorum, and Volvulus of the Small Intestine (Chapter 51).

Embolism and Thrombosis of Mesenteric Vessels (Chapter 51).

ACUTE NON-SPECIFIC ILEO-CAECAL MESENTERIC ADENITIS

Aetiology.—Non-specific mesenteric adenitis was so named to distinguish it from specific (tuberculous) mesenteric adenitis. It is now very much commoner than the tuberculous variety. Despite much investigation, the aetiology remains unknown. As so often happens in other inflammatory diseases when no causative bacterium can be found, an unidentified virus is blamed. In about 25% of cases a respiratory infection precedes an attack of acute non-specific mesenteric adenitis. In spite of the fact that the vermiform appendix is not diseased in this condition, which is definitely recurrent, appendicectomy does reduce the incidence of further attacks, perhaps by removing what is sometimes known as 'the abdominal tonsil'. This self-limiting disease is never fatal.

---

[1]*Seat Belt Syndrome.*— If a car accident occurs when a seat belt is worn, sudden deceleration can result in a torn mesentery. This possibility should be borne in mind particularly as multiple injuries may distract attention from this injury. If there is any bruising of the abdominal wall, or even marks of clothing impressed into the skin, laparotomy is indicated.

Living Pathology.—There is a small increase in the amount of peritoneal fluid. As seen and felt between the leaves of the mesentery, the ileo-caecal mesenteric lymph nodes are enlarged, being firmly elastic and usually about the size of a haricot bean. In very acute cases they are distinctly red, and many of them are the size of a walnut. The nodes nearest the attachment of the mesentery are the largest. They are not adherent to their peritoneal coats, and if a small incision is made through the overlying peritoneum, a node is extruded easily.

Clinical Features.—During childhood, acute non-specific mesenteric adenitis is a common condition, the ratio of acute appendicitis to acute non-specific adenitis being about 10:1. It is unusual after puberty, but is sometimes seen in teenage girls ('nurse's syndrome'). The typical history is one of short attacks of central abdominal pain lasting from 10–30 minutes, and associated with circumoral pallor. They tend to come on when the patient is tired. Vomiting is usual, but there is no alteration of bowel habit.

On Examination.—There are spasms of general abdominal colic, usually referred to the umbilicus, with intervals of complete freedom, which never appertains in obstructive appendicitis. The patient seldom looks ill. In more than half the cases the temperature is elevated; in severe examples it exceeds 38·3°C. Abdominal tenderness is greatest along the line of the mesentery. When present, shifting tenderness is a valuable sign for differentiating the condition from appendicitis. After laying the patient on the left side for a few minutes, the maximum tenderness moves to the left of the original site.

The pelvic peritoneum is tender to rectal palpation in 30% of cases. The neck, axillae, and groins should be palpated for enlarged lymph nodes—if these nodes are enlarged, brucellosis[1] should come to mind.

Leucocyte Count.—There is often a leucocytosis of 10–12,000/mm³ (10–12⁹/l) or more on the first day of the attack, but this falls on the second day.

Treatment.—When the diagnosis can be made with assurance, bed rest for a few days is the only treatment necessary. If at a second examination, an hour or two after confinement to bed, acute appendicitis cannot be excluded, it is safer to perform appendicectomy.

TUBERCULOSIS OF THE MESENTERIC LYMPH NODES

Tuberculous mesenteric lymphadenitis is considerably less common than acute non-specific lymphadenitis, and it has become increasingly less frequent in Britain during the past thirty years. Tubercle bacilli, usually but not necessarily bovine, are ingested, and enter the mesenteric lymph nodes by way of Peyer's patches. It is possible for one draught of raw milk to start the infection; it is equally possible that a toddler can become infected with human tubercle bacilli by placing one dust-covered small object in its mouth. Sometimes only one lymph node is infected; usually there are several; occasionally massive involvement occurs.

Presentation:

1. **Demonstrated Radiologically.**—The shadows cast by one or more calcified tuberculous lymph nodes are seen frequently in a plain radiograph of the abdomen. They must be distinguished from other calcified lesions, *e.g.* renal or ureteric stones. Their mobility on several plain abdominal radiographs can clinch the diagnosis, and urography can be employed in doubtful cases. Often the shadow cast by such a lymph node or nodes is situated in the ileo-caecal region, but nearly as many are displayed along the line of

---

[1] Sir David Bruce described Malta Fever ('brucellosis') in 1887.

Sir David Bruce, 1855–1931. Major-General, Royal Army Medical Service.
Johann Conrad Peyer, 1653–1712. Professor of Logic, Rhetoric and Medicine, Schaffhausen, Switzerland.

attachment of the mesentery. Usually the radiological characteristics are unmistakable. Each node is round or oval, not homogeneous, but mottled, and its outline is not regular, but bosselated like a blackberry. Calcification of these lymph nodes occurs at the earliest in eighteen months. It is often assumed, wrongly, that because a tuberculous lymph node is calcified, the infection is necessarily defunct. Especially in children, this assumption may not be valid.

2. **As a Cause of General Symptoms**—The patient, usually a child under ten years of age, loses appetite, looks pale, and there is some loss of weight; sometimes evening pyrexia occurs. In children with these symptoms, especially those who live in the country, if the Mantoux test is negative, brucellosis, the 'disease of mistakes', should be thought of, and an intradermal test with brucellin performed.

3. **As a Cause of Abdominal Pain.**—Sometimes abdominal pain is the cause of the patient being brought for advice; usually this pain is central, not severe, but rather a discomfort, and is often constant. On examination the abdomen is somewhat protuberant and there is tenderness on deep pressure to the right of the umbilicus. In these circumstances the condition resembles acute non-specific mesenteric lymphadenitis. On deep palpation inflamed mesenteric lymph nodes are sometimes palpable as firm, discrete, tender bean-like objects most frequently to the right of and near the umbilicus. In both conditions a normal leucocyte count favours tuberculosis, and in a child a positive Mantoux test is confirmatory evidence of tuberculosis.

4. **Symptoms Indistinguishable from those of Appendicitis.**—On occasions the abdominal pain is acute and may be accompanied by vomiting. This, combined with tenderness and some rigidity in the right iliac fossa, makes the diagnosis from subacute appendicitis almost impossible. When, as is sometimes the case, the tuberculous infection of the mesenteric lymph nodes become reactivated in adolescent or adult life, the diagnostic difficulties are even greater. A radiograph may show calcified lymph nodes, but as such a condition can co-exist with appendicitis, in some cases laparotomy for appendicectomy and visualisation of the lymph nodes is necessary. If the mesentery is found to be in an inflamed state with caseation of some of the lymph nodes, the diagnosis of active tuberculosis of the nodes is confirmed. Peritoneoscopy can help with the diagnosis in more 'chronic' cases.

Treatment is similar to that of other tuberculous infections (Chapter 4).

Most cases subside, but from time to time a local abscess forms, usually in the right iliac fossa, when the tuberculous pus should be evacuated and the abdomen closed without drainage (see Pseudo-mesenteric Cyst, below).

5. **As a Cause of Intestinal Obstruction.**—Remote, rather than recent, tuberculous mesenteric adenitis can be the cause of intestinal obstruction. For instance, a coil of small intestine becomes adherent to a caseating node, and is thereby angulated or a free coil may become imprisoned in the tunnel beneath the site of adherence and the mesentery.

6. **As a Cause of Pseudo-mesenteric Cyst.**—When tuberculous mesenteric lymph nodes break down, the tuberculous pus may remain confined between the leaves of the mesentery, and a cystic swelling having the characteristics of a mesenteric cyst is found. When such a condition is confirmed at operation the tuberculous pus should be aspirated without soiling the peritoneal cavity, the wound closed, the sensitivity of the organism should be sought and specific treatment continued until the infection has been overcome.

7. **As Ileo-caecal lymph nodes.**—At laparotomy hard enlarged lymph nodes may be found limited to the ileo-caecal mesentery as a result of previous tuberculous infection. If the nodes have a yellow colour, they arise from a carcinoid tumour of the appendix or ileum (see Chapter 50).

MESENTERIC CYSTS

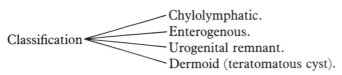

Classification
- Chylolymphatic.
- Enterogenous.
- Urogenital remnant.
- Dermoid (teratomatous cyst).

Chylolymphatic cyst, the commonest variety of mesenteric cyst, probably arises in congenitally misplaced lymphatic tissue that has no efferent communication with the lymphatic system: it arises most frequently in the mesentery of the ileum. The thin wall of the cyst, which is composed of connective tissue lined by flat endothelium, is filled with clear lymph or, less frequently, with chyle varying in consistency from watered milk to cream. Occasionally the cyst attains a great size. More often unilocular than multilocular, a chylolymphatic cyst is almost invariably solitary, although there is an extremely rare variety in which myriads of cysts are found in the various mesenteries of the abdomen. A chylolymphatic cyst has a blood supply independent of that of the adjacent intestine, thereby enucleation is possible without the necessity of resection of gut.

Enterogenous cyst is believed to be derived either from a diverticulum of the mesenteric border of the intestine which has become sequestrated from the intestinal canal during embryonic life, or from a duplication of the intestine. An enterogenous cyst has a thicker wall than a chylolymphatic cyst, and it is lined by mucous membrane, sometimes ciliated. The content is mucinous, and is either colourless or yellowish-brown from bygone haemorrhage into the cyst. As can be seen at operation, the muscle in the wall of an enterogenous cyst and the bowel with which it is in contact have a common blood supply; consequently removal of the cyst always entails resection of the related portion of intestine.

Clinical Features of a Mesenteric Cyst.—A mesenteric cyst is encountered most frequently in the second decade of life, less often between the ages of one and ten years, and exceptionally in infants under one year.

The patient presents on account of:

(*a*) *A painless abdominal swelling.*—A cyst of the mesentery presents characteristic physical signs.

1. There is a fluctuant swelling near the umbilicus.

2. The swelling moves freely in a plane at right angles to the attachment of the mesentery (fig. 1014).

3. There is a zone of resonance around and, classically, a belt of resonance across the cyst.

(*b*) *Recurrent attacks of abdominal pain* with or without vomiting. The pain results from recurring temporary impaction of a food bolus in a segment of bowel narrowed by the cyst, or possibly from torsion of the mesentery.

(*c*) *An acute abdominal catastrophe* arises as a result of (1) torsion of that portion of the mesentery containing the cyst; (2) rupture of the cyst, often due to a comparatively trivial accident; (3) haemorrhage into the cyst; (4) infection.

Radiography.—In most instances the patient should be submitted to x-ray after a barium meal. The hollow viscera will be found to be displaced around the cyst, and not infrequently some portion of the lumen of the small intestine will be narrowed. In order to exclude or confirm the diagnosis of a hydronephrosis an ultrasound examination or a urogram should not be omitted. In cases of painless enlargement of the abdomen this examination should be undertaken first. Needle aspiration combined with instillation of radio opaque water-soluble contrast media can transform doubt into certainty.

Treatment.—As has been indicated already, many chylolymphatic cysts can be enucleated *in toto*.

When, after aspiration of about half the contents of the cyst, the major portion of the cyst has been dissected free but one portion abutting on the intestine or a major blood-vessel seems too dangerous to remove, this portion can be left attached and its lining destroyed by careful diathermy.

In the case of an enterogenous cyst, enucleation must not be attempted. If a comparatively short segment of the intestine is involved, resection of the cyst with the adherent portion of the intestine, followed by intestinal anastomosis, is the correct course. Should a very large segment of small intestine be implicated, an anastomosis should be made between the apex of the coil of small intestine and the cyst wall which, in this instance, holds sutures well.

The older treatment of marsupialisation of a mesenteric cyst has nothing to recommend it, for a fistula or recurrence results. Occasionally, however, on account of its simplicity, it is advisable in a poor-risk subject in whom surgery is necessary, but this is usually not justified in such cases for an essentially benign condition.

Omental cyst occurs nearly as frequently as a mesenteric cyst. Preoperative differentiation is possible because a lateral radiograph shows the cyst in front of the intestines. Treatment is omentectomy.

Cyst of the mesocolon is uncommon, and it is differentiated from a mesenteric cyst only at operation. The treatment is similar.

Cysts arising from a urogenital (Wolffian or Müllerian) remnant are essentially retroperitoneal, but they are included in the classification because it is not impossible for such a cyst to project forward into the mesentery.

Kasper Friedrich Wolff, 1733–1794. Professor of Anatomy and Physiology, St. Petersburg (now Leningrad, USSR.)
Johannes Peter Müller, 1801–1858. Professor of Anatomy and Physiology, Berlin.

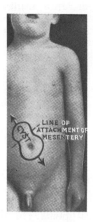

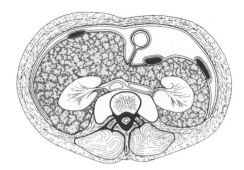

FIG. 1015.—Rapidly growing retroperitoneal liposarcoma.

FIG. 1014.—A mesenteric cyst moves freely in the direction of the arrows, *i.e.* at right angles to the attachment of the mesentery.

The following, while not being mesenteric cysts in the meaning of the term, give rise to the same physical signs, and, in practice, they *are* mesenteric cysts: (1) *Serosanguineous cyst* is probably traumatic in origin, but a history of an accident is seldom obtained. (2) *Tuberculous abscess of the mesentery.* (3)*Hydatid cyst of the mesentery.*

NEOPLASMS OF THE MESENTERY

Tumours situated in the mesentery give rise to physical signs similar to those of a mesenteric cyst, the sole exception being that they sometimes feel solid.

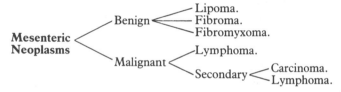

A benign tumour of the mesentery is excised in the same way as an enterogenous mesenteric cyst, *i.e.* with resection of the adjacent intestine. When possible, a malignant tumour of the mesentery is subjected to the same treatment. In inoperable cases radiotherapy can be employed if the biopsy specimen reveals that the growth is probably radiosensitive.

THE RETROPERITONEAL SPACE

Pus or blood in the retroperitoneal space tends to track to the corresponding iliac fossa. If a retroperitoneal abscess develops, it should be evacuated by the nearest route through the abdominal wall, avoiding opening the peritoneum. Should the retroperitoneal collection be found at laparotomy, it must be drained by a counter-incision in the flank. Pus frequently develops from a renal or spinal source, and is sometimes tuberculous ('cold abscess'): tracking can develop alongside the psoas muscle and appear in the groin, where it must be distinguished from other swellings (*e.g.* hernia—see Chapter 55). Retroperitoneal haematoma may be caused by fractured spine, a leaking abdominal aneurysm, acute pancreatitis or a ruptured kidney.

Retroperitoneal Cyst.—A cyst developing in the retroperitoneal space often attains very large dimensions, and has at first to be distinguished from a hydronephrosis. Even after the latter condition has been eliminated by urography, a retroperitoneal cyst can seldom be diagnosed with certainty from a retroperitoneal tumour, until displayed at operation. The cyst may be unilocular or multilocular. Many of these cysts are believed to be derived from a remnant of the Wolffian duct, in which case they are filled with clear fluid. Others are teratomatous, and are filled with sebaceous material.

Excision of these and other retroperitoneal swellings is best performed through a transperitoneal incision (see below).

Idiopathic Retroperitoneal Fibrosis.—See Chapter 57.

PRIMARY RETROPERITONEAL NEOPLASMS ARISING FROM CONNECTIVE TISSUES

Retroperitoneal lipoma, in the first instance, is usually mistaken for a hydronephrosis, a diagnosis which is ruled out by ultrasonography, CT scan and urography. Women are more often affected. These swellings sometimes reach an immense size. We have removed such a tumour weighing 2·5 kg, and much larger specimens have been recorded. A retroperitoneal lipoma sometimes undergoes myxomatous degeneration, a complication which does not occur in a lipoma in any other part of the body. Moreover, a retroperitoneal lipoma sometimes becomes malignant (liposarcoma) (fig. 1015).

Retroperitoneal sarcoma presents signs similar to a retroperitoneal lipoma. The patient may seek advice on account of a swelling or because of indefinite abdominal pain. On other occasions the tumour, by pressure on the colon, causes symptoms of subacute intestinal obstruction. On examination a smooth fixed mass, which is not tender, is palpated. The most probable original diagnosis is that of a neoplasm of the kidney. This is ruled out by scanning and urography. The ureter, however, is liable to become displaced by the tumour. Exploratory laparotomy should be performed, and when possible the tumour is removed. Often it is found widely disseminated in the retroperitoneal space, rendering complete removal impossible, in which case a portion is excised for microscopy. Even when excised at a comparatively early stage, recurrence always takes place, and these tumours must be looked upon as being necessarily fatal. Radiotherapy sometimes keeps recurrences in abeyance for a time.

Removal of a Retroperitoneal Cyst or Neoplasm.—After the anterior abdominal wall has been opened and the diagnosis of a retroperitoneal tumour has been confirmed, the incision is extended as necessary. The small intestine is packed away in the upper abdomen, and the caecum and the sigmoid are relegated to their respective fossae. The posterior peritoneum is then incised throughout its length over the area to be exposed, the incision parallel to the left border of the aorta. The peritoneum is dissected from the tumour which is removed as completely as possible, the intestines being kept out of the way with packs or exteriorised temporarily, depending on which manoeuvre is the more useful.

RETROPERITONEAL TUMOURS ARISING FROM SPECIFIC ORGANS

These may arise from:

LYMPH NODES (see Chapter 9)

ADRENAL GLAND (see Chapter 38)

KIDNEY & URETER (see Chapter 57)

NERVOUS TISSUE (see Chapter 28)

CHAPTER 50

THE SMALL AND LARGE INTESTINES

Abdominal pain arising from the Alimentary Canal is of two types:

1. *Visceral Pain.*—The alimentary tract is primarily a midline structure with a bilateral nerve supply. Although rotation about the midline occurs during development, nevertheless true visceral pain is referred to the midline as illustrated in fig. 1016. It is dull and poorly localised.

2. *Peritoneal Pain* however is of the somatic type—and is much more precise, more severe and localised to site of origin. These components account for the changes in character and site of pain which occurs in appendicitis (Chapter 52).

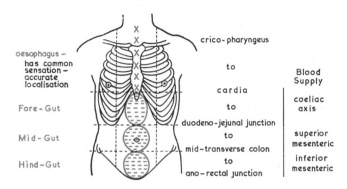

FIG. 1016.—Sites of origin of visceral pain.

Surgical Anatomy.—It is of great practical importance to be able:

1. To distinguish various portions of the intestinal canal at sight.

2. To know in which part of the abdomen the upper coils, as opposed to the lower coils, of the small intestine lie in relationship to the anterior abdominal wall.

3. To be able to decide which is the proximal and which the distal end of any coil under consideration.

4. To distinguish irrefutably large from small intestine.

For practical purposes these problems are settled as follows:

(*a*) The mesentery of the jejunum has only two series of arches of blood-vessels, whereas the lower ileum has several series of arches.

(*b*) The mesentery, after being made taut, is examined. As the mesenteric attachment runs from left to right, if palpation reveals that the mesentery is not twisted, then the upper end of the bowel in the wound is the proximal end.

(*c*) The large intestine is characterised by its taeniae coli and appendices epiploicae.

CONGENITAL MALFORMATIONS OF THE INTESTINES

Congenital Atresia of the Duodenum (Chapter 51).
Congenital Atresia of the Small Intestine (Chapter 51).
Volvulus Neonatorum (Chapter 51).
Vascular Anomalies (Angiodysplasia) (p. 1031).
Failure of Descent of the Caecum.—The caecum remains under the right lobe of the liver.

MEGACOLON

There are two varieties of this relatively uncommon condition (1) *primary* or true megacolon (*syn.* Hirschsprung's disease, congenital aganglionic megacolon) and (2) *secondary* or acquired megacolon.

Primary Megacolon.—Hirschsprung's disease:

Pathology.—This disease is characterised by enormous dilatation and hypertrophy of the pelvic colon, sometimes extending into the descending colon but rarely involving the more proximal parts of the large intestine. The pelvic mesocolon is elongated and thickened and its blood-vessels are large and prominent. All coats of the dilated intestine show gross pathological changes. The mucosa is chronically inflamed and frequently ulcerated. There is a terminal constricted, non-hypertrophied segment of bowel usually involving the anal canal, the rectum, and a variable part of the large intestine. In nine out of ten cases the upper limit of the contracted segment is the pelvi-rectal junction; occasionally the deficiency extends to a higher level. It is in this contracted segment that physiological obstruction lies,[1] and the dilatation hypertrophy of the colon above is due to absence of peristalsis in the spastic segment.

On histological examination the cause of the immotility of the spastic segment is evident; there is a complete absence of parasympathetic ganglion cells, and this ganglion deficiency extends for a distance of 1 to 5 cm into a transitional zone or cone between the terminal spastic segment and the hypertrophied portion. Above the transitional zone, parasympathetic ganglion cells are present as in normal intestine.

Clinical Features.—Hirschsprung's disease shows a familial tendency. It is much more common in males than females. In 90% of cases symptoms appear within three days following birth.

Constipation.[2]—The infant fails to pass meconium during the first two or three days of life, and then only after the insertion of a little finger or a tube into the rectum. Subsequently motions are toothpaste-like, and inadequate in amount; straining is in evidence during this passage.

Abdominal distension is usually unmistakable by the third day. In a proportion of cases the abdominal distension progresses, and sometimes it is evident that the colon is obstructed (fig. 1017); in others it is impossible clinically to differentiate large from small intestinal obstruction. Loud borborygmi and visible peristalsis are much in evidence.

Rectal Examination.—The anus is free from fissures and excoriation and there is no perianal soiling. The rectum is empty and *grips the examining finger*.

Complete intestinal obstruction occurs quite frequently within a few days of birth and may be fatal. As a rule, the attacks are recurring and relief is given by a small enema, by passing a greased examining finger or by the spontaneous passage of a large stool sometimes followed by diarrhoea. Owing to the enormous abdominal distension, chest infection may supervene. In any case, if the child survives, malnutrition and stunted growth are obvious features together with enormous abdominal distension.

Radiography. *Barium Enema.*—When the clinical findings are atypical a barium enema is often helpful in confirming the diagnosis. The objective is to demonstrate the contracted aganglionic segment, if such be present, and to this end preliminary wash-outs are with-

---

[1] In 1898 Treves attributed Hirschsprung's disease to congenital spasm of the distal segment, thus preceding the re-discovery of this concept by fifty years.

[2] *Diarrhoea*. It cannot be emphasised too strongly that these infants sometimes present with diarrhoea and abdominal distension, and unless a rectal tube is passed, the patient may rapidly succumb to what is mistakenly thought to be simple gastroenteritis.

Harald Hirschsprung, 1830–1916. Physician, Queen Louise Hospital for Children, Copenhagen.
Sir Frederick Treves, 1853–1923. Surgeon, The London Hospital.

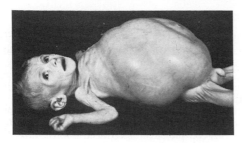

FIG. 1017.—Hirschsprung's disease showing enormous colonic dilatation and a wave of visible peristalsis.
(The late Sir Denis Browne, FRCS, London.)

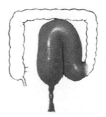

FIG. 1018.—Radiological appearances in Hirschsprung's disease; coning, as well as dilatation, is diagnostic.
(After B. C. H. Ward, London.)

held. For reasons explained below, the barium should be admixed with isotonic saline solution, not tap-water. By using only a little dilute barium emulsion—just sufficient to run over the faecal masses—a good outline of the bowel can be obtained (fig. 1018).

Biopsy of the ano-rectal wall is employed in order to prove or disprove the presence of ganglia. A piece of rectal wall 1 cm² is removed and searched for ganglia in the submucosa (Auerbach's plexus) and intermyenteric layer (Meissner's plexus). In centres with appropriate facilities, tests can be done to confirm that acetyl choline is not being produced from the aganglionic bowel: this test can replace biopsy as proof of Hirschsprung's disease.

Laparotomy is required when the patient has acute-on-chronic intestinal obstruction, and other causes cannot be eliminated. If the case proves to be one of Hirschsprung's disease it is advisable to establish a temporary transverse colostomy or, in the rare event of the whole colon being narrowed, an ileostomy.

Pre-operative Treatment.—Colonic lavage in Hirschsprung's disease is dangerous, because the use of tap-water in the enemas in this condition may cause water intoxication. The megacolon absorbs water much more rapidly than does a normal colon, and the disturbance of electrolytic balance, especially of sodium, may prove fatal. Provided the general condition is good, isotonic saline solution can be used with safety. In patients with impaired cardiac or renal reserve, 7% gelatine solution should be substituted. Unless measurements show that distension is increasing, four weeks' pre-operative preparation is desirable (Svenson). During the last five pre-operative days, metronidazole plus cefuroxamine are given for bowel sterilisation.

Treatment.—The only curative treatment of Hirschsprung's disease is excision of the entire aganglionic segment. No reparative operation should be done till the child is 8 kg in weight and thriving (Brown).

Modified Duhamel Operation.—This operation is designed to preserve rectal sensation and storage capacity. Preliminary colostomy and bowel preparation is carried out as above. The aganglionic segment is removed down to the level of the peritoneal reflection over the rectum. At this point the rectum is divided, turned in, and closed over. The sacral hollow is then opened up and the normal colon brought down to the posterior aspect of the rectal stump. The anus is now widely stretched and a transverse incision is made in the posterior wall just above the sphincter. Through this opening the colon lying behind the rectum is seized and brought down to present at the anus. The colon is then fixed to the rectum by a few catgut stitches to make a somewhat loose colo-rectal anastomosis. A special crushing clamp is now introduced to crush the spur between the rectum and the colon. It is left in position till the spur separates, when the clamp becomes loose and can be removed. The colostomy is closed a few weeks later. The crushing of the spur is now done by a stapling device in many hospitals: the GIA stapler is most often used for this purpose, which allows free communication between the colon and the rectum to be established immediately.

Abdomino-anal pull-through.—The patient is placed in a semi-lithotomy position, to give good access to the abdomen and the peri-anal region. Through a suitable incision the rectum, the contracted part of the adjoining colon, and the commencement of the hypertrophied portion are freed from their attachments as far downwards as possible

Georg Meissner, 1829–1905. Professor of Physiology, Göttingen, Germany.
Leopold Auerbach, 1828–1897. Professor of Neuropathology, Breslau, Germany (now Wrocław, Poland).
Orvar Svenson, Contemporary, Professor of Surgery, Northwestern University, Chicago, Illinois, U.S.A.
James Johnston Mason Brown, 1908–1964. Surgeon-in-Charge, Royal Hospital for Sick Children, Edinburgh.
Bernard Duhamel, Contemporary, Chief-Surgeon, Hôpital Saint-Denis, Saint-Denis, France.

towards the anal canal. In contrast to excision for carcinoma of the rectum, the dissection must be kept immediately outside the fascia propria. In this way the seminal vesicles and the autonomic nerve trunks to the bladder are protected. Should doubts exist as to whether the aganglionic segment has been encompassed, frozen section biopsy will provide the answer. The intestine is then transected proximally through normal colon, and the distal end is closed with a purse-string suture. The mobilised aganglionic segment is then everted through the anus. The mucosa thus exposed is painted with antiseptic solution, and dried. The anterior half of the junction of the inverted rectum with the anal canal is opened transversely, and the proximal colon is pulled through the opening. End-to-end anastomosis between the colon and the anal canal is carried out as the everted aganglionic segment is excised. The union having been completed, it is reduced into the anal canal. Gloves having been changed, the abdominal incision is repaired. By two teams working simultaneously, one abdominally and one perineally, the operation can be performed expeditiously. Cases of Hirschsprung's disease involving the entire colon have been treated successfully by total colectomy and ileoproctostomy.

Colo-anal Anastomosis.—A few patients with Hirschsprung's disease manage to lead reasonable lives until suddenly the colon 'decompensates' in adult life. Such cases can be treated by removing the abnormally dilated bowel, as well as the aganglionic segment down to the anus: normal colon can then be joined to the anus either directly or by a sleeve technique (Parks) with good functional results.

ACQUIRED OR SECONDARY MEGACOLON

Dilatation and hypertrophy of an otherwise normal large bowel extends to the anal canal. The obstruction is due to faecal impaction. Characteristically, there is a fissured anus, a spastic sphincter and much perianal soiling. As a rule, faulty bowel care and training are the sources of the trouble, and usually they can be traced to infancy; the onset, however, is never from birth. Sometimes the condition is encountered in the insane and the old.

Rectal Examination.—This is usually painful and the finger encounters a scybalous mass just inside the anus, which is contrary to the findings in Hirschsprung's disease.

Sigmoidoscopy.—Some patients may have taken aperients for many years to relieve their chronic constipation: these may eventually lead to a dark discoloration of the mucosa of the colon and rectum—'melanosis coli'.

Radiography.—In all cases of acquired megacolon the dilatation as shown by a barium enema ends at the anal canal (fig. 1019).

Biopsy of the Rectal Wall.—When acquired megacolon cannot be differentiated from Hirschsprung's disease by clinical and radiological means, biopsy is required. The presence of ganglion cells in the submucosa is the signal for conservative treatment.

Conservative Treatment.—Should an anal stricture or a fissure-in-ano be present, these lesions must be treated appropriately. The essential feature is bowel training so that a regular habit is established. It is wise to start with regular enemas and Senokot until the bowel is clean. The family environment must be thoroughly investigated. Upset of bowel habit in a child is a not uncommon result of domestic upheaval or emotional deprivation.

Redundant Colon.—Some constipated patients (usually female) are found on investigation by barium enema x-ray to have an elongated sigmoid colon (dolichocolon). Volvulus formation is a theoretical risk, but the wise surgeon avoids removing the redundant bowel for these patients may be neurotic, and will plague him after the operation with the same or other symptoms.

Cathartic Colon.—In some patients the dilatation and immobility of the colon is due

Sir Alan Parks, P.R.C.S., 1920–1982. Surgeon, St Marks and the London Hospitals, London.

to chronic poisoning ('intoxication') of the intestinal wall by large doses of purgatives taken over many years. The cascara and senna derivatives are the worst agents. In a few cases the generalised picture of dilated bowel is complicated by strictures (especially in the right colon). Melanosis coli is often observed on sigmoidoscopy. Such cases are grouped under the title of 'cathartic colon'. Conservative management is often successful in these patients.

VASCULAR ANOMALIES (ANGIODYSPLASIA)

Capillary or cavernous haemangiomas are a cause of haemorrhage from the colon at any age, presenting with haemorrhagic shock. In the middle aged or elderly patient the lesion needs to be distinguished from the other causes of sudden massive haemorrhage, viz. diverticulitis, ulcerative colitis, ischaemic colitis. In 50% of cases the bleeding arises in the ileocaecal region or right colon. Whereas a sigmoidoscopy will help to distinguish between an anorectal haemangioma (bluish subepithelial venous swellings) and colitis (acute mucosal inflammatory changes), a barium enema will only detect diverticular disease and ischaemic colitis, and a colonoscopy is disappointing. Selective superior and inferior mesenteric angiography alone suffices to show the site and extent of the lesion by a 'blush'. Recent evidence has implicated degeneration as the underlying cause of the condition, which accounts for its occurrence in the middle-aged and elderly.

The treatment may well involve an emergency total colectomy with ileorectal anastomosis if the site cannot be identified. This drastic step is preferable to a situation of continued massive-bleeding after a subtotal left or right sided colectomy.

TRAUMATIC RUPTURE OF THE INTESTINE

The intestine can be ruptured with or without an external wound. The most frequent cause of the latter is a blow on the abdomen which crushes the bowel against the promontory of the sacrum (see also seat belt syndrome in traffic accidents, Chapter 49). Rupture is particularly liable to occur in the presence of an irreducible inguinal hernia. Rupture typically occurs where a fixed part of the alimentary tract joins a mobile one, such as the duodenojejunal flexure, in which

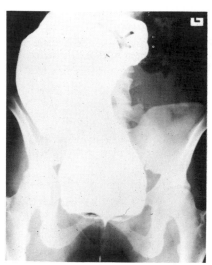

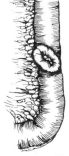

Fig. 1020.—Traumatic rupture of the ileum. Note the prolapse of the mucous membrane.

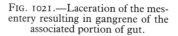

Fig. 1019.—Radiological appearances of acquired megacolon. Note that the 'contracted segment' is the anus.

Fig. 1021.—Laceration of the mesentery resulting in gangrene of the associated portion of gut.

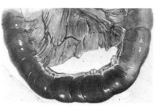

case the damage may be retroperitoneal and easily overlooked; this type of lesion is usually due to runover accidents.

In small perforations the mucosa prolapses and tends partially to seal the rent (fig. 1020); consequently the early signs are misleading. In general the signs simulate closely those of a perforated peptic ulcer.

Laceration of the mesentery is a frequent operative finding in the type of injury under consideration.

Traumatic rupture of the large intestine is much less frequent. Compressed-air rupture of the colon is sometimes the result of a damnable form of practical joke, whereby a hose, carrying air under considerable pressure, is turned on near the victim's anus.

Blast injuries of the abdomen sustained during air-raids resulted in a number of cases of traumatic rupture of the intestine. The pelvic colon was found to be injured more frequently than other segments of the intestine. Rupture of the upper reaches of the rectum is not unknown during sigmoidoscopy. In ulcerative lesions the air insufflation has been sufficient to perforate the intestinal wall.

Treatment.—In all cases of suspected rupture of the intestine immediate laparotomy must be performed. In many instances, simple closure of the perforation is all that is required. In others, *e.g.* where the mesentery is lacerated, resection may be necessary (fig. 1021). In the case of the large intestine, exteriorisation is the procedure of choice; if this is not feasible, the perforation is closed and proximal colostomy is performed. In the case of retroperitoneal portions of the intestine (*e.g.* duodenum) perforations may involve both the front and back walls, and the bowel has to be mobilised in order that a concealed tear is not overlooked (see duodenal injury, Chapter 44).

VASCULAR INSUFFICIENCY
(See Chapter 51)

THE BLIND LOOP SYNDROME

It has been shown in dogs that if a blind loop of the small intestine is made (fig. 1022) defects of absorption will appear. If this occurs in the upper intestine the defect is chiefly of fat absorption; if in the lower intestine there is vitamin B_{12} deficiency. This has been

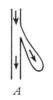

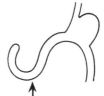

A   B

Experimental blind loops.

A. Self-filling: deficiency occurs.

B. Self-emptying: no deficiency occurs.

C. Long afferent loop stasis in Polya gastrectomy.

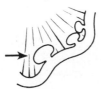
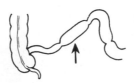
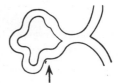

D. Jejunal diverticula.

E. Intestinal stricture causing stasis.

F. 'Stenosis-anastomosis loop' syndrome.

FIG. 1022.—Common types of blind loops.

found to occur in humans and is referred to as the blind loop syndrome, or the 'stenosis-anastomosis loop' syndrome (Witts).

Essentially, the stasis produces an abnormal bacterial flora, which prevent proper breakdown of the food (especially fat) and mop up the vitamins that are present. Sometimes the only manifestation is anaemia, due to Vitamin B_{12} deficiency, but if steatorrhoea appears, other serious malabsorption features follow. In general, high loops produce steatorrhoea, *etc.*, whereas low loops tend to produce anaemia.

Temporary improvement will follow the use of antibiotics to destroy the bacteria causing the trouble, but the main treatment is surgical extirpation of the cause of the stasis.

ALIMENTARY DIVERTICULA[1]

Diverticula occur from the stomach to the recto-sigmoid junction. There are two varieties:

(*a*) *Congenital.*—All three coats of the bowel are present in the wall of the diverticulum, *e.g.* Meckel's.

(*b*) *Acquired.*—The wall of the diverticulum lacks a proper muscular coat. Most alimentary diverticula are thought to be acquired.

DIVERTICULA OF THE SMALL INTESTINE

The belief that a diverticulum of the small intestine originates as a mucosal herniation through a point of entrance of blood-vessels is based on the fact that most of these diverticula arise from the mesenteric side of the bowel (fig. 1022).

FIG. 1023.—Primary diverticula of second and third parts of duodenum.

FIG. 1024.—Secondary diverticula of duodenal cap.

Duodenal Diverticulum.—There are two types.

1. *Primary.*—Mostly in older patients on the inner wall of the second and third parts, they are found incidentally on barium meal and usually do not cause symptoms.

2. *Secondary*, of the duodenal cap resulting from long standing duodenal ulceration.

Jejunal diverticula vary in size, are sometimes single (fig. 1022). More often several are present (figs. 1022 and 1025). Clinically they may (*a*) be symptomless (*b*) give rise to abdominal pain, flatulence and borborygmi or (*c*) produce a malabsorption syndrome. This latter consists of anaemia, steatorrhoea, hypoproteinaemia and avitaminosis. They are, in fact, examples of the blind loop syndrome (p. 1032). If the length of affected bowel is not too extensive, resection and end-to-end anastomosis give excellent results.

Meckel's diverticulum is present in 2% of the human race; it is situated upon the antimesenteric border of the small intestine, commonly 60 cm from the ileo-caecal valve, and it is usually 5 cm long. Many variations occur (2%—2 feet—2 inches is a useful *aide memoire*).

---

[1] Literally, a diverticulum means a wayside house of ill-fame, and these wayside houses certainly live up to their evil reputation.

Leslie John Witts, 1898–1982. Nuffield Professor of Clinical Medicine, Oxford, England.
Johann Friedrich Meckel (The Younger), 1781–1833. Professor of Anatomy and Surgery, Halle, Germany.

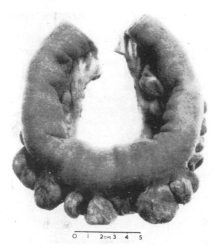

FIG. 1025.—Jejunal diverticula.

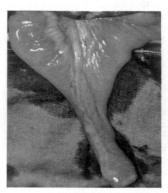

FIG. 1026.—Meckel's diverticulum.

In nearly 90% of cases the diverticulum arises from the antimesenteric border of the ileum, and, being congenital, it possesses all three coats of the intestinal wall. It will be noted in figs. 1026 and 1027 that it has its own blood supply (like the appendix) and this makes it vulnerable to infection and obstruction. In 20% of cases the mucosa contains heterotopic epithelium, viz. gastric, colonic, or sometimes pancreatic tissue. When present, heterotopic tissue lines the greater part of the proximal end of the pouch, and not infrequently extends for a short distance into the nearby ileum. Although Meckel's diverticulum occurs with equal frequency in both sexes, symptomatic cases, due almost entirely to the epithelium contained in the diverticulum, are predominant in males. In order of frequency, these symptoms are as follows:

1. **Severe haemorrhage per rectum**, due to peptic ulceration. The blood passed is maroon in colour. Although the patient frequently vomits, the vomitus contains no blood. Seldom is the haemorrhage preceded by pain; sometimes bleeding precedes perforation. When operation is required for serious progressive haemorrhage per rectum and no lesion in the stomach or duodenum is found, the next step should be the examination of the terminal 150 cm of ileum.

2. **Intussusception.**—In the majority of cases the apex of the intussusception is swollen, inflamed, heterotopic epithelium at the mouth of the diverticulum—not inversion of the diverticulum, as is commonly stated. Intussusception due to Meckel's diverticulum is discussed in Chapter 51.

3. **Meckelian diverticulitis** with or without perforation is usually due to lodgement of coarse food residue or a sharp foreign body. The symptoms of Meckelian diverticulitis without perforation are those of acute appendicitis, and unless the appendix has been removed the diagnosis is impossible before operation. When a diverticulum perforates, so rapid is the onset of peritonitis that the symptoms simulate those of a perforated duodenal ulcer. Whether or not the diverticulum has perforated, urgent operation is required. In non-perforated cases an inflamed diverticulum should be sought as soon as it has been ascertained that the vermiform appendix (and, in the case of a female, the Fallopian tubes) is not at fault.

4. **Chronic Peptic Ulceration.**—Because the diverticulum is part of the midgut, the pain, though related to meals, is felt around the umbilicus.

5. **Intestinal Obstruction.**—The presence of a band between the apex of the diverticulum and the umbilicus may cause obstruction either by the band itself or by a volvulus around it.

Gabriele Fallopio, 1523–1562. (See footnote, p. 211).

Radiography.—In cases of Meckel's diverticulum giving rise to symptoms, failure to visualise the diverticulum by radiography after a barium meal, which is very common, is of no significance, because so often the entrance of the diverticulum is blocked by oedema.

Technetium ($^{99}Tc^m$) Scanning.—When perforation or haemorrhage has occurred imaging of the abdomen with the gamma camera, after injection of 30–100 μCi $^{99}Tc^m$ intravenously may localise heterotopic gastric mucosa in a Meckel's diverticulum in 90% of cases. Uptake of isotope by the peptic mucosa may be enhanced by Pentagastrin 0·6 μ/Kg given subcutaneously.

'Silent' Meckel's Diverticulum.—A Meckel's diverticulum usually remains symptomless throughout life, and is found only at necropsy. When a silent Meckel's diverticulum is encountered in the course of an abdominal operation, and can be excised without appreciable additional risk, this should be done in order to exclude the possibility of subsequent complications.

Exceptionally a Meckel's diverticulum is found in an inguinal or femoral hernial sac, when it is known as a Littre's hernia.

Meckelian Diverticulectomy.—A Meckel's diverticulum which is broad based should not be amputated at its base and invaginated in the same way as a vermiform appendix, because of the risk of a stricture. Moreover, it does not remove heterotopic epithelium completely, if such be present. The steps of diverticulectomy are displayed in fig. 1027.

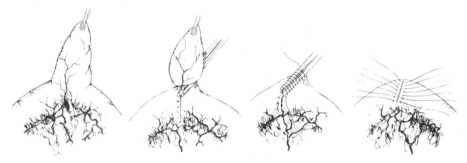

FIG. 1027.—Steps in the performance of Meckelian diverticulectomy.

Should there be considerable induration of the base of the diverticulum, and particularly when such induration extends into the neighbouring ileum, it is advisable to resect a short segment of the ileum containing the diverticulum, and to restore the continuity of the bowel by anastomosis.

DIVERTICULAR DISEASE OF THE COLON

Diverticula of the colon are acquired herniations of colonic mucosa, protruding through the circular muscle at the points where the blood vessels penetrate the colonic wall (fig. 1028). Thus they tend to occur in rows in between the strips of longitudinal muscle (taenia coli) (fig. 1029). The condition may be localised to one part of the colon, usually the sigmoid, but sometimes the entire large bowel is involved from the caecum to the rectosigmoid junction. The rectum with its complete muscle layers is not affected. In 90% of cases the sigmoid colon is involved and becomes almost always the site of inflammation, *i.e.* diverticulitis. Some 5% of patients have associated gallstones and hiatus hernia (Saint's triad).

Diverticular disease is rare in Africans and Asiatics who eat a diet which contains natural fibre. In Western countries, where the roughage has been removed from flour and sugar, diverticula are found in 5% of barium enemas over the age of 40, and the incidence increases with age.

Diverticulosis, the primary stage of the disease, is related to muscular incoordination and hypertrophy resulting in increased segmentation and intraluminal

Alexis Littre, 1658–1726. Surgeon and Anatomist, Paris.

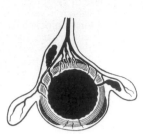

FIG. 1028.—The usual sites of
diverticulation of the colon.
(After Hamilton Drummond.)

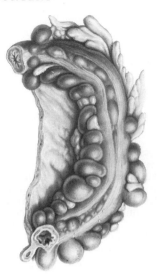

FIG. 1029.—Pelvic colon with
multiple diverticula.

pressure (fig. 1030 *a*, *b*, and *c*). This may lead to diverticulum formation (fig. 1030*d*). Segmentation plays an important part in colonic physiology. Emotion and drugs like morphine and prostigmine[1] increase segmentation and intracolonic pressure (see treatment). Muscular hypertrophy and increased elastin tissue are noted in colonic segments effected by diverticular changes.

Diverticulitis is the secondary state and is due to inflammation of one or more diverticula, usually with some pericolitis. Episodes of diverticulitis may be followed by years free of symptoms, but the condition is essentially progressive—the longer the duration, the worse are the symptoms and the greater the risk of complications. Diverticulitis is not a precancerous condition, but cancer may coexist.

The Complications are:

1. Recurrent periodic inflammation and pain.

2. Perforation leading to general peritonitis or local (pericolic) abscess formation.

3. Intestinal obstruction, due to progressive fibrosis leading to stenosis.

4. Haemorrhage: diverticulitis may present with *profuse* colonic haemorrhage in about 17% of cases, often requiring blood transfusion.

5. Fistula formation (vesico-colic, vagino-colic, entero-colic, colo-cutaneous) occurs in about 5% of cases.

Clinical Features—Diverticulosis may be asymptomatic, but the disordered colonic function may cause symptoms of distension, flatulence and a sensation of heaviness in the lower abdomen. Excessive colonic segmentation can cause severe colic pain in the left iliac fossa. This pain waxes and wanes too fast to be compatible with the onset and resolution of inflammation. Indeed, the sigmoid colon may only have thickened muscle. This condition is called *Painful Diverticular Disease* and is, in fact, due to spastic obstruction of the colon (Painter).

---

[1] Muscle relaxants of the curare type usually require the use of prostigmine at the end of an operation. This use of prostigmine may prejudice the safety of a colonic anastomosis.

Neil Stamford Painter, Contemporary. Surgeon, Manor House Hospital, London.

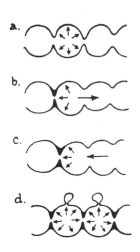

FIG. 1030.—Segmentation of the colon.

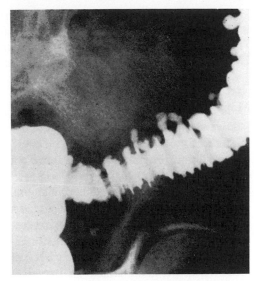

FIG. 1031.—Barium enema showing diverticular disease—'saw teeth' and diverticula.

Diverticulitis.—More persistent lower abdominal pain, usually in the left iliac fossa, or evidence of peritonitis, should always bring the diagnosis to mind in patients of either sex over the age of 40. Fever, malaise, and a leucocytosis help to differentiate diverticulitis from painful diverticular disease. The patient may pass loose stools or may be constipated. Abdominal distension may be relieved by flatus. The lower abdomen is tender especially on the left, occasionally in the right, iliac fossa. The sigmoid colon may be palpable, tender and thickened. Rectal examination may reveal a tender mass. The condition has been likened to left-sided appendicitis. Any urinary symptoms may herald the formation of a vesico-colic fistula, which leads to pneumaturia (flatus in the urine), and even faeces in the urine.

Diagnosis

Radiology.—Diverticulosis must never be blamed for symptoms unless all other diseases of the gastrointestinal tract have been excluded by barium meal, barium enema and by sigmoidoscopy. The diagnosis of acute diverticulitis is made on clinical grounds and is confirmed by barium enema and sigmoidoscopy *only when any acute inflammation has subsided* as an enema given in an acute attack may cause perforation and peritonitis. Diverticula may be revealed by a barium meal followed through the gut, but a barium enema must also be done to exclude a carcinoma and to assess the extent of the disease. Barium enema may show diverticula and the typical narrowed sigmoid. Sometimes no diverticula are seen but only the 'saw tooth' appearance of the 'pre-diverticular state' (fig. 1031). Such spastic strictures are sometimes relaxed by Probanthine and this may help to differentiate them from a neoplasm.

Sigmoidoscopy.—The mucosa may be normal. In acute attacks, sigmoidoscopy may be painful and the mucosa inflamed. The bowel may be rigid, narrow and acutely angled at about 15 cm so that the instrument cannot be passed further. The necks of diverticula are seldom seen. Sigmoidoscopy and colonoscopy excludes a neoplasm but diverticula are best diagnosed by barium enema.

Management

Diverticulosis should be treated with a high residue diet containing roughage in the form of wholemeal bread and flour, fruit and vegetables. Bulk formers such as bran, Celevac, Isogel, may be given until the stools are soft. Painful diverticular disease may require bed rest and antispasmodic drugs. Habitual liquid paraffin and purgative-taking should be avoided.

Acute diverticulitis is treated by bed rest, warmth to the abdomen, anti-spasmodic drugs and a 7–10 day course of broad-spectrum antibiotics (*e.g.* cefuroxamine) and metronidazole ('Flagyl'). Morphine and enemas are contraindicated. Probanthine rests the bowel but in large doses may cause ileus and retention of urine. After the acute attack has subsided the diagnosis must be confirmed by radiology and a carcinoma must be excluded.

Operative Procedures for Diverticular Disease.—About 10% of the patients require operation, either for recurrent attacks which make life a misery or for the complications:

1. *The ideal operation*, done as an interval procedure after careful preparation of the gut (p. 1058), is a *One Stage Resection*. This involves removal of the affected segment—10 to 20 cm long, and restoration of continuity by end-to-end anastomosis.

At operation the sigmoid loop is often found adherent in the pouch of Douglas. Patient yet persistent dissection, taking care to preserve the rectum in the retroperitoneal area, is rewarded by exposure of normal rectum and greater mobility.

2. *BUT, if there is obstruction, inflammatory oedema and adhesions or the bowel is loaded with faeces*, a preliminary transverse colostomy can be done as a first stage; the second stage of resection is performed after 3 weeks or when the inflammation has subsided. The colostomy is closed after a further 2 weeks. Because of a higher mortality associated with staged operations, experienced surgeons are now willing to do acute colectomies for emergency situations, but an immediate anastomosis should be avoided. In obstructed cases, the bowel can be decompressed by 'on-table' wash-throughs to make restoration of bowel continuity safer if an anastomosis is under consideration (Dudley).

3. *In acute perforation*, peritonitis which soon becomes general is usually purulent with a mortality of about 15%. Faecal peritonitis carries a 50% mortality. Pneumoperitoneum is present, but in this acute emergency often a diagnosis of peritonitis calling for urgent laparotomy is the only diagnosis which can be made. There is a choice of procedures:

(*a*) *Proximal colostomy* with suture of perforation.

(*b*) *Exteriorisation* of the affected bowel which is then opened as a colostomy.

(*c*) *Primary resection* of the inflamed bowel with immediate anastomosis in experienced hands. Primary resection removes the toxic tissues and may lower

Hugh F. Dudley, Contemporary. Professor of Surgery, St. Mary's Hospital, London.

the mortality of this desperate emergency. Permanent colostomy after excision with closure of bowel below the disease is safer (Hartmann's operation, see p. 1129).

All the above procedures must be accompanied by drainage of the abdomen. Simple drainage alone should be reserved for a localised pericolic abscess.

4. *Fistulas* can only be cured by resection of the diseased bowel and closure of the fistula. Ideally these procedures are done at the same operation but a staged procedure with a preliminary colostomy is sometimes necessary. Diverticular disease is a benign condition so the surgeon plays for safety even if it means staged procedures.

5. *Sigmoid Myotomy (Reilly).*—Resection of the thickened sigmoid colon may be avoided by sigmoid myotomy. The operation consists of a longitudinal incision through one taenia extending over the length of the affected colon. The incision is deepened until the mucosa bulges as in a Heller or Ramstedt's operation. This restores the colonic lumen and lowers the intracolonic pressures. The operation must never be used in acute diverticulitis. There is a risk of leakage post-operatively. The operation has not gained acceptance, and other types of myotomy are being tried out, *e.g.* multiple transverse myotomies of the taenia coli without much success.

DIFFERENTIATION OF DIVERTICULITIS FROM CARCINOMA OF THE COLON

These conditions co-exist in 12% of cases:

	Diverticulitis	Carcinoma
History	Long	Short
Pain	More common	
Mass	25% have tenderness	25% painless
Bleeding	17% often profuse, periodic	65%—usually small amounts persistently
X-ray	Diffuse change	Localised: no relaxation with Probanthine
Sigmoidoscopy	Inflammatory change over an area	No inflammation until ulcer reached
Colonoscopy	No carcinoma seen	Carcinoma seen & biopsied

Exploration may be necessary, but even then, differentiation may be difficult until histology is available. Weight loss, falling haemoglobin, and a persistently positive occult blood test are sinister features.

Solitary diverticulum of the caecum and ascending colon, is rare, and it is congenital for it has a complete muscular coat. it is usually situated just above the ileocaecal valve. Inflammation of such a diverticulum is indistinguishable from acute appendicitis. Recurrent diverticulitis may cause the formation of a mass whose nature can only be ascertained after resection of the caecum. An uninflamed caecal diverticulum found casually at laparotomy should be invaginated with a purse-string suture.

ULCERATIVE COLITIS

Aetiology.—The cause is unknown. In spite of intensive bacteriological studies, no organisms or group of organisms can be incriminated. Possibly the disease is linked with emotional stress. It may be related to the auto-immune diseases, but this is by no means certain. Some cases are allergic to milk protein. In cases of extensive ulceration secondary infection plays a large part. In some families there is a strong tendency for the disease to occur in successive generations: either a genetic predisposition is inherent in the members of these families, or an

Michael Charles Tempest Reilly, Contemporary. Previously Surgeon, Plymouth General Hospital, Plymouth, England.

unidentified environmental factor is present. The disease has been rare in Eastern populations, but is now being reported more commonly, suggesting an environmental cause that has developed as a result of increasing 'Westernisation' of diet and/or social habits and better access to medical care.

Pathology.—In 95% of cases the disease starts in the rectum and spreads proximally. When the ileocaecal valve is incompetent, retrograde ('backwash') ileitis involving the last foot (30 cm) of the ileum is liable to occur.

The disease is characterised by the appearance of multiple minute ulcers—sometimes the ulcers are discrete, in others there is a sea of ulceration. Microscopical evidence nearly always proves that the ulceration is more severe and extensive than the gross appearance indicates (Cuthbert Dukes). As time goes on the small ulcers are apt to coalesce to form larger ones, mainly due to the crypts of Lieberkühn becoming distended with pus and bursting into the bowel. When the ulceration extends into the submucosa it causes reflex muscle spasm,[1] and the appearance of a stricture. In long-standing cases there is always considerable intramural fibrosis, causing the affected part of the colon to become permanently contracted. In addition, attempts at healing may produce epithelial thickening between the ulcers—the so-called pseudopolyposis.

Clinical Features.—The onset of the disease, more common in women than men is the 3rd, 4th, and 2nd decade, in that order; exceptionally it is encountered in childhood. The first symptom is watery diarrhoea occurring day and night, in a person of previously normal bowel habit. A rectal discharge of mucus, sometimes blood-stained and sometimes purulent is very common. Pain as an early symptom is unusual. In the majority of cases, the disease is chronic, characterised by relapses and remissions. In general, a bad prognosis is indicated by (1) a severe initial attack; (2) disease involving the whole colon; (3) increasing age, especially after sixty years. If the disease remains confined to the left colon, the outlook is better.

Two types are encountered:

Fulminating type (5%) is ushered in with a temperature of 38·9° to 39·4°C and incessant diarrhoea containing blood, mucus, and pus; the patient looks and feels very ill. There may be abdominal distension due to toxic dilatation of the colon. Here immediate surgery is indicated. The condition must be differentiated from dysentery, typhoid and amoebic colitis (see below). A low serum albumin level is associated with the degree of severity of an attack and can influence the decision to operate.

Chronic Type (95%).—As a rule the initial attack is of moderate severity, but exacerbations occur at intervals of weeks, months or, in mild cases, years. As the disease progresses the patient becomes wasted from diarrhoea, and severely anaemic from loss of blood. Often during the attacks there are ten to twenty stools a day, accompanied by tenesmus. The frequency of the motions and the degree of invalidism go hand in hand, and are proportional to the extent of the involvement of the colon. Lesions of limited length are commonly found in milder cases. Sometimes the disease is confined entirely to the right hemi-colon. When the whole colon is involved the patient may be so weak as to be partially or wholly bed-ridden.

---

[1] Dilatation may occur in acute cases = acute toxic megacolon.

Cuthbert Esquire Dukes, 1890–1977. Pathologist, St. Mark's Hospital, London.
Johann Nathaniel Lieberkühn, 1711–1756. Anatomist, Berlin. He demonstrated his anatomical preparations in London, and was awarded the F.R.S.

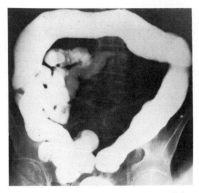

FIG. 1032.—Advanced ulcerative colitis. Showing tubular contraction and short-ening of the colon.
(*W. B. Gabriel, FRCS, London.*)

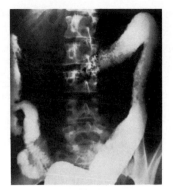

FIG. 1033.—Ulcerative colitis showing pseudopolyposis ('stippled' area in descending colon).
(*Dr. Clifford Hawkins, Birmingham.*)

Radiology after a barium enema[1] shows one of the following:

(1) The earliest sign is loss of haustration, especially in the distal colon. Embellished disease will show:

(2) A narrow contracted (pipe stem) colon (fig. 1032).

(3) Alteration in mucosal outline.

(4) Pseudopolyposis (fig. 1033) in 15% of cases.

Sigmoidoscopy is indispensable in the diagnosis of early cases and in mild cases when the pathological effects of the disease are insufficient to alter the barium shadow. The initial findings are those of proctitis—the mucosa is hypera-emic, bleeds on touch and there is considerable exudate. Later, tiny ulcers may be seen and appear to coalesce. This is very different from the picture seen in *amoebic dysentery*, where there are large deep ulcerations with the intervening mucosa comparatively healthy. As the disease progresses, the ulceration may become so severe that practically no normal mucous membrane remains.

A barium enema should be avoided during the fulminating phase. Rectal biopsy is valuable not only in establishing the diagnosis, but also as an index of the effect of therapy.

Local Complications

Pseudopolyposis 15% (see above).

Carcinoma.—Although this is an important complication, it must be seen in its true perspective. The overall risk is about 3·5%; this risk is much less in early cases but increases with the duration of the disease. Thus, after twenty years of the disease, the risk may be as much as 12%. Carcinoma is more liable to occur where the whole colon is involved and where the disease started in early life. Carcinomatous change may occur at many sites at once and these, often, are atypical. The colon is involved rather than the rectum and maximal incidence is during the 4th decade (Truelove). The golden rule is that after the disease has been present for more than ten years, regular radiological and colonoscopic checks must be done, even though the disease seems to be quiescent. It has been shown that the presence in a rectal biopsy of severe epithelial dysplasia denotes a pre-malignant potential, and may be the only sign that a carcinoma has already developed. At least one annual biopsy of all long-term cases of total colitis is indicated to enable this

---

[1] For safety reasons in acute cases it is best to avoid barium and use Gastrografin without bowel preparation = the 'instant enema' technique.

Sidney Charles Truelove, Contemporary. Physician, Radcliffe Infirmary, Oxford, England.

mucosal change to be detected (Morson and Peng). This precaution is also necessary after operations that have conserved the rectal stump.

Fibrous Stricture occurs in 6% of cases. The common sites are the rectosigmoid junction and the anal canal. Although they usually respond to simple dilation where the disease is confined to the distal colon, surgery may be advisable if the whole colon is involved.

Toxic Dilatation (1·5%) occurs in the fulminating type of the disease. It may result in perforation. Both require immediate surgery. Excessive steroid therapy may be a factor. Frequently the only sign the perforation has occurred is abdominal distension. This is a cardinal sign of impending doom.

Massive Haemorrhage (3%) usually arises from the rectum rather than the colon.

Recto-vaginal Fistulas[1] (3%), **Fistula in Ano** (4%), **Ischio-rectal Abscess** (4%), and **Haemorrhoids** (20%) also occur (Truelove).

General Complications

Liver Changes Abnormal liver function tests occur in 50% of patients at some time during the course of the disease. Cirrhosis occurs in 4% of patients.

Skin Lesions (18·5%) including Pyodermia Gangrenosum (0·5%) and Erythema Nodosum (2%).

Arthritis (5%) usually of small joints, may occur at any stage of the disease.

Iritis (7%), **Ankylosing Spondylitis** (2%), **Stomatitis** (10%), **Renal Disease** (5%) and **Anaemia** (20%) are also important complications. **Sclerosing cholangitis** (1%) and **Carcinoma of the bile duct** (1%) are other important complications.

Treatment

Several agents may induce a remission but it is difficult to predict the outcome in individual cases. The main *general principles* are:

(1) Maintenance of fluid and electrolyte balance.

(2) Anaemia must be speedily corrected.

(3) Adequate nutrition—at least 3000 C (12,560 kJ) per day—with high protein, carbohydrate and vitamin content and low fat.

(4) Sedatives and tranquillisers are useful. Antibiotics may precipitate moniliasis.

Specific Treatment

Quiescent Cases.—Are best maintained on Salazopyrin (2 g daily). This has been shown to reduce the incidence of relapse.

Mild to Moderate Relapses.—The dose of Salazopyrin is increased (4–6 g daily). Topical steroids are of real value particularly in the distal type of the disease. Retention enemas of prednisolone phosphate 20 mg in 100 ml daily are commenced. If the response is inadequate, treatment should be as in—

Acute Fulminating Cases.—Systemic prednisolone 20 mg or more daily may be required for up to three weeks.

Dangers of Prolonged Steroid Therapy.—1. Not only is there an increased risk of massive haemorrhage and of free perforation into the peritoneal cavity, but in patients who have not responded to a course of steroids over a period of four to six weeks, the colonic wall becomes excessively friable and in some areas disintegrates, its place being taken by the parietes or adjacent viscera, usually the small bowel. In such cases the surgeon may be unable to remove the colon (Brooke).

2. Steroid therapy renders the patient more susceptible to pyogenic infection.

---

[1] Recto-vaginal and anal fistulas usually mean that the underlying condition is Crohn's disease and not ulcerative colitis.

Basil Clifford Morson, Contemporary. Pathologist and Director of Research, St. Mark's Hospital for Diseases of the Rectum and Colon, London.
Lillian Shu Chao Peng, Contemporary. Histopathologist in Charge, Tumour Reference Collection, Imperial Cancer Research Fund, London.
Bryan Nicholas Brooke, Contemporary. Formerly Professor of Surgery, St. George's Hospital, London.

Indications for Surgery

(1) To save life—fulminating cases, toxic dilatation, severe haemorrhage, perforation.

(2) Local complications (p. 1041).

(3) General complications (p. 1042).

(4) Risk of neoplastic change—especially in pseudo-polyposis and colitis of long standing.

(5) Onset in children or adolescents.

(6) Chronic invalidism.

Between 15 and 20% of sufferers are recommended for surgical treatment by their physicians.

When surgical treatment is advised, about six days' intensive pre-operative preparation by the methods already enumerated is carried out.

Operations

(i) The classical procedure is *a one-stage total procto-colectomy with ileostomy*. If the disease is acute, it is wise to leave the rectal stump and either close it or bring it out as a midline colostomy or mucous fistula. The rectum can be removed about eight weeks later.

(ii) Some advocate *total colectomy* with immediate or subsequent *ileo-rectal anastomosis*. If the degree of rectal inflammation makes the ileo-rectal anastomosis unsound, a temporary loop ileostomy proximal to the anastomosis is employed. After the operation a physiological bowel frequency of three to five actions a day is to be expected. It should not be performed if peri-anal complications are present. Should ileo-rectal anastomosis fail because of recurrent severe disease, the rectal stump can be excised and a permanent ileostomy established. This operation can be done in many cases (Aylett) but all patients require regular post-operative checks in case a carcinoma develops in the retained rectum.

(iii) *Ileostomy alone* may sometimes be indicated for a gravely ill patient with fulminating disease and localised abscess around a perforation.

Colectomy is not a difficult operation when it is performed on an emaciated individual whose peritoneal cavity is free from adhesions. After a successful ileostomy both these desiderata are absent; firstly, the patient has gained weight and, secondly, adhesions are bound to be present, especially in the right iliac fossa.

(iv) *Total proctocolectomy and ileo-anal pouch*: this operation substitutes a 'pouch' of ileum for the rectum and allows for normal defaecation if successful: at present the operation is confined to special colo-proctological institutes: in many cases the 'pouch' needs

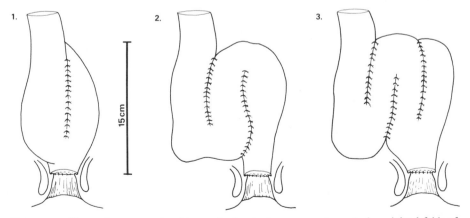

FIG. 1034.—Ileo-anal anastomosis with pouch. A substitute rectum is made from joined folds of ileum to form an expanded 'pouch' of small intestine. The pouch is then joined directly to the anus at the level of the dentate line, all other anal mucosa having been removed. Three ways of forming a pouch are illustrated: 1. A simple reversed 'J'; 2. An 'S' pouch; 3. A 'W' pouch.

Stanley Aylett, Contemporary. Consulting Surgeon, Westminster Hospital, London.

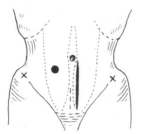

FIG. 1035.—Site of the ileostomy. The 'trephine' wound should be at least 5cm from all scars and bony points.

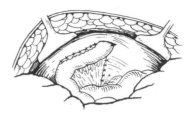

FIG. 1036.—Suture of the mesentery to the parietal peritoneum, to prevent prolapse.
(After J. C. Goligher, FRCS, Leeds.)

to be irrigated by the patient to achieve evacuation (fig. 1034). The techniques are highly specialised.

Ileostomy

As the ileostomy is nearly always permanent, the success of the operation lies in scrupulous attention to the details of technique in siting and fashioning the ideal 'spout'. It is best to arrange the position of the stoma beforehand with the patient (fig. 1035). The ileum should be brought through the lateral edge of the rectus abdominis muscle.

A disc of skin not more than 3 cm in diameter is removed at least 5 cm lateral to the umbilicus (fig. 1035). The abdomen is opened by a left paramedian incision and the ileum is divided near its termination, together with its mesentery. It may be necessary to divide the ileum more proximally if the terminal ileum is diseased also.

Important steps in the performance of ileostomy are (a) to close the peritoneal space on the external side of the ileostomy (otherwise a tunnel exists which invites intestinal obstruction), and (b) to anchor the anterior edge of the mesentery to the parietal peritoneum (fig. 1036). The latter prevents prolapse of the mucous membrane. The ileostomy opening must be prepared meticulously. A disc of tissue equal to the size of the skin disc should be removed from the anterior and posterior rectus sheath so that no stricture will occur in the parieties. The peritoneum is opened by a cruciform incision. About 7·5 cm of the divided ileum (closed temporarily with a noncrushing clamp) is brought through the opening and its periphery is stitched to the skin edges by interrupted catgut in such a way that it is everted to form a 'spout' projecting 4 cm from the skin surface. The greatest care must be taken in the construction of this projection (fig. 1037). A proctocolectomy is carried out and the abdomen is closed. A disposable plastic ileostomy bag (fig. 1038) is cut so that it exactly fits the skin at the muco-cutaneous junction and is fixed in position by latex rubber adhesive.

Care of Ileostomy.—During the first few post-operative days the fluid electrolyte balance must be adjusted with great care. For permanent use it is wise to fit a Chiron-type bag which has a firm rubber flange to be attached around the ileostomy spout. It is supported both by a waist strap and also made adherent to the skin by special double-sided adhesive plaster. The bag is attached to and detached from the flange which remains adherent to the skin for as long as is convenient. Great care must be taken that the lower rim of the bag does not press on and penetrate the lower margin of the ileostomy 'spout'. If soreness and excoriation of the skin occur as a result, a paste of aluminium 10 parts and zinc oxide 90 parts is helpful. Also a paste of Karaya gum (Goligher) acts as an adhesive and protective. The stools thicken in a few weeks and are semi-solid in a few months. A thin discharge from the stoma may indicate bolus obstruction and stenosis; digital dilatation will help to relieve this.

Continent Ileostomy (Koch).—Professor Nils Koch has recently developed an ileostomy with a 'reservoir' in the terminal ileum that opens to the surface by a one-way valve that prevents any escape of ileal effluent until a catheter is passed through the valve-spout

John Cedric Goligher, Contemporary. Emeritus Professor Surgery, Leeds, England.
Professor Nils Koch, Contemporary. Professor of Surgery, Malmo, Sweden.

Fig. 1037.—Suturing the free extremity of the proximal ileum to the skin edges.

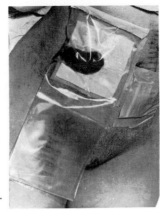

Fig. 1038.—Disposable ileostomy bag.
(Bryan N. Brooke, FRCS, London.)

to empty the ileal pouch. This type of ileostomy requires no bags or appliances and can be emptied at will by the patient. The ileostomy is called 'continent' for this reason. The continent ileostomy is not easy to construct, and has a considerable morbidity: even the occasional death has been reported. It should not be used routinely at present. An alternative procedure, that of construction of an ileal reservoir with endo-anal anastomosis has recently been launched. A satisfactory degree of continence and control of evacuation is claimed (Parks) (p. 1043).

INTESTINAL AMOEBIASIS

Amoebiasis denotes an infestation with *Entamoeba histolytica*. Contrary to general belief, *E. histolytica* is not strictly a tropical parasite: *it has a world-wide distribution*, and is found in Great Britain particularly in the southern counties. It is surprisingly common in overcrowded institutions. The reason why in some cases it becomes pathogenic is unknown.

Life History of the Parasite.—The active form of the parasite or trophozoite lives in the intestinal mucous membrane, where it ingests red blood corpuscles and other cells, and multiplies by mitosis. Should the parasite become pathogenic, it makes its way into the follicles of Lieberkühn, and, by dissolving interglandular tissue by cytolysins, submucous loculi are produced. Some of these burst through the mucous membrane to become amoebic ulcers. While the trophozoites continue their activities in the base of the ulcer, others cease to feed, migrate towards the surface, and become transformed into cysts (fig. 883), which pass into the outer world with the faeces. Amoebiasis is transmitted mainly in drinking water.

Pathology.—The ulcers, which have been described as 'bottle-necked' because of their considerably undermined edges, have a yellow necrotic floor, from which blood and pus exude. While on rare occasions the ulcers are scattered throughout the large intestine, in 75% they are confined to the lower sigmoid and the upper rectum.

Biopsy material is obtained by scraping the suspected area of mucosa with a long-handled Volkmann's spoon; this removes a thin slice of the diseased mucosa, which must be examined immediately. It should be noted particularly that the finding of *Entamoeba histolytica* is not conclusive evidence that the symptoms are due to amoebiasis. On numerous occasions a positive slide examination has caused the clinician to assume that the diagnosis has been established when there has been a proximal carcinoma of the colon and the *Entamoebae histolyticae* have been non-pathogenic and incidental.

Clinical Features.—Dysentery is only one manifestation of the disease. In various guises amoebiasis obtrudes itself into the surgeon's diagnostic arena:

Sir Alan Parks, P.R.C.S., 1920–1982. Surgeon, St. Mark's and the London Hospitals, London.
Richard von Volkmann, 1830–1889. Professor of Surgery, Halle, Germany.

Appendicitis or Amoebic Typhlitis[1]?—In tropical countries where amoebiasis is endemic, this is a constantly recurring problem. To operate upon a patient with amoebic dysentery without the precautions subsequently described is to invite an exacerbation of amoebiasis that may prove fatal. Especially in cases where a palpable mass is present, the bowel is friable and satisfactory closure of the appendix stump becomes difficult or impossible. The death-rate from peritonitis and wound infection in the notorious Chicago epidemic of amoebiasis in 1933 was appalling, which emphasises that surgeons in temperate climates should be familiar with the condition. In the case of amoebic typhlitis there is rarely rigidity, and pain commences in the right iliac fossa. In amoebic typhlitis there are two characteristic and localised zones of tenderness on deep palpation—one over the caecum and one over the sigmoid. The latter is sharply defined, and being comparable to McBurney's point on the right side, it has been aptly named '*the amoebic point*' by Sir Philip Manson-Bahr. Routine sigmoidoscopy is of great value. If doubt still exists, 60 mg of emetine hydrochloride in 20 ml of isotonic saline solution given intravenously very slowly is likely to ameliorate the symptoms within two hours (Andreasen).

Perforation.—The most common sites are the caecum and recto-sigmoid. Usually perforation occurs into a confined space where adhesions have previously formed, and a pericolic abscess results, which eventually needs draining. When there is sudden faecal flooding of the general peritoneal cavity, drainage of the region of the perforation, gastrointestinal aspiration, intravenous fluid replacement, antibiotic therapy, and a full course of emetine are sometimes successful.

Severe rectal haemorrhage due to the separation of sloughs is liable to occur.

Granuloma.—Progressive amoebic invasion of the wall of the rectum or colon, with secondary inflammation, may produce a granulomatous mass indistinguishable from a carcinoma. The exhibition of emetine as a therapeutic test will prevent mistakes in diagnosis. Amoebiasis and carcinoma occasionally co-exist.

Fibrous stricture may follow the healing of extensive amoebic ulcers.

Intestinal obstruction is a common complication of amoebiasis, and the obstruction is due to the adhesions associated with pericolitis and a large granuloma.

Paracolic abscess, ischio-rectal abscess, and fistula occur from perforation by amoebae of the intestinal wall followed by secondary infection.

Ulcerative colitis.—A search for amoebae should always be made in the stools of patients believed to be suffering from ulcerative colitis.

Treatment.—Metronidazole (Flagyl) is the first line drug, 800 mg t.d.s. for 7–10 days. The patient must avoid taking alcohol. Emetine hydrochloride, 60 mg daily s.c. for 4 days, is the alternative if metronidazole cannot be taken by mouth. The patient must be kept in bed during and for one day after the course of emetine. Diloxanide furoate 500 mg t.d.s. for 10 days is another intra-lumenal drug. Intestinal antibiotics, *e.g.* tetracycline, improve results in the chronic stages, probably by coping with superadded infection.

THE SURGICAL COMPLICATIONS OF TYPHOID AND PARATYPHOID

Chloromycetin exerts a rapidly curative effect on typhoid and paratyphoid infections; consequently complications are uncommon. When complications of typhoid arise, chloromycetin should be given in addition to other necessary treatment, not forgetting that this antibiotic destroys the organisms responsible for the production of vitamin B complex which must be replaced.

1. *Paralytic ileus* is the commonest complication of typhoid.

2. *Intestinal haemorrhage* may be the leading symptom. The condition must be distinguished from purpura with intestinal symptoms, and intussusception. A Widal reaction should be employed and, if negative, repeated in suspected cases. Urgent blood transfusion will be required.

3. *Perforation.*—Perforation of a typhoid ulcer usually occurs during the third week; occasionally it is the first intimation of the disease (ambulatory typhoid). The ulcer is parallel to the long axis of the gut, and is situated in the lower ileum. In paratyphoid B, perforation of the large intestine sometimes occurs. Formerly treatment was to perform laparotomy under local anaesthesia, and to close the perforation. The results were so poor that the conservative treatment of peritonitis plus chloromycetin yields better results.

---

[1] Typhlitis = inflammation of the caecum.

Charles McBurney, 1845–1913. Surgeon, Roosevelt Hospital, New York, U.S.A.
Sir Philip Manson-Bahr, 1881–1966. Physician to the Hospital for Tropical Diseases. London.
Anthony Turner Andreasen, Contemporary. (See footnote p. 942.)

4. *Cholecystitis.*—Acute typhoid cholecystitis is not uncommon and perforation can occur. Gallstones occasionally contain typhoid bacilli. Chronic typhoid cholecystitis can result in the patient becoming a typhoid carrier (Chapter 47).

5. *Phlebitis.*—Venous thrombosis, particularly of the left common iliac vein, is an occasional complication of typhoid fever.

6. *Genito-urinary Complications.*—Typhoid cystitis, pyelitis, bacilluria, and epididymo-orchitis all occur.

7. *Joints.*—All degrees of arthritis, from a mild effusion to suppuration, occur as a complication of this disease.

8. *Bone.*—Typhoid osteomyelitis and typhoid spine.

9. *Larynx.*—Typhoid perichondritis is met with occasionally, and typhoid laryngitis has been known to obstruct the airway.

CROHN'S DISEASE (Regional enteritis)

Aetiology.—No causative organism has been found in the lesion or in the stools although abnormal forms of *B. coli* have been discovered in most patients.

Electron microscope studies have shown that in Crohn's disease faecal bacteria enter the colonic wall. Whether it is these or something ingested or a metabolic product which acts as the hapten is not known, but granulomas develop (Aluwihare). There is evidence that heredity is a factor. Possibly Crohn's disease develops in patients with a relatively complete genotype. Ulcerative colitis is common in relatives of patients with Crohn's disease, but the converse is not common, suggesting that people with ulcerative colitis may have fewer of these genes. As with ulcerative colitis it is now believed that Crohn's disease is a pre-cancerous condition, but the incidence of malignant change is not as high as in ulcerative colitis, and is most manifest in the ileum.

Pathology.—It is essentially a cicatrising inflammation with ulceration of the mucosa. It usually commences at or near the ileo-caecal valve, and extends upwards along the ileum for about 30 cm, but as little as 5 cm, and, more often, as much as 1·2 metres may be implicated. In acute cases the affected intestine is seen to be swollen, bright pink in colour, and with a fibrinous exudate on its peritoneal surface; in chronic cases hyperaemia is less in evidence. On palpation the intestinal wall feels like a hose-pipe. The mesentery of the involved intestine is exceedingly thickened, oedematous, and contains enlarged and fleshy lymph nodes. Unlike tuberculosis, the affected lymph nodes neither break down nor calcify. Tracing the diseased ileum upwards, it terminates abruptly in normal intestine. Above this there is commonly another (short) area of diseased intestine; this is a so-called 'skip' lesion. Doubtless a comparatively inconspicuous additional lesion is sometimes overlooked, and is one cause of recurrence after resection. In 6% of cases there is an extension into the caecum and at times the ascending colon is implicated in the interrupted manner referred to. Examples of primary Crohn's disease of the colon, jejunum, duodenum, and even of the stomach and anus have been reported, which justifies the newer term, regional enteritis. Crohn's colitis is now nearly as common as the ileal form in some series.

Pathological Histology.—A characteristic finding is granulomatous infiltration of lymphatics of the submucosa with the presence of non-caseating giant-celled systems. In the late stages of the disease fibrosis extends into and obliterates the submucosa, but usually giant-celled systems can be found in the related mesenteric lymph nodes. An experienced histologist can easily distinguish the condition from tuberculosis.

Clinical Features.—The disease, which is independent of age, sex, social and economic conditions, or geographical location, is increasing in frequency. To some extent it is familial. Complications are the same as for ulcerative colitis (pp. 1041–1042) except that the cancer risk is very low.

Acute Crohn's disease occurs only in 5% of cases. The symptoms and signs resemble those of acute appendicitis, with one exception, *viz.* diarrhoea almost invariably precedes the acute attack. Exceptionally, perforation of the intestine resulting in local or diffuse peritonitis, occurs. Acute colitis with toxic megacolon can occur with Crohn's disease but is rarer than in ulcerative colitis.

Burrill Bernard Crohn, Contemporary. Gastroenterologist, Mount Sinai Hospital, New York. First described this disease in 1932.
A. P. R. Aluwihare, Contemporary. Professor of Surgery, Sri Lanka.

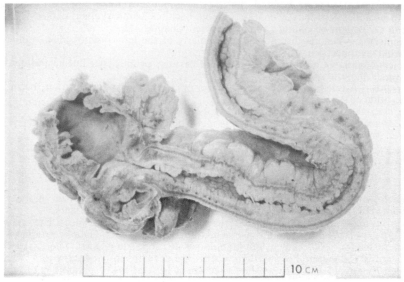

FIG. 1039.—Crohn's disease. Stage of cicatricial contracture.
(From the R.C.S. Museum, Professor G. Cunningham.)

Chronic Crohn's disease is the usual form of the disease. It can be divided into three stages, but sometimes the second stage is lacking.

First Stage.—There is a history of mild diarrhoea extending over months or years, occurring continuously or in bouts accompanied by intestinal colic, relieved by defaecation. Intermittent pyrexia, seldom more than 37.2°C is usual, but some patients are afebrile throughout. As a rule a tender mass can be felt in the right iliac fossa, and frequently by a pelvic examination also. There is often a moderate secondary anaemia. Occult blood and some mucus is present in the stools; two-thirds of the patients have some degree of steatorrhoea. *A perianal abscess* is a frequent accompaniment of early Crohn's disease. The cause is probably an infected anal crypt associated with the concomitant diarrhoea. The high incidence and diagnostic significance of perianal and perirectal abscesses and fistulas in patients with Crohn's disease is generally accepted.

Second stage.—Characterised by symptoms of acute or chronic intestinal obstruction. Cicatrisation of the granulomatous area has progressed to such an extent that the lumen of the affected portion of the intestine is narrowed (fig. 1039).

Third stage.—Adhesions form, sometimes accompanied by slow perforation of the intestinal wall. Adhesions are dense, abscess formation is common, and fistulous tracts are wont to develop:

(*a*) *Internally* into neighbouring hollow viscera, *e.g.* a redundant pelvic colon, or occasionally into the right side of the bladder. In all cases of enterocolic and vesico-intestinal fistulas the possibility of Crohn's disease should be considered.

(*b*) *Externally*, nearly always through the scar of a previous operation for the condition, *e.g.* appendicectomy.

Radiological Diagnosis.—X-ray examination after a barium meal often shows lack of segmentation and feeble or absent peristalsis in the affected portion of the intestine, the lumen of which remains constant in diameter. Radiologically, cases can be divided into stenosing and non-stenosing. In the non-stenosing phase straightening of the valvulae conniventes is characteristic. When ulceration has occurred multiple defects (cobblestone reticulation) can be seen after the barium has been evacuated from the segment in question. When cicatrisation has occurred the radiograph is particularly characteristic; sometimes the terminal ileum is so constricted that the 'string' sign of Kantor (fig. 1040) is seen. Characteristic linear fissures extending outwards through the bowel wall ('raspberry thorn' and 'rose thorn' types are very typical) are frequently seen outlined by the barium.

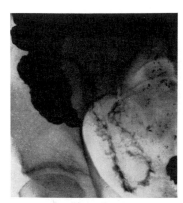

FIG. 1040.—The 'string' sign of Kantor. (Crohn's disease.)

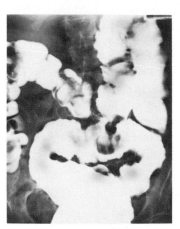

FIG. 1041.—Barium enema showing 'Scalloping' of the edges of the sigmoid in Pneumatosis Cystoides Intestinalis.

Treatment:

Medical Treatment.—In the early stages medical treatment is given an extended trial. It consists of rest in bed, a high protein diet with vitamin supplementation. Iron or blood transfusion may be required. Antibiotics—sulphaphthalidine is best—Salazopyrine or steroids (*e.g.* prednisone or A.C.T.H. depot) are used with caution. In the acute form of the disease, particularly acute colitis, azathioprine has proved effective in 5% of cases and may make colectomy unnecessary. It may also reduce fistula formation if operation is required. The drug may also have a place in the treatment of recurrences but not where obstruction is present. The response is less where the disease is chronic. Antibiotics are sometimes successful in abating an acute attack; gentamicin plus metronidazole are a good combination to try first of all. Malnourished patients can be improved by hyperalimentation regimes with either naso-gastric or parenteral feeding: in cases with fistulas a prolonged course of intra-venous feeding can sometimes cause the fistula to heal spontaneously (Williams).

Indications for Surgery.—These are: (1) failure to arrest the course of the disease by adequate medical treatment; (2) intestinal obstruction; (3) the presence of fistulas.

Operation.—Should the abdomen be opened on the mistaken diagnosis of acute appendicitis and Crohn's disease is found, the one thing *not* to do is to remove the appendix. Appendicectomy frequently determines the development of an external fistula. The correct procedure is to close the abdomen forthwith.

John Leonard Kantor, 1890–1947. Gastroenterologist, Presbyterian Hospital, New York, U.S.A.
John Alexander-Williams, Contemporary. Surgeon, Birmingham General Hospital, England.

Occasionally the condition resolves completely; more often chronic ileitis supervenes.

All operations have a high incidence of recurrence.

(i) *Right hemicolectomy.*—For ileo-caecal Crohn's disease, a right hemicolectomy with end-to-end ileo-transverse anastomosis is usually performed. In exceptional circumstances with unprepared bowel a defunctioning ileo-transverse bypass procedure can be justified.

(ii) *Segmental resection.*—Local segments of small or large bowel affected by Crohn's disease can be treated by a local resection.

(iii) *Colectomy and ileo-rectal anastomosis.*—This can be done for widespread colonic Crohn's disease.

(iv) *Temporary ileostomy.*—This may enable acute distal Crohn's disease to subside. In some cases this may allow consideration of restoration of bowel continuity later.

(v) *Strictureplasty.*—Multiple strictured areas of Crohn's disease have been treated by a local widening procedure (strictureplasty) (fig. 1042) to avoid excessive small bowel resection (see Chapter 57).

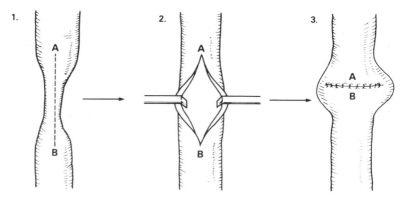

FIG. 1042.—Strictureplasty. 1. A strictured length of intestine is incised along its length. 2. The bowel is opened and the walls retracted as shown. 3. The bowel is resutured tranversely to widen the narrowed segment.

TUBERCULOSIS OF THE INTESTINE

1. **Ulcerative tuberculosis** is secondary to pulmonary tuberculosis, and arises as the result of swallowing tubercle bacilli. It is characterised by the presence of multiple ulcers in the terminal ileum, the long axis of each ulcer lying transversely. The serous coat overlying the ulcerated segment is thickened, injected, and sparsely bespattered with tubercles. Perforation is rare, but in patients who overcome the infection subsequent stricture or strictures of the ileum are rather frequent.

Clinical Features.—Diarrhoea is the predominant symptom; there is also loss of weight. The stools have a foetid odour, and contain pus and occult blood. Often the patient has received, or is receiving, treatment for pulmonary tuberculosis; more rarely pulmonary tuberculosis is detected for the first time in the course of the investigations.

Radiology.—A barium meal often discloses complete absence of filling of the lower ileum, the caecum, and most of the ascending colon, due to hypermotility of the ulcerated segment.

Treatment.—A course of chemotherapy is given (Chapter 4). Provided the intestinal ulceration is not a terminal event of advanced pulmonary tuberculosis, healing often occurs. Operation is required in the rare event of perforation. Occcasionally cicatrisation causes intestinal obstruction, and calls for surgical intervention.

2. **Hyperplastic tuberculosis** occurs most commonly in the ileo-caecal region, although solitary or multiple lesions of the lower ileum are met with occasionally. This form of intestinal tuberculosis is consequent upon the ingestion of *Mycobacterium tuberculosis* by a patient with a high resistance to the organism. In Western countries *Mycobacterium tuberculosis bovis* is often the causative organism, while in the East the human variety is the culprit (Toufeeq). The infection establishes itself in lymphoid follicles, and spreads to the submucous and subserous planes. The resulting chronic inflammation causes much thickening of the intestinal wall, and consequent narrowing of its lumen. There is early involvement of regional lymph nodes, which may caseate. Unlike Crohn's disease (which in many respects this disease simulates), abscess and fistula formation are rare.

Untreated, sooner or later subacute or acute intestinal obstruction supervenes, and in the East, not infrequently, impaction of an enterolith within the narrowed lumen is the precipitating cause.

Clinical Features.—Attacks of abdominal pain with intermittent diarrhoea are the premonitory symptoms. Frequently, the presenting picture is that of the 'blind loop' syndrome. The ileum above the partial obstruction is distended and the stasis and consequent infection lead to steatorrhoea, anaemia and loss of weight. Sometimes the presenting picture is that of a mass in the right iliac fossa in a patient with vague ill health. This finding raises the possibility of an appendix mass, a carcinoma of the caecum, Crohn's disease or a tuberculous or actinomycotic granuloma of the caecum. The problem can be quite perplexing.

Radiography.—In an established case a barium meal reveals a long, narrow filling defect consisting of the terminal ileum and ascending colon, lying vertically. The caecum may become subhepatic.

Treatment.—When the diagnosis is certain, and the patient has not yet developed obstructive symptoms, sanatorium treatment with chemotherapy is advised and may completely cure the condition. If obstruction is present, operative treatment is required. Right hemicolectomy with removal of the diseased segment of ileum is the treatment of choice. In patients with intestinal obstruction, and those in poor general condition, a defunctioning ileocolostomy similar to that recommended for Crohn's disease is advisable. If necessary resection can be undertaken later, for frequently striking improvement occurs after ileocolostomy and general treatment. However, without formal resection, there is always a considerable risk of further recrudescence of the disease, which may involve the recent by-pass anastomosis as well.

ACTINOMYCOSIS OF THE RIGHT ILIAC FOSSA

Abdominal actinomycosis is rare. Unlike intestinal tuberculosis, cicatrisation and consequent narrowing of the lumen of the intestine do not occur, neither do the mesenteric lymph nodes become involved. However, suppuration supervenes, and the disease spreads into the retroperitoneal tissues, the abdominal wall becomes the seat of multiple indurated discharging sinuses, and the liver becomes involved by way of the portal vein.

Clinical Features.—The usual history is that appendicectomy has been performed for appendicitis. About three weeks after the operation a mass forms in the right iliac fossa, and soon afterwards the wound commences to discharge. At first the purulent discharge is thin and watery; later, because of secondary infection, it becomes thicker and odorous. Other sinuses form, and faecal fistulae are liable to develop. At any stage of the disease, if pus is collected and allowed to trickle down the side of a test-tube, sulphur granules may be discovered. The pus should be sent for immediate bacteriological examination.

Another clinical type is that of a patient, most usually a young adult male, who presents with vague abdominal pain. On examination a firm, slightly tender mass is found in the right iliac fossa. Actinomycosis rarely gives rise to obstructive symptoms. There is loss of weight, anaemia, and occasional pyrexia. In most instances laparotomy is performed with one of the following findings: (*a*) an abscess is encountered and drained; (*b*) the mass is found to be densely adherent to the posterior abdominal wall, and irremovable—needing a by-pass ileo-transverse colostomy as for Crohn's disease.

Treatment (Chapter 4).

PNEUMATOSIS CYSTOIDES INTESTINALIS (fig. 1041)

Multiple gas cysts of the intestinal wall are pathological curiosities. Translucent, thin-walled cysts ranging from 1 or 2 or more centimeters in diameter, containing gas, mainly nitrogen, and having a lining of flattened cells of doubtful origin, occur in clusters under

Ahmed Khan Toufeeq, Contemporary. Professor of Surgery, Sir Ganga Ram Hospital, Lahore, Pakistan.

the serosa or in the mesenteries on the intestines. The condition nearly always affects the small intestine, but occasionally the colon, and even the rectum, are implicated. It is believed that air enters a breach in the mucosa, as would occur in the case, say, of a duodenal ulcer, and the air is driven onwards by peristalsis. The cysts, which are obvious on a plain radiograph, are usually symptomless, but occasionally they so occlude the lumen of the intestine that resection is necessary. A new treatment using an oxygen-enriched atmosphere for the patient to breathe over several weeks has been successful in causing the cysts to disappear, but they usually come back within a year of the treatment. The success of the treatment depends upon replacing the nitrogen in the cysts by oxygen, which is then re-absorbed with ensuing collapse of the cysts. Metronidazole has caused symptomatic improvement in some cases.

TUMOURS OF THE SMALL INTESTINE

Compared with the large intestine, the small intestine is rarely the seat of a neoplasm.

Benign.—Adenoma, submucous lipoma and leiomyoma occur from time to time, and sometimes reveal themselves by causing an intussusception. The second most common complication is intestinal bleeding from an adenoma, in which event the diagnosis is frequently long delayed because the tumour is overlooked at a radiological examination by barium meal, and often at operation as well, to be discovered perhaps only after a second or third operation.

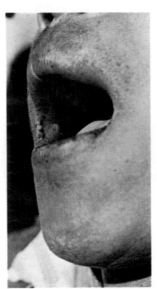

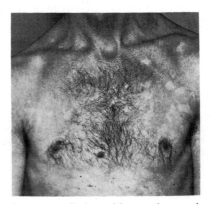

FIG. 1044.—Patient with secondary carcinoid tumour of the liver (primary in the terminal ileum) exhibiting flushing after a small dose of alcohol.
(Dr P. J. D. Snow, Manchester.)

FIG. 1043.—Melanin spots on the lips of a patient afflicted with Peutz-Jeghers syndrome.
(Major P. C. M. Mehta, Indian Medical Service.)

Peutz-Jeghers syndrome (small intestinal polyposis) consists of (a) familial intestinal hamartomatous polyposis affecting mainly jejunum, where it is a cause of haemorrhage, and often of intussusception, and (b) melanosis of the oral mucous membrane and the lips. The melanosis takes the form of melanin spots which are sometimes present on the digits and the peri-anal skin, but the pigmentation of the lips (fig. 1043) is the *sine qua non*.

Histology.—The polyps can be likened to trees. The trunk and branches are smooth muscle fibres and the foliage is virtually normal mucosa.

Treatment.—As a malignant change rarely occurs, resection is necessary only for serious bleeding or intussusception. Large single polyps can be removed by enterotomy, or short lengths of heavily involved intestine can be resected. It is now possible to snare these lesions by means of a fibrecolonoscope.

Malignant:

Sarcoma (40%).—Lymphosarcoma and spindle-cell sarcoma—more usually the

John Law Augustine Peutz, 1886–1957. Chief Specialist for Internal Medicine, St. John's Hospital, The Hague, Holland.
Harold Jos Jeghers, Contemporary. Professor of Internal Medicine, New Jersey College of Medicine and Dentistry, Jersey City, U.S.A.

former—occur in the first five decades, the average age of the patient being thirty-five years. There are usually multiple lesions and the disease may follow idiopathic steatorrhoea. The neoplasm tends to convert the affected intestine into a rigid tube without much interference with the size of its lumen until the disease is advanced. Loss of weight and anaemia are the chief early symptoms. Perforation into the peritoneal cavity occurs more often than is the case with other neoplasms of the small intestine.

Carcinoma (35%) occurs at the usual carcinoma age. The jejunum is affected three times more often than the ileum. The most frequent symptoms are melaena and those of intestinal obstruction, and in some cases a palpable tumour is present. It is unusual for malignant tumours to cause intussusception. Because the content of the small intestine is fluid, by the time intestinal obstruction has ensued metastases have occurred. Another train of symptoms is dyspepsia associated with melaena and increasing anaemia, in which case a tumour, often of the papilliferous variety, may be revealed radiologically at a barium meal.

Carcinoid (Argentaffin) Tumour (25%).—These tumours occur throughout the gastro-intestinal tract and also in the bronchus, testis and ovary. Of these, the appendix is the commonest site (65%). The next common site is the ileum (25%). They arise in the cells of Kulchitsky at the base of the crypts of Lieberkühn. The primary is usually less than 10 mm in diameter. When they metastasise, the liver is usually involved with numerous secondaries, larger and more yellow than the primary growth. When this has occurred the 'Carcinoid syndrome' may become evident.

The tumour produces 5-H.T. (hydroxytryptamine; serotonin) which may be present as 5 hydroxy indole-acetic acid in the urine during attacks. It also produces kinins, indoles, prostaglandins and perhaps histamine.

The clinical syndrome itself consists of reddish-blue cyanosis, flushing attacks, diarrhoea, borborygmi, asthmatic attacks, and eventually sometimes pulmonary and tricuspid stenosis. Classically the flushing attacks are induced by alcohol (fig. 1044).

The cyanotic flushing and asthmatic attacks have been attributed to 5-H.T. and histamine—the brick-red to kinins.

5-H.T. is responsible for the gastrointestinal symptoms. Prostaglandins may have similar effects to the kinins.

Treatment.—This tumour must be taken seriously. A radical operation is advisable where metastases are not found. For example, right hemicolectomy for lesions in the ileum or abdomino-perineal for lesions low in the rectum.

Where metastases have occurred, excision of the local lesion and, if feasible, partial hepatectomy should be considered. It should be borne in mind, however, that such patients may survive for up to 10 years having frequent carcinoid attacks. Medical measures include giving serotonin antagonists, long acting anti-histaminics and alphamethyl dopa which may help to reduce the severity of attacks. For hepatic metastases 5-fluoroura-cil given into the hepatic artery is under trial.

TUMOURS OF THE LARGE INTESTINE

Benign

Adenomatous Polyps are dark red pedunculated neoplasms (fig. 1045). A *villous adenoma* is simply a different morphological expression of the same pathological process, and is usually sessile, and may cause diarrhoea and hypokalaemia.

A solitary adenoma of the colon (fig. 1046) is acquired (see below for the multiple familial variety). It occurs in patients over forty years of age, and unless it is pedunculated, it cannot be distinguished macroscopically from a papilliferous carcinoma. In specimens of papilliferous carcinoma of the colon, often tiny adenomas are found adjacent to the parent tumour.

Treatment.—Because the lesions have a malignant potential they should be removed. Those beyond the reach of the sigmoidoscope require laparotomy, but this should only be undertaken if the lesion is larger than 1 cm in diameter and has been demonstrated on two barium enemas. Fibre endoscopic removal is available in an increasing number of centres. Multiple non-familial adenomas

---

Nicholas Kulchitsky, 1856–1925. Professor of Histology, Kharkov, Ukraine, USSR.

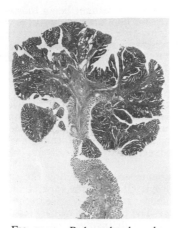

FIG. 1045.—Pedunculated adenomatous polyp of the large intestine.
Longitudinal section.
(J. H. Saint, FRCS, Santa Barbara, California.)

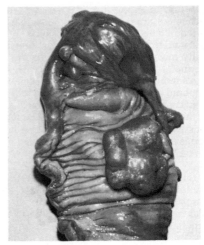

FIG. 1046.—Adenomatous polyp of the
colon.
(Max Pemberton, FRCS, Enfield, Middlesex.

may require a partial colectomy for their control. Any adenoma greater than 1 or
2 cm in size may be malignant and must be removed completely. Huge villous
adenomas of the rectum can be very difficult to remove totally without a proctectomy.

Familial Adenomatous Polyposis of the Colon, which must be distinguished from
Peutz-Jeghers syndrome, juvenile polyposis coli and pseudo-polyposis, is transmitted
from both sexes, though males are affected more frequently than females. Lockhart-
Mummery and Cuthbert Dukes studied 1069 members and 58 families; of these members
218 had polyposis, and 154 of them developed colonic carcinoma. The adenomatous
polyps are most frequently situated in the sigmoid and the rectum. Often hundreds of
tumours are present. The patient may have no symptoms or a few loose stools or may
have attacks of lower abdominal pain associated with loss of weight, diarrhoea, and
tenesmus, and the passage of blood and mucus, and sometimes pus—all symptoms very
like those of ulcerative colitis. A rectal examination may reveal one or more adenomatous
polypi. Sigmoidoscopy shows a variety of neoplasms ranging from small sessile pink
elevations to pedunculated tumours. A barium enema, especially a contrast barium enema,
outlines the larger polypi. Some patients develop adenomas and carcinomas of the gastro-
duodenal area.

Prevention.—(1) All members of the family should be examined at ten years. Repeat
every two years. (2) Most of those who are going to get polypi will have them at twenty
and these require operation. (3) If there are no polypi at twenty, continue with five-yearly
examination till fifty. If there are still no polypi there is no inherited gene. Carcinomatous
change may even occur before the age of twenty.

Treatment.—If operation is feasible, complete colectomy is advisable. A stump of
rectum can remain and the terminal ileum anastomosed to it, the reasons being (a) the
risk of carcinoma in the rectal stump is small if the patient is carefully followed-up and
the polyps burnt off before they can develop malignant change; (b) an artificial anus is
avoided; (c) other members of the family can be persuaded more easily to undergo the
operation before late symptoms develop. In America, protocolectomy with ileo-anal
'pouch' anastomosis is gaining ground as a procedure that eliminates any risk of rectal or
colon cancer but spares the patient a permanent ileostomy (Beart).

Hamartomatous Polyps.—Peutz-Jeghers polyps may occur in the colon either as solitary or multiple lesions. The other type of hamartomatous polyp is the juvenile or mucous
polyp which may occur as multiple lesions of the colon, often associated with a congenital
defect such as malrotation of the intestine, Meckel's diverticulum or congenital heart
lesions. They have minimal malignant potential and are only removed if they produce
troublesome pain, bleeding or hypoproteinaemia.

Sir Hugh Evelyn Lockhart-Mummery, Contemporary. Surgeon, St. Thomas's Hospital, London.
R. Beart, Contemporary. Surgeon, Mayo Clinic, Rochester, Minnesota, U.S.A.

Haemangioma.—A localised submucous telangiectasis is often the cause of bleeding, which may be profuse. When the lesion is beyond the sigmoidoscope often the only method of detecting it is to operate while the bleeding is in progress. The distribution of blood within the intestine is noted; scrutiny of the blood-containing portion of the intestine usually reveals a dilated leash of veins in one portion of the mesocolon. At this site the intestine is opened and the tumour is resected. Arteriography is being used in many centres with great success. Colonoscopy can also help.

Lipoma is less frequently encountered in the large than in the small intestine, and is almost confined to the caecum. The tumour is submucous and in more than half the cases it is the cause of an intussusception. Other symptoms to which it gives rise are almost impossible to distinguish from those of a carcinoma; even macroscopical or microscopical blood is found in the stools.

Malignant

CARCINOMA OF THE COLON

Pathology.—Microscopically, the neoplasm is a columnar-celled carcinoma originating in the epithelial cells that line the colon, or in the crypts of Lieberkühn. Macroscopically the growth takes one of four forms (fig. 1047):

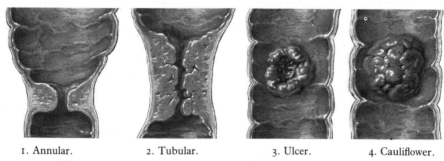

| 1. Annular. | 2. Tubular. | 3. Ulcer. | 4. Cauliflower. |

FIG. 1047.—The four macroscopical varieties of carcinoma of the colon.

Type 4 is the least malignant form. All types of carcinoma probably commence as a benign adenoma. The annular variety carries a relatively good prognosis, not because the growth is of low-grade malignancy, but because it gives rise to early obstructive symptoms, and therefore is often extirpated before metastases have occurred. Prognosis also relates to the differentiation of the tumour.

Site. The most frequent site is toward the termination of the colon, *viz.* the pelvic colon and the rectosigmoid junction.

The Spread of Carcinoma of the Colon.—Generally speaking, it is a comparatively slowly growing neoplasm, and if extirpated thoroughly at a reasonably early period a cure can be hopefully anticipated.

Local Spread.—The growth is limited to the bowel for a considerable time. It spreads round the intestinal wall, and to a certain extent longitudinally, but usually it causes intestinal obstruction before it has penetrated adjacent structures. Particularly in the ulcerative variety, penetration of the serous coat is apt to occur and, according to the segment involved, adjacent structures then become invaded by the growth. When a hollow viscus is thus implicated an internal fistula results; also the perforation may lead to the formation of a local abscess and an external faecal fistula.

Lymphatic Spread.—The lymph nodes draining the colon are grouped as follows:

1. *The epicolic lymph nodes*, situated in the immediate vicinity of the bowel wall.
2. *The paracolic lymph nodes*, lying in relationship to the leash of blood-vessels proceeding to the colonic walls.

3. *The intermediate lymph nodes*, arranged along the ileo-colic, right colic, mid colic, left colic, and the sigmoid arteries. In the last instance the paracolic lymph nodes are often absent.

4. *The main lymph nodes*, aggregated around the superior and inferior mesenteric vessels, where they take origin from the abdominal aorta.

Blood-stream Spread.—Spread by the blood-stream occurs late. Metastases are carried to the liver.

Clinical Features—Carcinoma of the colon usually occurs in patients over fifty years of age, but it is not rare earlier in adult life. Exceptionally it appears in childhood, when, owing to delayed diagnosis and a higher proportion of undifferentiated tumours, prognosis is poor. Twenty-five per cent of cases present as emergencies with intestinal obstruction or peritonitis. It must be remembered that in any case of colonic bleeding in patients over forty years of age, complete investigation of the colon is required.

Men are attacked more frequently than women (3:2), although carcinoma of the ascending colon is encountered more often in women.

While certain outstanding symptoms frequently prevail in all types and at all sites, it is instructive to contrast and to compare the symptoms produced by a carcinoma of the left side of the colon with that of the right, and to refer to the symptomatology of carcinoma of the sigmoid and that of the transverse colon.

Carcinoma of the Left Side of the Colon.—In about 75% of cases the neoplasm is situated on the left side of the colon. Neoplasms in this situation usually are of the stenosing variety (fig. 1047, 1 and 2) and as here the faecal content is relatively solid, and the lumen of the bowel comparatively narrow, the main symptoms are those of increasing intestinal obstruction in about 25% of cases.

Symptoms	*Right Colon*	*Left Colon*	*Sigmoid*
Abdominal pain	78	68	51
Alteration of bowel habit	30	58	70
Loss of weight	50	15	20
Vomiting (frequently with colic)	32	15	0
Anorexia	18	9	0
Faintness, breathlessness	20	9	6
Bleeding per rectum	8	9	29
Lump present	67	46	39
Indigestion	8	0	0
Acute-on-chronic obstruction	8	21	29

The duration of symptoms is extremely variable; 5·5 months is the average.

(*E. G. Muir's statistics—figures given are percentages.*)

Pain.—This is usually intestinal colic. If it becomes a constant ache, it suggests inoperability or pericolitis.

Alteration of Bowel Habit.—An adult who has had regular bowel movement all his life, in a short space of time develops irregularity. The patient often states that he has *increasing* difficulty in getting the bowels to move, and that he has to take *increasing* doses of purgatives. Because of the drastic purgation, or on account of irritation by the scybala causing excessive secretion of mucus above the constricting neoplasm, attacks of constipation are followed by diarrhoea.

Palpable Lump.—Very often the lump that is felt on abdominal, rectal, or abdomino-rectal examination, is not the growth itself, but impacted faeces above

Sir Edward Grainger Muir, P.R.C.S., 1906–1973. Surgeon, King's College Hospital, London. President, Royal College of Surgeons of England.

it. When the carcinoma is situated in a pendulous pelvic colon a hard movable swelling is often felt in the rectovesical pouch.

Distension.—Lower abdominal distension is not uncommon, and, like the pain, is relieved by passing flatus.

Carcinoma of the sigmoid follows the general pattern of the above, but there are differences.

Pain, when it occurs, is usually colicky from the commencement.

Tenesmus.—Growths of papilliferous type situated low in the colon are inclined to give rise to a feeling of the need for evacuation, which may result in tenesmus accompanied by the passage of mucus and blood, especially in the early morning.

Bladder symptoms are not unusual, and in some instances they herald colovesical fistula.

Carcinoma of the transverse colon may be mistaken for a carcinoma of the stomach because of the position of the tumour together wtih the anaemia and lassitude that it sometimes engenders.

Carcinoma of the caecum and ascending colon presents in several guises:

(*a*) Anaemia, severe and unyielding to treatment, is a frequent predominating feature. Should a palpable tumour be present, the diagnosis is, to some extent simplified.

(*b*) The presence of a mass in the right iliac fossa often proves a diagnostic conundrum. Colonoscopy makes diagnosis straightforward if the caecum can be reached.

(*c*) Caecal carcinoma sometimes is discovered unexpectedly at operation for acute appendicitis or for an appendix abscess that 'fails to resolve'. On rare occasions the appendix is inflamed, or even gangrenous, from obstruction to its lumen by the carcinoma.

(*d*) Less commonly a papilliferous growth is the apex of an intussuception. A lump, present at one time and smaller or absent at another (owing to partial reduction), associated with attacks of acute abdominal pain, is characteristic of this complication.

METHODS OF INVESTIGATION

Sigmoidoscopy should be performed in all cases where blood and mucus have been passed and also in suspected cases when a barium enema is negative, because early growths in the lower part of the pelvic colon are not always visualised by radiography. The flexible 60 cm colonoscope is being increasingly used as an alternative to sigmoidoscopy when available.

Radiography after a barium enema often shows a carcinoma of the colon as a constant, irregular filling defect (fig. 1048). On the other hand, negative radiography in comparatively early cases of carcinoma of the colon is not by any means conclusive evidence of the absence of a growth.

A tumour of the caecum is more likely to be discovered by a barium meal than a barium enema. As a rule, in suspected cases of carcinoma of the colon, a barium meal is inadvisable because inspissated barium can precipitate intestinal obstruction if the lumen of the bowel is narrowed.

Contrast Enema.—In cases of a neoplasm involving only the mucous membrane, a contrast enema is very valuable. The barium emulsion is partly evacuated and air is

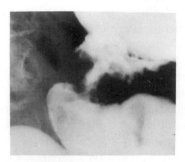

FIG. 1048.—Barium enema showing a carcinoma of the sigmoid colon. It may have an 'apple core' appearance.

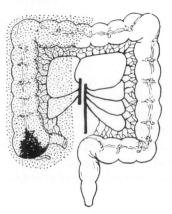

FIG. 1049.—Area to be resected when the growth is situated in the caecum.

injected into the colon. By this means the walls of the colon become delineated and a neoplasm that fails to alter the contour of the barium-filled colon may be demonstrated.

Exfoliative cytology.—In experienced hands colonic exfoliative cytology is a valuable adjunct in the diagnosis of obscure cases of carcinoma of the colon. To obtain satisfactory results, the patient must be prepared carefully by a somewhat laborious procedure. After an interval of 5 to 10 minutes, the returned fluid is collected and centrifuged. Films from the sediment are prepared and stained. Successful diagnoses have been made by this method if growth is situated in all parts of the colon.

Colonoscopy.—It has been shown already that this technique can supplement radiography in the diagnosis of both polyps and carcinoma of the colon. It can also help to prevent carcinomas arising by diagnosing and treating colonic polyps at an early stage (Williams). The technique is time consuming, and the apparatus is expensive.

TREATMENT

Pre-operative Treatment.—When there is no intestinal obstruction, blood transfusion to correct anaemia, if present, enemas to cleanse the bowel, a high caloric and low residue diet are required. Metronidazole (Flagyl) also suppresses anaerobic bacteria, and should be used in conjunction with gentamicin [250 mg given at the time of surgery, and a second dose 12 hours later]. The latest cephalosporins are also effective against all colonic bacteria.

Alternatively, whole gut irrigation using isotonic saline given via a nasogastric tube at a rate of 2–4 litres/hour for 3–4 hours has proved to be a satisfactory method of preparing the colon for surgery in the unobstructed patient.

When intestinal obstruction is present, preliminary drainage of the intestine proximal to the obstruction must be performed in advanced cases: right-sided obstructions rarely need such precautions, but left-sided obstructions are often treated in this way unless an experienced surgeon decides that immediate resection might be safe.

Operation.—*The Test of Operability.*—The abdomen having been opened in the first place through a short paramedian incision, which is extended if the growth is removable: (1) the liver is palpated for secondary deposits, the presence of which is not necessarily a contraindication to resection, as the best palliative treatment for carcinoma of the colon is removal of the tumour; (2) the perito-

Christopher Beverley Williams, Contemporary. Physician, St. Mark's Hospital for Diseases of Rectum and Colon, London.

neum, particularly the pelvic peritoneum, is inspected, if possible, and palpated for neoplastic implantations; (3) the various groups of lymph nodes that drain the involved segment are palpated. Their enlargement does not necessarily mean that they are invaded by metastases, for the enlargement may be inflammatory; (4) the neoplasm is examined with a view to ascertaining if it is fixed or free, and if it is operable. 'The whole colon above the last 7·5 cm of the pelvic portion is either mobile or can be mobilised' (Ogilvie).

The operations to be described are designed to remove both the primary as well as the lymph nodes which may be involved by metastases from the particular primary growth concerned. Lesser resections are indicated, however, should hepatic metastases render the condition incurable.

Carcinoma of the caecum or the ascending colon is treated, when resectable, by right hemicolectomy (fig. 1049).

The abdomen is opened through a right paramedian incision. The technique of right colectomy should include at the outset ligatures placed around the bowel to prevent intraluminal spread. The peritoneum 2·5 cm or more lateral to the ascending colon is incised and the incision is carried around the hepatic flexure. The right colon is elevated, with the leaf of peritoneum containing its vessels and lymph nodes, from the posterior abdominal wall, care being taken not to injure the ureter, spermatic vessels, or the duodenum. The peritoneum is separated medially to near the origin of the ileo-colic artery, which is divided between ligatures, as also is the right colic artery when that vessel has a separate origin from the superior mesenteric. The mesentery of the last 30 cm of ileum, and the leaf of raised peritoneum attached to the caecum, ascending colon and hepatic flexure, after ligation of the blood-vessels contained therein, is divided as far as the proximal third of the transverse colon (fig. 1049). The surgeon, having verified that the blood supply to the proposed intestinal stumps is adequate, forthwith clamps and divides the ileum and the transverse colon at the levels of their respective severed mesenteries, an excises the free intestine. And end-to-end anastomosis between the ileum and transverse colon is then carried out and their respective mesenteries approximated with catgut. The abdomen is then closed.

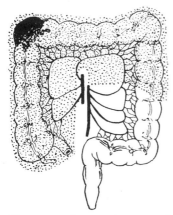

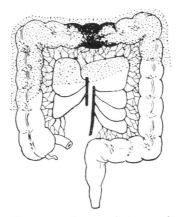

FIG. 1050.—Area to be resected when the growth is situated at the hepatic flexure.

FIG. 1051.—Area to be resected when the neoplasm is situated in the transverse colon.

Carcinoma of the Hepatic Flexure.—When the hepatic flexure is the seat of the neoplasm the resection must be extended correspondingly (fig. 1050).

Carcinoma of the Transverse colon.—When there is no obstruction, excision of the transverse colon and the two flexures (fig. 1051), together with the trans-

Sir Heneage Ogilvie, 1887–1971. Surgeon, Guy's Hospital, London.

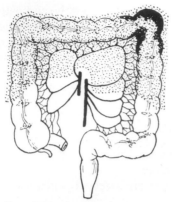

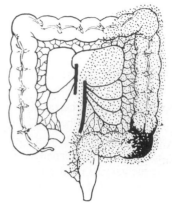

FIG. 1052.—Area to be resected when the neoplasm is situated at the splenic flexure, or the proximal part of the descending colon.

FIG. 1053.—Area to be resected in the case of a carcinoma of the pelvic colon.

verse mesocolon and the greater omentum, followed by end-to-end anastomosis, is a satisfactory procedure.

Carcinoma of the Splenic Flexure or descending colon. The extent of the resection is shown in fig. 1052. Sometimes removal of colon up to the ileum is preferable.

The phrenico-colic ligament is divided, and after incising the parietal peritoneum from the splenic flexure to the pelvic colon, the splenic flexure, descending colon, and pelvic colon are raised from the posterior abdominal wall in the same way as the ascending colon is raised on the right side. When this has been achieved, the left branch of the middle colic and the left colic arteries are ligated near their origins, and the peritoneal leaf with its contained lymph nodes is divided. Excision with end-to-end anastomosis is then carried out.

Carcinoma of the Pelvic Colon.—A left paramedian incision gives a good approach. The left half of the colon is mobilised completely (fig. 1053).

In order that the operation be rendered radical, the inferior mesenteric artery below its left colic branch, together with the related paracolic lymph nodes, must be included in the resection. This entails carrying the dissection as far as the upper third of the rectum, and accordingly the incision in the lateral leaf of peritoneum is extended downward to an appropriate level.

In every case of resection of the colon with anastomosis, drainage down to the site of anastomosis should be considered.

Modern methods of bowel preparation render one-stage resection and anastomosis reasonably safe in *non-obstructed* cases of colonic carcinoma but if any doubt exists a protective colostomy must be added. The methods of dealing with large bowel obstruction due to colonic carcinoma are described on p. 1073.

Post-operative Care following Colonic Resection.—Post-operative treatment includes the administration of antibiotics to guard against possible infection of the anastomotic area by *Cl. welchii*. Free fluids are not given by mouth after anastomotic operations until flatus is passed.

When a Growth is found to be Inoperable.—In the upper part of the left colon, transverse colostomy is performed. In the pelvic colon, left iliac colostomy is preferable. With an inoperable growth in the ascending colon, ileo-colostomy is the best procedure. However, about 90% of colonic carcinomas can be resected, if necessary at a 'second look' operation, when infection will have subsided follow-

William Henry Welch, 1850–1934. Professor of Pathology, Johns Hopkins University, Baltimore, Maryland, U.S.A.

ing the by-passing of faeces. As these are slow-growing neoplasms, after subsequent colostomy-closure, these patients often enjoy several years of trouble-free life.

Hepatic metastases

A solitary hepatic metastasis can be resected as the uninvolved lobe can be preserved: 50% of cases can be cured if selection is rigid. A right hepatic lobectomy is a technically severe procedure and requires experience.

Multiple painful hepatic metastases can be palliated by cytotoxic drugs or hepatic artery ligation.

FAECAL FISTULAS

An external fistula communicating with the caecum sometimes follows an operation for gangrenous appendicitis or the opening of an appendix abscess. A faecal fistula can occur from necrosis of a gangrenous patch of intestine after the relief of a strangulated hernia, or from a leak after an intestinal anastomosis. The opening of an abscess connected with chronic diverticulitis or carcinoma of the colon frequently results in faecal fistula. Tuberculous peritonitis, ileo-caecal actinomycosis, amoebiasis, and regional ileitis (in this instance nearly always following operation) are also causes of faecal fistulas, which may be multiple. About 4% of chronic faecal fistulas in hospital are kept open by patients pushing in knitting needles or other articles for reasons best known to themselves.

External faecal fistulas can be divided into three varieties: 1. A track lined by mucous membrane which protrudes above skin level. 2. A direct track lined by granulation tissue communicating with the exterior. 3. A long, tortuous track lined by fibrous tissue and partly epithelialised. The discharge from a fistula connected with the duodenum or jejunum is bile-stained and causes severe excoriation of the skin. When the ileum or caecum are concerned, the discharge is fluid faecal matter; when the distal colon is involved, it is solid or semi-solid faecal matter. In some cases, when the leak from the small intestine or caecum is small, it may be difficult to distinguish a faecal discharge from faeculent pus. If methylene blue is administered by mouth and a faecal leak is present, the blue colour will be distinguished easily in the discharge a few hours later. Often the site of the leak and the length of the fistula can be determined by radiography after a barium meal or barium enema. Should this fail to demonstrate the internal orifice, injection of lipiodol into the external opening will usually give the desired information.

Treatment.—Faecal fistulas, especially those in connection with the small intestine, tend to heal spontaneously, provided there is no obstruction beyond the fistulous opening. The abdominal wall must be protected from erosion by the use of a disposable ileostomy bag.

The higher the fistula in the intestinal canal the more skin excoriation must be expected. This reaches its zenith in the case of a duodenal fistula. A sump drain to remove the enzyme-laden discharge is a fundamental requirement. Such fistulas cause dehydration and hypoproteinaemia and intravenous parenteral feeding will be required. If there is no prospect of rapid healing, a feeding jejunostomy is often a life-saving measure.

A faecal fistula with mucosa visibly continuous with the skin edge will never close spontaneously. In some of these cases, where the opening is a large one, the intestine tends to prolapse upon the surface.

The operative treatment for closure of a faecal fistula consists in making an incision encircling the fistula and dissecting up the tract through the abdominal wall and the peritoneum. The base of the fistula, now free, is crushed, ligated and oversewn. The abdominal wall is then closed in layers. In the case of a colo-cutaneous fistula connected with colonic diverticulitis, if the fistula fails to heal after a few weeks, resection of the affected segment is usually advisable. Should the mass from which the fistula arises prove to be an inoperable carcinoma, a defunctioning colostomy should be performed at a higher level. In complicated fistulas, an operation to defunction the loop of intestine involved is probably the best procedure. When there is no obvious cause for the fistula, the discharge must be examined on several occasions for *actinomyces* or *Mycobacterium tuberculosis*. Before operating on an intestinal fistula a course of treatment with intra-venous hyperalimentation will improve the condition of the patient and may enable the fistula to close.

COLOSTOMY

A *colostomy* is an artificial opening made into the large bowel in order to divert faeces (and flatus) to the exterior, where they may be collected in an adhesive bag.

Depending on the purpose for which the diversion has been necessary, a colostomy may be *temporary* or *permanent*.

Temporary Colostomy

This is most commonly established to relieve a distal obstruction of the sigmoid colon either by a carcinoma or diverticulitis. Other indications include vesico-colic fistula, protection of a low colo-rectal anastomosis after anterior resection, to prevent faecal peritonitis developing after traumatic injury to the rectum or colon, and to facilitate the operative treatment of a high fistula-in-ano.

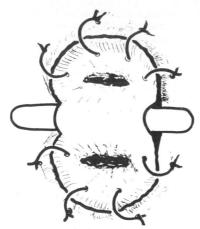

FIG. 1054.—Usual temporary (loop) colostomy opened over a rod, and immediate suture of colon wall to surrounding skin.

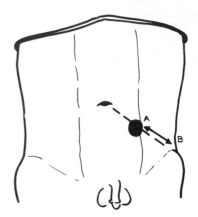

FIG. 1055.—Usual site of a permanent (end) colostomy in the left ilial fossa. Note distance A–B=2·5 cm at least.

A temporary colostomy is made by bringing a loop of bowel to the surface ('loop colostomy') where it is held in place by a glass rod passed through the mesentery. When firm adhesion of the colostomy to the abdominal wall has taken place after 7 days, the rod can be removed. As the colostomy has been established for obstruction (or other emergency situations) it is opened immediately at the end of the operation, and the edges of the colonic incision stitched to the surrounding skin margins (fig. 1054). Skin bridges and other techniques have been developed to replace the glass rod.

A loop of colon can be most easily brought to the surface by using large bowel that has a mesentery: most loop colostomies are made in the transverse colon, and if the disease involves the left side of the colon, the right half of the transverse colon is preferred so that the entire left side is left available for any subsequent formal operation, *e.g.* left hemicolectomy for a carcinoma of the sigmoid colon. The sigmoid colon is also suitable for a loop colostomy.

Following surgical cure of the distal lesion for which the temporary stoma was constructed, the colostomy is closed. Colostomy closure is most easily and safely accomplished when the stoma is 'mature', *i.e.* after the colostomy has been established for two months. Closure is usually performed nowadays by an *intraperitoneal* technique, as this has been shown to be safer than the *extraperitoneal* methods, and to be accompanied by fewer closure breakdowns with faecal fistulas.

Double-barrelled Colostomy.—This colostomy was designed so that it could be closed by crushing the intervening 'spur' by an enterotome. It is rarely used now, but occasionally the colon is divided so that both ends can be brought separately to the surface. This ensures that *absolute* rest is given to the distal segment of the colon and rectum (Devine).

Permanent Colostomy

This is usually formed after excision of the rectum for a carcinoma by the abdomino-perineal technique.

It is formed by bringing the distal end ('end colostomy') of the divided colon to the surface in the left iliac fossa, where it is stitched in place immediately by sutures placed between the colonic margin and the surrounding skin.

The point at which the colon is brought to the surface must be carefully selected to allow a colostomy bag to be applied without impinging on the bony prominence of the anterior superior ilial spine. The best site is usually through the lateral edge of the rectus sheath 6 cm above and medial to the bony prominence (fig. 1055).

An important point after the colostomy has been made is to close the 'lateral space' between the intraperitoneal segment of the sigmoid colon and the peritoneum of the pelvic wall to prevent internal herniation or strangulation of loops of small bowel through the deficiency. A retroperitoneal tunnel for the colostomy avoids creating a lateral space.

Colostomy bags and appliances.—Faeces from a permanent colostomy are collected in disposable adhesive bags. A wide range of such bags is currently available. An increasingly popular type employs a Karaya-gum seal (washer) that does not irritate the skin and needs to be changed less often than the regular 'stick-on' type (fig. 1056). Many now incorporate a 'stomahesive' backing.

In large district hospitals, stoma therapists and stoma clinics are being set up to offer advice to patients on stoma care, and to acquaint patients with the latest services.

An abdominal belt is commonly worn, but usually a light elastic 'roll-on' type rather than the heavy belts (St. Mark's pattern) previously advised.

Complications of Colostomies

The following complications can occur to *any* colostomy, but are more common after a badly performed technique:

Sir Hugh Berchmans Devine, 1878–1959. Surgeon, St. Vincent's Hospital, Melbourne, Australia.

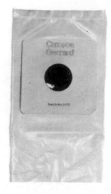 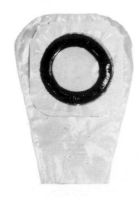

FIG. 1056.—The common *stick-on* bag and the alternative bag with a Karaya-gum seal (Hollister type).

1. *Prolapse.*
2. *Retraction.*
3. *Necrosis* of the distal end.
4. *Stenosis* of the orifice.
5. *Colostomy hernia.*
6. *Bleeding* (usually from granulomas around the margin of the colostomy).
7. *Colostomy 'diarrhoea'* (this is usually an infective enteritis and responds rapidly to treatment by metronidazole [200 mg B.D.]

Many of these complications necessitate that the colostomy should be reformed. Often this can only be done satisfactorily by re-opening the abdomen, freeing up the colostomy which is then re-established in a fresh spot.

CAECOSTOMY

In desperately ill patients with advanced obstruction, if the lesion is situated in the right half of the colon, a caecostomy may have to be performed. In late cases of obstruction, the caecum may become so distended that rupture of the caecal wall may be anticipated. This may occur spontaneously, giving rise to faecal peritonitis or at operation when an incision in the abdominal wall reduces its supportive role and allows the viscus to expand. In such cases the over-distended viscus should be decompressed by suction as soon as the peritoneum is opened. The caecum may then require partial mobilisation. In thin patients it may then be possible to carry out direct suture of the incised caecal wall to the abdominal skin of the right iliac fossa. More commonly, the decompression is performed by introducing a wide bore-tube (No. 22 Foley or Winsbury-White catheter) which is stitched in place by invaginating purse-string stitches—so placed as to 'inkwell' the site of entry.

A caecostomy is only a short-term measure to allow a few days for the condition of the patient to improve. Re-operation should normally be carried out within 7 days of establishing the caecostomy.

CHAPTER 51

INTESTINAL OBSTRUCTION

Intestinal obstruction is a common surgical emergency and because of its serious nature it demands early diagnosis and speedy relief. It may be classified into two types:

1. **Dynamic.**—Here there is peristalsis working against an obstructing agent, which may be in the *lumen*, such as a bolus of incompletely digested material, inspissated faeces, or a gallstone; *in the wall*, such as an inflammatory or malignant stricture; or *outside the wall*, as in hernias, adhesions, volvulus or intussusception.

2. **Adynamic.**—In this condition, peristalsis ceases and no true propulsive waves occur—as in paralytic ileus or mesenteric vascular occlusion.

DYNAMIC OBSTRUCTION

Is classified clinically into three types:

1. *Acute obstruction* favouring the small gut, with central abdominal pain, early vomiting, central abdominal distension, and constipation.

2. *Chronic obstruction* favouring the large bowel, with lower abdominal colic at first and absolute constipation and distension later.

3. *Acute-on-chronic obstruction* which spreads from the large bowel to involve the small intestine and gives early pain and constipation, followed by general distension and vomiting.

Pathology

The intestine above the point of obstruction endeavours at the outset to overcome the obstruction by vigorous peristalsis. Increased peristalsis continues for a period of from forty-eight hours to several days; the more distal the point of obstruction, the longer does it remain vigorous. If the obstruction is not relieved, a time is reached when increasing distension causes peristalsis to become less and less; finally, peristalsis ceases, and the obstructed intestine becomes flaccid and paralysed.

The intestine below the point of obstruction exhibits normal peristalsis, and absorption from it continues for two or three hours following the obstruction, until the residue of its contents has been passed onwards. Then the empty intestine becomes immobile, contracted, and pale, and so it remains, until the obstruction has been overcome, or death ensues.

Distension.—This occurs proximal to the obstruction, and begins immediately after the obstruction occurs. The cause of distension is two-fold:

(*a*) **Gas.**—This consists of swallowed atmospheric air (68%), diffusion from blood into the bowel lumen (22%), and the products of digestion and bacterial activity (10%). When the oxygen and carbon dioxide has been absorbed into the bloodstream, the resultant mixture is made up of nitrogen (90%), and hydrogen sulphide.

(*b*) **Fluid.**—This is made up by the various digestive juices—about 8000 ml per twenty-four hours.

Above pylorus.	4000 ml	Saliva 1500 ml
		Gastric 2500 ml
Below pylorus.	4000 ml	Bile and pancreatic 1000 ml
		Succus entericus 3000 ml

In obstruction, absorption from the gut is retarded but excretion of water and electrolytes into the lumen persists and may even be increased. Deprivation of water and electrolytes, therefore, is due to:

(*a*) Vomiting.
(*b*) Defective absorption.
(*c*) Sequestration in lumen of bowel.

The severity of depletion and speed with which it becomes manifest is dependent upon the level of obstruction. It is most severe and occurs early in high small intestinal obstruction, later in ileal obstruction, and is slow to appear in colon obstruction. (For effects of fluid and electrolyte loss, see Chapter 6.)

Intestinal Toxins.—It is well known that release of intestinal obstruction may be followed by death, particularly in cases of strangulation. In unrelieved strangulation, toxic substances appear in the peritoneal cavity only when the viability of the bowel wall is affected. However, when obstruction is relieved, these toxins may pass on to the bowel where absorption can occur. It is probable that the substances involved are endotoxins of Gram-negative bacilli. This factor stresses the need for intestinal decompression before and during operation, and for adequate prophylactic antibiotic cover against Gram-negative organisms (Chapter 3).

Strangulation of the bowel occurs when it is trapped by a hernia or a band, or involved in a volvulus or intussusception in such a way that its *blood supply is progressively interfered with.* It is a very dangerous condition and demands early treatment before gangrene of the bowel arises. Mesenteric vascular occlusion alone gives rise to gangrene without mechanical obstruction.

The Onset of Gangrene.—The first effect of strangulation is to compress the veins so as to cause the strangulated bowel, and its involved mesentery, to become blue and congested. Much depends on the tightness of the constricting agent. When the venous return is completely occluded, the colour of the intestine turns from purple to black. About this time, in many instances, owing to increased oedema at the point of obstruction, the arterial supply is jeopardised. Then the peritoneal coat loses its glistening appearance, the mucous membrane becomes ulcerated, and moist gangrene is imminent.

Loss of blood volume into the congested segment is proportional to the length of that segment. When, as is often the case in strangulated external hernia, only a few inches are involved, the amount of blood thus imprisoned is inconsequential; on the other hand, when a large coil of intestine becomes strangulated the loss of blood is sufficient to render the patient oligaemic; when several feet of small intestine are involved the volume of circulating blood is so reduced as to imperil the patient's life.

Distension.—For a considerable time the strangulated segment (fig. 1057) (B)) alone distends, the greatest distension occurring when the venous return is completely obstructed while the arterial supply remains unimpaired. Unlike non-strangulating obstruction, early distension of the proximal intestine (fig. 1057 (A)) is absent; indeed, for a time varying from a few minutes to several hours the proximal intestine contracts. After this varying interval, vigorous peristalsis

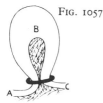

Fig. 1057

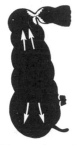

Fig. 1058.—Carcinomatous stricture of the hepatic flexure: closed-loop obstruction.

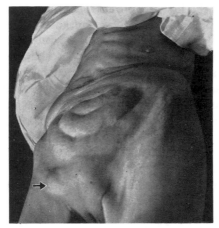

Fig. 1059.—Visible peristalsis. Intestinal obstruction due to the strangulated right femoral hernia, to which the arrow points.

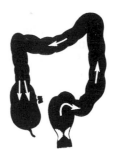

Fig. 1060.—Wherever the large intestine is obstructed the caecum bears the brunt.

occurs in the proximal segment, but is still unaccompanied by distension. By the time gangrene of the strangulated segment is imminent, retrograde thrombosis is proceeding along the related tributaries of the mesenteric vein. Distension then appears both on the proximal and distal sides of the strangulation (fig. 1057 (A) and (C)) (Chesterman).

Transmigration of Bacteria and Toxins.—When the wall of the intestine becomes partly devitalised, both bacterial toxins and the products of tissue autolysis pass into the peritoneal cavity, there to be absorbed into the circulation. This is followed by the migration of bacteria, and peritonitis follows. So it comes about that strangulation in an *external* hernia is far less dangerous than intraperitoneal strangulation, for in the former the transudate containing lethal toxins and bacteria is confined to the comparatively small absorptive area of the hernial sac.

Closed-loop obstruction is present in many cases of intestinal strangulation. In its typical form it is seen in carcinomatous stricture of the colon (fig. 1058). Distally the colon is occluded by the neoplasm, while in one-third of cases the ileo-caecal valve prevents regurgitation of the contents of the large intestine into the ileum, and consequently that part of the colon proximal to the neoplasm is closed at both ends (fig 1058). As a result of anti-peristalsis the pressure within the caecum becomes so high as to compress the blood-vessels within its walls. If the obstruction is unrelieved, stercoral ulceration, gangrene, and perforation of the caecum will eventually occur.

CLINICAL FEATURES OF ACUTE INTESTINAL OBSTRUCTION

There are four important symptoms and signs: pain, vomiting, distension, and constipation. These must be carefully looked for in each case.

Judson Tyndale Chesterman, Contemporary. Thoracic Surgeon, City General Hospital, Sheffield, England.

down, must be taken in the x-ray department as soon as possible. In cases of chronic obstruction, this should be preceded by an enema.

Gas Shadows.—When the jejunum, the ileum, or the colon is distended with gas, each has a characteristic appearance that allows it to be distinguished radiologically. The diameter of the viscus is no criterion as to whether it is small or large intestine. Obstructed small intestine is revealed by relatively straight segments that generally lie more or less transversely; obstructed large intestine is disclosed by its haustration markings; a distended caecum is shown by a rounded gas shadow.

Jejunum is characterised by its valvulae conniventes that pass from the antimesenteric to the mesenteric border, spaced regularly, giving rise to a concertina effect.

Ileum.—The distal ileum is piquantly described by Wangensteen as being 'characterless'.

Large intestine (the caecum excepted) shows haustral folds. Haustral folds, unlike the valvulae conniventes, are spaced irregularly and the indentations are not placed opposite one another.

Fluid Levels.—In infants under the age of two years a few fluid levels in the small intestine are a normal occurrence. In adults, two inconstant fluid levels must be regarded as physiological. One is at the duodenal cap; the other, which is more infrequent, is within the terminal ileum. In intestinal obstruction it takes a little time for the gas to separate from the fluid; consequently fluid levels appear later than gas shadows. When paralysis of the intestine has occurred, fluid levels become more conspicuous and more numerous. By the time fluid levels are pronounced, obstruction is advanced. The number of fluid levels is proportionate to the degree of obstruction and to its site in the small intestine; the nearer the obstruction is to the ileo-caecal valve, the larger the number of fluid levels (fig. 1061). Obstruction *low* in the colon does not commonly give rise to fluid levels in the small intestine, but in the case of obstruction *high* in the large intestine,

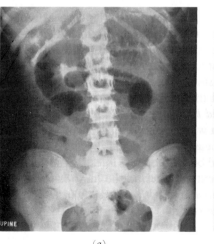 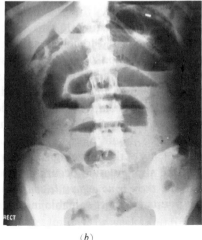

(a)   (b)

FIG. 1061.—(a) Gas-filled small bowel loops; patient supine. (b) Fluid levels with gas above; 'step-ladder' pattern. Small bowel obstruction by adhesions; patient erect.

Owen Harding Wangensteen, Contemporary. Emeritus Professor of Surgery, University of Minnesota, Minneapolis, U.S.A.

this phenomenon is not unusual, because in many individuals the ileo-caecal valve is incompetent.

In obstruction of the large intestine, a plain radiograph always shows a large amount of gas in the caecum. In most cases a barium enema is contraindicated during an attack of intestinal obstruction. A barium meal is also contra-indicated and can be disastrous.

Multiple gas-filled loops above fluid levels in both small and large bowel are also seen in established paralytic ileus. Here, however, bowel sounds are absent or much reduced.

TREATMENT OF ACUTE INTESTINAL OBSTRUCTION

There are four measures for combating and overcoming the effects of intestinal obstruction. They are: (1) gastro-duodenal or, when possible, gastro-intestinal suction drainage; (2) replacement of fluid and electrolytes; (3) relief of the obstruction, usually by operation; (4) antibiotics to prevent complications from associated sepsis, either locally (peritonitis) or peripherally (chest complications).

The first two are always necessary preliminaries to the relief of obstruction by operation, and they are also the mainstays of post-operative treatment. In some cases, as will be shown, they are used exclusively.

In every case of acute intestinal obstruction the first step is to empty the stomach by a transnasal aspirating tube and to keep the stomach empty by withdrawing the contents by continuous suction. The second step is to correct the fluid and electrolyte imbalance (Chapter 6). When, on clinical examination, the cause of the obstruction is not obvious, radiographs of the abdomen are taken and the clinical and radiographic data are correlated. The main indications for early operation (as soon as the fluid and electrolyte depletion has been corrected) are:

1. Obstructed or strangulated external hernia (Chapter 55).
2. Internal intestinal strangulation.
3. Acute or acute-on-chronic obstruction.

The most urgent of these is intestinal strangulation. Gastro-duodenal aspiration should be continued throughout the operation, and also in most instances the intravenous infusion, which, in cases of strangulation, should be supplemented by blood transfusion. The classic clinical advice that 'the sun should not both rise and set' on a case of unrelieved intestinal obstruction is sound, and should be followed unless there are positive reasons for delay.

Relief of Obstruction by Operation.—When the cause of the obstruction lies within the abdomen but its site is doubtful, a right lower paramedian incision is employed.

When the Obstruction lies in the Small Intestine.—The hand is passed to the caecum. In obstruction of the small intestine the caecum is collapsed. The site of obstruction may be obscured by dilated coils of intestine, in which event an unobstructed contracted coil of ileum is sought and followed upwards. This will guide the fingers to the site of obstruction which, if deeply placed, is exposed by displacing distended coils away from the site with warm, moist abdominal packs. Occasionally, it is necessary to withdraw several coils of distended intestine before the site of obstruction can be displayed satisfactorily. Eviscerated coils must be kept covered by abdominal packs. The obstruction is relieved by one of the various methods described under special forms of intestinal obstruction.

Emptying the Small Intestine at Operation.—If there is much distension, it is wise to deflate the bowel using Savage's decompressor. The tube is introduced into the lumen through a stab-wound in the bowel at its most distended part. The bowel is progressively emptied by threading it over the instrument for its full length (fig. 1062). The stab-wound is closed in two layers transversely. If this, or a similar instrument, is not available, an ordinary sucker or a rubber catheter attached to a sucker is an adequate substitute. By these means closure of the abdominal wall is facilitated and intestinal toxins mostly eliminated. Because the suction can withdraw large quantities of fluid and *electrolytes*, extra amounts of saline with potassium supplements should be given to compensate for the losses.

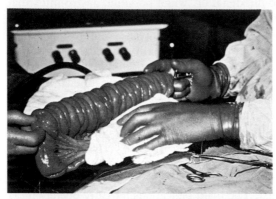

FIG. 1062.—Small intestinal obstruction. Savage's decompressor introduced into the small intestine which is plicated over it.

Measures to be taken when the Small Intestine is Strangulated.—If, as is frequently the case in intra-abdominal strangulation, blood-stained fluid is present in the peritoneal cavity, the fluid should be removed by suction or mopped up as completely as possible, for it is toxic and infected. After the relief of strangulation a decision must be reached as to whether the segment that was strangulated is viable. When it is black and the peritoneal coat has lost its sheen, when the mesentery shows a lack of arterial pulsation, or thrombosis of its veins, it is non-viable, if not already gangrenous, and, if practicable, resection followed by anastomosis is carried out. In doubtful cases when the intestine is blue, purple, or dark red, the effect of wrapping it in a warm moist abdominal pack is noted. At the same time the anaesthetist administers pure oxygen for three minutes. By these means viable is differentiated from non-viable intestine thus:

Intestine	Viable	Non-viable
Circulation	Dark colour becomes lighter; mesentery bleeds, if pricked.	Dark colour remains; no bleeding if mesentery is pricked.
Peritoneum	Shiny.	Dull and lustreless.
Intestinal musculature	Firm. Pressure rings may or may not disappear. Peristalsis may be observed.	Flabby, thin, and friable. Pressure rings persist. No peristalsis.

Paul Thwaites Savage, Contemporary. Surgeon, Whittington Hospital, London.

Special attention should always be paid to the sites of constriction ('pressure rings') at each end of the segment, which if of doubtful viability, should be enfolded by passing sutures through the sero-muscular coats and covering the area with omentum.

Pressure rings having received attention, viable intestine is returned to the abdominal cavity and the laparotomy incision is closed. When the strangulated intestine is deemed non-viable, it is resected and the continuity of the alimentary canal restored by end-to-end anastomosis.

When the obstruction occurs in the large intestine it is usually due to a carcinoma, or occasionally, in the case of the pelvic colon, to its imitator, diverticulitis, and the obstruction is of the acute-on-chronic variety. Acute-on-chronic obstruction of the large intestine should always be treated by early operation. In many cases it is possible to establish the diagnosis pre-operatively by *gentle* rigid or flexible colonoscopy which will reveal the carcinoma or confirm diverticulitis. If the patient's condition is good, laparotomy is performed through a right or left paramedian incision, according to the site of the obstruction. If the site is unknown, a right lower paramedian incision is employed. Distension of the caecum at once confirms that the obstruction lies in the large intestine. Palpation of the pelvic colon and, if that be collapsed, the transverse colon, will readily lead to the obstruction. When removable obstruction is present in the caecum, ascending colon, at the hepatic flexure, or in the proximal part of the transverse colon, emergency *right hemicolectomy* is the correct procedure. If the growth is irremovable or the patient extremely ill, an ileo-transverse enterostomy will relieve the obstruction. For an obstructing carcinoma of the hepatic flexure, an extended colectomy and ileum—descending colon re-anastomosis is 'best treatment'. For obstructing neoplasms of the left colon or recto-sigmoid junction immediate resection should be considered unless there are strong reasons against, *e.g.* inexperienced operator *or* very advanced disease *or* moribund patient. The proximal colon must be decompressed and cleaned by 'on-table' lavage (Dudley) before re-anastomosis is attempted: otherwise the proximal colon should be brought to the surface as a colostomy while the distal stump is closed and dropped back ('Hartmann procedure').

In very old or enfeebled patients when an obstructing carcinoma of the rectum is fixed and probably irremovable, left iliac colostomy is the best site for a permanent artificial anus, if the obstruction cannot be relieved by other ways, e.g. endoluminal electrocoagulation.

By placing the colostomy some inches proximal to the growth and excising it together with the growth at a second-stage operation, the number of operations and the length of hospitalisation can be reduced.

In rare circumstances, or if caecal perforation is judged imminent, time for improving the patient's condition can be bought by carrying out an emergency caecostomy through a small incision in the right iliac fossa.

GASTRO-INTESTINAL SUCTION DRAINAGE

When intestinal strangulation can be ruled out and the obstruction lies in the small intestine, a period of a few hours' gastro-intestinal suction drainage is the best form of

Hugh F. Dudley, Contemporary. Professor of Surgery, St. Mary's Hosital, London.

preliminary treatment.[1] Suction drainage should also be employed almost exclusively in paralytic ileus. In mechanical obstruction the combined effects of relieving distension by suction and the administration of fluid intravenously greatly improve the general condition of the patient for operation. Locally, diminution in size of the distended coils of intestine facilitates the operation and closure of the wound. Another most important consideration is that if highly toxic intestinal contents are aspirated before operation, it spares the patient the danger of absorbing this material after the obstruction has been relieved.

Maintenance of Fluid and Electrolytic Balance.—The fluid and the salt loss must be restored. Commonly as much as 3·5 litres of isotonic saline solution are required if the patient shows signs of severe dehydration, but considerably less if such signs are absent. A balance chart must be compiled, and the daily needs of the patient adjusted.

ACUTE INTESTINAL OBSTRUCTION OF THE NEWBORN

Congenital atresia[2] and stenosis[3] are the most common causes of intestinal obstruction in the newborn. The site of the obstruction is as follows:

Duodenum	33%
Jejunum.	15%
Ileum	25%
Ascending colon.	10%
Multiple sites	17%

The high incidence of multiple sites makes it imperative to examine the whole of the small intestine and the ascending colon at operation. Congenital abnormalities of the heart and great vessels are frequently associated with these lesions; only atresia below the duodenum escapes this association. Ileal atresia is commonly due to a vascular accident *in utero*.

Atresia and Stenosis of the Duodenum.—Atresia and stenosis occur with about equal frequency. Unless the obstruction is partial, persistent vomiting occurs from birth. The vomitus may or may not be bile-stained, depending on whether the septum lies below or above the duodenal papilla. Distension is often absent, but visible peristalsis is sometimes seen passing from left to right.

Radiography.—A plain film often confirms the diagnosis. The stomach and upper part of the duodenum are grossly distended with air, the so-called 'double stomach' (fig. 1063).

In cases of partial obstruction a small amount of Gastrografin injected through a gastric aspiration tube is useful for demonstrating the location of the obstruction; as soon as the films have been exposed, the medium must be aspirated.

Differential Diagnosis.—Suprapapillary duodenal atresia is distinguished from oesophageal atresia by the fact that there is no dribbling of saliva. The absence of a palpable lump serves to differentiate duodenal obstruction from infantile pyloric stenosis. Duodenal obstruction in infancy can also be caused by volvulus of the midgut (p. 1075), obstruction due to a band or to an annular pancreas.

Treatment.—Operation should be carried out as soon as dehydration has been combated. Duodeno-jejunostomy is the operation of choice. After completing the anastomosis, a stab incision is made through the wall of the pyloric antrum. Through this incision a rubber catheter is passed, and its tip guided through the anastomosis. A Witzel's valvular opening is constructed in the wall of the stomach and the tube is brought out through the laparotomy incision.

Atresia or Stenosis of the Ileum (less frequently of the jejunum).—The overriding importance of very early diagnosis of this condition lies in the fact that the distension immediately above the septum soon becomes so great that the vascular supply of the intestinal wall becomes jeopardised, and gangrene and perforation result. In atresia of the ileum (fig. 1064) the infant is either born with central distension of the abdomen, or distension appears within twenty-four hours of birth. In jejunal atresia early distension is lacking, but vomiting soon occurs. In both conditions some meconium is likely to be evacuated.

---

[1] Even when strangulation can be ruled out, not more than six or eight hours should be expended in this form of treatment. If operation is delayed over twenty-four hours, in spite of suction drainage, the mortality is nearly doubled.

[2] Atresia = imperforation.

[3] Stenosis = narrowing.

Friedrich Oskar Witzel, 1856–1925. Surgeon, Bonn, Germany.

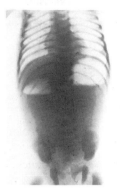

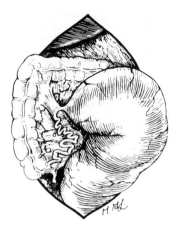

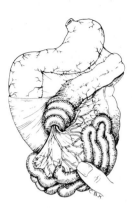

FIG. 1063. — Duodenal atresia. 'Double-stomach' appearance on erect film. Gas and fluid levels in both stomach and duodenum.

FIG. 1064.—Congenital atresia of the ileum.
(*V. Swain, FRCS, London.*)

FIG. 1065.—Volvulus of the midgut.

Radiography.—Obstruction of the small intestine cannot be diagnosed by plain x-rays unless fluid levels are seen in addition to the distended coils. By the time fluid levels are present, the obstruction is in an advanced state.

Operation.—If the stenosis is ileal, and the discrepancy in the diameters of the gut above and below the obstruction very great, the two limbs may be aligned and joined to make a spur (cf. Paul-Mikulicz operation for colonic volvulus), the apex of which is brought through the laparotomy wound or through a separate opening. After the abdomen has been closed, and the wound protected with a dressing, a small Paul's tube is tied into the proximal and a small catheter into the distal limb of the spur. Four days later the tubes are removed and a crushing clamp is applied to the septum. When the stenosis lies in the jejunum, so devastating are the effects of even a temporary jejunal fistula that primary end-to-end anastomosis, although a more difficult operation, must be recommended.

Arrested Rotation.—The caecum remains in the left hypochondrium, and a peritoneal band is found running from the caecum to the right side of the abdomen, and then across the second part of the duodenum. This is the transduodenal band of Ladd. The symptoms (repeated vomiting), due to pressure on the duodenum, and the radiographic appearances are identical with those of duodenal stenosis.

Treatment.—Early laparotomy is essential. The pressure on the duodenum can be relieved immediately by dividing the attachment of the band near the parietal peritoneum. Often there is a second peritoneal band, extending from the middle line to the commencement of the jejunum; this also must be divided. The caecum and colon are brushed over to the *left* side of the abdomen, leaving the small bowel on the right side (Nixon). The abdomen is closed. The results of timely operation in these cases are excellent.

Volvulus of the Midgut (*syn*. Volvulus Neonatorum).—Arrested rotation described above predisposes to volvulus of the midgut. The floating caecum, together with the whole of the small intestine, which has a narrow attachment, revolves. Broadly speaking, the clinical features are similar to, and the radiological findings are identical with, those of arrested rotation which, indeed, is present. The onset, however, is more catastrophic, and dehydration occurs more rapidly than in arrested rotation *per se*. In addition, abdominal distension is often evident.

Treatment.—When the abdomen is opened, only distended coils of small intestine (which may or may not be cyanotic) and the stomach are seen. The whole of the midgut must be delivered on to the surface, where the intestine is protected with warm, moist abdominal packs. Only after this step has been taken is it possible to see the volvulus (fig. 1065) which usually takes place in a clockwise direction. Untwisting is only half the operation; of equal importance is to divide the second obstructive lesion—the transduodenal band of Ladd—which is often present.

Meconium ileus is the neonatal manifestation of mucoviscidosis (fibrocystic disease of the pancreas). The terminal ileum becomes filled with meconium mixed with viscid mucus, notably from the pancreas, and during the latter months of foetal life this mixture

William Edwards Ladd, 1880–1967. Professor of Child Surgery, Harvard University, Boston, Massachusetts, U.S.A.
Harold Homewood Nixon, Contemporary. Surgeon, Hospital for Sick Children, Great Ormond Street, London.

becomes progressively inspissated. The infant is born with intestinal obstruction. At times the coil filled with inspissated meconium can be felt as a rubbery mass. A typical radiograph shows distended small intestine, some of which is mottled. Unlike ileal atresia, there is no abrupt termination of the gas-filled intestine.

Pathognomonic Test.—Into a bowl of vomitus is placed a piece of exposed x-ray film, and there it is left for half an hour. If trypsin is present, the gelatine that constitutes the sensitised coat of the film will be digested. In meconium ileus the film is merely rendered a little soft.

40% of cases are associated with complications, either volvulus neonatorum, atresia or meconium peritonitis (Dickson). When the physical signs of an acute intra-abdominal process are present, laparotomy must be carried out. When this is not so, however, a Gastrografin or Hypaque enema should be given to make the diagnosis. Since the colon is much reduced in size the radio-opaque fluid passes easily upwards to the ileum, and may on occasion disperse the obstructing meconium and relieve the condition. Gastrografin enema fluid also contains a wetting agent (Tween 80).

Treatment.—For laparotomy, adequate pre-operative preparation is essential. The only condition with which meconium ileus can be confounded is Hirschsprung's disease affecting the whole colon. The method of loosening the tenacious meconium from the mucous membrane by injections of 1% hydrogen peroxide through the bowel wall is not as satisfactory as believed previously. Recourse has to be made to a definitive resection of the most dilated segment. The proximal ileum is anastomosed end-to-side of collapsed colon beyond the obstruction (the Bishop-Koop operation). The distal ileal opening is formed into an ileostomy, through which the thick meconium can be eased postoperatively, assisted by irrigation of suitable lubricant solutions. The ileostomy becomes a mucous fistula which may need to be closed later.

Post-operative Complications.—In the section dealing with fibrocystic disease of the pancreas, attention has been directed to the susceptibility of infants with mucoviscidosis to pulmonary complications. Oxygen and antibiotic therapy, in addition to the usual post-operative regimen for intestinal obstruction, are given. Because the condition can recur, tube instillation of pancreatic enzymes can prevent this in some cases.

ACUTE INTUSSUSCEPTION

One portion of the gut becomes invaginated into another immediately adjacent; almost always it is the proximal into the distal. Very rarely indeed is an intussusception retrograde.

Aetiology.—In a few cases there is some obvious cause, *e.g.* a polypus, a papilliferous carcinoma, a submucous lipoma, or an inverted Meckel's diverticulum. Obviously such a protrusion invites intussusception (fig. 1066). In intussusception of infants it is generally agreed that:

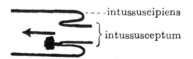

Fig. 1066.—The mechanism of the production of an intussusception.

1. Idiopathic intussusception occurs most often between the sixth and ninth months.
2. There is a change in diet—the infant is weaned.
3. An idiopathic intussusception usually commences in some part of the last 50 cm of the small intestine.
4. The maximum aggregation of Peyer's patches is in the lower ileum.

Theory—1. Change of diet brings about a change of intestinal flora. 2. This predisposes to inflammation of the intestinal tract. 3. Which in turn causes inflammation and swelling of Peyer's patches. 4. A swollen Peyer's patch produces an elevation protruding into the lumen of the gut comparable to one of the known causes of intussusception.

Another theory.—Intussusception often shows a seasonal incidence related to attacks of upper respiratory infection. After an operation for intussusception antibodies to certain viruses have been isolated and it is presumed that these cause swelling of Peyer's patches.

James Alexander Scott Dickson, Contemporary. Senior Lecturer in Paediatric Surgery, Institute of Child Health, University of London.
Harry Craden Bishop, Contemporary. Surgeon, Philadelphia, U.S.A.
Chas. Everett Koop, Contemporary. Surgeon, Philadelphia, U.S.A.
Johann Conrad Peyer, 1653–1712. Professor of Logic, Rhetoric, and Medicine, Schaffhausen, Switzerland.

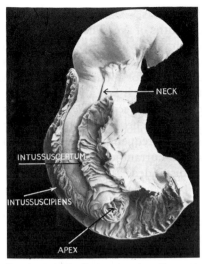

FIG. 1067.—An intussusception dissected to show its constituent parts.

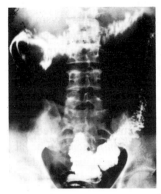

FIG. 1069.—'Claw' sign of ileo-colic intussusception. The barium in the intussuscipiens is seen as a claw around the negative shadow of the intussusception.
(R. S. Naik, M.S., Durg, India.)

FIG. 1068.— The physical signs recorded in a typical case of intussusception in an infant.

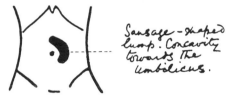

Sausage-shaped lump. Concavity towards the umbilicus.

In adults the hamartomatous polyps of 'Peutz-Jeghers syndrome' can cause intussusception which is recurring. The underlying condition is betrayed by the characteristic circumoral and lingual pigment patches (Chapter 50).

Pathology.—An intussusception is composed of three parts:

1. The entering, or inner, tube.
2. The returning, or middle, tube.
3. The sheath, or outer, tube.

The outer tube is called the *intussuscipiens*. The inner and middle tubes together form the *intussusceptum*. The neck is the junction of the entering layer with the mass. That part which advances is the apex, and the mass which constitutes the intussusception (fig. 1067) increases as it advances.

Types of Intussusception (After Gross) (In 702 cases)

	% of Series		% of Series
Ileo-ileal	5	Multiple	1
Ileo-colic	77	Retrograde	0·2
Ileo-ileo-colic	12	Others	2·8
Colo-colic	2		

A definite cause was found at operation in only 43 cases

The blood supply of the inner layers of the intussusception is liable to be impaired. The onset of early gangrene is dependent upon the tightness of the invagination. Because of the great pressure exerted upon it by passing through the ileo-caecal valve, an ileo-colic intussusception provides most examples of early gangrene.

Robert Edward Gross, Contemporary. Ladd Professor of Children's Surgery, Harvard University Medical School, Boston, Massachusetts, U.S.A.

Owing to earlier diagnosis, the number of irreducible intussusceptions is decreasing; and the mortality is correspondingly lower.

Methods of effecting Reduction in Difficult Cases

1. The little finger is inserted into the neck of the intussusception and an endeavour is made to separate adhesions between the intussuscipiens and intussusceptum, after which reduction is re-attempted (Cope's method).
2. The thumb and forefinger are placed as shown in fig. 1071, and gentle pressure is exerted. Gradually the pressure is increased. In this way oedema is squeezed from the region of the ileo-caecal valve.

Resection of an Irreducible or Gangrenous Intussusception.—Previous methods consisted of exteriorising the ileum and colon by various manoeuvres. With exact methods of electrolyte balance and of fluid replacement, these have been abandoned and resection with end-to-end anastomosis is the rule.

After-treatment.—Gastric aspiration should be continued for twelve to twenty-four hours and dextrose-saline administered intravenously, or subcutaneously with hyaluronidase. On the second day the gastric tube is removed and sips of water are given. A few hours later, feeding is commenced with the mother's milk if the infant is still being breast-fed. In cases where resection has been necessary, intravenous alimentation is required.

Recurrent intussusception occurs in only 2% of cases of idiopathic intussusception. If a second operation is necessary, the last few inches of the ileum should be anchored to the ascending colon by sutures in order to avoid further recurrence.

VOLVULUS

A volvulus results from axial rotation of a portion of the alimentary tract.

(*a*) **Volvulus Neonatorum.**

(*b*) **Volvulus of the small intestine,** other than the above, usually occurs in the lower ileum, and is favoured by the presence of an adhesion passing from the antimesenteric border of an intestinal loop (fig. 1072) to the parietes or to the female pelvic organs. In Africans, volvulus involving many feet of small intestine without causative adhesions occurs rather commonly. The consumption of a large meal of maize and vegetables seems to predispose to the condition.

Operation is to untwist the loop, if possible. The causative adhesion should be divided.

(*c*) **Volvulus of the caecum** can occur when the right half of the colon is lax and mobile. Volvulus of this part of the large intestine occurs nearly always in a clockwise direction. The first twist obstructs the ascending colon; if a second twist occurs, it obstructs the ileum also. Cases are recorded between 14 and 88 years. It is about twice as common in

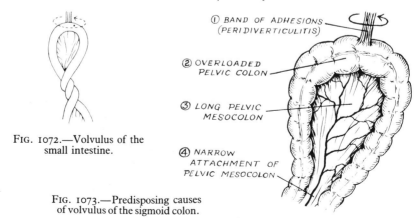

FIG. 1072.—Volvulus of the
small intestine.

① BAND OF ADHESIONS
(PERIDIVERTICULITIS)

② OVERLOADED
PELVIC COLON

③ LONG PELVIC
MESOCOLON

④ NARROW
ATTACHMENT OF
PELVIC MESOCOLON

FIG. 1073.—Predisposing causes
of volvulus of the sigmoid colon.

Sir Zachary Cope, 1881–1975. Surgeon, St. Mary's Hospital, London.

females. Presentation is usually acute with abdominal pain 90%, nausea and vomiting 70%, constipation 60%. In about 25% of cases there is a palpable tympanitic swelling not, as a rule, in the right iliac fossa, for in process of torsion the mobile caecum moves out of the right iliac fossa into the mid-abdomen, or even to the left side. A plain radiograph shows loops of gas-filled ileum, and sometimes an especially large gas shadow which can be recognised as the caecum. At first, the obstruction is not absolute; faeces and flatus may be expelled after an enema. Barium enema is most effective in diagnosis.

Operation.—In early cases it is usually possible to untwist the bowel. Sometimes before untwisting can be accomplished, it is necessary to deflate the ballooned caecum by the insertion of a needle. Untwisting should be followed by caecostomy, which serves two purposes—it relieves distension and it fixes the organ to the abdominal wall, thereby preventing a recurrence. If the caecum is gangrenous or its viability is not assured, right hemicolectomy is performed.

(d) **Volvulus of the pelvic colon** is common in Eastern Europe, India, Scandinavia, and Peru. The predisposing causes are indicated in fig. 1073. The loop may rotate half a turn, in which event spontaneous rectification sometimes occurs. After the loop has rotated 1½ turns the veins involved in the torsion are compressed, and the loop becomes greatly congested. If, as is sometimes the case, it rotates more than 1½ turns, the blood supply is cut off entirely and the loop becomes gangrenous. The rotation nearly always occurs in an *anti-clockwise* direction.

Clinical Features.—Males are more commonly affected than females, and the sufferers are usually middle-aged or elderly. There is often a history of acute attacks of left-sided abdominal pain, probably due to a partial volvulus, that untwists itself and is followed by the passage of large quantities of flatus and faeces. As a rule the onset of volvulus of the pelvic colon is sudden and is characterised by severe abdominal pain, often coming on while the patient is straining at stool. Abdominal distension soon follows; in no other condition does extreme abdominal distension, partly due to the diffusion of CO_2 from distended veins, occur so quickly. If the patient is examined two or three hours after the commencement of the attack, the distension is mainly left-sided. In a matter of six hours the whole abdomen becomes distended. Hiccough and retching occur early; vomiting is late. Constipation is absolute, but an enema may be returned blood stained. A plain x-ray film of the abdomen shows massive distension of the colon with gas.

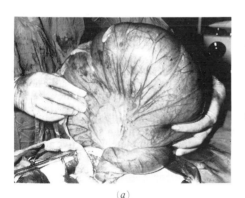 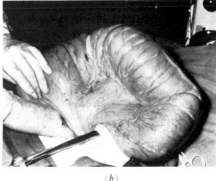

(a)   (b)

FIG. 1074.—Volvulus of the sigmoid colon (a) before and (b) after untwisting.
(S. U. Rahman, FRCS, Manchester.)

Treatment.—Sigmoidoscopy should be carried out and when the obstruction is reached an attempt is made to coax a soft rectal tube into the twisted gut. This will immediately deflate the gut and operation can be delayed for a few days until the patient is more fit. If deflation does not succeed, laparotomy must be performed immediately. At attempt is made to untwist the gas-filled viscus (fig. 1073); meanwhile a rectal tube is passed by a nurse and guided into position by the surgeon with his hand inside the abdomen. When the colon is deflated, a resection and end-to-end anastomosis can be carried out. Some surgeons prefer to exteriorise and resect the volvulus by the Paul-Mikulicz procedure. This method is specially valuable if there is any suggestion of impending gangrene. Redundancy of the colon makes the performance of this procedure simple (fig. 1075).

suffered direct compression by the band show any colour changes, they should be invaginated. Gangrenous intestine must be resected.

OBSTRUCTION DUE TO AN INTERNAL HERNIA

A portion of the small intestine passes into one of the retroperitoneal fossae or into a congenital defect of one of the mesenteries, there to be imprisoned. The potential internal hernias are as follows:

1. ***The Foramen of Winslow.**—The portal vein, common bile duct, and hepatic artery lie in its free border.
2. ***A Hole in the Mesentery.**
3. **A Hole in the Transverse Mesocolon.**
4. **A Defect in the Broad Ligament.**
5. **Congenital or Acquired Diaphragmatic Hernia.**
6. **One of the retroperitoneal fossae,** of which the following are most important:

Fossae about the Duodenum

(a) **The Left Paraduodenal Fossa.*—The inferior mesenteric vein lies in its free border.
(b) **The Right Duodeno-jejunal Fossa.*—The superior mesenteric artery runs in its free border.

Fossae about the Caecum and Appendix.

(a) *Superior Ileo-caecal Fossa.*—Between the general mesentery and a fold of peritoneum raised by the anterior caecal branch of the ileo-colic artery.
(b) *Inferior Ileo-caecal Fossa.*.—Between the 'bloodless' fold of Treves and the mesentery of the appendix.
(c) *The retro-caecal fossa* behind the caecum.
The intersigmoid fossa is situated in the base of the pelvic mesocolon.

An internal hernia is an uncommon cause of intestinal obstruction; a preoperative diagnosis can be only a guess.

Treatment.—In those herniae above marked with a * an important blood-vessel runs in the edge of the hernial orifice, and to divide the constricting agent (which is the correct treatment for the other varieties) may cause serious bleeding. When confronted with the difficult problem of how to release imprisoned intestine without dividing a vital constricting agent it becomes necessary, with adequate protection of the rest of the wound, to decompress the distended loop (see fig. 1062).

OBSTRUCTION FROM STRICTURE OF THE SMALL INTESTINE

Cicatricial contracture is usually an aftermath of tuberculous ulceration or Crohn's disease. Multiple strictures are usually present. Malignant stricture is rare, although both carcinoma and sarcoma occur from time to time. Gradual contraction of a stricture causes a chronic obstruction of the small intestine with dilatation and hypertrophy of the intestinal wall above. Clinically there is some colic and distension, associated with the features of the blind-loop syndrome, *i.e.* steatorrhoea, loss of weight, anaemia, avitaminosis, and cachexia.

Treatment.—Except in emergency, a simple stricture should never be by-passed by a lateral anastomosis. A blind-loop syndrome is sure to follow. A simple stricture should be excised locally, and a malignant stricture widely, and the continuity of the intestine restored by end-to-end anastomosis. In quiescent areas of Crohn's disease the strictures can be widened surgically ('stricture plasty') in order to avoid removing too much small intestine (fig. 1042, Chapter 50).

Jacob Benignus Winslow, 1669–1760. Professor of Anatomy, Physic and Surgery, Paris.
Sir Frederick Treves, 1853–1923. Surgeon, The London Hospital.

OBSTRUCTION BY OBTURATION OF THE SMALL INTESTINE

Obstruction by a gallstone[1] usually occurs in elderly obese women because the gallstone, which is 2·5 cm or more in diameter, requires some years to reach this dimension, and more years elapse before it ulcerates through the gall-bladder into the duodenum. It passes down the small bowel, becoming impacted about 60 cm above the ileo-caecal valve, because this is the narrowest part of the small gut. The symptoms are elusive. The patient has recurrent mild colic, accompanied by copious vomiting. As the obstruction is incomplete, there is often some result from an enema, and remissions of symptoms are frequent, but the vomiting returns, and by this time it is bilious; as time goes on it becomes faeculent. An x-ray may reveal the stone, and the small intestine will be seen to be distended with gas. It may actually be felt in the Pouch of Douglas on rectal examination. There is no abdominal distension until late, and late intestinal obstruction in an old person is an almost hopeless condition. Rarely, a large stone ulcerates into the transverse colon, and from time to time it remains in the large intestine long enough to increase in size, by the deposition of faecal matter upon it, so that eventually it becomes impacted in the rectum.

Treatment.—Through a lower right paramedian incision the loop containing the stone is delivered and packed off most carefully. Occasionally, it is possible to crush the stone between the fingers while it is still in the lumen. If not, the intestine is opened and the stone removed. It is an advantage to sew up the incision in the intestine transversely, to avoid constriction. A gallstone that causes intestinal obstruction is nearly always barrel-shaped and unfaceted. If there is a facet, it is essential to palpate the intestine above the obstruction for a possible fellow-calculus. The area of the gall bladder should be left strictly alone, as even gentle manipulation can break down a cholecyst-duodenal fistula.

Bolus obstruction due to food is particularly liable to occur after partial gastrectomy when insufficiently masticated articles of food will be hurried into the small intestine where they become impacted at the narrowest portion of the intestine, *i.e.* about 60 cm above the ileo-caecal valve. Normally they would be retained in the stomach until they had become partially digested. Unripe apples, coconut, Brussels sprouts, dried fruit, and, particularly, unmasticated orange pulp have caused intestinal obstruction in these circumstances.

Treatment.—Timely laparotomy is required. An attempt should be made to squeeze the bolus gently onward into the caecum, and there to break it up by kneading. Should the bolus be impacted so firmly that this manoeuvre proves impracticable—and such is likely only in cases of obstruction by dried fruit or when a stricture of the small intestine is present—enterotomy must be performed. After the obstructing material has been removed the opening in the intestine is sutured, the coil mechanically cleansed before returning it to the abdomen, which is then closed.

Obstruction by stercolith gives rise to symptoms identical with those of obstruction by a gallstone, for a stercolith, contrary to what might be expected, is usually formed and found in the small intestine, particularly in cases where a jejunal diverticulum or a stricture in the ileum is present. On careful dissection of a stercolith it is not unusual to find a nucleus of recognisable material, *e.g.* tomato skins.

Obstruction due to Worms. (fig. 1077).—An aggregation of *Ascaris lumbricoides* is sometimes the cause of low small intestinal obstruction in children, usually under ten

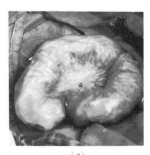
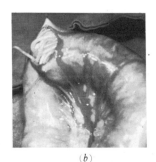
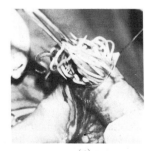

(a) (b) (c)

FIG. 1077.—Obstruction of the Small Intestine due to *Ascaris lumbricoides*
(Asal. Y. Izzidien, FRCS, Nenavah, Iraq.)

---

[1] Formerly called gallstone 'ileus'. Ileus, from ιλεοζ (Greek) = colic.

James Douglas, 1675–1742. Scottish Anatomist and Obstetrician.

years of age, and especially those living in or near the tropics. There is debility out of proportion to that produced by the obstruction. The obturation is inclined to follow the ingestion of an anti-helminthic. If it is not known that the patient is suffering from ascaris infestation, a worm in the vomitus or the presence of eosinophilia may be the means of making a correct pre-operative diagnosis. In this form of intestinal obstruction laparotomy must be performed, and if possible the tangled mass should be kneaded along the ileum into the caecum, if not it should be removed (fig. 1077).

PARALYTIC ILEUS

This has already been defined as a state in which the intestine fails to transmit peristaltic waves, and is due to failure in the neuromuscular mechanism—*i.e.* in the myenteric plexus (Auerbach) and the submucous plexus (Meissner). This results in a collection of fluid and gas in the intestine, with resulting distension, vomiting, absent or high 'tinkling' bowel sounds, and failure to pass flatus.

The following varieties are recognised:

1. *Post-operative.*—Some degree of ileus, either local or general, may follow any abdominal operation. In the absence of infection, it is not serious. Indeed, it has been shown that intestinal motility and absorption commonly returns to normal in about sixteen hours—well ahead of gastric and colonic activity. Post-operative ileus may be prolonged if there is hypoproteinaemia, or latent renal failure (*vide infra*), or if gastrointestinal suction is continued beyond the point at which effective bowel sounds have returned.

2. *Infective.*—Peritonitis gives rise to prolonged ileus, but several factors may be involved. At the outset, peristalsis ceases as a normal response to prevent dissemination, but afterwards, bacterial toxins prevent the normal activity of the nerve plexuses. When the bowel begins to recover, the early feeble peristaltic waves may not be able to overcome the obstructive effect of the newly formed slender adhesions between loops of intestines, and so further quiescence of activity follows. In this kind of ileus, there are therefore mechanical as well as neurogenic factors to be considered. Typhoid is associated with ileus in its acute form.

3. *Reflex.*—This form of ileus may occur following fractures of the spine or ribs, retroperitoneal haemorrhage, or even the application of a plaster jacket.

4. *Uraemia.*—This type, with distension, vomiting, and hiccoughs is well recognised, and is seen in renal failure. It may follow prostatectomy.

5. *Hypokalaemia.*—A low serum potassium may cause ileus.

Clinical Features.—Ileus is suspected if, 48 hours after laparotomy:

(*a*) There has been no passage of flatus.

(*b*) There is no return of normal bowel sounds on auscultation.

Abdominal distension becomes more marked and drum-like (tympanitic); in the absence of gastric aspiration, there is effortless vomiting of large volumes of dirty fluid. There is no colic, and often no abdominal pain at all. There may be respiratory distress from the abdominal distension and the pulse-rate increases. Prolonged distension increases the risk of wound dehiscence. Radiologically, the abdomen shows gas-filled loops of intestine with multiple fluid levels.

It is important to recognise three types of bowel sounds:
(1) The *normal* low-pitched borborygmi each lasting about a second and occurring every twenty seconds or so.
(2) The prolonged, rapidly recurring and noisy borborygmi of *dynamic obstruction*.

Leopold Auerbach, 1828–1897. Professor of Neuropathology, Breslau, Germany (now Wroclaw, Poland).
Georg Meissner, 1829–1905. Professor of Physiology, Göttingen, Germany.

(3) The high-pitched tinkling note 'like bells at evening pealing', which occurs every ten to thirty seconds, and is distinctive of *paralytic ileus*. It is due, not to peristalsis, but to the overflow of fluid from one distended loop to another.

Management.—The essence of this is prevention and the incidence has been greatly reduced by routine naso-gastric suction and withholding fluids by mouth after laparotomy until normal bowel sounds and/or the passage of flatus returns. Further, electrolyte balance should be achieved before, and maintained after operation. Specific treatment is directed to the cause, but there are some principles which have general application:

(1) The primary cause must be removed.

(2) Normal bowel activity will return if distension is relieved by adequate gastro-intestinal decompression. It is probably the distension of the gut (possibly exacerbated by the air swallowing of anxiety) that causes the ileus, rather than the ileus that causes the distension. Thorough decompression is therefore essential. If a naso-gastric tube is used after operation it must not be spigoted but be kept open to permit swallowed air to be evacuated.

(3) Morphine or pethidine in repeated small doses are well proved and valuable in these cases.

(4) Close attention to the fluid and electrolyte balance, especially the serum potassium and the blood urea, is essential (Chapter 6).

(5) Peristaltic stimulants have no place in treatment. The object is to *rest* the bowel, not to stimulate it, *i.e.* don't flog a tired horse!

Measurement of abdominal girth at the umbilicus is the only way of being certain of increase or decrease of distension. This should be done four- or six-hourly. As recovery occurs, segmentation returns before peristalsis. Bowel sounds commence and the patient feels hungry. 'Wind pains' are experienced but are soon followed by the passage of flatus.

Resolution is often accompanied by a short period of diarrhoea. No treatment is necessary for this.

If paralytic ileus is prolonged and threatens life, laparotomy should be carried out and the bowel decompressed with a Savage's sucker.

EMBOLISM AND THROMBOSIS OF THE MESENTERIC VESSELS

Arterial embolism is more common than spontaneous thrombosis, and the superior mesenteric vessels are implicated much more frequently than the inferior; the latter is often silent due to the better collateral circulation.

Embolism of the Superior Mesenteric Artery.—Possible sources of emboli include: the left auricle (especially in atrial fibrillation); a mural myocardial infarct; an atheromatous plaque of aneurysm of the aorta; a vegetation on the mitral valve; pulmonary vein thrombosis secondary to septic infarct; or from a left atrial myxoma.

Primary thrombosis of the superior mesenteric artery is the result either of arteriosclerosis or thrombo-angiitis obliterans.

Primary thrombosis of the superior mesenteric vein or its tributaries occurs occasionally in portal hypertension, portal pyaemia (pylephlebitis), sickle cell disease, and in women taking the contraceptive pill.

No matter whether the occlusion is arterial or venous, haemorrhagic infarction occurs although, in the case of embolism, a short-lived pallor has been observed at early laparotomy. The intestine and its mesentery become swollen and oedematous, demarcation between infarcted and healthy intestine being gradual. Blood-stained fluid is exuded into the peritoneal cavity and the lumen of the infarcted intestine becomes filled with blood.

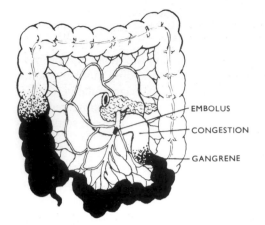

EMBOLUS

CONGESTION

GANGRENE

FIG. 1078.—Embolus lodged in the main trunk of the superior mesenteric artery. Showing the widespread gangrene that results.

When the main trunk of the superior mesenteric artery becomes occluded, infarction of nearly the whole of the small intestine, the caecum, and part of the ascending colon occurs (fig. 1078). More frequently a branch of the main vessel is implicated and the area of infarction is proportionately less.

Clinical Features.—(i) *Pain.* The most important clue to early diagnosis is the sudden onset of severe abdominal pain in a patient with atrial fibrillation or atherosclerosis. Pain is typically central abdominal and out of proportion to the physical findings.

(ii) *Gastro-intestinal emptying* with persistent vomiting and bowel evacuation occurs early. In late cases altered blood may be passed per rectum. Shock due to fluid and later actual blood loss into the bowel develops rapidly.

(iii) *Abdominal tenderness* may be mild initially but later rebound tenderness and rigidity supervene.

(iv) X-ray examination of the abdomen usually shows no gas in the small intestine. A neutrophilic leucocytosis occurs early and most always exceeds 15,000.

Provided that the predisposing factors are considered, the diagnosis of mesenteric thrombosis or embolism is not difficult. Mesenteric vascular occlusion carries a higher mortality than any other type of intestinal obstruction. This is not surprising when one considers the type of patient prone to this disaster.

Treatment.—In the early embolic case, when the diagnosis has been confirmed at laparotomy, superior mesenteric embolectomy should be attempted or the superior mesenteric artery re-anastomosed to the aorta at a fresh site after it has been divided below the obstruction. In the later cases the affected bowel should be resected. In all cases, blood transfusion is required and anti-coagulant treatment should be commenced twelve to twenty-four hours after operation. In patients who recover, intestinal obstruction secondary to ischaemic fibrosis of an area of small bowel may occur.

Infarction of the large intestine is rare. Lodgement of an embolus in the middle colic artery should be treated by resection of the transverse colon with exteriorisation of both ends. If the patient survives and is deemed fit for a further operation, the bowel ends can be joined; otherwise the colostomy must be permanent.

Ischaemic Colitis is the term given to describe the structural changes in the colon as a result of deprivation of blood. Such episodes are similar to those in the heart or brain and occur specially in the region of the splenic flexure whose blood supply is particularly

FIG. 1079.—Ischaemic colitis—site of lesion in a woman of 67 with six months' rectal bleeding; occasional colicky pain and vomiting. Lesion resected with recovery.
(Adrian Marston, FRCS, London.)

precarious. They are classified into gangrenous (see above), stricturing and transient forms (Marston). The presenting syndrome is lower abdominal pain of abrupt onset, vomiting,

Jeffrey Adrian Priestley Marston, Contemporary. Surgeon, Middlesex Hospital, London.

fever and the passage of bright red blood per rectum. The age is that expected in degenerative vascular disease and at operation the length of colon has the appearance of a haemorrhagic infarct which may require immediate resection. In the cases where no operation is performed, a stricture may appear on a barium enema as a tubular narrowing over several inches of bowel most often in the region of the splenic flexure. The differential diagnosis is from carcinoma, Crohn's disease and ulcerative colitis. An arteriogram is usually conclusive.

CHRONIC INTESTINAL OBSTRUCTION

The various abnormalities and diseases giving rise to chronic intestinal obstruction are described in Chapters 50 and 54. The bowel wall above a chronic obstruction becomes thickened as a result of muscular 'work hypertrophy'. There remains one condition to be considered here.

Faecal impaction in the rectum and the colon occurs principally in elderly, and often bed-ridden, patients. It is all too often overlooked, because a P.R. is not done because the patient is having 'diarrhoea', in which case the patient suffers unnecessary distress.

The symptoms are those of chronic intestinal obstruction, and attacks of spurious diarrhoea are a common accompaniment. A faecal accumulation may form a palpable abdominal mass which can be indented. When the mass is situated in the rectum, it can be indented by the palpating finger.

Treatment.—Enemas are usually insufficient. Repeated bowel washouts and the use of various proprietary faecal plasticisers (*e.g.* Dioctyl) by mouth or by enema, may result in disimpaction. Otherwise the anal sphincter must be dilated under general anaesthesia and the mass removed with the aid of fingers and a spoon ('disimpaction').

CHAPTER 52

THE VERMIFORM APPENDIX

SURGICAL ANATOMY

The vermiform appendix is present only in man, certain anthropoid apes, and the wombat.[1] Morphologically, it is the undeveloped distal end of the large caecum found in many lower animals.

The appendix varies considerably in length and circumference. The average length is between 7·5 cm and 10 cm. Specimens of over 30 cm in length have been recorded. The appendix averages 0·5 cm longer in the male than in the female. The lumen, which should admit a matchstick, is irregular, being encroached upon by the multiple longitudinal folds of mucous membrane.

The **mesoappendix** which springs from the lower surface of the mesentery is subject to great variations. Sometimes as much as the distal of one-third of the appendix is bereft of mesoappendix. Especially in childhood, the mesoappendix is so transparent that the contained blood-vessels can be seen. In many adults it becomes laden with fat, which obscures these vessels.

The **appendicular artery**, a branch of the lower division of the ileo-colic artery, passes behind the terminal ileum to enter the mesoappendix a short distance from the base of the appendix. It then comes to lie in the free border of the mesoappendix; but for a variable distance from the tip, where the mesoappendix is lacking, the artery lies directly on the muscle wall beneath the peritoneal coat. **An accessory appendicular artery** may be present, but in most people, once the appendicular artery reaches the wall of the appendix proper it becomes an 'end-artery': thrombosis of the artery as a result of appendicitis causes necrosis of the appendix (*syn.* 'gangrenous appendicitis').

Lymphatic Vessels.—Four, six, or more lymphatic channels traverse the mesoappendix to empty into the ileo-caecal lymph nodes.

MICROSCOPIC ANATOMY

The appendix is lined by columnar-cell intestinal mucosa of colonic type. Crypts are present but are not numerous: in the base of the crypts lie the special cells which give rise to carcinoid tumours. The appendix is the most frequent site for these rare tumours (see Chapter 50).

The submucosa contains numerous lymphatic aggregations ('follicles'). This profusion of lymph tissue has promoted the description of 'abdominal tonsil' for the appendix, and

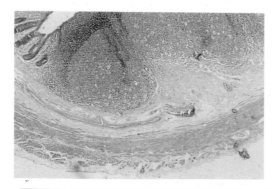

FIG. 1080.—Normal appendix. Low power view.
(*Courtesy of Dr D. Pollock, The London Hospital.*)

---

[1] Wombat—a nocturnal, burrowing Australian marsupial.

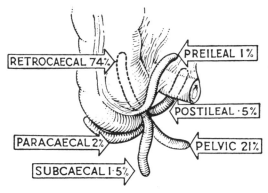

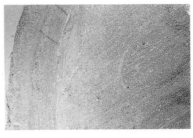

FIG. 1081.—The various positions of the appendix.
(After Sir Cecil Wakeley London, formerly PRCS)

FIG. 1082.—Acute appendicitis. Note how swollen the layers are in comparison with fig. 1080. The mucosal and submucosal layers are affected by an acute inflammatory exudate ('polymorphs'). Low power view.
(Courtesy of Dr D. Pollock, The London Hospital.)

draws attention to this feature as relevant to the causes of appendicitis. The lymphatic tissue is well-shown in fig. 1080. The muscular coat consists of two complete layers of smooth muscle—inner circular and outer longitudinal: the latter is formed by the joining together of the taenia coli at the base of the appendix.

The visceral layer of peritoneum envelops the appendix completely except for the narrow line of attachment of the meso-appendix.

McBurney's point lies at the junction of the lateral third with the medial two-thirds of a line joining the anterior superior iliac spine and the umbilicus. McBurney's point is the classical site of greatest tenderness in appendicitis, and also a most useful point to have in mind when a grid-iron incision is made.

LOCATION

Inconstancy of Position.—The relative frequency of the more usual positions occupied by the organ is depicted in fig. 1081. In addition, the appendix must necessarily share in abnormalities in position of the caecum. The most frequent of these is failure of the caecum to descend, which results in the base ofthe appendix being situated in the right hypochondrium. Very occasionally the caecum and appendix are situated in the left iliac fossa or in the left hypochondrium (see below).

Locating the Appendix.—The traditional method consists of following one of the taeniae coli downwards till the appendix is reached. If the organ is still not visible and it is certain that it has not been removed, it will probably be found adherent to the posterior caecal wall.

CONGENITAL ABNORMALITIES

Agenesis.—Once in 100,000 persons the vermiform appendix is absent.

Duplication.—A few cases of double appendix have been reported; in some instances one of the twin appendices has been found acutely inflamed and the other uninvolved.

Left-sided Appendix.—*Situs inversus viscerum*, a congenital abnormality where there is complete transposition of thoracic and abdominal viscera, occurs once in 35,000 individuals, and is more common in males. In such cases, of course, the vermiform appendix is situated on the left as it is also in some cases of non-rotation of the mid-gut.

ACUTE APPENDICITIS

During recent years the mortality from acute appendicitis has been falling. Earlier diagnosis and appendicectomy while the inflammation is still confined to

Charles McBurney, 1845–1913. Professor of Surgery, Columbia University College of Physicians and Surgeons, New York, U.S.A.

the appendix, the recognition by the general public that it is dangerous to take or give to a child a purgative in the presence of undiagnosed abdominal pain, more caution against performing immediate appendicectomy in late cases, a greater appreciation of the importance of accurate fluid and electrolytic balance, better anaesthesia, and the control of infection by antibiotics have all played a part in bringing about this improvement. Nevertheless, hospital statistics[1] show that in cases where the inflammation is no longer limited to the appendix, the mortality rate is 5% in males and 6% in females. In men over sixty-five the mortality may be as much as 25%.

All are agreed that early diagnosis with prompt appendicectomy is the goal. On the other hand, some patients fail to seek medical advice until a late hour. In such cases when and when not to operate becomes a matter of refined judgement (p. 1104). While there are no absolute rules, appendicectomy should be avoided in the presence of an established mass or a localised abscess, or if the history is more than 48 hours long. In cases of real doubt, infants and aged patients should influence the decision towards immediate appendicectomy.

Aetiology

Until the close of the nineteenth century appendicitis remained unrecognised. Unquestionably, before this time it was a comparatively rare disease, but there can be no doubt that it existed even in remote times, for an acutely inflamed, perforated appendix was found preserved in the mummy of a young royal princess of Egypt (Spencer).

The riddle of appendicitis—its actual cause and its meteoric rise from an insignificant disease to the most common serious intra-abdominal inflammatory affection of Western civilised races—has been a matter for much speculation. So far no satisfactory explanation has been forthcoming. The following aetiological factors are important, but for the most part they are purely contributory.

Race and Diet.—Appendicitis is particularly common in the highly civilised European, American, and Australasian countries, while it is rare in Asiatics, Africans, and Polynesians. Rendle Short showed that if individuals from the latter races migrate to countries where appendicitis is common, they soon acquire the local susceptibility to the disease. Even apes in captivity appear to acquire the human liability to appendicitis. These significant facts satisfy many that the rise of appendicitis amongst the highly civilised is due to departure from a simple diet rich in cellulose to one relatively rich in meat. But this cannot be the whole explanation, for acute appendicitis occurs in lifelong vegetarians and even in babes at the breast.

Social Status.—In England, acute appendicitis is more common among the upper and middle classes than in those belonging to the so-called working class. Thus the mortality from acute appendicitis is about 20% higher in men of social classes I and II (professional and managerial workers) than it is in social class V (unskilled labourers) (Registrar-General, 1954).

Familial Susceptibility.—This unusual but generally accepted fact can be accounted for by an hereditary abnormality in position of the organ, which predisposes to infection. Thus the whole family may have long rectrocaecal appendices with comparatively poor blood supply.

Obstruction of the Lumen of the Appendix. When an acutely inflamed appendix has been removed, some form of obstruction to its lumen can be demonstrated in a large percentage of cases. The obstructing agent is usually a faecolith or a stricture; exceptionally, a foreign body or a round worm or thread-worms are found.

Faecoliths (fig. 1083) vary in size and have a laminated structure. They are composed of inspissated faecal material, calcium and magnesium phosphates and carbonates, bacteria and epithelial debris; rarely, a foreign body is incorporated in the mass. The presence of a faecolith or faecoliths postulates some form of appendicular stasis.

---

[1] Statistics from the Social Medical Research Unit of the Medical Research Council, The London Hospital, 1957.

Arthur Morgan Spencer, Contemporary. Formerly Medical Superintendent, Powick Hospital, nr. Worcester, England.
Arthur Rendle Short, 1880–1953. Professor of Surgery, Bristol, England.

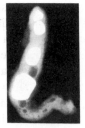

FIG. 1083.—Fae-
coliths. X-ray of
an appendix after
removal.

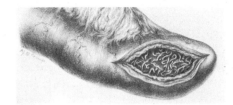

FIG. 1084.—An appendix filled with oxyuria vermicularis.

Worms.—Worms (fig. 1084) and other intestinal parasites can injure the appendicular mucous membrane and occasionally block its lumen.

Distal Obstruction of Colon.—Acute appendicitis can result from an obstructing (colon) carcinoma, usually of the right colon: these are usually elderly cases.

The Abuse of Purgatives.—It is abundantly clear that the ingestion of purgatives, particularly castor oil, by patients with 'stomach ache', and the violent peristaltic action which results, favours, and often determines, perforation of an inflamed appendix. 'Purgation means perforation' is a wise adage.

Bacteriology.—Cultures from inflamed appendices usually reveal that the infection is mixed and there is hardly a pyogenic organism which has not been isolated from such specimens. The most common organisms present are a mixture of *Esch. coli* (found in 85% of cases), enterococci (30%), non-haemolytic streptococci, anaerobic[1] streptococci, together with *Cl. welchii* (30%) and bacteroides. In most instances the infecting organisms are normal inhabitants of the lumen of the appendix.

Pathology.—The menace of acute appendicitis lies in the frequency with which the peritoneal cavity is infected from this focus, 1. By perforation, 2. By transmigration of bacteria through the appendicular wall.

The greater omentum, the 'abdominal policeman', attempts to arrest the spread of peritoneal invasion, whilst violent peristalsis from ingested purgatives tends to spread it. Obviously, if the inflamed appendix lies dangling amidst coils of small intestine, the threat of peritonitis is increased; should early perforation occur, diffusing peritonitis is inevitable.

It is of great importance to recognise two types of acute appendicitis.

(*a*) **Non-obstructive Acute Appendicitis.**—The inflammation usually commences in the mucous membrane; less often in the lymph follicles. Like any inflammatory process, it terminates in one of the following ways: (1) Resolution; (2) Ulceration; (3) Suppuration; (4) Fibrosis; (5) Gangrene. All grades of inflammation occur and once infection reaches the loose submucous tissues it progresses rapidly. The organ becomes turgid, dusky red, and haemorrhages occur into the mucous membrane. The vascular supply of the distal part of the appendix is often in jeopardy because it is intramural and liable to occlusion by inflammation or thrombosis. This may lead to gangrene of the tip. Non-obstructive appendicitis may progress sufficiently slowly for protective adhesions to form, and the resulting peritonitis is localised. In many instances the infection never progresses beyond the mucous lining (*i.e.* catarrhal inflammation) but although the attack passes off, it is unlikely that a *status quo ante* is ever regained.

---

[1] The foul odour of exudates connected with appendicitis with perforation is caused by anaerobic streptococci or anaerobic bacilli, and not by *Esch. coli*, as is so commonly believed.

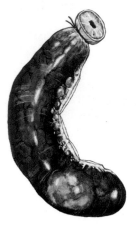

FIG. 1085.—Acute appendicitis. Perforation imminent.

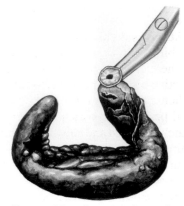

FIG. 1086.—Acute obstructive appendicitis with gangrene. There is a large faecal concretion impacted in the proximal end of the lumen of the organ.

Because the tip suffers most, after resolution of the acute attack, fibrosis usually occurs therein and this is a classical finding in recurrent appendicitis.

(b) **Obstructive Acute Appendicitis.**—About one-third of cases of acute appendicitis belong to this group. The obstruction can be in the lumen (faecolith, foreign body, or parasites); in the wall (almost invariably inflammatory, but exceptionally by direct occlusion by a carcinoma of the caecum); outside the wall (adhesions and kinking). Of these, much the most common is a faecolith Fibrosis of the wall from previous attacks of appendicitis can contribute by narrowing the lumen and promoting faecolith impaction and (rarely) appendicitis accompanies ileo-caecal Crohn's disease.

In obstructive appendicitis the products of inflammation become pent up so that the inflammation proceeds more rapidly and more certainly to gangrene or perforation. Often within twelve to eighteen hours the appendix distal to the obstruction becomes gangrenous (fig. 1086). Close examination of gangrenous appendices directly after their removal shows conclusively that they usually belong to the obstructive group (Wilkie). Perforation occurs most often at the site of an impacted faecolith before protective adhesions have had time to form. The escaping purulent and gaseous contents are under high pressure and early widespread peritonitis is liable to ensue.

Clinical Features (Fitz)

Age Incidence.—Rare before the age of two, acute appendicitis becomes increasingly common during childhood and adolescence. The maximum incidence is between the ages of twenty and thirty; thereafter there is a gradual decline, but no age is exempt.

The patient often gives a history of similar slight attacks. The attack can commence at any time, but frequently it does so in the early hours of the morning, awakening the patient from sleep. Recent constipation is usual.

Sir David Percival Dalbreck Wilkie, 1882–1938. Professor of Surgery, Edinburgh.
Reginald Heber Fitz, 1843–1913. Professor of Medicine, Harvard University, Boston, Massachusetts, U.S.A. Published a classical paper on appendicitis in 1886 which drew attention to the disease and framed the clinical features.

Non-obstructive Acute Appendicitis.—Typically there are three main features:

1. **Abdominal Pain which Shifts.**—Usually the first symptom is pain around the umbilicus, in the epigastrium, or it may be generalised. This is *visceral* pain and is therefore somewhat vague. It is due to distension of the appendix. In non-obstructive cases the pain is constant but in obstructive cases it is colicky. After a few hours the pain shifts to the point where the inflamed appendix irritates the parietal peritoneum, which is very sensitive. This pain is *somatic* or *peritoneal*, accurately localised and constant. A clinical and often valuable observation is that coughing causes pain in acute appendicitis but the pain is absent in the case of a stone in the ureter (p. 1099).

2. **Upset of Gastric Function.**—Protective pylorospasm occurs and this may be manifested by anorexia, nausea, vomiting, a brown-furred tongue, and a foul breath. Typically the vomiting is of short duration and stops as soon as the stomach is empty. In the majority of instances the patient is constipated but occasionally diarrhoea occurs, expecially in the very young or when the appendix lies in the post-ileal or pelvic position.

3. **Localised Tenderness at the Site of the Appendix.**—As soon as the pain has shifted, there is localised tenderness either at McBurney's point or elsewhere, as determined by the site of the appendix (fig. 1081). This tenderness may be confined to the pelvis and thus *rectal examination must be done in every case of lower abdominal pain.*[1] The identification of the site of the appendix is important; it will determine the operative approach. With the passage of time, accurate localisation becomes more difficult as muscular rigidity becomes evident in addition to the tenderness. Many surgeons stress the value of a positive 'release' sign as an indication of an acutely inflamed appendix adjacent to the parietal peritoneum of the right iliac foasa and operate if this sign is present.

General Features.—During the first six hours there is rarely any alteration in the temperature or pulse-rate; after that time slight pyrexia[2] ($37 \cdot 2°$ to $37 \cdot 7°C$) with corresponding increase in the pulse-rate to 80 or 90, is usual. In severe cases, as time passes the temperature rises to about $38 \cdot 3°C$ but seldom more, and the pulse-rate becomes correspondingly elevated. In 90% of cases the white cell count is greater than 10,000 cells per mm³ ($10 \times 10^9/l$). With experience, it is possible to recognise a special foetor oris associated with appendicitis.

In **Obstructive Appendicitis** the sequence of clinical events occurs much more quickly and early diagnosis and treatment are accordingly much more urgent. The onset is abrupt and there may be severe generalised abdominal colic from the start. The temperature is often normal, but vomiting is common, so that the clinical picture mimics acute intestinal obstruction. In a few hours, however, tenderness appears in the right iliac fossa and the diagnosis will become clear.

Special Features, according to position.

Retrocaecal.—Rigidity is often absent ('silent' appendix) and even on deep pressure tenderness may be lacking, the reason being that the caecum, distended

---

[1] 'If you don't put your finger in the rectum, you may put your foot in it.'
[2] In 20% of cases the temperature is 37°C or less.

with gas, prevents the pressure exerted by the hand from reaching the inflamed structure, and gurgling may even be elicited. However, deep tenderness is often present in the loin, and rigidity of the quadratus lumborum may be in evidence. Psoas spasm, due to the inflamed appendix being in contact with that muscle, may be sufficient to cause flexion of the hip joint; to extend the joint causes abdominal pain. Hyperextension of the hip joint may induce abdominal pain when a degree of psoas spasm is insufficient to cause flexion of the hip.

Pelvic.—When the appendix lies entirely within the pelvis there is usually complete absence of abdominal rigidity, and often tenderness over McBurney's point is lacking as well. In some instances deep tenderness can be made out just above and to the right of the symphysis pubis. In either event a rectal examination reveals tenderness in the recto-vesical pouch or the pouch of Douglas, especially on the right side. Psoas spasm may also be present when the appendix is in this position: alternatively, spasm of the obturator internus is sometimes demonstrable when the hip is flexed and internally rotated. If an inflamed appendix is in contact with the obturator internus, this manoeuvre will cause pain in the hypogastrium (Zachary Cope). An inflamed appendix in contact with the bladder may cause frequency of micturition. A child sometimes postpones micturition as this causes pain (McFadden). Occasionally early diarrhoea results from an inflamed appendix being in contact with the rectum.

Post-ileal.—Although this is rare, it accounts for some of the cases of 'missed appendix'. Here the inflamed appendix lies behind the terminal ileum. It presents the greatest difficulty in diagnosis because the pain may not shift, diarrhoea is a feature, marked retching may occur and tenderness, if any, is ill-defined, though it may be present immediately to the right of the umbilicus. As the appendix irritates the lower ileum, the patient usually passes small loose stools soon after eating or drinking.

Maldescended (*subhepatic*).—The tenderness is in the subhepatic region. It is sometimes mistaken for acute cholecystitis.

Special Features, according to age.

Acute Appendicitis in Infants.—In infants under thirty-six months of age the incidence of perforation is over 80% (Fields), and the mortality is considerably higher than the general mortality; indeed, when acute appendicitis occurs during the first year of life, only 50% of the patients reach their first birthday. One of the reasons for the rapid onset of diffuse peritonitis is that the greater omentum, being comparatively short and undeveloped, is unable to give much assistance in localising the infection.[1] Even more important is the difficulty in arriving at an early diagnosis, and particularly in differentiating the condition from enteritis; also acute appendicitis can complicate enteritis. In addition, acute appendicitis may be associated with acute respiratory infection or one of the exanthemas.

Acute Appendicitis in Children.—It is rare to find a child with appendicitis who has not vomited and they usually have complete aversion to food. In addition, they do not sleep during the attack and very often bowel sounds are completely absent in the early stages.

---

[1] The omentum is an apron of fat in the adult, but it is a mere bib in children.

James Douglas, 1675–1742. Anatomist and Obstetrician, London.
Sir Vincent Zachary Cope, 1881–1975. Surgeon, St. Mary's Hospital, London.
George Dixon Fisher McFadden, Contemporary, Late Senior Surgeon, Belfast City Hospital, Belfast, Northern Ireland.
Irving Anatole Fields, Contemporary. Associate Professor of Surgery, Loma Linda University, Los Angeles, U.S.A.

Acute Appendicitis in the Aged.—Gangrene and perforation occur much more frequently in elderly patients. Elderly patients with lax abdominal walls or obesity may harbour a gangrenous appendix with little evidence of it. In addition, the picture may simulate sub-acute intestinal obstruction and if enemas are given, peritonitis may be spread more widely.

Acute Appendicitis in the Obese

Obesity can obscure and diminish all the lcoal signs of acute appendicitis. It is safer to operate on such cases through a generous vertical incision rather than miss a gangrenous appendix.

Acute Appendicitis in Pregnancy

In pregnancy the appendix shifts to the upper abdomen, thus favouring peritonitis: the nearer to term, the greater the danger, even in cases without perforation, After the sixth month there is a maternal mortality of 20%—ten times greater than in the first three months (Parker). As pregnancy advances the pain becomes higher and more lateral. Microscopical examination of specimens of urine will help to exclude pyelonephritis, but in doubtful cases it is best to perform early appendicectomy. The pregnant patient with acute perforated appendicitis aborts or goes into premature labour in 50% of cases, while in acute non-perforated appendicitis this figure is reduced to 30%.

THE DIFFERENTIAL DIAGNOSIS OF ACUTE APPENDICITIS

Although acute appendicitis is the commonest abdominal emergency the diagnosis at times can be extremely difficult. It is wise to consider carefully possible diseases of the chest, the abdomen, the pelvis, the genito-urinary system, the central nervous system, and the spine.[1] For these purposes it is helpful to visualise the body as a house (fig. 1087) and compare seven parts of the house to the appropriate anatomical regions.

1. **The Attic** (*i.e. The Naso-pharynx and Thorax*)

TONSILLITIS. In children abdominal colic may arise from swallowed exudate ('Tonsil tummy').

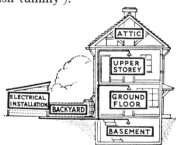

FIG. 1087.—See text. Note the water butt in the backyard (bladder).

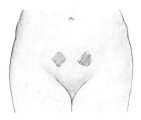

FIG. 1088..—Typical distribution of abdominal tenderness in acute salpingitis.

[1] 'Distension, rigidity, vomiting, pain,
Are actors abdominal which often deign
To act on behalf of the chest, spine or brain,
Or general ills of which typhoid's the main.'
From 'The Acute Abdomen in Rhyme' by 'Zeta' (Sir Zachary Cope)

Robert Bernard Parker, Contemporary. Obstetrician and Gynaecologist, Selly Oak Hospital, Birmingham, England.

PNEUMONIA AND PLEURISY, especially at the right base, give rise to right-sided abdominal pain, but they are associated with an increased respiration rate, and the pain prevents deep inspiration. Pleural friction or altered breath-sounds on auscultation, and a chest x-ray may be helpful.

2. The Upper Storey (i.e. Diaphragm to the level of the Umbilicus)

PERFORATED PEPTIC ULCER (notably a perforated duodenal ulcer with duodenal contents passing along the paracolic gutter to the right iliac fossa).—As a rule there is a history of dyspepsia and a very *sudden* onset of pain which starts in the epigastrium and passes down the right paracolic gutter. In appendicitis the pain starts in the umbilical region. Rigidity and tenderness in the right iliac fossa are present in both conditions, but in perforated duodenal ulcer the rigidity is usually greater in the right hypochondrium. X-ray may show gas under the diaphragm (fig. 854, Chapter 44).

ACUTE CHOLECYSTITIS.—Murphy's sign and especially the radiation of pain through to the right scapula are important features (Boas' sign). Retching and noisy vomiting are common. Jaundice may be present. In cases of difficulty in differentiating acute cholecystitis from acute appendicitis, the history and location of physical signs are of prime importance.

CYCLICAL VOMITING.—The patient is an infant or a young child, and there is a history of previous similar attacks. Rigidity is absent and acetone is found in the urine, but acetonuria may accompany starvation.

3. The Ground Floor (i.e. Umbilicus to the Brim of the Pelvis)

ENTERO-COLITIS.—In this condition there is intestinal colic together with diarrhoea and vomiting but localised tenderness does not usually occur. There is often a history of a local epidemic. Post-ileal appendicitis may mimic this condition almost completely and it is better to look and see than to wait and see.

NON-SPECIFIC MESENTERIC LYMPHADENITIS.—The patient, usually a child, is completely free from pain in between attacks, which last a few minutes. Cervical lymph nodes may be enlarged. Shifting tenderness when the child turns on to his left side, if present, is convincing evidence. This condition is a common difficulty in children and if doubt exists a laparotomy is advisable. Some hold the view that appendicectomy may help resolution of the lymph nodes.

INTESTINAL OBSTRUCTION.—Here there is persisting colicky pain around the umbilicus with vomiting first of the stomach, then of the intestinal contents. The bowel-sounds are noisy and a plain erect x-ray shows fluid levels.

REGIONAL ILEITIS in its acute form may be indistinguishable from acute appendicitis unless a doughy mass of inflamed ileum can be felt. A history of diarrhoea suggests regional ileitis rather than appendicitis.

CARCINOMA OF THE CAECUM, when obstructed, may very well mimic appendicitis in patients in the carcinoma age-group.

MECKEL'S DIVERTICULITIS.

4. The Basement (i.e. The Pelvis)

It is in women of the child-bearing age that pelvic disease so often mimics acute appendicitis:

SALPINGITIS.—Unlike early acute appendicitis, early salpingitis should be treated by non-operative measures. The history of a vaginal discharge, of menstrual irregularities and dysmenorrhoea, or burning pain on micturition, are all helpful

John Benjamin Murphy, 1857–1916. Professor of Surgery, Northwestern University, Chicago, U.S.A.
Ismar Isidor Boas, 1858–1938. Gastro-enterologist, Augusta Hospital, Berlin.

differential diagnostic points. The onset of symptoms usually follows a menstrual period and the pain *starts* low down and remains there (fig. 1088). On rectal or vaginal examination the enlarged tender Fallopian tubes may be palpated. A bacteriological cervical swab is cultured and will provide information about the sensitivity of the organism. When the condition is mainly right-sided, the differential diagnosis is so difficult that it is wiser to explore the abdomen through a midline or right paramedian incision.

ECTOPIC GESTATION.—It is unlikely that a *ruptured* ectopic pregnancy, with its well-defined signs of haemoperitoneum, will be mistaken for acute appendictis, but the same cannot be said for a right-sided tubal abortion, or still more for a right-sided unruptured tubal pregnancy. In the latter, the signs are very similar to those of acute appendicitis, except that the pain *commences* on the right side and stays there. The pain is severe and continues unabated till operation. Usually there is a history of a missed period. The cervix is softened and often severe pain is felt when it is moved on vaginal examination. In addition, in tubal abortion, the signs of intraperitoneal bleeding usually become obvious after a while. The patient should be questioned specifically regarding referred pain in the shoulder, especially a quarter of an hour after the foot of the bed has been raised on blocks.

RUPTURED OVARIAN FOLLICLE (*syn.* mittelschmerz) occurs about the fourteenth to the sixteenth day between a period, especially in early womanhood. The signs are similar to those of very early tubal abortion, but the history of a missed period and the sign of a soft cervix are absent. There is often a history of such attacks and the condition does not progress.

TWISTED RIGHT OVARIAN CYST.—Here the pain is severe, is often referred to the loin, and is made worse when the patient rolls over. The pulse-rate progressively rises while the temperature remains normal. Sometimes the cyst is not easy to feel. If examination of the pelvis under anaesthesia is practised preparatory to laparotomy, a mistake will seldom be made.

DIVERTICULUM OF CAECUM (solitary).—This is rare. When inflamed it is indistinguishable from acute appendicitis.

5. The Backyard (*i.e. The Retroperitoneal Structures*)

RIGHT URETERIC COLIC.—In typical ureteric colic, pain commences in the loin and passes to the groin; this symptom, combined with the presence of urinary symptoms, serves to distinguish many cases from acute appendicitis. When ureteric colic is due to a stone in the right ureter there is often considerable tenderness in the right iliac fossa. Coughing causes pain in acute appendicitis, but not with a ureteric calculus. A plain x-ray may show a stone in the line of the right ureter and microscopy of the urine will reveal red cells. If an intravenous pyelogram is done, it may show dilation or diminished excretion in the right urinary tract. However, if early acute retrocaecal appendicitis cannot be ruled out, it is safer to operate.

RIGHT-SIDED ACUTE PYELONEPHRITIS is accompanied and often preceded by increased frequency of micturition. It may cause difficulty in diagnosis, especially in women. The leading features are tenderness confined to the loin, fever (temperature 39°C) and possibly rigors and pyuria. It presents special difficulty in pregnancy.

6. The Electrical Installation (*i.e. Central Nervous System*)

Pre-herpetic pain of the right tenth and eleventh dorsal nerves is localised over the same area as that of appendicitis. It does not shift and is associated with marked hyperaesthesia. There is no intestinal upset nor rigidity. The herpetic eruption may be delayed for thirty-six to forty-eight hours.

Tabetic crises are now rare. Severe abdominal pain and vomiting usher in the crisis. Other signs of tabes confirm the diagnosis.

Spinal conditions are sometimes associated with acute abdominal pain especially in children and the elderly. These may include Pott's disease of the spine, secondary carcinomatous deposits, senile osteo-porosis, and myelomatosis. The pain is essentially due to compression of nerve roots and may be precipitated by movement. There is rigidity of the lumbar spine and intestinal symptoms are absent. In a doubtful case spinal x-rays will often be a guide.

7. Fuel Supply (*i.e. blood*)

Bleeding into appendicular and related structures can result from blood dyscrazias or the use of anti-coagulants. Peripheral purpuric manifestations should always be looked for in cases of 'appendicitis' in young people, especially with a recent history of sore throat (cf. Henoch-Shoenlein Syndrome).

Other conditions to be remembered are:

The abdominal crises of porphyria which may simulate appendicular colic are characterised by violent intestinal colic with constipation, and are liable to be precipitated by the administration of barbiturates, the symptoms being produced by areas of intestinal spasm. The urine of these patients is usually orange in colour, which is often dismissed as 'concentrated'. If the specimen of urine is left exposed to daylight for even a short space of time, it becomes amber in colour, particularly near the surface. There are several conclusive laboratory tests for porphyrinuria. A plain x-ray of the abdomen often displays short segments of intestinal spasm with related gaseous distension of the small and large intestine. In obscure cases of intestinal colic it is well to remember this condition, especially when it is associated with mental or neurological symptoms.[1]

'Diabetic abdomen' denotes the severe abdominal pain and vomiting which occasionally precedes coma. The urine should be tested in every abdominal emergency.

Acute Pancreatitis.—In early cases there may be vomiting and pain in the right iliac fossa.

PERFORATION AND GANGRENE

When perforation or gangrene occurs within twelve to twenty-four hours after the commencement of the attack, as is sometimes the case in acute appendicular obstruction, diffuse peritonitis is liable to occur. In non-obstructive appendicitis particularly, and in obstructive appendicitis when perforation or gangrene develops after a period of twenty-four hours, the resulting peritonitis often becomes localised, especially when the appendix lies in a relatively secluded portion of the peritoneal cavity.

LOCAL, DIFFUSING AND DIFFUSE PERITONITIS are discussed in Chapter 49.

THE APPENDIX MASS (*syn.* PERI-APPENDICULAR PHLEGMON)

On the third day (rarely sooner) after the commencement of an attack of acute appendicitis, a tender mass can frequently be felt in the right iliac fossa beneath some rigidity of the overlying musculature, the other quadrants of the abdomen being free from rigidity or tenderness. Alternatively, the mass is situated within the pelvis. The mass, which at this time is not yet an appendix abscess, and may never become one, is composed mainly of the greater omentum, oedematous caecal wall, and oedematous portions of the small intestine. In its midst is a

---

[1] It is almost certain that the bouts of mental instability from which King George III (who died in 1820) suffered were due to porphyria.

Percivall Pott, 1714–1788. Surgeon, St. Bartholomew's Hospital, London.

perforated or otherwise inflamed vermiform appendix. By the fourth or fifth day the mass becomes more circumscribed. As the rigidity passes off its periphery can be defined clearly and should be outlined with a skin pencil. During the ensuing days (fifth to tenth day) the swelling either becomes larger, and an appendix abscess results, or it becomes smaller, and subsides slowly as the inflammation resolves.

Appendix Abscess.—Accompanying an abscess there is variable pyrexia, but the pulse-rate is usually under 100. There is an increased leucocyte count with a relative increase of polymorphonuclear cells. To a great extent the location of the abscess is governed by the position of the appendix. Thus the commonest site of the abscess is in the lateral part of the iliac fossa (extension of retrocaecal suppuration) (fig. 1089) and the second most common is in the pelvis (fig. 1090). Notwithstanding, an abscess centred beneath McBurney's point is not so unusual as the percentages of the anatomical positions of the appendix would indicate. This is because perforation often implicates the proximal half of an inflamed appendix.

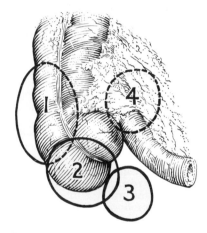

FIG. 1089.—Positions of an appendix abscess palpable from the abdomen. 1. Retrocaecal. 2. Subcaecal. 3. Retrorectus (behind the rectus abdominis muscle). 4. Post-ileal (pre-ileal occupies the same position as 4, but lies in front of the ileum). In positions 3 and 4 localisation is less secure and general peritonitis more likely to happen (cf. p. 1006).

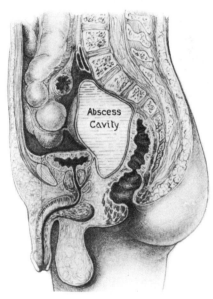

FIG. 1090.—Appendix abscess invading the pelvis. Note the relationship to the rectum.

Differential Diagnosis of an Appendix Mass

Carcinoma of the Caecum.—Here the lump is rarely tender, it has appeared slowly and there is usually a secondary anaemia with blood in the stools, which may be visible macroscopically or occult. There is often progressive deterioration in health over months. The liver may be enlarged and knobbly.

Crohn's Disease.—The diarrhoea, loss of weight, and a lump nearer the midline merits careful barium studies of the small bowel in order to make a firm diagnosis which may otherwise be difficult. Occult blood in the stools and a raised erythrocyte sedimentation rate may help, especially in a young adult.

Ovarian Carcinoma.—This is a common tumour of elderly women, and can be primary or secondary (Krukenberg tumour).

Parametritis.—Here there is usually a history of recent parturition, the lump is over the medial third of the inguinal ligament and appears to be continuous with it.

Actinomycosis (p. 1051).

Tuberculosis, Hyperplastic ileo-caecal tuberculosis is more commonly the cause of a mass in the right iliec fossa than Crohn's disease in Asian and Eastern populations.

Twisted Ovarian Cyst.—The essential step is diagnosis is the bimanual examination.

Iliac Lymphadenitis.—When right-sided, this condition sometimes simulates an appendix abscess. In the early stage psoas spasm is often in evidence. There is tenderness, some rigidity, and a palpable swelling above the inguinal ligament. Often the inguinal lymph nodes are unaffected. Suppuration of the iliac lymph nodes leads to an extraperitoneal abscess. There may be a focus of infection in the perineum or lower limb.

TREATMENT OF ACUTE APPENDICITIS

The treatment of acute appendicitis is appendicectomy.[1] If the diagnosis is made at an early stage in the attack, and particularly in the absence of a localised mass, all are agreed that the appendix should be removed urgently.

Appendicectomy.—When the diagnosis is certain the grid-iron incision is the best one to be employed. When the diagnosis is in doubt the lower right paramedian incision is preferable because it gives good access to the pelvic organs in the female and, if necessary, it can be readily extended upwards to deal with a perforated duodenal ulcer.

The Grid-iron[2] Incision.—An adequate incision, according to the age, musculature, or obesity of the patient, is made at right angles to a line joining the anterior superior iliac spine to the umbilicus, its centre being along the line at McBurney's point. In the subcutaneous tissues an arterial twig from the superficial circumflex iliac artery usually requires ligation. The external oblique is incised in the length of the incision. The fibres of the internal oblique and transversus abdominis are separated, and after suitable retraction the peritoneum is opened. If it is found that more room is required, it is better to cut the deeper muscles in the line of the incision thus converting the grid-iron into a Rutherford Morison incision (vide infra). The lowest complication rate following appendicectomy for acute appendicitis is associated with the grid-iron incision.

The paramedian incision is a vertical incision lying parallel to and 1·25 to 2·5 cm to the right of the middle line. It commences 2·5 cm below the level of the umbilicus and ends just above the pubis. The anterior rectus sheath is incised in the line of the incision and the rectus muscle is retracted laterally. Branches of the inferior epigastric vessels may require ligation. The transversalis fascia and the peritoneum are incised together, the peritoneal cavity being opened through the length of the incision. Care must be taken not to injure the bladder inferiorly. The advantages of the incision have been referred to already. Its disadvantages are (a) that it gives poor access to a retrocaecal appendix (it should be possible to diagnose retrocaecal appendicitis pre-operatively); (b) if the incision becomes infected its 'trap-door' nature harbours infection.

Rutherford Morison's incision is useful if the appendix is para- or retrocaecal and fixed. It is essentially an oblique muscle-cutting incision with its lower end over McBurney's point and extending obliquely upwards and laterally as necessary. All layers are divided in the line of the incision.

Removal of the Appendix.—It will be assumed that the abdomen has been opened by a grid-iron incision. A retractor is placed under the medial side of the

---

[1] The first surgeon to perform deliberate appendicectomy for acute appendicitis was Lawson Tait, in May 1880. The patient recovered. It is recorded in 1736 that Claudius Amyand successfully removed an acutely inflamed appendix from the hernial sac of a boy.

[2] Grid-iron—a frame of cross-beams to support a ship during repairs. The grid-iron incision was described first by McArthur.

Robert Lawson Tait, 1845–1899. Surgeon, Hospital for Diseases of Women, Birmingham, England.
Claudius Amyand, ?1685–1740. Surgeon, St. George's Hospital, London.
Lewis Linn McArthur, 1858–1934. Surgeon, St. Luke's Hospital, Chicago, U.S.A.
James Rutherford Morison, 1853–1939. Professor of Surgery, University of Durham, England.

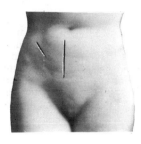

FIG. 1091.—Grid-iron incision
and paramedian incision.

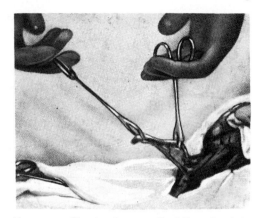

FIG. 1092.—Showing the appendix delivered and the
mesoappendix displayed.

peritoneum and the abdominal wall is lifted up. After removing any pus or serous exudate with a sucker, a pack is inserted into the wound on the medial side. Using a swab, the caecum is withdrawn. A finger may be inserted into the wound to aid delivery of the appendix. Once the appendix has been delivered the caecum is grasped by an assistant. A tissue-holding forceps (*e.g.* Lane's) are applied around the appendix in such a way as to encircle the organ and yet not damage it (fig. 1092). The base of the mesoappendix is clamped in a haemostat, tied and severed. Sometimes only one such manoeuvre frees the whole of the mesoappendix. When the mesoappendix is broad, the procedure must be repeated with a second, or rarely, a third haemostat. The appendix, now completely freed, is crushed near its junction with the caecum in a haemostat, which is removed and reapplied just distal to the crushed portion. A catgut ligature is tied around the crushed portion close to the caecum and an atraumatic catgut purse-string suture is inserted into the caecum about 1·25 cm from the base. This stitch passes through the muscle coat, especially picking up the taeniae coli. It is left untied

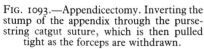

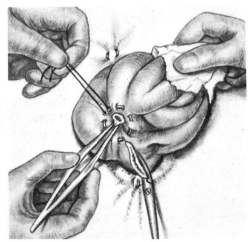

FIG. 1093.—Appendicectomy. Inverting the stump of the appendix through the purse-string catgut suture, which is then pulled tight as the forceps are withdrawn.

Sir William Arbuthnot Lane, 1856–1943. Surgeon, Guy's Hospital, London.

until the appendix has been amputated with a scalpel below the haemostat. The stump is invaginated (fig. 1093) while the purse-string suture is tied, thus burying the appendix stump.

Methods to be Adopted in Special Circumstances.—When the caecal wall is oedematous, the purse-string suture is in danger of cutting out. If the oedema is of limited extent, this can be overcome by inserting the purse-string suture into more healthy caecal wall at a greater distance from the base of the appendix. Occasions may arise when, because of the extensive oedema of the caecal wall, it is better not to attempt invagination, in which case the stump of the appendix should be ligated and the cut surface touched with the diathermy in an attempt to reduce infection.

When the base of the appendix is inflamed, it should not be crushed, for fear of distributing infection by way of the lymphatics or bloodstream. It should be ligated close to the caecal wall just tightly enough to occlude the lumen, after which the appendix is amputated and the stump invaginated.

Should the base of the appendix be gangrenous, neither crushing nor ligation must be attempted. Two stitches are placed through the caecal wall close to the base of the gangrenous appendix, which is amputated flush with the caecal wall, after which these stitches are tied. Further closure is effected by means of a second layer of interrupted seromuscular sutures.

Retrograde Appendicectomy.—When the appendix is retrocaecal and adherent, it is an advantage to divide the base of the organ between haemostats. After the vessels have been dealt with and the stump has been ligated and invaginated, gentle traction on the caecum will enable the surgeon to deliver the organ which is removed from base to tip.

Drainage of the Peritoneal Cavity.—This is usually unnecessary provided adequate peritoneal toilet has been done. If, however, there is considerable purulent fluid in the retrocaecal space or the pelvis, or if there is persistent oozing, it is wise to bring out a Penrose drain[1] through a separate stab incision.

Drainage of the Parietes.—This is indicated if there is any soiling of the wound, especially in the obese and in children.

The rule is: 'If in doubt drain, and especially the parietes.'

Antibiotics.—The use of prophylactic antibiotics active against aerobic and anaerobic organisms has been shown to reduce the incidence of post-operative wound infection. A short higher dose regimen involving only two doses—one at the time of surgery, and the next 8-12 hours later—has been shown to be as effective as longer courses of treatment.

THE MANAGEMENT OF AN APPENDIX MASS

If an appendix mass is present and the condition of the patient is satisfactory, the standard modern treatment is conservative, *i.e.* the *Ochsner-Sherren* regimen. This decision is based on the fact that Nature has already localised the lesion and it is foolish to disturb these barriers. Inadvertent surgery at this time is difficult, bloody, and dangerous. It may be impossible to find the appendix and, occasionally, a faecal fistula may form. For these reasons it is wise to observe a rigid non-operative programme, but to be prepared to operate at any time should Nature fail to control the infection.

The treatment is not merely a postponement of operation; it is not a substitute for operation, but a preparation for it—essentially a surgeon's treatment, to be undertaken only in a hospital, or a correspondingly equipped nursing home. Although the treatment should be conducted on the threshold of an operating theatre, there are circumstances—

---

[1] Penrose drain. Extremely thin (latex) rubber tubing with a gauze wick.

Charles Bingham Penrose, 1862–1925. Professor of Gynaecology, University of Pennsylvania, Philadelphia, U.S.A.
Albert John Ochsner, 1858–1925. Professor of Clinical Surgery, University of Illnois, Chicago, U.S.A.
James Sherren, 1872–1945. Surgeon, The London Hospital.

for instance, in an ill-equipped ship at sea—where conservative treatment would be less dangerous than to attempt operation.

The history is taken, and particular note is made of the number of hours since the onset. The history begins 'ten, twenty-six, fifty-five *hours* ago', not 'last Thursday' or 'three days ago'. The physical signs are then recorded in the clinical notes in diagrammatic form. The extent of the rigidity is marked by shading; the presence of a lump is drawn as near as possible to scale.

In this connection it should be noted especially that sometimes when a patient is first admitted overlying muscular rigidity renders an appendix mass indefinite, or even impalpable. In the majority of such instances, should a lump be present, if the patient is re-examined in two hours' time, lessened apprehension and the warmth of being in bed will reduce guarding of the abdominal wall sufficiently to permit the lump to be felt.

Charts.—As a routine, the pulse is recorded every hour on a special chart. Temperature is recorded every four hours. Instructions are given to the nurse to report if the patient vomits and to save the specimen for inspection. Unless the vomitus is a small quantity of clear fluid, no time should be lost in passing and retaining a transnasal gastric aspiration tube, in order to keep the stomach empty.

Diet.—Water, 30 ml hourly, may be given by mouth. Mouth-washes are given frequently. Desire for food, usually about the fourth or fifth day, is an indication that satisfactory progress is being made and that oral feeding may be started. The first feeds should be fluids only and progression to solid food can take place over the next few days.

Intravenous fluids with fluid balance chart and daily assay of electrolytes must be instituted.

Drugs.—It should be particularly noted that no morphine or its derivatives are given in border-line cases that are being watched closely for a few hours in order to observe whether the pulse-rate and other signs are tending to settle. Once it has been decided definitely to treat the patient by conservative measures, morphine may be given. Pain, as opposed to tenderness, is very seldom complained of after the first twelve hours of the treatment.

Antibiotic therapy is, of course, employed by both schools. Parenteral ampicillin, gentamicin and metronidazole are given. When the patient is permitted to receive nourishment by mouth, the antibiotic therapy is changed to the oral route.

Bowels.—If the bowels are not opened naturally by the fourth or fifth day, a glycerine suppository will encourage normal evacuation. No purgatives of any kind are given until resolution is complete—that is, until the temperature and pulse have been normal for a week and pain and physical signs are absent.

Criteria for Stopping 'Delayed' Treatment

(1) a rising pulse rate, (2) vomiting or copious gastric aspirate, (3) increasing or spreading abdominal pain, and, (4) increasing size of the abscess.

A rising pulse-rate in the early stages is the most reliable single sign that it is dangerous to proceed with the delayed method.

Vomiting (or copious gastric aspirate) after the first few hours should always be regarded seriously, and this by itself may be a sufficient indication to operate.

A patient undergoing delayed treatment should not complain of pain, as opposed to tenderness, after the first six hours of such treatment. If he does, there is usually something amiss, and there is a strong indication for operation.

Contraindications to the 'Delayed' Treatment

1. The diagnosis cannot be made between acute appendicitis and some other intra-abdominal catastrophe normally requiring immediate operation.

2. The signs indicate that the inflammation is still confined to the appendix.

3. When the patient is under ten years of age (poor development of the greater omentum and early perforation of the appendix).

4. When the patient is over the age of sixty-five years more than ordinary bias is directed towards immediate operation, because of the frequency of peritonitis with minimum clinical signs.

The outcome of cases suitable for delayed treatment is that 90% resolve without incident. The appendix, however, must be removed later to avoid further attacks. The originators of this treatment suggested that this should be done after an interval of three months. Present-day practice, however, favours appendicectomy as soon as convenient after *complete* resolution of the mass.

THE TREATMENT OF APPENDICITIS COMPLICATING REGIONAL ILEITIS (CROHN'S DISEASE)

Occasionally a patient is operated on for acute appendicitis who is found to have concomitant Crohn's disease of the ileo-caceal region. Providing the caceal wall is healthy at the base of the appendix, appendicectomy can be performed without increasing the risk of an entero-cutaneous fistula. Rarely, the appendix is involved with the Crohn's disease. A conservative approach is less likely to lead to post-operative complications than the aggressive style appropriate to a normal case of appendicitis: a tangled mass of Crohn's disease with adherent loops of small intestine can be the altar of sacrifice for a surgical reputation in unprepared circumstances.

THE TREATMENT OF APPENDIX ABSCESS

Failure of resolution of an appendix mass usually indicates that there is pus within the mass.

Indications for Opening an Appendix Abscess.[1]—(1) When the swelling is not diminishing in size after the fifth day of treatment; (2) when the temperature is swinging above 37·8C on several successive days; (3) a pelvic abscess seldom resolves—repeated rectal examinations are required to determine when it is ready for opening into the rectum (fig. 1005).

Opening an Appendix Abscess.—The swelling is palpated under the anaesthetic.

A retrocaecal appendix abscess should be opened extraperitoneally. An incision from 2·5 to 5 cm long, depending on the thickness of the abdominal wall, is made over the centre of the swelling, rather nearer the lateral than the medial aspect. The external oblique is incised and the fibres of the deeper muscles are divided, instead of being separated, so as to give freer exit to the contents of the abscess. When the peritoneum has been reached the extraperitoneal tissues are separated in an outward and backward direction, until the abscess cavity is entered. In cases where the abscess cavity lies at some distance from the incision, more direct drainage is afforded by a counter-incision in the flank, in which case the original incision is closed.

A subcaecal abscess can be opened in the same manner, the incision being placed nearer the anterior superior iliac spine.

A pre- or post-ileal abscess can be reached only through the peritoneal cavity. When the peritoneum has been opened, gauze packing is inserted so as to isolate the region from the general peritoneal cavity before opening the abscess.

A pelvic abscess is opened into the rectum as shown in fig. 1005.

When it is necessary to drain an appendix abscess, no prolonged attempt should be made to perform appendicectomy unless the appendix is lying free in the abscess cavity; usually the appendix is incorporated in the walls of the abscess.

Interval Appendicectomy.—Following successful drainage of an appendix abscess, arrangements should be made for the patient to return for appendicectomy three months after the wound has healed. It is highly important to explain to the patient that drainage of an appendix abscess is no safeguard against future

---

[1] The first recorded operation for an appendix abscess was by Henry Hancock (1809–1880) of Charing Cross Hospital, London, in 1848.

attacks of appendicitis. Sometimes carcinoma of the caecum may co-exist. In the carcinoma age group, all patients should have barium studies or colonoscopy to exclude this.

PERILS OF PROLONGED ANTIBIOTIC THERAPY

There are certain dangers peculiar to their use in intra-abdominal sepsis. These are:

1. The masking of the general signs (especially the raised temperature) of an intra-abdominal abscess behoves the clinician to make a daily abdominal and pelvic examination, lest an enlarging abscess bursts its confines, perhaps into the general peritoneal cavity.

2. Pus that has been sterilised by antibiotics remains and behaves as a foreign body, and as an irritant. For instance, cases have been reported where one or more sterile abscesses lay among the coils of small intestine, causing obscure subacute intestinal obstruction.

3. Cases have been reported whereby a pelvic abscess, by reason of antibiotic therapy, has been converted into granulation tissue, leading to a 'frozen' pelvis with consequent stricture of the rectum.

COMPLICATIONS AFTER APPENDICECTOMY FOR ACUTE APPENDICITIS

The complications vary with the degree of peritonitis that was present, and with the resistance of the patient to the infection. These complications include:

Early.—Ileus, Wound sepsis, Residual abscess (local, pelvic, paracolic, subphrenic), Intestinal obstruction from adhesions, Faecal fistula, Pylephlebitis, Post-operative thrombosis and embolism. Actinomycosis, Pulmonary complications (pulmonary collapse or pneumonitis).

Late.—Intestinal obstruction from adhesions, Incisional hernia, Right inguinal hernia following the grid-iron incision (especially if a drain is brought through the wound). Sterility in the female from 'frozen' pelvis.

★   ★   ★

It is advisable to include the following practical problem:

After an operation for acute appendicitis the condition of the patient is unsatisfactory. The temperature is swinging and the pulse rate is elevated—signs which foretell pocketing of pus. How would you investigate the case?

1. *Examine the wound and the abdominal wall* for an abscess.
2. *Consider a pelvic abscess, and perform a rectal examination.*
3. *Pulpate the left iliac fossa* for an abscess in this situation.
4. *Examine the loin* for retrocaecal swelling and tenderness.
5. *Examine the legs*—to exclude the possibility of venous thrombosis.
6. *Examine the conjunctivae for an icteric tinge and the liver for enlargement, and enquire if the patient has had rigors*—pylephlebitis.
7. *Examine the lungs*—pneumonitis or collapse.
8. *Examine the urine for organisms (pyelonephritis).*
9. *In children consider tonsillitis and otitis media.*
10. *Ensure that the i.v. apparatus is sterile. If you can't be sure, change it, needle and all.*
11. Lastly, *suspect the possibility of a subdiaphragmatic abscess* (fig. 1008, Chapter 49).

RECURRENT ACUTE APPENDICITIS

Appendicitis is notoriously recurrent. This is perhaps the commonest form of appendicitis—mild subacute attacks which are so often attributed to 'biliousness' or a 'chill on the liver' or dyspepsia which does not respond to alkalis. The attacks vary in intensity, may occur every few months, and the majority of cases ultimately culminate in severe acute appendicitis. If careful histories are taken from patients with acute appendicitis, over two-thirds remember having had milder but similar attacks of pain. The appendix in these cases shows obliterative appendicitis.

SUBACUTE APPENDICITIS

Subacute appendicitis is but a mild form of acute appendicitis, and requires no detailed consideration.

CHRONIC APPENDICITIS

Chronic appendicitis, *per se*, does not exist. Patients labelled thus are usually examples of the recurrent form of the disease.

LESS COMMON PATHOLOGICAL CONDITIONS OF THE APPENDIX

Mucocele of the appendix may occur when the proximal end of the lumen slowly becomes completely occluded, usually by a fibrous stricture, and the pent-up secretion remains sterile. The appendix is greatly enlarged; sometimes it contains several ounces of mucus. The symptoms produced are those of mild subacute appendicitis unless infection supervenes, when the mucocele is converted into an empyema. Rupture of a mucocele of the appendix is a cause of pseudomyxoma peritonei (Chapter 49). Occasionally the muco-cele is caused by a mucus secreting adeno-carcinoma: a right hemicolectomy is the correct treatment.

Diverticula of the Appendix.—Diverticulosis occurs once in about 200 appendices removed by operation (Edwards). These diverticula are not merely extensions of diverticu-losis of the colon; some are congenital (all coats); most are acquired (no muscularis layer). Diverticula of the appendix can occur in conjunction with a mucocele. The intramural pressure rises sufficiently to cause herniation of the mucous membrane through the muscle coat at several points. More often diverticula (fig. 1094) are not found in association with

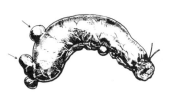

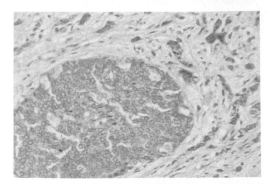

FIG. 1094.—Appendicular diverticulosis.

FIG. 1095.—Carcinoid tumour of appendix: this is a well-
differentiated type (high-power view).

a mucocele, and often there is no demonstrable obstruction to the lumen. Usually the patient gives a history of previous recurrent attacks of appendicitis. If encountered during the course of an operation for another condition, a diverticula-bearing appendix should always be removed, because if perchance such an appendix becomes the seat of inflam-mation, perforation will occur very easily.

Intussusception of the appendix is rare and occurs mostly in childhood. It can be diagnosed only at operation. The symptoms usually are not acute. Untreated, the con-dition may pass on to an appendiculo-colic intussusception. The appendix may slough,

Harold Clifford Edwards, Contemporary, Consulting Surgeon, King's College Hospital, London.

and this accounts for most of the very rare cases in which the appendix is absent. The treatment is appendicectomy.

Endometriosis of the Appendix.—About 150 cases have been reported. The tumour— a miniature uterus in so far as endometrium is concerned—gives rise to monthly melaena. The loss of blood per rectum may be severe.

Primary Crohn's Disease of the Appendix.—About 40 cases have been reported. Fistula has not been reported following appendicectomy in this location of the disease (see p. 1106 for the treatment of appendicitis in Crohn's disease).

Neoplasms of the Appendix

Carcinoid tumour (*syn*. Argentaffinoma), (fig. 1095) which arises in argentaffin tissue (Kulchitsky cells of the crypts of Lieberkühn) can occur anywhere in the gastro-intestinal tract, but most commonly it is situated in the vermiform appendix; indeed, the tumour is found once in about 300 to 400 appendices subjected to histological examination. Carcinoid tumours are distributed evenly among appendices removed from patients between the ages of ten and sixty years. Most of the patients are females (80%).

In many instances the appendix is removed because of symptoms of subacute or recurrent appendicitis. The tumour can occur in any part of the appendix, but it frequently does so in the distal third of the organ. The neoplasm feels moderately hard, and on slitting up the appendix it can be seen between the intact mucosa and the peritoneum, replacing the muscular coats. There is no mistaking it, because it is of a bright yellow colour, due to contained lipoid. Microscopically the chief cells are spheroidal in type and contain granules that stain with ammoniacal silver salts. Unlike carcinoid tumours arising in other parts of the intestinal tract in only 4% of cases does the tumour give rise to metastases, and it is most exceptional for metastases from an argentaffin carcinoma of the vermiform appendix to secrete sufficient hormone to produce the characteristic symptomatology described in Chapter 50. Carcinoid tumour is ten times more common than other forms of carcinoma of the vermiform appendix. Unless the caecal wall is involved, or the tumour is 2 cm or more in size, or involved lymph nodes are found, appendicectomy has been shown to be correct treatment (Moertel): otherwise a right hemicolectomy is indicated.

Primary Adenocarcinoma.—Less than 200 cases are recorded. These are mostly of the colonic type and should be treated by right hemicolectomy (as a second stage procedure if the condition is not recognised at the first operation). Less frequently, a malignant mucocele occurs and here appendicectomy alone is probably sufficient if the tumour is in the distal part of the viscus and is confined to the submucosa; otherwise right hemicolectomy is again indicated. The five-year survival rate after right hemicolectomy is of the order of 60%.

Nicholas Kulchitsky, 1856–1925. Professor of Histology, Kharkov, Ukraine, U.S.S.R.
C. G. Moertel, Contemporary. Surgeon, Mayo Clinic, U.S.A.

CHAPTER 53

THE RECTUM

Surgical Anatomy

The rectum has an ill-defined anatomical beginning, but *surgically* the rectosigmoid junction lies opposite the sacral promontory. From this point the rectum follows the curve of the sacrum to end at the ano-rectal junction. At this point the pubo-rectalis muscle encircles the posterior and lateral aspects of the junction, creating the ano-rectal angle (normally 120°). The rectum[1] has 3 lateral curvatures: the upper and lower are convex to the left, and the middle convex to the right: on the mucosal (lumen) aspect these three curves are marked by semicircular folds (Houston's valves) (fig. 1096). That part of the rectum that lies below the middle valve has a much wider diameter than the upper third, and is known as the Ampulla of the rectum.

The adult rectum is approximately 18–20 cm in length and is conveniently divided into 3 equal parts: the upper one third which is mobile and has a peritoneal coat except near to the middle third when the peritoneum only covers the anterior and part of the lateral surfaces; the middle third, which is the widest part of the rectum, and is confined within the diameter of the bony pelvis; the lowest one third which lies within the muscular floor of the pelvis and has important relations to fascial layers.

RELATIONS OF THE RECTUM

	MALE	FEMALE
ANTERIOR	BLADDER SEMINAL VESICLES URETERS PROSTATE URETHRA	POUCH OF DOUGLAS UTERUS CERVIX POSTERIOR VAGINAL WALL
LATERAL	LATERAL LIGAMENTS MIDDLE RECTAL ARTERY OBTURATOR INTERNUS MUSCLE SIDE WALL OF PELVIS LEVATOR ANI MUSCLE	LATERAL LIGAMENTS MIDDLE RECTAL ARTERY OBTURATOR INTERNUS MUSCLE SIDE WALL OF PELVIS LEVATOR ANI MUSCLE
POSTERIOR	SACRUM AND COCCYX LOOSE AREOLAR TISSUE FASCIAL CONDENSATION SUPERIOR RECTAL ARTERY LYMPHATICS	SACRUM AND COCCYX LOOSE AREOLAR TISSUE FASCIAL CONDENSATION SUPERIOR RECTAL ARTERY LYMPHATICS

[1] The word rectum means 'straight'. It is straight only in infants and the elderly.

John Houston, 1802–1845. Physician, City of Dublin Hospital and Lecturer in Surgery, Dublin.
James Douglas, 1675–1742. Anatomist and Obstetrician, London.

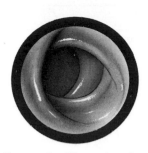
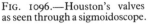

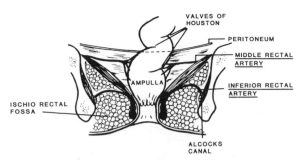

FIG. 1096.—Houston's valves as seen through a sigmoidoscope.

FIG. 1097.—To show the rectum lying in the pelvis (coronal view). Note the curvatures corresponding to Houston's valves.

The lowest part of the rectum is separated by a fascial condensation—Denonvilliers' fascia—from the prostate in front, and behind by another fascial layer—Waldeyer's fascia—from the coccyx and last two sacral vertebrae. *These fascial layers are surgically important as they are a barrier to malignant penetration, and are valuable guides at operation.*

Blood Supply

The superior rectal artery is the direct continuation of the inferior mesenteric artery and is the main arterial supply of the rectum. Opposite the third sacral vertebra the artery divides into a right and left branch: only the right branch subdivides again behind the lower third of the rectum into two—an anterior and a posterior branch. The arteries and their accompanying lymphatics are kept applied to the back of the rectum by dense connective tissue ('rectal fascia').

The middle rectal artery arises on each side from the internal iliac artery (fig. 1097) and passes to the rectum in the lateral ligaments. It is usually small and breaks up into several terminal branches.

The inferior rectal artery arises on each side from the internal pudendal artery as it enters Alcock's canal. It hugs the inferior surface of the levator ani muscle as it crosses the roof of the ischio-rectal fossa to enter the anal muscles (fig. 1097).

Venous Drainage

The superior haemorrhoidal veins draining the upper half of the anal canal above the dentate line pass upwards to become the rectal veins: these unite to form the *superior rectal vein* which later becomes the *inferior mesenteric vein*. This forms part of the portal venous system, and ultimately drains into the splenic vein. Middle rectal veins exist but are small unimportant channels unless the normal paths are blocked.

Lymphatic Drainage

The lymphatics of the mucosal lining of the rectum interchange freely with those of the muscular layers. The usual drainage flow is *upwards*, and only to a limited extent laterally and downwards. For this reason surgical ablation of malignant disease concentrates mainly on achieving wide clearance of proximal

Benjamin Alcock. Professor of Anatomy, Cork, Ireland (1849–1855). He was dismissed from his post for a breach of the Anatomy Acts, and disappeared in America.
Charles Pierre Denonvilliers, 1808–1872. French Surgeon.
Heinrich Wilhelm Gottfried Waldeyer-Hartz, 1836–1921. Professor of Pathological Anatomy, Berlin.

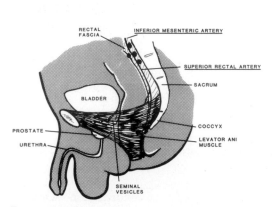

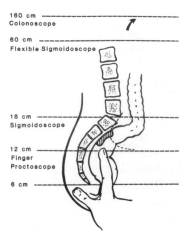

FIG. 1098.—To show the rectum lying in the male pelvis (sagittal view). Note the lymph nodes along the path of the superior rectal artery. (Gerota's nodes.)

FIG. 1099.—Shows how the various methods of examining the rectum reach different levels. Note that even cancers in the upper part of the rectum can be felt with the index finger, especially if the patient is asked to 'strain down'.

lymph nodes. However, if the usual upward routes are blocked (*e.g.* by carcinoma) flow can reverse, and it is then possible to find metastatic lymph nodes on the side walls of the pelvis (along the middle rectal vessels) or even in the inguinal region (along the inferior rectal artery). *Superior rectal nodes*: these are an important group of nodes on the back of the rectal ampulla above the levator ani muscle (fig. 1098): also known as the pararectal lymph glands of Gerota.

Middle rectal nodes.—These lie close to the middle rectal arteries and pass to lymph nodes around the internal iliac arteries. Recently, the Japanese have stressed the importance of removing these lymph glands when operating on rectal cancer.

Symptoms of Rectal Disease

Rectal disease is common, serious and can occur at any age. The symptoms of many of them overlap. In general, the inflammations affect younger age groups, while the tumours occur in the middle-aged and elderly. But no age is exempt from any of the diseases, however young: ulcerative colitis has been reported in the new-born, and rectal cancer is not rare in young people. The common symptoms of rectal disease are:

Bleeding.—This demands at least digital examination at any age.

Altered bowel habit.—Early morning stool frequency ('spurious diarrhoea') is a symptom of rectal carcinoma, while blood-stained frequent loose stools characterise the inflammatory diseases.

Discharge.—Mucus and pus are associated with rectal pathology.

Tenesmus.—Often described by the patient as 'I feel I want to go but nothing happens', this is normally an ominous symptom of rectal cancer.

Prolapse.—This usually indicates either mucosal (partial) or full-thickness (complete) rectal wall descent.

Dumitru Gerota, 1867–1939. Professor of Surgery, Bucharest, Rumania.

Pruritus.—This may be secondary to a rectal discharge.

Loss of weight.—This usually indicates serious or advanced disease (*e.g.* hepatic metastases).

Signs of Rectal Disease

Because the rectum is accessible via the anal orifice these can be elicited by systematic examination. The patient is positioned in either the left-lateral (Sims) position or is examined in the knee-elbow position.

Inspection.—Visual examination of the anus precedes rectal examination to exclude the presence of anal disease, *e.g.* fissure, haemorrhoids, fistula etc.

Digital examination.—The index finger used with gentleness and precision remains the most valuable test for rectal disease (fig. 1099). Tumours in the lower and middle thirds of the rectum can be felt and assessed; by asking the patient to strain, even some tumours in the upper third can be 'tipped' with the finger. After it is removed the finger should be examined for tell-tale traces of mucus, pus or blood. It is always useful to note the normal as well as the abnormal findings on digital examination, *e.g.* the prostate in the male. Digital findings can be recorded as *intra-luminal* (*e.g.* blood, pus etc.), *intra-mural* (*e.g.* tumours, granular areas, strictures etc.) or *extra-mural* (*e.g.* enlarged prostate, uterine fibroids etc).

Proctoscopy (fig. 1100).—This can be used to inspect the anus, ano-rectal junction and the lower rectum (up to 10 cm). Biopsy can be performed of any suspicious areas.

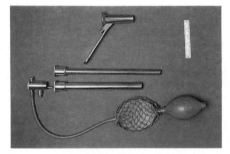

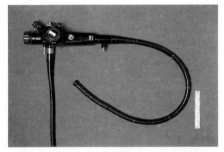

FIG. 1100.—A proctoscope and two Lloyd-Davies rigid sigmoidoscopes: note that there are two sigmoidoscope sizes—small (diam. 15 mm) and large (diam. 20 mm).

FIG. 1101.—The flexible (60 cm) endoscope: 'flexiscope'.

Sigmoidoscopy (fig. 1100).—The sigmoidoscope is a rigid stainless steel instrument of variable diameter and normally 25 cm in length. The rectum must be empty for proper inspection with a sigmoidoscope. Gentleness and skill are required for its use, and perforations can occur if care is not exercised.

Flexible sigmoidoscope (fig. 1101).—The 'flexiscope' can be used to supplement or replace rigid sigmoidoscopy. It requires special skill and experience and the lower bowel should be cleaned out with preliminary enemas. In addition to the rectum, the whole sigmoid colon is within visual reach of this instrument. The instrument is expensive and requires careful maintenance.

O. Lloyd-Davies, 1905–1987. Consultant Surgeon, St. Mark's Hospital, London.

INJURIES

The rectum or anal canal may be injured in a number of ways, all uncommon.

1. By falling in a sitting posture on to a spiked or blunt-pointed object. The up-turned leg of a chair, handle of a broom, floor-mop, pitch-fork, or a broken shooting-stick have all resulted in rectal impalement.

2. By the foetal head during childbirth.

3. During the administration of an enema by a syringe fitted with a bone, glass, or plastic nozzle.

4. During sigmoidoscopy, usually when examining a patient suffering from ulcerative procto-colitis or amoebic dysentery. Sigmoidoscopy performed under general anaesthesia is especially dangerous. In the lithotomy position perforation is usually anteriorly through the recto-sigmoid junctional zone.

5. 'Split Perineum'. A lacerated wound of the perineum, involving the anal canal, is an occasional pillion-riding accident.

6. Compressed-air rupture (as a result of a dreadful practical joke).

Diagnosis.—When there is a history of rectal impalement, the first interrogation should be, 'Has the patient passed urine since the accident?' The anus having been inspected, the abdomen should be palpated. If rigidity or tenderness is present, early laparotomy is imperative. Prior to the operation an urethral catheter is passed. If the urine is blood-stained and/or the quantity recovered is unexpectedly small, it is wise to suspect ruptured bladder or urethra (Chapters 58 and 60).

Treatment.—After the patient has been anaesthetised, the rectum is examined with a finger and a speculum, especial attention being directed to the anterior wall. Left lower laparotomy is then performed. If an intraperitoneal rupture of the rectum is found, the perforation is closed with sutures. Should blood be present beneath the pelvic peritoneum, it is necessary to mobilise the recto-sigmoid, which allows the rectum to be drawn upwards, thus permitting the perforation below the pelvic diaphragm to be closed securely. A perforation in the bladder also can be sutured *via* this avenue. After closing the laparotomy wound, a left iliac colostomy is performed through a separate grid-iron incision. In cases where the bladder has been injured a self-retaining urethral catheter is placed in position. If the rectal injury is below the pelvic floor, wide drainage from below is indicated. A 'protective' colostomy is advisable. Care must be taken to preserve sphincter function during the debridement of the perineal wounds. Antibiotic cover should be provided against both aerobic and anaerobic organisms.

FOREIGN BODIES IN THE RECTUM

The variety of foreign bodies which have found their way into the rectum is hardly less remarkable than the ingenuity displayed in their removal (fig. 1102). A turnip has been delivered *per anum* by the use of obstetric forceps. A stick firmly impacted has been withdrawn by inserting a gimlet into its lower end. A tumbler, mouth looking downwards, has been extracted by filling the interior with a wet plaster of Paris bandage, leaving the end of the bandage protruding, and allowing the plaster to set.

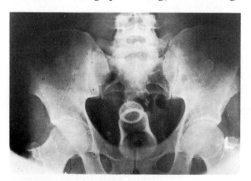

FIG. 1102.—Pepper-pot in the rectum. On removal it was found to be inscribed 'A present from Margate'!
(*Dr. L. S. Carstairs, Royal Northern Hospital, London.*)

If insurmountable difficulty is experienced in grasping any foreign body in the rectum, a left lower laparotomy is necessary, which allows that object to be pushed from above into the assistant's fingers in the rectum. If there is considerable laceration of the mucosa a temporary colostomy is advisable.

PROLAPSE OF THE RECTUM ⟵ Partial
Complete

Partial Prolapse.—The mucous membrane and submucosa of the rectum protrude outside the anus for not more than between 1·25 and 3·75 cm. When the prolapsed mucosa is palpated between the finger and thumb, it is evident that it is composed of no more than a double layer of mucous membrane (cf. complete prolapse). The condition occurs most often at the extremes of life—in children between one and three years of age, and in elderly people.

In Infants.—The direct downward course of the rectum, due to the as yet undeveloped sacral curve (fig. 1103) predisposes to this condition, as does the reduced resting anal tone which offers diminished support to the mucosal lining of the anal canal (Mann).

In children, partial prolapse often commences after an attack of diarrhoea, as a result of severe whooping cough, or from loss of weight and consequent diminution in the amount of fat in the ischio-rectal fossae.

In adults the condition is usually associated with third-degree haemorrhoids or a complete prolapse. In the female a torn perineum predisposes to prolapse, and in the male straining from urethral obstruction. In old age, both partial and complete prolapse are due to atony of the sphincter mechanism.

Partial prolapse may follow an operation for fistula-in-ano where a large portion of muscle has been divided. Here the prolapse is usually localised to the damaged quadrant and is seldom progressive.

Prolapsed mucous membrane is pink; prolapsed internal haemorrhoids are plum coloured, and more pedunculated.

FIG. 1103.—The absence of the normal sacral curve predisposes to rectal prolapse in an infant.

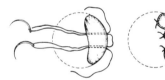

FIG. 1104.—Goodsall's ligature.

Treatment:

In Infants and Young Children: (1) *Digital Reposition.*—The mother must be taught to replace the protrusion. The distal two-thirds of the index finger is wrapped in Kleenex tissue. The finger is inserted into the protrusion and the mass is eased into place. Gently the finger is withdrawn, leaving the Kleenex tissue to disintegrate. In cases of malnutrition, dietetic adjustments are necessary.

(2) *Submucous Injections.*—If digital reposition fails after six weeks' trial, injections of 5% phenol in almond oil are carried out under general anaesthesia. As a result of the aseptic inflammation following these injections, the mucous membrane becomes tethered to the muscle coat.

Technique.—The submucosa at the apex of the prolapse is injected circularly, so as to form a raised ring, up to 10 ml of the solution being injected. A similar injection is made at the base of the prolapse. Alternatively, if the prolapse cannot be brought down, the injections are given through a proctoscope.

Charles Victor Mann, Contemporary. Surgeon, St. Mark's Hospital for Diseases of the Rectum and Colon, London.

(3) *Thiersch's Operation.*—When the prolapse persists in spite of these measures, Thiersch's operation (below) is almost certain to succeed. In infants, insertion of the little finger into the anus before the stitch is tied is recommended. In infants and young children, strong chromic catgut should be used for the stitch instead of silver wire: if wire were employed (or any other retained unabsorbable material) as growth proceeded the stitch would have to be removed or anal stenosis would result. Since the procedure is designed only as a *temporary* measure in the young, chromic catgut is adequate for the purpose.

In Adults: (1) *Submucous injections* of phenol in almond oil occasionally are successful in cases of early partial prolapse.

(2) *Excision of the Prolapsed Mucosa.*—When the prolapse is unilateral the redundant mucosa can be excised after inserting and tying Goodsall's ligature (fig. 1104) which, after the needles have been cut off, permits the base of the prolapsed mucous membrane to be ligated in three portions lying in juxtaposition. When necessary, the operation is combined with haemorrhoidectomy, and if the pedicle of one or more of the haemorrhoids is broad, Goodsall's ligature is applied.

Complete prolapse (*syn.* procidentia) is less common than the partial variety. The protrusion consists of all layers of the rectal wall and is a descending hernia-en-glissade of the rectum downward through the levator ani. As the rectum descends it intussuscepts upon itself. The process starts with the anterior wall of the rectum where the supporting tissues are weakest, especially in women. It is more than 3·75 cm and commonly as much as 10 to 15 cm in length. On palpation between the finger and the thumb the prolapse feels much thicker than a partial prolapse, and obviously consists of a double thickness of the entire wall of the rectum. Any prolapse over 5 cm in length contains anteriorly between its layers a pouch of peritoneum (fig. 1106). When large, the peritoneal pouch contains small intestine which returns to the general peritoneal cavity with a characteristic gurgle when the prolapse is reduced. The prolapsed mucous membrane (fig. 1105) is often arranged in a series of circular folds. The anal sphincter is characteristically patulous and gapes widely on straining to allow the rectum to prolapse. Complete prolapse is uncommon in children. In adults it can occur at any age, but is more common in the elderly. Women are six times more often affected than men. In women, prolapse of the rectum is commonly associated with prolapse of the uterus, or a past history of a gynaecological operation, *e.g.* hysterectomy. In the Middle East and Asia complete rectal prolapse is not uncommon in young males.

Differential Diagnosis.—In the case of a child with abdominal pain, prolapse of the rectum must be distinguished from **ileo-caecal intussusception** protruding from the anus. Figs. 1107 and 1008 make the differential diagnosis clear. In **recto-sigmoid intussusception** in the adult there is a deep groove (5 cm or more) between the emerging protruding mass and margin of the anus, into which the finger can be entered.

Treatment.—The Thiersch operation can be recommended in elderly patients, in those suffering from injury or disease of the spinal cord, and in the feeble-minded, in whom the condition is relatively common, as well as in very early life.

Karl Thiersch, 1822–1895. Professor of Surgery, Leipzig, Germany.
David Henry Goodsall, 1843–1906. Surgeon, St. Mark's Hospital for Diseases of the Rectum and Colon, London.

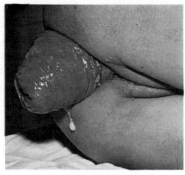

FIG. 1105.—Complete rectal prolapse.
(G. D. Adhia, FRCS, Bombay.)

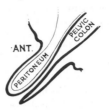

FIG. 1106.—Rectal prolapse containing pouch of peritoneum.

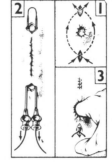

FIG. 1107.—Partial pro-   FIG. 1108.—Intussusception   FIG. 1109.—The Thiersch
lapse of the rectum.   protruding from the anus.   operation (Dodd's modifi-
                                                              cation).

The Thiersch Operation.—A short incision is made in the midline anteriorly and posteriorly about 1·25 cm from the anal verge. Large-bore hollow needles are inserted one at a time through the posterior wound, in such a way as to encircle the anus 1 cm from the orifice (fig. 1109 (1)), until their points emerge from the anterior wound (fig. 1109 (2)). A malleable silver wire, gauge 19 or 20, is introduced through the points of the needles. The needles are withdrawn. The assistant introduces his index finger into the anal canal (fig. 1109 (3)), and the surgeon tightens the wire around the finger by twisting the ends of the wire. The finger is withdrawn and the ends of the wire are clipped short, and bent back. Monofilament O nylon can be used instead of wire, and passed round the rectum two or three times to produce a 'watch-spring' effect when the stitch is tightened. The wounds are then closed. A glycerol suppository or a low-pressure enema is given as required post-operatively. Confinement to bed is unnecessary.

By and large, the results of Thiersch's operation are reasonable, but in about 50% of cases the wire breaks; it is, however, easily removed and the operation can be carried out several times, at intervals, on the same patient. Its main disadvantage is that spurious incontinence of faeces caused by faecal impaction is wont to occur in all age groups. Constipation must, therefore, be guarded against vigilantly.

If an abdominal repair must be avoided (*e.g.* in a young man in whom sexual potency must be preserved by avoiding damage to the pelvic nerves) more extensive perineal procedures are available. These include strengthening the pubo-rectalis and external anal sphincters by an approach through the inter-sphincteric plane (see above), the so-called *post-anal repair* (Parks).

Operative Suspension of the Prolapsed Bowel.—Of many operations designed to cure complete prolapse of the rectum, the following procedures are relatively simple. They are recommended in patients with complete prolapse who are otherwise in good health. All are abdominal procedures designed to replace and hold the rectum in its proper position. Many other procedures have been described incorporating the same principles illustrated by these operations, some of which are carried out through a perineal approach.

Harold Dodd, Contemporary. (See footnote, p. 192.)

Wells' Operation.—In this operation the rectum is fixed firmly to the sacrum by insert-ing a sheet of polyvinyl alcohol sponge between them. The rectum is separated from the sacrum in the usual way. The sponge is fixed by a series of sutures to the periosteum over the midline of the sacrum and is then wrapped loosely about the rectum covering all except the anterior wall. The free margins of the polyvinyl sponge are sutured to the lateral margins of the anterior wall of the rectum. The peritoneal floor is resutured so that the sponge is excluded from the peritoneal cavity. Polyvinyl sponge does not give rise to a foreign body reaction but it does produce very marked fibrous tissue formation. Many proctologists regard this as the method of choice. The results are excellent.

Ripstein's Operation.—In this operation, the recto-sigmoid junction is hitched up by a Teflon sling to the front of the sacrum just below the sacral promontory. The operation is very safe and simple and the results are good.

Lahaut's Operation.—This operation depends entirely upon mobilising the rectum and lower sigmoid colon and holding it up by extraperitonealising it through the rectus sheath. The results are moderate.

PROCTITIS

Inflammation is sometimes limited to the rectal mucosa; in others it is associ-ated with a similar condition in the colon (procto-colitis). The inflammation can be acute or chronic. The symptoms are tenesmus, the passage of blood and mucus and, in severe cases, of pus also. Although the patient has a frequent intense desire to defaecate, the amount of faeces passed at a time is small. Acute proctitis is usually accompanied by malaise and pyrexia. On rectal examination the mucosa feels swollen and is often exceedingly tender. Proctoscopy is seldom sufficient and sigmoidoscopy is the more valuable method of examination. Skilled pathological assistance is required to establish or exclude the diagnosis of specific infection by bacteriological examination and culture of the stools, examination of scrapings or swabs from ulcers, and serological tests. When early carcinoma cannot be excluded, biopsy is necessary.

Non-specific proctitis is an inflammatory condition affecting the mucosa, and to a lesser extent the submucosa, confined to the terminal rectum and anal canal. It is the most common variety. In 10% of cases the condition extends to involve the whole colon (= total or ulcerative colitis).

Aetiology is unknown. The concept that the condition is a mild and limited form of ulcerative colitis (although actual ulceration is not present) is the most acceptable hypothesis.

Clinical Features.—The patient is usually middle-aged, and complains of slight loss of blood in the motions. Often the complaint is one of diarrhoea, but on closer questioning it transpires that usually one relatively normal action of the bowels occurs each day, although it is accompanied by some blood. During the day the patient attempts to defaec-ate, with the passage of flatus and a little blood-stained faecal matter; which is mistakenly interpreted as diarrhoea. On rectal examination the mucosa feels warm and smooth. Often there is some blood on the examining finger. Proctoscopic and sigmoidoscopic examination shows inflamed mucous membrane of the rectum, but no ulceration. The inflammation extends for only 12·5–15 cm from the anus, the mucosa above this level being quite normal.

Treatment.—Although, fortunately, the condition is usually self-limiting, much relief may be obtained from the use of Salazopyrin, Acetarsol suppositories or Prednisolone retention enemas. Milk should be rigidly excluded from the diet and motions kept soft with Isogel or Celevac. In very severe resistant cases oral steroids may have to be used to obtain remission. Rarely, surgical treatment is used as a last resort (proctectomy) when the patient is desperate for relief of symptoms.

Ulcerative Procto-colitis.—Proctitis is present in a high percentage of cases of ulcer-ative colitis, and the degree of severity of the rectal involvement may influence the type of operative procedure.

Charles Alexander Wells, Contemporary. Professor Emeritus of Surgery, Liverpool, England.
Charles Benjamin Ripstein, Contemporary. Surgeon, Brookdale Hospital Center, New York, U.S.A.
Jules Lahaut. Contemporary. Surgeon-in-Chief, Hôpital du Pont Canal, Jemappes (Hainaut), Belgium.

Proctitis Due to Specific Infections:

Clostridium Difficile.—An acute form of procto-colitis by Cl. Difficile can follow broad-spectrum antibiotic administration (esp. lincomycin). A 'membrane' can sometimes be seen on proctoscopy ('pseudo-membranous' entero-colitis).

Bacillary Dysentery.—The appearance is that of an acute purulent proctitis with multiple small shallow ulcers. The examination of a swab taken from the ulcerated mucous membrane is more certainly diagnostic than is a microscopical examination of the stools. Proctological examination is painful; agglutination tests may render it unnecessary.

Amoebic Dysentery.—The infection is more liable to be chronic, and exacerbations after a long period of freedom from symptoms often occur. Proctoscopy and sigmoidoscopy are not painful. The appearance of an amoebic ulcer is described on p. 1046. Scrapings from the ulcer should be immersed in warm isotonic saline solution and sent to the laboratory for immediate microscopical examination.

Amoebic granuloma presents as a soft mass, usually in the recto-sigmoid region. This lesion is frequently mistaken for a carcinoma. Sigmoidoscopy shows an ulcerated surface, but the mass is less friable than a carcinoma. A scraping should be taken, preferably with a small sharp spoon on a long handle, and the material sent for immediate microscopical examination, as detailed above. If doubt exists, a provocative dose of emetine may cause cysts of the amoebae to appear in the stools. A biopsy is also required. Treatment is as described in Chapter 50.

Amoebic granuloma of the rectum is from time to time encountered in a patient who has never visited a country in which the disease is endemic. Persons living in old people's institutions are liable to harbour this deceptive lesion.

Tuberculous proctitis is nearly always associated with active pulmonary tuberculosis, and is often complicated by a tuberculous fistula-in-ano or tuberculous ulceration of the anus. Submucous rectal abscesses burst and leave ulcers with an undermined edge. A hypertrophic type of tuberculous proctitis occurs in association with tuberculous peritonitis or tuberculous salpingitis. This type of tuberculous proctitis requires biopsy for confirmation of the diagnosis.

Gonococcal proctitis occurs in both sexes as the result of rectal coitus, and in the female from direct spread from the vulva. In the acute stage the mucous membrane is hyperaemic and thick pus can be expressed as the proctoscope is withdrawn. In the early stages the diagnosis can be readily established by bacteriological examination, but later, when the infection is mixed, it is more difficult to recognise. Specific treatment is so effective that local treatment is unnecessary.

Lymphogranuloma Inguinale.—The modes of infection are similar to those of gonococcal proctitis, but in the female infection spreading from the cervix uteri via lymphatics to the pararectal lymph nodes is common. The proctological findings are similar to those of gonococcal proctitis. The diagnosis of lymphogranuloma inguinale should be suspected when the inguinal lymph nodes are greatly enlarged, although the enlargement may be subsiding by the time proctitis commences (Chapter 60).

Primary Syphilis.—A primary chancre may occur inside the anus (Chapter 57)—a paradox—'a painless anal fissure'.

'Strawberry' lesion of the recto-sigmoid is due to an infection by *Spirochaeta vincenti* and *Bacillus fusiformis*. The leading symptom is diarrhoea, often scantily blood-stained. Occasionally the diagnosis can be made by the demonstration of the specific organisms in the stools. More often sigmoidoscopy is required. The characteristic lesion is thickened, somewhat raised mucosa with superficial ulceration in the region of the recto-sigmoid. The inflamed mucous membrane oozes blood at numerous pin-points, giving the appearance of an over-ripe strawberry. A swab should be taken from the lesion and examined for Vincent's and fusiform organisms. Swabs from the gums and the throat are also advisable.

Treatment.—Acetarsol suppositories together with vitamin C is almost specific.

Rectal bilharziasis is caused by the *Schistosoma mansoni*, which is endemic in many tropical and subtropical countries, and particularly in the delta of the Nile.

Stage 1.—A cutaneous lesion develops at the site of entrance of the cercariae.[1]

Stage 2 is characterised by pyrexia, urticaria, and a high eosinophilia.

Both these stages are frequently overlooked.

Stage 3 is due to deposition of the ova in the rectum (much more rarely in the bladder, see Chapter 58) and is manifested by bilharzial dysentery. On examination in the later stages papillomas are frequently present. The papillomas, which are sessile or peduncu-

---

[1] Cercariae = a parasite of freshwater snails.

Jean Hyacinthe Vincent, 1862–1950. (See footnote, p. 574.)
Theodor Maximilian Bilharz, 1825–1862. Professor of Zoology, Cairo.

lated contain the ova of the trematode, the life-cycle of which resembles that of *Schistosoma haematobium*.

Untreated, the rectum becomes festooned, and prolapse of the diseased mucous membrane is usual. Multiple fistulas-in-ano are prone to develop.

General Treatment of Bilharziasis Mansoni.—(*a*) *Compounds not containing antimony* include niridazole (Ambilhar) in cases of infestation with *S. haematobium* or *S. mansoni* (**not** *S. japonicum* or in those with heart, mental or liver disease). Dose 25 mg/kg body wt. daily in two divided doses for 5–7 days. Hycanthone, lucanthone, oxamniquine are other compounds with weight related single doses given by deep i.m. injection, and all with toxic side effects. Metriphonate is an effective organophosphorus compound, also to be handled with great care.

(*b*) *Compounds containing antimony*, either as the salts, *tartar emetic* (antimony potassium tartrate) and the sodium salt given i.v., or antimony lithium thiomalate, sodium antimonylgluconate, stibogluconate and stibocaptate (Astiban) may still be required.

Local Treatment.—When the papillomas persist in spite of general treatment, they must be treated in the same manner as other papillomas.

Proctitis due to herbal enemas is a well-known clinical entity to those practising in tropical Africa. Following an enema consisting of a concoction of ginger, pepper, and tree-bark administered by a witch doctor, a most virulent proctitis sets in. Pelvic peritonitis frequently supervenes. Not infrequently a complete gelatinous cast of the mucous membrane of the rectum is extruded. Very large doses of morphine, together with streptomycin, often prevent a fatal issue if commenced early (Bowesman). Temporary colostomy is often advisable.

Treatment of severe proctitis that is due to a specific cause is treated by appropriate measures. General treatments should include bed rest in extreme cases. The stools should be kept soft with Isogel. Local instillations of 150 ml of olive oil are soothing. Suppositories of succinyl-sulphathiazole are often beneficial. The specific treatment for the dysenteries, tuberculosis, gonorrhoea, lymphogranuloma inguinale, and syphilis are described in the appropriate sections of this book.

SOLITARY ULCER

There is a rare condition that takes the form of an ulcer on the anterior wall of the rectum. It is thought to be traumatic in origin, either by sexual malpractices from below, or by intussusception of the anterior rectal wall into the anal sphincter from above. It is a benign condition that is clinically very easily confused with a carcinoma until repeated biopsies are performed. The clinico-pathological features have been well documented by Morson. The condition, although benign, is difficult to cure. The symptoms of bleeding and discharge can sometimes be ameliorated by topical hydrocortisone applications or by diathermy destruction of the ulcer (which usually returns). Some cases respond to perineal operations designed to prevent the downward intussusception, *e.g.* post-anal repair and even formal abdominal rectopexy in a few cases.

BENIGN TUMOURS OF THE RECTUM

The rectum along with the sigmoid colon is the most frequent site of polyps (and cancers) in the gastro-intestinal tract. All neoplastic polyps of the colon and rectum (with rare exceptions) have a tendency to become malignant. This tendency is greatly enhanced if the polyp is more than 1 cm in diameter, shows obvious signs of increasing size and has a sessile rather than a pedunculated shape. For these reasons, removal of all polyps is recommended, and *total* removal is mandatory. Only total removal will give complete histological examination and exclude (or confirm) localised carcinoma-in-situ, and also prevent local recur-

Sir Patrick Manson, 1844–1922. (See footnote, p. 947.)
Charles Bowesman, Contemporary. Formerly Surgical Specialist, Colonial Medical Service, Kumasi, Ghana.
Basil Clifford Morson, Contemporary. Pathologist, St. Mark's Hospital, London.

rence. For these reasons, destruction of anorectal tumours by fulguration is not the best treatment, and should be used for only the tiniest polyps. If one or more rectal polyps are discovered on sigmoidoscopic examination, an air contrast barium enema should be performed as further polyps are frequently found in the colon and treatment may be influenced. *No rectal tumour should be removed until the possibility of a proximal carcinoma has been ruled out, otherwise local implantation of cancer cells may occur in the distally situated rectal wound.*

The rectum shares substantially the same spectrum of polyps as the colon. Polyps are described chiefly in terms of their tissue organisation. For further clinical details the reader is referred to Chapter 50. Certain polyps which have features relevant to the rectum, are now described:

1. **Juvenile polyp.**—This is a bright red glistening pedunculated sphere ('cherry tumour') which is found in infants and children. Occasionally it persists into adult life. It can cause bleeding, or pain if it prolapses during defaecation. It often separates itself, but can be removed easily with forceps or a snare. It has virtually no tendency to malignant change but should be treated if it is causing symptoms. It has a unique histological structure of large mucous-filled spaces covered by a smooth surface of thin rectal cuboidal epithelium.

2. **Metaplastic polyps.**—These are small pinkish sessile polyps 2–4 mm in diameter and frequently multiple. They are harmless.

3. **Pseudo-polyps.**—These are actually oedematous bosses of mucous membrane. They are usually associated with colitis in the United Kingdom but most inflammatory diseases (including tropical diseases) can cause them. They are more likely to cause radiological difficulty as the sigmoidoscopic appearances are usually associated with obvious signs of the inflammatory cause.

4. **Villous adenomas.**—These have a characteristic frond-like appearance. They are often of very large size, and occasionally fill the entire rectum. The large tumours have an enhanced tendency to become malignant—a change that can be detected most easily by palpation with the finger; any hard area should be assumed to be malignant and should be biopsied.

Provided cancerous change has been excluded, these tumours can be removed either by submucous dissection per anum, or by sleeve resection from above. Only very unusually is rectal excision required, and then only when malignant change has occurred.

Rarely, the profuse mucous discharge from these tumours which is high in potassium content causes dangerous electrolyte and fluid losses.

All neoplastic polyps can be solitary or multiple. Small colonic polyps (<5 cm in size) can now be snared through the colonoscope. This new instrument has revolutionised the treatment of multiple polyps.

5. **Familial polyposis coli.**—This disease usually manifests itself by the development of multiple rectal polyps around puberty. An air-contrast barium enema will confirm the presence of multiple colonic polyps. As this condition is premalignant, a total colectomy must be performed, but sometimes the rectum can be preserved by regular fulguration of polyps before they develop carcinoma. The operation of proctocolectomy with ileo-anal anastomosis is now being used in some special centres of colo-proctology: the rectum is replaced by a 'pouch' of folded ileum (fig. 1034, Chapter 50).

Differential Diagnosis.—In patients who have lived in Egypt or any country where bilharzial infestation is rife, bilharzial papilloma must be excluded.

Treatment.—Diathermy coagulation is satisfactory in the case of a small papilloma, but the patient must be examined at regular intervals, for recurrence is common, as in the case of the bladder. For large papillomas, especially the sessile variety, excision of the rectum may be the only curative treatment. Some cases (not, as a rule, those invading the anal canal) are suitable for conservative resection of the rectum. In a few cases intestinal continuity can be restored by a low colo-anal 'sleeve' anastomosis achieved by the E.E.C. stapling gun.

Benign lymphoma, which occurs as a circumscribed movable nodule, firm but not hard, and greyish-white to pink in colour, is essentially submucosal. This neoplasm, which occurs at all ages and in both sexes, has no definite capsule. Notwithstanding, complete local excision is curative.

Endometrioma is not exceedingly rare, and as a rule it is diagnosed as a carcinoma. This neoplasm produces either a constricting lesion of the recto-sigmoid, or a tumour invading the rectum from the recto-vaginal septum. The latter variety gives rise to a very tender submucous elevation of the rectal wall. Endometrioma occurs usually between twenty and forty years of age; less often at the menopause. Dysmenorrhoea with rectal bleeding are the main symptoms. On sigmoidoscopy endometriosis involving the recto-sigmoid junction usually presents as a stricture with the mucous membrane intact. Bilateral öopherectomy may be followed by regression of the tumour, rendering resection unnecessary. The contraceptive 'Pill' is also effective as it inhibits ovulation.

Haemangioma of the rectum, which is an uncommon tumour, is a cause of serious and, if the neoplasm is large, sometimes fatal haemorrhage. When localised in the lower part of the rectum or anal canal, a haemangioma can be excised after applying Goodsall's ligature. When the neoplasm is diffuse, or lying in the upper part of the rectum, the symptoms simulate ulcerative colitis, and often the diagnosis is missed for a long period. At other times the neoplasm is mistaken for a vascular carcinoma, an error which, fortunately, is not often a cause for serious regret, because the correct treatment of an extensive haemangioma is excision of that portion of the ano-rectum bearing the neoplasm. Lesser procedures are followed nearly always by recurrence and renewed loss of blood.

Fibroma (*syn.* fibrous polypus) is not uncommon. *It is not a neoplasm*, but is due to fibrosis of a thrombosed haemorrhoid.

CARCINOMA OF THE RECTUM

This is the fourth most common variety of malignant tumour found in women, and its frequency in men is surpassed only by carcinoma of the bronchus and stomach.

Origin.—In many cases, operation specimens show that in some part of the bowel that has been removed, in addition to the carcinoma, there are one or more synchronous adenomas or papillomas, proof indeed that adenoma and papilloma of the rectum are pre-carcinomatous conditions. In approximately 3% of cases there is more than one carcinoma present. It is now believed that most rectal cancers start as an adenoma (the 'Adenoma–Carcinoma' sequence).

Pathological Histology.—Three types are recognised:

(1) Well differentiated adenocarcinoma; (2) Averagely differentiated adenocarcinoma; (3) Anaplastic, highly undifferentiated adenocarcinoma.

The more malignant varieties frequently contain large numbers of mucin producing cells. The prognosis after treatment is greatly influenced by the histological grading of the tumour (see below).

Usually these carcinomas present as an ulcer, but papilliferous and infiltrating types are not uncommon.

Local spread occurs circumferentially rather than in a longitudinal direction. Usually a period of six months is required for involvement of one-quarter of the circumference, and eighteen months to two years for complete encirclement, the annular variety being common at the recto-sigmoid junction. After the muscular coat has been penetrated the growth spreads into the underlying fat, but is still limited by the fascia propria (peri-rectal fascia). Eventually the fascia propria is penetrated but this occurrence is rare before eighteen months from the commencement of the disease. If penetration occurs anteriorly, the prostate, seminal vesicles, or the bladder become involved in the male; in the female the vagina or the uterus are invaded. In either sex, if the penetration is lateral, a ureter may become implicated, while posterior penetration involves the sacrum and the sacral plexus. Downward spread for more than a few centimetres is rare except in anaplastic tumours.

Lymphatic Spread.—Enlargement of lymph nodes from bacterial infection is more frequent than enlargement from metastasis, and microscopical examination is required to detect carcinomatous involvement of the nodes.

Lymphatic spread from a carcinoma of the rectum above the peritoneal reflexion occurs almost exclusively in an *upward* direction; below that level to within 1 to 2 cm of the anal orifice the lymphatic spread is still *upwards*, but the first halting place is in the para-rectal lymph nodes of Gerota. The exception to this rule is when the neoplasm lies within the field of the middle rectal artery, *i.e.* between 4 and 8 cm from the anus, in which case primary *lateral* spread along the lymphatics that accompany the middle rectal vein is not infrequent.

Downward spread is exceptional, drainage along the subcutaneous lymphatics to the groins being confined, for practical purposes, to the lymph nodes draining the perianal rosette and the epithelium lining the distal 1 to 2 cm of the anal canal.

Metastasis at a higher level than the main trunk of the superior rectal artery occurs only late in the disease. A radical operation should ensure that the high-lying lymph nodes are removed by ligating the inferior mesenteric artery and vein at the highest possible level.

Atypical and widespread lymphatic permeation can occur in highly undifferentiated neoplasms.

Venous Spread.—As a rule, spread via the venous system occurs late, except in that portion of the anal canal where the anoderm is firmly adherent to deeper structures. Anaplastic and rapidly growing tumours in younger patients are much more liable to spread in this way than tumours of relatively low malignancy. The principal sites for blood-borne metastases are: liver (34%), lungs (22%), adrenals (11%). The remaining 33% is divided among the many other locations where secondary carcinomatous deposits are wont to lodge, including the brain.

Peritoneal dissemination may follow penetration of the peritoneal coat by a high-lying rectal carcinoma.

Stages of Progression.—As a rule carcinoma of the rectum does not metastasise early. Dukes classified carcinoma of the rectum into three stages (fig. 1110).

A   The growth is limited to the rectal wall (15%). Prognosis excellent.

B   The growth is extended to the extra-rectal tissues, but no metastasis to the regional lymph nodes (35%). Prognosis good.

C   There are secondary deposits in the regional lymph nodes (50%). These are subdivided into C^1 where the local para-rectal lymph nodes alone are involved, and C^2 where the nodes accompanying the supplying blood-vessels are implicated up to the point of division. This does not take into account cases that have metastasised beyond the regional lymph nodes or by way of the venous system. Prognosis bad.

Cuthbert Esquire Dukes, 1890–1977. Pathologist, St. Mark's Hospital, London.

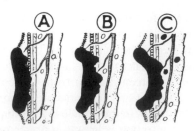

FIG. 1110.—The three cardinal stages of
progression of the neoplasm.
(After Cuthbert Dukes, FRCS.)

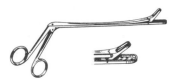

FIG. 1111.—Yeomans' biopsy
forceps.

Histological Grading.—In the great majority of cases carcinoma of the rectum is a columnar-celled adenocarcinoma. The more nearly the tumour cells approach normal shape and arrangement, the less malignant is the tumour. Conversely, the greater the percentage of cells of an embryonic or undifferentiated type, the more malignant is the tumour;

Low grade = well-differentiated tumours	11%	Prognosis good.
Average grade	64%	,, fair.
High grade = anaplastic tumours .	25%	,, poor.

Attempts to replace the Dukes grading system by more refined histopathological criteria are being made (e.g. by a T.N.M. system analogous to breast carcinoma: one such system, the Astler-Coller grading, has provoked wide interest).

Colloid carcinoma is present in 12% of cases. There are two forms—primary and secondary; much the more frequent is secondary mucoid degeneration of an adenocarcinoma. Histologically the glandular arrangement is preserved and mucus fills the acini. This type is of average malignancy. In a small number of cases the tumour is a primary mucoid carcinoma. The mucus lies within the cells, displacing the nucleus to the periphery, like the seal of a signet ring. Primary mucoid carcinoma gives rise to a rapidly growing bulky growth which metastasises very early and the prognosis of which is very bad.

Clinical Features.—Carcinoma of the rectum is not uncommon early in life, and when the disease commences in youth, in spite of radical treatment, death usually results within a year. Usually the early symptoms are so slight that the patient does not seek advice for six months or more.

Bleeding is the earliest and most constant symptom. There is nothing characteristic about the time at which it occurs, neither is the colour nor the amount of blood distinctive; often the bleeding is slight in amount, and occurs at the end of defaecation, or is noticed because it has stained underclothing. Indeed, more often than not, the bleeding in every respect simulates that of internal haemorrhoids[1], and it is lamentable that, in spite of oft-repeated exhortations, the patient's doctor sometimes fails to examine the rectum but prescribes a salve while the growth advances to inoperability (footnote, Chapter 52).

Sense of Incomplete Defaecation.—The patient has his bowels open but feels that there are more faeces to be passed. This is a very important early symptom[2] and is almost invariably present in tumours of the lower half of the rectum. The patient may endeavour to empty the rectum several times a day (spurious diarrhoea), often with the passage of flatus and a little blood-stained mucus ('bloody slime').

[1] Haemorrhoids and carcinoma sometimes co-exist (fig. 1128).
[2] *Tenesmus* is painful straining to empty the bowels without resultant evacuation.

Alteration in bowel habit is the next most frequent symptom, and the commonest deviation from normality is increasing constipation. The patient finds it necessary to start taking an aperient, or to supplement his usual dose, and as a result a tendency towards diarrhoea ensues. A patient who has to get up before the accustomed hour in order to defaecate, and one who passes blood and mucus in addition to faeces[1], is usually found to be suffering from carcinoma of the rectum. Usually it is the patient with an annular carcinoma at the pelvirectal junction who suffers with increasing constipation, and the one with a cauliflower growth in the ampulla of the rectum with early morning diarrhoea (Bruce).

Pain is a late symptom, but pain of a colicky character accompanies advanced growths of the recto-sigmoid and is due to some degree of intestinal obstruction. When a deep carcinomatous ulcer of the rectum erodes the prostate or bladder, there is severe pain. Pain in the back, or sciatica, occurs when the growth invades the sacral plexus. Weight loss is suggestive of hepatic metastases.

Abdominal examination is negative in early cases. Occasionally when an advanced annular growth is situated at the recto-sigmoid junction, signs of obstruction to the large intestine are likely to be present. By the time the patient seeks advice metastases in the liver may be palpable. When the peritoneum has become studded with secondary deposits, ascites results.

Rectal Examination.—In approximately 90% of cases the neoplasm can be felt digitally: in early cases as a plateau or as a nodule with an indurated base. When the centre ulcerates, a shallow depression will be found, the edges of which are raised and everted; this, combined with induration of the base of the ulcer, is a frequent and unmistakable finding. On bimanual examination it may be possible to feel the lower extremity of a carcinoma situated in the recto-sigmoid junction. After the finger has been withdrawn, if it has been in direct contact with a carcinoma, it is smeared with blood, or muco-purulent material tinged with blood. When a carcinomatous ulcer is situated in the lower third of the rectum, involved lymph nodes can sometimes be felt as one or more hard oval swellings in the extra-rectal tissues posteriorly or posterolaterally above the tumour. In females a vaginal examination should be performed, and when the neoplasm is situated on the anterior wall of the rectum, with one finger in the vagina and another in the rectum, very accurate palpation can be carried out.

Procto-sigmoidoscopy in the complete knee-elbow position (fig. 1123) will always show a carcinoma, if present—providing the rectum is emptied of faeces beforehand.

Biopsy.—Employing biopsy forceps (fig. 1111) by way of a rectoscope, a portion of the edge of the tumour is removed. If possible another specimen from the more central part of the growth is obtained also. Expert histological examination will not only enable the diagnosis of carcinoma to be confirmed, but the tumour can be graded as to its relative malignancy, although not always with complete accuracy.

Barium enema is required (*a*) in cases of suspected carcinoma of the pelvi-rectal junction when sigmoidoscopy fails to reveal the growth because of spasm of the bowel below it, (*b*) when multiple adenomatous polyposis of the colon must be excluded and (*c*) when practical, to exclude other synchronous carcinomas (5% of cases).

---

[1] 'Early morning bloody diarrhoea.'

Differential Diagnosis.—When a seemingly benign **papilloma** or **adenoma** shows evidence of induration or unusual friability, it is almost certain that malignancy has occurred, even in spite of biopsy findings to the contrary. On the other hand, biopsy is invaluable in distinguishing carcinoma from an **inflammatory stricture** or an **amoebic granuloma**, which simulates a carcinoma very closely. The possibility of a neoplasm being an **endometrioma** should always be entertained in patients with dysmenorrhoea. The possibility of a **carcinoid tumour** in atypical cases must be remembered. In the last four instances biopsy will establish the correct diagnosis. The **solitary ulcer** syndrome has already been alluded to above.

Treatment

Some form of excision of the rectum is essential, if at all possible, because of the extreme suffering entailed if the neoplasm remains.

Apart from co-existent disease or senile enfeeblement, the only prohibitions to excision of the rectum are widespread distant metastases and extensive peritoneal deposits. Many instances have been reported where a presumed solitary metastasis in the liver has been resected, either at the time of excision of the rectum, or subsequently with cure in many cases. Even when metastases in the liver are irremovable, resection of the rectum is often justifiable, and the patient may survive in comfort for a year or two.

A combined (abdominal and perineal) excision offers the best prospect of eradicating the disease for tumours in the lower third of the rectum. For those in the upper two-thirds of the rectum a restorative type of operation (anterior resection) is usually possible. Because of the much wider degree of local spread by anaplastic tumours and the high risk of local recurrence, restorative operations are not usually done for this group of lesions when they are in the lower half of the rectum, but the use of pre- and post-operative radiotherapy is allowing more cases than before to be handled by a sphincter-preserving type of operation. It is now known that well over half of rectal cancers can be satisfactorily treated by a restorative operation.

The combined operation can be carried out (1) as an abdomino-perineal procedure (Miles), by which is meant that the abdominal part of the operation is undertaken first, or (2) a perineo-abdominal (Gabriel), where the perineal stage is performed before the abdominal stage, or (3) as a synchronised procedure, where two operating teams work sumultaneously (Lloyd-Davies). The last is now the predominant method.

Pre-operative sterilisation of the alimentary tract.—This is usually achieved by a combination of mechanical cleansing (purgatives, enemas, or 'whole-gut irrigation') and antibiotics. The antibiotic regime must be active against both aerobic and anaerobic organisms. At present a suitable prescription would be gentamicin 80 mg plus metronidazole 200 mg one hour before surgery, plus another dose of each drug 12 hours after the operation. If a patient comes to surgery with a loaded-colon, peroperative washouts can be performed provided the rest of the wound is scrupulously protected. Detergent preparations are available for this.

Blood and electrolyte deficiencies are corrected. Before commencing the operation, an indwelling catheter is inserted into the bladder. In male patients a full size catheter is preferred as damage to the urethra is thereby made less likely during dissection anterior to the rectum.

Combined Synchronised Excision of the Rectum.—This is the operation which is

---

William Ernest Miles, 1869–1947. Surgeon, Royal Cancer Hospital (now the Royal Marsden Hospital), London.

now commonly performed. It combines the advantages of both the abdomino-perineal and the perineo-abdominal operations. A large catheter is passed and with the patient in Trendelenburg-lithotomy position, the legs being supported in special crutches designed by Lloyd-Davies, access is afforded to the abdomen and the perineum at the same time. Two surgeons operate simultaneously, one performing the perineal dissection and the other the abdominal portion of the operation. This considerably reduces the time expended in performing the operation, and obviates turning the patient. The resectability rate is increased by this operation.

The *Abdominal Surgeon* makes a left paramedian incision, extending it well above the umbilicus. The liver and the peritoneum are examined for metastases and the degree of fixity of the growth established. The small intestine is packed away from the pelvis. A self-retaining retractor is placed in the wound and the pelvic colon freed by dividing any congenital adhesions on the left side. The peritoneum and the pelvic floor are divided with a knife by an incision which runs from the colon at the proposed site of division over the mesocolon and across the base of the bladder or near the cervix on the peritoneal floor and then upwards on the right side of the mesocolon. The peritoneum is now raised, using the points of the scissors to expose the ureters and testicular or ovarian artery. The mesocolon is now divided at the site of the proposed division on the colon and the trunk of the inferior mesenteric artery (fig. 1112) ligated and divided distal to the first branch. (Some surgeons emphasise 'flush ligation' of the artery at its origin from the aorta.) The recto-sigmoid mesentery is further divided and separated from the sacrum by blunt dissection with the fingers. In this way the sacrum is cleared almost down to the coccyx. The peritoneal incision anterior to the rectum is now deepened and the seminal vesicles or the vaginal wall is identified so that Denonvilliers' fascia behind them is cleared by a dissection leading down to the prostate or perineal body. The middle rectal vessels usually lying anterior to the lateral ligaments on each side are now seized with clamps, divided and ligated. The site of division of the pelvic colon is cleared of fat and the colon divided between clamps with diathermy.

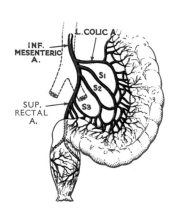

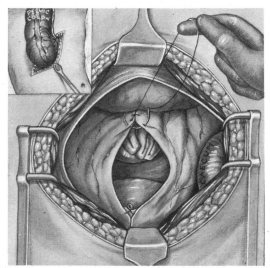

FIG. 1112.—The inferior mesenteric artery. S₁ S₂ S₃ = sigmoid branches.

FIG. 1113.—The cut edges of the pelvic peritoneum are being united over the space (filled by packing) where the 'perineal' surgeon is working. *Inset*: The rectum and pelvic colon drawn through the left iliac incision to form a terminal colostomy.

By this time the perineal surgeon working from below has mobilised the anus and the lower rectum so that the whole of the bowel below together with a clamp can be passed through the perineal wound by the abdominal surgeon. Haemostasis over the sacrum may be difficult but it is achieved by diathermy and a hot saline pack left in position for a few minutes. The pelvic peritoneum is now united by continuous catgut stitches from the bladder right back over the promontory of the sacrum (fig. 1113).

The site in the L.I.F. for the colostomy is then selected. This should be equidistant from the umbilicus and the left anterior superior iliac spine and is usually sited at the linea semi-lunaris about 2·5 cm above the spino-umbilical line. A circular piece of skin and fascia, about 3 cm in diameter, is incised and this hole deepened to excise similar layers of fascia and peritoneum. The protected end of the colon with the clamp is now passed through this incision and the colostomy performed by suturing the colon to the peritoneum and the mucosa directly to the skin. The paracolic gutter is closed with sutures—this will close the 'lateral space'. The abdomen is closed and the layers of the incision protected from the colostomy. An adherent plastic colostomy bag is then fitting in position and the dressings are placed on the abdominal wound.

Perineal Surgeon.—When the abdominal surgeon has made certain that the condition is operable, the perineal surgeon closes the anus with purse-string sutures of stout silk. An elliptical incision between the tip of the coccyx and the central perineal point is made around the anus and deepened. The left forefinger is insinuated into the levator ani which is divided lateral to the finger first on one side and then on the other. The dissection is deepened posteriorly by incising Waldeyer's fascia which is a thick condensation of pelvic fascia lying between the rectum and the sacrum. Contact is made with the abdominal surgeon. The apex of skin anterior to the anus is grasped in a haemostat, which serves as a retractor, and by scissors and gauze dissection the wound is deepened, when the catheter within the membranous urethra will be felt. Both in the male and the female a plane of cleavage will be found between the rectum and the prostate or the rectum and the vagina, respectively. This plane having been carefully determined, Denonvilliers' fascia is divided, after which the rectum can be stripped from the prostate or the vagina. The posterior wall of the vagina is frequently excised with the rectum. When the abdominal surgeon has cleared the rectum laterally, the whole of the anus and rectum can be drawn downwards and removed. Haemostasis must be secured and the perineal wound closed anteriorly and posteriorly in layers around a large drainage tube or closed entirely around suction drains. Large dressings of gauze and wool are applied over the area and a triangular bandage is used to keep the dressing in place. It is becoming a more common practice in some centres to employ *primary closure* of the perineal wound, and use laterally-situated suction drains brought out through each ischio-rectal fossa to keep the large perineal cavity from filling up with blood and serous exudate. These drains can be removed after 5 days.

After Treatment.—The patient is returned to bed, blood transfusion being continued as necessary. The catheter is connected to a closed drainage system and left in for five days. It may have to be re-inserted if voluntary micturition is not re-established; carbachol may be necessary to establish this.

Reactionary haemorrhage from the perineal wound may demand return to the theatre to open and pack the wound with gauze. The colour of the colostomy must be watched to make sure the blood supply is adequate. Small bowel obstruction may occur by herniation in the lateral space of the colostomy or through the pelvic peritoneal closure line. Discharge of urine from the perineal wound demands immediate investigation for bladder or ureteric damage.

Care of the Colostomy.—This is much the same as the care of an ileostomy (p. 1044). Within a very short time the colostomy acts once or twice a day. The patient soon learns which foods cause diarrhoea and therefore avoids them. Many patients are now taught to empty their lower colon by irrigations through the colostomy: this has many advantages for the patient who requires an inactive colostomy while at work.

Stenosis of the colostomy is usually avoided by the removal of the circle of skin and subcutaneous tissues at the colostomy site. Anal dilators may be necessary if there is any tendency for stenosis to occur.

Less Extensive Operations:

Abdominal Radical Restorative Resection (anterior resection).—In cases of carcinoma of the rectum situated above the peritoneal reflection, lymphatic spread is virtually confined to the upward paths, and wide resection of the bowel with its lymphatic field, followed by end-to-end anastomosis and preservation of the sphincter mechanism is both justifiable and highly desirable. The replace-

Heinrich Wilhelm Gottfried Waldeyer-Hartz, 1836–1921. Professor of Pathological Anatomy, Berlin.

ment of hand-suturing by staple-anastomosis has greatly assisted the safe performance of very low colo-anal unions (see Chapter 42).

This apparently ideal treatment was unpopular in many centres because it had been found that local recurrence occurred in a formidable percentage of cases. It has now been substantiated that the so-called recurrences are due, for the most part either to widespread pelvic recurrence 'breaking back' into the rectum through the anastomosis, or to local implantation of free malignant cells into the distal segment that is to be preserved, the survival and rooting of these cells being favoured by disinfection of the intestine by antibiotics. Naunton Morgan has shown that when a suitable clamp is placed at least 3 cm below the neoplasm, and the rectum is irrigated with buffered Dakin's solution (Chlorinated soda-0·5% available chlorine), and the lumen of the proximal end and the edges of both segments are swabbed with the same solution before anastomosis, the incidence of local recurrence is reduced considerably. The 5-year cure rate for rectal carcinoma treated by radical surgery (either by total rectal excision or a restorative procedure) is 50%.

Hartmann's Operation.—This is an excellent procedure in an old and feeble patient who would not stand an abdomino-perineal procedure. Through an abdominal incision the rectum is excised down to within an inch (2·5 cm) of the anus, a colostomy performed and the peritoneum oversewn to cover the pelvic defect in the usual way. The cavity below can be drained through the anus, which is divided posteriorly. In the old patient, where the neoplasm is usually slow growing and spread is late, this is a most useful operation.

Palliative colostomy is indicated *only* in cases giving rise to intestinal obstruction, or where there is gross infection of the neoplasm. It is often possible to resect the growth later.

Local Operations.—For small, low-grade mobile lesions, which are often Grade A tumours, local removal should be curative. For these tumours, especially in the unfit or patients who will not accept a colostomy, local removal has been used. Such operations are only suitable for lesions within 10 cm of the anal verge. Turnbull has advocated local diathermy removal while York-Mason has developed a trans-anal (trans-sphincteric) approach, but a peranal approach is usually suitable.

More Extensive Operations.—When the carcinoma of the rectum has spread to contiguous organs, the radical operation can often be extended to remove these structures. Thus in the male, where the spread is usually to the bladder, a total cystectomy and resection of the rectum can be affected. In the female the uterus acts as a barrier preventing spread from the rectum to the bladder. Accordingly, a total hysterectomy should be undertaken in addition to excision of the rectum. Should the bladder be involved, then pelvic evisceration must include that structure. Pelvic evisceration for carcinoma of the rectum is justifiable only when the surgeon is reasonably confident that the growth can be removed *in toto*.

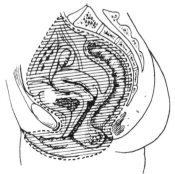

FIG. 1114.—Radical pelvic evisceration, indicating the extent of the dissection and the viscera removed.

Pelvic Evisceration (Brunschwig's operation).—The aim is to remove all the pelvic organs, together with the internal iliac and the obturator groups of lymph nodes (fig. 1114). The lithotomy-Trendelenburg position facilitates the procedure, and ligation of both internal iliac arteries diminishes the blood loss. The small intestine fills the empty pelvis. Especial care must therefore be taken to suture accurately the perineal skin, and to avoid pressure necrosis of the perineal incision by nursing the patient on alternate sides. Some form of urinary diversion is necessary (Chapter 58).

Henri Albert Charles Antoine Hartmann, 1860–1952. Professor of Surgery, Paris.
Sir Clifford Naunton Morgan, 1902–1986. Surgeon, St. Bartholomew's Hospital, London.
R. Turnbull, Contemporary. Surgeon, Cleveland Clinic, Cleveland, Ohio, U.S.A.
Aubrey York-Mason, Contemporary. Surgeon, St. Helier Hospital, Carshalton, Surrey.
Alexander Brunschwig. Formerly Surgeon, Memorial Hospital for the Treatment of Cancer, New York.

Radiotherapy.—With modern techniques (MV cobalt therapy or neutron beam irradiation) some adenocarcinomas now respond to radiotherapy. Some large tumours can be shrunk as a pre-operative measure to make removal easier, and palliative irradiation can be given for inoperable primary tumours or local recurrence especially when painful. Papillon has perfected a technique of intra-cavity radiation which applies the treatment direct to the tumour from the rectal lumen. In a selected series of early cases the results have been good (more than 70% 5-year survivals).

Cytotoxic and Chemotherapeutic Drugs.—These are still under evaluation, but have proved to be of little effect so far.

Carcinoid Tumour.—Carcinoid tumour of the rectum, as far as its lethal properties are concerned, can be looked upon as a gradation between a benign tumour and a carcinoma. A number of carcinoid tumours of the rectum have been reported during recent years so that a latter-day aphorism is 'keep carcinoid in mind when an atypical neoplasm of the rectum is encountered'. Like benign lymphoma, carcinoid tumour originates in the submucosa, the mucous membrane over it being intact. Consequently it seldom produces evidence of its presence in the early stages, when it appears as a small plaque-like elevation. The incidence of clinical malignancy, *i.e.* the occurrence of metastases, is 10%. This is much less than that for carcinoid tumour of the small intestine but it is greater than that of carcinoid tumour of the vermiform appendix. Multiple primary carcinoid tumours of the rectum are not infrequent. The neoplasm is slow of progression, and usually metastasises late. Large carcinoids (> 2 cm) are always malignant.

Treatment.—Resection of the rectum is advisable if the growth is more than 2·5 cm in diameter, if recurrence follows local excision, or if the growth is fixed to the peri-rectal tissues. Even when metastases are present, resection may prolong life.

J. Papillon, Contemporary. Professor of Radiotherapy, Lyons, France.

CHAPTER 54

THE ANUS AND ANAL CANAL

Surgical Anatomy

The anal canal commences at the level where the rectum passes through the pelvic diaphragm and ends at the anal verge.[1] The muscular junction between the rectum and anal canal can be felt with the finger as a thickened ridge—the anorectal 'bundle' or 'ring'.

Anal Canal Musculature:

The internal sphincter is a thickened continuation of the circular muscle coat of the rectum. This involuntary muscle commences where the rectum passes through the pelvic diaphragm, and ends at the anal orifice, where its lower border can be felt. The internal anal sphincter is 2·5 cm long and 2 to 5 mm thick. When exposed during life, it is pearly-white in colour, and its individual transversely placed fibres can be seen clearly. Spasm and contracture of this muscle play a major part in fissure and other anal affections.

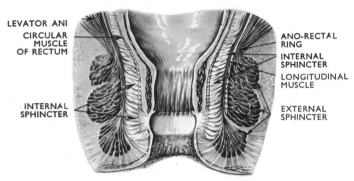

FIG. 1115.—The musculature of the anal canal.
(After Sir Clifford Naunton Morgan, FRCS, London.)

The longitudinal muscle is a continuation of the longitudinal muscle coat of the rectum intermingled with fibres from the pubo-rectalis. Its fibres fan out through the lowest part of the external sphincter, to be inserted into the true anal and perianal skin. The longitudinal muscle fibres that are attached to the epithelium provide pathways for the spread of perianal infections and mark out tight 'compartments' that are responsible for the intense pressure and pain that accompany many localised perianal lesions.

Beneath the anal skin lie the scanty fibres of the corrugator cutis ani muscle.

The external sphincter, formerly subdivided into a deep, superficial, and subcutaneous portion is now considered to be one muscle (Goligher). Some of its fibres are attached posteriorly to the coccyx, while anteriorly they are inserted into the mid-perineal joint in the male, whereas in the female they fuse with the sphincter vaginae. In life the external sphincter is pink in colour, and homogeneous. Unlike the pale internal sphincter muscle, which is involuntary, the red external sphincter is composed of voluntary (somatic) muscle.

Between the internal (involuntary) sphincter and the external (voluntary) sphincter muscle mass is found a potential space—*the intersphincteric plane.* This plane is important as it contains the basal parts of 8–12 apocrine glands, which can cause infections, and it is also a route for the spread of pus. It can also be opened up by a surgeon to provide access for operations on the sphincter muscles.

---

[1] Anal verge = the external or distal boundary of the anal canal.

John Cedric Goligher, Contemporary. Emeritus Professor of Surgery, Leeds, England.

A recent revision of the anorectal muscular anatomy (Shafik) has drawn attention to the close association between the pubo-rectalis portion of the levator ani and the external sphincter muscle, and gives a prime role to the pubo-rectalis in preserving continence and achieving satisfactory defaecation. Weakness or malfunction of this muscle can lead to rectal or vaginal prolapse.

The mucous membrane.—The *pink* columnar epithelium lining the rectum extends through the ano-rectal ring into the surgical anal canal. The mucosa of the upper anal canal is attached loosely to the underlying structures, and covers the internal rectal plexus. Passing downwards where it clothes the series of 8 to 12 longitudinal folds known as the columns of Morgagni, the mucous membrane becomes cubical, and *red* in colour (fig. 1116); above the anal valves the mucous membrane becomes *plum coloured*. Just below the level of the anal valves there is an abrupt, albeit wavy, transition to squamous epithelium, which is *parchment colour*. This wavy junction constitutes the dentate line. The squamous epithelium lining the lower anal canal is thin and shiny, and is known as the anoderm. This squamous epithelium differs from the true skin in that it has no epidermal appendages, *i.e.* hair, sweat glands. The anoderm passes imperceptibly into the pigmented skin of the anus. At the dentate line the anoderm is attached very firmly indeed to deeper structures.

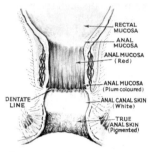

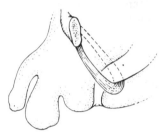

FIG. 1116.—The lining membrane of the anal canal.
(After Sir Clifford Naunton Morgan, FRCS, London.)

FIG. 1117.—Anal gland with duct opening into a crypt of Morgagni.

FIG. 1118.—The disposition of the pubo-rectalis muscle.

The dentate line is a most important landmark both morphologically and surgically. It represents (1) the site of fusion of the proctodaeum and post-allantoic gut, and (2) the position of the anal membrane, remnants of which may frequently be seen as anal papillae situated on the free margin of the anal valves. The dentate line separates:

Above	Below
Cubical epithelium	from squamous epithelium
Autonomic nerves (insensitive)	from spinal nerves (very sensitive)
Portal venous system	from systemic venous system

The anal valves of Ball are a series of transversely placed semilunar folds linking the columns of Morgagni. They lie along and actually constitute the waviness of the dentate line. They are functionless remnants of the fusion of the post-allantoic gut with the proctodaeum.

The crypts of Morgagni (*syn.* anal crypts) are small pockets between the inferior extremities of the columns of Morgagni. Into several of these crypts, mostly those situated posteriorly, opens one **anal gland** by a narrow duct. This duct bifurcates, and the branches pass outward to enter the internal sphincter muscle, in 60% of people (fig. 1117). Issuing from this ampulla there are three to six tubular sub-branches that extend into the intermuscular connective tissue, where they end blindly. In some lower animals these glands secrete an odoriferous substance during the rutting season; in man their function, if any, is obscure. Some of their cells have been shown to give a positive staining reaction for mucin, but as the lining epithelium is mainly cubical, the mucus-secreting propensity of the anal glands must be extremely small. Infection of an anal gland can give rise to an

A. Shafik, Contemporary. Professor of Surgery, Cairo.
Giovanni Battista Morgagni, 1682–1771. Professor of Anatomy, Padua, Italy.
Sir Charles Bent Ball, 1851–1916. Regius Professor of Surgery, Dublin.

abscess, and in the opinion of a number of surgeons, infection of an anal gland is the most common cause of ano-rectal abscesses and fistulas.

The anorectal ring marks the junction between the rectum and the anal canal. It is formed by the joining of the pubo-rectalis muscle (fig. 1118), the deep external sphincter, conjoined longitudinal muscle, and the highest part of the internal sphincter. The ano-rectal ring can be clearly felt digitally, especially on its posterior and lateral aspects. Division of the anorectal ring results in permanent incontinence of faeces. The position and length of the anal canal, as well as the angle of the anorectal junction, depends to a major extent on the integrity and strength of the pubo-rectalis muscle sling.

Arterial supply.—The anal canal is supplied by branches from the superior, middle and inferior haemorrhoidal arteries. The most important is the superior haemorrhoidal, whose left branch supplies the left half of the canal by a single terminal branch, while its right has two terminal branches. All the arteries contribute to a rich submucous and intramural plexus so that interruption of the arterial supply from above by division of the superior and middle rectal arteries does not deprive the anus of its blood supply.

Venous drainage.—The anal veins are distributed in similar fashion to the arterial supply. The superior and middle haemorrhoidal veins drain via the inferior mesenteric vein into the portal system, having become the superior rectal vein en-route. The superior haemorrhoidal vein drains the upper half of the anal canal. The inferior haemorrhoidal veins drain the lower half of the anal canal and the subcutaneous peri-anal plexus of veins: they eventually join the external iliac vein on each side.

Lymphatic drainage.—Lymph from the upper half of the anal canal flows upwards to drain into the post-rectal lymph nodes (fig. 1098, Chapter 53) and from there go to the para-aortic nodes via the inferior mesenteric chain. Lymph from the lower half of the anal canal drains on each side first into the superficial and then into the deep inguinal group of lymph glands. However, if the normal flow is blocked (*e.g.* by tumour) the lymph can be diverted into the alternative route.

Surgical Physiology of the Anal Muscles and Pelvic Floor

The function of the anal canal and pelvic floor muscles is to contain the contents of the rectum, but to allow effortless unimpeded voiding at defaecation. Interference with the integrity of the anatomy or physiology of the muscles of the anus and pelvic floor can lead to the extremes of intractable constipation or incontinence. If the muscles of the pelvic floor become too floppy, the entire ano-rectal mechanism can drop down ('perineal descent'), or alternatively can gape open, so allowing intussusception and prolapse of the rectum.

If the pubo-rectalis and anorectal ring of muscles fail to relax appropriately (so-called 'inappropriate function') to allow the rectum to empty at defaecation, obstructed defaecation ensues: this can usually be overcome by excessive voluntary straining efforts, but frequently ends in intractable constipation. Excessive straining can cause both partial and complete rectal prolapse. When a patient presents with incontinence caused by weak or damaged anorectal musculature, or if bizarre or extreme complaints of constipation are elicited, it is now possible to investigate these symptoms to obtain objective data on which to base a management protocol (Swash and Henry). The length, resting tone and the power to

M. Swash, Contemporary. Physician to the London Hospital and St. Mark's Hospital.
M. Henry, Contemporary Surgeon, Central Middlesex Hospital and St. Mark's Hospital.

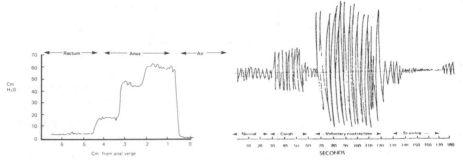

FIG. 1119.—A typical normal 'pull-through' manometric study of the anal canal (3·5 cm long: maximal pressure 60 cm H_2O approx.).

FIG. 1120.—A typical normal electromyographic study of the external sphincter during various activities.

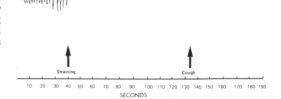

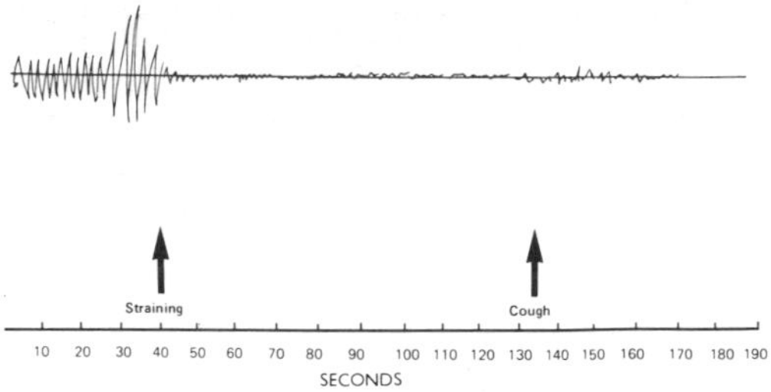

FIG. 1121.—An electromyographic study of the external sphincter showing prolonged inhibition on straining and absent cough reflex. This is typical of a denervated patulous sphincter.

relax and contract the anal sphincter muscles can be assessed by manometry and electromyography (figs 1119 and 1120): these studies can be combined with delineation of rectal sensibility and function by balloon-distention and radiology ('defaecatory proctography') and the abnormalities identified (fig. 1121). In addition to the intrinsic defects, mechanical deviations can also be mapped: the level and angle of the anorectal junction can be established by clinical observation, by an appliance ('perineometer') and radiologically (Williams). As a result of such combined clinical and laboratory methods, many patients can now be offered effective treatment for the curse of incontinence or constipation.

EXAMINATION OF THE ANUS

This requires careful attention to circumstances. The examining couch should be of sufficient height to allow easy inspection and access for any necessary manoeuvres. A good light is mandatory. The Sims (left lateral) or the Lithotomy position are satisfactory: the latter is less convenient for an elderly patient and can cause social embarassment to young women. A protective glove should be worn. The patient should be relaxed and able to co-operate. A few quiet words from the doctor can prevent many loud ones from the patient. The examination proceeds by:

1. **Inspection.**—With the buttocks opened, the anus is inspected. Note is made of any lesions, *e.g.* inflammatory skin changes, haemorrhoids, fissure ('sentinel pile'), fistula. The patient is asked to strain down before inspection is concluded.

2. **Digital examination with the index finger.**—A good lubricant is necess-

N. Williams, Contemporary. Professor of Surgery, The London Hospital.

ary—neither too little nor too much. Any secretions should be sampled prior to applying lubricant to the anal verge.

Extreme gentleness should be the rule so that pain is not caused. Painful spasm of the anal sphincters is confirmation of a hidden fissure if the history is suggestive.

The examination should check normal as well as abnormal structures according to the following plan:

Intraluminal——< normal: faeces
              abnormal: polyp or carcinoma

Intramural——< normal: sphincter muscles and anorectal angle
            abnormal: leiomyoma or carcinoma

Extramural——< normal: perianal structures
            abnormal: abscess

At the same examination, the rectum is examined according to the same system. Before withdrawing the finger, the patient is asked again to strain down, and a note is made regarding the prostate in a male patient and the cervix, uterus and pouch of Douglas in a female. *Discharge:* After withdrawal, the finger is examined for mucus, pus, blood and abnormal faecal material.

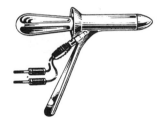

FIG. 1122.—An illuminated proctoscope.

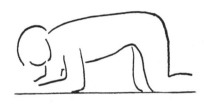

FIG. 1123.—Knee-elbow position for proctoscopy.

3. **Proctoscopy** (fig. 1122).—This examination is of great importance. Either the Sims position with the buttocks elevated on a small cushion, or the knee-elbow position (fig. 1123) may be used. The lower third of the rectum, the anorectal junction and the anal canal can be inspected as the instrument is withdrawn slowly. Minor procedures can be carried out through this instrument, e.g. treatment of haemorrhoids by injection or banding (pp. 1149/50) and biopsy.

4. **Sigmoidoscopy** (Chapter 53).—While this is strictly an examination of the rectum and lower sigmoid colon, it should be carried out even when an anal lesion has been confirmed. Rectal pathology, *e.g.* colitis or carcinoma is frequently the cause of an anal lesion, *e.g.* fissure or haemorrhoids. Not infrequently rectal pathology is found that is independent of the anal lesion and which requires treatment.

5. **Special investigations.**—These are discussed on p. 1134 and are not used routinely.

CONGENITAL ABNORMALITIES

Early in embryonic life there is a common chamber—the cloaca—into which open the hind gut and the allantois. The cloaca becomes separated into the bladder and postallantoic gut (rectum) by the down-growth of a septum. About this time an epiblastic bud, the proctodaeum, grows in towards the rectum. Normally fusion between these two structures occurs during the third month of intrauterine life.

Imperforate Anus.[1]—One infant in 4500 is born with an imperforate anus, or with imperfect fusion of the post-allantoic gut with the proctodaeum. The condition is divided into two main groups—the high and the low, depending on whether the termination of the bowel is above or below the pelvic floor. The low varieties are easy to diagnose, simple to treat, and the outlook is good. The high varieties often have a fistula into the urinary tract together with a deficient pelvic floor and the prognosis is not good.

Low Abnormalities (fig. 1124).—(*a*) The *covered anus*: the underlying anal canal is covered by a bar of skin with a track running forward to the perineal raphe. The track should be opened with scissors, followed by routine dilatation of the anus. (*b*) The *ectopic anus*: the anus is situated anteriorly and may open in the perineum in boys or more commonly in the vulva in girls, or rarely into the vagina. A plastic 'cut-back' operation is required. (*c*) The *stenosed anus*: the anus is microscopic but careful examination usually reveals a minute opening which responds to regular dilatation. (*d*) *Membranous stenosis*: here the anus is normally sited but is covered with a thin membrane which bulges with retained meconium. It is rare, and an incision will cure the condition.

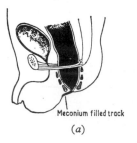 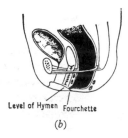 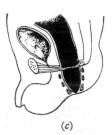

Meconium filled track   Level of Hymen Fourchette

(*a*)   (*b*)   (*c*)

FIG. 1124.—Low abnormalities of the anus: (*a*) covered anus, (*b*) vulval ectopic anus, (*c*) anal stenosis, (*d*) anal membrane.
(*J. P. Partridge, FRCS, Barnstaple, and M. H. Gough, FRCS, London.*)

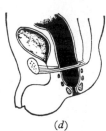

(*d*)

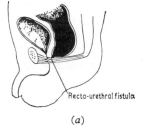 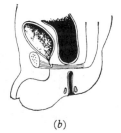

Recto-urethral fistula

(*a*)   (*b*)

FIG. 1125.—High abnormalities: (*a*) anorectal agenesis with recto-urethral fistula, (*b*) rectal atresia.
(*J. P. Partridge, FRCS, Barnstaple, and M. H. Gough, FRCS, London.*)

High Abnormalities (fig. 1125).—These are often associated with a fistulous connection between the blind rectal stump and the bladder, or other abnormali-

---

[1] The term imperforate anus is used as a well-recognised description. Strictly it should be 'agenesis' and 'atresia' of the rectum and anus.

ties of the pelvic structures. (1) *Anorectal Agenesis.*—A blind rectal pouch lies just above the pelvic floor—its anterior aspect in the male is attached to the bladder and often there is a recto-vesical fistula manifested by the passage of gas or meconium in the urine. In the female the fistula is usually into the posterior fornix. (2) *Rectal Atresia.*—The anal canal is normal but ends blindly at the level of the pelvic floor. The bowel also ends blindly above the pelvic floor without a fistulous opening. This anomaly is rare but must be treated by mobilisation of the rectum and excision of the stricture. After that, end-to-end anastomosis of the anus and rectum must be attempted. More conservative measures are followed by an intractable stricture. (3) *Cloaca.*—This occurs only in females and here the bowel, urinary and genital tracts all open into a common wide cavity. Commonly severe malformations of the area are associated with other developmental abnormalities (*e.g.* tracheo-bronchial fistula).

Clinical Management.—As congenital abnormalities are frequently multiple, very careful general examination of the baby must be made to exclude any other anomalies. It is urgent and important to determine whether the abnormality is high or low and an x-ray will help.

X-ray Examination.—Six hours after birth sufficient air may have collected in the large intestine to cast an x-ray shadow. With a metal button or a coin strapped to the site of the anus, or a metal bougie inserted into the blind anal canal, the infant is held upside down for three to four minutes and radiographed in the inverted position (fig. 1126). The gas in the rectum will rise to the top and indicate the distance between the site of the metal indicator and the blind end of the rectum. If the distance is over 2·5 cm, the abnormality is 'high'. This method, though useful, is sometimes vitiated by a plug of meconium in the rectum causing an apparent gap far in excess of that actually present. It may be necessary to wait until the baby is twenty-four hours old before rectal gas appears.

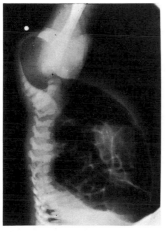

FIG. 1126.—X-ray of neonate while held upside down to show gas in rectum. Anal dimple marked by piece of lead shot.
(*Graham Airth, Bristol.*)

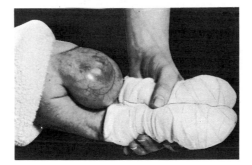

FIG. 1127.—Congenital sacro-coccygeal teratoma, excised successfully.
(*Maj. Gen. A. C. Bose, AVSM, MS, FACS, Senior Consultant (Surgery), Armed Forces, India.*)

Where a 'high' lesion is suspected an effort must be made to obtain a specimen of urine—the presence of *proteus* or *pyocyaneus* usually signifies that a fistula is present. An i.v. urogram is recommended by some, even though there is a definite radiation risk. There may be gas in the bladder. A diagnostic perineal exploration is usually unwise—it may prejudice the chances of further surgery.

Treatment.—In the *low* abnormalities this is usually simple and has been outlined when each condition was described above. The *high* abnormalities present a very difficult problem and each case must be considered on its merits. On the whole, newborn babies stand surgery very well, provided compatible blood is available and a clear airway is maintained post-operatively and inhalation of vomit prevented by naso-gastric suction. The presence of other congenital abnormalities is also a most important factor to consider. The possibilities are:

  1. Laparotomy, division of recto-urethral fistula, and transverse colostomy. A rectal 'pull-through' operation can be done later.
  2. Laparotomy, division of fistula, and 'pull-through' operation in one stage.
  3. Division of the fistula and rectal 'pull-down' operation through the (*a*) perineal or (*b*) sacral route (this method is now rarely used).
  4. Colostomy only (for the cloacal variety).
For the 'pull-through' operation the lower bowel is mobilised, and a new passage is created through the pelvic floor by passing a pair of curved forceps through it, keeping close to the urethra, to the site of the future anus. This is dilated by Hegar's dilators so that the bowel can be pulled down and its mucosa stitched to the skin of the newly formed anus. (For details the reader is referred to the standard textbooks of operative surgery and the publications of Swenson, Duhamel and Nixon.)

In general, daily dilatation will be required for at least three months and it may be necessary for years.

In a high percentage of cases, imperforate anus is associated with other congenital abnormalities, especially of the urinary organs, and nearly half the deaths in cases of imperforate anus are due to other malformations.

Sacro-coccygeal teratoma, although rare, is among the most common of the large tumours seen during the first three months of life. The frequency of the precoccygeal region for the development of a teratoma is explained by the fact that this area is the site of the 'primitive knot', a group of totipotent cells that retain their totipotentiality longer than any others save the sex anlage. Females are more often affected than males.

The tumour, which arises between the sacrum and the rectum, is firmly attached to the coccyx, and occasionally to the last piece of the sacrum. At the time of birth some of these tumours are huge, and in 20% of cases the infant is still-born. The tumour tends to be large (fig. 1127), but it can be small enough to pass unnoticed until it enlarges or a complication ensues. It is this variety that is prone to become malignant, usually at about ten months of age.

Treatment.—Removal soon after birth; delay is liable to result in fatal ulceration, infection, rectal or urinary obstruction, or malignant change.

Operation.—Excision is undertaken through a longitudinal elliptical incision, the coccygeal attachment being left until the last. The coccyx must always be excised; occasionally the last piece of the sacrum must be removed also. There may be a fistula between the tumour and the rectum but as a rule this is small, and can be closed safely without performing a colostomy. The dead space in the pelvis is drained, the skin is united, and a pressure dressing applied.

When the operation is undertaken soon after birth, the prognosis is good.

Post-anal Dermoid.—The space in front of the lower part of the sacrum and coccyx is occupied by a soft, cystic swelling—a post-anal dermoid cyst—which is regarded as a simple form of teratoma. Hidden in the hollow of the sacrum, it is unlikely to be discovered unless a sinus communicating with the exterior is present, or develops as a result of inflammation. Such a cyst usually remains symptomless until adult life, when it is prone to become infected. Exceptionally, by its very size, it gives rise to difficulty in defaecation. The cyst is easily palpable on rectal examination.

Differential Diagnosis.—Especially in a child, an anterior sacral meningocele must be excluded. The latter enlarges when the child cries, and is frequently associated with

Alfred Hegar, 1830–1914. Professor of Obstetrics and Gynaecology, Freiburg, Germany.
O. Swenson, Contemporary. Surgeon, U.S.A.
B. Duhamel, Contemporary. Surgeon, France.
H. H. Nixon, Contemporary. Surgeon, Royal Hospital for Sick Children, Great Ormond St., London.

paralysis of the lower limbs, and incontinence. When a discharging sinus is present, a post-anal dermoid will probably be mistaken for a pilonidal sinus, unless pressure over the sacro-coccygeal region with a finger in the rectum causes a flow of sebaceous material, and injection of contrast and radiography reveals a bottle-necked cyst in front of the coccyx.

Treatment is complete excision of the cyst, and sinus if present. In the case of large cysts it is necessary to remove the coccyx in order to gain access.

Post-anal Dimple (*syn.* Fovea Coccygea).—A dimple, sometimes amounting to a short, blind pit, in the skin beneath the tip of coccyx is noticed from time to time in the course of a clinical examination.

PILONIDAL[1] SINUS

Aetiology.—The army of supporters of the congenital theory of the origin of pilonidal sinus has become reduced to a corporal's guard.

That, in rare instances, a sinus in the ano-coccygeal area *is* congenital must be allowed, but in these cases of proven congenital origin the sinus is not necessarily pilonidal. It could be (*a*) a sinus connected with a post-anal dermoid, referred to above, or (*b*) a sinus resulting from a persistent caudal remnant of the original neural canal. The latter occurs in the sacral rather than the coccygeal region, and is definitely connected with the spinal theca. On this account, meningitis from an extradural abscess may occur in a child.

The reasons which support the acquired theory of origin of pilonidal sinus can be summarised thus:

1. Interdigital pilonidal sinus is an occupational disease of men's hairdressers, the hair within the interdigital cleft or clefts being the customers'. Also pilonidal sinuses of the axilla and umbilicus have been reported.

2. The age incidence of the appearance of pilonidal sinus (82% occur between the ages of twenty and twenty-nine years) is at variance with the age of onset of congenital lesions.

3. Hair follicles have almost never been demonstrated in the walls of the sinus.

4. The hairs projecting from the sinus are dead hairs, with their pointed ends directed towards the blind end of the sinus.

5. The disease mostly affects men, and hairy men most frequently.

6. Recurrence is common, even though adequate excision of the track is carried out.

The mode of origin of a pilonidal sinus is now believed to be as follows:
On sitting, the buttocks take the weight of the body, and move independently, or together. Hairs broken off by friction against clothing, and shed short hairs, whether originating from the nape of the neck, back, or buttocks, tend to collect in the cleft of the nates and/or a post-anal dimple. Furthermore, it is suggested that the use of toilet paper may contribute to hair entangled in faecal matter being swept into the cleft; pilonidal sinus is extremely rare in those races that employ ablution after defaecation. By reason of the shearing action of the buttocks, which is increased by sitting on a hard seat, and especially by vibration of a vehicle, loose hair travels down the intergluteal furrow, to penetrate the skin or the open mouth of a sudoriferous gland, such glands being more active in early manhood. It is not yet clear whether the initial entry of hairs through the skin is a primary event, or follows the softening of the skin due to pustular or other forms of dermatitis. Once a sinus has formed, intermittent negative pressure of the area may suck other loose hairs into the pit. So common was pilonidal sinus among jeep[2] riders in the 1939–45 war that it became known as 'jeep bottom'.

Pathology.—The sinus extends into the subcutaneous planes as an infected track. Branching side channels are not infrequent. A stratified squamous epi-

---

[1] Appertaining to a nest of hair. (Latin—*pilus* = hair, *nidus* = nest.)
[2] Jeep—U.S. Army reconnaissance motor vehicle.

thelial lining, of varying degrees of integrity, is found in about half the cases. Hair shafts are found either (a) laying loose in the sinus, (b) embedded in granulation tissue, or (c) deep in mature scar tissue in three-quarters of the cases. Foreign body giant cells are common.

Clinical Features.—There is a chronic or recurring sinus in the middle line about the level of the first piece of the coccyx. Typically a tuft of hairs projects from its mouth. The discharge from the sinus or sinuses is often blood-stained, contains foul sebum, and sometimes hairs. Secondary openings may be present on either side of the midline, often far out on to the buttocks or in the perineum.

As has been indicated already, symptoms usually commence during the third decade; patients presenting later in life nearly always give a history dating back to this period.

Males with this condition outnumber females by four to one, the females being on an average three years younger than the males; this corresponds to the earlier maturation of the female. The condition rarely occurs in blondes; many of the patients are exceptionally hairy and are usually obese. In spite of the preponderance in dark-haired persons, whose hair is stiffer than the silky blonde (Oldham), the condition is practically confined to white races. The complaint is of a discharge, pain, or a tender swelling at the bottom of the spine. Even at the height of an attack of inflammation the constitutional symptoms are slight. Often there is a history of repeated abscesses in the region that have discharged spontaneously or have been incised. The primary sinus may have one, or as many as six openings, all of which are strictly in the middle line between the level of the sacrococcygeal joint and the tip of the coccyx. Unlike a fistula-in-ano, the sinus passes upwards and forwards towards the sacrum. It does not reach bone, but ends blindly near the bone. When an abscess forms it may discharge through a primary sinus; more frequently it points and bursts, or is incised to one side of the middle line (usually the left), thus forming a secondary sinus.

Conservative Treatment.—Patients reporting for the first time with mild symptoms can sometimes be cured by conservative measures, which consist of cleaning out the track, removing all hairs from the area, followed by frequent washing of the parts with a detergent and water, and applying equal parts of witch hazel (Liq. Ext. Hamamelis) and alcohol. Long sitting, e.g. driving a car, is avoided if possible. These measures, tried on a large scale in the U.S. Army, proved tolerably successful—more successful than similar attempts in civil life, because the sufferer could be relegated to duties that were unlikely to aggravate the condition.

Treatment of an Acute Exacerbation (Abscess).—If rest, baths, local antiseptic dressings, and the administration of a broad spectrum antibiotic fail to bring about resolution, the abscess should be opened through a comparatively small incision. Provided all hairs and granulation tissue are removed from the abscess cavity, there is some prospect of curing the lesion (Millar). After it has been cleaned out, the track can be destroyed by careful instillation of pure phenol solution (Maurice). In all other circumstances an elective operation must be planned.

Operation should be performed only when the inflammation has been controlled by the measures indicated already.

The patient is placed on the operating table, for preference in the 'jack-knife' position.

James Bagot Oldham, 1899–1977. Surgeon, United Liverpool Hospitals, Liverpool, England.
Douglas Malcolm Millar, Contemporary. Surgeon, Essex County Hospital, Colchester.
Brian Armstead Maurice, Contemporary. Surgeon, Tunbridge Wells, Kent.

Methylene blue is injected into the sinus to colour all the tracks, the nozzle of the syringe being pressed against the opening to obtain some pressure. Variations in operative technique include the following:

1. Lay open the tracks, remove all debris and hair, and suture the edges to the skin, thus marsupializing the sinus. This procedure yields a good hairless scar.

2. Excise all the tracks, as stained by blue dye, meticulously secure haemostasis by diathermy and catgut ligature, and, using sutures coapt the subcutaneous fat and skin very accurately and institute a drain and suction (*i.e.* Redivac) for 48 hours to remove blood and serum. In cases of extensive sinus formation primary cover may be achieved by rotating a flap of skin and fat.

3. Excise all the tracks as stained by the blue dye and, after securing haemostasis as above, pack the wound. The following day the whole dressing is removed, and daily baths and moist dressings are instituted until the wound heals by granulation. Epithelialisation can sometimes be speeded up by skin grafting.

Immediately after operation the patient should avoid sitting on the wound. Subsequently, the scar may require protection from further incursions of hair by selective hair-trimming. The recurrence rate after primary closure may be as high as 50% without meticulous technique.

Recurrent Pilonidal Sinus.—Three possibilities account for this disappointment. (1) A diverticulum of the main channel has been overlooked at the primary operation. (2) New hairs enter the skin or the scar. (3) When the natal fold is deformed by scarring, the least trauma causes tearing of the scar, and the resulting crevice becomes contaminated with coliform and cutaneous bacteria. An alternative approach to circumvent the incidence of recurrence has been to ensure that the wound closure is to one side of the midline (Karydakis): this method has been reported as having a high rate of success.

ANAL INCONTINENCE

The origins of anal incontinence may derive from causes relating to Descent, Destruction, Debility, Deficiency, Damage, Denervation and Dementia.

Descent — prolapsing haemorrhoids — rectal prolapse

Destruction — malignant tumours — irradiation

Debility — illness — old age

Deficiency — congenital abnormalities

Damage — wounds — surgical procedures — childbirth

Denervation — spinal injuries — neuro-surgical procedures — spina bifida

Dementia — senility — psychological abnormality

Of these causes, geriatric; traumatic; and obstetric cases predominate—with anal surgical procedures an important contributor to the traumatic group.

Once the cause of the incontinence has been precisely defined by a careful history and meticulous examination, supported by special investigations as indicated (p. 1134), treatment may be possible. Surgical procedures have been developed to repair and support damaged or weak sphincter muscles. These may be classified as follows:

1. **Operations to re-unite divided sphincter muscles.**—The sphincter muscles may have been divided as a result of direct trauma, operations for fissure

Col. Dr Karydakis, Contemporary. Surgeon, Athens.

and fistula or by obstetrical injury. The ends of the divided muscle are found and re-united by a *double over-lap repair*.

2. **Operations to reef the external sphincter and pubo-rectalis muscle.**—If the sphincter muscles are stretched and patulous (as they often are in old age and cases of rectal prolapse) they may be tightened by a *post-anal repair*. These operations use darns of unabsorbable material to narrow down and plicate the external sphincter and the pubo-rectalis sling. They restore length to the anal canal, strength to the anal sphincter and angulation to the ano-rectal junction. The approach is usually through the intersphincteric plane.

3. **Operations to support the anal canal.**—If the anal canal is gaping and has feeble muscles that cannot be strengthened by direct means, support can be given by encircling stitches or Mersilene strands after the *Thiersch operation pattern* (see Chapter 53).

All these procedures achieve best results if the bowel habit is regulated and a normal defaecatory pattern established over the pre- and post-operative periods. The operations should be covered by antibiotics active against both aerobic and anaerobic organisms to reduce the risk of septic complications.

ANAL FISSURE (*syn.* FISSURE-IN-ANO)

Definition.—An elongated ulcer in the long axis of the lower anal canal.

Location.—The site of election for an anal fissure is the mid-line posteriorly. The next most frequent situation is the mid-line anteriorly.

Aetiology.—The cause of anal fissure, and particularly the reason why the midline posteriorly is so frequently affected, is not completely understood. A probable explaation is as follows: the posterior wall of the rectum curves forwards from the hollow of the sacrum to join the anal canal, which then turns sharply backwards. During defaecation the pressure of a hard faecal mass is mainly on the posterior anal tissues in which event the overlying epithelium is greatly stretched, and, being relatively unsupported by muscle, is placed in a vulnerable position when a scybalous mass is being expelled. Possibly some cases are due to tearing down of an anal valve of Ball. An anterior anal fissure is much more common in women, particularly in those who have borne children. This can be explained by the lack of support of the anal mucous membrane by a damaged pelvic floor and an attenuated perineal body.

Some causes of anal fissure are certain—(1) an incorrectly performed operation for haemorrhoids in which too much skin is removed. This results in anal stenosis and tearing of the scar when a hard motion is passed; (2) inflammatory bowel disease—colitis or Crohn's disease; (3) venereal infections.

Pathology.—An anal fissure is either acute or chronic. The upper internal end of the fissure stops at the dentate line. Because the fissure occurs in the stratified sensitive epithelium of the lower half of the anal canal, pain is the most prominent symptom (*vide infra*).

Acute anal fissure is a deep tear through the skin of the anal margin extending into the anal canal. There is little inflammatory induration or oedema of its edges. There is accompanying spasm of the anal sphincter muscle.

Chronic anal fissure is characterised by inflamed indurated margins, and a base consisting of either scar tissue or the lower border of the internal sphincter muscle. The ulcer is canoe-shaped, and at the inferior extremity frequently there is a tag of skin, usually oedematous. This tag is known picturesquely as a sentinel pile—'sentinel' because it guards the fissure. There may be spasm of the involuntary musculature of the internal sphincter. In long-standing cases this muscle becomes organically contracted by infiltration of fibrous tissue. Infection is common and may be severe, ending in abscess formation. A cutaneous fistula may follow.

Chronic fissure-in-ano may have a specific cause—often a granulomatous infection, *e.g.* Crohn's disease or syphilis. Biopsy examination is advisable of any tissue removed at operation for a chronic fissure. Specific fissures of this type are often less painful than the appearances of the lesion would suggest.

Clinical Features.—The condition is more common in women, and generally occurs during the meridian of life. It is uncommon in the aged, because of muscular atony; on the other hand anal fissure is not rare in children, is sometimes encountered during infancy, and may cause acquired mega-colon (Chapter 50).

Pain is *the* symptom—sharp agonising pain starting during defaecation, often overwhelming in intensity and lasting an hour or more. As a rule it ceases suddenly, and the sufferer is comfortable until the next action of the bowel. Periods of remission occur for days or weeks. The patient tends to become *constipated* rather than go through the agony of defaecation.[1]

Bleeding—this is usually slight and consists of bright streaks on the stools or the paper.

Discharge.—A slight discharge accompanies fully established cases.

On Examination.—In cases of some standing, a sentinel skin tag can usually be displayed. This, together with a typical history and a tightly closed, puckered anus, is almost pathognomonic of the condition. By gently parting the margins of the anus, the lower end of the fissure can be seen.

Because of the intense pain it causes, digital examination of the anal canal should not be attempted *at this stage* unless (*a*) the fissure cannot be seen or (*b*) it seems imperative to exclude major intrarectal pathology. In these circumstances the local application of a surface anaesthetic such as 5% xylocaine on a pledget of cotton-wool, left in place for about five minutes, will enable the necessary examination to be made. In early cases the edges of the fissure are impalpable; in fully established cases a characteristic crater which feels like a vertical buttonhole can be palpated. *The diagnosis must be established beyond doubt, for which a general anaesthetic may be required.*

Differential Diagnosis:

Carcinoma of the anus in its very early stages easily simulates a fissure. If real doubt exists, the lesion must be excised under general anaesthesia and submitted to histological examination.

Multiple fissures in the peri-anal skin are commonly seen as a complication of skin diseases, scratching and inflammatory bowel disease. Also homosexual practices (sodomy, fisting and the use of anorectal sex toys, fig. 1102) and ano-rectal venereal disease can cause multiple fissures in both sexes.

Anal chancre is becoming more common and may present as a *painful* rather than a painless ulcer. The serous discharge contains spirochaetes. A glass pipette is used to aspirate a few drops which are placed on a slide for examination by dark-ground illumination. Lubricating gel from the finger-stall may prevent adequate aspiration of serum

---

[1] One patient accustomed himself to take a generous dose of senna on Saturday night, and retire to the toilet on Sunday morning with a bottle of whisky and the newspaper.

from a chancre. All patients with anal venereal disease, and admitted homosexuals, should be tested for a positive serological response to HIV as they may have AIDS[1] (see Chapter 4).

Tuberculous ulcer has an undermined edge.

Proctalgia Fugax (below) causes severe episodic pain.

Treatment.—The pain of an anal fissure is so great that usually the patient demands relief, and consequently many patients with an acute fissure present early. The object of all treatment for this condition is to obtain *complete relaxation* of the internal sphincter. Provided the complications are dealt with, the fissure will slowly heal as soon as all spasm has disappeared.

Conservative Treatment.—In cases where the fissure is acute and superficial and where the inflammation is minimal, simple conservative measures will usually give relief. Xylocaine 5% in a water-soluble lubricant is introduced with a fine nozzle into the anal canal. After waiting a few minutes for the surface anaesthetic to act, relaxation may be sufficient to permit the passage of a well-lubricated finger into the canal. Following this a small anal dilator may be passed and, if the anaesthesia is adequate, it may be possible to introduce the largest dilator. Anal dilators are commonly made in three sizes and it may not be possible to use the largest dilator until several days have passed. The patient is supplied with xylocaine lubricant and instructed to pass a dilator twice a day for a month, by which time the fissure is usually healed. Laxatives are prescribed to ensure that the motions are soft, but the stools should not be made watery: Celevac 10 ml b.d. gives a soft stool of good bulk, which is ideal.

Operative Measures

The simplest procedure is wide forcible dilatation of the sphincter. Under general anaesthesia the index and middle finger of each hand are inserted simultaneously into the anus and pulled apart to give maximal dilatation. The patient can go home the same day but should be warned that there may be some faecal incontinence lasting possibly for a week or ten days.

Should these measures prove ineffective, or if the fissure is chronic with fibrosis, a skin tag, or a mucous polypus, then surgical measures are advisable. General anaesthesia is best, though some surgeons use a local anaesthetic in the form of xylocaine or proctocaine introduced into the ischiorectal fossa on each side, in order to anaesthetise the nerves passing towards the rectum. In other situations a caudal anaesthetic is suitable.

(i) *Lateral anal sphincterotomy* (Notaras). In this operation, the internal sphincter is divided away from the fissure itself—usually either in the right or the left lateral positions. The procedure can be done by an open or a closed method. Healing is usually complete within three weeks. The operation is more successful for acute than chronic fissures. 75% of cases are suitable for treatment by this method. The patients are able to leave hospital within three or four days, and the procedure can be done as an Out-Patient under local anaesthesia by an experienced surgeon.

(ii) *Dorsal fissurectomy and sphincterotomy*. The essential part of the operation is to divide the transverse fibres of the internal sphincter in the floor of the fissure. If a sentinel pile is present, this is excised. The ends of the divided muscle retract and a smooth wound is left. The after-treatment consists of attention to bowels, a daily bath, and the passage of an anal dilator until the wounds have healed, which usually takes about three weeks. Despite the presence of the wound there is little or no pain and the results are good. The disadvantage of this operation is the prolonged healing time—usually not less than three weeks and often longer—and occasionally a mild, persistent and permanent mucus discharge. It is now reserved only for the most chronic or recurrent anal fissures, the majority being treated by lateral sphincterotomy.

---

[1] AIDS = acquired immune deficiency syndrome (see Chapter 4). HIV = human immunodeficiency virus (see Chapter 4).

Mitchell James Notaras, Contemporary. Surgeon, Barnet General Hospital, London.

HYPERTROPHIED ANAL PAPILLA

Anal papillae occur at the dentate line, and are remnants of the ectodermal membrane that separated the hind-gut from the proctodaeum. As these papillae are present in fully 60% of patients examined proctologically, they should be regarded as normal structures. Anal papillae can become elongated, as they frequently do in the presence of an anal fissure. Occasionally an elongated anal papilla may be the cause of pruritus. An elongated anal papilla associated with pain and/or bleeding at defaecation is sometimes encountered in infancy. Haemorrhage into a hypertrophied anal papilla can cause sudden rectal pain. A prolapsed papilla may become nipped by contraction of the sphincter mechanism after defaecation. Occasionally a red oedematous papilla is encountered with local pain and a purulent discharge from the associated crypt. This condition of 'cryptitis' is more frequently seen abroad, but may be cured by laying open the mouth of the infected anal gland and removing the papilla.

Treatment.—Using a slotted proctoscope, elongated papillae without haemorrhoids should be crushed and excised after injecting the base with local anaesthetic. When large papillae complicate internal haemorrhoids, this is an indication for operative treatment of the haemorrhoids, as well as excision of the elongated papillae.

PROCTALGIA FUGAX

This disease is characterised by attacks of severe pain arising in the rectum, recurring at irregular intervals and apparently unrelated to organic disease. The pain is described as cramp-like, often occurs when the patient is in bed at night, lasts only a few minutes, and disappears spontaneously. It may follow straining at stool, sudden explosive bowel action or ejaculation. It seems to occur more commonly in patients suffering from anxiety or undue stress and also it is said to afflict young doctors. The pain may be unbearable—it is possibly due to segmental cramp in the pubo-coccygeus muscle. It is unpleasant, incurable, but fortunately harmless and gradually subsides. A more chronic form of the disease has been termed the 'levator syndrome' and can be associated with severe constipation. Bio-feedback techniques have been used to help such patients: some surgeons have been willing to sever the pubo-rectalis muscle but this can cause incontinence.

HAEMORRHOIDS[1, 2] (syn. PILES[3])

Haemorrhoids are veins occurring in relation to the anus. Such haemorrhoids may be **external** or **internal**—external or internal to the anal orifice. The external variety are covered by skin, while the internal variety lie beneath the anal mucous membrane. When the two varieties are associated, they are known as **interoexternal** haemorrhoids.

The veins which form internal haemorrhoids become engorged as the anal lining descends and is gripped by the anal sphincters. The mucosal lining is gathered prominently in three places (the 'anal cushions') which can be in the areas of the three terminal branches of the superior haemorrhoidal artery, but this is exceptional (Thomson). The anal cushions are present in embryonic life and are necessary for full continence. Straining causes these cushions to slide downwards, and internal haemorrhoids develop in the prolapsing tissues.

Haemorrhoids may be '*symptomatic*' of some other condition, and this important fact must be remembered. Symptomatic haemorrhoids may appear (*a*) in *carcinoma of rectum*. This, by compressing or causing thrombosis of the superior rectal vein, gives rise to haemorrhoids (fig. 1127) sufficiently often to warrant examination of the rectum and the recto-sigmoid junction for a neoplasm in every case of haemorrhoids. (*b*) During *pregnancy*. Pregnancy piles are due to compression of the superior rectal veins by the pregnant uterus and the relaxing effect of progesterone on the smooth muscle in the walls of the

---

[1] 'The common people call them piles, the aristocracy call them haemorrhoids, the French call them figs—what does it matter so long as you can cure them?'—John of Arderne, 1370.
[2] Greek—*haima* = blood, *rhoos* = flowing.
[3] Latin—*pila* = a ball.

John of Arderne, ?1306–?1390. The first English surgeon. He practised in Newark and later in London.
William Hamish Fearon Thomson, Contemporary. Surgeon, Gloucestershire Royal Hospital, Gloucester, England.

veins. (*c*) From *straining at micturition* consequent upon a stricture of the urethra—or an enlarged prostate. (*d*) From chronic constipation.

N.B. Contrary to the usual belief, in one hundred and twenty-eight consecutive cases of portal hypertension, Macpherson did not encounter a single example of haemorrhoids that could he attributed to portal cirrhosis, although bleeding oesophageal varices often complicate portal hypertension.

The great majority of haemorrhoids are not symptomatic. The description that follows concerns symptomatic haemorrhoids that are *not* secondary to an underlying cause.

INTERNAL HAEMORRHOIDS

Internal haemorrhoids, which include intero-external haemorrhoids, are exceedingly common. Essentially the condition is a dilation of the internal venous plexus within an enlarged displaced anal cushion. Because of the communication between the internal and external plexuses, if the former becomes engorged, the latter is liable to become involved also.

Aetiology: *Hereditary.*—The condition is so frequently seen in members of the same family that there must be a predisposing factor, such as a congenital weakness of the vein walls or an abnormally large arterial supply to the rectal plexus.

Varicose veins of the legs and haemorrhoids often occur concurrently.

Morphological.—In quadrupeds, gravity aids, or at any rate does not retard, return of venous blood from the rectum. Consequently venous valves are not required. In man, the weight of the column of blood unassisted by valves produces a high venous pressure in the lower rectum, unparallelled in the body. Except in a few fat old dogs, haemorrhoids are exceedingly rare in animals.

Anatomical.—(1) The collecting radicles of the superior haemorrhoidal vein lie unsupported in the very loose submucous connective tissue of the anorectum. (2) These veins pass through muscular tissue and are liable to be constricted by its contraction during defaecation. (3) The superior rectal veins, being tributaries of the portal vein, have no valves.

Exciting Causes.—Straining accompanying constipation or that induced by overpurgation is considered to be a potent cause of haemorrhoids. Less often the diarrhoea of enteritis, colitis, or the dysenteries aggravates latent haemorrhoids. In both instances descent and swelling of the anal cushions is a prominent feature.

Pathology.—Internal haemorrhoids are frequently arranged in three groups at 3, 7, and 11 o'clock with the patient in the lithotomy position (fig. 1129).[1] This distribution has been ascribed to the arterial supply of the anus whereby there are two subdivisions of the right branch of the superior rectal artery, but the left branch remains single but this is now known to be atypical. In between these three primary haemorrhoids there may be smaller secondary haemorrhoids. Each principal haemorrhoid can be divided into three parts:

(1) *The pedicle* is situated at the anorectal ring. As seen through a proctoscope, it is covered with pale pink mucosa. Occasionally a pulsating artery can be felt in this situation.

(2) *The internal haemorrhoid*, which commences just below the anorectal ring. It is bright red or purple, and covered by mucous membrane. It is of variable size.

(3) *An external associated haemorrhoid* lies between the dentate line and the anal

---

[1] Lithotomy position = the position in which patients used to be put for the classical operation of 'cutting' for bladder stone via the urethral or the perineal route (see Chapter 55).

Archibald Ian Stewart Macpherson, Contemporary. Surgeon, Royal Infirmary, Edinburgh.

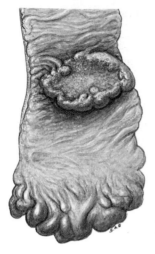

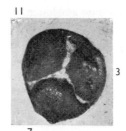

FIG. 1129.—Proctoscopy third-degree haemorrhoids. Note their 3, 7, and 11 o'clock positions.
(E. T. C. Milligan, FRCS, London.)

FIG. 1128.—Carcinoma of the rectum associated with haemorrhoids. A not infrequent diagnostic pitfall.

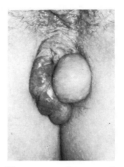

FIG. 1130.—An attack of piles. Prolapsed strangulated piles, as commonly seen, on the left. A less common mass on the right with a fibrofatty covering.

margin. It is covered by skin, through which blue veins can be seen, unless fibrosis has occurred. This associated haemorrhoid is present only in well-established cases.

Entering the pedicle of an internal haemorrhoid may be a branch of the superior rectal artery. Very occasionally there is a haemangiomatous condition of this artery—an 'arterial pile'—which leads to ferocious bleeding at operation.

Clinical Features.—*Bleeding*, as the name haemorrhoid implies, is the principal and earliest symptom. At first the bleeding is slight; it is bright red and occurs during defaecation (a 'splash in the pan'), and it may continue intermittently thus for months or years. Haemorrhoids that bleed but do not prolapse outside the anal canal are called *first-degree haemorrhoids*.

Prolapse is a much later symptom. In the beginning the protrusion is slight and occurs only at stool, and reduction is spontaneous. As time goes on the haemorrhoids do not reduce themselves, but have to be replaced digitally by the patient. Haemorrhoids that prolapse on defaecation but return or need to be replaced manually and then stay reduced are called *second-degree haemorrhoids*. Still later, prolapse occurs during the day, apart from defaecation, often when the patient is tired or exerts himself. Haemorrhoids that are permanently prolapsed are called *third-degree haemorrhoids*. By now, the haemorrhoids have become a source of great discomfort and cause a feeling of heaviness in the rectum but are not usually acutely painful.

Discharge.—A mucoid discharge is a frequent accompaniment of prolapsed haemorrhoids. It is composed of mucus from the engorged mucous membrane, sometimes augmented by leakage of ingested liquid paraffin. *Pruritus* will almost certainly follow this discharge.

Pain is absent unless complications supervene. For this reason any patient complaining of 'painful piles' must be suspected of having another condition (possibly serious) and examined accordingly.

Anaemia can be caused very rarely by persistent profuse bleeding from haemorrhoids.

On inspection there may be no evidence of internal haemorrhoids. In more advanced cases redundant folds or tags of skin can be see in the position of one or more of the three primary haemorrhoids. When the patient strains, internal haemorrhoids may come into view transiently, or if they are of the third degree they are and remain prolapsed.

Digital examination.—Internal haemorrhoids cannot be felt unless they are thrombosed.

Proctoscopy.—A proctoscope is passed to its fullest extent and the obturator is removed. The instrument is then slowly withdrawn. Just below the ano-rectal ring internal haemorrhoids, if present, will bulge into the lumen of the proctoscope.

Sigmoidoscopy.—Should be done as a precaution in every case (see Chapter 53 and fig. 1122).

Complications:

Profuse haemorrhage is not rare. Most often it occurs in the early stages of the second degree. The bleeding occurs mainly externally, but it may continue internally after the bleeding haemorrhoid has retracted or has been returned. In these circumstances the rectum is found to contain blood.

Strangulation.—One or more of the internal haemorrhoids prolapse and become gripped by the external sphincter. Further congestion follows because the venous return is impeded. Second-degree haemorrhoids are most often complicated in this way. Strangulation is accompanied by considerable pain, and is often spoken of by the patient as an 'acute attack of piles'.[1] Unless the internal haemorrhoids can be reduced within an hour or two, strangulation is followed by thrombosis.

Thrombosis.—The affected haemorrhoid or haemorrhoids become dark purple or black (fig. 1130) and feel solid. Considerable oedema of the anal margin accompanies thrombosis. Once the thrombosis has occurred the pain of strangulation largely passes off, but tenderness persists.

Ulceration.—Superficial ulceration of the exposed mucous membrane often accompanies strangulation with thrombosis.

Gangrene occurs when strangulation is sufficiently tight to constrict the arterial supply of the haemorrhoid. The resulting sloughing is usually superficial and localised. Occasionally a whole haemorrhoid sloughs off, leaving an ulcer which heals gradually. Very occasionally massive gangrene extends to the mucous membrane within the anal canal and rectum and can be the cause of spreading anaerobic infection and portal pyaemia.

Fibrosis.—After thrombosis, internal haemorrhoids sometimes become converted into fibrous tissue. The fibrosed haemorrhoid is at first sessile, but by repeated traction during prolapse at defaecation, it becomes pedunculated and constitutes a fibrous polypus that is readily distinguished by its white colour from an adenoma, which is bright red. Fibrosis following transient strangulation commonly occurs in the subcutaneous part of a primary haemorrhoid. Fibrosis in an external haemorrhoid favours prolapse of an associated internal haemorrhoid.

Suppuration is uncommon. It occurs as a result of infection of a thrombosed haemorrhoid. Throbbing pain is followed by perianal swelling, and a perianal or submucous abscess results.

Pylephlebitis (*syn.* Portal Pyaemia).—Theoretically, infected haemorrhoids should be a potent cause of portal pyaemia and liver abscesses (Chapter 45). Although cases do occur from time to time, this complication is surprisingly infrequent. It can occur when patients with strangulated haemorrhoids are subjected to ill-advised surgery, and has even been reported to follow banding (cf. p. 1150).

TREATMENT OF INTERNAL HAEMORRHOIDS

Non-operative treatment is recommended when the haemorrhoids are a symp-

---

[1] An 'acute attack of piles' also embraces a thrombotic pile (p. 1152) or an inflamed anal skin tag.

tom of some other condition or disease except, of course, when a carcinoma is present. The bowels are regulated by hydrophyllic colloids (Isogel etc.), and if necessary a small dose of Senokot at night. Various proprietary creams can be inserted into the rectum from a collapsible tube fitted with a nozzle, at night and before defaecation. Suppositories are also useful. **In cases of inflamed and permanently prolapsed haemorrhoids** with a patulous anus, once the oedema has been reduced by repeated dressings of glycerine and tannic acid B.P. (Eisenhammer) or Lotio Plumbi B.P., surgery offers the only hope of permanent cure. However, a severe stretching of the anal sphincter ('manual dilatation of the anus') is frequently successful in relieving symptoms even in advanced cases of piles, probably by preventing congestion of the anal cushions and its accompanying haemorrhoidal veins by a tight anal sphincter (Lord). This procedure is unsuitable for cases with a patulous sphincter. It requires a general anaesthetic and after-care by passing a special dilator to maintain sphincter relaxation; but the patient is usually hospitalised for less than 24 hours.

Active Treatment.—This consists of injection or treatment by elastic band applications to the base of each haemorrhoid or formal operation, each with specific indications. Treatment should not be withheld because the patient is elderly or infirm.

Injection Treatment[1].—*Indications.*—This is ideal for first-degree internal haemorrhoids which bleed. Early second degree haemorrhoids are often cured by this method but a proportion relapse.

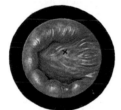

FIG. 1131.—Correct site for injecting a haemorrhoid.
(After W. B. Gabriel, FRCS, London.)

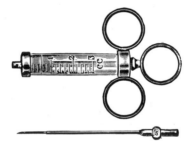

FIG. 1132.—Gabriel's syringe for injecting haemorrhoids.

Technique.—The patient should have an empty rectum, but no special preparation is necessary. A proctoscope is introduced, and the haemorrhoids are displayed. The proctoscope is introduced farther in until the haemorrhoid has almost disappeared from the lumen and only its upper end is visible. The injection is made at this point above the main mass of each haemorrhoid (fig. 1131) into the submucosa at or just above the ano-rectal ring. Using Gabriel's syringe (fig. 1132) with the bevel of the needle directed towards the rectal wall, from 3 to 5 ml of 5% phenol in almond oil is injected. The injection should produce elevation and pallor of the mucosa. The solution spreads in the submucosa upwards to the pedicle, and downwards to the internal haemorrhoid and to secondary haemorrhoids if present, but it is prevented by the intermuscular septum from reaching the external haemorrhoid. There is slight, transient bleeding from the point of puncture. The injection is painless, but a dull ache is common for a few hours. There is no special after-treatment. If there is only one haemorrhoid present, it may be cured by one injection; if all three haemorrhoids are equally enlarged, each is injected at the same session. Often

---

[1] In 1871, Mitchell of Clinton, Illinois, first used carbolic acid for injecting haemorrhoids. Itinerant irregular practitioners exploited the method.

Stephen Eisenhammer, Contemporary. Rectal Surgeon, Johannesburg, South Africa.
Peter Herent Lord, Contemporary. Surgeon, Wycombe General Hospital, High Wycombe, Bucks, England.
William Bashall Gabriel, 1893–1975. Surgeon, Royal Northern and St Mark's Hospitals, London.

three sessions at six-weekly intervals are required. Care should be taken not to inject into the prostate anteriorly, for the resulting prostatitis can be crippling.

Banding Treatment (Barron).—For second-degree haemorrhoids which are too large for successful handling by injections, treatment is available by slipping tight elastic bands on to the base of the pedicle of each haemorrhoid with a special instrument (fig. 1133). The bands cause ischaemic necrosis of the piles, which slough off within a few days. The procedure should be painless if done properly, and can be performed in the Out-Patient Department. Not more than two haemorrhoids should be banded at each session and three weeks at least should elapse between each treatment.

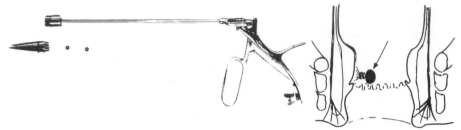

FIG. 1133.—Barron's banding apparatus with appearance of a typical 'banded' haemorrhoid.

Cryosurgery.—The application of *liquid nitrogen* is currently under active evaluation in some centres. The extreme cold (−196°C) of the application causes coagulation necrosis of the piles which subsequently separate and drop off. The procedure is painless and can be done in the Out-Patient Department. Some encouraging early reports have been issued (Lloyd-Williams).

Operation.—*Indications.*—The following cases are unsuitable for injection or banding treatment. (1) Third-degree haemorrhoids; (2) failure of non-operative treatments of second-degree haemorrhoids; (3) fibrosed haemorrhoids; (4) intero-external haemorrhoids when the external haemorrhoid is well defined. These are indications for haemorrhoidectomy.

HAEMORRHOIDECTOMY

Some pre-operative treatment is necessary. An aperient is given on the evening prior to the operation and a soap-and-water enema is administered. The anal region is shaved. On the morning of the operation the rectum is evacuated with the aid of a disposable enema.

Ligation and Excision.—With the patient in the lithotomy position the sphincter is widely stretched, a manoeuvre which greatly reduces post-operative pain. The internal haemorrhoids are then prolapsed by traction on the skin tags, or on the skin of the anal margin. Each haemorrhoid is dealt with as follows: It is picked up with dissecting forceps and traction is exerted. Traction displays a longitudinal fold (the pedicle) above the haemorrhoid. Each pedicle is grasped in a fine-pointed haemostat, as also is each external haemorrhoid or skin tag connected with each internal haemorrhoid. These pairs of haemostats, when held out by the assistants, form a triangle. The operator takes the left lateral pair of haemostats in the palm of his hand and places the extended forefinger in the anal canal to support the internal haemorrhoid. In this way traction is applied to the skin of the anal margin. With scissors, a V-shaped cut is made (fig. 1134 (A)), each limb of which is placed on either side of the skin-holding haemostat. This cut traverses the skin and the corrugator cutis ani. Exerting further traction a little blunt dissection exposes the lower border of the internal sphincter. A transfixion ligature of No. 3 chromic catgut is applied to the pedicle at this level (fig. 1134 (B)). Each haemorrhoid having been dealt with in this manner (fig. 1134 (C)), they are excised 1·25 cm distal to the ligature, the ends of which are cut about 1 cm from the knot. The stumps of the ligated haemorrhoids are returned to the rectum by tucking a piece of gauze into the anal canal with closed scissors.

The margins of the skin wounds are trimmed so as not to leave overhanging edges (fig. 1135). Bleeding subcutaneous arteries having been secured, the corners of three pieces of

John Barron, Contemporary. Surgeon, Chicago, Illinois, U.S.A.
Kenneth Lloyd-Williams, Contemporary. Surgeon, Royal United Hospitals, Bath, England.

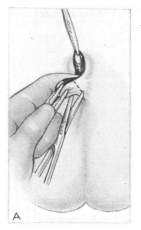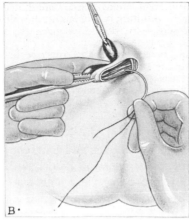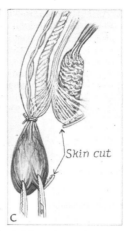

A   B·   C

FIG. 1134.—Ligation and excision of haemorrhoids: (A) The skin cut to the left lateral haemorrhoid; (B) Transfixion of the pedicle; (C) Ligation.

MUCO-
CUTANEOUS
JUNCTION

FIG. 1135.—The appearance of the anus at the conclusion of the operation. (Note: to avoid stricture formation it is necessary to ensure that a bridge of skin and mucous membrane remains between each wound.)

If it looks like a clover, the trouble is over,
If it looks like a dahlia, it's surely a failure.

petroleum-jelly gauze are tucked into the anus so as to cover the areas denuded of skin. A pad of gauze and wool, and a firmly applied T-bandage complete the operation.

Post-operative Treatment.—Twice daily baths are started from the first day and a hydrophyllic colloid (Isogel, Normacol) given in the evenings. The dressings float off in the bath; if not, they can be removed. An enema is rarely necessary as the bowels usually move on the fourth or fifth day. The baths and dry dressings (a sterile sanitary towel is best for this purpose) held in position by a T-bandage keep the area clean. On the seventh day a finger is passed into the rectum to assess the degree of spasm. If there is risk of stricture formation, a St. Mark's Hospital dilator is passed daily. The patient can leave hospital on the tenth to fourteenth day when the risk of secondary haemorrhage has passed. In the later stages a dry dressing is employed during the day and a zinc and castor oil dressing at night. Medicines should be stopped after the tenth day and the patient encouraged to pass solid motions in order to dilate the anal canal. The wounds heal in three to six weeks. Modifications of the haemorrhoidectomy operation have been described by Ferguson and Parks. In these modifications, the anal wound is closed completely or partly to reduce pain and healing time. They are now the preferred method of some specialist centres (Goldberg).

Post-operative complications may be early or late.

Early. *Pain* may demand repeated pethidine. Xylocaine jelly introduced through a fine nozzle into the rectum, as necessary, is of considerable value.

Retention of urine is not unusual after haemorrhoidectomy in male patients, and frequently it is precipitated by the presence of a rectal tube, or pack, or both. Before resorting to catheterisation, the patient should be reassured, given an analgesic, allowed to stand at the side of the bed in privacy or be assisted to a hot bath into which he may be able to void urine.

Reactionary haemorrhage is much more common than secondary haemorrhage. The haemorrhage may be mainly or entirely concealed, but will become evident on examining the rectum.

Treatment.—A suitable dose of morphine is given intravenously. If the bleeding persists, the patient must be taken to the operating theatre and the bleeding-point secured by diathermy or under-running with a ligature on a needle. Should a definite bleeding-point not be found, suspected areas are under-run in this way.

James A. Ferguson, Contemporary. Ferguson Clinic, Grand Rapids, Michigan, U.S.A.
Sir Alan Guyatt Parks, PRCS 1920–1982. Surgeon, The London Hospital and St. Mark's Hospital London.
Stanley Goldberg, Contemporary. Professor of Surgery, University of Minnesota, U.S.A.

Late.—**Secondary haemorrhage** is uncommon; when it occurs, it does so about the seventh or eighth day after operation. It is usually controlled by morphia but if the haemorrhage is severe, an anaesthetic should be given and a catgut stitch inserted to occlude the bleeding vessel.

Anal stricture.—This must be prevented at all costs (see fig. 1135 and legend). A rectal examination at the tenth day will indicate if stricturing is to be expected. It may then be necessary to give a general anaesthetic and dilate the anus to take four fingers. After that daily use of the dilator should give a satisfactory result.

Anal fissure and submucous abscess may also occur.

TREATMENT OF COMPLICATIONS OF HAEMORRHOIDS

In cases of strangulation, thrombosis, and gangrene, it was formerly believed that surgery would promote pylephlebitis. If adequate antibiotic cover is given from the start, this is not found to be so and immediate surgery can be justified in many patients. Besides adequate pain relief, bed rest with frequent hot sitz baths, warm saline compresses with firm pressure usually cause the pile mass to shrink considerably in three or four days when standard ligation and excision of the piles can be carried out. Some surgeons consider that the operation at this stage increases the risk of post-operative stenosis and delay surgery for a month or so. They then review the situation and only carry out haemorrhoidectomy if necessary. In spite of the low risk of pylephlebitis caution should dictate a 'non-interventionist' policy whenever this is practical. An anal dilation by Lord's technique can be used as a useful alternative treatment to surgery for painful 'strangulated' haemorrhoids.

In cases where the patient has been admitted because of severe haemorrhage the cause usually lies in a bleeding diathesis or the use of anticoagulants. If such are excluded, a local compress containing adrenaline solution, with an injection of morphine and blood transfusion if necessary, will usually control the haemorrhage. After blood replacement is adequate, ligation and excision of the piles may be required.

EXTERNAL HAEMORRHOIDS

Unlike internal haemorrhoids, external haemorrhoids comprise a conglomerate group of distinct clinical entities.

1. **A thrombosed external haemorrhoid** is commonly termed a *perianal haematoma*. It is a small clot occurring in the perianal subcutaneous connective tissue, usually superficial to the corrugator cutis ani muscle. The condition is due to back pressure on an anal venule consequent upon straining at stool, coughing, or lifting a heavy weight.

The condition appears suddenly and is very painful, and on examination a tense, tender swelling which resembles a semi-ripe blackcurrant is seen. The haematoma is usually situated in a lateral region of the anal margin. Untreated it may resolve, suppurate, fibrose, and give rise to a cutaneous tag, or burst and extrude the clot, or continue bleeding.

In the majority of cases resolution or fibrosis occurs. Indeed, this condition has been called 'a five-day, painful, self-curing lesion' (Milligan).

Provided it is seen within thirty-six hours of the onset, a perianal haematoma is best treated as an emergency. Under local anaesthesia the haemorrhoid is bisected and the two halves are excised together with 1·25 cm of adjacent skin.

Edward Thomas Campbell Milligan, 1886–1971. Surgeon, St. Mark's Hospital, London.

This leaves a pear-shaped wound which is allowed to granulate. The relief of pain is immediate and a permanent cure is certain. On the rare occasions in which a perianal haematoma is situated anteriorly or posteriorly, it should be treated conservatively because of the liability of a skin wound in these regions to become an anal fissure.

2. **Associated with internal haemorrhoids** = intero-external haemorrhoids. These have been discussed.

3. **Dilatation of the veins of the anal verge** becomes evident only if the patient strains, when a bluish cushion-like ring appears. This variety of external haemorrhoid is almost a perquisite of those who lead a sedentary life. The only treatment required is an adjustment in habits of the patient.

4. **A 'sentinel' pile** is associated with an anal fissure, (see above).

Genital Warts. See Chapter 60.

PRURITUS ANI

This is intractable itching around the anus. Usually the skin is reddened hyperkeratotic and may become cracked and moist. The causes are numerous.[1]

1. *Lack of cleanliness, excessive sweating, and wearing rough or woollen under-clothing* are common causes.
2. *An anal or perianal discharge* which renders the anus moist. The causative lesions include an anal fissure, fistula-in-ano, prolapsed internal or external haemorrhoids, genital warts and excessive ingestion of liquid paraffin. A mucous discharge is an intense pruritic agent and a polyp can be the cause.
3. *A vaginal discharge*, especially due to the trichomonas vaginalis.
4. *Parasitic causes.* Threadworms should be excluded, especially in young subjects.[2] Scabies and pediculosis pubis may infest the anal region.
5. *Epidermophytosis* is a common cause especially if the skin between the toes is infected also. Microscopic and cultural examinations are essential. Half-strength Whitfield's ointment quickly gives relief and is the sheet anchor of treatment.
6. *Allergy* is sometimes the cause, in which case there is likely to be a history of other allergic manifestations, such as urticaria, asthma, or hay-fever. Antibiotic therapy may be the precipitating factor.
7. *Skin diseases localised to the perianal skin*—Psoriasis, lichen planus and contact dermatitis.
8. *Bacterial infection.*—Intertrigo due to a mixed bacterial infection. Erythrasma due to *Corynebacterium minutissimum* is responsible for some cases and its presence is detected by ultra-violet light which induces a pink fluorescence.
9. *A psychoneurosis.*—It is alleged that in a few instances neurotic individuals become so immersed in their complaint that a pain-pleasure complex develops, the pleasure being the scratching. Possibly this is true, but such a syndrome should not be assumed without firm grounds for coming to this conclusion.

Treatment.—The cause is treated. Other methods include:

Hygienic Measures.—Cotton-wool should be substituted for toilet paper. Soap is avoided, and replaced by a detergent. These measures alone, combined with wearing cotton cellular underwear and applications of calamine lotion, are all that is necessary to cure some cases. If there is much anal hair trapping the moisture and discharge, shaving can be very helpful.

Hydrocortisone.—In cases with dermatitis, *and only in cases with dermatitis*, prednisolone, applied topically in a cream of 1% is often beneficial; sometimes after discontinuation of the therapy the pruritus is liable to return, in which event 5% Xylocaine ointment can be substituted for a time.

Strapping the buttocks apart is a most useful procedure, especially when the pruritus is

---

[1] A useful mnemonic is: 'Pus, Polypus, Parasites, Piles, Psyche'.
[2] Children suffering from threadworms should wear gloves at night, lest they scratch the perianal region and are reinfested with ova by nail biting—'Parasites lost, Parasites regained'.

Arthur Whitfield, 1868–1947. Professor of Dermatology, King's College Hospital, London.

acute, and in chronic cases when the opposing surfaces are moist. The strapping is worn so long as the patient finds it beneficial.

Operative Treatment.—This may be necessary for a concomitant lesion of the ano-rectum which is thought to initiate or contribute to the pruritis. Otherwise, surgery is not indicated and the older operations described for this condition are no longer performed.

ANO-RECTAL ABSCESSES

In 60% of cases the pus from the abscess yields a pure culture of *Esch. coli*; in 23% a pure culture of *Staphylococcus aureus* is obtained. In diminishing frequency, pure cultures of *Bacteroides*, a streptococcus, or B. *proteus* are found. In many cases the infection is mixed. In a high percentage of cases—some estimate it as high as 90%—the abscess commences as an infection of an anal gland (figs. 1136 and 1137). Other causes are penetration of the rectal wall, *e.g.* by a fish bone, a blood-borne infection, or an extension of a cutaneous boil.

A large percentage of anorectal abscesses coincide with a fistula-in-ano. For this reason, anorectal abscess becomes a highly important subject. Moreover, as antibiotics cannot reach the contents of an abscess in adequate concentration, no reliance can be placed on antibiotic therapy alone. A fistula is much more likely if bacterial culture of the pus discloses bowel (as opposed to skin) organisms (Grace.)

Differential Diagnosis.—The only conditions with which an anorectal abscess is likely to be confused are an abscess connected with a pilonidal sinus, Bartholin's gland, or Cowper's gland.

Classification of Ano-rectal Abscesses.—A clear understanding of suppuration in this area is dependent on a concise knowledge of the anatomy (figs. 1136 and 1137). There are four main varieties—perianal, ischiorectal, submucous, and pelvirectal.

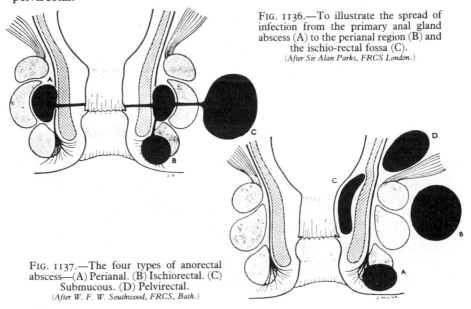

FIG. 1136.—To illustrate the spread of infection from the primary anal gland abscess (A) to the perianal region (B) and the ischio-rectal fossa (C).
(*After Sir Alan Parks, FRCS London.*)

FIG. 1137.—The four types of anorectal abscess—(A) Perianal. (B) Ischiorectal. (C) Submucous. (D) Pelvirectal.
(*After W. F. W. Southwood, FRCS, Bath.*)

Roger Grace, Contemporary. Surgeon, Wolverhampton, England.
Caspar Bartholin, 1655–1738. Professor of Medicine, Anatomy and Physics, Copenhagen.
William Cowper, 1666–1709. Surgeon, London.

1. **Perianal** (60%).—This usually occurs as the result of suppuration in an anal gland, which spreads superficially to lie in the region of the subcutaneous portion of the external sphincter (fig. 1137(A)). It may also occur as a result of a thrombosed external pile. If the haematoma is not evacuated, it may become infected and a perianal abscess results. This is the most common abscess of the region. Persons of all ages are affected, and the condition is not uncommon, even in infancy and childhood. The constitutional symptoms and the pain are less pronounced than in the ischiorectal abscess because the pus can expand the walls of this part of the intermuscular space comparatively easily. Early diagnosis is made by inspecting the anal margin when an acutely tender rounded cystic lump about the size of a cherry is seen and felt at the anal verge below the dentate line.

Treatment.—No time should be lost in evacuating the pus.

Operation.—Thorough drainage is achieved by making a cruciate incision over the abscess and excising the skin edges—this completely removes the 'roof' of the abscess. Healing commonly occurs within a few days.

2. **Ischiorectal abscess** (30%).—Commonly, this is due to an extension laterally through the external sphincter of a low intermuscular anal abscess (fig. 1012B). Rarely, the infection is either lymphatic or blood-borne. The fat, which fills the ischiorectal fossa (fig. 1138), is particularly vulnerable because it is poorly vascularised; consequently it is not long before the whole space becomes involved. The ischiorectal fossa communicates with that of the opposite side via the post-sphincteric space, and if an ischiorectal abscess is not evacuated early, involvement of the contralateral fossa is not uncommon. Should an internal opening into the anal canal ensue, a 'horseshoe' abscess develops enveloping the whole of the posterior part of the circumference of the anal canal (cf horseshoe fistula).

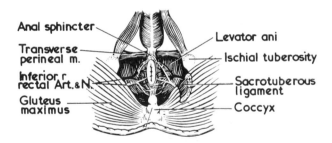

FIG. 1138.—The ischiorectal fossa.
(After V. C. Shah and Y. V. Shah.)

An ischiorectal abscess gives rise to a tender, brawny induration palpable on the corresponding side of the anal canal and the floor of the fossa. Constitutional symptoms are severe, the temperature often rising to 38·9°C. Men are affected more often than women.

Treatment.—Operation should be undertaken early—as soon as it is certain that an abscess is present in this area—remembering that antibiotic therapy often masks the general signs.

Operation.—*Stage 1.*—A cruciate incision (fig. 1139 inset) is made into the abscess. A portion of skin is sometimes excised (fig. 1139) but deroofing is not necessary in every case.

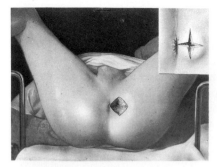

FIG. 1139.—Incision of ischiorectal abscess. The cavity is explored and, if septa exist, they should be broken down gently with a finger and the necrotic tissue lining the walls of the abscess is removed by the finger wrapped in gauze. Nothing further is done at this stage.

Stage 2.—As soon as the acute infection has subsided, the wound should be re-examined, preferably under general anaesthesia. A careful search is made for a fistulous opening communicating with the anal canal. If such is found, the treatment should be as for fistula. If no fistula is found, the cavity should be lightly packed with gauze wrung out in any weak antiseptic favoured by the operator. A T-bandage is applied. When the cavity has become covered with granulation tissue skin grafting may help to expedite final epithelialisation.

3. **Submucous abscess** (5%) occurs above the dentate line (fig. 1137C). When it occurs after the injection of haemorrhoids it always resolves. Otherwise, it can be opened with sinus forceps when adequately displayed by a proctoscope.

4. **Pelvirectal abscess** is situated between the upper surface of the levator ani and the pelvic peritoneum. It is nothing more or less than a pelvic abscess and as such is usually secondary to appendicitis, salpingitis, diverticulitis, or parametritis. *Abdominal Crohn's disease is an important cause of pelvic disease that can present as perianal sepsis (cf. fistula-in-ano).* A relevant point to remember is that rarely a supralevator abscess/fistula may be due to over-enthusiastic attempts to drain an ischiorectal abscess or to display a fistula, when a probe is forced through the levator ani/rectal wall from below.

5. **Fissure Abscess.**—This is the name given to a subcutaneous abscess lying in immediate association with an anal fissure. Drainage is achieved at the same time as the fissure is treated by sphincterotomy.

FISTULA-IN-ANO

A fistula-in-ano is a track, lined by granulation tissue which connects deeply in the anal canal or rectum and superficially on the skin around the anus. It usually results from an ano-rectal abscess which burst spontaneously or was opened inadequately (fig. 1136). The fistula continues to discharge and, because of constant reinfection from the anal canal or rectum, seldom, if ever, closes permanently without surgical aid. An anorectal abscess may produce a track the orifice of which has the appearance of a fistula, but it does not communicate with the anal canal or the rectum. By definition this is *not* a fistula, but a sinus.

TYPES OF ANAL FISTULAS

These are divided into two groups, according to whether their internal opening is below or above the anorectal ring.

Low Level.—These open into the anal canal below the anorectal ring.

For treating successfully Louis XIV's fistula-in-ano, Charles Félix, barber-surgeon to the Court, received a gift of a farm, 300,000 livres, and a title. 300,000 livres today would be worth about £25,000.

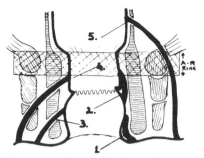

FIG. 1140.—Types of anal fistulas (standard classification). 1. Subcutaneous, 2. submucuous, 3. low anal, 4. high anal, 5. pelvirectal.

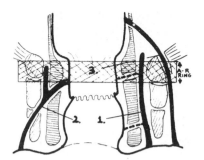

FIG. 1141.—Types of anal fistulas. 1. Intersphincteric, 2. transphincteric (which may be *high* or *low*), 3. supralevator.

(After Sir Alan Parks.)

High Level.—These open into the anal canal at or above the anorectal ring.

As an alternative to the common anatomical classification illustrated in fig. 1140, Parks produced another based on the origin of the fistula from an abscess in an anal gland situated on the plane between the internal and external sphincters (the 'anal intersphincteric plane') fig. 1141.

The importance of deciding whether a fistulas is a low- or a high-level type is that a low-level fistula can be laid open without fear of permanent incontinence (from damage to the anorectal bundle), while a high-level fistula can be treated only by 'staged' operations, often with the use of a protective colostomy to prevent septic complications and to shorten healing time between the stages.

In probing a high fistulous track, great care must be taken not to create an internal opening into the rectum where none existed previously. Such a disaster could convert a relatively straightforward 'intersphincteric' track into a high 'pelvi-rectal' fistula that might prove very difficult to cure.

By the standard classification, a *high* fistula refers to both a high anal (No. 4, fig. 1140) and a pelvirectal fistula (No. 5, fig. 1140). By the Parks classification, both a high transphincteric or a supralevator fistula would qualify as high, with the intersphincteric falling into either category depending on whether an internal opening was present at all, and at what level it entered the anal canal (see No. 1, fig. 1141).

Low-level Fistulas

Clinical Features.—Commonly, the principal symptom is a persistent sero-purulent discharge that irritates the skin in the neighbourhood and causes discomfort. Often the history dates back for years. So long as the opening is large enough for the pus to escape, pain is not a symptom, but if the orifice is occluded pain increases until the discharge erupts. Frequently there is a solitary external opening, usually situated within 3·75 cm of the anus, presenting as a small elevation with granulation tissue pouting from the mouth of the opening. Sometimes superficial healing occurs, pus accumulates and an abscess reforms and discharges through the same opening, or a new opening. Thus there may be two or more external openings, usually grouped together on the right or left of the middle line, but occasionally, when both ischiorectal fossae are involved, an opening is

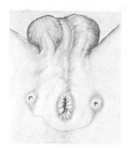

FIG. 1142.— Horse-shoe fistula-in-ano. Both ischio-rectal fossae involved. Usually there is only one internal orifice.

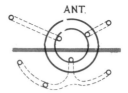

FIG. 1143.—Illustrating Goodsall's rule.

seen on each side, in which case there is often intercommunication between them (fig. 1142). As a rule there is much induration of the skin and subcutaneous tissues around the fistula.

Goodsall's Rule.—Fistulas with an external opening in relation to the anterior half of the anus tend to be of the direct type (fig. 1143). Those with an external opening or openings in relation to the posterior half of the anus, which are much more common, usually have curving tracks, and may be of the horseshoe-variety. Note that posteriorly situated fistulas may have multiple external openings which always connect to a solitary internal orifice (fig. 1143).

Digital Examination.—Not infrequently an internal opening can be felt as a nodule on the wall of the anal canal. Irrespective of the number of external openings, there is almost invariably but one internal opening.

Proctoscopy sometimes will reveal the internal opening of the fistula. A hypertrophied papilla is suggestive that the internal orifice lies within the crypt related to the papilla (fig. 1144).

Probing.—In the past it was the universal practice to probe a fistula in the ward or the out-patient department. *Such manoeuvres accomplish nothing*, are painful, and are liable to reawaken dormant infection. Furthermore, if probing is performed without the utmost gentleness, or if the patient, experiencing pain, makes a sudden jerk, a false passage may result which complicates the condition still further. Probing should be postponed until the patient is under an anaesthetic in the operating theatre.

The injection of lipiodol, or other opaque medium, along the sinus, 'prior to radiography, *has little to recommend it*. The radiographs thus obtained are seldom illuminating, and the procedure is likely to cause a recrudescence of inflammation.

Radiography of the thorax should be undertaken and the possibility of pulmonary tuberculosis considered, despite the fact that today it will be found in only a small proportion of patients with fistula-in-ano—usually of Asian origin (see 3. below).

Special Clinical Types of Fistulas-in-ano:

1. **Fistula connected with an Anal Fissure.**—Unlike the usual fistula-in-ano, pain (due to the fissure) is a leading symptom. The fistula is very near the anal orifice, usually posterior, and the external opening is often hidden by the sentinel pile.

2. **Fistula with an internal opening above the ano-rectal ring** is due, almost invariably, to penetration by a foreign body or probing and interference with a high abscess. A supralevator fistula arising spontaneously will be seen only once or at most twice in a surgical career.

3. **Granulomatous infections.**—If induration around a fistula is lacking, if the opening is ragged and flush with the surface, if the surrounding skin is discoloured and the discharge is watery, it strongly suggests that the fistula is due to a tuberculous infection. In more than 30% of patients suffering from pulmonary tuberculosis, virulent tubercle bacilli

David Henry Goodsall, 1843–1906. (See footnote p. 1116.)

are present in the rectum. About 2–3% of fistulas-in-ano are tuberculous, but in sanatoria and settlements for tuberculous patients the incidence is higher. Histopathological examination supplies the only criterion of importance as to whether the tissue removed is tuberculous. The fistula will usually respond to anti-tuberculous drugs alone. The differential diagnosis is from Crohn's disease. In Crohn's disease the rectal mucosa is often involved.

4. **Fistulas with many external openings** may arise from tuberculous proctitis, ulcerative proctocolitis, Crohn's disease of colon or ileum, bilharziasis, and lymphogranuloma inguinale with a fibrous rectal stricture. Colloid carcinoma may complicate fistulas-in-ano. *Crohn's disease* is the most frequent cause seen in this country from this group.

5. **Carcinoma arising within Perianal Fistulas.**—Colloid carcinoma of the rectum is notoriously liable to be complicated by perianal fistulas. In some instances the fistulous condition, with its discharge of colloid material, overshadows the primary carcinoma, and not a few unfortunate patients have had their condition diagnosed for a time as an inflammatory fistula-in-ano. If a primary tumour is present in the rectum, usually it can be detected and its nature established by biopsy. Dukes has established conclusively that colloid carcinomatous fistulas can develop without a primary neoplasm in the rectum. He regards such cases as examples of colloid carcinoma developing in a reduplicated portion of the intestinal tract. Both adenocarcinoma and squamous-cell carcinoma are known to arise within chronic fistulous tracks. The former can develop from the anal glandular tissue: the latter is an example of true malignant change of squamous epithelium lining the wall of the track.

Hidradenitis Suppurativa.—This is a chronic infection of the apocrine glands around the anal margin giving rise to numerous sinuses. The mons pubis and groin also can be affected. After excision of the area, granulation and healing is accelerated by using Silastic foam dressings (L. Hughes).

Treatment.—That the fistulous track must be laid open from its termination to its source was a rule promulgated by John of Arderne more than 500 years ago.

The operation can best be described in stages:

Step 1.—Pre-operate cleansing enemas are necessary. When the patient has been anaesthetised, he is placed in the lithotomy position or in the prone jack-knife position, according to the preference of the operator. Using bidigital palpation under anaesthesia, it is often possible to obtain more information concerning a fistula than can be learned from probing; it is surprisingly easy to perforate a probe through the wall of the track. Unfortunately, many inexperienced operators find it more reassuring to create a false passage than to risk criticism for not being able to demonstrate the internal opening. Careful bidigital palpation of the perianal tissue will often reveal a cord-like induration, representing the track, which will lead the intra-anal finger towards the proximal opening. Rather than insert a probe through the distal orifice at this stage, it is better to endeavour to find the internal opening via a proctoscope. If the internal opening still cannot be seen, the insertion of a probe retrogradely into an anal crypt, especially one with a nearby hypertrophied papilla, often reveals the internal portion of the track (fig. 1144). The injection of diluted methylene blue or other dye into the external mouth of the fistula to establish the site of the internal opening is occasionally necessary, but is not recommended as a routine.

Step 2.—A probe-pointed director (fig. 1145) is inserted into the distal orifice, and it is

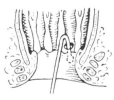

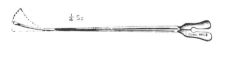

FIG. 1144.— Retrograde probing of an anal crypt sometimes reveals the internal orifice of the fistula.

FIG. 1145.—A director with a probe-pointed malleable extremity is a useful instrument.

Burrill Bernard Crohn, Contemporary. Gastro-enterologist, Mount Sinai Hospital, New York, U.S.A.
Cuthbert Esquire Dukes, 1890–1977. Pathologist, St. Mark's Hospital, London.
Leslie Ernest Hughes, Contemporary. Professor of Surgery, Welsh National School of Medicine, Cardiff, Wales.

advanced delicately until it reaches a point where it does not pass readily. The track is opened along the director, and bleeding is controlled.

Step 3.—If it is not at once evident in which direction the track passes, granulations are wiped away with gauze (it is seldom necessary to use a curette). Often this will leave a granulation-filled spot at one site only. Gentle probing at this spot frequently will give the clue to the continuation of the fistula. The director is reinserted, and again followed with the knife for a short distance. This procedure is repeated until the entire track, and any side channels, are laid open. As far as possible, all muscle is divided at right angles to its fibres. In the rare event of the track passing above the ano-rectal ring, cutting should cease at the level of the dentate line, and from thenceforth the operation is conducted as suggested below. In most instances probing and laying open the track can be repeated until the entire track is laid open. Pursuing this course, if there is no internal opening the track will become bereft of granulations on wiping it. As a rule the internal opening can be demonstrated either by direct inspection through a proctoscope, or by a bent probe inserted into an anal crypt. In the latter circumstance, the internal portion of the track is excised in continuity.

Step 4.—The edges of the track are trimmed, 1 to 3 mm of tissue being removed—a step that makes post-operative packing unnecessary after the first twenty-four to thirty-six hours. E. Hughes advocates primary split skin grafting of the wound resulting from fistulotomy. The grafts are taken from the inner aspect of the thigh and applied to the anal wound, being stitched to the skin edges and to each other in the depths of the wound. Tulle gras is then superimposed, and a firm pack of cottonwool applied. The first dressing is done on the fifth post-operative day.

When skin grafting is not employed, digital dilatation of the anus, or the passage of a St. Mark's Hospital dilator every other day, prevents pocketing or bridging of the granulating wound.

Biopsy.—Always send a piece of track for biopsy.

High-level Fistulas

The treatment of these cases is difficult. If the track is laid open as for low-level fistulas, incontinence will follow. There are three types (Parks):

(1) *Supralevator fistula—secondary* to local disease (type 3, fig. 1141).—It occurs as a result of Crohn's disease, ulcerative colitis, carcinoma, foreign body perforating the rectal ampulla from above, or trauma. This fistula is quite unrelated to the ordinary type and the treatment is that of the cause. A traumatic fistula usually needs a colostomy. None of these fistulas requires to be laid open, which would in any case cause incontinence.

(2) *Transphincteric fistula* (type 3, fig. 1141) with *perforating secondary track.*— The condition starts as an *intersphincteric* track (type 2, fig. 1141), often with a high secondary track in the ischiorectal fossa up to the levator ani. Here lies the danger. Although the anal opening may be low, during exploration of the high secondary track, unless great care is taken, the probe can be pushed through the levator ani into the rectal ampulla, thus converting a low fistula into a high-level type. Treatment should first of all be directed to the low transphincteric fistula and healing of the upper track may follow. If it fails to do so, or if the opening into the rectum is of any size or near the anorectal bundle a colostomy must be done before complete healing will take place.

A *seton*—a time-honoured device—(*i.e.*, a ligature of silk or linen) is helpful when the internal opening is near the anorectal ring. Insertion of a seton and subsequent re-examination of the patient without anaesthesia will establish whether the internal opening is situated so near to the anorectal ring that incontinence would result if the track was laid open. Under these conditions, a staged operation and a covering colostomy would be the proper treatment. While the

Sir Edward Stuart Reginald Hughes, PRACS, Contemporary. Surgeon, Melbourne, Victoria, Australia.
St. Mark's Hospital for Diseases of the Rectum and Colon, London, founded in 1835 as St. Mark's Hospital for Fistula.

seton remains in-situ it acts as a wick/drain and allows the acute inflammatory reaction around the track to subside: this can greatly simplify subsequent surgery. In expert hands, primary repair of divided sphincter muscle can preserve continence when a high level track is laid open.

(3) *High Intersphincteric Fistula.*—The track starts as a primary anal gland abscess (type A, fig. 1136), and it runs between the internal and external sphincter along the plane of the longitudinal muscle fibres. It may have an opening into the rectum above the anorectal ring and below at the site of a perianal abscess (type B, fig. 1136). Providing it is recognised it is easy to treat. The internal sphincter is divided and the whole track is laid open without fear of incontinence.

NON-MALIGNANT STRICTURES

1. Congenital:

(*a*) A stricture at the level of the anal valves, due to incomplete obliteration of the proctodeal membrane, sometimes does not give rise to symptoms until early childhood.

(*b*) Patients who have had an operation for imperforate anus in infancy may require periodic anorectal dilatation.

2. Spasmodic:

(*a*) An anal fissure causes spasm of the internal sphincter, which in time becomes fibrotic.

(*b*) Rarely, a spasmodic stricture accompanies Secondary Megacolon (Chapter 50), possibly due to chronic use of laxatives.

3. Organic:

(*a*) *Post-operative stricture* sometimes follows haemorrhoidectomy performed incorrectly. Low colo-anal anastomoses, especially if a stapling gun is used, can narrow down post-operatively.

(*b*) *Irradiation stricture* is an aftermath of irradiation.

(*c*) *Senile Anal Stenosis.*—A condition of chronic internal sphincter contraction is sometimes seen in the aged. Increasing constipation is present with pronounced straining at stool. Faecal impaction is liable to occur. The muscle is rigid and feels like a tight umbrella-ring. There is no evidence of a fissure-in-ano. The treatment is internal sphincterotomy or dilation at frequent intervals.

(*d*) *Lymphogranuloma Inguinale* (Chapter 60).—This is by far the most frequent cause of a *tubular* inflammatory stricture of the rectum, and 80% of the sufferers are women. Frei's reaction is usually positive. This variety of rectal stricture is particularly common in Negro races, and may be accompanied by elephantiasis of the labia majora. In the early stages, antibiotic treatment may lead to cure. In advanced cases excision of the rectum is required.

(*e*) *Ulcerative Colitis.*—Stricture of the anorectum also complicates ulcerative proctocolitis and large bowel Crohn's disease; in this instance the stricture is *annular*, and often more than one are present. A carcinoma should be suspected if a stricture is found, until a biopsy is obtained.

(*f*) *Endometriosis* of the rectovaginal septum may present as a stricture. There is usually a history of frequent menstrual periods with the appearance of severe pain during the first two days of the menstrual flow.

Wilhelm Siegmund Frei, 1885–1943. Professor of Dermatology, Berlin, who later settled in New York, U.S.A.

(g) *Neoplastic*.—When free bleeding occurs after dilatation of a supposed inflammatory stricture, carcinoma should be suspected (Grey Turner), and a portion of the stricture should be removed for biopsy. Sometimes, in these cases, repeated biopsies show inflammatory tissue only. If, however, the symptoms show a marked progression, malignancy should be strongly suspected.

Clinical Features.—Increasing difficulty in defaecation is the leading symptom. The patient finds that increasingly large doses of aperients are required, and if the stools are formed, they are 'pipe-stem' in shape. In cases of inflammatory stricture, tenesmus, bleeding, and the passage of mucopus are superadded. Sometimes the patient comes under observation only when subacute or acute intestinal obstruction has supervened.

Rectal Examination.—The finger encounters a sharply defined shelf-like interruption of the lumen. If the calibre is large enough to admit the finger, it should be noted whether the stricture is annular or tubular. Sometimes this point can be determined only after dilatation. A biopsy of the stricture must be taken.

Treatment:

Prophylactic.—The passage of an anal dilator during convalescence after haemorrhoidectomy greatly reduces the incidence of post-operative stricture. Efficient treatment of lymphogranuloma inguinale in its early stages should lessen the frequency of stricture from that cause.

Dilatation by Bougies.—For anal and many rectal strictures dilatation by bougies at regular intervals is all that is required.

Incision and Primary Free Skin Graft.—For post-operative and senile strictures this operation gives by far the best results.

The stricture is exposed and divided posteriorly so as to remove about 1 cm of the fibrosed ring. A 'back cut' is made and a triangular piece of skin removed with its apex above in such a way as to ensure complete and adequate enlargement of the strictured region. A split skin graft is then taken from the inner side of the thigh, laid firmly into the defect, and sutured into position with fine catgut sutures. Dressings are applied to keep it firmly in position and renewed on about the fourth day when the bowels are allowed to act. The percentage 'take' is high and the results surprisingly good.

Colostomy must be undertaken when a stricture is causing intestinal obstruction, and in advanced cases of stricture complicated by fistulas-in-ano. In selected cases this can be followed by restorative resection of the stricture-bearing area. If this step is anticipated, the colostomy is placed in the transverse colon.

Rectal Excision and Colo-anal anastomosis.—When the strictures are at or just above the anal-rectal junction and are associated with a normal anal canal, but irreversible changes necessitate removal of the area, excision can be followed by a colo-anal anastomosis with good functional results. A similar procedure can be done for an otherwise incurable supra-levator fistula.

MALIGNANT TUMOURS OF THE ANUS AND ANAL CANAL

Carcinoma of the anus differs from carcinoma of the rectum in histological structure, behaviour, and types of treatment. This is mainly because of its accessibility, its sensitivity and its abundant lymph drainage, both superficial and deep.

George Grey Turner, 1877–1951. Professor of Surgery, Postgraduate Medical School, London. Formerly Professor of Surgery, University of Durham.

70% of anal tumours arise in the anal canal: 30% are squamous cell carcinomas of the anal verge.

A. **Squamous-celled Carcinoma.**—Because of its superficial situation the presence of this lesion is frequently recognised by the patient, who often presents early. However, there are exceptions (1) radiation carcinoma sometimes develops in the anal and perianal skin of a patient unwisely treated with lightly filtered x-rays for pruritus ani. The chronic radiation dermatitis becomes so familiar to the patient that too often he does not perceive the superimposition of carcinoma. (2) Simple papillomas (anal warts) sometimes take on a carcinomatous change (fig. 1146). (3) Occasionally a squamous cell carcinoma develops in the track of a long-standing fistula-in-ano.

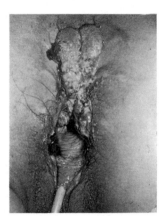

FIG. 1146.—Neglected papillomas of the anus which have become malignant.

Other malignant tumours of the anal canal are also found, but they are rare:

B.   **Basaloid carcinoma.**—This is also known as cloacogenic carcinoma and is a form of non-keratinising squamous carcinoma. It can metastasise to lymph nodes, and can be highly malignant. It is not very sensitive to irradiation.

C.   **Muco-epidermoid carcinoma.**—This tumour arises near the squamo-columnar cell junction and is of average malignancy. It is not well keratinised and is radio-sensitive.

D.   **Basal-cell carcinoma.**—Like the true squamous cell carcinomas of the anal verge and lower anal canal these are 'skin tumours' and behave accordingly.

E.   **Melanoma.**—Melanoma of the anus presents as a bluish-black soft mass that is apt to be confused with a thrombotic pile, and therefore unfortunately incised. Such trauma, followed by the trauma of defaecation, incites the tumour to rapid metastasis. Left undisturbed, it ulcerates, and the colour of the tumour changes from blue to black. The inguinal lymph nodes are soon involved. Unless a melanoma is excised at an early stage, it disseminates by the blood-stream. The tumour is radio-resistant and has a very poor prognosis.

Treatment

Operation.—For small squamous cell lesions of the anal verge and lower anal canal wide local excision leaving a margin of at least 2·5 cm of tissue all round is sufficient to effect a cure. Lymphatic dissemination will be to the inguinal nodes, which should be watched carefully. If they become involved, block dissection removal of the glands of one or both groins will be necessary and carries a fair prognosis for cure. Unless selected for treatment by radiotherapy all other cases, including the basaloid carcinomas, should be treated by:

An abdominoperineal excision, removing the growth and perianal area widely. If and when the inguinal lymph nodes become involved, a radical dissection of the groins is carried out. This formidable operation, which is founded on sound premises based on pathology, gives more favourable results than has been generally believed. It should be noted that dissection of the lymph nodes of the groin or groins, is carried out only when involvement of the nodes can be recognised clinically, or when a doubtful lymph node, submitted to frozen section at the time of the operation, proves to be involved. As has been emphasised already, patients with carcinoma of the anus often present early, and in many patients the inguinal lymph nodes are not involved clinically. Should they become so later, dissection of the groin is carried out.

A Super-radical operation comprises removal of perianal and groin skin together with a block dissection of the inguinal lymph nodes and a radical abdominoperineal excision of the rectum. This operation is very formidable and causes considerable morbidity and the nursing care of such patients can only be described as highly demanding.

Radiotherapy.—Radiotherapy can also be used for these tumours, but requires special techniques: if the specialised equipment and expertise is available, radiotherapy can offer a similar prognosis to local surgical excision with less damage to the anal sphincters: also, the poorly differentiated tumours carry such a bad prognosis that provided local disease can be eradicated or controlled, the patient is often best left to die in comfort without a colostomy. However, few centres at present can offer as effective treatment as surgical intervention using local excision for small tumours of good outlook, and radical rectal excision for the advanced or highly malignant cases. Either external beam or needles, 2 mC each, placed 1·5 cm apart at the base of a small tumour, can be used for the following types of cases (Pack):

1. Early papillary or basal-celled carcinoma of low-grade malignancy.
2. Advanced lesions that have recurred after operation.
3. In an inoperable case, with the hope of converting an inoperable carcinoma into one that is resectable.

However, with modern techniques higher 'curative' doses of irradiation are being employed as an alternative to surgery, with an acceptably low complication rate.

Chemotherapy.—For highly malignant tumours (poorly differentiated or anaplastic histological features) 'combination treatments' with chemical cytotoxics have proved effective for providing good palliation, and even cure (Quan). Radiotherapy has also been used in tandem with cytotoxic agents (Nigro). The long-term outlook with such treatments is not yet known, and they involve formidably frequent programmes of hospital attendances and expensive drugs. They cannot be recommended for wide use at the present time, but in specialist centres impressive results have been achieved.

George Thomas Pack. Formerly Clinical Professor of Surgery, New York Medical College, New York
S. H. Q. Quan, Contemporary. Surgeon, Memorial and Sloan-Kettering Cancer Centre, New York, U.S.A.
N. Nigro, Contemporary. Surgeon, Wayne State University, Detroit, U.S.A.

CHAPTER 55

HERNIAS. UMBILICUS. ABDOMINAL WALL

HERNIA

A hernia is the protrusion of a viscus or part of a viscus through an abnormal opening in the walls of its containing cavity. The external abdominal hernia is the commonest form and mostly of the inguinal, femoral and umbilical varieties, respectively 73, 17 and 8·5% (fig. 1147). This leaves 1·5% for the rarer forms and excludes post-operative incisional hernia.

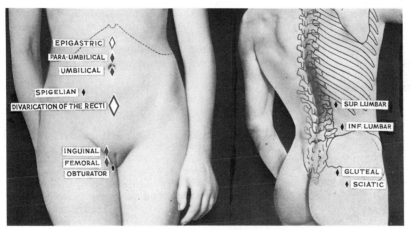

FIG. 1147.—External hernias. Red = common. White = not unusual. Black = rare,

GENERAL FEATURES COMMON TO ALL HERNIAS

Aetiology.—A powerful muscular effort or strain occasioned by lifting a heavy weight, indeed any condition which raises intra-abdominal pressure is liable to be followed by a hernia. Whooping cough is a predisposing cause in childhood, whilst a chronic cough, straining on micturition because of urethral obstruction and straining on defaecation may precipitate a hernia in an adult. It should be remembered that the appearance of a hernia in an adult can be a sign of intra-abdominal malignancy.

Stretching of the abdominal musculature because of an increase in contents, as in obesity and in pregnancy, can be another factor. Fat acts as a kind of 'pile-driver' for it separates muscle bundles and layers, weakens aponeuroses, and favours the appearance of paraumbilical, direct inguinal, and hiatus hernias. A femoral hernia is more common in women than in men due to the differences in pelvic anatomy. An indirect inguinal hernia may occur in a congenital preformed sac—the remains of the processus vaginalis.

Composition of a hernia.—As a rule, a hernia consists of three parts—the sac, the coverings of the sac, and the contents of the sac.

The sac is a diverticulum of peritoneum consisting of mouth, neck, body and fundus. The neck is usually well-defined, but in some direct inguinal hernias and in many incisional hernias there is no actual neck. The diameter of the neck is important, because strangulation of bowel is a likely complication where the neck is narrow as in femoral and umbilical hernia.

The body of the sac varies greatly in size and is not necessarily occupied. In cases occurring in infancy and childhood the sac is gossamer thin. In long-standing cases, especially after years of pressure by a truss, the wall of the sac is comparatively thick.

Coverings are derived from the layers of the abdominal wall through which the sac passes. In long-standing cases they become atrophied from stretching and so amalgamated that they are indistinguishable one from another.

Contents.—These can be:

1. Omentum = omentocele (*syn*. epiplocele).
2. Intestine = enterocele. Usually small intestine, but, in some instances, large intestine or the vermiform appendix.
3. A portion of the circumference of the intestine = Richter's hernia.
4. A portion of the bladder, or a diverticulum of the bladder, is sometimes present in addition to other contents in a direct inguinal, a sliding inguinal, and in a femoral hernia.
5. Ovary with or without the corresponding Fallopian tube.
6. A Meckel's diverticulum = Littré's hernia.
7. Fluid. As a part of ascites, or as a residuum thereof. Blood-stained fluid accompanies strangulation.

Classification.—Irrespective of site, a hernia can be:

      1. *Reducible.*
      2. *Irreducible.*   *(Complication of 1.)*
      3. *Obstructed*[1]. }
      4. *Strangulated.* }   *(Complications of 2.)*
      5. *Inflamed.*

Reducible Hernia.—The hernia either reduces itself when the patient lies down, or can be reduced by the patient or by the surgeon. Note that *intestine* gurgles on reduction, and the first portion is more difficult to reduce than the last. *Omentum* is doughy, and the last portion is more difficult to reduce than the first. A reducible hernia imparts an *expansile* impulse on coughing.

Irreducible Hernia.—When the contents cannot be returned to the abdomen and there is no evidence of other complications. It is brought about by adhesions between the sac and its contents or from overcrowding within the sac. Irreducibility without other symptoms is almost diagnostic of an omentocele especially in femoral and umbilical hernia. *Note:*. Any degree of irreducibility predisposes to strangulation.

Obstructed Hernia.—This is an irreducible hernia containing intestine which is obstructed from without or from within; but there is no interference to the blood-supply to the bowel. The symptoms are less severe and the onset more gradual than is the case in strangulation, but more often than not the obstruction culminates in strangulation. Usually no clear distinction can be made between obstruction and strangulation in hernias, so the safe course is to assume that strangulation is imminent and to treat accordingly.

Incarcerated Hernia.—The term 'incarceration' is often used loosely as an alternative

---

[1] The term 'incarcerated' should be reserved for impaction of faeces within large intestine.

August Gottlieb Richter, 1742–1812. Lecturer on Surgery, Göttingen, Germany.
Gabriele Fallopio (Fallopius), 1523–1563. Professor of Anatomy, Surgery and Botany, Padua, Italy.
Johann Friedrich Meckel (The Younger), 1781–1833. Professor of Anatomy and Surgery, Halle, Germany.
Alexis Littré, 1658–1726. Surgeon and Anatomist, Paris. Littré described 'Meckel's' diverticulum in a hernial sac in 1700, 81 years before Meckel was born.

to obstruction or strangulation. As emphasised already, the term 'incarceration' should be employed only when it is considered that the lumen of that portion of the *colon* occupying a hernial sac is blocked with faeces. In that event the scybalous contents of the bowel should be capable of being indented with the finger, like putty.

Strangulated Hernia.—A hernia becomes strangulated when the blood-supply of its contents is seriously impaired, rendering gangrene imminent. Gangrene may occur as early as five or six hours after the onset of the first symptoms of strangulation. Although inguinal hernia is four times more common than femoral hernia, a femoral hernia is more likely to strangulate because of the narrowness of the neck of the sac and its rigid walls.

Pathology.—The intestine is obstructed, and in addition its blood supply is constricted. At first only the venous return is impeded. The wall of the intestine becomes congested and bright red, and serous fluid is poured out into the sac. As the congestion increases, the intestine becomes purple in colour. As a result of increased intestinal pressure the strangulated loop becomes distended, often to twice its normal diameter. As venous stasis increases, the arterial supply becomes more and more impaired. Blood is extravasated (an ecchymosis) under the serosa and is effused into the lumen. The fluid in the sac becomes bloodstained. The shining serosa becomes dull and covered by a fibrinous, sticky exudate. By this time the walls of the intestine have lost their tone; they are flabby, and are very friable. The lowered vitality of the intestine favours migration of bacteria through the intestinal wall, and the fluid in the sac teems with bacteria. Gangrene appears at the rings of constriction (fig. 1148), which become deeply furrowed and grey

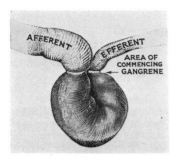

FIG. 1148.—Gangrene commences at the areas of constriction and then at the antimesenteric border.

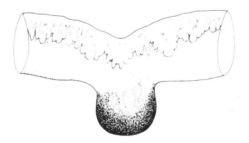

FIG. 1149.—Gangrenous Richter's hernia from a case of strangulated femoral hernia.

in colour, and then it appears in the antimesenteric border and spreads upwards, the colour varying from black to green according to the decomposition of blood in the subserosa. The mesentery involved by strangulation also becomes gangrenous. If the strangulation is unrelieved, perforation of the wall of the intestine occurs, either on the convexity of the loop or at the seat of constriction. Peritonitis spreads from the sac to the peritoneal cavity.

Clinical Features.—Sudden pain at first situated over the hernia is followed by generalised abdominal pain, paroxysmal in character and often located mainly at the umbilicus. Vomiting is forcible and usually oft-repeated. The patient may say that the hernia has recently become larger. *On examination, the hernia is tense, extremely tender, irreducible and there is no expansile impulse on coughing.*

Unless the strangulation is relieved by operation, the paroxysms of pain continue until peristaltic contractions cease with the onset of gangrene when paralytic ileus (often the result of peritonitis) and endotoxic shock (Chapter 5) develop. Spontaneous cessation of pain is therefore of grave significance.

Richter's Hernia is a hernia in which the sac contains only a portion of the circumference of the intestine (usually small intestine). It usually complicates femoral and, rarely, obturator hernias.

Strangulated Richter's Hernia (fig. 1149) is particularly dangerous as operation is frequently delayed because the clinical features mimic gastro-enteritis. The local signs of strangulation are often not obvious, the patient may not vomit, or vomits only once or twice. Intestinal colic occurs, but the bowels are often opened normally or there may be diarrhoea; absolute constipation is delayed until paralytic ileus supervenes. For these reasons gangrene of the knuckle of bowel and peritonitis often have occurred before operation is undertaken.

Strangulated Omentocele.—The initial symptoms are in general similar to those of strangulated bowel. Vomiting and constipation may be absent. Unlike intestine, omentum can exist on a very meagre blood-supply. The onset of gangrene is therefore correspondingly delayed, and it occurs first in the centre of the fatty mass. Unrelieved, a bacterial invasion of the dying contents of the sac will almost certainly occur. Infection is limited to the sac for days, and sometimes for weeks. In an inguinal hernia infection usually terminates as a scrotal abscess, but extension of peritonitis from the sac to the general peritoneal cavity is always a possibility.

Inflamed Hernia.—Inflammation can occur from inflammation of the contents within the sac, *e.g.* acute appendicitis or salpingitis, also from external causes, e.g. from a sore caused by an ill-fitting truss. The hernia is tender but *not* tense, and the overlying skin becomes red and oedematous. Operation is necessary to deal with the cause.

INDIVIDUAL FEATURES OF HERNIAS

Inguinal Hernia

Surgical Anatomy.—**The superficial inguinal ring** is a triangular aperture in the aponeurosis of the external oblique, and lies 1·25 cm above the pubic tubercle. The ring is bounded by a superomedial and an inferolateral crus joined by criss-cross intercrural fibres. Normally the ring will not admit the tip of the little finger (fig. 1150).

The deep inguinal ring is a U-shaped condensation of the transversalis fascia and it lies 1·25 cm above the inguinal (Poupart's) ligament, midway between the symphysis pubis and the anterior superior iliac spine. The transversalis fascia is the fascial envelope of the abdomen, and the competency of the deep inguinal ring depends upon the integrity of this fascia.

The Inguinal Canal.—In infants the superficial and deep inguinal rings are almost superimposed, and the obliquity of the canal is slight. In adults the inguinal canal, which is about 3·75 cm long, is directed downwards and medially from the deep to the superficial inguinal ring. In the male the inguinal canal transmits the spermatic cord, the ilio-inguinal nerve, and the genital branch of the genito-femoral nerve. In the female the round ligament replaces the spermatic cord.

Boundaries of the Inguinal Canal.—The best way to understand these is to study fig. 1150 (viewing the canal from the superficial to the deep layers as is seen at operation):

Thus, the boundaries of the inguinal canal are as follows:

Anteriorly.—fig. 1150A and B). External oblique aponeurosis. The conjoined muscle (mainly internal oblique) laterally.

Posteriorly.—Inferior epigastric artery; fascia transversalis; conjoined tendon (internal oblique and transversus-medially) (fig. 1150C and B).

Superiorly.—Conjoined muscles (internal oblique and transversus), (fig. 1150B).

Inferiorly.—Inguinal ligament (fig. 1150A, B and C).

An indirect inguinal hernia travels down the canal on the outer (lateral and anterior) side of the spermatic cord. A direct hernia comes out directly forwards through the posterior wall of the inguinal canal. While the neck of the indirect hernia is lateral to the

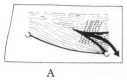 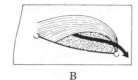 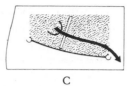

A   B   C

FIG. 1150.—The boundaries of the right inguinal canal. The inguinal ligament passes between the anterior superior iliac spine laterally, and the pubic tubercle medially. A depicts the superficial layer, the external oblique aponeurosis, the crura of the external ring and the intercrural fibres. B shows the conjoined muscle (internal oblique and transversus) arching over the cord. Laterally the conjoined muscle lies superficial to the cord and the internal ring, then above the cord and medially, as the conjoined tendon, behind the cord. C shows the deepest layer which is the transversalis fascia (the fascial envelope of the abdomen). The inferior epigastric artery is shown lying medial to the internal ring.

inferior epigastric vessels, the direct hernia usually emerges medial to this except in the saddle-bag or pantaloon type, which has both a lateral and a medial component. An inguinal hernia can be differentiated from a femoral hernia by ascertaining the relation of the neck of the sac to the medial end of the inguinal ligament and the pubic tubercle, *i.e.* in the case of an inguinal hernia the neck is above and medial, while that of a femoral hernia is below and lateral (fig. 1159). Digital control of the internal ring will help in distinguishing between an indirect inguinal hernia and a direct inguinal hernia.

Indirect (*syn.* **Oblique**) **Inguinal Hernia.**—This is the most common of all forms of hernia (and see Aetiology). It is most common in the young whereas a direct hernia is most common in the old. In the first decade of life inguinal hernia is more common on the right side in the male. This is no doubt associated with the later descent of the right testis. After the second decade left inguinal hernias are as frequent as right. The hernia is bilateral in nearly 30% of cases.[1]

Three types of oblique inguinal hernia occur (fig. 1151):
1. **Bubonocele.**—When the hernia is limited to the inguinal canal.
2. **Funicular.**—The processus vaginalis is closed just above the epididymis. The contents of the sac can be felt separately from the testis, which lies below the hernia.
3. **Complete** (*syn.* Scrotal).—A complete inguinal hernia is rarely present at birth but is commonly encountered in infancy. It also occurs in adolescence or adult life. The testis appears to lie within the lower part of the hernia.

Clinical Features[2]—Occurring at any age, males are twenty times more com-

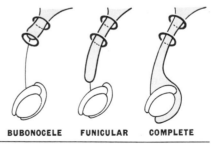

FIG. 1151.—Types of oblique inguinal hernia. Boubon. Gr. = the groin. Bubo = an enlarged lymph node in the groin or axilla. Funiculus. L. = a small cord.

BUBONOCELE   FUNICULAR   COMPLETE

[1] If both sides are explored in an infant presenting with one hernia, the incidence of a patent processus vaginalis on the other side is 60%.

[2] *Notes on the clinical examination.*—The clinician is seated in front of the patient who stands with his legs apart. He is instructed to look at the ceiling and to cough at the ceiling. If the hernia will come down it usually does. The examiner looks for the impulse and feels for the impulse and then satisfies himself on the following points: (1) Is the hernia right, or left, or bilateral? (2) Is it an inguinal or a femoral hernia? (see p. 1176). (3) Is it a direct or an indirect inguinal hernia? (4) Is it reducible or irreducible? (patient has to lie down for this to be ascertained). (5) Is the inguinal hernia incomplete (bubonocele) or complete (scrotal)? (6) What are the contents—bowel (enterocele), or omentum (omentocele or epiplocele)?

monly affected than females. The patient complains of pain in the groin or pain referred to the testicle when he is performing heavy work, or taking strenuous exercise. When he is asked to cough a small transient bulging may be seen and felt together with an expansile impulse. When the sac is still limited to the inguinal canal, the bulge may be better seen by observing the inguinal region from the side or even looking down the abdominal wall while standing slightly behind the respective shoulder of the patient.

As an oblique inguinal hernia increases in size it becomes apparent when the patient coughs, and persists until reduced (fig. 1152). As time goes on the hernia comes down as soon as the patient assumes the upright position. In large hernias there is a sensation of weight, and dragging on the mesentery may produce epigastric pain. If the contents of the sac are reducible, the inguinal canal will be found to be commodious (fig. 1153).

In infants the swelling appears when the child cries. It can be translucent in infancy and early childhood, but never in an adult. In girls an ovary may prolapse into the sac.

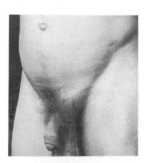

Fig. 1152.—Oblique left inguinal hernia which became apparent when the patient coughed, and persisted until it was reduced when he lay down.

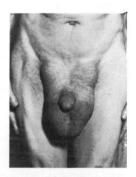

Fig. 1153.—Bilateral oblique inguinal herniae which have descended into the scrotum. The presence of bowel is confirmed by gurgling on reduction, or by the presence of bowel sounds on auscultation.

Differential Diagnosis in the Male.—(a) A vaginal hydrocele. (b) An encysted hydrocele of the cord. (c) Spermatocele. (d) A femoral hernia. (e) An incompletely descended testis in the inguinal canal. An inguinal hernia is often associated with this condition. (f) A lipoma of the cord. This is often a difficult, but unimportant, diagnosis. It is usually not settled until the parts are displayed by operation. N.B. Examination using finger and thumb across the neck of the scrotum will help to distinguish between a swelling of inguinal origin and one which is entirely intrascrotal.

Differential Diagnosis in the Female.—(a) A hydrocele of the canal of Nuck is the commonest differential diagnostic problem. (b) A femoral hernia.

Treatment of Indirect Inguinal Hernia

Operative Treatment.—*Operation is the treatment of choice.* It must be remembered that patients who have a bad cough from chronic bronchitis should not necessarily be denied operation, for these are the very people who are in danger of getting a strangulated hernia. In adults, local, epidural or spinal, as well as general anaesthesia can be used.

Inguinal Herniotomy is the basic operation which entails dissecting out and opening the hernial sac, reducing any contents and then transfixing the neck of the sac and removing the remainder. It is employed either by itself or as the first step in a repair procedure (herniorrhaphy). By itself it is sufficient for the treatment of hernia in infants, adolescents and young or fit adults who have

Anton Nuck, 1650–1692. Professor of Anatomy and Medicine, Leiden, Netherlands.

good inguinal musculature. In fact, any attempts at repair in such cases are meddlesome and do more harm than good.

In infants it is not necessary to open the canal, as the internal and external rings are superimposed. Excellent results are obtained. The operation should be done in the morning and the child allowed home in the evening. Usually there is no need for the child to stay in hospital. 'The best nurse is the mother.'

Herniotomy and Repair (Herniorrhapy).—This operation consists of (1) excision of the hernial sac (above) plus (2) repair of the stretched internal inguinal ring and the transversalis fascia and (3) further reinforcement of the posterior wall of the inguinal canal. (2) and (3) must be achieved without tension resulting in the wound, usually by darning with a monofilament suture material such as polypropylene. Fascial flaps, or Dacron mesh implants, are employed when the deficiency of the posterior wall is extensive.

OPERATIVE PROCEDURES

1. Excision of the Hernial Sac (Adult Herniotomy).—An incision[1] is made in the skin and subcutaneous tissues 1·25 cm above and parallel to the medial two-thirds of the inguinal ligament. In large irreducible herniae the incision is extended into the upper part of the scrotum. After dividing the superficial fascia and securing complete haemostasis, the external oblique aponeurosis and the superficial inguinal ring are identified. The external oblique aponeurosis is incised in the line of its fibres, and the structures beneath are carefully separated from its deep surface before completing the incision through the superficial inguinal ring. In this way the ilio-inguinal nerve is safeguarded. With the inguinal canal thus opened, the upper leaf of the external oblique aponeurosis is separated by blunt dissection from the internal oblique. The lower leaf is likewise dissected until the inner aspect of the inguinal ligament is seen. The cremasteric muscle fibres are divided longitudinally to open up the subcremasteric space and display the spermatic cord, which is then lifted out.

Excision of the sac. The indirect sac is easily distinguished as a pearly white structure lying on the outer side of the cord and, when the internal spermatic fascia has been incised longitudinally, it can be dissected out and then opened between haemostats.

Variations in Dissection.—If the sac is small (*e.g.* bubonocele) it can be freed *in toto*. If it is of the long funicular or scrotal type, or is extremely thickened and adherent, the fundus need not be sought. The sac is freed and divided in the inguinal canal. Care must be taken to avoid damage to the vas and the spermatic artery, including the blood supply to the epididymis.

An adherent sac can be separated from the cord by first injecting saline under the posterior wall from within. A similar tactic is used when dissecting the gossamer sac of infants and children.

Reduction of Contents.—Intestine or omentum is returned to the peritoneal cavity. Omentum is often adherent to neck or fundus of the sac; if to the neck, it is freed, and if to the fundus of a large sac, it may be transfixed, ligated and cut across at a suitable site. The distal part of omentum, like the distal part of a large scrotal sac, can be left *in situ* (the fundus should not, however, be ligated).

Isolation and Ligation of the Neck of the Sac.—Whatever type of sac is encountered, it is necessary to free its neck by blunt and gauze dissection until the parietal peritoneum can be seen on all sides. Only when the extraperitoneal fat is encountered and the inferior epigastric vessels are seen on the medial side has the dissection reached the required limit. If it has not been done already, the sac is opened. The finger is passed through the mouth of the sac in order to make sure that no bowel or omentum is adherent. The neck of the sac is transfixed and ligated as high as possible, and the sac is excised 1·25 cm below the ligature.

2. Repair of the Transversalis Fascia and the Internal Ring.—When the internal

---

[1] Prior to the skin incision in large inguino-scrotal hernias, the usual antiseptic preparation of the skin should not be extended to the perineal aspect of the scrotum, for, by so doing, severe bacterial contamination of the operation site is likely.

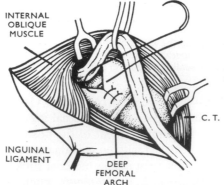

INTERNAL
OBLIQUE
MUSCLE

INGUINAL
LIGAMENT

DEEP
FEMORAL
ARCH

C. T.

FIG. 1154.—The Lytle method of repair of the stretched internal inguinal ring which should be narrowed to admit the tip of the little finger. Lateral displacement of the cord is often advantageous. C.T. = Conjoined Tendon.
(After F. S. A. Doran, FRCS, Bromsgrove.)

ring is weak and stretched, and the transversalis fascia is bulging, the repair should include the *Lytle method* of repairing and narrowing the ring with lateral displacement of the cord (fig. 1154), or the **Toronto (Shouldice) method**, whereby the ring and fascia are incised and carefully separated from the deep inferior epigastric vessels and extraperitoneal fat before an overlapping repair ('double breasting') of the lower flap behind the upper flap is effected. This repair using monofilament continuous suturing or darning materials (*e.g.* polypropylene, polyamide, wire) and avoiding tension is the basis for obtaining good results (p. 1188).

3. Reinforcement of the Posterior Inguinal Wall is achieved by approximating without tension the tendinous and aponeurotic part of the conjoined muscle to the pubic tubercle (and, according to some, to Astley Cooper's iliopectineal ligament) and to the under surface of the inguinal ligament. Care is taken not to pick up the same tendinous bundle for each suture. Suturing of muscle bundles is of no value. The suturing method includes (*a*) simple interrupted (Bassini type), (*b*) darning (fig. 1155), (*c*) a rectus relaxing incision (Halsted-Tanner), (*d*) a Dacron mesh implant (fig. 1156). Other techniques include overlapping the external oblique behind the cord (making it lie subcutaneously). Special care is needed to avoid excessive narrowing of the new external ring which would jeopardise the vascular supply to and the venous return from the testis.

4. Completion of Operation.—If possible the cremasteric muscle should be reconstituted: the external oblique is directly sutured or overlapped leaving a new external ring which will accommodate the tip of the little finger.

A Truss: A truss is used when operation is contraindicated because of cardiac, pulmonary, or other systemic disease, or when operation is refused. The hernia must be reducible. A rat-tailed spring truss with a perineal band to prevent the truss slipping will, with due care and attention, contrcl a small or moderate-sized inguinal hernia. A truss must be worn continuously during waking hours, kept clean, and in proper repair, and renewed when it shows signs of wear. It must be applied before the patient gets up and while the hernia is reduced. A properly-fitting truss must control the hernia when the patient stands with his legs wide apart, stoops, and coughs violently. If it does not it is a menace, for it increases the risk of strangulation.

Infants and Trusses.—Special inflatable rubber trusses, formerly popular for the control of an infant's hernia, are rarely used. Provided urgent admission is not required for sudden irreducibility, the parents are advised to wait until operation is performed when the infant is at least three months old.

Direct Inguinal Hernia.—Between 10 and 15% of inguinal hernias are direct. Over half of these are bilateral.

A direct inguinal hernia is always acquired. The sac passes through a weakness or defect of the transversalis fascia in the posterior wall of the inguinal canal. In some cases the defect is small and closely related to the insertion of the conjoint tendon, while in others there is a generalised bulge. Often the patient has poor lower abdominal musculature, as shown by the presence of elongated bulgings (Malgaigne's bulges). Women practically never develop a direct inguinal hernia

William James Lytle, 1896–1986. Surgeon, Royal Infirmary, Sheffield, England.
Edoardo Bassini, 1844–1924. Professor of Surgery of Padua, Italy.
William Stewart Halsted, 1852–19. Surgeon, Johns Hopkins Hospital, Baltimore, Maryland, U.S.A.
Joseph François Malgaigne, 1806–1865. Professor of Surgery, Paris.
Norman Cecil Tanner, 1906–1982. Surgeon, Charing Cross Hospital, London.

(Brown). Predisposing factors are a chronic cough, straining, and heavy work. Damage to the ilioinguinal nerve (previous appendicectomy) is another possible cause.

Direct hernias rarely attain a large size or descend into the scrotum. In contradistinction to an oblique inguinal hernia, a direct inguinal hernia lies behind the spermatic cord. The sac is often smaller than the hernial mass would indicate, the protruding mass mainly consisting of extraperitoneal fat. As the neck of the sac is wide, direct inguinal hernias rarely strangulate.

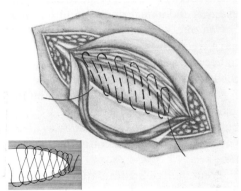

FIG. 1155.—The first layer of the two-layer darn of the posterior wall of the inguinal canal. The darning is conducted from the pubic tubercle up to and above the deep inguinal ring and back to the starting point. The darning is kept fairly loose, and it forms a lattice upon which fibrous tissue is laid down. The external oblique aponeurosis is reunited either in front or behind the cord. Meticulous asepsis is essential. Inset: An alternative lattice darn.

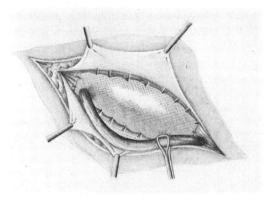

FIG. 1156.—Dacron mesh reinforcement. The mesh is attached to the inguinal ligament, the coverings of the pubis, the rectus sheath and the conjoined aponeurosis and tendon. It is also fashioned by a slot laterally above and below the cord at the internal ring.

Funicular direct inguinal hernia (*syn.* prevesical hernia) is a narrow-necked hernia with prevesical fat and a portion of the bladder that occurs through a small oval defect in the medial part of the conjoined tendon just above the pubic tubercle. It occurs principally in elderly males, and occasionally it becomes strangulated. Unless there are definite contraindications, operation should always be advised.

Dual (*syn.* **Saddle-bag; Pantaloon**) **Hernia.**—Here there are two sacs which straddle the inferior epigastric artery, one sac being medial and the other lateral to this vessel. The condition is not a rarity, and is a cause of recurrence, one of the sacs having been overlooked at the time of operation.

Operation for Direct Hernia.—The principles of repair of direct hernia are the same as those of an indirect hernia with the exception that the hernial sac need not be removed, for after it has been dissected free from surrounding structures it is inverted into the abdomen and the transversalis fascia repaired in front of it. Some form of reconstruction of the posterior wall of the inguinal canal is necessary, Polypropylene darns, and Dacron mesh implantations are popular (figs. 1155 and 1156).

Francis Robert Brown, 1889–1967. Surgeon, Royal Infirmary, Dundee, Scotland.

Strangulated Inguinal Hernia

(**Pathological and Clinical Features** are described on pp. 1167–1168.)

Strangulation of an inguinal hernia occurs at any time during life, and in both sexes. Oblique inguinal hernias strangulate commonly; the direct variety but rarely owing to the wide neck of the sac. Sometimes a hernia strangulates on the first occasion that it descends; more often strangulation occurs in patients who have worn a truss for a long time, and in those with a partially reducible or irreducible hernia.

In order of frequency, the constricting agent is: (*a*) the neck of the sac; (*b*) the external abdominal ring in children; (*c*) rarely adhesions within the sac.

Contents.—Usually small intestine is involved in the strangulation; the next most frequent is omentum; sometimes both are implicated. For large intestine to become strangulated in an inguinal hernia is of the utmost rarity, even when the hernia is of the sliding variety.

Strangulation during Infancy.—The incidence of strangulation is 4% (Gross), and the ratio of females to males is 5:1. More frequently the hernia is irreducible but not strangulated. In most cases of strangulated inguinal hernia occurring in female infants the content of the sac is an ovary, or an ovary plus its Fallopian tube.

Treatment of Strangulated Inguinal Hernia.—The treatment of strangulated hernia is by *emergency operation.*[1]

If dehydration and collapse are present, intravenous fluid replacement (Chapter 6) and gastric aspiration for one to three hours are invaluable. It is *absolutely essential* to make sure that the stomach is emptied just before commencing the anaesthetic. The passing of a large-bore stomach tube is the best way of prevening vomiting, drowning, and cardiac arrest during the induction. The bladder must also be emptied, if necessary by a catheter. Suitable broad spectrum antimicrobials (Chapter 3) are given i.v.

Inguinal Herniotomy for Strangulation.—An incision is made over the most prominent part of the swelling. The external oblique aponeurosis is exposed, and the sac, with its coverings, is seen issuing from the superficial inguinal ring. In all but very large hernias it is possible to deliver the body and fundus of the sac together with its coverings and (in the male) the testis on to the surface. Each layer covering the anterior surface of the body of the sac near the fundus is incised, and if possible it is stripped off the sac. The sac is then incised, the fluid therein is mopped up or aspirated very thoroughly, for it can be highly infected. The external oblique aponeurosis and the superficial inguinal ring are divided. Returning to the sac, a finger is passed into the opening, and employing the finger as a guide, the sac is slit along its length. If the constriction lies at the superficial inguinal ring or in the inguinal canal, it is readily divided by this procedure. When the constricting agent is at the deep inguinal ring, by applying haemostats to the cut edge of the neck of the sac and drawing them downwards, and at the same time retracting the internal oblique upwards, it may be possible to continue slitting up the sac over the finger beyond the point of constriction. When the constriction is too tight to admit a finger, a grooved director is inserted and the neck of the sac is divided with a hernia knife in an upward and inward direction, *i.e.* parallel to the inferior epigastric artery, under vision. Once the constricting agent has been divided, the strangulated contents can be drawn down. Devitalised omentum is excised after being securely ligated, by interlocking stitches if bulky. Viable intestine is returned to the peritoneal cavity. Doubtfully viable and gangrenous intestine is dealt with as described on p. 1072. If the hernial sac is of moderate size and can be separated easily from its coverings, it is excised and closed by a purse-

---

'The danger is in the delay, not in the operation'—Astley Cooper.

Robert Edward Gross, Contemporary, Ladd Professor of Children's Surgery, Harvard University Medical School, Boston, Mass., U.S.A. Sir Astley Paston Cooper, 1768–1841. Surgeon, Guy's Hospital, London.

string suture. When the sac is large and adherent, much time is saved by cutting across the sac as described (p. 1171). Having tied or sutured the neck of the sac a repair can be made if the condition of the patient permits.

Conservative Measures.—These are only indicated in infants. The child is given a sedative and then slung to a Balkan beam[1] or to the bedrail by his feet (the judgment of Solomon[2] position) for no longer than three hours. In 75% of cases reduction is effected and there appears to be no danger of gangrenous intestine being reduced (Irvine Smith).

N.B.—Vigorous manipulation (taxis) has no place in modern surgery, and is mentioned only to be condemned. Its dangers include: 1. *Contusion or rupture of the intestinal wall.* 2. *Reduction-en-masse.* 'The sac together with its contents, is pushed forcibly back into the abdomen; and as the bowel will still be strangulated by the neck of the sac, the symptoms are in no way relieved' (Treves). 3. *Reduction into a loculus of the sac.* 4. The sac may rupture at its neck and its contents are reduced, not into the peritoneal cavity, but extraperitoneally.

Maydl's hernia(*syn.* Hernia-in-W) is rare. The strangulated loop of the W lies within the abdomen, thus local tenderness over the hernia is not marked. At operation two comparatively normal-looking loops of intestine are present in the sac. After the obstruction has been relieved, the strangulated loop will become apparent if traction is exerted on the middle of the loops occupying the sac.

Results of Operations for Inguinal Hernia. Recurrence.—Only by using a meticulous technique, principally concentrating on the repair of the transversalis fascia and the internal ring, can a recurrence rate of less than 2% be achieved. Recurrences through the repair tend to occur within 2 years. In a few cases false recurrences occur, i.e. another type of hernia occurs—direct after indirect, femoral after direct or indirect. To the patient it is a recurrence! In elderly men orchiectomy facilitates a secure repair.

The Spermatic Cord as a Barrier to Effective Closure of the Inguinal Canal.—In the elderly patient, removal of the testis and cord aids in an effective repair in the case of recurrent inguinal hernia, sliding hernia, and some large direct hernias. The signed permission of the patient must always be obtained beforehand.

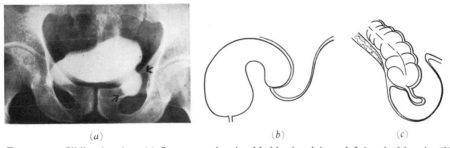

(a)   *(b)*   *(c)*

FIG. 1157.—Sliding hernia.—(*a*) Cystogram showing bladder involving a left inguinal hernia. (*b*) Diagram of the same. (*c*) Caecum and appendix in right sliding hernia.

Sliding Hernia (*syn.* **Hernie-en-Glissade**) (**fig. 1157**).—As a result of slipping of the posterior parietal peritoneum on the underlying retroperitoneal structures, the posterior wall of the sac is not formed of peritoneum alone, but by the sigmoid colon and its mesentery on the left, the caecum on the right and, sometimes, on either side by a portion of the bladder. It should be clearly understood that the caecum, appendix, or a portion of the colon *wholly within* a hernial sac does not constitute a sliding hernia. A small bowel sliding hernia occurs once in 2000 cases; a sacless sliding hernia once in 8000 cases.

---

[1] An overhead beam or bar for applying traction to a fractured femur, first used in the Balkan theatre of war, 1914–1918.

[2] Solomon, King of Israel. The story of the judgment of Solomon is told in the Bible 1 Kings III, 16–28.

Karel Maydl, 1853–1903. Professor of Surgery, Prague, Czechoslovakia.
Irvine Battinson Smith, Contemporary. Surgeon, Burton-on-Trent General Hospital, Staffs., England.
Sir Frederick Treves, 1853–1923. Surgeon, The London Hospital.

Clinical Features.—A sliding hernia occurs almost exclusively in males. Five out of six sliding herniae are situated on the left side; bilateral sliding herniae are exceedingly rare. The patient is nearly always over forty, the incidence rising with the weight of years. There are no clinical findings that are pathognomonic of a sliding hernia, but it should be suspected in every large globular inguinal hernia descending well into the scrotum.

Occasionally large intestine is strangulated in a sliding hernia; more often non-strangulated large intestine is present behind the sac containing strangulated small intestine.

Treatment.—A sliding hernia is impossible to control with a truss, and as a rule the hernia is a cause of considerable discomfort. Consequently operation is indicated, and the results generally are good.

Operation.—It is unnecessary to remove any of the sliding hernial sac provided it is freed completely from the cord and the abdominal wall, and that it is replaced deep to the repaired fascia transversalis. In many instances it is desirable to perform orchiectomy (p. 1175) in order to effect a secure repair. No attempt should be made to dissect the caecum or colon free from the peritoneum under the impression that these are adhesions, in which case peritonitis or a faecal fistula resulting from necrosis of a devascularised portion of the bowel may occur. This is specially liable to occur on the left side, as vessels in the meso-colon may be injured.

Femoral Hernia

Femoral hernia is the third most common type of hernia (incisional hernia comes second). It accounts for about 20% of herniae in women, and 5% in men. The overriding importance of femoral hernia lies in the facts that it cannot be controlled by a truss, and that of all hernias it is the most liable to become strangulated mainly because of the narrowness of the neck of the sac and the rigidity of the femoral ring.

Surgical Anatomy.—The femoral canal occupies the most medial compartment of the femoral sheath, and it extends from the femoral ring above to the saphenous opening below. It is 1·25 cm long, and 1·25 cm wide at its base, which is directed upwards. The femoral canal contains fat, lymphatic vessels, and the lymph node of Cloquet. It is closed above by the septum crurale, a condensation of extraperitoneal tissue pierced by lymphatic vessels, and below by the cribriform fascia.

The femoral ring is bounded;
Anteriorly by the inguinal ligament.
Posteriorly by Astley Cooper's (ilio-pectineal) ligament, the pubic bone, and the fascia over the pectineus muscle.
Medially by the concave knife-like edge of Gimbernat's (lacunar) ligament, which is also prolonged along the ilio-pectineal line as Astley Cooper's ligament.
Laterally by a thin septum separating it from the femoral vein.

Sex Incidence.—The female to male ratio is about 2:1, but it is interesting that whereas the female patients are frequently elderly, the male patients are usually between thirty to forty-five years. The condition is more prevalent in women who have borne children than in nulliparae.

Pathology.—A hernia passing down the femoral canal descends vertically as far as the saphenous opening. While it is confined to the inelastic walls of the femoral canal the hernia is necessarily narrow, but once it escapes through the saphenous opening into the loose areolar tissue of the groin, it expands, sometimes considerably. A fully distended femoral hernia assumes the shape of a retort, and its bulbous extremity may be above the inguinal ligament. By the time the contents have pursued so tortuous a path they are usually irreducible and apt to strangulate.

Clinical Features.—Femoral hernia is rare before puberty. Between twenty

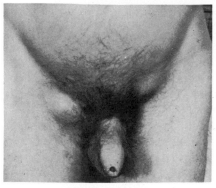

FIG. 1158.—The patient has a left inguinal and a right femoral hernia.

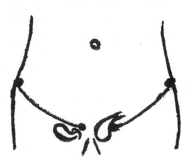

FIG. 1159.—The essentials of differential diagnosis between a femoral and an inguinal hernia (see text).

and forty years of age the prevalence rises, and continues to old age. The right side (fig. 1158) is affected twice as often as the left, and in 20% of cases the condition is bilateral. The symptoms to which a femoral hernia gives rise are less pronounced than those of an inguinal hernia; indeed, a small femoral hernia may be unnoticed by the patient or disregarded for years, until perhaps the day it strangulates. Adherence of greater omentum sometimes causes a dragging pain. Rarely, a large sac is present.

Differential Diagnosis—A Femoral Hernia has to be distinguished from:
(i) *An Inguinal Hernia.*—An inguinal hernia lies above and medial to the medial end of the inguinal ligament at its attachment to the pubic tubercle. The femoral hernia lies below this (fig. 1159). Occasionally the fundus of a femoral hernia sac overlies the inguinal ligament.
(2) *A Saphena Varix.*—A saphena varix is a saccular enlargement of the termination of the long saphenous vein and it is usually accompanied by other signs of varicose veins. The swelling disappears completely when the patient lies down, while a femoral hernia sac usually is still palpable. In both there is an impulse on coughing. A saphena varix will, however, impart a fluid thrill to the examining fingers when the patient coughs, or when the saphenous vein below the varix is tapped with the fingers of the other hand. Sometimes a venous hum can be heard when a stethoscope is applied over a saphena varix.
(3) *An Enlarged Femoral Lymph Node.*—If there are other enlarged lymph nodes in the region the diagnosis is tolerably simple, but when Cloquet's lymph node alone is affected the diagnosis may be impossible unless there is a clue, such as an infected wound or abrasion on the corresponding limb or on the perineum.
(4) *Lipoma.*
(5) *A Femoral Aneurysm.*—(Chapter 14).
(6) *A Psoas Abscess.*—There is often a fluctuating swelling—an iliac abscess—which communicates with the swelling in question. Examination of the spine and an x-ray will settle the diagnosis.
(7) *A distended Psoas Bursa.*—The swelling diminishes when the hip is flexed, and osteoarthrosis of the hip is present.
(8) *Rupture of the adductor longus* with haematoma.
Hydrocele of a Femoral Hernial Sac.—The neck of the sac becomes plugged with omentum or by adhesions, and a hydrocele of the hernial sac results.
Laugier's femoral hernia is a hernia through a gap in the lacunar (Gimbernat's) ligament. The diagnosis is based on unusual medial position of a small femoral hernial sac. Nearly always the hernia has strangulated.
Narath's femoral hernia occurs only in patients with congenital dislocation of the hip and is due to lateral displacement of the psoas muscle. The hernia lies hidden behind the femoral vessels.

Stanislas Laugier, 1799–1872. Surgeon, Hôtel Dieu, Paris.
Albert Narath, 1864–1924. Professor of Surgery, Heidelberg, Germany.

Cloquet's hernia is one in which the sac lies under the fascia covering the pectineus muscle. Strangulation is likely. The sac may coexist with the usual type of femoral sac.

Strangulated Femoral Hernia.—*A femoral hernia strangulates frequently and gangrene develops rapidly.* This is accounted for by the narrow, unyielding femoral ring. In 40% of cases the obstructing agent is not Gimbernat's (lacunar) ligament but the narrow neck of the femoral sac itself (Henry Souttar). The frequent occurrence of a *Richter's hernia* also must be stressed (p. 1168).

Treatment of Femoral Hernia. The constant risk of strangulation is sufficient reason for urging operation. A truss is contraindicated because of this risk.

Operative Treatment.—The low operation (Lockwood), the high operation (McEvedy), and the inguinal operation (Lotheissen) all have their advocates. In all cases the bladder *must* be emptied immediately before commencing the operation.

The Low Operation (Lockwood).—The sac is dissected out below the inguinal ligament via a groin-crease incision. It is essential to peel off all the anatomical layers which cover the sac. These are often thick and fatty. After dealing with the contents (*e.g.* freeing adherent omentum) the neck of the sac is pulled down, ligated as high as possible and allowed to retract through the femoral canal. The canal is closed by suturing the inguinal ligament to the ilio-pectineal line using three unabsorbable sutures.

The High (McEvedy) Operation.—A vertical incision is made over the femoral canal and continued upwards above the inguinal ligament. Through the lower part of the incision the sac is dissected out. The upper part of the incision exposes the inguinal ligament and the rectus sheath. The superficial inguinal ring is identified, and an incision 2·5 cm above the ring and parallel to the outer border of the rectus muscle is deepened until the extraperitoneal space is found. By gauze dissection in this space the hernial sac entering the femoral canal can be easily identified. Should the sac be empty and small, it can be drawn upwards; if it is large, the fundus is opened below, and its contents, if any, dealt with appropriately before delivering the sac upwards from its canal. The sac is then freed from the extraperitoneal tissue and its neck is ligated. An excellent view of the iliopectineal ligament is obtained and the conjoined tendon is sutured to it with non-absorbable sutures (fig. 1160).

Strangulation.—An advantage of the operation is that if resection of intestine is required, ample room can be obtained by opening the peritoneum. The disadvantage of the operation is that if infection occurs incisional hernia is not very unusual.

Lotheissen's Operation.—The inguinal canal is opened as for *inguinal* herniorrhaphy. The transversalis fascia is incised to the medial side of the epigastric vessels and the opening is enlarged. The peritoneum is now in view; one must be certain that it *is* the peritoneum and not the bladder or a diverticulum thereof. The peritoneum is picked up with dissecting forceps, and incised. It is now possible to ascertain if any intraperitoneal structure is entering the femoral sac. Should the sac be empty, haemostats are placed upon the edges of the opening into the peritoneum, and by gauze dissection the sac is withdrawn from the femoral canal. An empty sac can be delivered easily; in the event of the sac being occupied, the technique described below for strangulation should be followed.

The Lotheissen Repair.—The conjoined tendon is sutured to the iliopectineal line to form a shutter. While protecting the external iliac/femoral vein with the forefinger, unabsorbable sutures are passed through the periosteum and Cooper's ligament overlying the iliopectineal line (fig. 1161). The retractor having been removed, the long ends of the sutures are passed from within, outwards, through the conjoined tendon, and tied, thus approximating the conjoined tendon to the iliopectineal line. If there is any tension, a Tanner's slide will facilitate this step. The incised external oblique is sutured.

Strangulation. Modified Lotheissen Operation.—As soon as the external oblique has been exposed, the inferior margin of the wound is retracted strongly, thereby displaying the swelling. The coverings of the sac are incised and peeled off, until the sac, dark from contained bloodstained fluid, is apparent. The sac is incised, and the fluid that escapes is mopped up with great care. The retractor is removed and the operation is continued above the inguinal ligament in the same way as described already. Once the peritoneum has been

Sir Henry Sessions Souttar, 1875–1964. Surgeon, The London Hospital.
Charles Barret Lockwood, 1856–1914. Surgeon, St. Bartholomew's Hospital, London.
Peter George McEvedy, 1890–1941. Surgeon, Ancoats Hospital, Manchester, England.
Georg Lotheissen, 1868–1941. Surgeon, Kaiser Franz Joseph Hospital, Vienna.

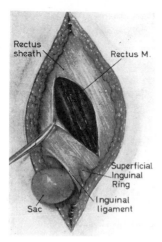

FIG. 1160.—McEvedy's
operation. Right side.

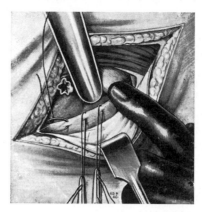

FIG. 1161.—Method of placing the deep
sutures (see text). The finger is protecting
the left external iliac/femoral vein.

opened above the inguinal ligament, one can see exactly what is entering the sac. Should the obstruction lie in a narrow neck of the sac, the beak of a haemostat is insinuated, and with great care the neck is stretched.[1] The contents of the sac are delivered, and dealt with. Sometimes, in order to facilitate reduction of the hernial contents, it becomes necessary to divide or digitally to avulse part of Gimbernat's ligament.

N.B.—It must be repeated that throughout operations for the repair of a femoral hernia, *on the lateral side*, the external iliac/femoral vein must be protected, and *on the medial side* great care must be taken not to injure the bladder, particularly since a portion of the bladder may form part of the wall of the sac (a sliding femoral hernia).

Umbilical Hernia

Exomphalos (*syn.* omphalocele) occurs once in every 6000 births; it is due to failure of all or part of the mid-gut to return to the coelom during early fetal life. Sometimes a large sac ruptures during birth (fig 1162). When the sac remains unruptured, it is semi-translucent, and although very thin it consists of three

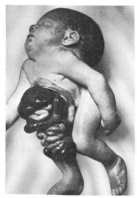

FIG. 1162.— Exomphalos.
The delicate sac burst during
delivery.

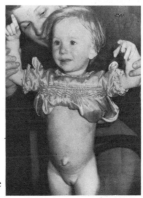

FIG. 1163.—Infantile
umbilical hernia.

---

[1] An abnormal obturator artery is present either on the medial or the lateral side of the neck of the sac in 28% of cases.

layers—an outer layer of amniotic membrane, a middle layer of Wharton's jelly, and an inner layer of peritoneum. There are two varieties of exomphalos:

Exomphalos Minor.—The sac is relatively small and to its summit is attached the umbilical cord. Inadvertently a loop of small intestine or a Meckel's diverticulum can be included in the ligature applied to the base of an umbilical cord containing this protrusion.

Exomphalos Major.—The umbilical cord is attached to the inferior aspect of the swelling, which contains small and large intestine, and nearly always a portion of the liver. Half the cases belong to this group.

Treatment: (*a*) *Exomphalos Minor.*—It is necessary only to twist the cord, so as to reduce the contents of the sac through the narrow umbilical opening into the peritoneal cavity, and to retain them by firm strapping. Despite a sero-purulent discharge on no account must the strapping be removed for fourteen days.

(*b*) *Exomphalos Major.*—Operation within the first few hours of life is the only hope, otherwise the sac will burst. In order to prevent further distension of the contents of the sac, the infant should not be fed. A few newborn infants with a ruptured sac have survived following immediate operation and antibiotic therapy.

Operation.—It must be realised that most of the contents of the sac have never been housed within the abdominal cavity; consequently that cavity is unduly small, and to attempt to replace the contents of the sac is like endeavouring to put 2 kg of sugar into a 1 kg bag—a feat that so often results in respiratory embarrassment, compromise of venous return, and possibly intestinal obstruction. It is necessary to create flaps of skin by undermining the subcutaneous tissue on either side, so that the flaps can be brought together over the sac. If necessary relaxing incisions must be made in the loins to permit closure. For several days following the operation it is advisable to carry out aspiration through an indwelling gastric tube, in order to relieve or prevent distension. If the patient survives the construction of this protective cutaneous coverage, repair of the hernia can be delayed for months, or even years. At the second operation, it is surprising to find that the peritoneum and the muscles can be drawn together and closed in layers.

Congenital Umbilical Hernia.—Rarely, a fully developed umbilical hernia is present at birth presumably due to intra-uterine epithelialisation of a small exomphalos.

Umbilical Hernia of Infants and Children.—This is a hernia through a weak umbilical scar usually the result of neonatal sepsis. The ratio of males to females is 2:1 The hernia is often symptomless, but increases in the size of the hernia by crying causes pain, which makes the infant cry the more. Small hernias are spherical; those that increase in size tend to assume a conical shape (fig. 1163) and are present apart from crying. Obstruction or strangulation below the age of three years is extremely uncommon.

Treatment.—Conservative treatment by *masterly inactivity* is successful in about 93% of cases. When the hernia is symptomless, reassurances of the parents is all that is necessary, for in a very high percentage of cases the hernia will be found to disappear spontaneously during the first few months of life. Cure may also be hastened by pulling the skin and abdominal musculature together by adhesive strapping placed across the abdomen.

Herniorrhaphy.—In cases where masterly inactivity fails, operation is required, and it should be carried out, preferably, about the age of two years.

Operation.—In infants a small curved incision is made immediately below the umbilicus. The skin cicatrix is dissected upwards, and the neck of the sac is isolated. After ensuring that the sac is empty of contents, it is either inverted into the abdomen or it is ligated by transfixion and excised. The defect in the linea alba is closed with two unabsorbable sutures.

Para-umbilical Hernia of Adults (*syn.* supra-, infra-umbilical hernia).—In adults the hernia does *not* occur through the umbilical scar. It is a protrusion

---

Thomas Wharton, 1614–1673. Physician, St. Thomas's Hospital, London.

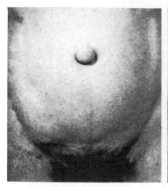

FIG. 1164.—Small.

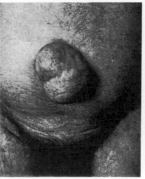

FIG. 1165.—Large.
Para-umbilical hernias

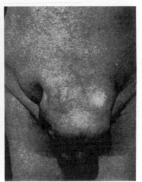

FIG. 1166..—Very large.

through the linea alba just above or sometimes just below the umbilicus (fig.1164). As it enlarges, it becomes rounded or oval in shape (fig. 1165) with a tendency to sag downwards. Para-umbilical hernias can become very large (fig. 1166). The neck of the sac is often remarkably narrow as compared with the size of the sac and the volume of its contents, which consist of greater omentum often accompanied by small intestine and, alternatively or in addition, a portion of the transverse colon. In old-standing cases the sac sometimes becomes loculated due to adherence of omentum to its fundus.

Clinical Features.—Women are affected five times more frequently than men. The patient is usually corpulent and between the ages of thirty-five and fifty. Increasing obesity, with flabbiness of the abdominal muscles, and repeated pregnancy are important factors. These hernias soon become irreducible because of omental adhesions within the sac. A large umbilical hernia causes a local dragging pain by its weight. Gastro-intestinal symptoms are common and are probably due to traction on the stomach or transverse colon. Often there are transient attacks of intestinal colic due to subacute intestinal obstruction. In old-standing cases intertrigo of the adjacent surfaces of the skin is a troublesome complication.

Treatment.—Untreated, the hernia increases in size, and more and more of its contents become irreducible. Eventually, strangulation may occur. Therefore without undue delay operation should be advised in nearly all cases. If the patient is obese and the hernia is symptomless, operation can be postponed with advantage until weight has been reduced.

Mayo's Operation.—A transverse elliptical incision is made around the umbilicus. The subcutaneous tissues are dissected off the rectus sheath to expose the neck of the sac. The neck is incised to expose the contents. Intestine is returned to the abdomen. Any adherent omentum is freed, and ligated by transfixion if it is bleeding. Excess adherent omentum can be removed with the sac if necessary. The sac is then removed and the peritoneum of the neck closed with catgut. The aponeurosis on both sides of the umbilical ring is incised transversely for 2·5 cm or more—sufficiently to allow an overlap of 5 or 7.5 cm. Three to five mattress sutures are then inserted into the aponeurosis as shown in fig. 1167. When this row of mattress sutures has been tied, the over-lapping upper margin is stitched to the sheath of the rectus abdominis and the midline aponeurosis. In fat patients, who ooze blood and liquid fat, a drain is provided at each end of the wound. The subcutaneous fat and skin are then approximated with deep sutures. If the patient has a tendency to bronchitis, it is wise to prescribe antibiotic therapy and breathing exercises.

William James Mayo, 1861–1939. Surgeon, The Mayo Clinic, Rochester, Minnesota, U.S.A., described this operation in 1901.

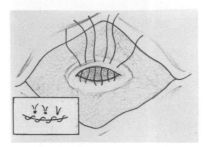

Fig. 1167.—Mayo's operation for umbilical hernia. Interrupted sutures to provide an overlap are first inserted. Inset.—The overlap has been made and completed with a continuous suture. It is important to denude the area of fat before stitching the flap in position.

Additional Lipectomy.—In patients with a para-umbilical hernia associated with a large, pendulous, fat-laden abdominal wall the operation can, with great advantage, be combined with lipectomy by fashioning the incisions to embrace a larger area of the fat-laden superficial layers of the abdominal wall.

Strangulation is a frequent complication of a large para-umbilical hernia in adults. Owing to the narrow neck and the fibrous edge of the linea alba, gangrene is liable to supervene unless early operation is carried out. Also it should be remembered that in large hernias, the presence of loculi may result in a strangulated knuckle of the bowel in one part of an otherwise soft and non-tender hernia.

Operation.—In early cases the operation does not differ from that for non-strangulated cases. Gangrenous contents are dealt with as in other situations. If a portion of the transverse colon is gangrenous, it should be exteriorised by the Paul-Mikulicz method (fig. 1075) and the gangrenous portion excised. If the ring is large enough to transmit the colon unhampered, it is left alone; otherwise it is enlarged. It is important that the small intestine be thoroughly scrutinised as a small loop may have been trapped and slipped back when the constriction was relieved. If non-viable gut is overlooked, peritonitis quietly supervenes, and the symptoms are ascribed to 'post-operative discomfort'. The condition of the patient steadily deteriorates until she succumbs after a few days (Franklin).

Epigastric Hernia (*syn.* Fatty Hernia of the Linea Alba)

An epigastric hernia occurs through the linea alba anywhere between the xiphoid process and the umbilicus, usually midway between these structures. Such a hernia commences as a protrusion of extra-peritoneal fat through the linea alba, where the latter is pierced by a small blood-vessel. Sometimes more than one hernia is present.

A swelling the size of a pea consists of a protrusion of extraperitoneal fat only (fatty hernia of the linea alba). If the protrusion enlarges, it drags a pouch of peritoneum after it, and so becomes a true epigastric hernia. The mouth of the hernia is rarely large enough to permit a portion of hollow viscus to enter it; consequently, either the sac is empty or it contains a small portion of greater omentum.

It is probable that an epigastric hernia is the direct result of a sudden strain tearing the interlacing fibres of the linea alba. The patients are often manual workers between thirty and forty-five years of age.

Clinical Features.—(*a*) *Symptomless.*—A small fatty hernia of the linea alba can be felt better than it can be seen, and may be symptomless, being discovered only in the course of routine abdominal palpation.

(*b*) *Painful.*—Sometimes such a hernia gives rise to attacks of local pain, worse

Richard Harrington Franklin, Contemporary. Consulting Surgeon, Royal Postgraduate Medical School, London.

on physical exertion, and tenderness to touch and tight clothing, possibly because the fatty contents become nipped sufficiently to produce partial strangulation.

(c) *Referred Pain* (Peptic ulcer cases).—It is not uncommon to find that the patient, who may not have noticed the hernia, complains of pain suggestive of a peptic ulcer.

Treatment.—If the hernia is giving rise to symptoms, operation should be undertaken.

Operation.—An adequate vertical or transverse incision is made over the swelling, exposing the linea alba. The protruding extraperitoneal fat is cleared from the hernial orifice by gauze dissection. If the pedicle passing through the linea alba is slender, it is separated on all sides of the opening by blunt dissection. After ligating the pedicle, the small opening in the linea alba is closed by unabsorbable sutures. When a hernial sac is present it is opened and any contents reduced, after which the sac is excised before repairing the linea alba. Sometimes smaller protrusions of fat are found above and below the hernia. These should also be dealt with.

RARE EXTERNAL HERNIAS

Interparietal Hernia (*syn.* Interstitial Hernia).—An interparietal hernia has a hernial sac that passes between the layers of the anterior abdominal wall. The sac may be associated with, or communicate with, the sac of a concomitant inguinal or femoral hernia. Lack of knowledge of this condition is the cause of misdiagnosis and mismanagement.

Other Varieties (fig. 1168): 1. *Properitoneal* (20%).—Usually the sac takes the form of a diverticulum from a femoral or inguinal hernia.

2. *Intermuscular* (60%).—The sac passes between the muscular layers of the anterior abdominal wall, usually between the external oblique and internal oblique muscles. The sac is nearly always bilocular, and is associated with an inguinal hernia.

3. *Inguino-superficial* (20%).—The sac expands beneath the superficial fascia of the abdominal wall or the thigh. This type is commonly associated with an incompletely descended testis.

Clinical Features.—The patients (mostly male) present with intestinal obstruction, due to obstruction or strangulation of the hernia. In the pro-peritoneal variety, as no

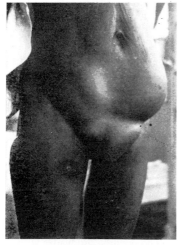

FIG. 1168.—Bilateral interstitial and bilateral inguinal hernias. The interstitial hernias were between the external and internal oblique muscles, the left containing several feet of small bowel.
(*V. J. Hartfield, formerly S.E. Nigeria.*)

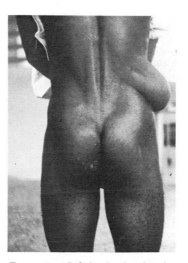

FIG. 1169.—Inferior lumbar hernia. It contained caecum, appendix and small bowel. Note filarial skin rash on buttocks.
(*V. J. Hartfield*)

swelling is likely to be apparent, delays in diagnosis occur and consequently the mortality in this variety is high.

Treatment.—Operation is imperative because of intestinal obstruction.

A Spigelian hernia is a variety of interparietal hernia occurring commonly at the level of the arcuate line. The fundus of the sac, clothed by extraperitoneal fat, may lie beneath the internal oblique muscle, where it is virtually impalpable. More often it advances through that muscle and spreads out like a mushroom between the external and internal obliques and gives rise to a more evident swelling. The patient is often corpulent and usually over fifty years of age, men and women being affected equally. Typically, a soft, reducible mass will be encountered lateral to the rectus muscle and below the umbilicus. Because of the rigid fascia surrounding its neck, strangulation may occur.

Treatment.—Operation. The external oblique aponeurosis is split. After isolating the sac, dealing with any contents, and ligating and excising it, the transversus, internal oblique, and external oblique muscles are repaired.

Lumbar Hernia.—Most primary lumbar herniae gain exit through the inferior lumbar triangle of Petit (fig. 1169), bounded below by the crest of the ilium, laterally by the external oblique, and medially by the latissimus dorsi. Some come through the superior lumbar triangle, which is bounded by the twelfth rib above, medially by the sacrospinalis, and laterally by the posterior border of the internal oblique. An extensive incisional lumbar hernia sometimes follows an operation upon an infected kidney.

Differential Diagnosis.—A lumbar hernia must be distinguished from: (*a*) Lipoma. (*b*) A cold abscess pointing to this position. (*c*) Phantom hernia due to local muscular paralysis. Lumbar phantom herniae can result from any interference with the nerve-supply of the affected muscles (*e.g.* poliomyelitis).

Treatment.—A primary lumbar hernia, being small, is easily repaired. A post-operative lumbar hernia may be large, and the defect is impossible to repair unless fascial flaps are used. The area can be reinforced still further by stitching in place a piece of tantalum gauze or Dacron mesh.

Perineal hernia (*syn.* hernia through the pelvic floor) is rare:

(*a*) *Post-operative hernia through a perineal scar* may occur after excision of the rectum.

(*b*) *Median sliding perineal hernia* is a complete prolapse of the rectum (Chapter 53).

(*c*) *Antero-lateral perineal hernia* occurs in women and presents as a swelling of the labium majus.

(*d*) *Postero-lateral perineal hernia*, which passes through the levator ani to enter the ischiorectal fossa.

Treatment.—A combined operation is generally the most satisfactory for (*c*) or (*d*). The hernia is exposed by an incision directly over it. The sac is opened and its contents are reduced. The sac is cleared from surrounding structures and the wound is closed. With the patients in semi-Trendelenburg position, the abdomen is opened and the mouth of the sac is exposed. The sac is inverted, ligated, and excised, and the pelvic floor is repaired as adequately as possible.

Obturator Hernia.—The hernia, which passes through the obturator canal, occurs six times more frequently in women than in men. Most of the patients are over sixty years of age. The swelling is liable to be overlooked because it is covered by the pectineus. It seldom causes a definite swelling in Scarpa's triangle, but if the limb is flexed, abducted, and rotated outwards, sometimes the hernia becomes more apparent. The leg is usually kept in a semi-flexed position and movement increases the pain. In more than 50% of cases of strangulated obturator hernia pain is referred along the obturator nerve by its geniculate branch to the knee. On vaginal or rectal examination the hernia sometimes can be felt as a tender swelling in the region of the obturator foramen.

Cases of obturator hernia which present themselves have usually undergone strangulation, which is often of the Richter type.

Treatment.—(*a*) Perform lower laparotomy (on the side of the lesion, if known). Confirm the diagnosis and then adopt full Trendelenburg's position; (*b*) the constricting agent is the obturator fascia. Taking every precaution to avoid spilling infected fluid from the hernial sac into the peritoneal cavity, this fascia can be stretched to allow reduction by inserting suitable forceps through the gap in the fascia and opening the blades with care. If incision of the fascia is required, it is made parallel to the obturator vessels and nerve; (*c*) the contents of the sac are dealt with; (*d*) the broad ligament is stitched over the opening to prevent recurrence.

Gluteal and Sciatic Hernias.—A *gluteal hernia* passes through the greater sciatic foramen, either above or below the piriformis. A *sciatic hernia* passes through the lesser sciatic

Adrien Van der Spieghel (Spigelius), 1578–1625. Professor of Anatomy, Padua, Italy.
Jean Louis Petit, 1664–1750. Director of the Academy of Surgery, Paris.
Frierich Trendelenburg, 1844–1924. Professor of Surgery, Leipzig, Germany.
Antonio Scarpa, 1747–1832. Professor of Anatomy, Pavia, Italy. Elected F.R.S. in 1791.

foramen. *Differential diagnosis* must be made between these conditions and (*a*) A lipoma or fibro-sarcoma beneath the gluteus maximus. (*b*) A tuberculous abscess. (*c*) A gluteal aneurysm. All doubtful swellings in this situation should be explored by operation.

UMBILICUS

DISEASES OF THE UMBILICUS

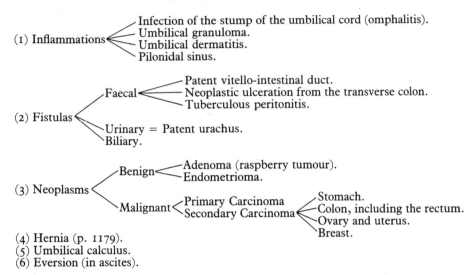

(1) Inflammations
- Infection of the stump of the umbilical cord (omphalitis).
- Umbilical granuloma.
- Umbilical dermatitis.
- Pilonidal sinus.

(2) Fistulas
- Faecal
  - Patent vitello-intestinal duct.
  - Neoplastic ulceration from the transverse colon.
  - Tuberculous peritonitis.
- Urinary = Patent urachus.
- Biliary.

(3) Neoplasms
- Benign
  - Adenoma (raspberry tumour).
  - Endometrioma.
- Malignant
  - Primary Carcinoma
  - Secondary Carcinoma
    - Stomach.
    - Colon, including the rectum.
    - Ovary and uterus.
    - Breast.

(4) Hernia (p. 1179).
(5) Umbilical calculus.
(6) Eversion (in ascites).

INFLAMMATIONS OF THE UMBILICUS

Infection of the Umbilical Cord.—By the third or fourth day of life the stump of the umbilical cord is found to be carrying staphylococci in over 50% of babies born in maternity hospitals. Less commonly the stump of the cord harbours streptococci, and epidemics of puerperal sepsis in maternity hospitals have been traced to the umbilical cord of one infant in the nursery thus infected. *Esch. coli* and *Cl. tetani* (causing neonatal tetanus) are other possible invaders. The chief prophylaxis is strict asepsis during severance of the cord, and the use of 0·1% chlorhexidine locally, for a few days.

Omphalitis.—The incidence of an infected umbilicus is much higher in communities that do not practise aseptic severance of the umbilical cord. When the stump of the umbilical cord becomes inflamed, antibiotic therapy usually localises the inflammation. By employing warm moist dressings the crusts separate, giving exit to pus. Exuberant granulation tissue requires a touch of silver nitrate. In more serious cases infection is liable to spread along the defunct hypogastric arteries or umbilical vein, when, in all probability, one or other of the following complications will supervene:

1. **Abscess of the Abdominal Wall.**—If gentle pressure is exerted below or above the navel, and a bead of pus exudes at the umbilicus, a deep abscess associated with one of the defunct umbilical vessels is present. This must be opened. A probe is passed into the sinus to determine its direction and this is followed by a grooved director on to which the skin and overlying tissues are incised in the middle line.

2. **Extensive ulceration of the abdominal wall,** due to a synergic infection, is treated in the same way as post-operative subcutaneous gangrene (see p. 1191).

3. **Septicaemia** can occur from organisms entering the blood-stream via the umbilical vein. Jaundice is often the first sign. An abscess in the abdominal wall above the umbilicus should be sought. In other respects the treatment of this grave complication follows the usual lines (Chapter 4).

4. **Jaundice in the Newborn.**—Infection reaching the liver via the umbilical vein may cause a stenosing intrahepatic cholangiolitis, appearing some three to six weeks after birth.

5. **Portal vein thrombosis** and subsequent portal hypertension.

6. **Peritonitis** carries a particularly bad prognosis.

7. **Umbilical Hernia.**

Umbilical Granuloma.—Chronic infection of the umbilical cicatrix which continues for weeks causes granulation tissue to pout at the umbilicus. There is no certain means of distinguishing this condition from an adenoma. Usually an umbilical granuloma can be destroyed by one application of a silver nitrate stick followed by dry dressings but an adenoma soon recurs in spite of these measures.

Dermatitis of and around the umbilicus is common at all times of life. Fungus and parasitic infections are more difficult to eradicate from the umbilicus than from the skin of the abdomen. Sometimes the dermatitis is consequent upon a discharge from the umbilicus, as is the case when an umbilical fistula or a sinus is present. In fat women intertrigo occurs.

A deep, tender swelling in the midline below the umbilicus signifies an abscess present in the extraperitoneal fat, and is usually due to an *infected urachal remnant*. Exploration and proper drainage is necessary.

Pilonidal sinus (a sinus containing a sheaf of hairs) is sometimes encountered. It should be excised.

Umbilical calculus (umbolith), often black in colour, is composed of desquamated epithelium which becomes inspissated and collects in the deep recess of the umbilicus. Eventually it gives rise to inflammation, and often a blood-stained discharge. The treatment is to dilate the orifice and extract the calculus, but, to prevent recurrence, it may be better to excise the umbilicus.

UMBILICAL FISTULAS

The umbilicus being a central abdominal scar, it is understandable that a slow leak from any viscus is liable to track to the surface at this point. Added to this, very occasionally, the vitello-intestinal duct or the urachus remains patent; consequently it has been remarked aptly that the umbilicus is a creek into which many fistulous streams may open.

For instance, an enlarged inflamed gallbladder perforating at its fundus may discharge gallstones through the umbilicus. Again, an unremitting flow of pus from a fistula at the umbilicus of a middle-aged women led to the discovery of a length of gauze overlooked during hysterectomy five years previously.

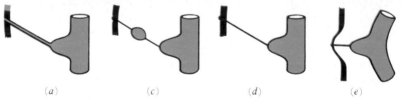

(a)   (c)   (d)   (e)

FIG. 1170.—Anomalies connected with the vitello-intestinal duct; (a) umbilical fistula; (b) umbilical sinus (not illustrated); (c) intra-abdominal cyst; (d) intraperitoneal band; (e) Meckel's diverticulum adherent to the sac of a congenital umbilical hernia.

The vitello-intestinal duct occasionally persists, and gives rise to one of the following conditions:

1. It remains patent (fig. 1170 (a)). The resulting umbilical fistula discharges mucus and, rarely, faeces.

Often a small portion only of the duct near the umbilicus remains unobliterated (fig. 1170(b)). This gives rise to a sinus that discharges mucus. The epithelial lining of the sinus often becomes everted to form an adenoma.

2. Sometimes both the umbilical and the intestinal ends of the duct close, but the mucous membrane of the intervening portion remains, and an intra-abdominal cyst develops (fig. 1170 (c)).

3. With its lumen obliterated or unobliterated, the vitello-intestinal duct provides an intraperitoneal band (fig. 1170 (d)) which is a potential danger, for intestinal obstruction is liable to occur. The obstruction results from a coil of small intestine passing under or over, or becoming twisted around the band.

4. Such a band may contract and pull a Meckel's diverticulum into a congenital umbilical hernia (fig. 1170 (e)).

5. A vitello-intestinal cord connected to Meckel's diverticulum, but not attached to the umbilicus, becomes adherent to, or knotted around, another loop of small intestine, and so causes intestinal obstruction.

6. Sometimes a band extending from the umbilicus is attached to the mesentery near its junction with a distal part of the ileum. In this case the band is probably an obliterated vitelline artery, and is not necessarily associated with a Meckel's diverticulum.

Treatment.—A patent vitello-intestinal duct should be excised, together with a Meckel's diverticulum, if such be present, preferably when the child is about six months old. When a vitello-intestinal band gives rise to acute intestinal obstruction, after removing the obstruction by division of the band, it is expedient, when possible, to excise the band and to bury the cut ends.

A patent urachus seldom reveals itself until maturity, or even old age. This is because the contractions of the bladder commence at the apex of the organ and pass towards the base. A patent urachus, because it opens into the apex of the bladder, is closed temporarily during micturition, and so the potential urinary stream to the umbilicus is cut off. Therefore the fistula remains unobtrusive until a time when the organ is overfull, usually due to some form of obstruction.

Treatment.—Usually treatment is directed to removing the obstruction to the lower urinary tract. If, after this is remedied, the leak continues or a cyst develops in connection with the urachus, umbilectomy and excision of the urachus down to its insertion into the apex of the bladder, with closure of the latter organ, is indicated.

Abscess in a urachal remnant, causing persistent umbilical dermatitis and discharge, is described above.

NEOPLASMS OF THE UMBILICUS

Umbilical adenoma or **Raspberry tumour** is commonly seen in infants (fig. 1171), but only occasionally later in life. It is due to a partially (occasionally a completely) unobliterated vitello-intestinal duct. Mucosa prolapsing through the

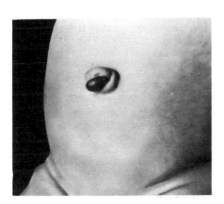

FIG. 1171.—Adenoma (raspberry tumour) of the umbilicus.

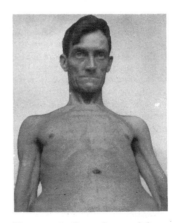

FIG. 1172.—Secondary nodule at the umbilicus in a case of carcinoma of the stomach.

umbilicus gives rise to a raspberry-like tumour, which is moist with mucus and tends to bleed.

Treatment.—If the tumour is pedunculated, a ligature is tied around it, and in a few days the polypus drops off. Should the tumour reappear after this procedure, umbilectomy is indicated. Sometimes a patent vitello-intestinal duct, or more often a vitello-intestinal band, will be found associated with a Meckel's

Johann Freidrich Meckel (The Younger), 1781–1833. Professor of Anatomy and Surgery, Halle, Germany.

diverticulum. The Meckel's diverticulum and the attached cord or duct should be excised at the same time as the umbilicus. Histologically, the tumour at the umbilicus consists of columnar epithelium rich in goblet cells.

Endometrioma occurs in women between the ages of twenty and forty-five. On histological examination it is found to consist of endometrial glands occupying the same plane in the dermis as the sudoriferous glands, and opening on to the surface in the same way. The umbilicus becomes painful and bleeds at each menstruation, when the small fleshy tumour between the folds of the umbilicus becomes more apparent. Occasionally an umbilical endometrioma is accompanied by endometriomas in the uterus or ovary. When, as is usually the case, the tumour is solitary, umbilectomy will cure the condition.

Secondary carcinoma at the umbilicus[1] (fig. 1172) is not very uncommon, but it is always a late manifestation of the disease. The primary neoplasm is often situated in the stomach, colon or ovary, but a metastasis from the breast, probably transmitted along the lymphatics of the round ligament of the liver, is sometimes located here.

THE ABDOMINAL WALL

BURST ABDOMEN (*syn*. Abdominal dehiscence) **AND INCISIONAL HERNIA** (*syn*. Ventral Hernia)

In 1 to 2% of cases, mostly between the sixth and eighth day after operation, a laparotomy wound bursts open and viscera are extruded. The disruption of the wound tends to occur a few days beforehand when the sutures opposing the deep layers (peritoneum, posterior rectus sheath) tear through or even become untied. An incisional hernia usually starts as a symptomless partial disruption of the deeper layers during the immediate or early post-operative period, the event passing unnoticed if the skin wound remains intact after the skin sutures have been removed.

Factors relating to the incidence of Burst Abdomen and Incisional Hernia

1. *Factors relating to wound closure* (*a*) Choice of suture materials:—Catgut leads to a higher incidence of bursts than the use of non-absorbably monofiliament polypropylene, polyamide, wire. (*b*) Method of closure:—Interrupted suturing has a low incidence. Thru' and Thru' suturing is good for the obstructed case: A one layer closure has a low incidence but it is higher than that following a two layered closure. When continuous suturing of layers (one or two) is performed a particular fault is the use of a short length of material, pulled tightly, for in an anaesthetised relaxed patient the incision is shortened thereby, and made taut so that the material will become as it were a cheese wire cutter when the patient is conscious and coughing. The golden rule is to insert a length of suture *at least* 2 times the length of the incision so as comfortably to coapt the layers. (*c*) Drainage through a wound leads to a higher incidence of 'bursts' than employing drainage through a separate ('stab') incision.

2. *Factors relating to incisions.*—Upper midline and vertical are descriptive of those incisions with a tendency to burst which is higher than those which are called 'transverse'.

3. *Reason for operation.*—Peritonitis is linked to burst abdomen and incisional hernia because the wound usually becomes infected. Operations on the pancreas, with leakage of enzymes, and obstructed cases are other reasons for disruption.

4. *Coughing. Vomiting. Distension:*—At the completion of an operation any violent coughing set off by the removal of an endotracheal tube and suction of the laryngopharynx strains the sutures. Likewise cough, vomiting and distension (*e.g.* due to ileus) in the early post-operative period.

5. *General condition of the Patient.*—Obesity, jaundice, malignant disease, hypoproteinaemia, anaemia are all factors conducive to disruption of a laparotomy wound (see Chapter 1).

---

[1] The neoplastic nodule so caused is known as Sister Joseph's nodule. Sister Joseph of the Mayo Clinic imparted this clinical observation to the late Dr. William Mayo.

Burst Abdomen

Clinical Features.—A serosanguineous (pink) discharge from the wound is a forerunner of disruption in fully 50% of cases. It is the most pathognomonic sign of impending wound disruption, and it signifies that intraperitoneal contents are lying extraperitoneally. The patient often volunteers the information that he 'felt something give way'. If skin sutures have been removed, omentum or coils of intestine may be forced through the wound and will be found lying on the skin. Pain and shock are often absent. It is important to note that there may be symptoms and signs of intestinal obstruction.

Treatment.—An emergency operation is required to replace the bowel, relieve any obstruction, and to resuture the wound. While awaiting operation, reassure the patient and cover the wound with a sterile towel. The stomach is emptied by a gastric tube and intravenous fluid therapy commenced.

Operation.—Each protruding coil of intestine is washed gently with saline solution, and returned to the abdominal cavity. Then protruding greater omentum is treated similarly and spread over the intestine. The abdominal wall having been cleansed, all layers are approximated by through-and-through sutures of braided nylon each passed through a soft rubber or plastic tube collar. The abdominal wall may be supported by strips of adhesive plaster encircling the anterior two-thirds of the circumference of the trunk. Antibiotic therapy is started.

Contrary to what might be thought, peritonitis rarely supervenes and, though the skin wound beomes infected, healing is satisfactory. Also a second dehiscence rarely occurs. There is biochemical evidence that healing after disruption produces a stronger wound. This is due to the improvement in collagen metabolism under these circumstances.

Incisional Hernia (*syn.* **Ventral Hernia: Post-operative Hernia**)

Aetiology.—Incisional hernia occurs most often in obese individuals, and a persistent post-operative cough and post-operative abdominal distension are its precursors. There is a high incidence of incisional hernia following operations for peritonitis because, as a rule, the wound becomes infected. The accommodation of a drainage tube in a stab incision, as opposed to placing such a tube through the laparotomy wound, reduces the frequency.

An incisional hernia usually starts as a symptomless partial disruption of the deeper layers of a laparotomy wound during the immediate or very early post-operative period. Often the event passes unnoticed if the skin wound remains intact after the stitches have been removed. A serosanguinous discharge is often the signal of dehiscence, and resuture of the deeper disrupted layers of the incision obviates the more difficult repair of an established hernia later on.

Clinical Features.—There are great variations in the degree of herniation. The hernia may occur through a small portion of the scar, often the lower end. More frequently there is a diffuse bulging of the whole length of the incision. A post-operative hernia, especially one through a lower abdominal scar, usually increases steadily in size, and more and more of its contents become irreducible. Sometimes the skin overlying it is so thin and atrophic that normal peristalsis can be seen in the underlying coils of intestine. Attacks of subacute intestinal obstruction are common, and strangulation is liable to occur at the neck of a small sac or in a loculus of a large one.

Treatment.—(i) *Palliative.*—An abdominal belt is sometimes satisfactory, especially in cases of a hernia through an upper abdominal incision.

(ii) *Operation.*—Many procedures are advocated.

Pre-operative Measures.—In order to obtain a lasting repair, very special preparation is required. If the patient is obese, reduction by dieting should precede the operation. To attempt to return the contents of a very large hernia to the main abdominal cavity if they have not been there for several years is to court danger, unless weight reduction has been effected. In these circumstances, not only is there a risk of failure of the hernioplasty, but there is a greatly increased risk of paralytic ileus from visceral compression, and of pulmonary complications from elevation of the diaphragm.

Principles of the Operation—The hernial sac is dissected. It is then formally, if not already inadvertently, opened and the contents are reduced. Adherent omentum and bowel have to be freed by dissection before the mouth of the sac can be defined. The layers are repaired usually with nonabsorbable sutures: 1. The peritoneum from the sac. 2. The fascial (apneurotic) layers. The lateral edges of the fascia are freed from the overlying muscles for some distance, and this fascial layer is approximated with interrupted sutures at the upper and lower ends of the wound. 3. The muscles and the remaining fascial layer are approximated. Tension-relaxing incisions may be required and should be placed well laterally.

Plastic Fibre Mesh or Net closures.—These are becoming increasingly popular. The sac and the layers are dealt with as above. Any deficiency in the abdominal wall can very easily be bridged without tension by laying and sewing on a sheet of tantalum gauze, or a mesh or net made of Nylon or Dacron, cut to well oversize and tacked down to the aponeurosis.

Careful haemostasis and meticulous asepsis are essential during these operations. Post-operative collections of serum can be removed by drainage, using plastic tubing led, via skin punctures lateral to the wound, into closed suction drainage bottles (*e.g.* Redi-vac).

Post-operative Treatment.—Gastric decompression and intravenous fluids are employed, and nothing by mouth allowed until the bowels have functioned. Early ambulation is to be discouraged, but exercises, especially of the legs, are to be encouraged. The patient should not resume strenuous exercise for three months.

DIVARICATION OF THE RECTI ABDOMINIS

Divarication of the recti abdominis is seen principally in elderly multiparae. When the patient strains, a gap can be seen between the recti abdominis through which gap the abdominal contents bulge. When the abdomen is relaxed the fingers can be introduced between the recti.

Treatment.—An abdominal belt is all that is required.

A similar condition is met with in babies, only the divarication exists above the umbilicus. No treatment is necessary; as the child develops a spontaneous cure results.

TEARING OF THE INFERIOR EPIGASTRIC ARTERY

Tearing of the inferior epigastric artery occurs in three dissimilar types of individual, viz. elderly women, often thin and feeble; athletic, muscular men, usually below middle age; and pregnant women, mainly multiparae late in pregnancy. The site of the haematoma is usually at the level of the arcuate line, where the posterior sheath of the rectus abdominis is lacking.

Clinical Features.—The possibility of tearing of the epigastric vessels should always be considered when, following a bout of coughing, or a sudden blow to the abdominal wall, an exquisitely tender lump appears in relation to the rectus abdominis. Occasionally, a haematoma occurs within the muscles lateral to the rectus sheath. Unless there is bruising of the overlying skin the diagnosis may be difficult.

Differential Diagnosis.—The conditions for which the haematoma is frequently mistaken are, in the female, a twisted ovarian cyst, and in both sexes, when the lump is on the right side, an appendix abscess. The sign most likely to be of value in differentiating a haematoma of the abdominal wall from these conditions, namely tensing the abdominal musculature, is often unsatisfactory because of the pain it causes. Again, the differential diagnosis between the haematoma and a strangulated Spigelian hernia may be difficult. The absence of vomiting suggests a haematoma, and the presence of resonance over the swelling favours a Spigelian hernia, while a plain radiograph of the abdomen sometimes gives positive evidence of the latter.

As a Complication of Pregnancy.—Rupture of the inferior epigastric artery occurs occasionally during pregnancy. Surprising to relate, the haemorrhage into this closed space from this comparatively small artery has proved fatal.

Treatment.—With rest, a comparatively small haematoma may resolve, but sometimes renewed haemorrhage causes the haematoma to rupture into the peritoneal cavity. Therefore it is safer to operate early, evacuate the clot, and ligate the artery.

INFECTIONS

Cellulitis can occur in any of the planes of the abdominal wall.

Superficial cellulitis is usually discovered when an abdominal wound is inspected following pyrexia. The earliest sign is when the stitches become embedded in the oedematous skin. Later there is a blush extending for a variable distance from the incision or the stitch holes. On palpation with the gloved hand usually one area is found to be more indurated and tender than the remainder. A stitch should be removed from the immediate vicinity, and if pus or sero-pus escapes it is sent for bacteriological examination, meanwhile a broad spectrum antibiotic is administered.

Deep cellulitis is characterised by brawny oedema towards one or both flanks, and not infrequently of the scrotum or vulva as well. Antibiotic therapy is the mainstay of treatment. When tenderness persists, an anatomical incision dividing the muscles carefully, layer by layer, until pus or purulent fluid is encountered, is often advisable.

Progressive post-operative bacterial synergistic gangrene is fortunately a rare complication after laparotomy, usually for a perforated viscus (notably perforated appendicitis). It has also occurred after gallbladder operations, colectomy for ulcerative colitis, and even after drainage of an empyema thoracis. The condition is due to the synergic action of microaerophilic non-haemolytic streptococci and, usually, a staphylococcus. The skin in the immediate vicinity of the wound exhibits signs of cellulitis. Within a few days a central purplish zone with an outer brilliant red zone can be distinguished, and the whole region is extremely tender. Slowly the condition advances (fig. 1173). The gangrenous skin liquefies, exposing underlying granulation tissue. If the condition persists, the general condition deteriorates.

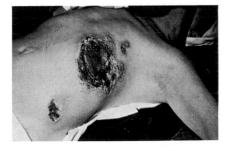

FIG. 1173.—Bacterial synergistic gangrene of the chest and abdominal wall. The area has become gangrenous and looks like suede leather. Beware of amoebiasis cutis (see below).

Treatment.—Identification of the organisms and a report on their sensitivity to antibiotics is essential Metronidazole should be given with an antistaphylococcal antibiotic (Chapter 3). Bacitracin zinc can be effective (10,000 to 20,000 units I.M., every six hours with local application of 500 units per ml, 4 times daily). Without vigorous and effective treatment the gangrene spreads to the flanks and the patient may die of toxaemia. Hyperbaric oxygen, if available, can be life-saving. Cellulitis due to bacteroides may give no bacteriological growth by conventional techniques and may be missed. **Amoebiasis cutis** (Chapter 45). The possibility of this potentially lethal complication of amoebic colitis, liver abscess or empyema being present should always be considered. Confirmation may be difficult and an immunofluorescence test necessary (Turner).

Subcutaneous gas infection.—This is described in Chapter 4.

NEOPLASMS OF THE ABDOMINAL MUSCULATURE

Desmoid tumour is a tumour arising in the musculo-aponeurotic structures of the abdominal wall, especially below the level of the umbilicus. It is a completely unencapsulated fibroma, and is so hard that it creaks when it is cut. Some cases recur repeatedly in spite of apparently adequate excision.

Aetiology.—80% of cases occur in women, many of whom have borne children, and the neoplasm occurs occasionally in scars of old hernial or other abdominal operation wounds. Consequently, trauma—*e.g.* the stretching of the muscle fibres during pregnancy or possibly a small haematoma of the abdominal wall—appears to be an aetiological factor. They can occur in cases of familial polyposis coli (Gardner's syndrome).

Pathology.—The tumour is composed of fibrous tissue containing multinucleated plasmodial masses resembling foreign-body gaint-cells. Usually of very slow growth, it tends to infiltrate muscle in the immediate neighbourhood. Eventually it undergoes a myxomatous change: it then increases in size more rapidly. Metastasis does not occur. Unlike fibroma elsewhere, no sarcomatous change occurs.

Treatment.—Unless the tumour is excised widely, with a surrounding margin of at least 2·5 cm of healthy tissue, recurrence commonly takes place. After removal of a large tumour, repair of the defect in the abdominal wall by tantalum gauze or nylon mesh is required. These tumours are moderately radio-sensitive.

Fibrosarcoma of the abdominal wall is rare. It is resistant to radiotherapy and only in some cases can a wide excision, with tantalum or nylon net repair, offer hope of a cure.

Adenocarcinoma of the colon or of other viscera may invade the abdominal wall. In such cases the resection of this extension, along with the primary growth, may require special repair of the resulting defect.

Secondary implantation in the wound may follow any abdominal operation for carcinoma.

Leslie Turner, Contemporary. Consultant Surgeon, Withington Hospital, Manchester.

CHAPTER 56

URINARY SYMPTOMS. INVESTIGATION OF THE URINARY TRACT. ANURIA

URINARY SYMPTOMS

The three most common symptoms accompanying diseases of the urinary tract are *pain, urinary frequency* and *haematuria*. Of these by far the most important is haematuria (the presence of blood in the urine), a symptom that cannot be ignored and one that requires complete investigation of the urinary tract.

Haematuria

It is interesting how many variations can occur with what appears to be one single symptom, namely haematuria. The patients may describe initial haematuria, blood throughout the urinary stream, terminal haematuria, bleeding with clots and perhaps pieces, and sometimes that their urine looks rather like stale tea. Whilst many of these individual variations may give one an indicator as to the site of the bleeding, the end result is the same—complete investigation is indicated. An indicator of some of the main causes of haematuria is illustrated diagramatically in fig. 1174.

Pain

A number of quite different forms of pain arise from the urinary tract.

Renal pain.—Pain arising from the kidney whether associated with inflammation or obstruction at the level of the pelviureteric junction is usually well localised. The pain if simply due to obstruction will be described as an ache; the presence of infection is often recognised by an added postural element and perhaps some irritation of the psoas muscle. There may be tenderness on palpation in the costovertebral angle; tenderness is usually also elicited anteriorly in the right hypochondrium.

Ureteric colic.[1]—The pain associated with the passage of a stone is totally different. It is usually sudden in onset and severe in quality. The patient is quite unable to get comfortable and prefers to pace about or thrash around. This is quite unlike someone with peritonism when the slightest movement causes exacerbation of the pain. Careful history taking can often site the stone; the pain is restricted to the loin when the stone is just coming out of the kidney. As the stone moves into the upper ureter so the pain moves into the upper abdomen and gradually down towards the groin. With a stone in the lower ureter pain may radiate into the perineum, or to the vulva in a woman and sometimes the base of the penis in a man; it may also go down the inner thigh.

Vesical pain is usually sited suprapubically. It is made worse by the bladder

---

[1] Renal colic is a term that is deeply rooted. Pain passing from loin to groin is more accurately termed ureteric colic.

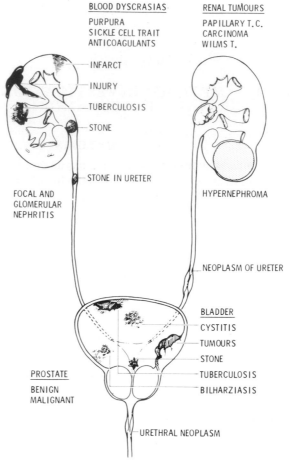

BLOOD DYSCRASIAS
PURPURA
SICKLE CELL TRAIT
ANTICOAGULANTS

RENAL TUMOURS
PAPILLARY T.C.
CARCINOMA
WILMS T.

INFARCT

INJURY

TUBERCULOSIS

STONE

STONE IN URETER

FOCAL AND
GLOMERULAR
NEPHRITIS

HYPERNEPHROMA

NEOPLASM OF URETER

BLADDER
CYSTITIS
TUMOURS
STONE
TUBERCULOSIS
BILHARZIASIS

PROSTATE
BENIGN
MALIGNANT

URETHRAL NEOPLASM

FIG. 1174.—The more common causes of haematuria.[1]

filling or emptying and sometimes by defaecation particularly with an impending colovesical fistula.

Prostatic and seminal vesicle pain is usually deep seated either in the rectum or the perineum. It is usually described as an ache which may also occur both in the suprapubic region and in one or both iliac fossae.

Urethral pain is typically scalding in nature and associated with active cystitis. Pain may also be experienced in the base of the penis particularly with the presence of a vesical calculus when the stone is forced onto the bladder neck as the detrusor contraction empties the bladder.

Frequency may be due to incomplete emptying, as in prostatism, to irritability of the bladder as by inflammation or stone, to a contracted bladder, to a diuresis, or to sphincter weakness.

---

[1] Pink or red urine may occur after eating beetroot, while many drugs, *e.g.* Dindevan®, Pyridium®, and Furadantin® may make the urine a deep orange red. Actual bleeding occurring while a patient is on anticoagulants should make the practitioner consider the possibility of unsuspected renal or vesical pathology.

INVESTIGATION OF THE URINARY TRACT

A complete history and physical examination of the patient is of course mandatory before investigation of any condition. One has to remember that the systemic complications of renal disease are legion. It is also of paramount importance to remember that haematuria may not arise from primary disease of the urinary tract but because of some other systemic illness. The presence of lymphadenopathy and hepatosplenomegaly may herald the fact that the bleeding is secondary to thrombocytopenia caused by a leukaemia. A broad approach to the investigation of any patient must therefore be adopted and obviously the haemoglobin, sometimes a blood film, liver function test and a chest x-ray may all be appropriate. If one looks more closely at the urinary tract much information can be obtained by initial examination of the urine.

    1. The Urine.—The urine may be examined:
  (i) Microscopically—for the presence of red cells, white cells, bacteria crystals and casts.
 (ii) Biochemically—for electrolytes, glucose, bilirubin and its products and the breakdown products of haemo- and myoglobin.
(iii) pH.
(iv) Bacteriologically—simple culture may be used to reveal infection. Taking a mid-stream specimen is desirable because (*a*) it avoids contamination and (*b*) it is without the risks of catheterisation. Occasionally specialised media and anaerobic conditions are required for the isolation of some organisms. Early morning specimens should be cultured on a Lowenstein Jensen medium when looking for tuberculosis.
 (v) Malignancy—the Papanicolaou stain used for demonstrating the presence of carcinoma in situ of the uterine cervix has been adopted for cells exfoliating from the urinary tract. This has a place in the detection of urothelial malignancy.

    2. Tests of Renal Function.—Because of the large reserve of renal tissue, considerable structural damage can occur before functional damage becomes apparent. Kidney function can be impaired in three principal ways: the renal plasma-flow may be reduced, the glomeruli damaged, or the function of the tubules impaired. In essential hypertension the chief fault lies in the renal plasma-flow. In glomerulonephritis the main effect is reduction in the glomerular filtration rate, while in pyelonephritis the brunt falls on tubular function. In back pressure due to obstruction all become impaired.

    Range of Specific Gravity (concentration dilution test).—The power of the kidneys to concentrate and dilute urine is a good test of their functional integrity. Fluid is withheld for twelve hours overnight. The specific gravity of the first two morning specimens should reach 1·020; a specific gravity of 1·025 in a urine free of protein indicates good renal function. A litre of water is given by mouth. Within four hours the specific gravity should be as low as 1·002. A fixed specific gravity of 1·010 under these varying circumstances is good presumptive evidence of impaired function of the distal renal tubules.
    The blood urea (or non-protein nitrogen) is normally between 2·5–6·5 mmol/l (15–40 mg/100 ml) of blood.

Creatinine (42–130 mmol/l (0·2–1·5 mg/100 ml) is a more sensitive test of renal function.

Creatinine Clearance.—This is a convenient method of measuring the glomerular filtration rate. One sample of blood and an accurately timed collection of urine for a period of about twenty-four hours are all that is required. The normal clearance is between 90 and 130 ml/min. It decreases in old age.

3. Radiology—Contrast studies

A plain film of the abdomen can reveal a wealth of information about the patient. One should adopt a routine for insuring initially the film is correctly orientated right to left, remembering that the liver is on the right and a gastric air bubble on the left. A glance at the spine and the bony structures may reveal the presence of scoliosis, spina bifida, degenerative disease of the lumbar spine, the presence of a previous pelvic fracture and arthritis affecting the hips. All of these may have serious implications with respect to the urinary tract. The soft tissue shadows should be inspected looking at the outline of the psoas muscles and the soft tissue shadow of the kidneys, and the bladder can usually be appreciated. Thirdly one should look for the presence of calculi along the line of the urinary tract.

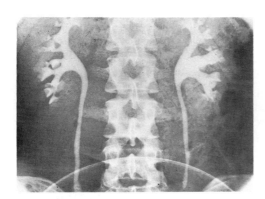

Fig. 1175.—Normal intravenous (excretory) urogram. Compression applied to the abdomen by a strap enhances the clarity of the pyelographs, because it delays emptying of the renal pelvis. The concentration reaches its maximum in 15 to 30 minutes.

Intravenous Urogram[1] (fig. 1175).—Radiological examination of the urinary tract has been the mainstay of investigation since the introduction of contrast media in the early 1930's The process relies on the glomerular filtration of sodium diatrizoate. One has to remember that this is allergenic.

Prior to any injection of contrast it behoves the administrator to enquire about a general history of allergy, atopy or eczema. It is also important to know if contrast has previously been administered and if any reaction occurred. A reaction should it occur may simply be a sensation of flushing. It may of course be more pronounced with the development of wheals and in its most extreme form the development of laryngeal oedema and circulatory collapse. It is therefore vital that the equipment and drugs for resuscitation of the patient are available in the room at the time of any of these investigations. Only limited information will be gained from an IVU in the presence of poor renal function.

Preparation.—A laxative is usually given prior to the investigation and the patient requested not to drink for 6–8 hours prior to the study. It is vital that

---

[1] Intravenous urogram (urography)=Intravenous pyelogram (pyelography) IVP.

patients with multiple myeloma are not dehydrated as acute renal failure may be precipitated.

Technique.—The contrast (45% Hypaque) is then injected into a suitable fore-arm vein. Careful observation for the presence of a reaction should be maintained during the circulation of the first few mls injected. Early films may be taken to demonstrate the nephrogram phase. Here comparison between the two kidneys can be made, a delay on one side signifying the presence of perhaps renal artery stenosis or the presence of unilateral obstructive uropathy. After a few minutes the contrast is excreted into the collecting system appearing in the calyces and the renal pelvis. Later films will demonstrate the ureters and the bladder. At the end of the study the patient is asked to micturate and a final film is then taken of the bladder area. It is important to remember that an intravenous urogram is simply the topographical representation of a dynamic event. Sometimes the radi-ologist will require to apply compression to the lower abdomen in order to achieve good delineation of the upper tract anatomy (see fig. 1175). It is important to remember that this is often uncomfortable for the patient.

Infusion Urography.—In patients with a blood urea of 16·6–33·2 mmol/l (100 to 200 mg/100 ml), an infusion of 50% Hypaque 2 ml/kg in an equal volume of isotonic saline, over a period of 10 minutes, may produce useful urograms, but is rarely used nowadays.

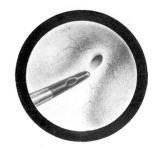

FIG. 1176.—A ureteric catheter about to enter the left ureteric orifice. Cysto-scopic view.

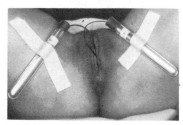

FIG. 1177.—Specimens of urine being collected after ureteric catheterisation. The test-tubes are capped with rubber finger-stalls.

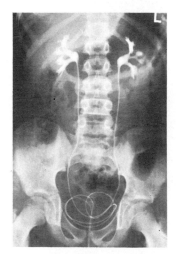

FIG. 1178.—Normal retrograde pyelogram. The definition is much clearer, consequently this pro-cedure is invaluable in confirming doubtful abnormalities visualised by the excretory method, or where excretion is poor.

Retrograde Ureteropyelography (fig. 1178).—This investigation which requires initially the passage of a cystoscope and subsequently the passing of a fine ureteric catheter (fig. 1057) into the ureteric orifice normally requires a general anaesthetic, particularly in a male. Contrast media may be injected up the ureter if there is doubt about the presence of an intraluminal lesion. It is also important to display the upper ureter prior to performing a pyeloplasty for an obstructed pelviureteric junction (see p. 1221). The anatomy during this investigation can be displayed using an image intensifier but of course a permanent record should be obtained if possible. In some unusual circumstances it is of value to collect urine from each individual orifice (fig. 1177). The induction of a diuresis may hasten this part of the test. A new application of this approach allows the passage of a catheter from which a small brush can be projected. This permits brushings to be obtained from a suspected urothelial tumour and by using this technique not only may the diagnosis be confirmed but also the grade of the tumour be reported by an experienced cytologist.

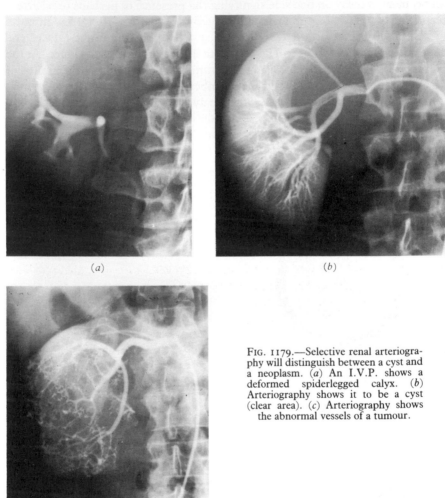

(a)

(b)

(c)

FIG. 1179.—Selective renal arteriography will distinguish between a cyst and a neoplasm. (a) An I.V.P. shows a deformed spiderlegged calyx. (b) Arteriography shows it to be a cyst (clear area). (c) Arteriography shows the abnormal vessels of a tumour.

Renal Arteriography (fig. 1179).—Renal arteriography initially was developed as a diagnostic tool. More recently some theraputic applications have been added. The interarterial injection of contrast may be of value to demonstrate the pathological anatomy of the renal artery when considering the diagnosis of renal artery stenosis, severe atheroma or renal artery aneurysm. It may be useful to confirm the diagnosis of a renal cell carcinoma and most recently it has been used to delineate the site of bleeding whether from renal trauma or a suspected arteriovenous malformation. In these cases it may be possible to demonstrate a bleeding vessel or fistula which then can be embolized using a small plug of gel foam or similar material. A recent vogue for embolising kidneys prior to nephrectomy for renal cell carcinoma seems to be losing popularity. The second therapeutic application is that of transluminal angioplasty for renal artery stenosis; here a balloon is blown up inside the narrowed artery.

There are two methods of performing arteriography:

(a) *Translumbar aortography* is carried out under general anaesthesia. A needle is passed into the abdominal aorta just above the renal arteries (level of L.I.), the contrast medium is injected and four films are taken in rapid succession. To minimise accidents a small quantity of medium is injected and a film taken to ensure that the needle is in its correct position (see 'dangers' below).

(b) *Retrograde Arteriography.*—A Seldinger's needle is used (Chapter 14). The needle is passed into the femoral artery. The stilette is removed. A guide wire (a 'leader') with a supple tip is passed into the artery and the needle is removed. The artery is compressed to avoid bleeding while a radio-opaque arterial catheter is threaded on to the leader and so guided through the skin and arterial puncture into the artery. The catheter is advanced to the desired level. The contrast fluid (Hypaque) is then injected. *Selective Renal Arteriography* can be achieved by using a hooked catheter, and guiding it into the renal artery (fig. 1179).

6–7 ml of contrast fluid are usually sufficient for selective arteriography; 30 ml for a free flush into the aorta. *The dangers of the procedure* (a) tubular necrosis of the kidneys, (b) paraplegia, often temporary, have been eliminated with modern contrast fluids, but damage to a plaque of atheroma, embolism, and dissecting aneurysm can occur.

Cystography.—Simple cystography involving the injection of contrast material through a catheter introduced into the bladder is rarely necessary these days except in the investigation of children, or when one suspects a fistulous tract or vesical trauma. A micturating cystogram is used when looking for the presence of vesico-ureteric reflux. The patient who is often a child should have a tiny catheter passed and the bladder then filled in calm and quiet surroundings. The catheter is then removed and the patient screened under the x-ray tube during the voiding phase, looking particularly at the function of the bladderneck and for the presence of reflux. With the addition of bladder pressure monitoring equipment much more useful information can be added to this test and ideally a full urodynamic assessment would be more appropriate (Chapter 58).

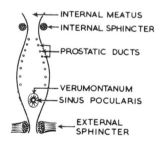

Fig. 1180.—Structures on the floor of the posterior urethra.
(*After J. C. Ainsworth-Davis, FRCS, London.*)

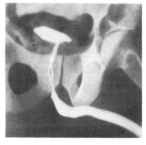

Fig. 1181.—Normal urethrograph.

Urethrography.—Urethrography (fig. 1181) is especially valuable for gaining information concerning the length of a urethral stricture, of dilatation or diverticulum formation above a stricture, or of failure of the medium to pass a stricture. It also reveals dilated prostatic ducts in chronic prostatitis and especially in tuberculous prostatitis. The one contraindication to its use is the presence of urethral haemorrhage. The medium employed must be chosen with great care, for should there be a breach in the continuity of the lining membrane of the urethra, the medium may enter the circulation.

Lipiodol brings with it the danger of oil embolus and this medium should never be employed. Even worse is to inject barium emulsion, and deaths have occurred from its use in cases of ruptured urethra.

The medium must therefore be harmless should some of it enter the circulation, and the injection must not be rapid or forceful. For general purposes the most satisfactory medium is Umbradil viscous V. This is a jelly which is squeezed from a tube into the butt end of a urethral syringe. It is injected easily and contains the local anaesthetic lignocaine. The injection is made most satisfactorily by employing Knutsson's apparatus which has a penile clamp attached.

Venography.—This has been used to show whether a renal carcinoma has spread into the renal vein or even the inferior vena cava. This information can usually be best obtained by either ultrasound or a CT scan thus avoiding an invasive procedure.

4. Ultrasonography

The quality of image achieved by ultrasound scanning has revolutionised the investigation of the urinary tract. Fluid can be differentiated from solid tissue hence cyst from tumour. The size of the kidney and the thickness of the cortex can be delineated. Individual calyces can be demonstrated and the width of the collecting system (hence hydronephrosis can be diagnosed within seconds). This has taken away the agonising hours spent performing tomograms and perhaps infusion urograms when dealing with acute renal failure.

Only limited views can be obtained of the ureter as the pelvic bones tend to get in the way. The bladder may be scanned looking for the presence of a residual urine or perhaps even the presence of a filling defect. Intracavity probes are now available which can be placed per urethram for investigation of the bladder and prostate or per rectum for demonstrating the architecture of the prostate. Their precise role in clinical practice has yet to be evaluated.

5. Computed Tomography (CT) (fig. 1183)

The computerised assessment and display of a cross section, or images, of the body at the selected levels has almost eliminated the need for arteriography, certainly as a diagnostic tool. The images obtained are particularly useful when doubt exists about a lump in the kidney; the different tissues of the body having a designated Hounsfield unit. CT can also be applied to the staging of bladder cancer and prostate cancer. Perhaps its most useful role has been in the initial staging and follow up of young men with testis cancer.

6. Radioisotope Scanning

A further new dimension has been added with the use of radioisotopes (fig. 1182). Gamma camera scanning following the injection of Technetium 99m labelled DMSA[1] (99m TC) will give information about the renal plasma flow and

---

[1] DMSA = dimercaptosuccinic acid.

Folke Knutsson, Contemporary. Director Roentgen Department, University Hospital, Uppsala, Sweden.
Sir Godfrey Hounsfield, FRS, Contemporary. The pioneer of CT scanning at EMI.

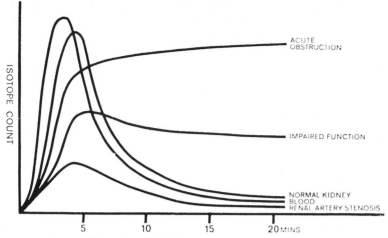

FIG. 1182.—Radioisotope renogram (see text).

its handling in the glomerulus; the majority being reabsorbed in the proximal tubules. Hence a comparative value of renal contribution can be obtained. Similarly 99m DTPA[1] is excreted earlier giving a good image of the renal outline. Considerable interest has centred over the last few years in the injection of DTPA and adding Frusemide when looking at cases of suspected pelviureteric junction obstruction. Despite the most scientific measurements a clear answer is not obtained in a small proportion of cases. When this exists an antegrade pressure perfusion test will be required as devised by Whitaker. Whitaker's test involves the fine needle puncture of the collecting system which is then perfused at varying rates. During this inflow continuous monitoring of the intra pelvic pressure is made. A urethral catheter needs to be in situ to eliminate artefact caused by raised intravesical pressure. An abnormal rise in the pressure will suggest obstruction.

7. Endoscopy

Since the introduction of the cystoscope in 1877 by Nitze, surgeons have appreciated the importance of visual inspection of the bladder. The range of instruments now available would have surpassed even his wildest dreams.

Cystourethroscopy can be performed under local anaesthetic but with a rigid instrument it is often kinder for men to be given a short general anaesthetic.

Preparation.—The external genitalia are cleaned with a soapy antiseptic. 1% Lignocaine with 0·25% Chlorhexidine gluconate jelly is injected into the urethra to provide anaesthesia and lubrication. This must be allowed to act and should be left in situ for 5–10 minutes.

A. Cystoscopy.—Having entered the bladder one usually uses a telescope with a wider field of vision (30° or 70°). Systematic inspection of the urothelium is made. The recent use of fibreoptic instruments for cystoscopy has made the procedure very much more comfortable, often saving the need for hospitalisation.

Instruments are now available for direct inspection of the ureter (ureteroscope) and the kidney (nephroscope).

---

[1]DTPA = diethylene triamine penta-acetic acid.

Robert Whitaker, Contemporary. Consultant Urologist, Addenbrooke's Hospital, Cambridge.

In countries where x-ray facilities are not available, information about renal function can be obtained by injecting 7 ml of 0·4% (adult dose) of indigocarmine intravenously. A careful watch is made for the appearance of dye at each ureteric orifice. Unilateral delay is indicative of obstruction or disease on that side, whereas if the delay is on both sides there is bilateral renal impairment.

B. Urethroscopy.—(*a*) *Anterior urethroscopy* is employed when the presence of a urethral stricture (fig. 1174) or strictures is suspected, or in cases of chronic urethritis, in order to exclude or confirm the presence of an infected urethral crypt or a granuloma (a 'soft' stricture).

(*b*) *Posterior urethroscopy* permits inspection of the prostatic and membranous urethras. It is carried out with an irrigating urethroscope with an end-viewing optical system (0°). The most notable normal spectacle of posterior urethroscopy is the verumontanum, which presents as an eminence on the floor of the prostatic urethra. On the summit of this projection is the sinus pocularis (fig. 1180), with the ejaculatory ducts opening on either side. The verumontanum is reddened and enlarged in cases of chronic vesiculitis. In cases of chronic prostatitis, one or more of the numerous prostatic ducts, which normally are difficult to visualise, may be seen exuding pus. When the prostate is enlarged, the lateral lobes project into the intestinal meatus producing an inverted V; a middle lobe or bar can be easily seen.

ANURIA (*syn.* SUPPRESSION OF URINE)

Oliguria should be defined as an excretion of less than 300 ml of urine in twenty-four hours. Anuria is an absence of excretion for twelve hours.

The most helpful classification of anuria is into pre-renal, renal, and post-renal. Although suppression of urine is commonly and conveniently referred to as anuria, except in post-renal (ureteric obstruction) cases the suppression is seldom absolutely complete.

Pre-renal Anuria

The blood pressure in the glomeruli is normally about 90 mmHg (12 kPa); when the systolic blood pressure falls below 70 mm (9·3 kPa), filtration from

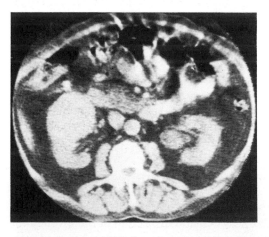

FIG. 1183.—CT scan showing hypernephroma. (N.B. CT scans are read from the feet of the patient. Here there is a right-sided renal swelling on the left of the picture.)

glomeruli ceases. If the glomeruli are diseased, a higher pressure (up to 100 mmHg (13.3 kPa)) may be inadequate to maintain filtration. The causes of pre-renal anuria are traumatic shock, severe haemorrhage, spinal anaesthesia, extensive burns, dehydration from vomiting, diarrhoea, or excessive sweating, and cardiac failure.

Treatment.—Blood transfusion in the case of haemorrhage, the treatment of shock if that be the cause of the fall in the blood-pressure, or in cases of dehydration the administration of dextrose-saline solution intravenously often restores urinary excretion. If hypotension is long maintained, damage to the renal epithelium results, and the condition passes on to one of renal anuria, due to tubular necrosis.

Acute Renal Anuria (Acute tubular necrosis)

Acute renal anuria results from damage to, or ischaemia of, the renal tubular epithelium. The principal causes met with in surgical practice are:

1. Severe shock (hypotension) lasting two hours or more.
2. Incompatible blood transfusion.
3. Bilateral pyelonephritis.
4. The crush syndrome (Chapter 5).
5. Concealed accidental haemorrhage and abortion.
6. Certain poisons. The most important are (*a*) media used for aortography, (*b*) the toxin of eclampsia, (*c*) chemicals—mercury salts, carbon tetrachloride.
7. Acute pancreatitis.
8. Operations on jaundiced patients.
9. Bacteraemic shock.
10. Drugs. Aminoglycosides, cephalosporines (especially if used in a patient on frusemide).

When renal anuria is reversible, and it is treated correctly, the condition is divided into three phases: 1. *The oliguric phase.* 2. *The phase of diuresis.* 3. *The phase of recovery.*

Clinical Features.—The average duration of the oliguric phase is ten to twelve days. Dark urine in small amounts and with a specific gravity of 1·010 is passed, or will be found on catheterisation. Anorexia is an early symptom which is followed by hiccough. Within four or five days there is copious effortless vomiting. Abdominal distension is common. Untreated, or treated incorrectly, the blood urea mounts by 20 to 30 mg (3·3–5·0 mmol) daily. The systolic bloodpressure may be elevated—200 mmHg (26·6 kPa) after two or three days.

Still untreated, or treated incorrectly, about the sixth day increasing drowsiness, thirst, a dry skin, and a dry brown tongue are characteristic findings. The respiratory and pulse-rates become slower and irregular, and Cheyne-Stokes' respirations are often in evidence. The final stages are usually characterised by muttering delirium followed by coma.

Treatment: Special Early Measures.—(a) If there is any doubt as to the cause, post-renal (obstructive) anuria must be eliminated by plain radiography and renal ultrasound. (b) In cases of incompatible blood transfusion, renal damage can sometimes be prevented by provoking a diuresis within an hour of the reaction—500 ml of Rheomacrodex or mannitol (Chapter 4) is given intravenously. If no urine is secreted (the bladder is emptied naturally—or via a catheter), all fluids are restricted forthwith.

In all other circumstances of acute renal anuria it is imperative not to force fluids. The important substances in the genesis of uraemic coma are not urea and

John Cheyne, 1777–1836, and William Stokes, 1804–1878. (See footnote, p. 88.)

other end products of nitrogen metabolism, but water and electrolytes, such as potassium.

Management of an established case

Oliguric phase.—The most important aspect in the early management of oliguric renal failure is the careful attention that is required to the water and electrolyte balance.

A. *Water balance.*—In the absence of vomiting the elimination of water by an anuric patient is limited to extra renal routes, i.e. lung, skin and faeces. The daily fluid intake therefore should be limited to 500 ml plus an amount equal to that of the volume vomited or lost by gastric aspiration, diarrhoea or through fistulas. Additions may be made for excessive sweating; an extra 200 ml is allowed for each $0·5°$ of the patient's temperature above $37·0°C$. When the weather is exceedingly hot the allowance is increased but even in these circumstances it should rarely exceed 1,000 ml per 24 hours.

Bedside evaluation.—Moisture of the tongue and the skin turgor are excellent guides to the state of hydration. It is also helpful to weigh the patient daily.

B. *Electrolyte balance.*—It is preferable to avoid the use of intravenous fluids at this stage for risk of creating a state of fluid overload. It is particularly important therefore not to infuse large volumes of sodium chloride. These patients develop a marked acidosis and there is often a temptation to give sodium bicarbonate or lactate intravenously. On the whole this is best avoided. *At this stage the greatest danger to the patient lies from a rising serum potassium.* It is important to have regular estimations of the potassium and also to watch for electrocardiograph changes. Should the potassium rise to dangerous levels a calcium resonium enema is the simplest remedy. These ion exchange resins can also be used orally. Another way of reducing the serum potassium is by the cautious use of intravenous dextrose and insulin. Should there be a state of absolute emergency potassium can be forced into the cells by the administration of sodium bicarbonate or lactate given i.v.

C. *Nitrogen metabolism.*—The simplest method of reducing any excess protein load that occurs is by the administration of a diet high in carbohydrates. The aim is to administer approximately 2,000 calories per 24 hours and this can normally be achieved with the use of products taken orally, *e.g.* Hycal. Occasionally if there is excessive vomiting a nasogastric tube may be used or intravenous feeding may have to be introduced.

D. *Infection.*—These patients are at an increased risk of developing generalised infections and a careful vigil must be maintained. Swabs are taken from the nose and throat, and sputum and urine should be sent for culture. With the detection of an infection antibiotics should be commenced, particular care being taken to avoid if possible those with nephrotoxic properties. Should one of these be required administration at the appropriate reduced dosage must be instituted and monitored by frequent blood levels.

E. *General nursing care.*—Meticulous records must be made of the fluid balance as patients are often tempted to cheat if they can gain access to extra fluid. For those who are more ill and perhaps even stuporose regular turning and care to pressure areas is important. Regular physiotherapy is recommended.

F. *Dialysis*.—Should the urea rise to dangerously high levels, or there is a problem with hyperkalaemia or fluid overload, it may be necessary to dispose of fluid and waste products artificially by dialysis. The method of dialysis adopted should be determined by the predicted need and the facilities available.

(i) **Peritoneal dialysis**.—The placement of a fenestrated peritoneal dialysis catheter into the peritoneal cavity can be simply done with local anaesthetic. It should be passed just below the umbilicus in the midline. For long term dialysis a Tenckhoff catheter is used – Chronic Ambulatory Peritoneal dialysis.

(ii) **Haemodialysis**.—When the back up of a renal unit is available, a few sessions of haemodialysis may be life saving. For patients with chronic renal failure a Cimino fistula (A-V shunt) is surgically created to give easy vascular access (Chapter 62).

Diuretic Phase.—In reversible lesions, usually about the eighth day, the epithelium of the lower nephrons regenerates sufficiently to prevent resorption of the glomerular filtrate, and a little urine is passed. This is a most hopeful sign, and given correct management and previously healthy kidneys an increasing twenty-four-hourly output during the subsequent week is usual. When diuresis commences, an amount of water equal to the output of urine for the previous twenty-four hours is added to the daily allowance. It is more difficult to estimate an appropriate allowance of electrolytes, for the restitution of renal electrolyte-regulating function returns slowly. A heavy loss of sodium and potassium may occur and must be replaced. Estimation and quantitative replacement of the loss in the previous twenty-four hours is the most accurate way of management. Only when renal excretion reaches 1 litre per day does the blood-urea level commence to fall. Once diuresis exceeds 1 litre in twenty-four hours, the intragastric tube (if one has been used because of vomiting or to control input in a semi-comatose patient) is removed and the patient is fed on a high-calorie, low-protein diet containing an adequate daily amount of mineral salts.

Post-renal (*syn*. Obstructive) Anuria

1. **Calculus anuria** arises in one of the following ways:

(*a*) A calculus becomes impacted in the ureter of the only functioning kidney, the other kidney being congenitally absent, previously removed, or destroyed by disease.

(*b*) Both ureters become obstructed by stones or crystals.

Clinical Features.—Usually the patient is a man between forty and sixty years of age with a long history of urinary lithiasis, but in about 20% of cases calculous anuria arises without previous symptoms.

Onset.—Typically an attack of renal colic precedes the anuria, the onset of which is sudden. This pain may disappear and be replaced by a constant severe pain in the loin. In a few cases there is little, if any, pain, and the anuria is preceded by several days of increasing oliguria.

Stage of tolerance usually lasts from three to six days. The patient feels comparatively well and may continue his work. During this time the blood urea mounts steadily, and as it does so headache, sleeplessness, constipation, and lassitude supervene.

Stage of uraemia follows, and is characterised by the same clinical features described in late renal anuria.

Examination.—The obstructed kidney is tender and there is guarding by the overlying muscles. A large palpable kidney is probably functionless and the seat of a hydronephrosis or pyonephrosis; a recently obstructed kidney is not usually palpable.

Action to be taken:

(i) *Pass a catheter* to exclude retention. A few ounces of blood-stained urine may be obtained.

(ii) *Plain x-ray* may show the obstructing calculus, but more often visualisation is difficult. This is because the small size of the stone (it is seldom larger than an orange-pip), makes it difficult to see against super-imposed bone and intestinal gas shadows. Disparity in the size of the kidneys may be apparent. *Ultrasound* will demonstrate a dilated pelvis and dilated calyces.

(iii) *Cystoscopy.*—Pass a catheter up both ureters. This may pass or dislodge the stone and the emergency is over. Leave the catheter in position to drain, and when the general condition of the patient is satisfactory, remove the calculus by open uretero-lithotomy. (Just prior to this, further radiographs *must* be taken to confirm the site of the stone. An I.V.U. is permissible and helpful when the blood urea has fallen to within normal limits.) Occasionally at cystoscopy a stone is seen wedged in the ureteric orifice (fig. 1184) whereupon attempts should be made to dislodge the stone with a ureteric catheter, or by meatotomy of the orifice.

(iv) *Percutaneous nephrostomy.*—An alternative is for a radiologist to puncture the collecting system of the obstructed kidney under ultrasound control. A guide wire is then passed down the needle. A series of small dilators are then passed and a BF pigtail nephrostomy tube inserted. This permits drainage of urine, or pus, allowing the general condition of the patient to improve prior to definitive stone removal.

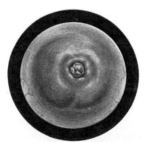

FIG. 1184.—Stone impacted in the ureteric orifice as seen by cystoscopy.

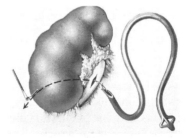

FIG. 1185.—Cabot's method of performing nephrostomy.

(v) If this fails and no stone is visualised by the x-ray, then the kidney on the side which was more painful should be explored. Pyelostomy, or nephrostomy (figs. 1185 and 1186) may be necessary. If the kidney is explored and found to be hopelessly diseased, nephrostomy must be performed on the other side.

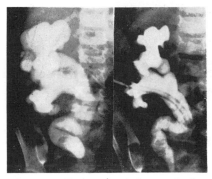

FIG. 1186.—Pyelograms before and after nephrostomy.

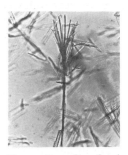

FIG. 1187.—Acetylated sulphapyridine crystals resemble small wheat sheaves.

Through and Through, Loop, Ring, Nephrostomy (Tresidder).—a useful alternative to Cabot's method is to lead a single length of suitable tubing to the surface through the opening in the renal pelvis as well as through the kidney substance. Two holes are cut halfway along the tube where it is positioned in the pelvis. The ends of the tube are anchored to the surface or secured together and connected to the drainage bag. This is advantageous in affording (*a*) double drainage, (*b*) security against inadvertent removal, and (*c*) the continuous facility for replacement of the tube simply by railroading another into position.

(vi) *When the obstruction has been relieved* either by ureteric catheterisation or percutaneous nephrostomy, and until diuresis is established, the general treatment is similar to that described above. In cases where surgical nephrostomy has been necessary, preparations should be made for blood transfusion, for sometimes the haemorrhage from the incised oedematous kidney is excessive.

2. **Anuria due to Sulphonamide Crystalluria**.—Sulphapyridine, sulphadiazine, and occasionally sulphathiazole in the presence of an acid medium are changed into acetyl salts which are insoluble. Crystals (fig. 1187) are desposited in the kidney tubules and ureters. The condition is now infrequent, and occurs mainly in patients with partial obstruction to the kidneys, and in those who are dehydrated. Acetazolamide used in the oral treatment of acute glaucoma can cause crystalluria.

Treatment.—When a patient undergoing sulphonamide therapy develops renal colic and oliguria, the drug should be withheld and the high fluid intake further increased, and frusemide 80 mg given i.v. Should anuria supervene there should be no delay in performing cystoscopy and attempting to catheterise the ureters. Provided the catheters can be inserted, the kidney pelves are washed out with 2·5% sodium bicarbonate solution. The crystalline mass can, on occasions, be dislodged with a stone dislodger (Chapter 57). If these measures are unsuccessful, unilateral or bilateral pyelostomy may be performed.

3. **Anuria due to Uric Acid Crystalluria** can occur in rapidly breaking-down neoplasms—more particularly lymphomas. The pelvis and ureters can become completely blocked by uric acid and urate crystals. Serum uric acid estimations should be performed on such cases having radiotherapy and/or cytotoxic chemotherapy, and the urine should be kept alkaline. (The solubility of uric acid is vastly increased at pH 7–8.)

4. **Anuria due to Accidental Ligation of the Ureters**.—This is a hazard mainly of hysterectomy. Immediate exploration to divide the ligatures encircling the ureters should follow once the site of the obstruction has been determined by passing ureteric catheters. Pyelostomy should be reserved for cases unfit for this.

5. **Anuria due to Involvement of both Ureters in a Neoplastic Process,** *e.g.* **Carcinoma of the Cervix and Prostate are the most common**.—Percutaneous nephrostomy is the most appropriate form of immediate relief of the obstructed upper urinary tracts.

6. **Anuria due to Involvement of Ureters in Retroperitoneal Fibrosis** (Chapter 57).

Hugh Cabot, 1872–1945. Professor of Surgery, Minnesota Graduate School of Medicine, Rochester, Minnesota, U.S.A.
Gerald Charles Tresidder, Contemporary. Senior Lecturer in Human Morphology, Southampton University, England.

THE KIDNEYS AND URETERS

Embryology.—A bud from the lower end of the mesonephric (Wolffian) duct grows backwards behind the peritoneum to the sacral region. The stalk of the bud forms the ureter and its dilated extremity the pelvis. Sometimes the bud is duplicated or the stalk becomes bifurcated, giving rise to congenital anomalies (see below). From six weeks to eight months, the primitive pelvis divides repeatedly to form generations of collecting tubules, the early (4th to 5th) generations ultimately forming the pelvis and calyces.

Later generations form the collecting tubules, and adjacent mesoblast produces a glomerular apparatus and nephric tubules which establish continuity with the collecting system. It is failure of this junction which has been postulated as one cause for the development of polycystic kidneys. Between the fifth and eighth week of this development the kidney ascends on the posterior abdominal wall to reach its subcostal position. it also rotates so that the previously forward facing hilum faces medially.

The fetal kidney is at first lobulated, but in the human the lobules become welded together by the growth of a new cortex and the capsule. In some mammals, *e.g.* oxen and bears, fetal lobulation is retained throughout life.

Surgical Anatomy.—Usually the parenchyma of each kidney is drained by seven pairs of calyces, three in the upper and two each in the middle and lower segments. Each of the three segments represents an anatomical and physiological unit with its own blood supply, an important point in view of the increased indications for partial nephrectomy (Carl Semb).

Surgical Physiology.—Cine-pyelography indicates that there are sphincters at the junction of the minor and major calyces, and at the pelvi-ureteric junction. Each segment of the calyceal system fills before its contents are passed into the next chamber.

CONGENITAL ABNORMALITIES OF THE KIDNEY

Absence of One Kidney.—Sometimes pyelography reveals only one functioning kidney, and at cystoscopy only one ureteric orifice is present; alternatively a ureter and pelvis are present on the non-functioning side, but the parenchyma is almost or entirely absent. In either case the functioning kidney is hypertrophied. An absent or congenitally atrophic kidney is present in about 1:1,400 individuals.

Renal ectopia occurs once in 1000 cases. The kidney is arrested in some part of its normal ascent, usually at the brim of the pelvis. As a rule the kidney of the opposite side is present and in its normal position. The left kidney is ectopic far more often than the right; the reason is unknown. Ectopia may present a diagnostic problem when acute disease develops in the ectopic kidney.

Horse-shoe Kidney.—The most medial subdivisions of the primary mesonephric bud of each side fuse and the kidneys fail to ascend completely. The adrenal glands, being developed separately, are in their normal positions. The abnormality (found once in every 1000 necropsies) is more common in the male. Usually the bridge joining the lower poles lies in front of the fourth lumbar vertebra. Fusions occurs very early, when the embryo is but thirty to forty days old, at which time the two masses of mesoblast destined to form the kidneys lie very close together. Exceptionally, it is the upper poles that are fused.

Clinical Features.—Horse-shoe kidneys are prone to become diseased, largely because the ureters are angulated as they pass over the fused isthmus (fig. 1188). This produces urinary stasis; consequently simple infection, tuberculosis, and

Kaspar Friedrich Wolff, 1733–1794. Professor of Anatomy and Physiology, St. Petersburg (now Leningrad, U.S.S.R.).
Carl Boye Semb, 1895–1971. Professor of Surgery, University of Oslo.

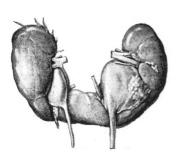

FIG. 1188.—Horse-shoe kidney. Note the ureters passing in front of the fused lower poles.

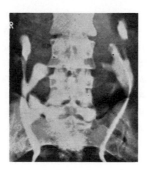

FIG. 1189.—Urogram of a horse-shoe kidney. Only rarely are all the calyces directed towards the spinal column.

(*A. Jacobs, FRCS, Glasgow.*)

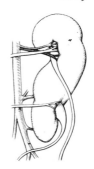

FIG. 1190.—Unilateral S-fusion of the kidneys.

calculus formation are common complications. Although a fixed mass below the umbilicus may suggest a horse-shoe kidney, the final diagnosis is established by urography. The most characteristic finding is that the lowest calyx on each side is reversed in position (*i.e.* directed towards the vertebral column). Rarely most, or all, of the calyces are reversed (fig. 1189). In a large percentage of cases the ureters curve like a flower vase. While horse-shoe kidney is not a contraindication to pregnancy, urinary complications are more frequent.

There was once a vogue for dividing the isthmus of the kidney. The only reason for doing this today is at surgery for abdominal aortic aneurysm.

Unilateral fusion (*syn.* crossed dystopia) is rare. Both kidneys are situated in one loin. One kidney, carrying its own blood-vessels and with the ureter opening into the bladder in a normal position, crosses the middle line, and its upper pole fuses with the lower pole of the normally placed kidney. In this instance both kidney pelves are situated one above the other medial to the renal parenchyma (unilateral long kidney). In some cases the pelvis of the crossed kidney faces laterally (unilateral S-shaped kidney (fig. 1190)) (See also fig. 1197).

Congenital Cystic Kidneys (*syn.* Polycystic Kidneys)

In 18% of cases there is a congenital cystic liver: occasionally the pancreas and lung are affected similarly. The disease is hereditary and can be transmitted by either parent. This is important in relation to genetic counselling as the risk of transmitting the autosomal dominant trait is very high. The disease is not easily demonstrable on urography before the late 'teens' and rarely gives clinical manifestations until the fourth decade.

Pathology.—The organs may become enormously enlarged. The surface gives an appearance of many bubbles. On section the renal parenchyma is riddled with cysts of varying sizes, some containing clear fluid, others thick brown material, and still others coagulated blood.

Clinical Features in the Adult.—The condition is slightly more common in women than in men. There are six clinical features:

(1) *Renal Enlargement.*—The large knobbly kidneys when discovered in the course of a routine examination can hardly be mistaken. Sometimes congenital

cystic kidneys are revealed only at laparotomy for some other condition. *Unilateral Renal Swelling.*—One kidney contains larger cysts than the other, and the physical signs are similar to those of a renal neoplasm.

Patients with congenital cystic kidneys pass abundant urine of low specific gravity (1·010 or less) containing a slight trace of albumin but neither casts nor cells. On cystoscopy there is often considerable delay in the excretion of indigocarmine, even in cases with a normal or only slightly elevated blood urea.

(2) *Pain* is due either to the weight of the organ dragging upon its pedicle or to tension within the cysts. Often the pain is a dull ache in the loin; sometimes it takes the form of renal colic, when a calculus, which is not rare in this condition, should be suspected.

(3) *Haematuria.*—In about 25% of cases, as a result of over-distension, one of the cysts ruptures into the renal pelvis and causes haematuria. Usually moderate haematuria lasts for a few days, and recurs at varying intervals; sometimes it is profuse.

(4) *Infection.*—The most common complication of congenital cystic kidneys in adult life is pyelonephritis.

(5) *Hypertension.*—About 75% of patients with congenital cystic kidneys above the age of twenty have hypertension. Why some escape this complication is not clear. Possibly the high blood pressure is due to a separate genetic factor frequently linked with congenital cystic kidneys.

(6) *Uraemia.*—The patient complains of anorexia, headache, and vague gastric symptoms, and is frequently given a placebo, until persistent symptoms demand a complete clinical examination. Later drowsiness and vomiting occur. Signs of uraemia often commence suddenly during middle life; only one quarter of patients with this condition survive the age of fifty-five years. Severe anaemia is common.

Urography.[1]—Excretory urography is the best way of confirming the diagnosis. The shadows of the kidneys are enlarged in all directions. The renal pelvis is elongated and may be compressed. The calyces are stretched over the cysts and are often narrow (like the legs of a spider) or bell-like (fig. 1193). Ultrasound (fig. 1191) will confirm the presence of multiple renal cysts, some of which may contain turbid fluid or altered blood from haemorrhage. This appearance can be contrasted with the scan of a solitary (acquired) cyst (fig. 1192). The nature of the cyst fluid can be determined by simultaneous aspiration of the cyst(s) using fluoroscopy.

Treatment:

(a) *Expectant.*—Routinely the patient should drink large quantities of water, have a low-protein diet, and take iron to prevent anaemia. Infection, when it occurs, should be treated by an appropriate drug.

(b) *Operative.*—By relieving pressure on the remaining renal parenchyma, Rovsing's operation, if performed early, has been claimed to improve renal function. Few surgeons advocate this operation now.

Rovsing's Operation.—One kidney and then the other is exposed. The cysts are incised

---

[1] See footnote p. 1196.

Nils Thorkild Rovsing, 1862–1927. Professor of Surgery, Copenhagen.

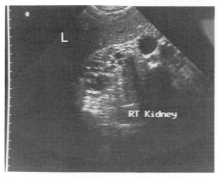
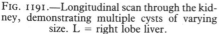

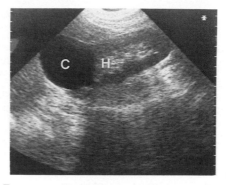

FIG. 1191.—Longitudinal scan through the kidney, demonstrating multiple cysts of varying size. L = right lobe liver.

FIG. 1192.—Longitudinal scan of kidney. Large cyst (C) at the upper pole of the kidney. H = hilum of the kidney.

with a narrow-bladed scalpel, first on the convex border, then on the posterior surface and, finally, as the kidney becomes more manageable in size, the peritoneum is peeled away and the anterior surface is dealt with similarly.

(c) *Renal Failure* should be treated by dialysis, possibly bilateral nephrectomy and kidney transplantation.

Infantile Polycystic Disease is an unrelated condition—autosomal recessive— and much rarer. The kidneys are large, may obstruct birth and many cases are stillborn. Most others die in early life from renal failure.

Unilateral Multicystic Disease is much commoner. It presents as a mass in the flank. No function is detectable on urography, and exploration and removal is the treatment of choice. In the differential diagnosis, Wilms's tumour (p. 1247), neuroblastoma and hydronephrosis are all rarer conditions.

Solitary Renal Cyst. (fig. 1192)

While the term 'solitary' serves to distinguish the condition from congenital cystic disease of the kidneys, it is found that not infrequently one or two similar but smaller cysts are also present.

Aetiology.—The origin of the cyst may be identical (but on a smaller scale) with that of congenital cystic kidney (above), or it could arise from bygone trauma or infection causing blockage of a tubule. The mature age at which the cyst is usually found is in favour of the latter supposition.

Clinical Features.—There are no pathognomonic symptoms or signs. Sometimes there are no symptoms until a swelling is noticed, at others there is a dull ache in the loin. The cyst can become infected and if a swelling is palpable, and particularly if the swelling is tender, the creditable diagnosis of pyonephrosis will be made. A spontaneous haemorrhage into the cyst occurs from time to time, in which case sudden renal pain is likely to be experienced. Occasionally the cyst presses on the pelvi-ureteric junction and causes urinary symptoms.

Radiology.—(a) Urography reveals a filling defect with one of more calyces stretched over it, simulating the deformity produced by a neoplasm, but typically more rounded. (b) It is possible to distinguish a renal cyst from a renal neoplasm by ultrasound in many cases, by percutaneous puncture, and by arteriography (fig. 1179).

Treatment.—Today a simple cyst, completely free of 'echos' on ultrasound, should be left untouched. When there is doubt cyst puncture with examination of the fluid bacteriologically and for malignant cells can be done. Exploration used to be advised. Renal cysts can rarely be caused by a tumour blocking tubules and interfering with the vascular supply to the same area of the kidney. Having displayed the kidney the operation is varied according to circumstances.

(*a*) *Kirwin's Method.*—When the cyst is blue-domed and aspiration reveals clear fluid, that portion of the cyst wall lying above the surface is excised. The cavity is filled with perinephric fat and after securing haemostasis of the cut edges, a corrugated drain is left down to the area, the fascia of Gerota closed over it, and the wound closed in layers.

(*b*) *Partial nephrectomy* is performed if the contents of the cyst are blood-stained (one-third of such cysts contain a papilliferous neoplasm).

(*c*) *Nephrectomy* is performed if there are indications that the cyst is a malignant degeneration of a neoplasm, *e.g.* irregular induration at the periphery of the cyst.

Differential Diagnosis.—In sheep-raising districts, *hydatid cyst of the kidney* is common. On the right side (if hydatid disease is suspected) the swelling is liable to be mistaken for a hydatid cyst of the liver. Occasionally the patient complains of passing 'grape skins' (ruptured daughter cysts) in the urine. The treatment is excision of the cyst but in many cases the cyst is so large that nephrectomy is advisable.

Aberrant renal vessels

These are found on the left side more frequently than on the right; in females more often than males; unilateral examples are three times more common than bilateral. Aberrant renal vessels can cause hydronephrosis (fig. 1205). More frequently, however, aberrant vessels accentuate a hydronephrosis present on account of another reason (fig. 1204).

Usually the aberrant artery is small; occasionally it is comparatively large, supplying one-quarter of the renal parenchyma. Division will cause infarction of the corresponding portion of renal tissue. On the other hand, an obstructing aberrant renal *vein* can be divided with impunity, because the venous collateral circulation is very generous.

CONGENITAL ABNORMALITIES OF THE RENAL PELVIS AND URETER

Duplication of a renal pelvis is the most common congenital anomaly of the upper renal tract and is found in about 4% of patients. It is usually unilateral, and is somewhat more common on the left side than on the right. The upper renal pelvis is comparatively small (fig. 1194) and drains the upper group of calyces; the larger lower renal pelvis drains the middle and lower groups of calyces.

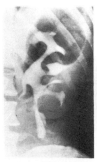

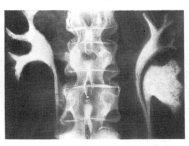

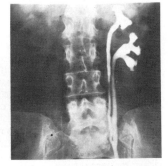

FIG. 1193. — Poly-cystic kidney. Uro-graphic appearance. Note length of kid-ney and elongated bell-like calyces stretched over cysts.

FIG. 1194.—Urogram showing a kidney with double pelvis.

FIG. 1195.—Double ureter. Retrograde pyelogram.

Thomas Joseph Kirwin, 1889–1959. Director of Department of Urology, Fourth and Fifth Avenue Hospitals, New York, U.S.A. Dumitra Gerota, 1867–1939. Professor of Surgery, Bucharest, Rumania.

Reno-renal reflux, from one segment of a duplex kidney to the other may be a cause of pain. It is usually associated with pyelonephritis changes in the segment affected by the reflux.

Duplication of a Ureter.—Double ureters are present in addition to double renal pelves in about 3% of cases submitted to urography. The ureters often join, usually in the lower third of their course (fig. 1195), and have a common orifice into the bladder. Less frequently the ureters open independently into the bladder (fig. 1196), in which case the ureter draining the upper pelvis crosses its fellow, and opens below and medial to it.

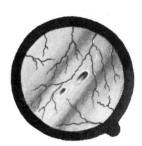

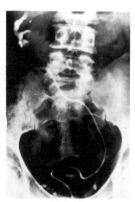

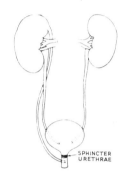

FIG. 1196.— Complete duplication of the left ureter as seen through the cystoscope.

FIG. 1197.—Crossed dystopia. The ureteric orifices are situated normally.
(R. K. Garg, FRCS, Bombay.)

FIG. 1198.—Ectopic ureter in a female.

Clinical Features.—In many instances a double renal pelvis or a double ureter is found by chance in the course of an investigation of the urinary organs. A double pelvis is more liable to become the seat of infection, calculus formation, or hydronephrosis than a normal pelvis. Initially such disease is confined to one part of the duplication. In cases of complete duplication of the ureter the lower ureteric orifice is sometimes the site of congenital atresia.

Treatment.—Ureteric meatotomy can be performed in some early cases of stricture of a ureteric meatus. Difficulty is encountered in cases of Y-shaped bifid ureter, because a ureteric catheter cannot be made to enter the smaller orifice. Heminephrectomy with removal of its ureter is eminently satisfactory when disease normally requiring total nephrectomy is confined strictly to one half of a kidney that has a double pelvis. The exception to the rule is, of course, a neoplasm.

Ectopic Ureteric Orifice.—Should a second ureteric bud arise from the mesonephric duct later than usual, the orifice of the accessory ureter is prone to occupy a grossly abnormal position. This is a rare anomaly. In both sexes the existence of double ureter is determined by excretory urography.

In the female an ectopic ureter opens either into the urethra below the sphincter urethrae (fig. 1198) or into the vagina, and causes an intractable incontinence of urine. The diagnosis can nearly always be made from the history alone. A girl or woman who has dribbled for as long as she can remember, despite the fact that she has a desire to void, and does urinate, has an ectopic ureteric orifice. The demonstration of this orifice is often extremely difficult, because it is guarded by a valve. The diagnosis may be established by giving an intravenous injection of indigocarmine, and placing one swab into the vestibule and another in the vagina; the one coloured blue signifies the position of the ectopic orifice. Sometimes laparotomy is the only way of finding or excluding the additional ureter.

In the male the aberrant opening may be situated at the apex of the trigone, in the posterior urethra, in a seminal vesicle, or in an ejaculatory duct. As in all these diverse situations, the ectopic ureteric orifice is situated above the sphincter urethrae, the male

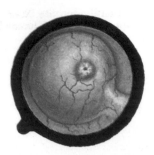

FIG. 1199.—Right-sided ureterocele.
(After J. C. Ainsworth-Davies, FRCS, London.)

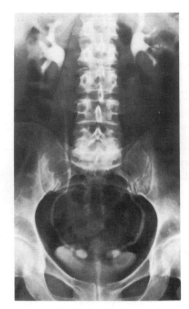

FIG. 1200.—Intravenous urographic appearance of ureterocele. Typical adder-head appearance of lower ureters which remain filled with Hypaque (diatrizoate).

patient is continent, but recurrent acute or chronic pyelonephritis is apt to supervene in the renal tissue served by the ectopic ureter. Posterior urethroscopy, after the intravenous injection of indigocarmine, may be of help in demonstrating that a male patient has an ectopic ureter.

Treatment.—*In the female* excision of that segment of the kidney served by the ectopic ureter is usually advisable, because it is so often hydronephrotic and chronically infected. In the rare event of the urine draining from it being sterile, the ectopic ureter can be implanted into the bladder, or joined to its fellow.

In the male—Often no treatment is required. Should urinary infection supervene hemi-nephrectomy is indicated.

Congenital Megaureter may be unilateral or bilateral, and in late stages is accompanied by hydronephrosis. Other congenital abnormalities may be manifest. Commoner in males the condition is often symptomless until infection has occurred. If, however, the patient experiences pain, a diagnosis can be made before the onset of infection. The lower end of the ureter and orifice appear normal but constitute an obstruction. Reflux is not present; a ureteric catheter passes easily. Vigorous peristaltic activity can be seen in the dilated ureter under the image intensifier, but efflux is small, while marked delay in emptying of the pelvis and ureter is seen in late films many hours after.

Treatment.—In infected cases, percystoscopic meatotomy and drainage of the dilated ureter with a ureteric catheter for about six weeks has been found to be effective in clearing up the infection. Reflux afterwards is likely however, and the condition is better treated by initial nephrostomy and then when the infection is completely controlled, by open excision of the lower ureter, followed by excision of excessive length of tortuous ureter, refastening the end by wedge excision to narrow the lumen, and tunnel reimplantation to prevent reflux. When the renal parenchyma is severely damaged, nephroureterectomy is curative. In bilateral cases where function is diminishing, cutaneous ureterostomy should be considered.

Post-caval Ureter.—The right ureter passes behind the inferior vena cava instead of lying to the right of it. This may cause obstructive symptoms. Should these symptoms warrant it, the ureter can be divided in the dilated portion and reanastomosed in front of the cava. Occasionally the retrocaval portion of the ureter is fibrotic and must be excised. A long oblique anastomosis should be made of the normal lower ureter to the dilated upper portion.

Ureterocele is due to congenital atresia of a ureteric orifice which causes a cystic enlargement of the intramural portion of the ureter. Usually the wall of the cyst is composed of mucous membrane only; infrequently the muscle coat is included. This condition may be discovered in childhood; often it is not recognised until adult life. Women are more often affected than men, and in 10% of cases the condition is bilateral. The condition, producing some obstruction, does render the patient more liable to stone formation and recurrent infection. The cystoscopic findings are characteristic: when the wall consists of mucous membrane there is a translucent cyst over which blood-vessels radiate (fig. 1199); in the rare variety containing muscle in the wall, the cyst is opaque. In either case the sac is seen to enlarge rapidly with each efflux of urine, and then slowly to collapse. The urographic findings are characteristic (fig. 1200).

Treatment.—Many cases are symptomless and no treatment is required. Hydronephrosis, stone, or recurrent infection may necessitate treatment. Cauterising a hole through the wall of the cyst with a diathermy electrode is a simple and satisfactory procedure. A micturating cystogram should be performed three months later to exclude urinary reflux. In advanced unilateral cases associated with a hydro- or pyonephrosis and dilatation of the whole of the ureter, nephrectomy is needed.

INJURIES TO THE KIDNEY

In civil life blows or falls upon the loin are the most fruitful sources of such injuries, while blows from in front and crushing accidents add their quota (road traffic accidents). Haematuria following minor injuries should suggest the possibility of pre-existing renal abnormality, *e.g.* stone, hydronephrosis, or tuberculosis.

The degree of injury varies considerably from a small subcapsular haematoma to a complete tear involving the whole thickness of the kidney (fig. 1201); in addition, the kidney may be partially or wholly avulsed from its pedicle. Tears of the renal parenchyma follow the lines of the uriniferous tubules. The whole of one pole may be detached.

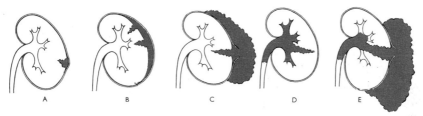

FIG. 1201.—Various types of renal injuries: A, small subcapsular haemorrhage; B, large subcapsular haemorrhage; C, cortical laceration with perinephric haematoma; D, medullary laceration with bleeding into the renal pelvis; E, complete rupture.
(After P. Adams.)

The injury is extraperitoneal, except very occasionally in children in whom there is little perinephric fat; in these cases the peritoneum, being intimately related to the kidney, is liable to be torn in addition to the renal capsule, allowing blood and, perhaps, urine to escape into the peritoneal cavity.

Clinical Features.—Rarely is there superficial bruising, but there is likely to be local pain and tenderness.

Haematuria is a cardinal sign of a damaged kidney, but it may not make its appearance until some hours after the accident. If the haemorrhage is profuse, it may be followed by clot colic.

Severe Delayed Haematuria.—Sudden profuse haematuria can occur between the third day and the third week after the accident in a patient who appears to be progressing favourably. It is due to a clot becoming dislodged.

Meteorism.—In many cases of renal injury, abdominal distension comes on about twenty-four to forty-eight hours after the accident. In all probability it is caused by a retroperitoneal haematoma implicating splanchnic nerves.

A perinephric haematoma should be suspected if there is even a slight flattening of the normal contour of the loin, always provided there is no scoliosis.

Management and Treatment

Conservative treatment is usually successful and must be instituted at once. However, it must be remembered that injury to other organs may be associated with injury to the kidney.

1. The patient must rest flat in bed until macroscopic haematuria has been absent for one week.

2. Morphine should be given for pain, and as a sedative.

3. Hourly pulse and blood-pressure charts must be kept.

4. Give an antibiotic to prevent infection of the haematoma.

5. Save a sample of each specimen of urine passed.

6. Group and cross-match blood. A transfusion may be required for shock or continuing haemorrhage.

7. An intravenous urogram (I.V.P.) should be obtained urgently to show that the other kidney is normal. A leak of urine on the damaged side is often demonstrated.

Under this regimen the haematuria should diminish, pain and guarding decrease, and pulse and colour of the patient improve.

Exploration is necessary in 20 to 25% and is undertaken if: 1. There are signs of progressive blood loss. 2. A swelling develops in the loin. 3. Signs of perirenal infection develop. The aim is to conserve the kidney or part of it if possible.

Before proceeding to surgical exploration for bleeding a renal arteriogram should be performed if possible. If the bleeding vessel is visualised it may be embolised with small starch microspheres to stop the bleeding.

In all cases the peritoneum should be opened to exclude damage to other organs.

Should the necessity for an urgent operation arise and facilities for urography not be available, the presence of a functioning kidney on the contralateral side can often be confirmed by chromo-cystoscopy (Chapter 56). When the kidney is found to be ruptured in several places, or the kidney pedicle is damaged, nephrectomy must be undertaken. Small tears can be sutured over Oxycel or a piece of detached muscle, either of which promotes haemostasis. Larger single rents in the middle of the kidney are best dealt with by performing nephrostomy through the rent and suturing the kidney on either side of the tube. If laceration is confined to one pole of the kidney, partial nephrectomy may be practicable.

When a sole existing kidney is sufficiently damaged to necessitate exploration, it must be repaired. Failing this, the wound is packed firmly with gauze in the hope that not only will the bleeding be controlled but that the ruptured kidney may heal.

Multiple Injuries.—Simultaneous splenectomy and left nephrectomy have been carried out successfully when both organs have been ruptured. The mortality of cases of rupture of the kidney with damage to the liver or hollow organs, often complicated by fractured ribs, pelvis, or vertebrae, is high.

Complications.—1. Clot retention in the bladder can be cleared with a urethral catheter and bladder washout. Sometimes the washout must be done via a cystoscope.

2. Pararenal pseudo-hydronephrosis may occur in the course of a few weeks, due to combination of a complete tear of the renal cortex and ureteric obstruction.

3. Hypertension may follow fibrosis of the kidney, usually after three months or more. Nephrectomy will be necessary.

4. **Aneurysm of a renal artery** (fig. 1202) is a rare complication of injury to a kidney. The most frequent symptom is pain in the renal region, and, when the aneurysm is large, a non-tender swelling will be felt. Only occasionally is it pulsatile, and a bruit may be heard. An x-ray may show a shadow in relation to the pelvis of the kidney. An intravenous urogram demonstrates that the swelling is extrarenal with the renal pelvis displaced laterally. Aortography will confirm the diagnosis. Attacks of haematuria occur, and are probably due to congestion of the renal parenchyma. The aneurysm may rupture into the peritoneal cavity or into the perirenal tissues, with fatal results.

Treatment by nephrectomy and excision of the aneurysm is usually required. In a few cases a saccular aneurysm has been resected with preservation of the renal vessels and the kidney.

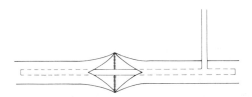

FIG. 1203.—Repair of the ureter using a T-tube.

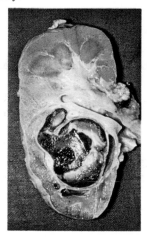

FIG. 1202.—Aneurysm of the renal artery containing laminated thrombus.

INJURIES TO THE URETER

Rupture of a ureter can occur as the result of an accident causing hyperextension of the spine. The clinical diagnosis is impossible until a diminished quantity of urine is passed, followed by a swelling in the loin or iliac fossa. An I.V. urogram shows a diffuse shadow below the kidney on the injured side.

Injury of one or both ureters during a pelvic operation is considerably more common than the foregoing and occurs most often during the course of a difficult hysterectomy. Preliminary catheterisation of the ureters prevents such accidents, for with catheters within them, the ureters can be felt and seen unmistakably. The accidents include division of the ureter, ligating it, crushing it in forceps or removing a portion of its wall.

Injury recognised at the Time of the Operation.—The uretero-vesical continuity should be restored by one of the methods described below, unless the patient's condition is poor, when ligation of the proximal end of the ureter is the best course. If the patient rallies within two days, temporary nephrostomy is carried out, and a reparative operation undertaken later.

Injury not recognised at the Time of the Operation:

(*a*) **Unilateral Injuries.**—There are three possibilities:

1. *No Symptoms.*—If one ureter is ligated securely with unabsorbable material and the contralateral kidney and ureter are normal, in 68% of cases the kidney on the obstructed side undergoes silent atrophy. Thus the accident remains unsuspected unless the patient, some time later, undergoes a urological examination.

2. *Development of loin pain and a fever*, possibly proceeding to a pyonephrosis, occurs in less than a half of the remainder. Excretory urography reveals no excretion on the side of the lesion. If this is discovered early, and the patient is fit, re-exploration to free the ureter is best: alternatively, nephrostomy and, later, repair of the ureter.

3. *A urinary fistula develops* through the abdominal incision or, following hysterectomy,

through the vagina. Again, a temporary nephrostomy may be performed, and a reparative operation postponed until oedema and infection have abated after an interval of about six weeks. However, this tradition of delay only leaves the poor patient continually wet and dissatisfied. Early repair is now regarded as safe, providing the patient is fit and the surgeon experienced.

(b) **Bilateral Injury.**—In cases of anuria following ligation of both ureters during hysterectomy an attempt is made to pass ureteric catheters, when both ureters will be found to be occluded. The wound should be explored and ligatures removed.

Repair of the Injured Ureter

1. If the ends are clean cut and no length is lost, each end should be split for 1·5 cm and the edges united as a flat ribbon (fig. 1203). A soft latex T-tube may be left with one limb across the gap for two weeks. This is to be preferred to end-to-end suture which frequently results in stricture formation, although internal splintage is probably more satisfactory, using a double-J pigtail catheter[1] if one is available.

2. In division low down, it may be possible to reimplant the ureter into the bladder.

3. The ureter can often be implanted end-to-side into the opposite ureter.

4. *Boari's Operation.*—A flap of bladder is turned up to replace the lower ureter.

5. Occasionally, where conservation of all renal tissue is vital, replacement by a segment of ileum is necessary.

Nephrectomy may be the best course, for example, in the elderly patient with a malignant condition, the other kidney being normal.

HYDRONEPHROSIS

A hydronephrosis is an aseptic dilatation of the whole or part of the kidney due to a partial or intermittent obstruction to the outflow of urine.

A hydronephrosis may be unilateral or bilateral.

Unilateral hydronephrosis is due to some form of *ureteral* obstruction, often at the pelvi-ureteric junction; any length of ureter above the obstruction is dilated also. The causes are:

Extramural.—1. 'Aberrant Vessels'. In a number of cases of pelvic hydronephrosis a lower polar artery or vein arising from the main vessels in an aberrant position appears to obstruct the upper ureter where it crosses in front of it. The pyelographic appearance is shown in fig. 1205(b). In many more instances this is not an aberrant vessel, but a normal inferior renal artery or vein that has been displaced downwards by the enlarged renal pelvis. This displaced vessel, while adding considerably to the rapid increase in the size of the hydronephrosis, is not the cause thereof (fig. 1204).

2. Involvement of ureter by growth outside it, *e.g.* carcinoma of the cervix, prostate, rectum, colon, or caecum.

3. Idiopathic retroperitoneal fibrosis.

Intramural.—1. Congenital stenosis, physiological narrowing, or achalasia at the pelvi-ureteric junction.

2. Ureterocele and congenital small ureteric orifice.

3. Inflammatory stricture of the ureter following removal of a stone that was lodged in one portion of the ureter for a considerable time, or tuberculosis of the ureter. Stricture of the ureter may follow uretero-ureteric anastomosis or trauma to the ureter during a pelvic operation.

4. Neoplasm of a ureter, or the bladder involving a ureteric orifice.

Intraluminal.—A calculus in the ureter or small calculus in the renal pelvis. The latter often gives rise to intermittent hydronephrosis.

---

[1] A pigtail catheter is a fine 'spring' of plastic tubing: when inserted, the ends are retained in position by residual coils at top and bottom while the centre is stretched and straight.

Achille Boari. Nineteenth-century Italian surgeon.

Bilateral hydronephrosis is generally the result of some form of *urethral* obstruction, but it can also be caused by one of the lesions described above occurring on both sides.

When due to lower urinary obstruction, the cause may be:

(*a*) *Congenital:*

1. Congenital stricture of the urethral meatus or, very rarely, phimosis.

2. Congenital valves of the posterior urethra, or congenital contracture of the bladder neck.

(*b*) *Acquired:*

1. A neoplasm of the bladder which involves both ureteric orifices.

2. Prostatic enlargement or carcinoma; acquired contracture of the bladder neck.

3. Carcinoma of the cervix (occasionally carcinoma of the rectum), involving both ureters.

4. Inflammatory or traumatic urethral stricture. Phimosis.

When the obstruction lies in the urethra, muscular hypertrophy of the bladder occurs, and the ureters, by reason of this hypertrophy, become partially obstructed in the intra-mural portion of their course.

Pathology.—The pathological changes differ in some respects according to whether the kidney has an extrarenal or an intrarenal pelvis, the former being much more common. In a kidney with an extrarenal pelvis, at first the pelvis alone becomes dilated (pelvic hydronephrosis) (fig. 1204). As time goes on, if the

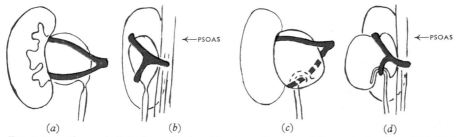

(*a*)   (*b*)   (*c*)   (*d*)

FIG. 1204.—'Congenital' hydronephrosis with obstruction at pelvi-ureteric junction. (*a*) Initial arrangement. (*b*) Lateral view of the hilum. (*c*) and (*d*) show pelvis of kidney prolapsing forward between branches of the renal artery.

obstruction is not relieved the calyces become increasingly dilated and the renal parenchyma is progressively destroyed by pressure atrophy. In a kidney with an intrarenal pelvis the destruction of the parenchyma occurs more rapidly. In either case, it may be a matter of years before the diagnosis is made, by which time the kidney may be merely a lobulated sac containing pale uriniferous fluid of low specific gravity. On bisecting the specimen longitudinally a series of compartments representing the dilated calyces will be found. Rarely is the renal parenchyma destroyed in its entirety, although in advanced cases the amount remaining is very small.

CLINICAL FEATURES

Unilateral Hydronephrosis

The female/male ratio is 2:1; the right side is more commonly affected. Presenting features include:

1. *Insidious.*—Pain is slight; often there is only a dull ache or a sense of weight in the loin which may be brought on by alcohol or excessive fluid intake. On examination an enlarged, sometimes a greatly enlarged, kidney is found. In these cases the obstruction is usually at the pelvi-ureteric junction.

2. *Attacks of renal colic* occur. Often there is no palpable swelling.

3. *Intermittent Hydronephrosis.*—After an attack of renal colic with its accompanying abdominal rigidity passes off, a swelling in the loin is found. Some hours later, or on the next day, following the passage of a large quantity of urine due also to some reflex polyuria, the pain is relieved and the swelling disappears (Dietl's crisis).

Bilateral Hydronephrosis

1. *Due to Lower Urinary Obstruction.*—There is little to call attention to the hydronephrosis except, perhaps, a dull ache in the loins. The symptoms are overshadowed by those of the causative lesion (above). Symptoms of uraemia— thirst, loss of appetite are commoner than loin pain. There is often polyuria of low specific gravity containing a small quantity of albumin. The kidneys are unlikely to be palpable because before the hydronephroses became large enough to be felt, renal failure will have occurred.

2. *Due to Bilateral Upper Urinary Obstruction.*—This is rare compared with a unilateral lesion. Symptoms may be bilateral, but more frequently are on one side, a urogram revealing hydronephrosis on the other side.

3. *Due to Pregnancy.*—Dilatation of the ureters and renal pelves occurs in every pregnancy. Both renal pelves and ureters are affected, but the right side to a much greater extent than the left. The dilatation commences during the first few weeks of gestation, and reaches its zenith between the fifth and sixth months. It then remains stationary until after delivery, when involution occurs within two to twelve weeks. The condition is due to atony of the ureteric musculature brought about by the hormone progesterone. Possibly pressure of the fetal head on the ureters plays some part during the last months of pregnancy. The main importance of the condition is an increased liability to infection. Exceptionally the hydronephrosis persists.

Urography (I.V.P.).—Except during pregnancy, when x-rays are contraindi-cated for fear of causing a congenital malformation, the diagnosis is made by *excretory urography.* When the hydronephrosis is advanced, films taken six to twenty-four hours after the injection of the medium may show a hydronephrotic kidney which was imperceptible on films taken at the routine times. As a rule the earliest pyelographic manifestation of a hydronephrosis is dilatation of the renal pelvis, for in the majority of cases the pelvis is extrarenal. The next change is decreasing concavity and then flattening of the minor calyces and dilatation of the major calyces, which are the first changes when the pelvis is intrarenal. In moderate-sized hydronephroses the minor calyces become convex and finally club-shaped and the major calyces considerably broadened. In advanced cases there is extreme dilatation of the renal pelvis and the calyces (fig. 1205), or no excretion of opaque media. Doubtful cases may be clarified on occasion by inducing a diuresis during excretion pyelography which may 'blow up' a hydrone-

---

Joseph Dietl, 1804–1878. Professor of Pathology and Therapeutics, Cracow. In his later years he achieved fame as a politician.

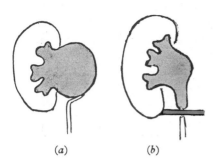

FIG. 1205.—(a) Urographic appearance in 'congenital' hydronephrosis with obstruction at the pelvi-ureteric junction. (b) Urographic appearance in obstruction due to a polar vessel.

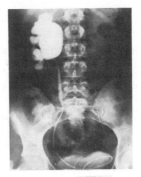

FIG. 1206. — Retrograde pyelogram of a hydronephrosis showing a greatly enlarged pelvis and dilated calyces.

FIG. 1207.—Kidney hydronephrosis. Longitudinal scan through the kidney (coronal) showing dilated renal pelvis (P) and dilated calyces (C). A = aorta.

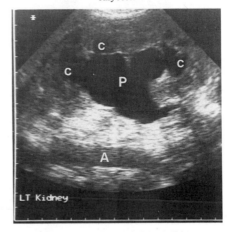

phrosis. Just occasionally there remains an element of doubt as to whether a kidney is obstructed or not. If this situation arises an answer can usually be obtained by administering Lasix during a radioisotope renogram. When this fails to clarify the situation a *Whitaker test* is indicated. A fine needle puncture of the kidney through the loin is made and the kidney perfused at a constant rate up to 10 ml per minute with continuous monitoring of the intrapelvic pressure. An abnormal rise in the pressure will confirm obstruction. *Retrograde pyelography* (fig. 1206) is required only when the results of excretory pyelography are inconclusive or before surgical reconstruction of a damaged or divided ureter. Delay in emptying may be shown by a film taken ten minutes after the pelvis has been filled retrogradely; by this time a normal pelvis should have emptied.

Ultrasound scan (fig. 1207): confirmation of hydronephrosis can be obtained by an ultrasound scan.

Treatment.—The indications for operation are bouts of renal pain, increasing dilation of the renal pelvis and calyces, or evidence of infection. *Conservation* of renal tissue is the aim. Nephrectomy should only be performed when the renal parenchyma has been largely destroyed. Mild bilateral cases with few symptoms should be followed up, but only operated upon if dilatation is increasing.

Robert Whitaker, Contemporary. Consultant Urologist, Addenbrooke's Hospital, Cambridge.

Careful freeing of the ureters (ureterolysis) is an essential preliminary to specific procedures;

Ligation and division of an obstructing blood-vessel, together with clearance of adhesions in the neighbourhood of the pelvi-ureteric junction, gives a lasting cure in the few cases due to this cause. The objection to dividing the obstructing artery is that ischaemic infarction ensues in the portion of kidney supplied, and is nowadays regarded as 'unacceptable practice' since a plastic reconstruction is possible in front of such a vessel (see below).

Reconstruction of a hydronephrosis is employed in cases of advanced pelvic hydronephrosis providing a reasonable thickness of renal parenchyma remains. The Anderson-Hynes operation (fig. 1208) is probably the best. The affected kidney is displayed and the

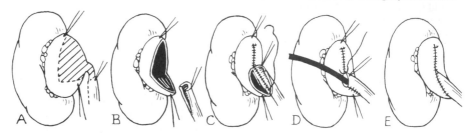

FIG. 1208..—The Anderson-Hynes plastic reconstruction of a hydronephrosis. Note the placement of the stay sutures.

upper third of the ureter and the renal pelvis are mobilised. A renal vein overlying the pelvi-ureteric junction can be divided, but an artery in this situation, whether aberrant or not, should be preserved. The anastomosis is made in front of such an artery. The upper end of the ureter is divided a short distance below the pelvi-ureteric junction, or any narrow segment of ureter. The redundant part of the renal pelvis, together with the ureteropelvic junction is resected as shown in fig. 1208 A, a flap of the lower part of the pelvis being retained. The upper two-thirds of the opening thus created in the renal pelvis is closed with a 0000 chromic catgut suture traversing all coats (fig. 1208 B). The upper end of the ureter is slit for 2–3 cm and its anterior edge is anastomosed to the anterior edge of the pelvic flap by a continuous suture of 0000 plain catgut (fig. 1208 C). A ureteric catheter is passed into the ureter for a short distance; this is merely a temporary expedient to keep the deep sutured layer out of the way while the superficial edges are drawn together (fig. 1208 D) in the same manner as were the deep. The catheter is withdrawn just before the anastomosis is completed (fig. 1208E).

Intubated Ureterostomy (Davis).—Longitudinal incision of a narrowed segment of ureter, leaving a T-tube across the split to allow regrowth round the tube is a simple and effective treatment when the pelvis is not greatly enlarged.

RENAL CALCULUS

Aetiology.—The subject is a complicated one, and the following is an epitome of current opinion. (Compare with the aetiology of gallstones, Chapter 47).

1. **Dietetic.**—A deficiency of vitamin A causes a desquamation of epithelium. The cells form a nidus around which the stone is deposited. From a study of economic conditions in districts where urinary calculi are common, it is evident that the inhabitants suffer from dietetic imbalance. This is more applicable to bladder calculi.

2. **Altered Urinary Solutes and Colloids.**—In hot climates the concentration of solutes will rise. It has been postulated that any reduction of the urinary colloids which adsorb solutes, or excess of muco-proteins which may chelate[1] calcium, predispose to the formation of an insoluble complex.

3. **Decreased Urinary Output of Citrate.**—The presence of citrate in the urine, 300–900 mg/24h (1·6–4·7 mmol/24h as citric acid), tends to maintain in solution otherwise relatively insoluble calcium phosphate and carbonate. The excretion of citrate is under hormonal control and decreases during menstruation.

---

[1] Chelate—to seize hold of. Chētē, Gr. = the prehensile claw of a crab or scorpion.

James Christie Anderson, Contemporary. Consulting Surgeon, Royal Hostpial, Sheffield, England.
Wilfred Hynes, Contemporary. Surgeon, Plastic and Jaw Department, United Sheffield Hospitals, Sheffield, England.
David Melvin Davis, Contemporary. Professor Emeritus of Urology, Jefferson Medical College, Philadelphia, U.S.A.

4. **Renal Infection.**—Infection favours the formation of urinary calculi. Both clinical and experimental stone formation is common when the urine is infected with a urea-splitting streptococcus, staphylococcus, or proteus. The predominant bacteria found in the nuclei of urinary calculi are a staphylococcus and *Esch. coli.*

5. **Inadequate Urinary Drainage.**—Stones are prone to occur in patients with obstruction to the free passage of urine.

6. **Prolonged immobilisation** form any cause, *e.g.* paraplegia, is prone to result in skeletal decalcification and an increased output of calcium in the urine. This, combined with the mechanical effects of recumbency on renal drainage, favours the deposition of calcium phosphate calculi. In uninfected cases spontaneous dissolution sometimes occurs.

7. **Hyperparathyroidism,** although rare, occurring perhaps in 5% of cases, should always receive consideration. In cases of multiple or recurrent urinary calculi this cause should be eliminated by biochemical tests (chapter 38). Hyperparathyroidism results in a great increase in the elimination of calcium in the urine. It has been aptly remarked that these patients pass their skeleton in their urine. A parathyroid adenoma should be removed before the urinary calculi are treated.

8. **Randall's Plaque. Microliths.**—Randall showed that the initial lesion in many cases of renal calculus is an erosion at the apex of one of the renal papillae. On this erosion are deposited urinary salts=Randall's plaque. It has further been shown that minute concretions (microliths) occur normally in the renal parenchyma and Carr postulates that these particles are carried away, like carbon particles from the bronchi, by lymphatics. Should some of the renal lymphatic vessels become blocked by inflammatory exudate, a subendothelial calculus may form. Later the endothelium becomes ulcerated, leaving the calculus in contact with the urine.

Varieties of Renal Calculi

Oxalate Calculus (Calcium Oxalate).—Popularly known as the mulberry stone, it is covered with sharp projections (fig. 1209). These cause the kidney to bleed, and altered blood is precipitated on the surface of the stone.

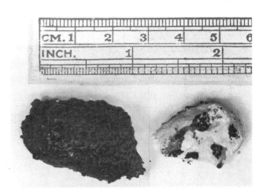

FIG. 1209.—Two oxalate calculi. The larger one removed from the right kidney and the small from the left of the same individual. The larger is black, owing to altered blood. The smaller is beginning to be discoloured around its sharp projections. These specimens illustrate clearly the process by which the oxalate calculus changes its complexion.

An oxalate calculus, which is usually single, casts an exceptionally good shadow radiologically, and this is fortunate, for often by virtue of its rough surface it gives rise to symptoms when comparatively small. A calcium oxalate stone is very hard, and on section is laminated concentrically. 'Envelope' crystals can be identified in the urine.

Phosphatic calculus (usually calcium phosphate, although sometimes combined with ammonium magnesium phosphate and, rarely, composed of the latter only) is smooth and dirty white. In an alkaline urine it enlarges rapidly, and often fills the renal calyces, taking on their shape (staghorn calculus, fig. 1210). Because it is smooth, a phosphatic calculus gives rise to few symptoms until it has

Alexander Randall, 1883–1951. Professor of Urology, University of Pennsylvania, Philadelphia, U.S.A.
Reginald Joseph Carr, Contemporary, Radiologist, Bradford Royal Infirmary, Bradford, England.

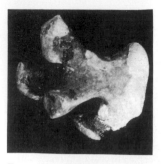

Fig. 1210.—Phosphatic calculus (actual size). Note its branched nature (staghorn calculus).

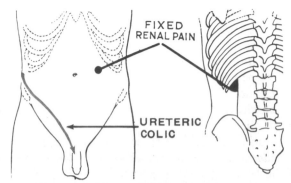

Fig. 1211.—The usual distribution of renal pain.

attained a large size. By reason of its size rather than its density, it is demonstrated readily by x-rays.

Uric acid and urate calculi are hard and smooth and, because they are usually multiple, they are typically faceted. Their colour varies from yellow to reddish brown. Pure uric acid calculi are not opaque to x-rays, but absolutely pure uric acid calculi are uncommon; the majority contain enough calcium oxalate crystals to render them opaque. Calculi of ammonium and sodium urate are sometimes found in children. Such stones are yellow, soft, and friable, and unless they contain impurities they do not cast an x-ray shadow.

Cystine calculi are wont to appear in the urinary tract of patients with cystinuria and are sometimes encountered in young girls. Cystinuria results from a greatly diminished or absent resorption of cystine from the renal tubules. Cystine crystals are hexagonal, white, translucent, and appear only in acid urine. Cystine calculi are usually multiple and may assume a cast of the renal pelvis and calyces. These calculi are soft, like beeswax, and pink or yellow when first removed. On exposure the colour changes to a greenish hue. They are radio-opaque to the sulphur they contain.

Xanthine calculi are extremely rare. They are smooth and round, brick red in colour, and show a lamellar structure.

Indigo calculi are curiosities. Blue in colour, they are derived from indican.

Clinical Features.—Fifty per cent of patients with renal calculus present between the ages of thirty and fifty. The male/female ratio is 4:3.

The symptoms are not stereotyped and sometimes the diagnosis remains obscure until a radiological examination has been made.

Quiescent Calculus.—Some stones, especially those composed mainly of phosphates, lie dormant for a long period, during which time there is progressive destruction of the renal parenchyma, and uraemia may be the first indication. Secondary infection usually supervenes.

Pain is the leading symptom in 75% of cases.

Fixed renal pain is located in the renal angle posteriorly (fig. 1211), in the hypochondrium anteriorly, or in both situations simultaneously. It is often worse on movement, particularly on walking upstairs. (See Chapter 56 for fuller description of the various types of renal pain.)

Ureteric[1] *colic* is an agonising pain passing from the loin to the groin, coming on suddenly, causing the patient to draw up his knees and roll about. It is often accompanied by vomiting and profuse sweating. Strangury[2] may occur if the stone is in the intramural ureter. The pulse quickens, and as the attack progresses the temperature becomes subnormal. An attack of colic rarely lasts more than eight hours. The condition is often due to a stone entering the ureter, but also occurs when a stone in the renal pelvis temporarily blocks the pelviureteric junction. Colic may also be caused by the passage of a shower of oxalate crystals, *e.g.* after eating an excess of strawberries or rhubarb.

Abdominal Examination:—During an attack of ureteric colic there is rigidity of the lateral abdominal muscles but not, as a rule, of the rectus abdominis. Percussion over the kidney produces a sharp stab of pain; tenderness of the kidney may be apparent on bimanual palpation. Only when a calculus-containing kidney becomes the seat of hydronephrosis or pyonephrosis of considerable size does it give rise to a palpable swelling.

Haematuria.—Infrequently, haematuria is a leading, or the only symptom. As a rule haematuria occurs in small amounts (enough to render the urine 'smoky') during or after an attack of pain.

Pyuria.—Infection of the kidney is liable to supervene, and pus will be found in the urine in varying amounts. Stones lead to an increase in the number of white cells in the urine even in the absence of infection.

Investigation of a suspected case of Renal Calculus

Radiography.—Before the examination the bowels should be emptied by giving a *vegetable* laxative, for minerals in the intestine cast a shadow (fig. 1212).

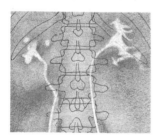

FIG. 1212.—The two shadows in the region of the right kidney were mistaken for calculi. They were due to enteric-coated pills of ammonium chloride.

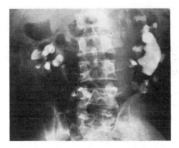

FIG. 1213.—Plain radiograph showing horse-shoe kidney full of stones. The patient, a man of forty-two, stated that he had enjoyed good health until one week previously.

Radiographs of both kidneys, ureters, and the bladder are taken. When a renal calculus is branched, there is no doubt concerning the shadow it casts. If a shadow *may* be a calculus in the kidney, exposures are made during full inspiration and full expiration. If the opacity moves with the kidney, and measurements from the lower pole of the kidney to the opacity remain constant, then the shadow is intrarenal.

---

[1] See footnote p. 1193.
[2] Strangury is the passage of a few drops of urine, often blood-stained, after painful straining.

The following structures and substances from time to time cast a shadow which at first sight may appear to be a renal calculus:

    (i) A calcified lumbar or mesenteric lymph node.
    (ii) A gallstone or a concretion in the appendix.
    (iii) Drugs (*e.g.* Navidrex-K and fersolate) or foreign bodies in the alimentary canal.
    (iv) Phleboliths.
    (v) The ossified tip of the twelfth rib.
    (iv) A chip fracture of the transverse process of a lumbar vertebra.
    (vii) Calcified tuberculous lesion of the kidney.
    (viii) A calcified suprarenal gland.

A doubtful shadow in relation to the kidney can often be proved to be extrarenal by a *lateral radiograph*. When the shadow can be shown to lie anterior to the bodies of the vertebrae, *ipso facto* it is anterior to the kidney. Such is the finding in calcified mesenteric lymph nodes, gallstones, and opacities in the alimentary tract.

Excretory urography is of value in confirming that the opacity is intrarenal, in determining in which part of the kidney the stone is situated (fig. 1214), and in revealing the function of the other kidney.

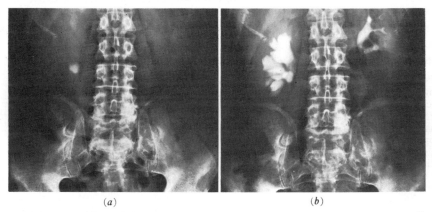

(*a*)   (*b*)

FIG. 1214.—(*a*) Plain x-ray showing a renal calculus. In which part of the kidney is it situated? (*b*) Same case. Excretory urogram. The stone is obstructing the pelvi-ureteric junction. Pyelolithotomy is needed urgently.

The presence of a non-opaque calculus also can be demonstrated by urography, for it causes a filling defect in the shadow cast by the medium. A similar defect is seen in papilloma of the renal pelvis. Retrograde pyelography may be required to give a clearer delineation.

  Cystoscopy.—A urethral stricture or prostatic obstruction, both of which may be a predisposing factor in renal stone formation, will be revealed by instrumental examination. Unless cystitis is present, the bladder wall looks normal.

  Treatment of Ureteric Colic (p. 1232).

OPERATIONS FOR THE REMOVAL OF RENAL CALCULI

Pre-operative Treatment.—If urinary infection is present, antibiotic treatment is instituted, and continued after operation as necessary. A bacteriology swab for culture should be taken of urine in the renal pelvis.

Operation—General Remarks.—All the operations about to be described have certain features in common. Via a lumbar incision the kidney is exposed and mobilised. When delivery is impossible, the choice of procedure is more limited and the operation more difficult. An x-ray showing the calculus or calculi clearly should be displayed in an illuminated viewing-box in the operation theatre. The stone or stones removed should coincide in every respect with the x-ray findings.

It is advisable to x-ray the exposed kidney (using a special film encased in a sterile plastic cover). This ensures that no stone or portion of stone within the kidney has been overlooked, and reduces the number of so-called recurrences.

Nephroscopy.—The inspection of the interior of the pelvis and calyces by means of a urethroscope is feasible in some kidneys. The development of rod lens systems, and glass fibres for transmission of increased light, has enabled the production of a nephroscope with flushing system and small forceps with which the interior of calyces can be examined, small calculi picked off, and subepithelial plaque visualised. This teaches one that even a clear x-ray is not proof that kidneys are cleared of foci on which other calculi can form.

At the conclusion of all the operations to be described the kidney is replaced in its bed, the fascia of Gerota repaired, and the lumbar wound closed with drainage of the perinephric space. If nephrostomy has been performed, the tube is either brought through the lumbar incision or through a stab incision.

Pyelolithotomy is indicated when a stone (it is usually solitary) lies in the renal pelvis, provided the pelvis is extrarenal. In nearly 50% of cases a renal calculus is so situated. The posterior wall of the renal pelvis is dissected free from its surrounding fat. The kidney is grasped in the left hand so that the tops of the index and middle fingers lie beneath the renal pelvis, making it more prominent, while the thumb anteriorly prevents the stone slipping into one of the calyces. An incision is made on to the stone in the long axis of the renal pelvis. The stone is removed with gallstone or suitable forceps, care being taken to avoid breaking it. If pyelography showed a stone in a calyx and the renal pelvis is large, the stone can be located by the little finger introduced into the renal pelvis. Should the stone be accessible, it can be grasped in forceps and removed by this route. After a stone has been removed via the renal pelvis, a bougie is passed through the pelvi-ureteric junction to calibrate it and to exclude any obstruction lower down. If the kidney is known to be uninfected, the incision in the renal pelvis is closed by interrupted sutures of fine plain catgut. If the kidney is grossly infected, nephrostomy (Chapter 56) is performed before closing the incision in the renal pelvis.

Extended Pyelolithotomy (Gil-Vernet).—By dissecting in the renal sinus posteriorly, a plane between the pelvis and calyces and the renal vessels leads to the necks of the calyces. Incisions continued into the calyces enable a direct view into the calyx to be obtained in many cases, facilitating the removal of large and small stones. Thermocouple-regulated cooling of the kidney, by ice chips in polythene bags, or liquid nitrogen circulating through coils placed around the kidney, enables the renal pedicle to be clamped to provide a bloodless field and unhurried surgery.

Nephrolithotomy[1] is frequently indicated if extended pyelolithotomy is employed. It may be necessary when there has been previous surgery, with adhesions making approach to the pelvis difficult. The kidney is cooled, and the renal pedicle is clamped as an incision into the renal parenchyma is accompanied by considerable haemorrhage. The incision is made just behind and parallel to the most prominent part of the convex border of the kidney (Brödel's line). As the terminal branches of the anterior and posterior renal arteries meet along this line, no large artery is divided, thereby minimising the amount of sub-

---

[1] The first operation of nephrolithotomy was performed by Ambroise Paré (1510–1590). His patient was a criminal condemned to death by hanging, instead of which Paré removed two stones from his kidney. Fifteen days later the patient was cured, secured his remission, and was given a grant of money.

Gil-Vernet, Contemporary. Surgeon, Madrid, Spain.
Max Brödel, 1870–1941. Artist of Pathology and Founder and Director of the Department of Art as Applied to Medicine (the first school of its kind in the world), Johns Hopkins University, Baltimore, U.S.A.

sequent cortical necrosis. Mapping the intra- and extra-renal vessels at operation with a Doppler (ultrasound) probe may be helpful. The incision, usually about 2·5 cm long, is made over that calyx containing the stone or stones, which are removed with lithotomy forceps. All bleeding points are underrun and tied with 0000 chromic gut, the edges of the opened calyx closed if necessary. The renal incision can be closed by interrupted catgut sutures passing through the kidney substance but not penetrating the calyx, and tied over a piece of Oxycel or muscle to enhance haemostasis. If infection is present, nephrostomy is carried out by placing a small self-retaining catheter through the incision into the renal pelvis. The incision is then closed on either side of the tube in the manner just described.

Partial Nephrectomy.—When the stone is in the lowermost calyx—a fairly common position—and there is considerable damage to the calyx, as in multiple stones, or 'grit' in the renal substance, then lower partial nephrectomy is the best operation (p. 1253). If the damaged calyx is not removed, its dependent position encourages further stone formation.

Nephrectomy is indicated when the contralateral organ has been proved to be perfectly healthy and the stone or stones have destroyed much of the renal parenchyma. Large branched calculi are notorious for recurring, so nephrectomy is often the best treatment in such cases, especially in the elderly.

Post-operative Treatment.—The patient should lie on the side of the operation or on his back to encourage drainage and obliteration of dead space in the wound. Wound drains should be shortened after 36–48 hours and removed as soon as any leak has ceased.

If a nephrostomy tube has been inserted then it is wise to give a broad spectrum antibiotic to decrease the risk of infection and possible secondary haemorrhage.

PERCUTANEOUS METHODS OF STONE REMOVAL

The last few years has seen a dramatic change in the need for open surgery for renal stones.

Percutaneous approach.—This involves the initial passage of a needle through the loin, transgressing the renal cortex, into the pelvis of the kidney. This is usually performed through a lower calyx. A guide wire is then passed through the needle and a series of dilators passed over the guide so that a nephroscope can be introduced into the collecting system. Stones may then be visualized and if small enough extracted whole. If the stones are too large for this they can be broken up with either an ultrasonic lithotriptor or an electro-hydraulic probe. When this is done the fragments can then be removed or excreted.

Dornier lithotriptor.—This can be used in combination or to substitute for other methods. The ingenious development of this 'stone banger' saves the need for instrumental penetration of the body. A shock wave is generated within an ellipse and if the kidney stone is placed where the waves focus it will be broken up. This all occurs with the patient anaesthetised lying in a water bath (to aid the physical principles underlying the method) and the stone is fragmented by repeated shocks into sand or tiny pieces. These bits have then to be passed which may result in some ureteric colic. In some intances passage of the fragments has to be assisted with a ureteroscope. If rarely severe hydronephrosis occurs or infection of the kidney, a temporary nephrostomy tube may be necessary.

The combined use of percutaneous surgery and the Dornier lithotriptor is gradually replacing the need for open surgery in many patients.

Treatment of Bilateral Renal Calculi.—Usually the kidney with the better function is operated upon first, the operation on the contralateral side being postponed for two or three months. Exceptions to this rule are (a) if there is pain on one side, that side is operated upon first, for pain usually signifies that the stone is obstructing the outflow of urine from the kidney, the function of which will become increasingly impaired; (*b*) if there is a pyonephrosis on one side this should be treated by nephrectomy, or, if the patient's condition is poor, by nephrostomy. In cases of bilateral staghorn calculi without infection and with few symptoms especially in the elderly, it is probably wiser not to operate. The patient should drink large amounts of fluid.

Prevention of Recurrence

Frère Jacques, that famous lithotomist of the Middle Ages, used to say, 'I have removed the stone, but God will cure the patient.' With the advance of knowledge our responsibilities do not end with the removal of the stone; provision must be made to prevent recurrence. Recurrent calculi can be divided into two varieties:

(*a*) *False Recurrence.*—Even a tiny fragment overlooked at the time of the operation is liable to become the nucleus of a new stone. Similarly infection and obstruction are factors in recurrence and should be eliminated in the treatment of the first stone.

(*b*) *True Recurrence.*—Ideally all stone formers should be investigated to exclude metabolic factors. The following investigations in bilateral and recurrent stone formers are essential:

(i) Serum Calcium, measured starving on three occasions to exclude hyperparathyroidism. This series may need to be repeated (Chapter 38).

(ii) Serum Uric Acic to exclude gout. Elevated serum uric acid levels can predispose to the formation of calcium phosphate stones.

(iii) Urinary urate and calcium and phosphate excretions in 24-hour urine, and screening for cystine.

(iv) Analysis of any stone passed.

(*c*) *Dietary Advice:*

(i) There should be a high fluid intake at all times, regardless of the chemistry of the stones. This is clearly indicated in cystinuria where the liability to stone formation is directly related to the concentration of the cystine in the urine. It is equally important to keep the urine dilute at night. Avoidance of milk, cheese and other items of the diet containing a great deal of calcium and, if renal function is satisfactory, the use of bran or sodium cellulose phosphate (5 g t.d.s. with meals) to reduce calcium absorbtion may be considered.

(ii) **Uric-acid and Urate Calculi.**—Red meats, offal, and fish which are rich in purine should be avoided. Sufficient sodium citrate and sodium bicarbonate are given to keep the urine alkaline. Allopurinol in doses sufficient to overcome a high serum uric acid is essential.

(iii) **Calcium Oxalate Calculi.**—Rhubarb, strawberries, plums, spinach, and asparagus, which are rich in oxalate, should only be taken if they are accompanied by cream or milk, as then oxalates are precipitated as an insoluble calcium salt in the intestine, and are not absorbed. At all times a diet adequate in magnesium is necessary; calcium oxalate is rendered less soluble in the presence of magnesium ions.

(iv) **Phosphate Calculi.**—Excessive alkalinity of the urine should be treated by giving ammonium chloride or another urinary acidifier. Phosphates in the diet should be restricted. Aluminium gel, 40 ml t.d.s., p.c. and at bedtime, drastically reduces the incidence of recurrence.

(v) **Cystine Calculi.**—Sulphur-containing proteins such as eggs, meat, or fish are restricted, and proteins with a low sulphur content substituted. Carbohydrates and fats are unrestricted. The urine must be kept dilute at all times as the formation of calculi is directly related to the concentration of cystine in the urine. Fluids must be drunk during the night as well as during the day. Solubility is increased by keeping the urine strongly alkaline, but this is often difficult to achieve. Penicillamine is a costly and by no means always successful drug in preventing recurrent cystine calculi.

(vi) **Recumbency Calculi.**—In patients doomed to long recumbency, sodium phytate taken by mouth forms insoluble calcium phytate, thus removing by the bowel one source of hypercalcuria. Regular timing is essential.

(vii) **Idiopathic Hypercalcuria.**—A strict low calcium diet (400 mg daily) should be tried first. 5 mg Bendrofluazide reduces calcium loss in the urine. Water softening to remove calcium in the local water may be required in order to allow a high fluid intake. Indomethacin 25 mg t.d.s. has been found to reduce calcium secretion. The mode of

Frère Jacques, 1651–1719. Itinerant Italian lithotomist, after serving as a trooper in the French army, adopted semi-religious habit and cut for stone in the bladder.

action is unknown. Sodium phytate taken orally at regular intervals is the last line of treatment.

URETERIC CALCULUS

A stone in the ureter nearly always has its birth in the kidney. When it enters the ureter the calculus is rounded or oval in shape. Should it become arrested in its descent to the bladder, in time it becomes enlarged and elongated, resembling in shape a date stone (fig. 1215): In 90% of cases the stone is single.

Clinical Features.—When a stone descends into the ureter there is an attack of ureteric colic, which is repeated at longer or shorter intervals, until the stone is ejected into the bladder or becomes impacted in the ureter. There are five sites of anatomical narrowing of the ureter where a stone may be arrested (fig. 1216).

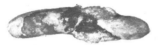

FIG. 1215.— Ureteric calculus removed by operation (3 cm long)

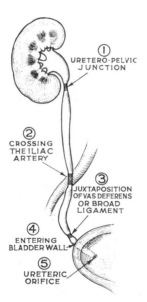

FIG. 1216.—Normal anatomical narrowings of the ureter.
(*After C. C. Higgins.*)

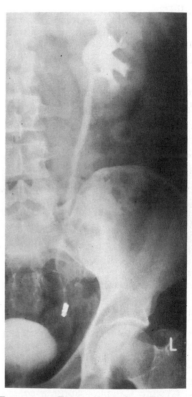

FIG. 1217.—Excretory pyelogram revealing hydronephrosis and hydro-ureter due to stone in lower ureter.

Ureteric Colic.—A stone in the upper third of the ureter produces symptoms identical with those of a stone blocking the pelvi-ureteric junction. When a calculus enters the lower third of the ureter, the colic it produces often commences anteriorly at a lower level than the kidney, and is frequently accompanied by pain referred along the two branches of the genito-femoral nerve, to the testis in the male, the labium majus in the female, and to the anterior surface of the thigh in both sexes. The testis usually becomes retracted by spasm of the cremaster, and tender, the tenderness persisting for some time after the colic has ceased. When the stone enters the intramural portion of the ureter, the pain is referred to the tip of the penis in the male. In both sexes there is strangury. In more than 50% of cases the stone is passed spontaneously.

Impaction.—When the stone becomes impacted the attacks of colic pass off and give place to a dull pain, usually in the iliac fossa, for impaction usually occurs in the pelvic portion of the ureter. The pain is increased by exercise, and relieved by rest. Such pain varies in intensity and is often associated with back-ache due to distension of the renal pelvis. Cessation of pain sometimes occurs by the stone forming for itself a false diverticulum in the wall of the ureter by a process of pressure necrosis; perforation or extravasation is very rare from this situation. Severe renal pain persisting for one or two days and then gradually subsiding suggests that complete obstruction has occurred. If urography (IVP) performed one or two weeks later shows no function, the stone must be removed, otherwise complete atrophy of the kidney will occur.

Haematuria.—Some degree of haematuria occurs after an attack of ureteric colic, and it lasts for a few hours or a day. It is sometimes so slight as to require microscopic identification.

Abdominal Examination.—There is tenderness and often rigidity over some part of the course of the ureter. On rare occasions a stone in the lower end of the ureter can be felt on rectal or vaginal examination. The principal difficulty on the right side is distinguishing the symptoms and signs produced by a ureteric calculus from those of acute appendicitis. The presence of blood in the urine does not necessarily rule out appendicitis, for an inflamed appendix lying in juxtaposition to the ureter can give rise to ureteritis which may cause a small amount of red cells in the urine. Pain on percussion over the kidney is unlikely in acute appendicitis.

Radiography.—Occasionally a typical elongated shadow in the line of the ureter confirms the diagnosis; more often either no shadow is seen, owing to the small size of the stone and the presence of intestinal gas shadows, or a shadow is seen which may or may not be a ureteric calculus.

Intravenous Urography.—In, and for some time after, an attack of renal colic there is either no excretion or greatly delayed excretion on the affected side. Films taken later, even up to forty-eight hours after the intravenous injection of Hypaque (diatrizoate) may outline the ureter down to the site of obstruction. A stone not visible in the plain x-ray may become outlined in the ureter by the contrast solution. After a stone has been impacted for a week or more, a varying degree of hydronephrosis and dilatation of the ureter is often apparent (fig. 1217).

If urograms taken during an attack of pain show normal excretion on the affected side, then the patient has not got ureteric colic.

Cystoscopy.—When a calculus is in the upper part or the ureter, the ureteric orifice shows no abnormality. When a calculus has reached the lower third of the ureter, or sometimes when it is in the middle third, the ureteric orifice becomes patulous and its immediate vicinity bespattered with minute petechial haemorrhages. As the calculus descends to just above the bladder wall, these haemorrhagic spots coalesce to form larger, bright-red extravasations. The stone having entered the intramural portion of the ureter, the ureteric orifice becomes grossly oedematous. Finally, the pouting calculus may be seen (fig. 1184).

The passage of a ureteric catheter provides much information, and in conjunction with radiography confirms the diagnosis. Usually a catheter fails to pass the obstruction and a radiograph shows the tip of the catheter abutting on the lower margin of the calculus. However, when the urinary efflux is increased, a catheter sometimes passes into the renal pelvis without hindrance, or, if arrested, after partial withdrawal and reinsertion (fig. 1218).

Retrograde pyelography is seldom required. The only indications for its employment are when there is doubt concerning a shadow being a ureteric calculus and excretory urography shows absence or ineffective delineation of the corresponding renal pelvis and the ureter. It sometimes proves a means of displaying the presence of a ureteric calculus non-opaque to x-rays.

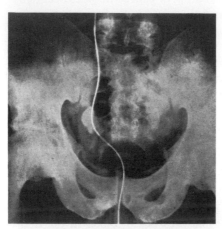

FIG. 1218.—Stone in the ureter. Catheter passed alongside the stone.

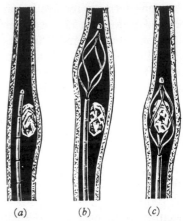

(a)   (b)   (c)

FIG. 1219.—Dormia stone-catching basket in use. (a) basket introduced past stone. (b) opened and (c) enclosing stone ready for withdrawal.
(*Porgès, Paris.*)

Treatment.—1. **Of the Colic.** Morphia (15 mg) is the best drug to relieve severe pain and is reputed not to produce spasm in ureteric muscle. The stone produces spasm and one dose of probanthine (15 mg) should be given at the same time. Repeated doses of probanthine can easily produce retention of urine by paralysis of the detrusor muscle of the bladder.

2. **Of the Stone.**

(i) **Expectant.** Provided the urine is sterile, most small calculi will pass naturally. This may take many months. Progress of the stone is observed by plain x-rays every six to eight weeks, and occasional urography to see that the function and appearance of the kidneys are satisfactory.

(ii) **Removal of the stone** may be required if:

(*a*) Repeated attacks of colic produce no advance of the stone.

(*b*) The stone is enlarging but not moving.

(*c*) Complete obstruction of the kidney occurs, or a hydronephrosis is increasing.

(*d*) The urine is infected.

(*e*) The stone when first seen is thought to be too large to pass.

Instrumental Treatment

(*a*) *Ureteric catheterisation.*—A small stone half a centimetre or less in dia-

Dormia, Contemporary. Assistant Professor of Urology, University of Milan, Italy.

meter arrested in any part of the ureter often passes after ureteric catheterisation (fig. 1218).

(b) *Dormia Basket* (fig. 1219).—This can be used for stones in the lower third of the ureter.

(c) *Ureteric Meatotomy.*—The ureteric orifice is the narrowest part of the whole ureter. By enlarging the opening a stone is often enabled to pass. However, this procedure almost invariably leads to urinary reflux afterwards and should therefore be avoided.

(d) *Intra-ureteric Manipulation.*—Rigid ureteroscopes are now available to inspect the whole length of the ureter and it is sometimes possible to remove a stone by forceps or by basket under direct vision.

(e) *Push-bang.*—In some instances it may be appropriate to push the stone back into the renal pelvis with a ureteric catheter, so relieving the hydro or pyo-nephrosis. The stone can then be fragmented in the Dornier waterbath providing a double-J stent is left in situ to prevent the stone from re-entering the ureter.

Operative Treatment

Uretero-lithotomy.—The patient should be submitted to radiography just prior to the operation, in order to detect any change in the position of the calculus.

(a) **Stone Impacted in the Upper Third of the Ureter.**—An incision similar to that for exposing the kidney (p. 1252) is made; it can be prolonged downwards if necessary.

(b) **Stone Impacted in the Lower Two-thirds of the Ureter, but above the Spine of the Ischium.**—With the patient in the dorsal position, an incision is made from a point 4 cm above the anterior superior iliac spine to the middle of the inguinal ligament. The flank muscles are divided in the direction of their fibres. The peritoneum is displaced medially by gauze dissection until the dilated ureter is found adhering to its under-surface. The stone is sought by palpation, and, if possible, is milked upwards or downwards to a convenient point for extraction. The ureter is incised longitudinally and the stone with-drawn by a scoop or forceps. If the stone is impacted firmly, the only course is to incise the ureter directly over it, a practice to be avoided whenever possible, for the mucous lining is ulcerated at the size of impaction, and healing is impaired. The incision in the ureter is closed by sutures of 0000 plain catgut passing through the muscular coats only. The lower end of the wound is drained down to the incision in the ureter.

(c) **Stone Impacted in the Juxtavesical or Intramural Portions of the Ureter.**—A midline, sub-umbilical extraperitoneal approach is employed, with the patient in Trende-lenburg's position. The peritoneum is stripped from the dome of the bladder and from the side wall of the pelvis. A dissection is then made between the posterior surface of the bladder and the wall of the pelvis with division of the superior vesical vascular pedicle. Often at this stage the stone will be felt. If this is not possible, the ureter must be identified where it crosses the iliac vessels, and traced downwards. Once the stone has been located it is removed as described above.

After removal of a stone at any site, a ureteric catheter or bougie should be passed to prove the patency of the distal ureter.

Idiopathic retroperitoneal fibrosis

This condition is rare. The patient, who typically has complained of backache for many months, suddenly becomes anuric. In other circumstances when kidney disease has been suspected pyelography reveals rapidly developing unilateral or bilateral hydronephrosis associated with a rising blood urea. Characteristically the ureters are nearer the mid-line than normally and this is due to an area of fibrosis centred over the bifurcation of the aorta which strangulates the ureters. The cause is largely unknown. Some cases have been noted followed the use of methysergide for the treatment of migraine, and methyl-dopa may also cause the condition.

Treatment.—In the anuric patient, if an attempt at ureteric catheterisation is success-ful, the catheters should be left *in situ* to relieve the obstruction. If this fails, bilateral nephrostomy is necessary although dialysis (Chapter 56) may be indicated. Steroids may be considered.

Friedrich Trendelenburg, 1844–1924. Professor of Surgery, Leipzig, Germany.

In non-urgent cases the involved ureter or ureters should be freed from the fibrous mass by sharp dissection and fixed laterally to the psoas muscles or wrapped in omentum to prevent recurrence. Should this prove impossible an ileal loop ureter should be constructed.

INFECTIONS OF THE KIDNEY

Aetiology.—Renal infections arise in the following ways:

1. *Haematogenous.*—From infected tonsils, carious teeth, or from cutaneous infections, particularly boils or a carbuncle, and in the case of tuberculosis from affected lymph nodes in the neck, chest or abdomen.

2. *Ascending the peri-ureteral lymphatics* from the cervix or the prostate.

3. *Ascending the lumen of the ureter* from the bladder is the commonest route. It may occur in lower urinary tract obstruction with dilated ureters as a result of vesicourethral reflux. This is an important route also in children with recurrent urinary tract infection.

On complete urinary investigation, which should always be undertaken after the acute phase of the infection has subsided, about 30% of males and a smaller number of females will be found to have an obstructive lesion in some part of the urinary tract. Moreover, with or without such a lesion, a focus of infection in the genital organs may be demonstrable.

Bacteriology.—By far the most common organisms responsible are *E. coli* and other Gram-negative bacilli. When *Strept. faecalis* is present it is usually associated with another organism. In *E. coli* and streptococcal infections the urine is acid. Both Proteus and Staphylococci split urea into ammonia, rendering the urine alkaline and so may promote stone formation.

PYELONEPHRITIS

Renal infection, by whatever route it originates, is never confined to the renal pelvis. In haematogenous infection the renal parenchyma is attacked first, and the infection spreads to the renal pelvis. In ascending infection the bacterial inflammation is not limited to the renal pelvis; it implicates the calyces, the pyramids, and at least some part of the adjacent parenchyma. It is, therefore, more correct to discard the term 'pyelitis' in connection with the latter type of infection, in favour of the more accurate designation 'pyelonephritis'.

ACUTE PYELONEPHRITIS

Acute pyelonephritis is more common in females, especially during childhood, at puberty, soon after marriage ('honeymoon pyelitis'), during pregnancy, and the menopause. It occurs more often on the right side than on the left, and is frequently bilateral.

Clinical Features.—While there may be prodromal symptoms of headache, lassitude, and nausea, the onset is usually sudden, often commencing with a rigor and even vomiting. There is acute pain in the flank and the hypochondrium. In a few cases the pain radiates from the loin to the groin (ureteric colic). The temperature rises to 38·8° or 39·5°C, and is remitting. Soon after the onset, increased frequency of micturition, due to cystitis, sets in, and when, as is often the case, the urine is acid, micturition is accompanied by a scalding pain in the urethra. On examination there is tenderness in the hypochondrium and in the angle between the last rib and the sacrospinalis, accompanied by a varying degree of muscular rigidity. In the early stages, when it is imperative to make a correct diagnosis, the urine is clear macroscopically.

In cases of severe bilateral pyelonephritis, particularly when there is an associated obstruction, there are likely to be symptoms of uraemia.

Bacteriological Examination of the urine.—A mid-stream specimen should be collected in a sterile bottle; the urine is centrifuged and examined microscopically. In early acute pyelonephritis there are typically a few pus cells and many bacteria. When pyelonephritis has been present for twenty-four hours or more, the urine is often cloudy and pus cells abound. Quantiative estimations of the cells and bacteria in the specimen are of real value, whereas vague impression reported as . . . 'many, some, a few' are usually misleading. In all cases the investigation includes an examination of the sediment stained by Gram's method, culture of the specimen, and an investigation of the sensitivity of the organism or organisms to various antibiotics and chemotherapeutic agents.

Severe Cases.—There are repeated rigors and the temperature rises to 40° or 40·5°C, often without a corresponding rise in the pulse-rate. There is vomiting, sweating, and great thirst, and the patient looks and feels ill. The blood culture, if the specimen is taken soon after a rigor, often gives a positive result. After some hours the pain is localised in one or, rarely, both loins. Urine is scanty and highly concentrated, and is frequently teeming with coliform organisms and pus cells, in which case the diagnosis is simplified. In blood-borne infections the organisms and pus cells do not appear in the urine until the infection has spread from the cortex to the medulla—a matter of many hours, or even days. As the abdominal rigidity abates, the enlarged affected kidney may be palpable.

Differential Diagnosis.—When the symptoms and signs are typical the diagnosis is straightforward. In other circumstances there may be difficulty in distinguishing the condition from pneumonia, acute appendicitis, and acute cholecystitis. The urgent need is to differentiate acute appendicitis from right-sided pyelonephritis. The fact that the pain commenced in, and did not pass to the right side, greatly favours the latter condition. Excretory urography may prove of assistance, for in an early acute pyelonephritis limited to the right kidney the concentration of medium in the renal pelvis and calyces on the affected side may be so poor that no shadow, or a very indefinite shadow, is cast. A radioisotope renogram using Chlormerodrin (^{203}Hg) 3·7–11·1 Bq (100–300μCi) will show scattered areas of diminished uptake (fig. 1182).

Pyelonephritis of Pregnancy.—The condition usually develops between the fourth and sixth months of gestation. It is commoner in women who have had recurrent bouts of cystitis or pyelonephritis in the past. In 90% of cases the right side alone is affected. The initiating causes are often chronic urethritis or a cervical erosion. The symptoms do not differ from those of pyelonephritis occurring in the non-pregnant. In about 10% of cases the disease runs a more severe and protracted course, and occasionally it results in abortion or premature birth. In all patients who have had pyelonephritis of pregnancy, periodic examinations of the urine are necessary during the rest of the pregnancy, the puerperium and for several months afterwards, for if the infection has not been eradicated, recrudescence is liable to occur during this period.

Urinary infection in childhood is not uncommon, and is important to recognise because it frequently involves the kidneys. If recurrent it may lead to severe renal impairment or renal failure in early adult life. In young children there may be no urinary symptoms, although the mother may notice a cloudy or offensive urine. If a child fails to thrive, refuses to eat, has a high fever (temp. 39-40°C) with *rigors or convulsions*, the possibility must always be considered. Pain or screaming on micturition may occur. The older child may complain of loin pain, or suddenly develop frequency and enuresis.

Many cases (50%) are associated with an underlying anatomical or congenital abnor-

Hans Christian Joachim Gram, 1853–1938. Professor of Medicine, Copenhagen.

mality. Once the diagnosis has been confirmed by a clean catch specimen or by a specimen obtained by suprapubic needle puncture of the bladder, a full urological investigation is essential.

Reflux of urine occurs up the ureters during micturition in about 35% of cases with a proven urinary infection. It may be intermittent and is certainly more frequent when infection is present. It can only be demonstrated clearly by micturating ciné-cystography, but this does necessitate catheterisation: this must be performed gently and with strict asepsis, and it is wise to leave a solution of neomycin (50 ml 0·5% freshly made) in the bladder afterwards. Renal function tests and full blood analysis should be done.

Reflux also occurs when the intravesical pressure is high, and the obliquity of the intramural ureter is lost. A thin bladder wall and the presence of a saccule near the ureteric orifice may lead to funnelling of the orifice during ureteric peristaltic retraction. Renal damage associated with reflux usually occurs when the urine is infected or if the reflux is under high pressure secondary to neurogenic bladder dysfunction. Once the diagnosis has been made the urine must be cleared of infection with the appropriate antibiotic. In the case of recurrent infections a low dose non-toxic antibiotic taken prophylactically may be of benefit. Surgery with reimplantation of the ureter into the bladder is usually reserved for patients where there is evidence of progressive renal scarring indicating failure of conservative measures. Ureteric reimplantation into a neurogenic bladder is always doomed to failure.

Urinary infection must be treated with the appropriate drug until the clean catch specimen is sterile on culture. A repeat urine sample 10—14 days after cessation of treatment must be examined to exclude recurring infection.

ACUTE PYELONEPHRITIS ASSOCIATED WITH RETENTION OF BLADDER URINE

Acute Pyelonephritis with retention of bladder urine occurs most frequently in men suffering from prostatic obstruction or stricture of the urethra, and in case of fracture of the spine with injury to the spinal cord (Chapter 27). The retention is not necessarily complete and the patient may be able to urinate, but there is a varying amount of residual urine, from a few ounces to several pints. In most cases the infection is bilateral. Often it follows the passage of a catheter or other instrument, or operations on the lower urinary tract, but it may arise spontaneously. The old name for this condition was 'surgical kidneys', and in the days of unsterile catheterisation it was frequent and dreaded. At post-mortem examination the kidneys are enlarged and miliary abscesses can be seen beneath the capsules. On bisection there are numerous yellow streaks of pus in the parenchyma radiating from the medulla to the convex border. The renal calyces, pelves, and ureters are dilated.

Treatment of Acute Pyelonephritis

The essential factors in curing pyelonephritis are *early*, *correct* and *prolonged* treatment, and careful follow-up with repeat cultures and white cell counts of the urine after treatment has finished. A full investigation to exclude abnormalities in the urinary tract should be undertaken when the acute attack is controlled.

A mid-stream specimen of urine should be taken and sent for culture and tests of the sensitivity of the organisms to antibiotics. Bed rest is important.

If the urine is acid, as it is in the common coliform infections, alkalinisation of the urine has a most beneficial effect in relieving the symptoms and in inhibiting the growth of these organisms. Mist. Pot. Cit. et Hyocyamus, 10 ml 6 hourly is an old but useful treatment.

When pain is severe, an antispasmodic is given and heat is applied to the affected loin. Morphia, in addition, may be necessary sometimes.

The patient should be instructed to drink large quantities of bland fluid, at least 3 litres in the twenty-four hours. In severe cases with vomiting or dehydration, intravenous dextrose-saline is given until the dehydration has been rectified and the vomiting has ceased.

While awaiting the bacteriological report and the result of the sensitivity tests, in comparatively mild cases an antimicrobial with a wide range of activity, *e.g.* co-trimoxazole or amoxycillin, should be given, pending the bacteriological report.

Three and seven days after commencing the treatment of pyelonephritis the urine must be sent for culture. Even when a full initial course (ten days) of an antibiotic or chemotherapeutic agent has rendered the urine sterile, it may be advisable to continue treatment with another drug for a further two or three weeks, or until the hourly white cell excretion rate has fallen to normal levels (less than 200,000 per hour). During this treatment further investigations to rule out abnormalities in the urinary tract should be carried out. Despite the undoubted efficacy of modern antibacterial drugs, none is likely to succeed in sterilising the urine of a patient with an abnormality of the urinary tract. A history of previous urinary infection also reduces the likelihood of a cure, although to a lesser extent (Garrod).

Colomycin, Gentamicin and *Carbenicillin* are the best drugs currently available for combating infections with the more resistant strains of *Pseudomonas pyocyanea*, Proteus, and Klebsiella.

Chemotherapeutic and Antibiotic Agents

Sulphonamides: *Sulphafurazole* (Gantrisin) is capable of high urinary concentration without risk of crystalluria, and is of low toxicity. It is capable of controlling many *Esch. coli* infections and some strains of *proteus* and *Ps. aeruginosa*. The dose is 3 g *statim* followed by 1 g six-hourly until the temperature has remained normal for three days, and cultures of the urine have proved sterile on three consecutive occasions.

Sulphamethizole (Urolucosil) has similar properties, but unlike other sulphonamides it is unnecessary to insist on a high fluid intake while the patient is taking this drug. The dose is 100 mg four times daily. *Septrin* is a sulphonamide mixed with trimethoprim. The combination has proved most effective.

Antibacterial Nitrofuran: *Nitrofurantoin* (Furadantin) is a synthetic antibacterial agent. Although when taken by mouth the blood levels remain low, the concentration in the urine is significant; hence it is of value only in genito-urinary infections. It is particularly effective against *Esch. coli*, A. *aerogenes* and *proteus*; often it has proved lethal to antibiotic-resistant strains of these organisms. The average dose by mouth is 5 to 8 mg per kg of body weight. One-quarter of this dose is administered immediately after food three times daily and a further dose with cold milk last thing at night. If nausea or vomiting occurs, the dose must be reduced.

Antibiotics: *Broad Spectrum Antibiotics.*—While these are effective if employed in accordance with bacteriological findings, when it is necessary to continue treatment for a prolonged period (which is not unusual) a number of dangers loom large. Firstly, there are the toxic properties, producing nausea, vomiting, and diarrhoea. Secondly, there is the alteration in the intestinal micro-flora these antibiotics produce, sometimes leading to moniliasis or staphylococcal enterocolitis. Thirdly, the frequency with which resistant variants emerge, often in a comparatively short time, is disturbing.

CHRONIC PYELONEPHRITIS

Chronic pyelonephritis is an important, common, and dangerous disease. It is still a frequent cause of death from uraemia. Like its acute counterpart it can be primary, or secondary to abnormality of the urinary tract.

Pathology.—The inflammation is interstitial, and microscopically scars resulting from the destruction of adjacent parenchyma can be seen. These scars are unevenly distributed and nearly always are more evident in one kidney than in the other. Histologically it can be seen that the brunt of the onslaught has been

Lawrence Paul Garrod, 1895–1979. Professor of Bacteriology, St. Bartholomew's Hospital, London.
Theodor Albrecht Edwin Klebs, 1834–1913. Professor of Bacteriology successively at Prague, Zurich and Rush Medical College, Chicago, Illinois, U.S.A.

borne by the renal tubules; they are atrophic, often dilated, and sometimes cystic. In time many of them are destroyed and disappear in scar tissue. On the other hand, the glomeruli retain their normal structure until late in the disease. Chronic pyelonephritis is almost three times as common in females as it is in males. Two-thirds of the affected females are under forty years of age, while 60% of the males are over forty.

Clinical Features.—It is possible, but unusual, for chronic pyelonephritis to remain asymptomatic until advanced renal insufficiency appears.

Lumbar pain, dull in character, is present in 60% of cases.

Increased frequency and dysuria are leading symptoms in most cases.

Hypertension is present in 40% of cases, being more common in primary than in secondary pyelonephritis. It develops slowly and thus is more in evidence in long-standing cases. In 20% of cases the hypertension is of the accelerated ('malignant') type.

Constitutional symptoms comprising lassitude, malaise, anorexia, nausea, and headache constitute the main complaint in 30% of cases. The disease often remains unrecognised in these sufferers, perhaps for years.

Pyrexia. Attacks of pyrexia exceeding 37·8°C are the main symptoms in 20% of cases. The need to explain these attacks often leads to a thorough investigation including the urinary tract, and the disease is then brought to light.

Anaemia.—A normochromic anaemia due to unsuspected renal impairment may be the presenting feature.

The urine. *Proteinuria.*—On account of the late destruction of the glomeruli, contrary to glomerulonephritis, the amount of protein passed in the urine is small (less than 3 g daily).

Casts are found infrequently.

White cells are numerous. A fresh three-hour urine should be examined and a count of over 200,000 per hour is abnormal—often it may be as high as several million. Ureteric specimens may reveal considerable difference in this respect between the kidneys, and on the ability of the individual kidney to concentrate and acidify urine.

Bacteriological Examination of the Urine.—Commonly found are *Esch. coli*, *Streptococcus faecalis*, *proteus* and *pseudomonas*.

Treatment is not easy. Two principles must be followed: (1) to eradicate predisposing causes such as obstructions or stones, and (2) by repeated cultures and sensitivity tests to control and, it is hoped, ultimately to eradicate the infection with repeated courses of suitable drugs. In secondary cases, even if the cause can be removed, the renal pelves have frequently lost their musculature and are fibrotic and non-contractile. Moreover, once the parenchyma has been damaged it is a locus of predilection for blood-borne organisms. Consequently chemotherapy and antibiotics confer as a rule only temporary benefit. The longer the infection has persisted, the more difficult is it to eradicate. When prolonged treatment is required, there is a definite place for the following inexpensive drug.

Mandelic acid and its salts are often curative in coliform infections and those caused by *Streptococcus faecalis*. Ammonium mandelate 3 g (or better, mandamine, which is mandelic acid and hexamine combined), together with a capsule of 2 g ammonium chloride, is given six-hourly. Fluids are restricted to 1·5 litres in the twenty-four hours. It is essential that the urine be kept acid (pH 5·3 or less). Contraindications to this form of therapy are impairment of renal function and infections producing ammoniacal decomposition of the urine.

In nearly 50% of patients with pyelonephritis due to infection by one organism only, in whom infection persists in spite of treatment with antibacterial drugs, it is found that the original organism has been replaced by another, *e.g. Streptococcus faecalis*, instead of *Esch. coli*.

It is highly important to eradicate distant foci of infection whenever possible. In occasional cases when the disease is unilateral and associated with the accelerated type of hypertension, nephrectomy is sometimes curative. Partial nephrectomy, removing a badly damaged portion of renal tissue, may be necessary by helping to sterilise the urine and free the patient of pain.

Recurrent Dialysis.—In advanced cases, diminishing renal function may require institution of recurrent dialysis using an artificial kidney. Difficulty in controlling hypertension or renal infection may necessitate bilateral nephrectomy.

Transplantation of a kidney from a donor or a cadaver may be possible (Chapter 62).

Follow-up Investigation of a case of Pyelonephritis

The following investigations are carried out in chronic cases a week or more after treatment with antibacterial drugs, and in acute cases after the infection has subsided with treatment. These investigations are to discover any cause of obstruction to the upper or lower urinary tract, and/or a source of infection, which is present most often in the genital organs or the urethra.

(a) *The Clinical Examination is Repeated.*—The kidneys are palpated for tenderness and enlargement, and the bladder for chronic retention of urine. In middle-aged or elderly males the prostate is examined for enlargement or fibrosis. In male children, atresia of the meatus or meatitis is sought. Inspection of the cervix uteri often displays cervicitis or cervical erosion. Examination of the secretion expressed by prostatic massage sometimes accounts for the presence of infection. If no infection is found in these situations, a possible focus in carious teeth or infected tonsils is sought.

(b) *Renal Function Tests.*—To assess the glomerular and tubular function.

(c) *Intravenous Urography.*—The plain film of the urinary tract may reveal the presence of a urinary calculus. In chronic pyelonephritis, and after an attack of severe acute or recurring acute pyelonephritis, changes in the pyelographic shadow or shadows will be manifest. Some of these are similar to those of early hydronephrosis, but they are more unequally distributed. Although the calyces become flattened or clubbed, this is more in evidence in one part of the kidney than another. Persistent poor definition in one group of calyces is presumptive evidence of chronic infection. In cases of longer standing the renal pelvis becomes slightly dilated, but, unlike hydronephrosis, the dilatation of the calyces predominates. The most important x-ray sign is narrowing of the cortex, often localised, and giving rise to depressed scars seen as notches in the outline, or considerable contracture of one pole. Nephrotomography can be very helpful in demonstrating these scars.

(d) *Cysto-urethroscopy.*—After the instrument has been passed, residual urine, if any, is measured. Examination of the urethra may show chronic urethritis or the presence of a stricture. In the female urethro-trigonitis is commonly found. Hitherto unconfirmed obstruction to the prostatic urethra by an enlarged middle lobe or contracture of the bladder neck may be demonstrated. Evidence of cystitis is the most common finding. Sometimes the ureteric orifice, or orifices in bilateral cases, is seen pouting, oedematous, or gaping. Delay in efflux is usual on the affected or more affected side. Ureteric catheters are passed and specimens collected from each kidney. These specimens are examined for cells and bacteria. By these means it is ascertained whether the infection is bilateral or unilateral. In male children valves in the posterior urethra, or a contracture of the bladder neck, are sometimes revealed.

(*e*) *Micturating Cine-cystography*, using a cine-camera coupled to an x-ray image inten-sifier, may reveal reflux of urine up one or both ureters. This can be a transient phenomena due to infection. It is commonly a factor in childhood.

HYPERTENSION AND A UNILATERAL RENAL LESION

Renal ischaemia regularly produces increased arterial tension, as ischaemia of the renal parenchyma leads to the formation of a vasopressor substance. Too often cases are labelled essential hypertension without thorough investigation. Sometimes in a case of hyperten-sion a unilateral diseased kidney is demonstrated and nephrectomy is followed by perma-nent lowering of the blood pressure. Renal artery stenosis sometimes is a cause of hypertension (fig. 165). Direct arterial surgery and now transluminal angioplasty (Chapter 14) may be curative.

PYONEPHROSIS

The kidney is converted into a multilocular sac containing pus or purulent urine, with a varying amount of renal parenchyma in its walls. A pyonephrosis can result from infection of a hydronephrosis, follow acute pyelonephritis or, most commonly, arise as a complication of renal calculus (calculus pyonephrosis). As a rule the condition is unilateral.

Clinical Features.—The classical triad of pyonephrosis is anaemia, fever, and a loin swelling. When the condition arises as an infection of a hydronephrosis the swelling may be a large one. When the pyonephrosis is open, an evening rise of temperature to 37·2° or 37·7°C is usual; if the pyonephrosis becomes closed, the temperature is higher. Pyuria, when present, gives rise to cystitis, and sometimes symptoms of that condition are the chief complaint.

Investigation.—A plain x-ray may show a calculus. Intravenous urography shows the same vagaries as advanced hydronephrosis, in that the appearance of the shadow of the dilated renal pelvis and calyces is long delayed and may be absent. Cystoscopy often reveals cystitis with a purulent efflux from the ureter of the affected side. In closed cases the bladder may be normal and a ureteric catheter either becomes arrested, usually at the pelvi-ureteric junction, or passes the obstruction and gives exit to pent-up purulent urine.

Treatment.—Infection in an obstructed hydronephrotic kidney should be tre-ated as an emergency. Antibiotics should be given, and the kidney drained by inserting a large percutaneous nephrostomy tube. If this is unsatisfactory an open nephrostomy may be necessary. In cases known to be due to stone, the stone should be removed. Where obstruction is known to have destroyed most of the renal substance, and function on the other side is good, nephrectomy should be performed. Should the capsule prove to be densely adherent to the surrounding structures subcapsular nephrectomy is performed. When a pyonephrosis arises in a single kidney, or the condition is bilateral, permanent nephrostomy may be the best possible measure. Drainage by an 'ileal conduit' to bladder or the skin is another possibility (Chapter 58).

CARBUNCLE OF THE KIDNEY

The source of origin of the organism is usually a cutaneous lesion, such as a boil, carbuncle, whitlow, or an abscess of the breast, and the *Staphylococcus aureus* is conveyed to the kidney via the blood-stream. Occasionally a blow on the loin determines the issue, when injury to the kidney produces a small haematoma. Coliforms are now the most common infecting organisms.

Morbid Anatomy.—On splitting open the kidney there is a necrotic mass of tissue, usually localised, involving the parenchyma.

Clinical Features.—There is an ill-defined, tender swelling in the loin, persistent pyrexia and leucocytosis, signs that closely simulate a perinephric abscess. In early cases the urine contains neither pus cells nor organisms, but after a few days staphylococci can sometimes be isolated. Urography often shows compression or obliteration of a group of calyces, an appearance that does not differ from adenocarcinoma of the kidney.

Treatment.—Antibiotics have cured some early cases. When the response to antibiotic therapy is not dramatic the kidney must be exposed, the carbuncle incised, and the necrotic material removed. Haemorrhage is not excessive and can be controlled by pressure with a moist warm pack. A drainage tube is passed down to, but not into, the resultant cavity and the wound is closed around the tube. Antibiotics are continued for at least ten days. Primary nephrectomy is indicated only when the major part of the kidney is involved by the carbuncle.

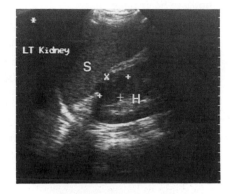

FIG. 1220.—Longitudinal scan through the upper pole of the left kidney demonstrates a renal carbuncle, outlined by the crosses. S = spleen; H = hilum of kidney.
(Dr T. Naunton-Morgan)

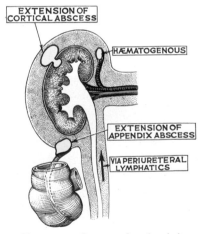

FIG. 1221.—Sources of perinephric abscess.

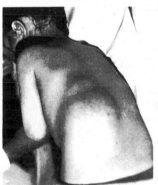

FIG. 1222.—A large perinephric abscess.

PERINEPHRIC ABSCESS

The most common causes are depicted in fig. 1221. Other causes are infection of a perirenal haematoma, and perforation of the renal capsule from undue delay in operating upon a pyonephrosis or a renal carbuncle. A tuberculous perinephric abscess can arise from an advanced pyonephrosis or from tuberculosis of a nearby vertebra.

Clinical Features.—The classical symptoms and signs of a perinephric abscess are a high, swinging temperature, rigidity, tenderness, and fullness in the loin (fig. 1222). If the suppuration commences in the lower part of the perinephric fat, local signs present early, but when the suppuration is confined to the upper portion of the perinephric fat which lies beneath the lower ribs, it produces no visible swelling, and even rigidity and tenderness may be absent. The leucocyte count is always raised, often to 20,000/mm³ (20 × 10⁹/l). As a rule no pus or organisms are present in the urine.

Radiography shows obscurating of the psoas shadow, with one or more of the following additional signs—scoliosis with concavity towards the abscess, and elevation and immobility of the diaphragm on the affected side.

Mathé's Sign.—Absence of the downward displacement that occurs in the erect posture in every normal kidney. Two radiographs, one in the lying posture and one in the erect posture, during excretory urography are required. In established cases the kidney can be shown to be displaced forwards if a lateral view is obtained.

Treatment.—Under antibiotic cover a lumbar incision is made large enough to enable the surgeon to open up pockets both above and below the kidney. The surface of the kidney is palpated for an unruptured cortical abscess, which, if present, should be incised. A specimen of pus having been obtained for bacteriological examination, the wound is closed with ample drainage. Appropriate antibiotic treatment follows.

RENAL TUBERCULOSIS

Aetiology and Pathology.—Tuberculosis of the urinary tract cannot arise except as a blood-borne infection from a distant focus, which, in many cases, is impossible to locate.

When clinically recognisable, in the great majority of cases renal tuberculosis

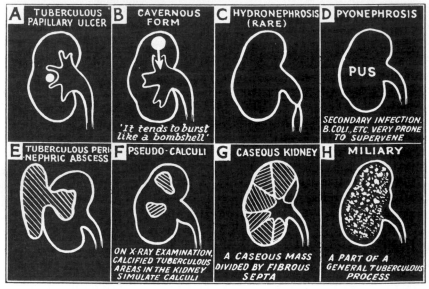

FIG. 1223.—Blackboard sketches of types of tuberculous kidney (macroscopic pathology).[1]

---

[1] G is known also as the 'putty kidney' and by the French as the 'cement kidney'. It is nature's method of performing (ineffective!) autonephrectomy.

Charles Pierre Louis Mathé, Contemporary. Formerly Urologist-in-Chief, St. Mary's Hospital, San Francisco, California, U.S.A.

is apparently confined to one kidney. A group of microscopical lesions coalesce and discharge pus and tubercle bacilli along one set of tubules, and the pyramid which gives exit to the discharge becomes ulcerated (fig. 1223A).

Course: *Tuberculous bacilluria* is a convenient term to designate a very early lesion of the renal cortex when no abnormality in the affected kidney can be detected, even by retrograde pyelography. It indicates the presence of active tuberculous disease which may progress, and as such must be treated in the same way as the demonstrable lesions.

A *macroscopical lesion* progresses rather slowly, and other similar lesions appear in the same kidney. The infection can be confined to the affected kidney for months or years, causing one or other of the changes depicted in fig. 1223 C to G. More often the disease spreads along the ureter (tuberculous ureteritis) to give rise to tuberculous cystitis in both sexes and prostatitis, vesiculitis and later epididymitis in the male.

In the male, renal and genital tuberculosis can be associated before the bladder and posterior urethra are involved, in which event the genital infection probably occurs in the following way. An urgent desire to micturate causes the internal sphincter to open, while at the same time, because there are no immediate facilities for emptying the bladder, voluntary closure of the external sphincter is called into play. At that moment infected urine is forced under pressure into the mucosal crypts of the prostate and the common ejaculatory ducts (Wells).

Clinical Features.—Renal tuberculosis usually occurs between twenty and forty years of age. Men are affected twice as commonly as women, and the right kidney somewhat more commonly than the left.

Frequency.—The earliest symptom is increased frequency of micturition. Often this is the only symptom. It is progressive, the patient complaining that (over a period of months) the frequency has increased both by day and night. Frequency is occasionally due to polyuria as the result of the renal tubular inflammation: it is usually due to patchy tuberculous cystitis.

Pyuria.—In early cases the urine is pale and slightly opalescent. The presence of pus cells without organisms in an acid urine is very suggestive of tuberculous urinary infection.

Painful Micturition.—Once tuberculous cystitis has set in, micturition becomes increasingly painful. First there is suprapubic pain if the bladder cannot be emptied immediately; later a burning pain accompanies micturition, and when secondary infection has occurred there is superadded agonising pain after micturition referred to the tip of the penis or the vulva, often associated with terminal haematuria (strangury).

Renal pain is often absent, but sometimes the patient complains of a dull ache in the loin.

Haematuria.—In 5% of cases the disease is ushered in with painless haematuria occurring from an ulcer situated on a renal papilla. During the haemorrhage, and after it has ceased, investigations may or may not demonstrate the presence of a renal lesion and tubercle bacilli in the urine. In the latter event more typical symptoms commence some months later. Apart from a few drops of blood at the end of micturition in cases complicated by severe cystitis, macroscopic haematuria occurs only occasionally.

A tuberculous kidney is oedematous and friable, and is therefore more likely to be damaged by trauma than is the normal pliable kidney.

Constitutional Symptoms.—A continuous slight loss of weight is usual. Evening pyrexia to 37·3°C occurs when the disease is fully established. A high temperature is indicative of a secondary infection of disseminating tuberculosis.

Charles Alexander Wells, Contemporary. Professor Emeritus of Surgery, Liverpool, England.

On Examination.—It is unusual for a tuberculous kidney to be palpable.

When a patient with renal tuberculosis has an enlarged kidney which can be felt, it is by no means certain that this kidney is the one that is diseased, for compensatory hypertrophy sometimes renders the healthy kidney both large and tender.

The prostate, vesicles, each vas, and epididymis should be examined for nodules or thickening, which may indicate tuberculous invasion.

Investigation:

Bacteriological Examination of the urine.—Prompt examination must be made of an early morning specimen before contaminants can overgrow. When, after staining a specimen of the sediment with Ziehl-Neelsen's stain, acid-fast bacilli are found, it is highly probable that they are tubercle bacilli, but the proof lies in culture or guinea-pig inoculation, either of which is reliable. **Most important—specific therapy should never be started until a positive culture has been obtained.** If this precaution is neglected, an exacting course of treatment may be started for a non-tuberculous condition, and at a later stage it is impossible to prove or disprove the diagnosis.

In few fields of medicine is the diagnosis more exact. The microscope demonstrates tubercle bacilli in 72%, the guinea-pig test in 94%, and the culture medium in 98% of cases.

A Plain x-ray may show calcification in healing foci. In gross disease this may be a rim around a caseous mass, or complete dense spheres. In minimal lesions specks of calcification may be scattered in one part of the cortex or pyramid. Ureteric calcification is late except at the lower end, and here, in males, the vesicles may also show patchy calcification.

Intravenous Urography (fig. 1224).

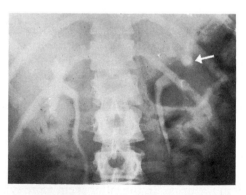

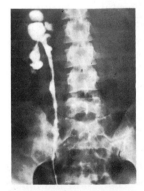

FIG. 1224.—Intravenous urogram showing a small localised lesion with hydrocalyx. Healing took place under conservative treatment. (*Professor E. Wildbolz, Berne.*)

FIG. 1225. — Retrograde pyelogram showing advanced tuberculosis of the right kidney and ureter.

Changes in the urogram commence with loss or dysfunction of one or more calyces, and irregular density in the nephrogram. Spasm or oedema may obliterate a calyceal neck, and if this becomes severe a hydrocalyx will develop. Complete obstruction leads to an abscess displacing adjacent calyces and the

Franz Heinrich Paul Ziehl, 1857–1926. Neurologist, Lübeck, Germany.
Friedrich Carl Adolf Neelsen, 1854–1894. Prosector, Stadt-Krankenhaus, Dresden, Germany.

appearance of a space-occupying lesion. The bladder tends to become round and spastic when involved, and ulceration may produce spasm and flattening of the bladder in this area. Ureteric fibrosis leads to loss of the natural curves of the ureter, and a wider, straighter and shorter line between kidney and bladder.

In late cases, the contralateral ureter becomes dilated also; this is not necessarily an indication of disease on the opposite side, for the dilation may be due to the cicatrised bladder causing obstruction to the ureter in its intramural course.

Cystoscopy.—When increased frequency is the only symptom and it has not been present long, the bladder and the ureteric orifices are normal.

A unilateral cloudy efflux is sometimes observed. Either more frequent efflux or a delay in excretion of indigo-carmine is indicative of the side that is diseased. In 10% of cases there is an absence of efflux on the affected side, and no pathological changes in the bladder. These are examples of a closed ureter leading to so-called autonephrectomy, or a pyonephrosis.

Oedema causes pallor around a ureteric orifice and is the earliest cystoscopic sign of vesical involvement. Infiltration follows, and the mucous membrane of the affected ureteric orifice pouts. Tubercles appear, usually lateral to the ureteric orifice, and later in the dome of the same half of the bladder. By confluence of a circumscribed group of tubercles, a tuberculous ulcer, which has an irregular periphery, may form. In long-standing cases, as a result of sclerosing peri-ureteritis, which causes shortening of the ureter, the ureteric orifice becomes displaced upwards and its mouth remains open (the so-called 'golf-hole' ureteric orifice). As the disease progresses, the capacity of the bladder steadily diminishes. At any stage, if a secondary infection supervenes, the intense generalised inflammation of the bladder wall obliterates many of the characteristic features of urinary tuberculosis just described above.

Retrograde pyelography may be necessary when investigating a suspicious pyuria if renal function is poor and tubercle bacilli have not been seen in the Ziehl-Neelsen film. Appearances, such as shagginess of a calyx or an abscess of the parenchyma connected to a calyx by a narrow neck, are often displayed by this method when excretory urograms appear normal. Retrograde pyelography is also of great assistance in cases of unilateral renal tuberculosis too advanced to concentrate contrast given intravenously (fig. 1225). Remember, however, that the diagnosis depends on finding bacilli and *not* on the pyelographic appearances.

Examination of the Lungs.—A radiograph is necessary to exclude active or previous pulmonary tuberculosis.

Treatment.—It is desirable to have the patient under observation when commencing treatment. The liability to serious side-effects from the drugs used will usually become obvious within the first three weeks.

The drug regimes used in the treatment of renal tuberculosis have depended to some extent on the cost and availability of the drugs, and the difficulty in some parts of the world in keeping contact with the patients to ensure that treatment regimes are followed through. The guidelines have been discussed in Chapter 4.

Prognosis in renal tuberculosis has improved enormously since the advent of chemotherapy and antibiotic treatment, and if the regimen detailed is carried out properly there should be a very low incidence of recrudescence of infection.

Operative Treatment.—Some lesions are surrounded by so much necrotic and fibrous tissue that antibiotic agents do not reach the organisms in sufficient concentration to kill them. Unilateral lesions of this character, and those in which the disease is more advanced, call for operative treatment, the optimum time for which is after six to twelve weeks of antibiotic treatment.

According to circumstances one of several operations is carried out. It must be emphasised that conservative surgery should be the aim, and several conservative procedures may prove necessary on one or both kidneys and ureters during the course of the disease. The fact that a horseshoe kidney is involved does not alter this principle, neither does the fact that one kidney may have been removed already.

1. **Renal Cavernostomy** (Hanley).—As the primary lesion of the calyx heals (fig. 1223A and B) fibrosis tends to cause a stricture at the neck of the calyx. Radiological disappearance of such a cavity should be viewed with suspicion, and usually indicates that there is a closed pyocalyx which remains infected, as its avascularity prevents the drugs from reaching the tubercle bacilli present. Sometimes such a pyocalyx will re-open and discharge its contents some six months after starting treatment, but if this does not occur after a year and a calyx is radiologically 'missing', a drainage operation must be undertaken.

The kidney is approached as described on p. 1252 and after clearing the perinephric fat, the abscess is aspirated with a syringe and wide-bore needle. The roof of the abscess is removed with scissors and its caseous contents swabbed out until healthy granulation tissue is reached. Any bleeding from the cut edges is controlled with fine catgut stitches (fig. 1226). The wound is closed without drainage. As the cavity is closed off from the pelvis (if it is not, the operation is unnecessary), there is no leakage of urine. Multiple abscesses in both kidneys can be dealt with in this way.

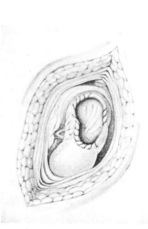

FIG. 1226.—Renal cavernostomy completed
(After H. G. Hanley, London.)

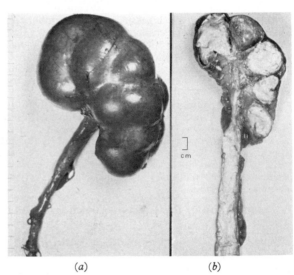

(a)   (b)

FIG. 1227.—(*a* and *b*)—Nephro-ureterectomy. Tuberculous pyonephrosis.

2. **Nephro-ureterectomy.**—The indication is a unilateral lesion with gross impairment of renal function on the affected side.

In such advanced cases the ureter as well as the kidney usually proves to be diseased, and nephroureterectomy (fig. 1227), in which, through a separate incision, the ureter is divided and ligated at its entrance to the bladder before commencing lumbar nephrectomy, is the operation of choice. By total removal of the ureter a possible source of continued infection of the bladder is removed, and the incidence of post-operative wound infection and sinus formation is reduced.

3. **For Hydronephrosis.**—This is due to tuberculous cicatricial contracture and healing of the bladder around the lower end of the ureter or at the pelvi-ureteric junction. A procedure similar to the Anderson-Hynes operation should be performed (p. 1222).

4. **For Systolic bladder** (*syn.* 'thimble bladder' (fig. 1256)).—This is due to healing by fibrosis and often leads to extreme frequency of micturition. The best operation is the type of ileo-cystoplasty, described by Hanley, in which a 15 cm opened-out loop of terminal ileum is sutured to the bladder, from which the dome has been removed to provide a maximum opening (fig. 1257).

Howard Granville Hanley, Contemporary. Consulting Surgeon, St. Paul's Hospital, London.

ABACTERIAL PYURIA

That sterile pyuria indicates urinary tuberculosis is almost axiomatic. Nevertheless, a small group of cases of abacterial pyuria is definitely non-tuberculous. The symptoms simulate renal tuberculosis very closely, and it is only when repeated examinations of the urine, and in the male the seminal fluid, fail to reveal *Mycobacterium tuberculosis* or other bacteria, and cultures and guinea-pig inoculations are negative, that the diagnosis can be made. Urography occasionally shows slight dilatation of the renal pelvis and ureter of one or both sides; more usually this examination is negative. Cystoscopy reveals a severe cystitis and often diminished bladder capacity. Occasionally amoebiasis is responsible.

Treatment.—Aureomycin usually cures the condition in three days. In cases resistant to this treatment 0·3 g of neoarsphenamine intravenously weekly for four weeks is often successful. In rare instances, when amoebiasis is responsible, treatment with emetine hydrochloride will eradicate the infection.

NEOPLASMS OF THE KIDNEY

Benign Neoplasms

Adenoma.—Pea-like cortical adenomas are sometimes found at necropsy. They give rise to no symptoms, and are only of academic interest.

Angioma may give rise to profuse haematuria.

Truly benign tumours of the kidney are so rare that a good rule is that *all neoplasms of the kidney which can be recognised clinically should be considered malignant and treated as such.*

Malignant Neoplasms

Clinically neoplasms of the kidney are divided into two classes:

In children between the ages of one and seven.

In adults after the age of forty.

Between the ages of seven and forty malignant neoplasms are unusual.

RENAL NEOPLASMS IN CHILDREN

Wilms's tumour (*syn.* nephroblastoma) is a mixed tumour containing epithelial and connective tissue elements arising from embryonic nephrogenic tissue, situated originally in one or other pole of the kidney. In infancy such tumours are very occasionally bilateral. Far more common is a unilateral tumour. They usually occur during the first four years of life. Cases arising under one year seen to have a much better prognosis.

Pathology.—*Macroscopically.*—On section the neoplasm is a greyish-white or pinkish-white colour; its consistence varies with the rapidity of the growth, *i.e.* the more rapid the growth, the softer the tumour (fig. 1228).

Microscopically it is composed mainly of two types of cells—epithelial and connective—tissue. Cartilage, bone, and smooth or striped muscle fibres are occasional findings. The epithelial and connective-tissue cells exist side by side, but one type is usually predominant. Thus the tumour is composed of mixed cellular elements, some of which are radio-sensitive and some radio-resistant. Consequently, the radio-resistant elements show a continuance of activity in spite of radiotherapy.

Clinical Features:

Abdominal Tumour.—The symptomatology is always the same. An abdominal tumour appears and progresses rapidly, while the general health deteriorates. Examination of the abdomen reveals a mass which may be enormous; the bulk

Max Wilms, 1867–1918. Professor of Surgery, Heidelberg, Germany.

of the tumour is on one side of the abdomen. Wilms's tumour tends to grow within a capsule, pushing the rest of the kidney aside; thus the reniform shape of the kidney is lost early.

Pyrexia.—Half these patients have some elevation of temperature, which disappears if the tumour is removed.

Haematuria is a sign of ill omen. It denotes that the previously encapsulated tumour has burst into the renal pelvis, and all patients suffering from a Wilms's tumour with this sign die within nine months (Scott).

Urography shows gross deformity of some of the calyces.

Metastases.—Wilms's tumour metastasises early, mainly by the bloodstream to the lungs, less commonly to the liver, rarely to bones, and exceptionally to the brain. Lymphatic dissemination is much less common.

Differential Diagnosis.—From a practical standpoint there is but one swelling with which Wilms's tumour can be confused, and that is retroperitoneal neuroblastoma, but as the treatment is precisely the same such differentiation is an academic exercise. However, if radiography reveals bone metastases, this distinctly favours a neuroblastoma. Although these abdominal tumours arouse considerable diagnostic interest, multiple examination by, for instance, a class of students, must be forbidden for fear of accelerating dissemination.

Treatment.—*Immediate nephrectomy and post-operative radiotherapy.* The earlier nephrectomy can be carried out, the better. A few hours may be necessary to correct anaemia by transfusion. Radiotherapy should be commenced immediately after operation, and 200 rad given daily to a total of 4000 to 4500 rad.

Prognosis.—Under the age of one year 80% survive five years, over this age it drops to 30%. Recurrences usually occur within a year, so a child surviving eighteen months is probably cured.

Bilateral Cases and Inoperable Cases.—Radiotherapy should be given to the renal areas. There is some hope that chemotherapeutic agents and particularly actinomycin D may prove of value in these cases.

RENAL NEOPLASMS IN ADULTS

1. **Hypernephroma** (*syn.* Grawitz tumour) is an adenocarcinoma and is the commonest neoplasm of the kidney (75%). It arises in the cortex, possibly from a pre-existing adenoma, probably *per primam* in cells of the uriniferous tubules.

Pathology.—A tumour of moderate size is spherical in shape, and it often occupies one or other pole, the seat of election being the upper pole; less often it is in the central portion of the kidney. On section it is characteristically yellow (due to lipoid); less often it is dull white, or semi-transparent. Haemorrhagic areas are often seen. The tumour is divided into numerous lobules by fibrous septa (fig. 1229). The larger the tumour the more extensive is central haemorrhage and necrosis.

Microscopical Structure.—The most common appearance is solid alveoli of cubical or polyhedral clear cells, with deeply stained small rounded nuclei and abundant cytoplasm containing lipoids, cholesterol, and glycogen. The cells may also be arranged in the form of papillary cysts or tubules. In a much smaller percentage the cells are granular (dark). Clear and dark cells can co-exist in different parts of the same tumour. In all cases the stroma is scanty but rich in large blood-vessels, the walls of which often appear, in places, to consist of tumour cells.

Lyall Stuart Scott, Contemporary. Surgeon, Urology Department, Victoria Infirmary, Glasgow, Scotland.
Paul Albert Grawitz, 1850–1932. Professor of Pathology, Greifswald, Germany.

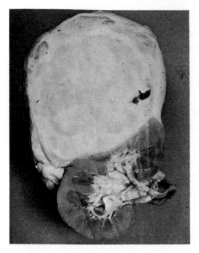

FIG. 1228.—Wilms's tumour.

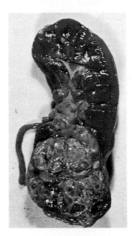

FIG. 1229.—Adenocarcinoma of the kidney.

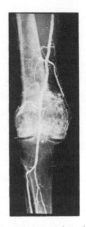

FIG. 1230.—Arteriogram showing vascular 'blush' due to a metastasis from a Grawitz tumour.

Spread.—As the tumour enlarges, it encroaches upon a group of calyces and is prone to grow into the renal veins. Pieces of growth becoming detached are swept into the circulation, to become arrested particularly in the lungs to produce 'cannon ball' secondary deposits (fig. 1232), and in bones. Occasionally, when a secondary growth appears in a long bone, it remains the only metastasis for perhaps a year or more.

While spread by the blood-stream predominates, spread by lymphatics occurs also. If the tumour bursts through the renal capsule into the perirenal tissues, it then metastasises to the lymph nodes in relation to the hilum of the kidney, and from there to the para-aortic and other lymph nodes.

Clinical Features.—Men are more often affected than women, the ratio being 2:1. Typically the first sign is intermittent haematuria. Clot colic may follow. Dragging pain in the loin is sometimes a leading symptom. Occasionally the first manifestation is a palpable renal swelling. In the adult male a rapidly developing varicocele is a rare but impressive sign.[1]

Atypical Cases.—(*a*) In 25% of cases the primary growth remains 'silent', the patient presenting because of secondary deposits such as a painful enlargement of a bone (fig. 1230), a spontaneous fracture, persistent cough, or haemoptysis.

(*b*) Occasionally persistent pyrexia (37·8°-38·9°C) is the only symptom, there being no infection to account for the temperature. It is presumably due to absorption of blood and necrotic material. Such pyrexia usually disappears after nephrectomy: should it persist metastases are present.

(*c*) In a small group of cases the patient presents on account of lassitude and is found to be extremely anaemic, the anaemia being out of proportion to that which could be expected from the haematuria, if such be present.

(*d*) 'Polycythaemia' occurs in 4% of cases. The sedimentation rate is *always raised* above the 1 to 2 mm found in idiopathic polycythaemia vera. The blood

---

[1] A left-sided varicocele is more likely, as the left spermatic vein joins the left renal vein.

count will return to normal after nephrectomy, but a return of the polycythaemia has been known with development of metastases.

(*e*) A nephrotic syndrome has been the presenting feature in some cases of hypernephroma.

(*f*) Endocrine disturbances. Renin secreting tumours producing hypertension have been recorded. Hypercalcaemia can occur.

Early Diagnosis.—By the time a patient has the classical triad of symptoms, *viz.* haematuria, pain, and a palpable renal tumour, he nearly always has metastases. It is therefore of paramount importance to endeavour to make an early diagnosis, and any one of these symptoms calls for a thorough renal investigation. Patients with haematuria should be examined cystoscopically while the bleeding is in progress. If blood is seen issuing from one ureteric orifice, and there is a clear efflux from the other, the information gained is of considerable importance, but is by no means conclusive evidence of a renal neoplasm. Extremely suggestive is bleeding occurring from a palpable kidney. When blood is not seen issuing from a ureter, but an enlarged middle lobe of the prostate or a papilloma of the bladder is discovered, it must not be assumed that the source of the haemorrhage has been found. Investigation must proceed until each kidney has been proved either to be normal or culpable.

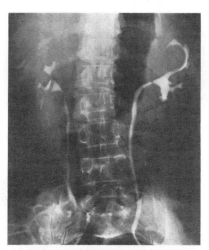

Fig. 1231.—Urogram is a case of hypernephroma of the left kidney. The only symptom was one attack of painless haematuria.

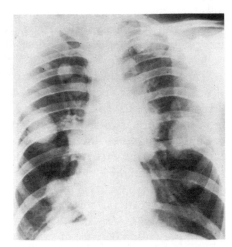

Fig. 1232.—Cannon ball secondaries from a hypernephroma.

Intravenous Urography.—(fig. 1231). The early diagnosis rests almost entirely on urography, but it may be inconclusive in early cases, because of lack of precise definition, and in late cases because there is poor or absent concentration of the medium, but at all times it is of great value in determining the function of the contralateral kidney. The presence of a projection in the cortical outline is important.

Tomography during the nephrogram phase can be helpful in outlining the periphery and may distinguish between cyst and tumour.

Ultrasound and CT scanning are helpful when the kidney functions poorly. *Retrograde pyelography* may help if these are not available.

Aortography is widely used as a final diagnostic measure, followed by *embolism of the renal artery* (Chapter 14, p. 212). This can be helpful in reducing the vascularity of large tumours, and, by some, is believed to enhance the immune response to the tumour.

Chest x-ray.—A radiograph of the thorax should always be taken before deciding the best course of treatment. It is not rare for a hitherto unsuspected metastasis or metastases in a lung to be revealed in this way (fig. 1232).

Bone Scans should, if possible, be carried out as this may reveal metastases which fail to show on x-ray.

Differential Diagnosis.—(*a*) Haemorrhage into a hydronephrosis, (*b*) congenital cystic kidney with haematuria, or (*c*) a solitary cyst of the kidney can closely simulate a renal neoplasm, or (*d*) aneurysm of a renal artery.

Treatment.—In cases without metastases the treatment is nephrectomy with removal of the perinephric fat.

The incision is a matter of personal preference, the objective being to gain wide exposure of the enlarged kidney and especially of its pedicle. The abdominal approach (p. 1253) is best for accomplishing the following manoeuvre.

Preliminary Division of the Renal Pedicle.—It is advisable to deal with the renal pedicle before manipulating the kidney, otherwise blood-borne metastases may occur as a direct result of the operation. Before undertaking ligation and division of the renal pedicle the renal vein and vena cava should be palpated delicately between the finger and thumb for a tumour-thrombus which, if present, calls for opening the vein and extracting the thrombus.

In other respects the details of the operation are those described below.

When an extremely large tumour is encountered a paramedian incision is easily enlarged by a transverse cut.

Radiotherapy.—In general terms these tumours are resistant to irradiation, and some series suggest that post-operative radiotherapy makes things worse.

Drug Treatment.—There is some suggestion that preliminary infarction of the kidney enhances the immune response and improves the response to drug treatment (vinblastine and progesterone) of the secondary deposits existing at the time of presentation.

Prognosis.—Even some of the largest neoplasms have been followed by a permanent cure. In operable cases 44% of the patients are alive and well after three years, and 30% after five years. If there is macroscopic involvement of the renal vein or its branches, the prognosis is poor.

2. **Papillary Transitional Cell Tumours of the renal pelvis** (fig. 1233) resemble those in the bladder but are less common. They tend to invade the kidney proper, and to take on malignant characteristics. Spread downwards by seeding may give rise to multiple ureteric and bladder tumours, but a diffuse metaplasia may be the result of some carcinogenic agents in the urine.

Clinical Features.—Haematuria is often continued for months at a time. A renal swelling is absent, except in rare cases where the pelvi-ureteric junction becomes occluded and hydronephrosis results, in which event there is lumbar pain. Clot colic may occur.

Cytology—examination of the urine may reveal the presence of malignant cells.

Urography reveals a characteristic filling defect of the renal pelvis (fig. 1234).

Treatment.—Nephrectomy with extended ureterectomy is the correct treat-

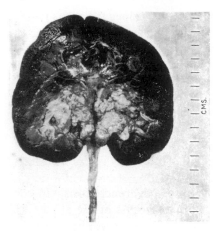

FIG. 1233.—Papillary tumour of the renal pelvis.

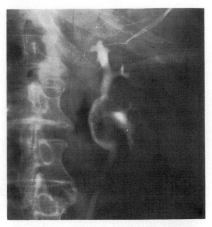

FIG. 1234.—Urogram showing a filling defect of the renal pelvis due to papilloma.

ment. The intramural portion of the ureter along with the ureteric orifice must be excised in continuity by sleeve resection of the bladder wall.

3. **Squamous-celled carcinoma of the renal pelvis** is the least common variety of malignant disease of the kidney. In some instances it appears to be preceded by leucoplakia, and in most cases a stone or stones are present.

Unless the stone gives rise to symptoms, this is the most elusive of all renal neoplasms, for it causes indefinite abdominal pain which finally becomes localised in the region of the involved kidney. Haematuria is slight, or to be found only on microscopical examination of the urine. Intravenous urogram shows a kidney excreting little or no medium. Retrograde pyelography sometimes reveals a deformed renal pelvis. Owing to diagnostic difficulties, by the time nephrectomy is performed there are often widespread metastases that are radio-resistant. This neoplasm has the worst prognosis of any renal neoplasm.

Primary neoplasms of the ureter are rare, and similar to those of the renal pelvis. The symptoms are identical with those of a neoplasm of the renal pelvis, although hydronephrosis, haemonephrosis, and pyonephrosis are more frequent accompaniments. Occasionally a portion of a papillomatous growth can be seen protruding from a ureteric orifice. Usually the diagnosis is made by pyelography.

Papillary tumours of the ureter should be treated by nephro-ureterectomy, as the epithelium frequently shows changes of carcinoma in situ at many sites. The intra-mural ureter should be removed, or the epithelium destroyed by fulguration. Only rarely is it justifiable, because of reduced renal reserve to perform resection of the ureter, and replacement by an ileal conduit. On the whole, the prognosis of tumours of the ureter is very poor, largely on account of late diagnosis.

Experience has shown that one half of the patients with 'upper tract' transitional cell tumours have, or will develop bladder tumours. Cystoscopy is therefore essential at the onset of treatment and follow up 'check cystoscopies' should be performed.

EXPOSURE AND REMOVAL OF THE KIDNEY

The kidney lies in a deep recess beneath the rigid bulwarks of the thoracic cage and, having regard to the possibility of a short renal pedicle, no single incision will meet all requirements.

The Oblique Lumbar Incision (Morris).—The patient is placed in the lateral 'kidney' position (fig. 1235), and is held in this position by a broad band of adhesive strapping, which is fixed to one side of the table and passed over the pelvis to the other side. The armrest also steadies the patient and relieves the chest of the weight of the arm, which would otherwise embarrass respiration. Morris's classical incision commences 1·25 cm

Sir Henry Morris, 1844–1926. Surgeon, Middlesex Hospital, London.

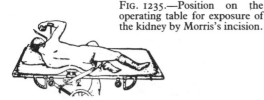

FIG. 1235.—Position on the operating table for exposure of the kidney by Morris's incision.

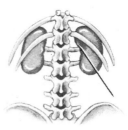

FIG. 1236.—Morris's incision.

below and lateral to the angle made by the twelfth rib with the outer border of the sacrospinalis, and it passes downwards and upwards towards the anterior superior iliac spine (fig. 1236) and all muscular layers are incised until the extraperitoneal fat is reached. An alternative and more favoured approach is to make the incision over the 12th rib and then either to resect the rib or, by displacing the upper half of the periosteum, to 'drop' it into the lower part of the wound. Care must be taken when removing periosteum not to open the pleural cavity. The pleura will be seen lying on the diaphragm after removing the rib. The extraperitoneal fat has a free posterior border and this is displaced forwards to display the perinephric fascia, which is then incised to reveal the perinephric fat surrounding the kidney. To perform nephrectomy the kidney is lifted from the posterior leaf of the perinephric fat, the fingers of one hand being inserted behind the pelvis and the vessels. Fat and fascia are dissected away from these structures as they lie on the operators' fingers. The vessels are ligated individually and the ureter is divided as low as possible. The wound is closed in layers with a corrugated drain placed beside the pedicle.

If the pleura has been breached, the anaesthetist should expand the lung fully before the pleura is closed, at the end of the operation. An x-ray should be taken to check that the lung is re-expanded. Any residual pneumothorax may need to be aspirated.

Transabdominal nephrectomy is frequently employed for the removal of renal tumours, as it gives an unrivalled approach to the renal vessels which must be tied before the tumour is handled, in order to prevent cells being displaced into the circulation by the manipulations. A transverse or paramedian incision is used.

Subcapsular Nephrectomy.—In order to prevent damage to densely adherent structures such as the duodenum, colon, and spleen, the kidney may be removed by incising the capsule along the convex border and dissecting it free to the hilum, where it is again incised to allow access to the renal pedicle.

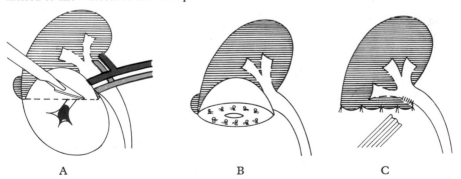

A   B   C

FIG. 1237.—Partial nephrectomy. (A) Capsule preserved and reflected; clean cut across parenchyma. Isolation of the affected calyx. (b) Haemostasis by suture of individual vessels. (C) No attempt to approximate the cut surface of the renal parenchyma, just cover the surface with the capsule.

Partial Nephrectomy (Semb).—A wide lumbar exposure with resection of the twelfth rib is required. Bleeding is controlled by compression of the appropriate branches of the renal vessels. The stages of the excision are shown in fig. 1237.

Carl Boye Semb, 1895–1971. Professor of Surgery, University of Oslo.

CHAPTER 58

THE URINARY BLADDER

SURGICAL ANATOMY AND PHYSIOLOGY

Surgical Anatomy.—Possessing an anterior, superior and posterior surface and being lined by transitional epithelium, the average bladder is capable of holding between 400 and 500 ml of urine without over-distension. The bladder wall is made up of a muscular coat of smooth muscle, known as the **detrusor muscle**, the fibres of which are arranged in three more or less distinct strata. *The internal layer* is thin, and its fasciculi have a reticular[1] arrangement. *The middle layer* is thicker than the others, and consists of densely interlaced fasciculi running mainly in a circular direction. When hypertrophy of the musculature of the bladder occurs it is the fasciculi of this layer that stand out and give rise to the characteristic trabeculation of the bladder wall (fig. 1279). While this layer is virtually absent within the limits of the trigone, its fibres are so well marked below that structure as to warrant their being accorded the dignity of the term **sphincter vesicae**. The **trigonal muscle** is a separate entity derived from a prolongation of the longitudinal layer of each ureter. In the trigone the muscular strands from each side decussate, and eventually are inserted into the wall of the posterior urethra. *The external layer* is composed mainly of longitudinal fibres. Some of the fibres of this layer are prolonged in the pubo-prostatic ligaments (see below).

Supports of the Bladder.—Several parts of the surrounding pelvic fascia are described as **true ligaments of the bladder**. The rectovesical portion of the pelvic fascia supports the bladder posteriorly. At the base of the bladder this fascia is united closely to the muscular tunic, but it thins out rapidly as it is reflected upwards. The two lateral true ligaments of the bladder are indistinct, but the anterior, or **pubo-prostatic ligaments**, are well defined, and are of great surgical importance. Each stretches from the front of the prostate and adjacent portion of the bladder to the lower part of the periosteum of the pubis.

The urachus and obliterated hypogastric arteries, together with the folds of peritoneum overlying these structures, are called the **false (median and lateral umbilical) ligaments of the bladder**. Condensations of fascia around the blood-vessels passing to the bladder are known as the **superior and inferior vascular pedicles**.

Arteries.—The superior and inferior vesical arteries are derived from the anterior trunk of the internal iliac artery. Branches from the obturator and inferior gluteal arteries (and in the female from the uterine and vaginal arteries) also help to nourish the bladder.

Veins form a plexus on the antero-inferior surface of the bladder; in the male the prostatic plexus is continuous with the vesical plexus, which drains into the internal iliac vein.

Lymphatics accompany the veins, and drain into the lymph nodes along the internal iliac vessels. Some lymphatics from the fundus pass to lymph nodes situated at the promontory of the sacrum.

Physiology (fig. 1238).—The nerves concerned in micturition are:

The sympathetic fibres, which arise in segments eleventh dorsal to second lumbar. These fibres pass via the presacral hypogastric nerve and the sympathetic chains to the inferior hypogastric plexus, and thence to the bladder.

The parasympathetic innervation, which is derived from the anterior primary divisions of the second, third and fourth sacral segments. These fibres pass through the pelvic splanchnic nerves to the inferior hypogastric plexus, from which they are distributed to the bladder.

The somatic innervation also comes from the second, third and fourth sacral segments as the pudendal nerves which pass, not to the bladder itself, but to the sphincter urethrae (striated muscle).

---

[1] Reticular (Lat. *reticularis*) = resembling a net.

While the sympathetic nerves convey afferent painful stimuli of over-distension *from* the bladder to the brain, it is unlikely that either set of autonomic nerves convey *to* the bladder any cortical impulses, such impulses being transmitted via the pudendal nerves to the sphincter urethrae, relaxing the latter. At the same time stretching of the muscle fibres by distension of the bladder initiates a reflex which is mediated through the parasympathetic nerves, and causes the detrusor muscle to contract. The neurogenic theory therefore ascribes the act of micturition to a stretch reflex which, if the time or place are not propitious, can be inhibited by cerebral control (fig. 1238).

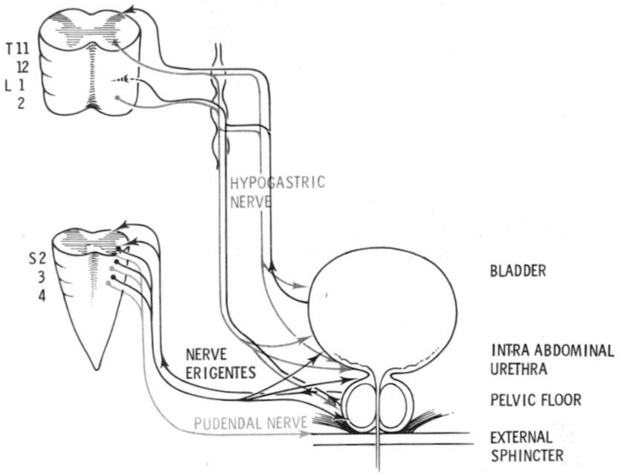

FIG. 1238.—The nervous control of the bladder. Micturition is partly a reflex and partly a voluntary act.

ECTOPIA VESICAE (*syn.* EXSTROPHY OF THE BLADDER)

Aetiology.—Incomplete development of the infra-umbilical part of the anterior abdominal wall, associated with incomplete development of the anterior wall of the bladder, is the embryological origin of the condition.

Clinical Features.—Ectopia vesicae occurs once in 50,000 births, and may be complete or incomplete. In the more common complete variety, because of the pressure of the viscera behind it, the deep-red posterior bladder wall protrudes through the defect (fig. 1239). If the exposed mucous membrane, which bleeds readily, is drawn gently upwards, the paler, wet trigone is displayed, and effluxes of urine from the ureteric orifices can be seen. There is a well-defined line of demarcation between the protruding mucous membrane and the adjacent skin, and, especially after reducing the extruded bladder wall beneath the mucocutaneous junction, the firm edge of the hernial ring can be felt. Usually the umbilicus is absent. There may be umbilical and inguinal herniae. The rectal sphincter is often lax. The sex ratio is about four males to one female.

In the male, the completely epispadiac penis is broader and shorter than normal, and not infrequently bilateral inguinal herniae are present; the prostate and seminal vesicles are rudimentary or absent, whereas the testes are normal and have descended more often than not. *In the female*, the clitoris is cleft and the labia minora are separated anteriorly, exposing the vaginal orifice. In both sexes there is separation of the pubic bones (fig. 1240), which are connected by a strong ligament, and, except for the fact that the patient has a waddling gait, this bony defect causes no disability; indeed, in those female sufferers who become pregnant, it facilitates delivery. The linea alba is as wide as the separation of the pubic bones. In the rare incomplete form the pubes are united and the external genitalia are almost normal.

The lot of a patient with ectopia vesicae is particularly unfortunate. A portable urinal seldom keeps him dry for long, and the odour of urine always accompanies him. Frequently the everted vesical mucous membrane becomes ulcerated and painful. It undergoes metaplastic changes, and sometimes becomes the seat of an adenocarcinoma.

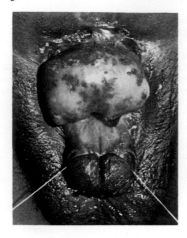

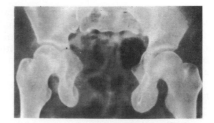

FIG. 1240.—Showing the separation of the pubes in a case of ectopia vesicae.
(*The late Professor Grey Turner, London.*)

FIG. 1239.—Ectopia vesicae in a male. A drop of urine is seen at the left ureteric orifice, the corona glandis being retracted by threads.
(*G. D. Adhia, FRCS, Bombay.*)

Attempts to prevent recurrent attacks of ascending pyelonephritis by chemotherapeutic and antibiotic agents are only partially successful; 50% of those afflicted die of renal failure before the age of thirty.

Treatment

(*a*) *Diversion of urine* into the colon or isolated rectum, followed some months later by cystectomy. The operation is undertaken between four and six years of age.

(*b*) The best long term results would seem to follow diversion into an *ileal conduit, with excision of the bladder*, at the age mentioned. Renal function is likely to be better maintained than following uretero-colic anastomosis, and there are no problems of rectal control (see clinical features).

(*c*) *Iliac Osteotomy and closure of abdominal wall.*—In recent years, attempts to reconstruct the bladder and sphincters by operation within the first year of life have shown that it is possible to obtain a sound mid-line abdominal scar by commencing the operation with osteotomy of both iliac bones just lateral to the sacro-iliac joints. The bladder can be closed, and the reconstructed urethra displaced behind the pubis, which now meets in the mid-line. However, the ultimate results in respect of continence, freedom from urinary infection and stone formation are disappointing, though in males the procedure may be a useful method of keeping the patient dry with an appliance. It is better, if this is the intention, to make no attempt to produce continence at the bladder neck.

Results.—Comparatively few who have undergone successful uretero-sigmoidal implantation for ectopia vesicae live for twenty years. The causes of the untimely demise are (1) stricture at the site of anastomosis and bilateral hydronephroses, (2) recurrent pyelonephritis and (3) hyperchloraemic acidosis. Many different methods of implanting the ureters have been devised (fig. 1275); all aim at reducing the risks of stenosis and reflux.

RUPTURE OF THE BLADDER ⟨ Intraperitoneal 20% / Extraperitoneal 80%

As the bladder has intraperitoneal and extraperioneal relations it follows that rupture or perforation results in either intraperitoneal or extraperitoneal extravasation of urine (figs. 1241 and 1242). Intraperitoneal rupture may be due to a blow, kick or fall on to a fully distended bladder and it is more common in the male than in the female. Extraperitoneal rupture is usually caused by a fractured pelvis, occasioned by the all too common road traffic accidents of today. Other causes of rupture or perforation of either type include gunshot wounds, stab wounds, the passage of instruments, endoscopic resection, or diathermy coagulation of bladder tumours.

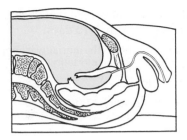

FIG. 1241.—Intraperitoneal extravasation of urine.

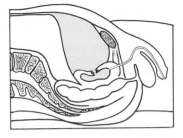

FIG. 1242.—Extraperitoneal extravasation of urine.

Intraperitoneal Rupture.—There is sudden, agonising pain in the hypogastrium, often accompanied by severe shock and perhaps syncope. However, especially if the patient was 'drunk and distended', in a few minutes the shock subsides and the pain lessens, so that the patient may continue with his orgies, but the abdomen commences to distend. Usually the patient has no desire to micturate. On examination varying degrees of abdominal rigidity and, after a few hours, abdominal distension are present. In spite of the fact that the patient has not passed urine since the accident, there is no dullness above the pubis corresponding to a distended bladder. Usually there is tenderness in the hypogastrium. If the amount of urine in the peritoneal cavity is considerable, shifting dullness can be elicited. Rectal examination often reveals a bulging of the rectovesical pouch. When the urine is sterile, symptoms and signs of peritonitis are delayed for hours.

Extraperitoneal Rupture.—As in many cases this cannot be differentiated from a rupture of the posterior urethra and as the treatment is the same, this injury is dealt with in Chapter 60.

Confirming a Suspected Diagnosis.—A plain x-ray taken in the erect position may show the ground glass appearance of fluid in the lower abdomen. Intravenous urography may confirm a leak from the bladder. A peritoneal 'tap' may be of value. If doubt still exists and if there is no sign of fracture then retrograde cystography can be performed safely. With careful asepsis a small (14F) catheter is passed. Usually some blood-stained urine will drain. A solution made from 60 ml of 35% Hypaque or Conray with 120 ml of sterile isotonic saline is injected into the bladder and radiographs taken.

Treatment.—When there are reasonable grounds for suspecting rupture of the bladder, operation should be undertaken without delay.

Intraperitoneal Rupture.—Lower laparotomy is performed. Urine is removed by suction, after which the patient is placed in Trendelenburg's position. The edges of the rent, which are usually situated in the posterior part of the dome of the bladder are trimmed and sutured by two layers of interrupted catgut stitches, and the operation completed by stitching a large Malécot catheter into an extraperitoneal suprapubic incision in the bladder. The latter ensures intravesical tension being kept at a minimum during healing of the sutured tear. Unless obvious infection is present the peritoneum can be closed without drainage. The abdominal wall is repaired around the Malécot catheter, not omitting drainage

Friedrich Trendelenburg, 1844–1924. Professor of Surgery, Leipzig, Germany.
In 1839 Dr. Walther, a General Practitioner of Pittsburg, successfully sutured an intraperitoneal rupture of the bladder of a blacksmith.
Achille-Etienne Malécot, 1852–?. He invented his catheter while Interne des Hôpitaux de Paris.

of the prevesical space. Following the operation, antibiotic therapy is given until the urine is proved sterile after removal of the catheter in 8–10 days.

Prognosis.—When operation is performed within twelve hours the mortality is approximately 11%; when operation is delayed to twenty-four hours the mortality rises to 55%. Without operation the mortality is 100%.

WOUNDING OF THE BLADDER DURING OPERATION

Operations in which the bladder is liable to be injured are (1) inguinal or femoral herniotomy (especially during the performance of the low operation for strangulated femoral hernia); (2) hysterectomy (particularly panhysterectomy) by either the abdominal or vaginal route and (3) excision of the rectum. In all these operations, to minimise this accident the bladder must be emptied *after* the patient has been anaesthetised. If the injury is recognised at the time of its infliction, the bladder must be repaired in two layers and urethral catheter drainage maintained for seven days. If it is not so recognised, the treatment is similar to that of rupture of the bladder.

When accidental perforation of the bladder occurs during endoscopic resection of a bladder tumour, or the prostatic capsule is perforated during transurethral prostatectomy, for practical purposes the perforation is always extraperitoneal. When the accident is recognised at the time, drainage of the bladder with a large urethral catheter, and the administration of antibiotics, usually suffice.

RETENTION OF URINE

Retention of urine is either acute or chronic, the latter leading ultimately to retention-with-overflow.

Acute retention

Aetiology.—The most frequent causes are:

In the male	*In the female*	*In the male child*
Prostatic enlargement. Urethral stricture. Post-operative.	Retroverted gravid uterus. Multiple sclerosis. Hysteria.	Meatal ulcer with scabbing.

Other causes:

Following spinal anaesthesia.	Acute urethritis or prostatitis.
Blood-clot in the bladder.	Urethral calculus.
Rupture of the urethra.	Phimosis.
Neurogenic (injury or disease of the spinal cord).	Certain drugs
	Muscular atony from advanced age.
Faecal impaction in the rectum.	Anal pain (haemorrhoidectomy).

Clinical Features.—The patient has not passed urine for some hours, and is unable to do so. Often the swelling caused by a full bladder can be seen in a thin person; it is somewhat tender to palpation, and dull to percussion above the symphysis pubis. Spasms of acute pain occur periodically as the muscle of the bladder contracts. An attempt is made to elicit the cause of the retention; this is most frequently due to vascular engorgement of an already enlarged prostate, but the floor of the urethra should be palpated for the induration characteristic of a stricture, and the reflexes in the lower limb and perianal sensation should be tested to exclude spinal (neurogenic) causes.

Treatment.—It is of paramount importance never to relieve, or attempt to relieve, acute retention and forthwith send the patient home. He must always be admitted and kept under observation for at least twenty-four hours. Once the patient is in suitable surroundings, the effect of administering a dose of Omnopon to relieve anxiety, and a hot bath to diminish internal congestion, in many cases enables the patient to void. If the patient gives a good history of bladder outflow obstruction there seems little point attempting conservative measures and a catheter should be passed; this should be done using full aseptic technique. Following a thorough wash of the hands and arms sterile gloves should be donned. The external genitalia are gently cleaned using a soapy antiseptic solution (Savlon). A tube of local anaesthetic (Lidothesin) is then carefully inserted down the urethra warning the patient that this will create a strange sensation but if the jelly is injected slowly through the plastic nozzle it should cause no pain. A few minutes should be allowed to elapse while this takes effect. A small (14 French[1]) Foley self-retaining catheter should then gently be passed down the urethra while the penis is held taut. In a female patient the labia should be parted using the middle and index finger of the left hand which should not be moved once the cleaning process has been performed, to prevent contamination. Providing a stricture is not the cause of the retention the catheter should normally pass freely into the bladder and the self-retaining balloon can then be gently inflated. *Force should not be necessary.* Occasionally a large obstructing middle lobe of the prostate may prevent a simple catheter entering the bladder; in this instance a Coudé[2] catheter should pass without difficulty. The bladder is then allowed to drain and the catheter attached to a closed drainage system. In the male, if the catheter will not pass into the bladder, it is usually due to poor technique, traumatisation of the urethra, or because there is a urethral stricture. If the latter is suspected the simplest method of solving the problem is to use a set of filiform and 'follower' bougies. A fine filiform with a dog-leg bend created at the tip is gently passed down the urethra and this will normally negotiate any stricture. Should the filiform not pass with ease the procedure should be abandoned. Once a filiform is in the bladder a series of follower bougies can be screwed on to it and the stricture dilated. A small catheter can be passed after satisfactory dilatation. The use of a catheter introducer in the acute situation rarely helps and usually results in unnecessary urethral trauma.

If, after a reasonable attempt with catheters, the bladder has not been entered, one of four courses may be adopted according to circumstances.

1. **Suprapubic Puncture.**—Suprapubic puncture with a lumbar puncture needle or an 'Abbocath' is a useful method of relieving acute retention when catheterisation has failed. If the bladder is allowed to refill after it has been punctured, leakage into the prevesical space may follow.

2. **Suprapubic Catheterisation** (Riches' Technique).—A catheter is inserted into the bladder suprapubically through a 1·25 cm incision made under local anaesthesia 2·5 cm below the level at which the anterior surface of the bladder curves upwards and backwards

---

[1] The French scale is also known as Charrière's scale, so called after Joseph Charrière (1803–1876), a Paris surgical-instrument maker.
[2] coudé (adjective) = bent; coude (noun) = elbow.

Frederic Eugene Baisal Foley, 1891–1966. Urologist and Ancker Hospitals, St. Paul, U.S.A.
Sir Eric William Riches, 1897–1987. Surgeon and Urologist, The Middlesex Hospital, London.

to form the dome. The fibres of the linea alba are divided up to the length of the incision. After the special catheter has been mounted on its introducer it is passed through the incision until its sharp point touches the surface of the bladder, and the instrument is passed into the bladder with a short, sharp thrust directed backwards and downwards. The introducer is removed and the advancer is passed down the lumen of the catheter and its expander is opened. Thus the catheter is carried towards the trigone, and the advancer is removed. A stitch secures the catheter to the skin, and this is reinforced with a strip of adhesive plaster.

3. **Immediate Prostatectomy.**—Occasionally immediate prostatectomy in cases of benign enlargement of the prostate in fit patients who may have been worked-up previously, can be performed.

4. **Urethral instrumentation** (Chapter 60), in the case of a urethral stricture.

Whenever the bladder is catheterised for urinary retention it is important to record the volume drained and also to examine the patient's abdomen a few minutes after the procedure, for occasionally the retention may mask some other intra abdominal pathology.

Chronic Retention

In such cases the distension of the bladder is painless. The blood urea must be estimated before any attempt is made to relieve the retention. If it is below 70 mg% (12 mmol/l), treatment is as outlined for retention. Above this figure slow decompression is advisable (Chapter 59).

Retention with Overflow

In this condition the patient has no control of his urine, small amounts passing involuntarily from time to time from an overflowing bladder. It may follow a neglected acute retention, or chronic retention.

Retention with overflow is referred to also under 'incontinence' and 'prostatic enlargement'. The general principles which govern the treatment of this condition are similar to those of acute retention, but decompression of the bladder must be carried out very slowly (Chapter 60).

THE INDWELLING CATHETER AND THE CLOSED SYSTEM OF CATHETER DRAINAGE (fig. 1243)

The incidence of ascending infection is nearly halved by connecting the catheter (urethral, suprapubic or perineal) to sterile tubing conducted to a sterile collecting bottle, and employing irrigations only if clot retention occurs. When a catheter has been *in situ* for five or more days, some degree of urethritis is likely to supervene, though this has been much reduced by the use of catheters made from various non-irritant plastic substitutes for rubber *e.g.* Silastic. To change the catheter in the presence of urethritis entails a grave risk of infection spreading from the anterior to the posterior urethra, and thence to other parts of the urogenital system (fig. 1244).

SPECIAL FORMS OF RETENTION OF URINE

Post-operative Retention of Urine

Retention of urine can be encountered after any operation. It is common after operations on the anal canal and perineal region, and is due to reflex spasm of the urinary sphincters. After operations on the pelvic viscera, retention of urine is so common that it is usual to forestall it by inserting a catheter before or at the conclusion of the operation.

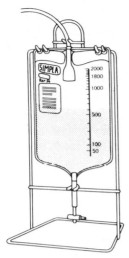

FIG. 1243.—Modern 'Simpla' bag[1] used for continuous bladder drainage. (The nurse who is emptying the bag should be wearing a disposable glove to avoid contaminating her hands with organisms.) A disadvantage is that the tube may be too stiff to 'milk'.

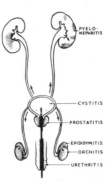

FIG. 1244.—Complications liable to follow changing a urethral catheter in the presence of urethritis.
(After C. G. Scorer, FRCS, London.)

When the patient is an elderly male, prostatic obstruction, hitherto latent, should be suspected. Many patients cannot urinate while lying or sitting in bed.

Treatment.—First of all, reassure the patient. Provide privacy. If the male patient, while supported, is permitted to sit on the edge of his bed, he is often able to empty his bladder. The sound of running water is often helpful. When circumstances permit (*e.g.* after haemorrhoidectomy) a warm bath is often helpful. If after a reasonable trial the patient cannot pass urine, he or she must be catheterised.

Acute Retention due to Drugs.—A number of drugs are prone to induce or precipitate retention of urine. Antihistamine drugs, antihypertensive drugs, anticholinergics, tricyclic antidepressants and I.N.A.H. compounds (chemotherapeutic agents for tuberculosis) have all been responsible for producing acute retention of urine. Indeed, 'drug retention' has become a clinical entity.

Management of the Bladder in Spinal Injuries (Chapter 27).

Immediately after a spinal cord injury *spinal shock* occurs, which may last for days, weeks or even months, and in this state the detrusor is paralysed, the bladder distends and overflow incontinence will occur. This will lead to *atony*, infection and ultimately renal failure. To manage this:

1. The bladder must be kept empty either by intermittent catheterisation with an aseptic technique performed two or three times daily or by the use of an indwelling Gibbon catheter (fig. 1245) on continuous drainage together with sulphamethizole (Urolucosil) and a high urinary output (3 litres daily) to combat infection.

2. The upper level of the neurological lesion must be assessed by the level of

---

[1] Simpla Plastics Ltd., Cardiff, Wales, U.K.

Norman Otway Knight Gibbon, Contemporary. Surgeon, Sefton Hospital, Liverpool, England.

sensory and motor loss. Ischaemic necrosis of the cord may extend a variable distance below the upper level of injury, but will indicate whether any section of the nerve supply to the bladder is likely to be involved. The sacral roots S2, 3, 4 will be at or about vertebrae level T12, L1.

Where sensory loss below the level is total, recovery is unlikely. Incomplete lesions on the other hand may recover somatic and particularly bladder function.

3. Demonstration of intact bulbo-cavernosus and anal reflexes indicates an intact sacral cord, and ultimately a *reflex or automatic bladder* will result. If these reflexes are absent and there is total loss of perineal sensation recovery is unlikely and the bladder will behave in an *autonomous* fashion.

In cauda equina lesions there may be sensory, motor or mixed loss.

4. Full assessment of the bladder lesion should be undertaken about three months after the injury (p. 1264).

With the help of *urodynamic techniques*, including electromyography where possible, much more accurate assessment of the detrusor and sphincter activity and the sensory side of the reflexes controlling micturition can be obtained. N. K. Gibbon of Liverpool has pleaded for the assessment of the three functions, *storage*, *evacuation* and *control of urine*, carefully related to the neurological damage which at this time has stabilised. Many types of bladder dysfunction can occur in the absence of detectable neurological abnormality (fig. 1248).

The urethral pressure profile (U.P.P.) is helpful in demonstrating resistance to outflow at the bladder neck, external sphincter and along the urethra. Evidence is accumulating that the smooth muscle elements of the posterior urethra and external sphincter may play a larger part than previously supposed in the increased peripheral resistance which is so often the main factor in poor bladder emptying. Block of the alpha adrenergic receptors (with i.v. phentolamine 10 mg) and repeating the U.P.P. will demonstrate this. In addition to this effect which is common to all complete cord lesions, Gibbon and his associates have suggested that damage to the sympathetic outflow can lead to a hypersensitivity of the smooth muscle of the posterior urethra to circulating catecholamines—thus patients have increased difficulty in emptying the bladder in the erect posture.

The results of these studies should enable decisions to be made as to the further management of the bladder, the aim being to produce good emptying and to avoid infection.

Lesions above cord segment D10 = Upper motor neurone bladder with all reflexes intact but separated from higher control and inhibition.

Emptying.—Detrusor contractions are present but are normally inappropriate and of a high pressure. These contractions are often associated with spasm of the external sphincter giving rise to what has now become known as detrusor sphincter dyssynergia. The bladder neck itself in these patients normally opens widely associated with a contraction. If left untreated the upper tracts suffer at the hands of the chronically raised intravesical pressure and the pressure that develops at the time of these 'isometric contractions'. Hydronephrosis and renal failure may result.

Capacity.—This tends to reduce as the years pass by. Trabeculation and the 'fir-tree' appearance of the bladder on x-ray seems to be progressive.

Control.—Continence in these patients is rarely complete due to the uninhibited contractions. When the intravesical pressure is raised endoscopic sphincterotomy is necessary to protect the upper tracts. In men a condom appliance may then be worn.

Constant vigilance is required of these patients, a watch being kept for hydronephrosis. This may be by serial intravenous urography or ultrasound scanning. Follow up urodynamic investigations are necessary to ensure that the sphincterotomy has been complete.

Lesions involving the sympathetic outflow, D11, 12, L1, L2 = Essentially an upper motor neurone bladder but with the additional loss of the sympathetic afferents and sensory efferents from the bladder.

There is less smooth muscle element in the urethral resistance as shown by phentolamine

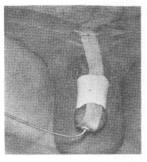
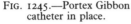

FIG. 1245.—Portex Gibbon
catheter in place.

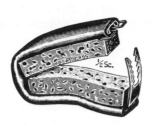

FIG. 1246.—Cunningham's
penile clamp.

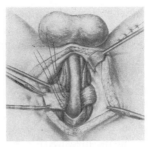

FIG. 1247.—Transplantation of
the gracilis muscle to make a
new sphincter urethrae.

block but a greater response to posture and these patients may have difficulty in emptying in the erect posture. 'Alpha-blockers' may nevertheless be a help in cutting out the effect of circulating catecholamines in the erect posture.

Damage to the sacral centre S2, 3, 4 and Cauda Equina lesions. = Essentially a lower motor neurone bladder.

Emptying.— The detrusor is paralysed (parasympathetic injury). Abdominal straining and pressure on the bladder through the abdominal wall can produce reasonable emptying. Sensation through the hypogastric nerves if D11, 12 is intact may enable the patient to know when the bladder is getting full. Intermittent catheterisation is also frequently used, as developed at Stoke Mandeville Hospital.

Capacity.— Quite a good capacity.

Control.— Reasonable in the early stages if there is no infection but liable to leak on straining. The bladder neck is usually open. The external sphincter may be paralysed but if the motor nerves are intact incoordination may be present and sphincterotomy is needed to enable emptying to occur. Reflux is more common with the lower motor neurone bladder.

Persistent Retention of Urine following Excision of the Rectum.—In 10% of cases retention of urine persists for three months or more. Probably, owing to the absence of cystometric substantiation of damage to the parasympathetic nerve supply to the bladder, the retention is due to mechanical factors, notably sagging of the bladder into the space formerly occupied by the rectum. In most cases the retention can be cured by conservative transurethral resection of the prostate. Usually the prostate is not enlarged, and consequently the resection can be carried out easily and quickly. Therefore, if after two weeks the patient is unable to empty his bladder and his general condition is satisfactory, transurethral prostatic resection should not be postponed. Thus the patient is spared what would probably be a long period of invalidism and the risk of urinary infection.

INCONTINENCE OF URINE

Continence of urine is dependent on a fine balance between the bladder having a storage capacity, the brain being aware of fullness and the subsequent coordination of the detrusor and the urethral sphincters to perform the act of voiding. Due to the multifactorial sources that can affect this fine balance it is hard to adopt a simple classification for the causes of urinary incontinence. The basic pre-requisites of urinary incontinence include anatomical integrity, cerebral awareness, a degree of mobility and competent sphincter control.

A careful history and physical examination will usually be sufficient to elucidate the cause. Nevertheless investigation of the urinary tract as a whole is nearly always indicated. The urine should be cultured for evidence of infection and biochemical estimation of the blood to assess renal function. It may be appropriate to have anatomical visualisation of the urinary tract with intravenous urography although ultrasound examination will often provide adequate details.

Urodynamic Testing

The key to lower urinary tract function lies with urodynamic investigation. The principle is to artificially simulate bladder filling and emptying whilst obtaining scientific measurements of the various functions involved.

The test involves the aseptic passage of a small pair of catheters or a twin lumen catheter into the bladder; this allows the bladder to be filled with saline or constrast medium whilst a continuous recording of the intravesical pressure is made via a transducer. To obtain true detrusor pressure a second pressure channel is required which is connected to a small balloon carefully inserted into the rectum. Modern equipment has the facility to subtract this value from that recorded in the bladder, thus removing artefacts associated with changes in intra-abdominal pressure. Initially the residual urine volume is measured and then the bladder filled at 50ml per minute with a note being kept of the patient's awareness of fullness. The Urethral Pressure Profile (UPP) can be measured by withdrawing a catheter perfused at a constant rate across the sphincter complex. The requirement for the latter measurement has largely been superseded now that combined pressure and x-ray facilities are increasingly available. Once the bladder has been filled to comfortable capacity the filling catheter is removed and the patient is asked to void preferably in discreet surroundings. Information can be acquired of the voiding pressure, the flow rate and the whole process can be visualised on an x-ray monitor (fig. 1248). Electro-myography of the pelvic floor and urethral sphincter can also be obtained with the careful placement of fine bi-polar needle electrodes.

Should sophisticated equipment not be available simple bedside measurements can be obtained by filling the bladder and making recordings of intravesical pressure with a CVP side arm. Then ask the patient to void while observing the process.

The normal bladder will accept approximately 400 ml of fluid without undue distress and the rise in intravesical pressure should not exceed 15 cm of water. The normal voiding pressure should not exceed 60 cm of water in a man and 40 cm of water in a woman, with the flow rate between 20 and 25 ml per second. The ability of the bladder to accept an enormous volume (in excess of a litre) with very little awareness would indicate the presence of flaccidity. This may be associated with chronic over-distension or neuropathy from diabetes mellitus, acute multiple sclerosis, tertiary syphilis or pernicious anaemia. Disorders associated with reduced capacity and a hypertonic bladder can usually be diagnosed quite simply although this is not always so easy in ladies suffering from 'sensory frequency'. An abnormal rise in intravesical pressure may simply arise from hypertonicity or (particularly in the presence of neurogenic dysfunction) from unstable excessive contractions. These can be associated with incontinence of urine. When incontinence does result they are called *uninhibited detrusor contractions*.

Causes of Incontinence

The common causes may be classified into male, female or mixed sex groups.

Male.—Chronic urinary retention with overflow is a common cause of incontinence. This may be secondary to benign prostatic hypertrophy but *there may be coexistent carcinoma of the prostate*. Hypertrophy of the bladder neck usually occurs in a younger age group and rarely the cause may be a urethral stricture. The key to the diagnosis lies with the history of prolonged hesitancy and a poor urinary stream with both daytime and nocturnal 'dribbling incontinence'. Examination may reveal that the bladder is visibly distended, the transverse suprapubic crease is lost and the painless distension of the bladder may be palpated or percussed. The treatment is discussed in Chapter 59 and below.

Post-prostatectomy.—Post-prostatectomy incontinence may result from injury to the external sphincter mechanism caused by clumsy surgery. Urodynamic evaluation will demonstrate this but may also reveal the presence of uninhibited contractions which occasionally develop secondary to bladder outflow obstruction. If these do not subside following relief of the obstruction *urge incontinence* may result, (see Chapter 59 and below).

Female.—The commonest cause of leakage of urine in women is stress incontinence. This occurs secondary to laxity of the pelvic floor with incompetence of the bladderneck and sphincter mechanism. It most commonly occurs in the late multiparous group although a minor degree of stress incontinence is experienced by many young women. The patient complains of loss of urine associated with coughing, laughing or sneezing and this may also occur with changes in posture. Urinary frequency and urgency may coexist and it is important to establish if urgency is associated with flooding, as this may indicate the presence of unstable bladder contractions. Apart from the overall assessment of the patient an appreciation of the psyche is necessary. Physical examination should ensure that the bladder is not palpably distended and the presence or absence of a cystocele should be determined. The demonstration of incontinence associated with coughing and its subsequent control applying Bonney's test (a finger either side of the urethra pushed upwards to support the pelvic floor) is important. A simple urodynamic assessment is often indicated. Minor degrees of stress urinary incontinence can be controlled using alpha adrenergic drugs which will tone up the bladder neck muscle. This combined with pelvic floor exercises and faradism may be sufficient. When a significant cystocele is present, surgical correction may be necessary by an anterior colporrhaphy with buttress sutures inserted to support the bladder neck.

In the presence of gross descent of the pelvic floor a suprapubic approach is preferable to reduce what is in fact simply herniation of the bladder neck through the pelvic floor. A *Marshall Marchetti* type procedure is usually preferred with insertion of chromic catgut sutures into the paraurethral tissues of the lateral fornices which are then hitched up on to the retropubic ligaments. This operation performed correctly should carry a 95% long term cure rate.

Common to Both Sexes

Congenital.—Ectopia vesicae and severe epispadias. The abnormal entry of a ureter beneath the sphincter complex or into the vagina in a female results in total urinary incontinence. This is discussed in Chapter 57.

Trauma.—Trauma whether from pelvic surgery or associated with pelvic fracture may result in disruption of the nerve supply to the urethra.

Infection.—Simple cystitis will often be sufficient, particularly in a woman, to induce urinary incontinence. A history of frequency, burning and a fever should alert one to the diagnosis. The bladder may be tender whether palpated suprapubically or per vaginam. Symptoms will usually settle with a course of antibiotics but in the case of recurrent infection further investigation of the urinary tract will clearly be indicated.

Endocrine.—Occasionally women suffering from thyrotoxicosis will experience urinary frequency and some incontinence. Appropriate treatment of the thyroid gland will usually result in a complete cure.

Neoplasia.—Locally advanced cancers in the pelvis, particularly carcinoma of the cervix in a woman and prostate in a man, may result in direct invasion of the sphincter mechanism causing incontinence; occasionally fistula formation may occur in women.

Other causes can be classified into neurogenic, psychogenic, capacitance or drug-induced incontinence.

Neurogenic Incontinence

Causes: *Myelodysplasia*
Multiple sclerosis
Spinal cord injuries
Cerebral dysfunction (CVA, dementia)
Parkinson's disease (paralysis agitans)

These conditions lead to a combination of neurogenic vesical dysfunction associated frequently with loss of mobility. Careful investigation of the whole urinary tract is always required and the treatment depends on the attempt to strike a fine balance between preventing hydronephrosis from abnormally high bladder pressures yet at the same time maintaining continence. The two are frequently not compatible. Intermittent self-catheterisation, surgical sphincter ablation and occasionally a chronic indwelling catheter provide the basis of management often in association with the use of anticholinergic type drugs. If all else fails urinary diversion (ileal conduit) may be necessary particularly in women where no adequate collecting device is available to prevent the dreadful bed sores that can occur associated with recumbency and urinary incontinence. Prostatectomy for males after severe strokes and in the presence of dementia is associated with a high incontinence rate. In the case of men with Parkinson's disease it is usually best to wait until they develop retention before advising a prostatectomy.

Psychogenic Incontinence

With every incontinent patient careful thought must be paid to the psychological status of the patient; retention can occur particularly in women suffering from hysteria and in both sexes incontinence may herald a depressive illness.

Capacity Disorders

The capacity of the bladder may be considerably reduced causing crippling urinary frequency and also incontinence. This may occur following tuberculosis when the bladder can be severely contracted from the ensuing fibrosis. Radiotherapy for pelvic cancer can also cause both early irritative symptoms and later a reduction in capacity causing incontinence.

Drug Induced

The detrusor muscle is basically under post-ganglionic parasympathetic control and its transmitter is cholinergic. Recent studies have established the presence of a number of alpha adrenergic fibres in the region of the bladderneck. A knowledge of these transmitters can allow one to manipulate the bladder pharmacologically. A number of drugs can induce urinary retention (anticholinergic agents, tricyclic antidepressants, lithium, some antihypertensives). Overflow may ensue. Drugs giving extra pyramidal side affects may induce urinary frequency and incontinence, e.g. phenothiazines.

Frequency Urge Syndrome.—This relatively uncommon condition consists of urinary frequency, urgency, sometimes urge incontinence and enuresis. Neurological examination is usually normal although occasionally the lack of fusion of the vertebral arch of L5 or S1 may lead one to suspect the diagnosis of spina bifida occulta. Urodynamic testing usually reveals the presence of an unstable bladder but a cause is not found in the majority of patients. The treatment consists of anticholinergic and tricyclic drugs in the hope of reducing the height of the unstable contractions and so the frequency and incontinence they cause.

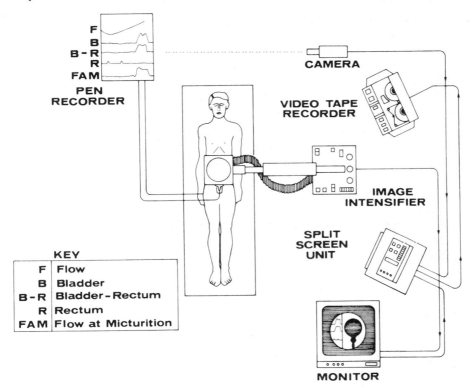

FIG. 1248.—Urodynamic study.

Urodynamic study (fig. 1248) has thrown a great deal of light on cases of urgency and incontinence. The principle is to record the pressure within the bladder during filling, and emptying, and at the same time to record the patient's subjective symptoms, and observe the activity of the bladder with an image intensifier. A catheter is passed along the urethra into the bladder together with a small fine pressure tube. A similar pressure tube is placed in the rectum to record intra-abdominal pressure. Via transducers the pressures in the bladder and abdomen are recorded as waves on heat sensitive paper. A third pen records true intravesical pressure by a subtraction performed electronically (see also Spinal Injuries and Urodynamic Testing).

TREATMENTS OF INCONTINENCE

These are exceedingly numerous, and are listed below:

Management of Incontinence.—The aim is to keep the patient dry, free of odour, to lessen the incidence of skin excoriation, and to protect the kidneys from the effects of infection and back pressure.

Appliances in women are usually unsatisfactory. An indwelling catheter drained constantly into a leg urinal is usually a satisfactory solution although in some instances diversion via an ileal conduit is necessary.

In men, a condom urinal or a Cunningham penile clamp (fig. 1246) may be satisfactory, and they avoid an indwelling catheter. Regular pyelographic checks to confirm the absence of retention and back pressure effects are essential.

Some of the conditions below may be amenable to specific surgical treatment. Thus a gracilis muscle sling may be attempted for epispadias (fig. 1247). This usually needs to be activated by an electrical stimulator for complete success.

In neurological disease it is usually necessary to divert the urine into an ileal loop if there is evidence of increasing dilation of the upper tract, particularly in the presence of recurrent infections. The bladder need not be removed but should be washed out after the operation and 1 g neomycin instilled. It should also be washed out two or three times in the post-operative period; after this it rarely produces any symptoms.

TREATMENTS AVAILABLE FOR FUNCTIONAL INCONTINENCE

1. **Drugs**
   - to increase to strength of bladder neck (= adrenergic agonists)
   - to decrease strength of bladder neck (= adrenergic blockers)
   - mixed action on bladder neck and CNS (= tricyclic drugs)

2. **Intermittent self-catheterisation**

3. **Devices for collection or control**
   - external penile condom
   - indwelling catheter
   - penile clamps (Cunningham device)

4. **Outlet surgery**
   - prostatectomy
   - bladder neck widening
   - sphincterotomy

5. **Denervation of bladder**
   - neurectomy procedures
   - transection of bladder neck

6. **Augmentation of bladder capacity**
   - ileo-cystoplasty
   - caeco cystoplasty

7. **Artificial sphincter**

8. **Urinary diversion** —— uretero-ileostomy

9. **Correction of bladder neck distortion**
   - raising bladder neck (Marshall Marchetti manoeuvre)
   - correction of cystocele (Manchester repair)
   - levatorplasty procedures

10. **Control of infection**

Uretero-ileostomy.—The collection of urine from an artificial bladder into an ileostomy bag especially if the ileostomy has been given a spout 2·5 cm long, is much more water-tight than a portable urinal worn over the genitalia. The incidence of pyelonephritis is so much less, that the substitution of an artificial for a normal non-functioning bladder is a change for the better, not only for the patient but for those with whom he or she lives (the uriniferous odour is reduced, sometimes to vanishing point). The operation is particularly successful in cases of incontinence due to spina bifida (Wells).

Everard Williams' operation for stress incontinence is simple, and gives as good results as more complicated procedures. A Foley's catheter having been introduced into the bladder, the bladder neck and adjoining portion of the urethra are exposed via the retropubic route. The lower part of the bladder and the intrapelvic portion of the urethra are mobilised, but there is no necessity to separate the urethra from the vagina. Three chromic catgut sutures are introduced on either side, each traversing the wall of the

Charles Alexander Wells, Contemporary. Professor Emeritus of Surgery, Liverpool, England.
Harry George Everard Williams, 1892–1970. Obstetrician and Gynaecologist, Charing Cross Hospital, London.

urethra or the bladder neck, being careful not to penetrate the mucous membrane. The sutures are then passed through the fascia covering the deep surface of the pubic bones near the symphysis. When the sutures are tied they suspend the bladder neck and the proximal part of the urethra.

Dribbling of Urine and Normal Micturition

This occurs when there is a ureteric fistula or an aberrant ureter opening into the urethra beyond the sphincters (in male), or into the vagina in females. The history is diagnostic, and intravenous pyelography may reveal the absent upper calyces on one side. These segments are very liable to infection. Treatment is by excision of the aberrant ureter and portion of kidney which feeds it.

Nocturnal Enuresis

Enuresis of lifelong origin often heralds some abnormality of the urinary tract. The majority of children suffering from this condition in fact usually have secondary enuresis (i.e. have previously been dry for a period of time). Usually in these children no organic lesion can be demonstrated and apart from excluding urinary infection more detailed examination of the urinary tract is probably not indicated. Discreet enquiry into the home and environmental circumstances will often reveal some factor behind the condition which is usually psychological in origin. For children the treatment consists of a 'star reward' system initially. If this fails a buzzer alarm often breaks the habit and one should only introduce the tricyclic drugs as a last resort. Enuresis is also seen in teenagers and young adults. Urodynamic testing will reveal unstable contractions in approximately half of this age group. Another contributing factor is that many of them appear to be very deep sleepers. The treatment consists of an attempt to quieten unstable contractions and to use drugs which might lighten the depth of sleep.

VESICAL CALCULUS

Definition.—*A primary vesical calculus* is one that develops in sterile urine; it often, but not necessarily, originates in a kidney and passes down the ureter to the bladder, where it enlarges.

A secondary vesical calculus occurs in the presence of infection.

A vesical calculus can occur also by the deposition of urinary salts upon a foreign body in the bladder.

Incidence.—Until the twentieth century vesical calculus was one of the most prevalent disorders among the poorer classes, and the incidence was especially high in childhood and adolescence. Owing to improved diet, especially an increased protein-carbohydrate ratio, primary vesical calculus is comparatively rarely encountered. The most remarkable fall in incidence is among children.

Composition and Cystoscopic Appearance.—Most vesical calculi are composite, but have one component in excess, and assume the appearance of that variety.

1. *Oxalate calculus* is a primary calculus that grows slowly. Usually it is of moderate size, and is solitary. Its surface is uneven (mulberry type); sometimes it bristles with spines (fig. 1249). Although calcium oxalate is white, the stone is usually dark brown or black because of the incorporation of blood pigment into it.

2. *Uric acid and urate calculi* are round or oval, fairly smooth, and vary in colour from pale yellow to light brown: they may be single or multiple. These stones also are primary: they are not opaque to x-rays.

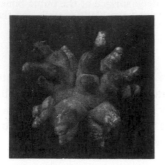

FIG. 1249.—'Jack-stone'[1] calculus. This type of vesical calculus is typically found in a post-prostatic pouch.

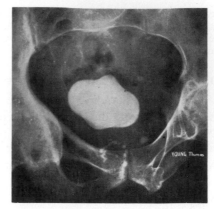

FIG. 1250.—Radiograph showing a vesical calculus.

3. *Cystine calculus* occurs only in the presence of cystinuria, and is radio-opaque due to its high sulphur content.

4. *Triple Phosphate calculus* is composed of ammonium, magnesium and calcium phosphates and occurs in urine infected with urea-splitting organisms. It tends to grow rapidly. In some instances it occurs on a nucleus of one of the foregoing types of calculus; much more rarely on a foreign body. In others the nucleus is composed of desquamated epithelium and bacteria. It is dirty white in colour, and of chalky consistency.

A vesical calculus is usually free to move in the bladder. It gravitates to the lowest part of the organ, which, when the patient is erect or sitting, is the bladder outlet. In the recumbent position (as also at cystoscopy) the stone occupies a position behind the interureteric ridge. Less commonly the stone is wholly or partially in a diverticulum or a post-prostatic pouch, and in either case the stone may be partially or completely hidden from view.

Clinical Features.—Males are eight times more often affected than females.

(*a*) *Latent.*—When a stone is situated in a post-prostatic pouch or a diverticulum of the bladder, it is usually discovered unexpectedly at cystoscopy or on x-ray examination.

(*b*) *Typical.*—*Frequency* is the earliest symptom. Unlike other forms of frequent micturition, it is not much in evidence during the night. After micturition the patient does not feel satisfied that the bladder is empty.

Pain is most in evidence in cases of spiculated oxalate calculus. It occurs at the end of micturition, and is usually referred to the tip of the penis or to the labia majora; more rarely to the perineum or suprapubic region. Pain and discomfort are much in evidence during exertion, and are aggravated by jolting movements (*e.g.* riding in a vehicle). If the patient lies down, the symptoms tend to pass off because the stone falls away from the sensitive portion of the bladder, the trigone. Thus he usually sleeps peacefully through the night. In young boys, screaming and pulling at the penis with the hand at the end of micturition are indicative of vesical calculus.

Haematuria is characterised by the passage of a few drops of bright red blood at the end of micturition, and is due to the stone abrading the vascular trigone—a fact that also accounts for the pain.

---

[1] 'Jack-stone' = the kernel of the fruit of the jack tree. These fruit stones are used for a game played by children in the U.S.A.

Interruption of the urinary stream by the stone blocking the internal meatus, occurs occasionally, and may be remedied by a change of posture.

Acute retention of urine from a vesical calculus is extremely uncommon in adults, but not so in children.

(c) *Masked.*—The symptoms of a concomitant persistent cystitis may over-shadow those that might be occasioned by the stone.

Rectal or vaginal examination, when accompanied by abdominal palpation, occasionally enables a vesical calculus to be felt. Unless the stone is large, rectal examination is negative in the adult male, but in a female or child a calculus of moderate size may be palpable.

Examination of the urine will reveal blood, and possibly pus or crystals typical of the calculus, *e.g.* envelope-like in the case of an oxalate stone, or hexagonal plates with cystine calculi.

Radiography.—In at least 92% of cases vesical calculus can be demonstrated on an x-ray film (fig. 1250). If the stone is not opaque, a filling defect may be visualised. Radiographs of the whole of the urinary tract should be taken, after which excretory pyelography is carried out; the former will reveal or disprove the presence of opaque renal or ureteric calculi, while the latter will help to determine the normality or otherwise of the kidneys.

Cystoscopy is essential for evaluation of the case. Frequently, on introducing the sheath of the cystoscope, a significant 'click' will be felt when a free-lying stone comes in contact with the instrument. As described already, cystoscopy usually reveals the composition of the calculus. Stones which are non-opaque to x-rays (*e.g.* uric acid) can be seen.

In all cases the whole of the bladder wall is inspected: in primary calculus, aseptic cystitis is basal; in secondary calculus, bacterial cystitis is universal. In appropriate cases the exit of the bladder is examined for prostatic enlargement or contracture of the bladder neck.

Treatment:

Litholapaxy.—In most cases crushing the stone with a lithotrite is highly satisfactory. However, the contraindications to the method are as follows:

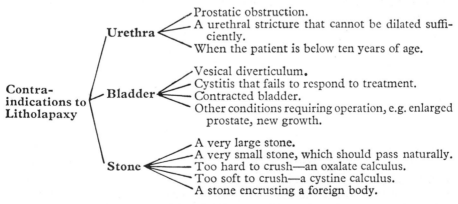

Contra-indications to Litholapaxy

Urethra
- Prostatic obstruction.
- A urethral stricture that cannot be dilated sufficiently.
- When the patient is below ten years of age.

Bladder
- Vesical diverticulum.
- Cystitis that fails to respond to treatment.
- Contracted bladder.
- Other conditions requiring operation, e.g. enlarged prostate, new growth.

Stone
- A very large stone.
- A very small stone, which should pass naturally.
- Too hard to crush—an oxalate calculus.
- Too soft to crush—a cystine calculus.
- A stone encrusting a foreign body.

Technique.—For several days before the operation a suitable drug is administered to reduce infection. While blind litholapaxy is preferred by those who have had much experience with the solid lithotrite, its only advantage is that, by reason of its solidity and greater strength, harder stones can be crushed than is the case with an instrument that contains a light and telescope incorporated in its shaft. A cystoscopic lithotrite (Canny Ryall, Riches) enables the stone, and such fragments as are necessary, to be seized under vision. The instrument, with its obturator in place, is introduced into the bladder, and rotated so that its closed jaws point downwards. The obturator is removed and the bladder is irrigated with water or glycine solution by means of two 200-ml syringes until the solution is returned clear. The bladder is then filled with not more than 300 ml of the solution, and after inserting the telescope, the stone is seen. The screw on the handle of the instrument is turned, and the jaws thereby opened. The distal blade is hooked over the centre of the stone and by rotating the screw handle the proximal movable blade is advanced so that the stone is grasped firmly. The ocular end of the lithotrite is depressed, thereby lifting the calculus away from the bladder wall. After withdrawing the telescope slightly, to prevent damage to the light bulb, the screw is turned slowly, breaking the stone. Large fragents are crushed into small ones by repeating the manoeuvre. With the jaws closed, the lithotrite is rotated so that the jaws point upwards, and after removing the telescope and allowing the solution to escape, the instrument is withdrawn.

Evacuation of the Fragments.—An evacuating cannula, the largest that the urethra will take, is passed, and 200 ml of solution are introduced into the bladder. The evacuator, filled with solution and with its tap closed, is fitted on to the cannula. The tap is opened and the bulb is elevated so as to depress the beak of the cannula towards the base of the bladder, after which the bulb is compressed slowly. The bulb is then permitted to expand, and the returning solution carries with it sand and fragments of the stone which, being heavier than the solution, drop into the glass receptacle. Alternate compression of the bulb and aspiration is continued until no further fragments fall. The beak of the cannula is turned to the left and to the right, and suction is applied in these situations. To save time in emptying and refilling two evacuators can be used. If at any time the bulb fails to expand, this may be due to blocking the eye by bladder mucosa, in which event release can be effected by further compression of the bulb and slight rotation of the instrument. Blockage of the cannula by fragments of the stone can sometimes be remedied in the same way, but more often they must be dislodged by detaching the evacuator and passing the obturator of the cannula. When no more fragments can be aspirated, the evacuator is detached and the bladder is irrigated until the fluid is returned clear. The cystoscopic lithotrite is reintroduced, and if no fragments remain, a Foley's catheter is passed. After the patient has been returned to bed the catheter is connected to a sterile bottle. Usually the catheter can be removed in twenty-four hours. As soon as it is assured that the patient is passing urine without difficulty, he can return home. Suitable drugs should be given until the urine is sterile.

Suprapubic Lithotomy.—The alternative to litholapaxy is removal of the stone through a suprapubic incision, after which the bladder is closed and drained by a urethral catheter.

Lithotomy in Special Circumstances.—A stone associated with an enlarged prostate can be removed in the course of a suprapubic or retropubic prostatectomy. When the stone is associated with contracture of the bladder neck, it can be removed in the course of an open operation for that condition.

A very small stone sometimes can be removed by means of an evacuator after passing the largest-sized cannula commensurate with the calibre of the urethra. For stones too large to pass through the cannula but small enough to pass through the urethra, removal by seizing the stone in the jaws of a cystoscopic rongeur is ideal.

FOREIGN BODIES IN THE BLADDER

A piece of catheter or bougie may become broken and remain in the bladder. The variety of foreign bodies which have been removed from the bladder is astonishing, *e.g.* manicure sticks, hair-clasps, hairpins and candle-grease. The presence of such objects in the bladder is usually accounted for by urethral masturbation, or attempts to produce a miscarriage. Occasionally a foreign body enters through the wall of the bladder, *e.g.* a piece of rubber tubing after cystostomy; unabsorbable sutures used in an extravesical pelvic operation. The diagnosis rests on cystoscopy, and in the case of radio-opaque foreign bodies on radiography.

Frère Jacques de Beaulieu, 1651–1714, was the most famous Journeyman Lithotomist; he mainly practised the perineal operation using a bread-knife.
Edward Canny Ryall, 1865–1934. Surgeon, All Saint's Hospital, London.

Complications of a Foreign Body in the Bladder:

1. Cystitis, which is the most common-complication.
2. Perforation of the bladder wall.
3. Vesical calculus.

Treatment.—A small foreign body can be removed per urethram by means of an operating cystoscope or Young's cystoscopic rongeur. When the foreign body is heavily encrusted, penetrating the bladder wall, or accompanied by severe cystitis, the suprapubic route should be chosen. Paraffin wax can be dissolved by the introduction of equal parts of xylol and water into the bladder for half an hour.

DIVERTICULUM OF THE BLADDER

Definition.—It is most important to distinguish a saccule from a diverticulum of the bladder. The normal intravesical pressure at the commencement of micturition is about 35 cm of water (25·7 mmHg or 3·4 kPa). Pressures as great as 100 cm (73·5 mmHg or 9·8 kPa) are reached by a hypertrophied (trabeculated) bladder (fig. 1279) endeavouring to force urine past an obstruction. This pressure causes the mucous lining between the inner layer of hypertrophied muscle bundles to protrude, so forming multiple saccules. If one or more, but usually one, saccule is forced through the whole thickness of the musculature of the bladder wall it becomes a diverticulum.

Aetiology

(*a*) **Congenital diverticulum** is rare. It may be situated in the middle line anteriosuperiorly, and represent the unobliterated vesical end of the urachus. It empties with the bladder, and is symptomless. Others in the usual situation on the base of the bladder can occur without obstruction and may require excision because of the risk of chronic infection or stone formation in a young adult.

(*b*) **Pulsion Diverticulum.**—The causative obstructive lesion, in order of frequency, is contracture of the bladder neck, benign enlargement of the prostate, fibrous prostate, urethral stricture and congenital valves of the posterior urethra.

Pathology.—Usually the mouth of the diverticulum is situated above and to the outer side of one ureteric orifice. Exceptionally, it is near the middle line behind the interureteric ridge. The size varies from 2–5 cm, but may be larger. It is lined by bladder mucosa and the wall is composed of fibrous tissue only (compare traction diverticulum). A diverticulum enlarges in a downward direction and sometimes may obstruct a ureter.

Complications

1. **Recurrent Cystitis.**—As the pouch cannot empty itself there remains a stagnant pool of urine within it. Once infected, the infection persists and continues to reinfect the bladder. In long-standing cases peridiverticulitis causes dense adhesions between the diverticulum and surrounding structures. Squamous cell metaplasia and leukoplakia occur in 15–20% of cases.

2. **Vesical calculus** due to stagnation and infection is present in 20% of cases, most often in the bladder, sometimes in the diverticulum as well, less often in the diverticulum only. On rare occasions a dumb-bell calculus fills the diverticulum and projects into the bladder.

3. **Hydronephrosis and hydroureter,** consequent upon compression of the lower end of the corresponding ureter, are liable to be followed by pyelonephritis and pyonephrosis.

4. **Neoplasm** arising in a diverticulum is an uncommon complication (7–8%). Unless

Hugh Hampton Young, 1870–1945. Director, James Buchanan Brady Urological Institute, Baltimore, Maryland, U.S.A.

the diagnosis is made at a very early stage, the prognosis is poor, because extra-vesical invasion through the thin wall of the sac occurs so readily.

Clinical Features.—An uninfected diverticulum of the bladder may cause no symptoms whatsoever. The patient is nearly always a male (95% of cases), usually over fifty years of age.

There are no pathognomonic symptoms of a vesical diverticulum; they are those of lower urinary tract obstruction, recurrent cystitis, and pyelonephritis. Haematuria (due to cystitis, vesical calculus, or, rarely, a neoplasm) is a leading symptom in one-third of cases. In a few cases micturition occurs twice in rapid succession (the second act may follow a change of posture), and when the first specimen is clear and the second cloudy, diverticulum of the bladder should be strongly suspected. In cases of chronic retention of urine, two swellings may be recognised rising out of the pelvis, one being the bladder and the other the diverticulum.

Cystoscopy is the usual means of discovering the diverticulum. Most often its orifice is seen as a clear-cut hole about the diameter of a lead pencil, the depths of which are black and unilluminated (fig. 1251). With inadequate distension of the bladder, sometimes the mouth of the diverticulum is seen closed, when the mucous membrane around the potential orifice is thrown into radiating pleats (fig. 1252); therefore, when searching for a diverticulum, it is important to have

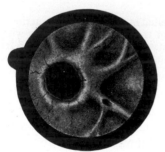

FIG. 1251.—Cystoscopic appearance of the orifice of a diverticulum and trabeculation of the bladder.

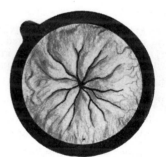

FIG. 1252.—Occasional appearance with inadequate distension of the bladder.

the bladder fully distended. In heavily infected cases much irrigation is necessary before a clear view of the bladder wall can be obtained. The differential diagnosis of a diverticulum from sacculation of a trabeculated bladder is not difficult, for the orifice of the saccule is relatively large, and the shallow interior can be seen. It is sometimes possible to pass an endoscope into a diverticulum and examine its interior.

Intravenous urography will not only exclude or reveal implication of the upper urinary tract, but in many instances the accompanying cystogram will give information regarding the size of the diverticulum.

Retrograde cystography is employed only when the former fails to show the pouch clearly. The bladder is emptied of urine, and filled with a non-irritating radio-opaque medium. Radiographs taken before and after micturition show the dimensions and position of the diverticulum clearly.

Ultrasonography (fig. 1253).—This can sometimes be helpful in making the diagnosis when other methods are either unhelpful and must be avoided (*e.g.* patient is not fit for cystoscopy or is sensitive to contrast media).

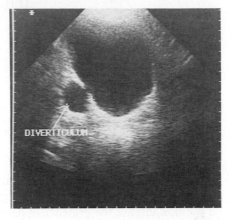

FIG. 1253.—Bladder diverticulum demonstrated by ultrasound.

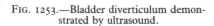

Indications for Operation.—A vesical diverticulum gradually increases in size, and once infected the infection cannot be permanently eradicated. Therefore, unless the pouch is small and uninfected, it should be removed, usually when the associated lower urinary tract obstructive lesion is treated.

Pre-operative Treatment.—When the urine is infected, suitable pre-operative antibiotic treatment is given. In the presence of gross sepsis and retention of urine, it is necessary to resort to an indwelling urethral catheter, and to give bladder washes.

Combined intravesical and extravesical diverticulectomy is the operation that is practised most frequently. Cystoscopy is performed, and a large ureteric catheter is passed up the ureter on the affected side, and left in place, 240 ml of solution remaining in the bladder. With the patient in the Trendelenburg position, the anterior bladder wall is exposed through a suprapubic incision. The peritoneum is dissected upwards, and that side of the bladder bearing the diverticulum is cleared from surrounding structures with the fingers until some part of the pouch is brought into view. The bladder is then incised in the middle line near its dome, and emptied by suction. The interior of the diverticulum is packed with a strip of gauze, and with the fingers of one hand in the bladder and the rectus muscles retracted widely, the diverticulum is freed from surrounding structures by gauze and sharp dissection. Usually the neck of the diverticulum can be separated from the ureter, and when the pouch is free it is severed from its attachment to the bladder with a diathermy knife. The resulting defect is closed in two layers. The cystostomy incision is sutured around a Malécot catheter, and the abdominal wall is closed, leaving a drainage tube in the extravesical space which housed the sac.

An alternative method, if the sac is densely adherent, is to carry the incision in the bladder down to the rim of the diverticular orifice, then to detach the diverticulum, together with its fibrous rim. The incision in the bladder is closed and the diverticulum left in position with a corrugated drain into it for two to three days. The track fibroses rapidly after removal of the drain.

If outlet obstruction is part of the picture, *e.g.* by an enlarged prostate, a prostatectomy should be done at the same time as the diverticulectomy.

TRACTION DIVERTICULUM OF THE BLADDER (*syn*, HERNIA OF THE BLADDER)

A portion of the bladder protruding through the inguinal or femoral hernial orifice occurs in 1·5% of such herniae treated by operation (Sir Cecil Wakeley). The condition

Sir Cecil Pembrey Grey Wakeley, 1892–1980. Surgeon, King's College Hospital, London.

is relatively frequent in femoral and direct inguinal herniae. The disposition of the diverticulum in the hernia varies, and in order of frequency is:

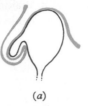 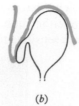 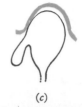

(*a*)   (*b*)   (*c*)

FIG. 1254.—(*a*) Intraperitoneal   (*b*) paraperitoneal   (*c*) extraperitoneal hernia of the bladder.

Clinical Features.—In a few cases, in order to empty the bladder completely, the patient finds it necessary to exert pressure on the hernia. Suspicion of a bladder hernia can be confirmed by cystoscopy or cystography.

URINARY FISTULAS

A urinary fistula is an abnormal communication between any part of the urinary system and the skin or some internal hollow viscus. The persistence of a fistula on the skin implies the presence of distal obstruction or the presence of chronic infection such as tuberculosis or a foreign body, *e.g.* stone, or non-absorbable ligature.

Congenital Urinary Fistula.—(1) *Ectopia vesicae.* (2) *From patent urachus.*—If present at birth or commencing soon after, the possibility of obstruction at the bladder neck or urethra must be investigated. In later life infection in a urachal cyst may produce a fistula. Carcinoma in such instances is not uncommon. Treatment in each case is excision of the urachal tract and closure of the bladder once distal obstruction has been dealt with or excluded.

(3) *In association with imperforate anus* (Chapter 54).

Traumatic Urinary Fistula.—Perforating or penetrating wounds, damage not recognised during surgery, or poor healing and avascular necrosis following a combination of radiotherapy and surgery may lead to leakage of urine from ureter or bladder through the wound. Also a clot retention occurring after a transvesical prostatectomy or diverticulectomy may lead to dehiscence of the bladder wound and a temporary fistula, which will heal quickly, provided the bladder is kept empty with an indwelling catheter.

Vesico-vaginal fistula 'is the greatest misfortune that can happen to a woman, the more so because she is condemned to live with it, and cannot hope to die from it' (Dieffenbach).

Aetiology:1. *Obstetrical Causes.*—From time immemorial the usual cause has been protracted or neglected labour.

2. *Gynaecological Causes.*—The operations chiefly concerned with this complication are total hysterectomy and anterior colporrhaphy.

3. *Radiotherapeutic Causes.*—First and foremost is the radium treatment of carcinoma of the cervix uteri; to a lesser extent irradiation of the pelvic viscera for other reasons is responsible.

4. *Direct Neoplastic Infiltration.*—Exceptionally carcinoma of the cervix uteri ulcerates through the anterior fornix to implicate the bladder.

Johann Friedrich Dieffenbach, 1792–1847. Director of the Surgical Division of the Charité Krankenhaus, Berlin.
James Marion Sims, 1813–1883, while a country Practitioner at Montgomery, Alabama, was the first to succeed in closing a vesico-vaginal fistula.

When a wound of the bladder is recognised and repaired at once, leakage is uncommon, but escape of urine will quickly follow if such damage passes unnoticed. However, most vesico-vaginal fistulas are the result of ischaemic necrosis of the bladder wall due to prolonged pressure of the fetal head in obstetric cases. In gynaecological cases the ischaemia is brought about by grasping the bladder wall in a haemostat, including the bladder wall in a suture, or perhaps even by local oedema or haematoma. Leakage due to necrosis of tissue seldom manifests itself before seven days after the operation.

An intractable fistula following radium treatment of carcinoma of the cervix uteri may arise from avascular necrosis years after the apparent cure of the original lesion.

Clinical Features.—There is leakage of urine from the vagina, and, as a consequence, excoriation of the vulva. Digital examination of the vagina reveals a localised thickening on its anterior wall or in the vault in the case of post-hysterectomy fistula. On inserting a vaginal speculum, urine will be seen escaping from an opening in the anterior vaginal wall. It is usually possible to pass a bent probe from the vagina into the bladder. Cystoscopy is often difficult, owing to the contraction of the bladder from cystitis and the escape of urine from the fistula; however, usually the tip of the probe that has been passed can be seen emerging through an area of granulation tissue.

Differential Diagnosis between a Uretero-vaginal and Vesico-vaginal Fistula.—If a swab is placed in the vagina and a solution of methylene blue is injected through the urethra, the vaginal swab becomes coloured blue. In the case of a uretero-vaginal fistula the vaginal swab is not so coloured. With the advent of good portable x-ray image intensifiers, a cystoscopy and bilateral retrograde ureterograms provide more reliable demonstration of the anatomy. Uretero-vaginal fistula is discussed in Chapter 57.

Treatment.—Just occasionally conservative management of a vesico-vaginal fistula following hysterectomy by urethral bladder drainage is successful. Usually operative treatment is required and the traditional teaching has been to delay surgery for some months. This has recently been questioned. The low fistula is best repaired per vaginam. The fistula is exposed with dissection of the edges which are freshened. The bladder is then closed using absorbable sutures and the vagina subsequently closed with a separate layer. A urethral catheter should be left in situ for at least ten days. For the higher fistula a transvaginal approach can be extremely difficult. These patients should always be cystoscoped prior to any repair procedure and bilateral ureterograms performed as occasionally one of the ureters is also injured. For the high fistula the Pfannensteil incision should be reopened. The bladder should be dissected free from the peritoneum and bisected posteriorly in the midline down to the level of the fistula. The bladder is then separated from the vagina and occasionally careful dissection from the rectum is also required. The vagina is then closed with a heavy catgut suture and omentum brought down to lie between the closed vagina and the bladder anteriorly. This is lightly sutured in place and the bladder then closed. A urethral and suprapubic catheter should be left in situ for 10–14 days.

For the patient with a uretero-vaginal fistula an extraperitoneal approach to the ureter via the previous Pfannensteil incision is made. Considerable adhesions will be encountered but the ureter can usually be found above the level of the injury and followed down. Fibrosed or strictured ureter should be discarded and then reimplantation into the bladder is required. Depending on the amount of ureter lost it may be possible to achieve a simple reimplantation with a Psoas hitch procedure. If the gap is too large to be bridged by this manoevre a Boari flap of anterior bladder wall should be cut and brought over to meet the ureter and a reimplant performed. The most important principle of ureteric reimplantation is that there should be no tension on the anastomosis. Results from these repairs need to be 100%, for a failure will only cause despair and further enrage the already litiginous patient.

Fistula from Renal Pelvis to Skin or Gut.—Tuberculosis of a kidney may result in destruction of the kidney by caseation, and a chronic sinus leading to duodenum or colon and/or the skin, usually in the iliac fossa, or in the lumbar triangle of Petit. Similarly pyonephrosis and stone may spontaneously discharge into the gut or by a fistula to the skin. Cases of duodenal ulcer involving the pelvis of the right kidney are also on record.

Fistulas Arising as a Result of Infection.—The commonest cause is diverticulitis of the colon. It may also follow Crohn's disease, appendix abscess, or pelvic sepsis in association with acute salpingitis, or as a result of surgery and radiotherapy within the pelvis.

The onset may not be dramatic and may well be treated as acute cystitis. The diagnosis can be difficult to make because the acute signs subside, but on cystoscopy a patch of oedema on the left side of the vault is suggestive and bubbles of gas may be seen (fig. 1255). A cystogram may reveal the fistula. However, as the track is not always patent a

Burrill Bernard Crohn, Contemporary. Gastro-enterologist, Mount Sinai Hospital, New York, U.S.A.

negative result may be obtained. If this is so, a water-soluble contrast study of the large bowel may not only demonstrate the fistula but also define the cause. The passage of gas per urethram in a patient who has cystitis is most suggestive (providing diabetes is excluded).

Treatment.—In some cases, a defunctioning colostomy is made above the fistula as the first step. Inflammation is allowed to subside over two to three months. At laparotomy the communication is separated, the hole in the bladder being closed and patched with omentum, and the segment of diseased bowel resected. The bladder is drained by a urethral catheter. The colostomy is closed about 3 weeks later provided a barium enema reveals no leaks.

Cases due to Carcinoma.—By the time a fistula between the bowel and the bladder has developed, as a rule the growth is inoperable or requires pelvic evisceration for its attempted eradication. As so often these patients are unfitted for this major procedure, it is best to leave the patient with the defunctioning colostomy performed in the first instance. Exceptions do occur, and occasionally it is warranted to undertake segmental resection of the colon and a partial or complete cystectomy.

Urethral Fistulas occur as the result of infection above a stricture producing a per-urethral abscess which rupturing into the urethra allows extravasation to occur suddenly into the scrotum and perineum. Urine and infection extend into the upper 2·5 cm of thigh and lower abdominal wall. Widespread cellulitis and tissue necrosis will occur unless diversion of urine is achieved by suprapubic cystotomy, and the tissue planes are freely drained by inguinal and scrotal incisions.

Neoplastic Fistulas.—Primary bladder tumours may fungate through the abdominal wall when neglected. Only palliative treatment is possible in most of such cases. Involvement of the bladder by growths of cervix, uterus and colon and rectum do produce fistulas, as may lymphosarcoma of small gut. Carcinoma of the prostate rarely produces a rectal fistula. Treatment in most such cases is difficult and prolonged and in most only palliative relief can be given. It is rarely in the patient's interest to divert the ureters.

CYSTITIS

Until after middle age, cystitis is very much commoner in women than in men. Cystitis occurs in some healthy women after intercourse, without any demonstrable abnormality of the urinary tract. Repeated attacks of cystitis in women, or a single attack in a man or a child of either sex, should always be followed by investigation to discover and treat the predisposing cause; sometimes, however, no cause can be found.

Predisposing causes

1. Incomplete emptying of the bladder such as in prostatic obstruction, urethral stricture, stenosis of the external urinary meatus, diverticulum of the bladder, pregnancy or puerperium, also injuries or diseases of the spinal cord.

2. The presence in the bladder of a calculus, foreign body or neoplasm. Cystitis is sometimes associated with vesico-ureteral reflux causing attacks of pyelonephritis. It is especially important to detect and treat this in childhood and so prevent serious permanent damage to the kidney.

3. Lowered general resistance from intercurrent disease and avitaminosis.

Avenues of Infection

Ascending infection from the urethra is much the commonest (see Chapter 60). The organisms, especially *E. coli*, originate in the bowel, contaminate the vulva and reach the bladder because of the shortness of the female urethra. The passage of urethral instruments may cause cystitis in either sex, especially when the bladder contains residual urine. This may happen even when the instrument is sterile because it carries organisms from the urethra into the bladder (fig. 1244).

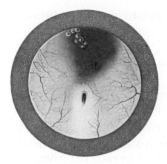

FIG. 1255.—Cystoscopic view of a vesico-intestinal fistula. Bubbles of gas can be seen issuing from the orifice of the fistula.

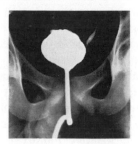

FIG. 1256.—Retrograde cystograph showing exceedingly contracted ('thimble') bladder in a case of tuberculous cystitis.

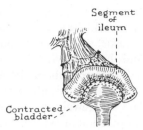

FIG. 1257.—Ileocystoplasty using a 6-inch segment of ileum.
(After D. O. Ferris.)

Other routes *e.g. descending* from the kidney, *haematogenous, lymphogenous,* and from *adjoining structures* (Fallopian tube, vagina, or intestine, especially fistulas) are less common.

Bacteriology.—*E. coli* is the commonest organism, followed by *Proteus mirabilis* and (in young women), *Staphylococcus saprophyticus* (formerly called 'Micrococcus'). Other organisms, sometimes mixed, and found especially in cystitis complicating underlying lesions of the urinary tract, include Pseudomonas, klebsiellae, *Staph. aureus, Staph. albus* and various streptococci. Tuberculous cystitis is considered under 'special forms of cystitis'.

The presence of pus cells without organism calls for repeated examination for *M. tuberculosis* and the gonococcus (very rare cause of cystitis). Having eliminated these possibilities, the condition may be abacterial cystitis, or a bladder tumour.

Clinical Features.—The severity of the symptoms varies greatly; those of acute cystitis are usually the more distressing.

Frequency is the outstanding symptom, both during the day and at night. The desire to urinate occurs from every hour to every few minutes, and often it is so urgent that if the bladder cannot be emptied forthwith, incontinence results. In severe cases, because of infection and loss of sleep, the patient looks drawn and haggard.

Pain varies from mild to agonising.[1] When the inflammation is situated in the dome of the bladder, pain is referred to the suprapubic region, while when, as is often the case, the inflammation involves the trigone, pain is referred to the tip of the penis, the labia majora, and the perineum.

Haematuria.—The passage of a few drops of blood-stained urine or blood-stained debris at the end of micturition is a frequent accompaniment. Less often the whole specimen is blood-stained, but more so at the end.

Pyuria is always present, except in some cases of trigonitis and interstitial cystitis (p. 1281). If urine is passed into two glasses, the second is the more cloudy.

On examination there is tenderness over the bladder suprapubically, per rectum, or per vaginam.

---

[1] An Irish surgeon, long since dead, always finished his evening prayers—'Please God, when you take me, may it not be through the bladder'.

Initial and midstream urine specimens should be collected in a male as prostatitis may be present, in which case threads will be seen clearly in the initial specimen. In a female, and when the initial urine in the male does not contain threads, a midstream specimen must be subjected to microscopy and culture, and the sensitivity of any organisms assessed.

Treatment should be commenced forthwith, and modified if necessary when the bacteriological report is to hand. The patient is urged to drink plentifully, and while awaiting sensitivity results, one should prescribe either a sulphonamide preparation or amoxycillin (250 mg t.d.s.) together with Mist. pot. cit et hyocyamus 10 ml t.d.s. as a bladder sedative. Failure to respond, or early recurrence of infection, indicates the necessity for further investigation to exclude predisposing factors.

Cystoscopy to confirm the diagnosis may be performed in women during the acute phase. The benefits of doing this are few and the procedure will cause considerable discomfort. The appearances may vary from hyperaemia, sometimes with mucosal haemorrhages, to severe sloughing and ulceration of the mucosa. In men, cystoscopy to exclude predisposing causes should be delayed until the infection has been controlled.

SPECIAL FORMS OF CYSTITIS

Acute Abacterial Cystitis (*syn.* Acute Haemorrhagic Cystitis).—The patient, a young man or woman, presents with symptoms of severe cystitis. Pus is present in the urine, but no organism can be cultured therefrom. The condition, which sometimes is associated with abacterial urethritis, commonly follows recent venereal exposure. While tuberculous cystitis always must be ruled out by cultural or biological tests, the fact that excretory pyelography shows normal excretion on both sides strongly favours acute abacterial cystitis. In 60% of cases, by special cultural methods the pleuro-pneumonia-like organism, which frequently accompanies acute abacterial urethritis, is found.

Although this is a self-limiting disease its course can be shortened by the antibiotic therapy recommended for abacterial urethritis. When cystoscopy is performed after the acute symptoms have abated, abundant mucosal haemorrhages are seen, and presumably at its height the infection causes a haemorrhagic cystitis.

Urethro-trigonitis is a common form of recurrent lower urinary tract infection in women. Cystoscopy shows increased vascularity of the trigone, oedema of its mucous membrane (most marked towards the apex) and, in severe cases, there is a pseudo-membrane limited to the trigone. Inflammatory polypi may be present at the bladder neck. Later the urethra becomes narrowed. A cystocele is frequently present.

A primary focus of infection must be sought; the most common being (*a*) the cervix uteri (chronic cervicitis or a cervical erosion) or (*b*) the intestinal tract, notably chronic diverticulitis. No examination is complete without examining the cervix with a speculum, and if the cervix is healthy a barium enema is necessary for evidence of diverticulitis.

Treatment.—In addition to the usual measures, namely treatment of the acute infection, a prolonged course of a low dose antibiotic (e.g. trimethoprim) may be indicated. Benefit may be achieved by dilating the urethra. Cervicitis or a cervical erosion is treated by excising the glandular tissue of the cervix with a diathermy loop. Diverticulitis is discussed in Chapter 50.

Tuberculous cystitis is always secondary to renal tuberculosis, and unless treated early is a particularly relentless form of chronic cystitis.

Cystoscopy shows that early tuberculosis of the bladder commences around one ureteric orifice or in the neighbourhood of the trigone, the earliest evidence being pallor of the mucosa, due to submucous oedema. Subsequently tubercles may be seen, and in long-standing cases there is much fibrosis, and the capacity of the bladder is so much reduced that it has earned the name of 'thimble' bladder. This feature can be well shown by cystography (fig. 1256).

Treatment.—Tuberculous cystitis usually responds rapidly to antituberculous drugs (Chapter 4), but occasionally, in cases with advanced renal changes, may not subside until the involved kidney and ureter have been removed. Local treatment of persistent tuberculous cystitis consists of instillations of a substance inimical to *M. tuberculosis*. Among the best is B53,[1] a soap derived from a branched fatty acid, having a high inhibitory index for the *M. tuberculosis*. A correctly buffered 0·5% solution containing local anaesthetic is instilled and retained for one hour daily. A fortnight's course can be repeated after an interval of a week.

When the bladder is considerably contracted, but free from ulceration, remarkable relief from the distressing frequency can be achieved by ileocystoplasty (fig. 1257), which is an extremely efficacious method of increasing the capacity of a contracted bladder. When, in addition, tuberculous contracture threatens to implicate the remaining kidney by back pressure, as shown by dilatation of the ureter on excretory pyelography, the ureter is implanted into the newly constructed pouch of intestine with every hope of conserving renal function as well as rendering the patient symptom-free.

Ileocystoplasty.—After pre-operative preparation of the intestines (Chapter 50) a 15-cm segment of ileum with an ample blood supply as demonstrated by transillumination is disconnected, leaving its mesentery intact, and the continuity of the intestine is restored by anastomosis. After closing the ends of the donor segment and opening it longitudinally it is anastomosed to the dome of the contracted bladder (fig. 1257).

Interstitial Cystitis (*syn.* **Hunner's Ulcer**; Elusive Ulcer).—For practical purposes Hunner's ulcer can be said to be a condition peculiar to women. The symptoms commence in the early forties. It can cause more pain, mental anguish and associated neurosis than does carcinoma of the bladder; as a consequence, the incessant painful micturition it occasions sometimes leads to drug addiction and even suicide.

Aetiology is still as obscure as it was when Guy Hunner first described the condition in 1914. Certainly it does not commence as an ordinary pyogenic infection of the mucous membrane, but rather as an infection of the paravesical tissues secondary, it is suggested, to infection of the adnexae, or even to infection from a more distant focus such as the nasopharynx. Some believe the condition is due to an attenuated *M. tuberculosis* which so far has defied isolation. In a number of instances the symptoms have commenced three or four months after a pelvic operation.

Pathology.—As a result of the paracystitis, fibrosis of the vesical musculature ensues, leading to contracture of the bladder and areas of avascular atrophy of the mucous membrane. Finally, ulceration of the mucosa occurs in the least vascular portion of the bladder, namely the fundus. Often the capacity of the bladder is reduced to 30 to 60 ml. The characteristic linear bleeding ulcer is a crack due to splitting of the mucous membrane when the bladder is distended under anaesthesia for cystoscopy.

Microscopically, inflammation of all coats of the bladder is present with granulation tissue in the submucosa underlying the ulcer. The muscularis is hypertrophied and the peritoneum in proximity to the area of maximum disease is thickened.

Clinical Features.—Bladder capacity becoming much reduced, increased frequency, eventually every hour both day and night, is the leading symptom. Pain, relieved by micturition and aggravated by jarring and overdistension of the bladder is the second and most characteristic symptom. In early cases the urine is crystal clear and sterile; in later cases it contains ordinary pyogenic bacteria in under half the specimens examined; in the remainder the urine remains sterile. In 60% of cases haematuria is a leading symptom.

Cystoscopy.—The lesion appears in the roof of the bladder as a star-shaped area of intense congestion in which a fissure can be seen when the bladder is distended. The ulcer, if ulcer it can be called, bleeds readily. This is seen characteristically as the bladder is decompressed.

---

[1] B53 (Hinconstarch) is produced in the laboratories of the Irish Medical Research Council.

Guy Leroy Hunner, 1868–1951. Gynaecological Surgeon, Johns Hopkins University, Baltimore, U.S.A.

Treatment is difficult and unsatisfactory. Local hydrocortisone and irrigation of the bladder with various sedatives rarely prove valuable. Hydrostatic dilatation under anaesthesia may give relief for some months. Light diathermy fulguration of the ulcer may help. Recently considerable relief of both suprapubic pain, and urinary frequency have been achieved with the intravesical instillation of dimethylsulphoxide (Rimso 50). Complete relief may be obtained by urinary diversion, while ileo-cystoplasty after excision of the affected bladder wall, though frequently very satisfactory, is not always permanently successful in relieving all symptoms.

Alkaline encrusting cystitis is due to urea-splitting organisms causing phosphatic encrustations on the bladder mucosa of elderly women. There are symptoms of chronic cystitis and a plain x-ray shows the bladder outline. The encrustations may be curetted and removed via a cystoscope or a suprapubic cystotomy, or controlled by tidal lavage using a dissolvent solution such as 0·5% acetic acid.

Cystitis Cystica.—Glands are not found in the normal vesical mucosa. Under the influence of chronic inflammation, the surface epithelium sends down buds, resulting in minute cysts filled with clear fluid, most abundant on the trigone. Most of the cases are seen in women, and the urine usually contains pus, and commonly *E. coli*. An adenocarcinoma may originate in one of these cysts.

BILHARZIASIS OF THE BLADDER

Geographical Distribution.—The disease is endemic in the greater part of Africa, throughout Israël, Syria, Arabia, Iran and Iraq. It is met with frequently in Portugal and in Greece, and in the islands of Madagascar, Mauritius and Cyprus. Dwellers along the valley of the Nile[1] have suffered from time immemorial. The condition also occurs along the shores of some of China's great lakes. Marshes or slow-running fresh water provide a favourable habitat for the particular freshwater snail (*Bullinus contortus*), which is the intermediate host.

Mode of Infestation.—The disease is acquired while bathing or standing in infected water. The free-swimming bifid-tailed embryos (cercariae) of the trematode *Schistosoma haematobium* penetrate the skin by their motile and erosive secretory powers. Shedding their tails, which enabled them to swim, they enter blood-vessels and are swept by the blood-stream into all parts of the body. All perish save those that are carried to the liver. Once within the liver the survivors flourish by sustaining themselves on erythrocytes, and they develop into male and female worms. The female is long, smooth and slender and is furnished with two weak suckers anteriorly. The male is broader, shorter (11 mm in length), bosselated and provided with a strong sucker at either end. Sexual maturity having been attained, the nematodes leave the hepatic nursery and enter the portal vein. Here the male bends into the shape of a canoe and in so doing a gutter (the gynaecophoric canal) is formed along its length. Into the groove a female nestles and, thus conjugating, the pair paddle their way against the stream towards the inferior mesenteric vein. The long journey is accomplished in short stages, the male's suckers serving as anchors to the vein wall during periods of rest. *Schistosoma haematobium* worms have an affinity for the vesical venous plexus, and to reach it they must pass along the portal-systemic anastomotic channels, the most important in this respect being the venules in relation to the lumbar lymph nodes (Makar); other communications being venules in relation to the lower part of the ureters.

Having reached one of the smaller radicles of the vesical plexus the pair can go no further coupled, so the female, now pregnant but still comparatively slender, parts from the male and moves forward until she enters a submucous venule so small that she completely blocks it. She now proceeds to lay about twenty ova in a chain, and after each is deposited, by slightly withdrawing herself, the venule contracts upon the ovum. Each ovum is provided with a terminal spine which penetrates the vessel wall. Aided by muscular contraction of the bladder, and perhaps by secreting lytic fluid, some of the ova reach the lumen of the bladder; others die incarcerated in the mucous membrane. A heavily infected subject passes many hundreds of ova a day. If the ova reach fresh water, the low osmotic pressure of the new environment causes their envelope to burst, and thus emerges the miracidium, which is ciliated. To survive, the miracidium must reach and penetrate the intermediate host within thirty-six hours. Within the snail's liver the miracidium

---

[1] Napoleon's troops who served in his march to the Pyramids suffered from haematuria.

Theodor Maximilian Bilharz, 1825–1862. Professor of Zoology, Cairo.
Naguib Makar, Contemporary. Emeritus Professor of Urology, Cairo University, Cairo, Egypt.

enlarges and gives rise to myriads of daughter cysts, broods of which are set free on the death of the snail. A single miracidium begets thousands of cercariae to complete the life-cycle.

Clinical Features.—After penetration of the skin there may arise urticaria, which lasts for about five days and sometimes recurs (swimmer's itch). After an incubation period ranging from four to twelve weeks, high evening temperature, sweating, and asthma, together with leucocytosis and eosinophilia of over 10%, sometimes last several weeks. Usually an asymptomatic period of several months supervenes before the ova laid in the bladder wall find egress and cause the typical early sign and symptom of intermittent, painless, terminal haematuria. Men are three times more often affected than women. Native patients of the peasant class rarely consult a doctor for this haematuria *per se*, so that many late cases are encountered.

Examination of the urine.—The last few millitres of an early-morning specimen of urine are collected and centrifuged. It is essential that all receptacles be absolutely dry. The ovum is recognised without staining under the low-powered microscope. Examination on several consecutive days may be required. Even so, a negative result does not exclude bilharziasis, especially in patients no longer resident in bilharzial districts.

Cystoscopy.—Dependent on the length of time the disease has remained untreated, cystoscopy will reveal one or more of the following:

1. *Bilharzial pseudo-tubercles* are the earliest specific appearance. The pseudo-tubercles are larger, more prominent, more numerous, more yellow and more distinctly grouped (fig. 1258) than those of tuberculosis.

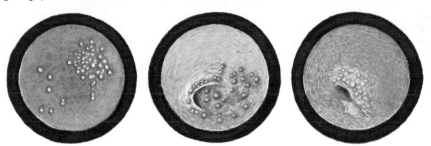

FIGS. 1258.—Bilharzial tubercles; 1259 Bilharzial nodules; 1260 'Sandy patches'.
(After N. Makar.)

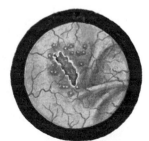

FIG. 1261.—Bilharzial ulcer.
(After N. Makar.)

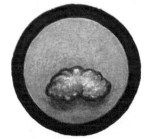

FIG. 1262.—Bilharzial papilloma.
(After N. Makar.)

2. *Bilharzial nodules* (fig. 1259) are due to the fusion of tubercles in the presence of secondary infection. They are larger and greyer than the foregoing.

3. *'Sandy patches'* are the result of calcified dead ova with degeneration of the overlying epithelium. They occur in the first instance around one or both ureteric orifices (fig. 1260). Considerable calcification of this nature is visible on the radiograph.

4. *Ulceration* is the result of sloughing of mucous membrane containing dead ova, or what is even more common, sloughing of a bilharzial papilloma. The ulcer is shallow (fig. 1261), bleeds readily, and its common position is the posterior wall of the bladder.

5. *Fibrosis* is mainly the result of secondary infection. The capacity of the bladder

becomes much reduced. Contracture of the bladder neck is also a common result of bilharzial fibrosis.

6. *Granulomas.*—Bilharzial masses are due to an aggregation of nodules. They are sessile, soft and bleed readily when touched.

7. *Papillomas* are distinguished from the foregoing by being more pedunculated (fig. 1262). They vary in size from that of a pea to that of a walnut, and they may be single or multiple.

8. *Carcinoma* is a common end-result in grossly infected bilharziasis of the bladder which has been neglected for years. It usually commences, not in a papilloma, but in an ulcer, and is therefore a squamous-celled carcinoma.

Treatment[1].—Lesions 1 to 6 inclusive can be expected to heal under general treatment by antimony and other preparations (*e.g.* praziquantel and metrifonate). It takes many months for dead ova to be expelled, and even after repeated courses and healing of the bladder lesion, living bilharzial worms have been found at necropsy in the portal system. In addition to general treatment, healing of bilharzial ulcers and granulomas is expedited by light diathermy coagulation. Bilharzial papillomas and, of course, carcinoma do not respond to general treatment: these lesions require the same surgical measures as non-bilharzial papillomas and carcinomas, in addition to general treatment.

Other Complications and their Treatment:

(*a*) *Secondary bacterial cystitis is commonly present in cases of long standing and the treatment of it must be thorough and prolonged.*

(*b*) *Urinary calculi*, especially vesical and ureteric, occur more frequently when bilharzial lesions of the bladder are present. Litholapaxy is contraindicated in cases where there is ulceration of the bladder wall.

(*c*) *Stricture of the ureters* affects the last inch of the ureters. These strictures often respond to dilatation, but sometimes transplantation of the affected ureter into another part of the bladder is necessary.

(*d*) *Prostato-seminal vesiculitis*, like tuberculosis of these structures, is made worse by prostatic massage, and general treatment alone must be employed.

(*e*) *Contracture of the bladder, and contracture of the bladder neck* (fig. 1263), must be treated in the same way as similar contractures of non-bilharzial origin.

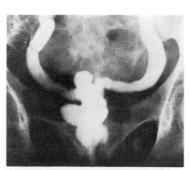

FIG. 1263.—Bilharzial contracture of the bladder, with ureteric reflux.
(*H. Talib, FRCS, Baghdad.*)

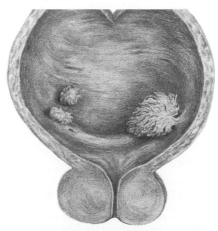

FIG. 1264.—Papillary tumour with daughter implantations ('kiss' cancer).

---

[1] John Brian Christopherson, 1868–1955. Introduced the treatment of bilharziasis by the intravenous injection of tartar emetic in 1918 whilst he was Director of Civil Hospitals at Khartoum and Omdurman, Sudan.

(f) *Bilharzial urethral strictures* are often accompanied by fistulas, and can be cured only by excision of the fistulous tracks and urethroplasty.

NEOPLASMS OF THE BLADDER

More than 95% of primary tumours of the bladder originate in its mucous membrane; the remainder are connective-tissue growths—angioma (the least uncommon), myoma, fibroma, and sarcoma. These are too rare to merit further description, as also is a phaeochromocytoma arising in the bladder wall from accessory adrenal tissue.

Another uncommon benign bladder tumour is an **endometrioma**, characterised by a localised, smooth, vascular projection on the bladder wall, sometimes containing chocolate-coloured cysts; and at other times translucent cysts of a bluish hue. The tumour enlarges and bleeds during menstruation. Treatment is partial cystectomy.

Secondary involvement of the bladder can occur from extension of a malignant neoplasm of a neighbouring organ, particularly the large intestine (sigmoid and rectum), the uterus or an ovary.

On rare occasions the first symptoms of a carcinoma of the pelvic colon are those of cystitis. Cytoscopy reveals a circumscribed area of intense inflammation, usually on the left side of the fundus. If the diagnosis is not made and treatment carried out at this stage, a vesico-intestinal fistula results.

Aetiology.—The first suspicion of a chemical cause for bladder tumours was raised by Rehn in 1894 when he recorded a series of tumours in workers in aniline dye factories. Subsequent investigation has exonerated aniline itself—It was the impurity of beta-naphthylamine. It is now recognised that benzidine, alpha-naphthylamine, xylenamine, dichlorbenzidine, auramine and magenta are all carcinogenic. The particular industries involved are the dyeing industry, gas workers, the rubber and cable industries and the printing industry. More recently also found to be at risk are sewage workers and rodent exterminators. People working in the leather industry with textiles and hairdressers are also now recognised to have a higher incidence of bladder cancer[1]. Bladder cancer became a prescribed industrial disease (No. 39) in 1953. Tumours occurring in workers in these industries are accepted for compensation. Epidemiological studies over the last few years have quite clearly indicated the association between cigarette smoking and bladder cancer. In areas where *Schistosoma haematobium* is endemic (particularly Arabia and North East Africa) bladder cancer is more common, and this tends to be squamous in type[2].

Phenacetin, cyclophosphamide, saccharin and excessive caffeine intake have all been implicated in the aetiology. Balkan nephropathy has been clearly associated with an increased incidence of upper track urothelial tumours.

Pathology

Benign Papillary Tumours.—A papilloma of the bladder commences as a single frond with a central vascular core—later it becomes tufted. From the tufts spring villi—long, finger-like projections composed of three or four layers of transitional epithelium surrounding a capillary vessel with a minimum amount

---

[1] Workers exposed to this hazard should have a sample of urine centrifuged and examined for red cells and neoplastic cells at three-monthly intervals.

[2] It has been suggested that nitrosamines excreted in the urine of agricultural workers may be an essential factor in the development of carcinoma in those bladders which are affected by bilharzia.

Ludwig Rehn, 1849–1930. Surgeon, Frankfurt on Main, Germany.

of supporting fibrous tissue. Thus the fully developed papilloma appears like a red sea anemone with delicate tentacles eddying to and fro with each and every movement of the bladder contents.

CARCINOMA OF THE BLADDER

Carcinoma arising within the bladder may be of three cell types: transitional, squamous, adenocarcinoma. The vast majority (greater than 90%) is transitional in origin. Squamous carcinoma is uncommon, apart from areas where Bilharzia is endemic. Primary adenocarcinoma, which usually arises from the urachal remnant, accounts for less than 1% of bladder cancer.

Transitional Cell Carcinoma

Examination of the biological behaviour of transitional cell cancers of the bladder shows that they basically fall into three groups. (1) *The papillary tumour* which can be single or multiple in which histological examination may reveal invasion of the lamina propria but not of the muscle; these tend to carry a relatively good prognosis. (2) When there is evidence of *muscle invasion*; the outlook changes dramatically because one is dealing with a much more aggressive growth. (3) The group consisting of *carcinoma in-situ* which has really only been recognised over the last three decades, and carries an intermediate prognosis.

(1) Superficial Bladder Cancer

These are papillary tumours which grow in an exophytic fashion into the bladder lumen. They may be single or multiple at the time of presentation. They sometimes are relatively pedunculated arising on a stalk with a narrow base but may, particularly with the less well differentiated tumour, begin to appear rather more solid with a wider base. The area around the tumour within the bladder is often rather oedematous with angry-looking dilated blood vessels.

A proportion of bladder cancers are infected and there may be evidence of frank cystitis within the bladder. Occasionally calcium salts are deposited on these tumours giving them a crusted exterior. The urothelium elsewhere in the bladder may also appear rather oedematous and velvety; this suggests a generalised 'field change' with the presence of widespread carcinoma in-situ.

The most common sites for these superficial tumours to develop is in the region around the trigone and over the lateral walls of the bladder (fig. 1266). Careful examination of the natural history of this condition shows that despite surgical removal of these growths between 50% and 70% of patients will develop a further tumour or tumours. This provides the rationale for performing check cystoscopies. The single most important factor affecting the prognosis is the degree of differentiation of the cells ('the grade'). This is sub-divided into G1, 2 and 3, corresponding to well, moderately and poorly differentiated tumour. If treated carefully the prognosis for patients with G1 and for the majority of those with G2 tumours is excellent and on the whole this group of patients are as likely to die from intercurrent illness as from their bladder cancer. The pattern begins to change with the poorly differentiated tumours. The disease can advance beyond the lamina propria with muscle invasion; there may be invasion of the lymphatics

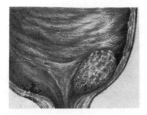

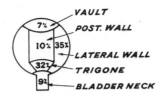

FIG. 1265.—Nodular carci-
noma of the bladder, sometimes known as the 'bun-
shaped' tumour.

FIG. 1266.—Sites of carcinoma
of the bladder.
(American Urological Association Statistics.)

with the subsequent development of metastases and the tumour may also begin
to grow in the prostatic ducts. These features all indicate a worsening in the
outlook.

(2) Invasive Transitional Cell Carcinoma

The tumour with muscle invasion is always solid (fig. 1265) in its consistency
although there may be a low tufted exterior. These tumours are often large,
broad based, having an irregular ugly sometimes ulcerated appearance within the
bladder. The incidence of metastases, whether from lymphatic invasion in the
pelvis or blood-borne to the lung, liver or bones, is much more common and will
cause the demise of 30% of these patients.

(3) In-situ Carcinoma

The histological appearance of irregularly arranged cells with large nuclei and
a high mitotic index replacing the normally well ordered urothelium is now
known as carcinoma in-situ. This may occur alone or in association with a demonstrable tumour. This change may be appreciated macroscopically at the time of
cystoscopy, although often is only diagnosed when a biopsy is examined under
the microscope. The association of in-situ carcinoma with papillary tumours
increases the chance of recurrent disease. Worldwide experience of this condition
seems to indicate that it carries a high malignant potential. 50% of the patients
will die of their bladder cancer.

Squamous Cell Carcinoma of the Bladder.—Squamous cell tumours tend to
be solid in consistency and are nearly always associated with muscle invasion.
This is the most prevalent form of bladder cancer in areas where Bilharzia is
endemic. Squamous cell tumours may arise secondary to chronic irritation caused
by stone disease in the bladder.

Adenocarcinoma.—This accounts for approximately 1% of bladder cancer. It
usually arises in the fundus of the bladder at the site of the urachal remnant.
Occasionally primary adenocarcinomas arise at other sites but are as likely to be
secondary in origin. The prognosis is generally poor.

Clinical Features

Painless haematuria is by far the most common symptom and should be
regarded as indicative of a bladder carcinoma until proven otherwise. The haema-

turia may occur on only one or two occasions and because the urine once again becomes clear patients only too often fail to declare the symptom to their practitioner. Many months may elapse before it recurs and causes concern. The bleeding if more severe may give rise to clot formation in the bladder and subsequent clot retention. It is fairly uncommon for the bleeding to be so profuse that emergency admission to hospital and blood transfusion is necessary. Occasionally a pedunculated tumour may occlude the bladder neck during the passage of urine thus shutting off the flow; following a change in posture further micturition is often possible. The development of recurrent urinary tract infections particularly in women in the later decades of life should also arouse one's suspicions.

For patients with more solid tumours pain in the pelvis usually heralds extravesical spread. There is often also frequency and discomfort associated with urination. Pain in the loin or pyelonephritis may suggest the presence of ureteric obstruction with the development of hydronephrosis. A late manifestation due to nerve involvement is pain referred to the suprapubic region, the groins, perineum, the anus and into the thighs.

It is also important to assess the patient as a whole. Many of these patients are elderly men who have been lifelong smokers and suffer from chronic obstructive airways disease. Their suitability for anaesthesia must be borne in mind.

Investigation

Urine.—Bacteriological culture of the urine is essential. The urine may also be examined for the presence of malignant cells which can be demonstrated using the Papanicoloau stain. This tends not to be a good screening test for patients with haematuria as particularly with low grade tumours malignant cells may not be identified unless a specimen obtained at bladder washout is examined. False positive results occur infrequently and are usually associated with stone disease.

Blood.—Estimation of the haemoglobin and the serum electrolytes and urea need little justification.

Intravenous Urography.—This should be performed on all patients who complain of haematuria. Occasionally the preliminary film shows a faint shadow of an encrusted neoplasm of the bladder. The most common radiological confirmation of a bladder cancer is the presence of a filling defect distorting the uniform distribution of contrast. Occasionally irregularity of the bladder wall may herald the presence of an invasive tumour (fig. 1268). Hydronephrosis may occur if there is a large tumour adjacent to the ureteric orifice or more commonly with direct invasion of the ureter. If this is longstanding the kidney may not be functioning.

Cystourethroscopy.—Cystourethroscopy is the mainstay of diagnosis and should always be performed on patients with haematuria. The urethra is inspected at the initial insertion of the instrument (urethroscopy). In a small proportion of males a tumour will be present. The bladder is then examined in a systematic fashion.

Bimanual Examination (fig. 1267).—A bimanual examination with the patient fully relaxed under general anaesthesia should be performed both before and after endoscopic surgical treatment of these tumours. The bladder should be

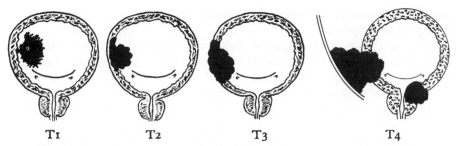

T1   T2   T3   T4

FIG. 1267.—Clinical assessment of the stage of progression of a bladder tumour by bimanual palpation.

(After D. M. Wallace.)

Staging by the **TNM** classification (cf. Chapter 8). *Stage T1*—involving subepithelial connective tissue. *Stage T2*—infiltration of muscle superficially. *Stage T3*—full thickness of muscle and possibly perivesical tissues affected, but mobile. *Stage T4*—fixed to adjoining organs or involving prostate.

empty and the bimanual examination is executed with the right index finger in the rectum of a male and placed per vaginam in a female. The four fingers of the left hand push down on the anterior abdominal wall in the suprapubic region. Occasionally a very large superficial frondy tumour may be felt as a soft but mobile thickening. On the whole these tumours are not palpable bimanually at the beginning and by definition not after surgical resection. Once there is muscle invasion the differentiation between T2 and T3 disease lies between whether a mass is palpable bimanually at the end of the procedure (T3). Where invasion has spread into the prostate in a male or the vagina in a woman it is classified as T4a. If the tumour is fixed to the lateral pelvic sidewall it is staged as T4b. (UICC classification, Chapter 8).

TREATMENT

Non-invasive Tumours

Endoscopic Surgery.—It is no longer acceptable to take a tiny biopsy from the top of a papillary tumour and apply a fulgurating coagulation current to the rest of the growth (fig. 1269) unless a small recurrence is being dealt with. The

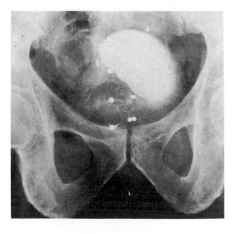

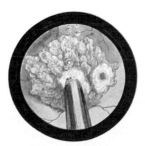

FIG. 1268.—Cystograph in a case of malignant tumour of the right side of the bladder.

FIG. 1269.—Cystodiathermy of a papilloma of the bladder.

treatment of this cancer has become highly specialised with proven therapeutic benefit for the patients.

Endoscopic surgical techniques now allow one to provide the histopathologist with the appropriate material to help stage the cancer and therefore one can develop a rational approach to treatment.

If a papillary tumour is found in the bladder, three or four random biopsies of the urothelium should be taken from sites away from the growth; a further biopsy should probably be taken of the urothelium adjacent to the tumour. A resectoscope is then introduced per urethram and with an isotonic irrigating fluid (1·5% Glycine) the tumour can then be resected under direct vision. The resection should be completed with the material placed in a formalin pot. After removal of the main mass of tumour, two or three further loops of tissue should be sent separately so that the pathologist can accurately determine whether there is muscle invasion. The base of the tumour is then coagulated so achieving haemostasis. The appearance of pale yellow glistening fat will indicate a perforation of the bladder. Should this occur before the resection is complete it may be prudent to stop the resection and place a catheter in the bladder for a few days. In this instance the procedure could be completed some two weeks later. The bimanual is repeated at the end of each endoscopic procedure.

Patients with solid tumours should have adequate material resected for histological staging and grading. These patients will usually need some other form of treatment. It is at present undetermined whether a debulking resection or a radical resection of T3 tumours is helpful. Following these procedures an irrigating catheter is left in-situ for 48 hours to prevent clot retention of urine.

Follow-up.—As more than half of the patients with superficial bladder cancer will develop single or multiple recurrence whether at the original site of the tumour or at other parts of the bladder, follow up cystoscopies are essential. These should initially be performed at three monthly intervals over the first year; following this the time interval between cystoscopies can be determined according to the presence or absence of further disease. 30% of patients will never develop another tumour so that after two years if the bladder has remained clear annual inspection may be adequate. For patients who go on to develop multiple recurrences within the bladder at each examination the cystoscopies need to be maintained at frequent intervals so that the growths can be resected. These patients are at a greater risk from developing progression of their disease and experience has shown that the introduction of intravesical chemotherapeutic agents has been of benefit in reducing the number of recurrences.

Intravesical Chemotherapy.—Thiotepa using the Orovisto regime (30 mg in 30 ml of water) can be instilled into the bladder; this is done thrice on alternate days, the solution being kept in for one hour. The incidence of side affects is low but all the tumour bulk needs to have been resected to avoid systemic absorption of the drug which may otherwise cause myelosuppression. Mitomycin (30 mg) instilled for one hour leaving the catheter in-situ to allow subsequent drainage of the drug can not only reduce the number of recurrences but cause lesions to regress. Contact with the urethra should be avoided as it can be the cause of a urethral stricture. More recently adriamycin and BCG have also been shown to be effective.

Should the random biopsies show evidence of in-situ carcinoma the chance of early recurrence is enhanced and the use of one of these intravesical agents is advised.

Transvesical Excision of a Large Villous Growth.—This should rarely be performed now as resectoscopes and diathermy machines are so much improved. The bladder is distended with 1:2000 silver nitrate solution and the viscus is exposed by a suprapubic incision. The contents of the bladder having been evacuated by a trocar and cannula (which permits suction of the fluid contents so that none is spilled), the edges of the abdominal wall are covered with packs soaked in silver nitrate solution or 60% alcohol, as a precaution against contamination of the wound by detached tumour cells. The bladder is opened, and the surface of the tumour is lightly coagulated (with the object of preventing detachment of cells). It is then picked up with Fergusson's cupped forceps which surround the tumour. An innocent tumour can be elevated so that there is a substantial pedicle of normal mucous membrane. This is transected with the diathermy needle. After coagulating bleeding-points, the area from which the papilloma sprang is electro-coagulated. In the case of a sessile neoplasm, a diathermy loop electrode (fig. 1270) allows excision of the tumour including a fraction of the muscle layer. This accomplished, the cut surface is lightly fulgurated. The bladder can then be closed with indwelling urethral catheter drainage. Drainage of the prevesical space is necessary.

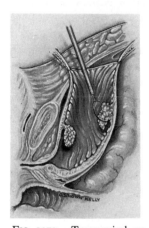

FIG. 1270.—Transvesical excision of a bladder tumour with diathermy loop electrode.
(After A. R. C. Higham.)

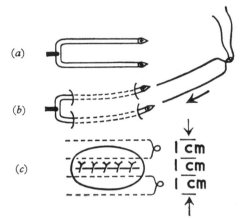

FIG. 1271.—Insertion of radioactive tantalum wire. (*a*) The curved twin hollow needles. (*b*) Insertion of the wire loop via the curved needles, (*c*) Position of wires relative to site of tumour pedicle.

Invasive Tumours

The treatment of cancer with proven muscle invasion remains a subject for debate. Whatever the modality of treatment employed few centres have survival figures of more than 40% of the patients alive at 5 years. The controversy is centred around whether primary surgery (total cystectomy), radical radiotherapy or a combination of the two, provides the best result.

Radiotherapy

Local radiotherapy.—For small invasive lesions local radiotherapy can be delivered by the open placement of a radioactive tantalum wire (^{192}Ta) or the implantation of gold grains (^{198}Au). Historically these methods have been successful for small tumours but the patients are subjected to the discomfort of an open surgical procedure.

(a) **Implantation of Radioactive Gold Grains (^{198}Au).**—The gold grains are inserted by means of a repeater gun, which is loaded with a cartridge containing fourteen grains. This isotope has a half life of two and a half days. The grains are implanted according to physical rules depending on the area to be irradiated. Stereoscopic films taken subsequently enable the physicist to determine the dosage the tumour will receive.

(b) **Radioactive tantalum wire (^{192}Ta) (Wallace) (fig. 1271)** has a long half-life (four months), and it therefore can be stored in the hospital ready for use when required, instead of having to be obtained from an atomic pile for each patient. The wire is bent hair-pin fashion with a loop provided at the blunt end. Through the opened bladder the sharp ends of the wire are drawn beneath the base of the tumour by means of twin, hollow needles, mounted on a boomerang needle introducer which enters and emerges some millimetres from the periphery of the neoplasm. The wire having been inserted, a plastic or rubber catheter is passed from the external urinary meatus and its tip is attached to the loop of wire by a stitch. The bladder is then closed. Again, stereo-radiographs enable the physicist to determine how long the wires should be allowed to remain in position. They are removed by withdrawing the catheter.

Deep external beam x-ray therapy.—The introduction of external beam radiotherapy with cobalt 60 has now been extended by the implementation of a series of high powered machines (linear accelerators) which deliver the radiotherapy. Radical radiotherapy giving 60Gy over a 4-6 week period will cause the cancer to melt away in just over half of the patients. In the face of complete response to radiation the prognosis is reasonable. For patients whose tumour does not respond the outlook is hopeless but is marginally improved by performing a salvage cystectomy. The protagonists of radiotherapy would claim that for most patients it saves the need to remove the bladder and allows the men to retain potency. Radiotherapy is not always without complications and during the course of treatment will cause some urinary frequency and also some frequency of stool. Late complications can leave the bladder contracted and fibrosed, in which case the bladder may need to be removed for palliative reasons. Late complications affecting the rectum should be uncommon.

Surgery

Partial cystectomy.—Partial cystectomy for invasive disease ensuring removal of a 2 cm margin of normal bladder around the tumour has a limited place in the repertoire of options. This is largely because relatively few of these tumours are in the dome of the bladder which is the most suitable site. For lesions near the trigone partial cystectomy should not be contemplated for attempts to preserve the anatomy of the ureters will inevitably compromise one's chances of obtaining an adequate margin of clearance away from the tumour.

Radical cystectomy.—Before contemplating radical surgery to remove the bladder it is important to have evidence that surgical cure is attainable. A CT scan of the pelvis will show how advanced the tumour is locally and may also reveal the presence of enlarged lymph nodes along the iliac and paraortic chains. As ultrasound of the liver should show whether there are hepatic metastases and a bonescan (99 m Technetium) will help show if there is spread to bone.

Controversy continues to exist over the place for cystectomy. There are still many surgeons who perform this as their primary treatment for invasive disease. Some precede this by a palliative cause of radiotherapy (20 Gy). If one accepts radiotherapy as one's prime treatment for this condition cystectomy should only be necessary in the event of tumour not responding or the bladder becoming so contracted that urinary frequency and incontinence develop. Should there be recurrence following a partial cystectomy removal of the remainder of the bladder may be necessary. Cystectomy for multiple papillary superficial disease should rarely be necessary with modern endoscopic procedures. Uncertainty still exists as to the malignant potential of carcinoma in-situ.

Experience from some centres certainly suggests that a substantial proportion of these patients die of their disease and therefore advocate cystectomy. As mentioned earlier control can usually be achieved with the judicious use of chemotherapeutic agents (intravenous cyclophosphamide or intravesical mitomycin or adriamycin) but should these fail the bladder should probably be removed.

Operation.

Alternative drainage for the urine is necessary following removal of the bladder. Most surgeons perform an ileal conduit. It is sensible to place an ileostomy bag filled with water over the proposed site for the stoma. This ensures that the correct site is chosen and that one does not end up with the disaster of a leaking urinary ileostomy. Preoperatively the bowel is prepared with suitable antibiotics, purgatives and enemas. The abdomen is opened through a lower midline incision extending down to the symphysis pubis. The liver and the retroperitoneum are checked for evidence of metastases and the operability of the bladder is assessed. The ureters should first be isolated and followed down to the level of the bladder. The bladder is then mobilised from the pubic arch so creating the plane anteriorly. This is usually quite easy even when the patient has previously had radical radiotherapy. The peritoneum is then incised laterally on each side round to the internal iliac vessels. A pelvic lymph node dissection should then be performed particularly in patients who have not had radiotherapy; its value after radiotherapy is less clear. The peritoneum is then divided transversely behind the bladder allowing one to create a plane between the bladder and the rectum. This reveals the lateral vascular pedicles on each side. The superior and inferior vesical arteries are divided and ligated with linen. Following complete mobilisation of the bladder and the prostate the specimen is removed en bloc. In women the uterus and anterior vaginal wall need to be included.

An isolated loop of ileum is then prepared on its own mesentery and continuity of the small bowel restored. The ureters are then implanted into the bowel and the ileostomy created. Meticulous care must be taken to close all mesenteric windows thus avoiding internal hernias.

The operative mortality associated with cystectomy was considerable until a few years ago. The use of prophylactic antibiotics (a cephalosporin or aminoglycoside and metronidazole) have probably been the single most important factor in improving mortality.

In men there is a 10% local recurrence rate if the urethra is left in-situ; many surgeons advocate its removal through a separate perineal incision.

URINARY DIVERSION

This chapter closes with an account of the principles of this important subject, and includes indications, the methods employed and their attendant problems, and some operative details.

Indications.—Diversion of the urine may be either (a) a temporary expedient to relieve distal obstruction, or (b) a permanent procedure when (1) the bladder has been removed, (2) the sphincters of the bladder have been damaged or have lost their normal neurological control, (3) there is an incurable vesico-vaginal fistula, (4) there is an irremovable obstruction, and (5) in cases of ectopia vesicae.

Methods of Urinary Diversion (fig. 1273)

The diversion may be achieved by any of the following methods, but the choice in each case will be decided largely by the primary disease.

Pyelostomy or nephrostomy (Chapter 57), or urethrostomy (with indwelling catheters).

Cutaneous ureterostomy.

Suprapubic cystostomy (with indwelling catheter).

Cutaneous vesicostomy (cystostomy).

Suprapubic displacement of the urethra.

Uretero-sigmoidostomy (*a*) in continuity, (*b*) making a rectal bladder and colostomy.

Trigono-colostomy (*a*) in continuity, (*b*) into an isolated conduit.

Ureteric transplantation into an isolated ileal or colonic conduit.

Diversion of urine immediately raises the following problems: 1. the collection of the urine, 2. stricture-formation at any anastomosis, and 3. reflux and reabsorption of urinary solutes. The problems of infection are intimately related to all three.

Collection of the Urine

(*a*) **Catheters.**—In the past, indwelling catheters have been used for permanent diversion. They invariably result in infection and they often become blocked by phosphatic encrustation. There is now *no place for permanent catheter drainage* of the kidneys or ureters. For temporary drainage the tubes should be of latex or soft Silastic. Polyvinyl plastics are irritant and predispose to a stricture.

Bladder Drainage.—In elderly patients unfit for prostatectomy and in some terminal cases of carcinoma of the prostate, an indwelling Foley catheter changed every three weeks is a satisfactory method of drainage. Alternatively, a St. Peter's Hospital suprapubic drainage apparatus (fig. 1272) incorporating a straight catheter which the patient or nurse changes daily is acceptable.

(*b*) **Cutaneous Stomas:** *Suprapubic Vesicostomy or Urethrostomy.*—Collection from a formal suprapubic vesicostomy (cystostomy), or from the urethra displaced on to the abdominal wall (*e.g.* for cases of multiple sclerosis in a woman), may be unsatisfactory because the local incisions result in creases which make it difficult to apply a water-tight collecting appliance.

Cutaneous ureterostomies are very liable to stricture formation. In addition two openings (fig. 1273) and appliances add to the patient's burden. Mobilisation of the ureters and the making of a central abdominal stoma (fig. 1273(e)) can be successful, but such a degree of mobilisation is attended by the high risk of sloughing of the distal ureters due to impairment of blood-supply.

Ileal or Colonic Conduit.—At present the most generally useful form of diversion is to implant each ureter with as little mobilisation as possible into an isolated segment of gut (ileum or colon), which conducts the urine onwards to a cutaneous stoma (fig. 1273(a)). Urine is then collected in an ileostomy bag. This form of diversion limits infection and avoids the problems of reabsorption of urine as contact-time with the mucosa is minimal. In some cases in which the pelvis has been subjected to radiation the lower ureters may be unhealthy. A high division with insertion of the ureters into an ileal loop above the roof of the mesentery may be wiser (fig. 1274), (Wallace).

Siting of Stoma.—The site for the stoma must be chosen before operation. The

St. Peter's Hospital for Stone, London, founded in 1860.
David M. Wallace, Contemporary. Former surgeon to St. Peter's Hospital and Professor of Urology, University of Riyadh, Saudi Arabia.

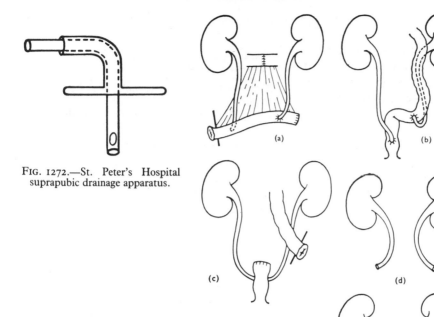

FIG. 1272.—St. Peter's Hospital suprapubic drainage apparatus.

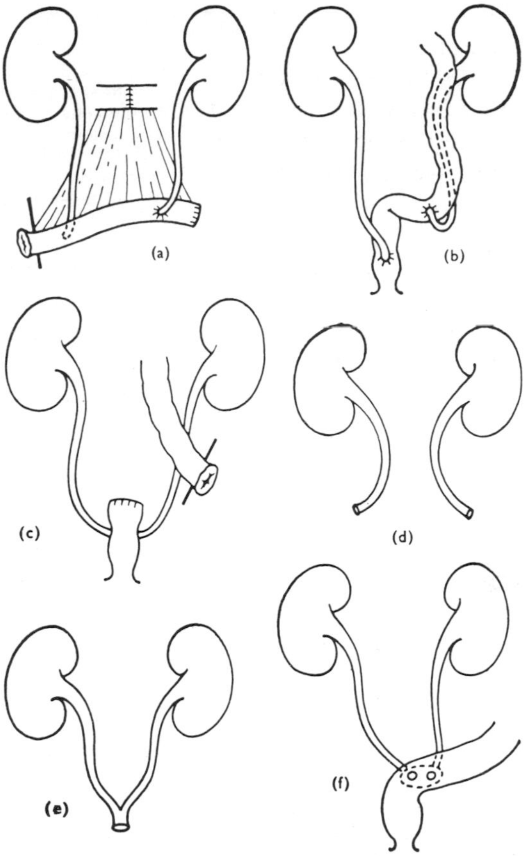

FIG. 1273.—Diversion of urine. Favoured methods: (*a*) Ileal conduit, (*b*) Uretero-sigmoidostomy. (*c*) Rectal bladder with terminal colostomy, (*d*) Bilateral cutaneous ureterostomies, (*e*) Joined ureters—cutaneous opening, (*f*) Trigono-colostomy.

ileostomy ring and bag are applied to the abdominal wall, and by trial and error the point at which the belt can support the ring and bag at all times and in all positions is found. Having checked this by sticking on a bag full of water and asking the patient to perform the type of movements which his work will entail, the site of the future stoma is marked indelibly on the skin.

(*c*) **Colon and Rectum.**—The advantage of diverting urine into the colon is that no collecting apparatus is necessary (fig. 1273(b) and (f)). Clearly, however, the rectal sphincter must be competent. Before any uretero-sigmoidostomy is undertaken, the patient must prove that he can control at least 200 ml of fluid in the rectum. The disadvantage of the operation is that the renal tract is exposed continuously to infection from the faeces. This can be avoided by establishing a terminal left iliac colostomy, and closing the upper rectum to make a rectal bladder (fig. 1273c)). It prevents the urine refluxing retrogradely round the colon to the caecum, diminishes reabsorption (see below), and protects renal function. Cancer can develop at long-standing uretero-colic junctions.

Stricture Formation

Uretero-sigmoidostomy was first used by Chaput (1894). Subsequent modifications included those made by Coffey and Grey Turner. In these methods the ureters were cut obliquely and pulled into the gut by a stitch—the ends were not stitched to the gut wall.

Henri Chaput, 1857–1919. French Surgeon.
Robert Calvin Coffey, 1869–1933. American Surgeon.
George Grey Turner, 1877–1951. Professor of Surgery, Postgraduate Medical School, London. Formerly Professor of Surgery, University of Durham.

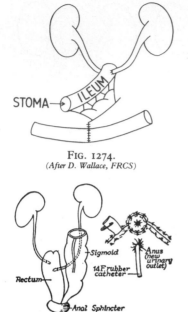

FIG. 1274.
(*After D. Wallace, FRCS*)

FIG. 1276.—Lowsley's operation.

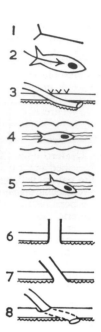

FIG. 1275.—Methods of uret-ero-colic anastomosis. 1. Incision in the sero-muscular layer, which, on dissection, exposes an area of submucosa and mucosa which looks rather like a fish. 2. The ureter is laid along the 'fish' and inserted through the opening into the lumen made in the 'fish's head'. 3. Lateral view of completed anastomosis. 4. Coffey type. 5. Grey Turner type. 6. Nesbit, 7. Cordonnier, and 8. Leadbetter types entail a careful mucosa to mucosa anastomosis. The last named includes a submucosal tunnel, and is probably the best anastomosis for preventing stricture formation and reflux.

Stenosis was not uncommon. Nesbit, Cordonnier, and Leadbetter all recognised that these strictures could be prevented by anastomosing mucosa to mucosa (fig. 1275).

Reflux of Urine and Reabsorption of Urinary Solutes

Reflux of Urine.—Pressure within the colon can interfere with drainage, and so force air, faeces, and organisms up to the renal pelvis. Daniel has demonstrated that a high intra-colonic pressure (over 24 cm water) results in all these complications being more likely. For many years it had been noted that the left kidney was much more likely to cease functioning after uretero-sigmoidostomy than the right kidney. As the left ureter is implanted into the sigmoid and the right often in the upper rectum, the former is more likely to be subjected to higher intra-colonic pressures. A sigmoid myotomy performed from the upper rectum to the splenic flexure may help to overcome this problem.

Reabsorption of Urinary solutes depends upon two factors, (1) reflux of urine round the colon and even into the terminal ileum (fig. 1273 (b) and (f)), (2) because the colon is acting as a reservoir, the urine is in contact with gut wall for a longer period. Biochemical disturbances are rare, if a rectal bladder is made (see above).

The biochemical changes associated with transplantation into the colon are due to a combination of reabsorption of chloride and urea, and progressively diminishing tubular function as a result of chronic pyelonephritis. Diarrhoea with loss of potassium-containing mucus may exacerbate the loss of potassium.

The typical changes are a hyperchloraemic acidosis with potassium depletion, and they occur in every patient with a uretero-sigmoid diversion. When severe, the patient develops loss of appetite, weakness, thirst, and diarrhoea. He becomes listless, and respirations are rapid, deep, and unremittent. Coma may ensue. Mild acidosis, unrecognised over a long period, produces osteomalacia from calcium reabsorption. Bone pain and even pathological fractures occur.

Renal impairment from pyelonephritis and reabsorption from the mucosa are infrequent complications if the diversion is into an ileal or colonic conduit.

Treatment.—(*a*) *Prevention.*—Patients should be instructed to empty the rectum two-hourly by day, and in cases where acidosis is present, a rectal tube should be inserted at night to drain the urine continuously. The patient should avoid added salt in the diet, and he should take a mixture of potassium citrate and sodium bicarbonate, t.d.s. (two grams

Reed M. Nesbit. Formerly Professor of Surgery, University of Michigan Medical School, Ann Arbor, U.S.A.
Justin Joseph Cordonnier, Contemporary. Professor of Urology, Washington University School of Medicine, St. Louis, Missouri, U.S.A.
Wyland F. Leadbetter, Contemporary. Clinical Professor of Surgery, Harvard Medical School, Boston, U.S.A.

of each, either as crystals or tablets). Regular biochemical analyses, including calcium, are required. The patient should be told to report if he loses his appetite or develops weakness.

(b) *In established hyperchloraemic acidosis*, the patient should be given suitable doses of sodium bicarbonate ($8 \cdot 4\% = 1$ mmol/ml = molar) intravenously to correct the pH with suitable amounts of potassium, also intravenously, if necessary. Furadantin, ampicillin, or the appropriate antibiotic should be given to correct the inevitable pyelonephritis which will be present. Later, conversion to an ileal conduit should be considered.

Operative Details

Uretero-colic Anastomosis.—The preparation of the colon is the same as that described in Chapter 50. The abdomen is opened by a right lower paramedian incision. The patient is then placed in the Trendelenburg position and the right ureter is sought as it crosses above the bifurcation of the common iliac artery. An incision is made through the peritoneum overlying the medial side of the ureter, thus avoiding damage to the ureteric vessels which always approach the duct from the outer side (Daniel), and the ureter is identified and dissected from its bed towards its entry into the bladder. The ureter is then divided and its distal stump ligated. The proximal end is trimmed obliquely and split upwards for one centimetre. An incision 3 cm long is made in the anterior wall of the colon and the peritoneal and muscular coats are divided, but not the mucous membrane (fig. 1275(3)). An incision is made into the extreme lower end of the exposed mucous membrane and the full thickness of the ureteric wall is joined by interrupted 4/0 chromic catgut sutures to the mucosal opening. The incision in the outer coats of the bowel is approximated over the ureter (Leadbetter anastomosis). Suturing the peritoneal incision around the ureteric implant extraperitonealises the site, and a drain is left down to the area. The left ureter is implanted into the colon above in a similar manner. A full-sized Foley's catheter is inserted through the anus no farther than the rectal ampulla, the balloon then being inflated. This permits all urine to be measured until the third day, when the catheter is removed. There must be a full fluid intake. If oliguria or anuria supervene, treatment is as described in Chapter 56.

Uretero-ileostomy (Ileal Loop Conduit).—A coil of ileum, approximately 15–25 cm long, and one foot from the ileo-caecal valve, with its blood supply intact, is isolated. The left ureter is brought through the pelvic mesocolon, and after the ureter has been cut obliquely, end-to-side anastomosis is performed between the ureter and the intestine. The right ureter is also cut obliquely, and it is joined to an elliptical opening made in the side of the coil. In each case the anastomosis may be effected by the method of Nesbit (fig. 1275(6)). The coil of intestine is tacked lightly to the peritoneum of the anterior abdominal wall at the level of the pelvic brim. The distal end of the coil is brought out through a stab incision in the right lower abdomen, and, because of the anchoring of the intestine to the peritoneum, the opening is made a little lower than is the case when ileostomy is performed for ulcerative colitis. The method of anchoring the ileostomy opening to the abdominal wall, and the after-care of the orifice so formed, in no way differs from that described in Chapter 50.

Lowsley's Operation.—The rectosigmoid junction is divided completely and its lower end closed. The ureters or the trigone are implanted into the excluded lower segment, so that the rectum functions as a bladder. The sigmoid colon is mobilised sufficiently for it to be drawn through the perineum immediately anterior to the anus. Thus both the original anal canal and the new anal canal are encompassed by the external sphincter ani muscle (fig. 1276).

Owen Daniel, Contemporary. Consultant Surgeon, Royal Alexandra Hospital, Rhyl, Wales.
Oswald S. Lowsley, 1884–1955. Director of Urology, James Buchanan Brady Foundation, New York Hospital.

CHAPTER 59

THE PROSTATE AND SEMINAL VESICLES

Embryology.—The prostate arises from the primitive urethra as a series of solid buds; in a matter of weeks these become canalised. The surrounding mesenchyme becomes the muscular and connective tissue of the gland. The buds are arranged into five groups—anterior, middle, posterior, and two lateral. These are the fore-runners of the lobes of the prostate.

Skene's tubules opening on either side of the female urethral orifice are the homologues of the prostate.

Surgical Anatomy.—The prostatic glands (fig. 1277) lie in the fibromuscular stroma and their ducts open into the posterolateral grooves on either side of the verumontanum. The epithelium is columnar. Commencing peripherally, and passing centrally, beneath the anatomical capsule lie the long branched **prostatic glands proper**. This region is named the carcinomatous zone. Beneath this envelope, and separated from it by an indefinite capsule, lies another mass of secreting elements, also branched. These are the **submucosal glands**—and the zone that they occupy is known as the adenomatous zone. Still nearer the urethra are the unbranched **urethral glands** whose mouths open directly into the urethra.

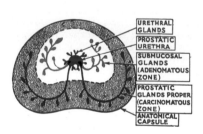

FIG. 1277.—Distribution of the normal glands of the prostate, transverse section.
(After J. C. B. Grant.)

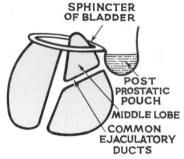

FIG. 1278.—The surgical subdivisions and relationships of the prostate.

Into the prostatic urethra, therefore, open the prostatic ducts proper, the ducts of the submucosal and mucosal glands, as well as the common ejaculatory ducts and the prostatic utricle. No wonder that chronic infection of the prostatic urethra is difficult to eradicate!

Certain relationships and divisions of the prostate as seen in sagittal section are set out in fig. 1278. The middle lobe is that part of the prostate included between the common ejaculatory ducts and the prostatic urethra: it contains more secretory glandular element (subcervical glands, as opposed to muscle and fibrous tissue) than the lateral lobes.

An enlarged prostate is invested with three capsules: (1) The compressed outer zone = *the false capsule*; (2) The anatomical capsule = *the true capsule*; and external to this (3) *The prostatic sheath of pelvic fascia*. Between the anatomical capsule and the prostatic sheath lies the prostatic venous plexus. The prostatic sheath is contiguous with the strong fascia of Denonvilliers that separate the prostate and its coverings from the rectum.

Physiology.—That the prostate is purely a genital organ is evinced by the fact that in such animals as manifest a seasonal sexual life, the organ is rudimentary except during the rutting season. That normal adult prostatic epithelium undergoes atrophy after castration was known to John Hunter.

Hormonal Influences.—The prostate is governed by two testicular hormones, one male (androgenic) and the other female (oestrogenic). Normally the preponderant testicular

Alexander Johnston Chalmers Skene, 1838–1900. Professor of Gynaecology, Long Island College Hospital, New York, U.S.A.
Charles Pierre Denonvilliers, 1808–1872. Professor of Anatomy, and later of Surgery, Paris.
John Hunter, 1728–1793. Surgeon, St. George's Hospital, London.

hormone is androgen, which is supplemented by androgens secreted by the adrenal glands.

Oestrogens cause retrogressive changes in the testes and prostate glands. For example, most capons are produced by implanting oestrogen pellets into the neck of the bird rather than by castration.

Elaboration and Secretion of Acid Phosphatases.—Enzymes that split organic phosphates and are most active about pH5, are present in many human tissues, but their concentration in the adult prostate is several hundred times greater than in any other organ or tissue. This high level is not achieved until after puberty. While the function of this enzyme is speculative, it is highly suggestive that the acidity which is most favourable for its action corresponds to that of the vagina at the time of ovulation. Most of the acid phosphatase secreted by the prostate drains along the prostatic ducts into the urethra, so that the blood level of this enzyme remains low. When the cells producing this enzyme cannot discharge their products externally, the serum acid phosphatase rises.

Acid phosphatase estimations are made on plasma or serum, free from haemolysis. The blood sample must be taken in the morning before breakfast, and on no account after a heavy meal, since lipoid-rich serum gives inaccurate estimations. Digital rectal examination has now been shown not to affect the acid phosphatase level in the blood. The normal range of findings is 0–5 King-Armstrong units per 100 ml of serum.

The serum acid phosphatase is usually raised in carcinoma of the prostate *with metastases*, but is seldom above normal if the growth is confined to the gland, and almost never in benign prostatic hyperplasia. On the other hand, slightly increased values are not uncommon in (1) acute prostatitis, (2) Paget's disease of bone, (3) hepatic cirrhosis.

BENIGN ENLARGEMENT OF THE PROSTATE

'When the hair becomes grey and scanty, when specks of earthy matter begin to be deposited in the tunics of the artery, and when a white zone is formed at the margin of the cornea, at this same period the prostate gland usually—I might perhaps say invariably—becomes increased in size.' (SIR BENJAMIN BRODIE.)

Benign enlargement of the prostate usually occurs in men over fifty years of age; most often between sixty and seventy. In Indians prostatic enlargement is less frequent, and occurs more often in a younger age-group; in Negroes it is rare. The reason for these discrepancies is unknown.

Theories of causation of benign enlargement of the prostate:

The Hormonic Theory.—As age advances the male hormone diminishes while the quantity of the oestrogenic hormone is not decreased equally. According to this theory the prostate enlarges because of predominance of the oestrogenic hormone. Prostatic enlargement can be regarded as involuntary hyperplasia akin to fibroadenosis of the breast, due to a disturbance of the ratio and quantity of the circulating androgens and oestrogens.

The Neoplastic Theory postulates that the enlargement is a benign neoplasm. As the prostate is composed essentially of fibrous tissue, muscle tissue, and glandular tissue, the neoplasm is a *fibro-myo-adenoma*.

Pathology.—Hyperplasia affects the glandular elements and connective tissue, but in variable degrees. In this respect the changes are very similar to those occurring in breast dysplasia (Chapter 39), where adenosis, epitheliosis, and stromal proliferation are seen in differing proportions. Benign adenomatous hyperplasia affects the submucous group of glands, forming a nodular enlargement—the typical 'lateral' lobes—which compresses the external group of glands into a false capsule (fig. 1277).

As the prostate enlarges extravesically, it tends to displace the seminal vesicles, so that instead of lying on the base of the bladder, these structures become a direct posterior relation of the upper limit of the prostate. When the hyperplasia affects the subcervical glands a 'middle' lobe develops which projects up into the bladder within the internal sphincter (fig. 1278). Sometimes both lateral lobes

Earl J. King, 1901–1962. Professor of Chemical Pathology, University of London (Postgraduate Medical School), and Arthur Riley Armstrong, Contemporary. Director of Laboratories, Hamilton Health Association, Ontario, formerly co-workers at the Department of Medical Research, Banting Institute, University of Toronto.
Sir James Paget, 1814–1899. Surgeon, St. Bartholomew's Hospital, London.
Sir Benjamin Collins Brodie, 1783–1862. Surgeon, St. George's Hospital, London.

also project into the bladder, so that when viewed from within, the sides and back of the internal urinary meatus are surrounded by an intravesical prostatic collar.

SECONDARY EFFECTS OF PROSTATIC ENLARGEMENT

Urethra.—That portion of the urethra lying above the verumontanum becomes elongated, sometimes to as much as twice its normal length. The canal is compressed laterally, so that it tends to become an antero-posterior slit. The normal posterior curve may be so exaggerated that it requires a coudé, bicoudé, or even a fully curved metal catheter to negotiate it. When one lateral lobe is enlarged predominantly, lateral distortion of the prostatic urethra occurs.

Bladder.—The musculature of the bladder hypertrophies to overcome the obstruction (fig. 1279). When the middle lobe projects upwards into the bladder it acts as a dam to the last ounce or more of urine, which remains in the post-prostatic pouch. Calculi are prone to form in this stagnant pool of urine.

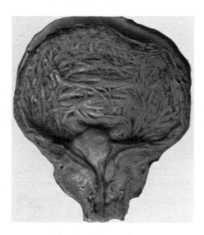

FIG. 1279.—Trabeculation of the bladder from prostatic obstruction. When viewed from within, bands of muscle fibres can be seen—*trabeculation*. Between these hypertrophied bundles there are shallow depressions, *i.e. sacculations*. Sometimes one of the saccules (rarely two or more) continues to enlarge, and forms a *diverticulum*.
(The late Professor K. A. L. Aschoff, Freiburg.)

The enlarged prostate may compress the prostatic venous plexus; the resulting congested veins (vesical 'piles') at the base of the bladder are apt to cause haematuria.

Unless the obstruction is relieved, a time is reached when bladder hypertrophy gives place to atony, the tired muscle making no attempt to overcome the obstruction.

Ureters and Kidneys.—Increasing intravesical pressure, or in some cases direct pressure of the intravesical portion of the prostate on the ureteric orifices, causes gradual dilation of the ureters, followed by some degree of bilateral hydronephrosis. When bladder hypertrophy wanes, the sphincter mechanism around the ureteric orifices ceases to function, permitting reflux of urine from the bladder into the dilated ureters, with increasing damage to the renal parenchyma. As a result of ascending infection, or more rarely from the blood-stream, acute or chronic pyelonephritis supervenes.

Sexual Organs.—In the early stages of prostatic enlargement there is increased libido. Later, impotence is the rule.

Clinical features are variable and depend upon the lobes affected. *Frequency* is the earliest symptom. At first it is nocturnal, the patient being obliged to get up to micturate twice or more during the night, usually commencing at 2 or 3 a.m. Frequent micturition at this stage is probably due to vesical introversion of the sensitive prostatic mucous membrane by the intravesical enlargement of the prostate. The frequency becomes progressive, and is then present both by night and by day. When the vesical sphincter becomes stretched, a little urine escapes into the normally empty prostatic urethra, causing an intense reflex desire to void, and *urgency* is added to the frequency. Later, as residual urine increases, frequency becomes more and more in evidence, and there is terminal dribbling. Finally, in neglected cases, frequency is further encouraged by cystitis, and polyuria due to renal insufficiency.

Difficulty in Micturition.—The patient notices that he must wait patiently for urination to start; it is useless to strain (cf. urethral stricture and fibrous prostate).

The stream is variable, often weak, tending to stop and start, and dribble towards the end of micturition.

Pain occurs with cystitis or acute retention of urine. When hydronephrosis commences there may be a dull pain in the loins. A feeling of weight in the perineum, or a fullness in the rectum, are occasional complaints.

Acute retention of urine is sometimes the first symptom to compel the patient to seek relief because of the intense pain it produces. The postponement of micturition is a common precipitating cause (*e.g.* a non-corridor train), as also is indulgence in alcoholic liquors, particularly when he goes out of doors on a cold night. Confinement to bed on account of some intercurrent illness or operation is another cause of acute retention of urine.

Retention with Overflow.—The patient complains that urine constantly dribbles away. Nocturnal enuresis should be a warning sign. It is exceptional for him to have noticed the swelling caused by the distended bladder and he experiences no pain.

Haematuria.—A drop of blood at the beginning or end of micturition is not unusual. Occasionally alarming haematuria occurs from a ruptured prostatic vein, or from an erosion on the enlarged prostate itself. Incrimination of an enlarged prostate as the source of haematuria before excluding other causes has resulted in the term 'decoy' prostate.

Renal Insufficiency.—The patient presents himself with signs of renal failure (Chapter 56).

Examination.—The patient lies on a couch and the abdomen is examined. In patients with a long history, varying degrees of chronic retention of urine will be found on palpation, percussion, and sometimes on inspection with loss of the transverse suprapubic skin crease. The renal areas are palpated for tenderness and possible enlargement of the kidneys. The state of the tongue is noted; a dry brown tongue and a urine of low specific gravity indicate a considerable degree of renal insufficiency. The external urinary meatus is examined to exclude stenosis, and the epididymes are palpated for signs of inflammation.

Rectal examination is carried out and, in the absence of a full bladder, bimanually in the dorsal position. In benign enlargement of the lateral lobes, increase in their size is evident. They are smooth, convex, and typically elastic, but the fibrous element may give the prostate a firm consistency. The rectal mucosa can be made to move over the prostate. On bimanual palpation an intravesical lobe can sometimes be felt. By exerting pressure on the apex of the prostate by the finger in the rectum, it will be found that a gland which is the seat of benign enlargement possesses a definite degree of mobility. Residual urine may be felt as a fluctuating swelling above the prostate. It should be noted that if there is a considerable amount of residual urine present, it pushes the prostate downwards, making it appear larger than it is.

When possible, the act of micturition should be watched. Loss of projectile power is significant. The urine is passed into two glasses; mere inspection of it is often helpful. It is later examined chemically, and a mid-stream specimen may be sent for bacteriological examination.

The nervous system is examined to eliminate a neurogenic lesion. Diabetes mellitus, tabes, disseminated sclerosis, cervical spondylosis, Parkinson's disease and other neurological states may give symptoms that mimic prostatic obstruction.

The Micturograph.—A graphic recording of a patient's stream rate and volume of urine can be obtained and is most helpful in determining the degree of outflow obstruction.

Examination of the Blood.—A blood urea estimation, a blood count, and a Wasserman reaction are all important, the first two being essential.

Examination of the Urine.—The urine should be examined for evidence of infection, and cultured and tested for the presence of glucose.

Intravenous Urography.—It has been the tradition to perform an intravenous urogram when investigating patients with bladder outflow obstruction. The plain film may show the presence of a calculus whether in the kidney or in the bladder. It will also show if there is degenerative disease of the lumbar spine and sometimes the characteristic features of a sclerotic bony metastasis from carcinoma of the prostate. The urogram itself may reveal evidence of hydronephrosis. It will show the contour of the bladder and whether trabeculation, sacculation or a diverticulum is present. A film after micturition may reveal a significant residual urine. In the presence of renal failure urography is unlikely to be helpful. With the progress made in the quality of ultrasound examination over the last few years much of this information can be obtained without the need for the intravenous injection of contrast and the exposure of the patient to radiation. However, a plain abdominal x-ray should never be omitted. Should doubt exist following ultrasound examination the topography of the urinary tract may then be demonstrated with a urogram.

Urodynamics.—When a clear diagnosis has not been reached or if neuropathy is suspected a urodynamic investigation can usually establish whether bladder outflow obstruction is present. Recordings of the residual volume, the intravesical pressure, the bladder capacity and the sensation of fullness can all be obtained quite simply. The voiding pressure and the flow rate should then be measured and if a video unit is available the bladder outlet can be visualised (p. 1267).

Cystourethroscopy.—Inspection of the urethra, the prostate and the urothelium of the bladder should always be made before prostatectomy whether it is being done transurethrally or by the open route, it being important to exclude the presence of a urethral stricture, a bladder carcinoma and the occasional non-radio opaque vesical calculus. The decision whether or not to perform a prostatectomy

---

August von Wassermann, 1866–1925. Director of the Kaiser Wilhelm Institute for Experimental Therapeutics, Berlin.

should usually have been made before the cystoscopy. This should be based on the patient's symptoms, signs and the results of the investigations. Direct inspection of the prostate itself is a poor indicator of bladder outflow obstruction and the need for surgery.

The Management of Retention

Acute urinary retention is distressing and painful. It requires decompression of the bladder by the passage of a urethral catheter. For patients with chronic urinary retention, which is painless, careful assessment is necessary; patients who do not have symptoms suggestive of co-existent infection and who have a normal serum creatinine do not necessarily require a catheter before proceeding with a prostatectomy. For those who are uraemic, decompression of the bladder is mandatory. Controversy exists over whether the bladder should be drained completely or decompressed slowly when dealing with chronic retention. Occasionally bleeding can occur from rapid decompression of a chronically over-distended bladder but regrettably the diligent management necessary for slow bladder decompression is often not exercised and the patient is left in a state of continuing retention under the misapprehension that good is being done. The use of a 'gate' clip is only to be condemned.

Uraemic patients with chronic retention are often dehydrated at the time of admission. Due to the chronic back pressure on the distal tubules within the kidney there is loss of their ability to reabsorb salt and water. The result, following release of this pressure, is an enormous outflow of salt and water which has become known as a post obstructive diuresis. It is for this reason that a careful fluid chart, daily measurements of the patient's weight and serial estimations of the urea and electrolytes are mandatory. Intravenous fluid replacement is required if the patient is unable to keep up with this fluid loss. It is indeed sad to see patients becoming increasing uraemic and dehydrated when this condition is poorly managed. These patients are usually anaemic and require a blood transfusion once the fluid balance is stabilised.

Catheterisation.—For catheterisation of the bladder the patient should be placed in a quiet and clean environment. The external genitalia should be carefully washed with a soap based antiseptic and strict adherence to aseptic technique needs to be employed. 1% Lignocaine hydrochloride with 0·25% chlorhexidine in a jelly base should be gently inserted into the urethra. This should then be held in place for several minutes allowing it to take effect. The catheter can then be gently advanced along the urethra with the penis being held taut and upright. A simple Jacques catheter may be used if drainage and catheter removal is all that is intended. More usually a catheter is left in situ; therefore a Foley catheter size 12 or 14F should be used and the self-retaining balloon inflated. There is no benefit gained from using a larger catheter unless blood clots are present. It will only increase the risk of irritation, urethritis and subsequent stricture formation. It is also preferable to only use a 5ml balloon to retain the catheter as larger volumes will increase the risk of the patient developing unpleasant bladder spasms caused by the detrusor contracting in an attempt to expel the foreign body. The catheter is then connected to a closed system drainage bag.

Suprapubic Puncture.—If a urethral catheter fails to pass into the bladder because of a urethral stricture, the creation of a false passage from clumsy instrumentation or regrettably so often poor technique, it is then safer to insert a small suprapubic tube than to risk further damage to the urethra (Chapter 60).

Indications for Operation

(1) *Prostatism.*—Increasing difficulty in micturition, with considerable frequency day and night, delay in starting, and a poor stream—such are the usual symptoms for which prostatectomy is advised. It must be stressed that *frequency alone* is never an indication for prostatectomy, and also that the natural progression of benign prostatic enlargement is variable and rarely gets worse after ten years. A patient with symptoms for nine years is unlikely to get much more severe symptoms, while a similar degree of symptoms reached in three years is a greater indication for surgery. This fact may be helpful when considering the correct advice to give to elderly patients possibly suffering from other disease.

(2) *Acute retention which is unrelieved* by passing a catheter, emptying the bladder, and immediately removing the catheter.[1]

(3) *Chronic Retention.*—A residual urine of 200 ml or more. A raised blood urea, hydroureter, or hydronephrosis demonstrated on urography, and uraemic manifestations.

(4) *Complications.*—Stone, infection, and diverticulum formation, which are often present in varying combinations.

(5) *Haemorrhage.*—Occasionally venous bleeding from a ruptured vein overlying the prostate will not stop with catheter drainage, so prostatectomy must be performed as an emergency measure.

Operative Treatment

Until the commencement of the present century the accepted treatment of prostatic obstruction was a catheter-life. The patient passed the instrument himself, often lubricating it with saliva. The more affluent sufferers carried their catheters in their top hats. Nearly 20% of all sufferers died within three months. Some of the remainder acquired partial immunity to recurring bouts of infection.

Nowadays a permanent catheter, either urethral or suprapubic, is a rarity. Prostatectomy, or more correctly the removal of the adenomatous hyperplasia, by one of the four routes, is practicable in the great majority of cases.

The prostate can be approached (1) through the bladder (transvesical), (2) retropubically, (3) from the perineum, or (4) trans(per)urethrally (fig. 1280).

Preliminary Vasectomy.—In the operations described, bilateral vasectomy may be performed. It prevents infection from the prostatic bed spreading to the epididymes. This minor procedure can be undertaken as a preliminary step, or at the conclusion of prostatectomy. With the improvement in aseptic procedure and the availability of broad spectrum antibiotics vasectomy is now rarely necessary. *Technique.*—Through a small incision over each superficial abdominal ring the vas deferens is isolated from the spermatic cord and a small piece resected, the ends being ligated with catgut.

Transurethral (Perurethral) Resection of the Prostate (T.U.R.P. (P.U.R.P.)) has largely replaced other methods unless diverticulectomy or the removal of large stones

---

[1] Wilson Hey recommended immediate prostatectomy as the treatment of choice in such patients who are usually fit, thus avoiding the dangers of infection by instrumentation and the increased liability to venous thrombosis if catheter drainage and bed-rest are instituted.

Wilson Harold Hey, 1882–1956. Surgeon, Royal Infirmary, Manchester, England.

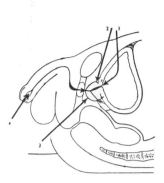

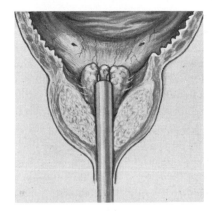

FIG. 1280.—The surgical approaches to the prostate.

FIG. 1281.—Transurethral resection showing the loop commencing to remove a strip from the middle lobe of the prostate.
(After R. M. Nesbit.)

necessitate open operation. The earlier instruments designed by McCarthy have been replaced by single hand operated instruments. Perhaps the greatest advance in the history of transurethral surgery is marked by the development of the rigid rod lens system by Professor Harold Hopkins. His lenses illuminated by a fibreoptic light source now permit unparallel visualisation of the working field.

Strips of tissue are cut from the bladderneck down to the level of the verumontanum. Cutting is established by a high frequency diathermy current which is applied across a loop mounted on the hand-held trigger of the resectoscope. Coagulation of bleeding points can be accurately achieved and damage to the external sphincter is avoided provided one uses the verumontanum as a guide to the most distal point of the resection. The 'chips' of prostate are then removed from the bladder using an Ellik evacuator. Hyponatraemia is avoided by using 1.5% isotonic glycine for irrigation and the recent introduction of continuous flow resectoscopes makes the procedure swift and safe in experienced hands. A three way self-retaining catheter irrigated with isotonic saline is then introduced into the bladder at the end of the procedure to prevent any further bleeding from forming blood clots. Irrigation is continued until the outflow is pale pink and the catheter usually removed on the third post-operative day.

After treatment

Following open operations practice varies concerning the need to irrigate the bladder. If good haemostasis is achieved a self-retaining catheter can be attached to a sterile drainage bag and 'washout' achieved with the use of intravenous fluids and the induction of a diuresis by the injection of frusemide. Care must always be executed when doing this as so many elderly gentlemen have compromised cardiac function and therefore run the risk of developing congestive cardiac failure if intravenous fluids are given too liberally.

It is perhaps safer to use a three way catheter thus allowing continuous irrigation to wash out any continuing blood loss.

If the urine is infected, or a catheter has been in situ for a number of days it is wise to cover the surgery with a broad spectrum antibiotic. Patients with valve disease of the heart, prostheses or grafts of foreign material should all be given antibiotics prophylactically (amoxycillin and gentamicin).

Complications

Local.—*Haemorrhage.*—Reactionary haemorrhage is the most tiresome complication following prostatectomy whatever the surgical approach. If the blood is not adequately washed out clot retention will ensue. In the recovery room one should check that the bladder is adequately decompressed, for the distended bladder and a catheter that is not draining indicate that a clot is blocking the eye of the catheter. This is the only indication for interruption of the closed drainage system. The bladder should be promptly washed out using strict aseptic technique. The catheter should never be changed except by the surgeon himself. Only rarely is it necessary to return the patient to the operating room.

Secondary haemorrhage tends to occur around the tenth post-operative day and is usually associated with the patient over-exerting himself or the presence of a urinary infection. If the bleeding is not severe and there are no clots the patient is simply advised to rest, encouraged to have a high fluid intake and is given a broad spectrum antibiotic. If clot retention occurs a catheter will have to be passed and the bladder washed out.

Perforation.—Perforation of the bladder or the prostatic capsule can occur at the time of transurethral surgery. This usually occurs in association with a large prostate or heavy blood loss. If the field of vision becomes obscured by heavy blood loss it is often prudent to achieve adequate haemostasis and abandon the operation, swallowing one's pride on the understanding that a second attempt may be necessary.

Infection.—Infection whether in the bladder, epididymis or the kidneys should be treated with the appropriate antibiotic. Wound infection following open prostatectomy is common if a urethral catheter has been in-situ for a number of days before the operation. Perhaps the most worrying aspect of infection is the early rigor following surgery. If left undetected and untreated this may progress to frank septicaemia with profound hypotension. A blood culture should be taken and powerful antibiotics given parenterally, e.g. gentamicin.

Incontinence.—Incontinence is inevitable if the external sphincter mechanism is damaged. The bladder neck is rendered incompetent by these operations and therefore an intact external mechanism is essential for continence. Damage to the sphincter may occur at open prostatectomy and following transurethral surgery if the resection extends beyond the verumontanum. The outcome for these patients is naturally disastrous. Urodynamic investigation has shown that not all of these patients with incontinence have sphincter damage. Some will have unstable bladders with inappropriate bladder contractions contributing to the incontinence. The use of powerful anticholinergic agents or imipramine may help.

Retrograde ejaculation and impotence.—All patients having a prostatectomy should be warned that they are likely to suffer from retrograde ejaculation; this occurs once the bladder neck is rendered incompetent. A proportion of men will also claim that the operation is the final insult on their already waning sex life.

Stricture.—Stricture may occur secondary to prolonged catheterisation, the use of an unnecessarily large catheter, clumsy instrumentation or secondary to the presence of the resectoscope in the urethra for too long a period. These strictures arise either just inside the meatus or in the bulbar urethra. An early stricture can usually be managed by simple bouginage but later on it may be necessary to cut the densely fibrotic stricture with the optical urethrotome. Many surgeons claim the routine use of an Otis urethrotomy reduces the incidence of post-operative stricture.

Bladder neck contracture.—Just occasionally a dense fibrotic stenosis of the bladder neck occurs following the resection of a small prostate. It may be due to the over use of the coagulating diathermy. Re-resection of the scar tissue is necessary.

General.—*Cardio-vascular.*—Pulmonary atelectasis, pneumonia, myocardial infarction, congestive cardiac failure, and deep venous thrombosis are all potentially life threatening conditions that can effect this elderly and often frail group of gentlemen. It is particularly for this group of complications that the transurethral route of surgery which saves the need for a painful abdominal scar and permits early ambulation, has proved of benefit.

Water intoxication.—The absorption of water into the circulation at the time of a transurethral resection can give rise to congestive cardiac failure, hyponatraemia and haemolysis. Accompanying this there is frequently confusion and other cerebral events often mimicking a stroke. The incidence of this condition has been reduced since the introduction of isotonic glycine for performing the resections and the use of isotonic saline for post-operative irrigation. The treatment consists of diuretics for the fluid overload and digoxin may be necessary. Cautious replacement of intravenous fluids should be with isotonic saline.

Osteitis pubis is rare. It is possibly due to pricking of the periosteum during operation, or to infection in the prevesical space. The symptoms do not appear until two or more weeks after the operation. There is pain and tenderness over the pubes, with inability to walk more than a few steps owing to painful spasms of the adductor muscles. An x-ray shows irregular rarefaction of the ischio-pubic rami and widening of the symphysis. This exceedingly painful state continues for many weeks. Spontaneous cure with recalcification of the rarefied bone occurs after several months.

Transvesical Prostatectomy.—The bladder is opened, the prostate enucleated by putting a finger into the urethra, pushing forwards towards the pubes to separate the lateral lobes, and then working the finger between the adenoma and the false capsule. In **Freyer's operation** (1901) the bladder was left open widely and drained by a suprapubic tube with a 16-mm lumen, in order to allow free drainage of blood and urine. **Harris** (1934) advocated control of the prostatic arteries by lateral stitches inserted with his boomerang needle (figs. 1282 and 1283), and closure of the raw areas by stitching the mucosa of the posterior

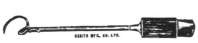

FIG. 1282.—A boomerang needle.   FIG. 1283.—Harris's ligature carrier.

lip of the internal meatus to the urethral mucosa, and narrowing the cavity with stitches in front of the urethral catheter which was left in to drain the bladder. The bladder wall was left completely closed and the wound drained. **Wilson Hey** (1944) also advocated a transvesical prostatectomy, stressing the importance of careful asepsis in this as in any other surgery. The catheter for drainage was passed retrogradely to avoid carrying urethral organisms up into the raw prostatic cavity. Mass ligatures of tissue for haemostasis was replaced by careful diathermy of bleeding points with insulated haemostats. Careful closure of the bladder enabled the urethral catheter to be removed on the fourth day.

Retropubic Prostatectomy (Millin, 1945).—Using a low, curved transverse suprapubic incision, which includes the rectus sheath, the recti are retracted to expose the bladder with its typical appearance of pale brown muscle bundles with a loose covering of fatty tissue and veins. With the patient in the Trendelenburg position the surgeon separates the bladder and the prostate from the posterior aspect of the pubis. In the space thus obtained the anterior capsule of the prostate is incised with diathermy below the bladder neck, care being taken to obtain complete control of bleeding from divided prostatic veins. The prostatic adenoma is exposed and enucleated with a finger. A wedge is taken out of

Sir Peter Johnston Freyer, 1852–1921. Surgeon, St. Peter's Hospital for Stone, London.
Samuel Harry Harris, 1881–1937. Urologist, Lewisham Hospital, Sydney, Australia.
Terence John Millin, 1903–1980. Surgeon, Westminster Hospital, London.

the posterior lip of the bladder neck to prevent secondary stricture in this region. The exposure of the inside of the prostatic cavity is good, and control of haemorrhage is achieved with diathermy and stitching before closure of the capsule over a Porges catheter (inserted per urethram) draining the bladder.

Perineal Prostatectomy (Young).—A ∧-shaped incision is made in the perineum in front of the anus. The rectum is retracted backwards to expose the posterior aspect of the prostate above the triangular ligament. This is incised and the adenoma enucleated. This operation is not popular in Britain because of the incidence of incontinence.

CONTRACTURE OF THE BLADDER NECK

Aetiology.—The condition occurs in children of both sexes and in women as well as men. It may be due to a congenital muscular hypertrophy, or fibrosis of the tissues at the bladder neck (and is then an aftermath of chronic prostatitis in men, or urethro-trigonitis in women). The former cause may give rise to symptoms at any age, usually in young children or early adult life, the latter cause after the age of forty-five.

Clinical Syndromes:

(a) *Due to Muscle Hypertrophy.*—Marion described a series of cases in which muscular hypertrophy of the internal sphincter in a young person had resulted in the development of a vesical diverticulum *or* hydronephrosis (Marion's Disease, or *prostatism sans prostate*). Milder degrees of obstruction can occur without the development of these secondary effects. These patients have difficulty in micturition or may present with recurrent urinary infections.

A severe degree of obstruction produces symptoms at birth or in early childhood. A distended bladder may be visible or easily felt. Many cases develop urinary infection. Ureteric reflux of urine associated with high intravesical pressure during micturition leads to loin pain and severe pyelonephritis with gross scarring and contraction of the renal cortex.

(b) *Due to Fibrosis.*—The symptoms are similar to those of prostatic enlargement, but straining helps to expel the urine, and as a consequence an inguinal hernia may develop. There is no prostatic enlargement. Secondary effects of the obstruction are in all respects similar to those seen in prostatic enlargement. Contracture of the bladder neck is the most common cause of a diverticulum of the bladder.

Treatment

The management of these patients depends on achieving an accurate diagnosis. For this a urodynamic investigation is often necessary. Some of the men will have features of obstruction with raised intravesical pressure and diminished flow rate, yet in others the intravesical pressure may be low, with a poor bladder contraction.

Drugs.—The demonstration of alpha adrenergic receptors in the region of the bladder neck allows pharmacological manipulation of the outflow to the bladder. Alpha blocking drugs (phenoxybenzamine) can be very useful, causing relaxation of the bladder neck. One has to remember that these drugs are not target specific and the patients must be warned of the possibility of postural hypotension.

Porges. Surgical Instrument Manufacturers, Paris, France.
Hugh Hampton Young, 1870–1945. Director, James Buchanan Brady Urological Institute, Baltimore, Maryland. U.S.A.
Jean Baptiste Camille Georges Marion, 1869–1960. Professor of Urology, Faculty of Medicine, Paris.

Dilatation.—Just occasionally temporary benfit can be achieved following the passage of a urethral sound.

Transurethral resection.—Transurethral resection of the bladder neck or bladder neck incision are the operations of choice. Sometimes symptoms recur but this is usually due to inadequate division of the fibres of the bladder neck. It is now uncommon to have to resort to the open procedures that so many young people were subjected to over the last two or three decades.

Open Operation.—The principle of open operative treatments, like that of Johanson's operation for urethral stricture (Chapter 60), is to establish in the strictured portion of the canal one part of the circumference that is non-fibrotic and pliant.

Sphincteroplasty is conducted through a retropubic incision.

Bonnin's operation is suitable for adult male patients. A V-shaped flap in the bladder (muscle and mucosa) is introduced into the anterior aspect of the vesical outlet, and the steps of the operation are shown in fig. 1284. When severe vesical atony is present, which is usual in cases of some standing, it is desirable to resect a large portion of the bladder. This is accomplished by mobilising the antero-superior aspect of the bladder before incising it. To have the viscus well distended is most important.

Congenital Valves of the Prostatic Urethra (Chapter 60).

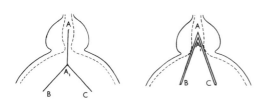

FIG. 1284.—Bonnin's operation for contracture of the bladder neck in the male.

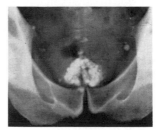

FIG. 1285.—Endogenous prostatic calculi.

PROSTATIC CALCULI

Prostatic calculi are of two varieties—endogenous, which are common, and exogenous, which are comparatively rare.

An *exogenous* prostatic calculus is a urinary (commonly ureteric) calculus that becomes arrested in the prostatic urethra. This is considered in Chapter 60.

Endogenous prostatic calculi are usually composed of calcium phosphate combined with about 20% of organic material.

Clinical Features.—Quite often prostatic calculi are symptomless, being discovered on radiography of the pelvis, during prostatectomy, or associated with carcinoma of the prostate or chronic prostatitis. The symptoms vary in severity and are at first those of chronic prostatitis, or of prostatic obstruction. On rectal examination it is difficult to differentiate from carcinoma. On x-ray these stones often form a horseshoe (fig. 1285) or a circle.

Treatment of Prostatic Calculi

Conservative Measures.—When the calculi are small and the symptoms are mild, the treatment of chronic prostatitis by a course of sulphonamide may keep the patient free from symptoms for months at a time.

Transurethral resection of the fibrous prostate will release small calculi as the strips of prostatic tissue are excised, and many more are removed by the irrigation inseparable from transurethral resection. Others are passed per urethram at a later date.

Noel James Bonnin, Contemporary. Surgeon, Queen Elizabeth Hospital, Adelaide, Australia.

Retropubic Prostato-lithotomy.—After incising the capsule of the prostate, the incision is deepened until the prostatic urethra is opened. Using a sharp curette, all the calculi and as much as possible of the infected prostatic tissue is removed. The bladder neck is then exposed, and a generous wedge of the posterior lip is resected with curved scissors. The operation is concluded in a manner similar to that of retropubic prostatectomy. Total prostatectomy may be necessary in cases where there are frequent acute exacerbations of a chronic prostatitis.

Corpora amylaceae

Corpora amylaceae are found in the prostates of elderly men and apes, but not in the prostates of animals lower in the phylogenetic scale than anthropoids. Corpora amylaceae occur also in the homologue of the prostate—the tubules of the bladder neck of women (Skene's tubules). These bodies consist of amorphous debris and desquamated epithelium. Often an intact epithelial wall of a prostatic duct forms their outer coat. They are always deeply pigmented, and are variously described as like poppy seeds, black pepper, or coal dust. Neither the composition nor the origin of the pigment is known. Probably corpora amylaceae are the forerunners of endogenous prostatic calculi.

CARCINOMA OF THE PROSTATE

Carcinoma of the prostate is the commonest malignant condition in men over the age of sixty-five years. About 20% of cases of prostatic obstruction prove to be due to carcinoma, to which must be added a substantial number in whom the first and main symptoms are due to metastases. The incidence of carcinoma of the prostate has been increasing, due to an increasingly ageing population as well as to improved methods of diagnosis. It is less common in the Japanese while its incidence is higher and its behaviour more aggressive in American negroes compared with the Caucasian population. Carcinoma of the prostate usually originates in the external group of glands (fig. 1277), so 'prostatectomy' for benign enlargement of the gland confers little protection from the subsequent development of carcinoma.

Latent Carcinoma of the Prostate.—Serial sections of prostates obtained at routine necropsy has revealed carcinoma in that organ in no less than 15% of men over fifty years of age. True, many of these neoplasms are tiny and (if life had continued) might have remained latent for years. In men over ninety years of age, over three-quarters of the prostates are involved (Franks).

Histological Appearance.—The prostate is a glandular structure consisting of ducts and acini; therefore the histological pattern is one of an adenocarcinoma. The prostatic glands are surrounded by a layer of myoepithelial cells. The first change associated with carcinoma is the loss of this layer with the glands appearing in confluence. As the cell type becomes less differentiated more solid sheets of carcinoma cells are seen. A classification of the histological pattern based on the degree of glandular dedifferentiation and its relation to the prostatic stroma has been devised by Gleeson; this appears to correlate with the likelihood of spread and so of prognosis.

Local Spread.—A growth *commencing in the posterior zone of the gland* is prevented (at least temporarily) from extending backwards by the strong fascia of Denonvilliers. Consequently it tends to grow upwards to involve the seminal vesicles. Further upward extension obstructs the lower end of one or both ureters, the latter terminating in anuria. Carcinoma *commencing in a lateral lobe* involves the prostatic urethra early: in advanced cases the base of the bladder is invaded.

Leonard Maurice Franks, Contemporary. Research Pathologist, Imperial Cancer Research Fund, Royal College of Surgeons of England, London.
Donald F. Gleeson, Contemporary. Pathologist, V.A. Hospital, Minneapolis, Minnesota. U.S.A.

The rectum may become stenosed by growth infiltrating round it, but direct involvement is very late, and the mucosa does not ulcerate unless traumatised, *e.g.* by transrectal biopsy.

Spread by the blood-stream occurs particularly to bones; indeed, the prostate is the most common site of origin for skeletal metastases, being followed in turn by the breasts, the kidneys, the bronchial tree, and the thyroid gland. The bones involved most frequently by metastases of carcinoma of the prostate are the pelvic bones and the lower lumbar vertebrae. Femoral head, rib cage and skull are other favoured sites. The frequent proximity of skeletal metastases to the primary growth has been attributed to reversed flow from the vesical venous plexus to the emissary veins of the pelvic bones during coughing, sneezing, *etc.*

Lymphatic Spread.—(*a*) Via lymphatic vessels passing along the sides of the rectum to the lymph nodes along the internal iliac vein and in the hollow of the sacrum. (*b*) Via lymphatics which pass over the seminal vesicles and follow the vas deferens for a short distance to drain into the external iliac lymph nodes. From both these situations the retroperitoneal lymph nodes, later the mediastinal nodes, and occasionally the supraclavicular lymph nodes, become implicated.

Clinical Features.—Carcinoma of the prostate occurs in the older man. Incontinence, a short history of up to six months, and pain on micturition are suggestive features of carcinoma in a patient with a history of prostatism.

Type 1.—Discovered only on histological examination of tissue removed at prostatectomy.

Type 2.—Rectal findings of a hard nodule or extension outside the capsule; investigated by perineal biopsy (see below) (fig. 1287).

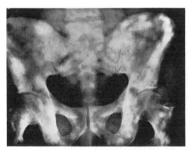

FIG. 1286.—Osseous metastases of the pelvic bones in carcinoma of the prostate.
(*L. N. Pyrah, FRCS, Leeds.*)

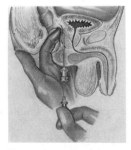

FIG. 1287.—Obtaining a specimen of prostatic tissue by means of Turkel's needle.

Type 3.—The primary may be tiny and occult, the patient presenting with 'rheumatism' or 'arthritis', with blood acid phosphatase levels often very high. Urinary symptoms are absent or slight.

Type 4.—Pain in the back, or sciatica, is the main symptom. Bilateral sciatica in an elderly man is most often due to metastases in the spine from carcinoma of the prostate. Oedema of one or both legs, paraplegia, or a spontaneous fracture are occasionally due to metastases from a carcinoma of the prostate. Anaemia may be the presenting symptom.

Eric Francis Turkel, Contemporary. Urological Surgeon, Pomona Valley Community Hospital, Pomona, California, U.S.A.

On account of destruction of bone marrow, bone metastases from carcinoma of the prostate can give rise to a haemorrhagic diathesis, and the patient suffers haemorrhage, often severe, not necessarily from the urinary tract.

Rectal Examination.—Bimanual examination under anaesthesia, together with cystoscopy and needle biopsy are essential in order to asses the local stage of growth. Irregular induration, characteristically stony hard in part or in the whole of the gland—with obliteration of the median sulcus suggests carcinoma. Extension beyond the capsule up into the bladder base and vesicles is diagnostic, as is deformity and projection outwards of the capsule.

T.N.M. Classification
  Tumour:

    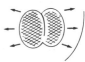

To. Clinically unsuspected   T1. Local nodule   T2. Diffuse or deforming capsule   T3. Outside capsule or extension into vesicle   T4. Fixed to other tissue

Nodes: No = No evidence of involvement of regional nodes.
      N1 = Involvement of one regional node.
      N2 = Involvement of several regional nodes.
      N3 = Fixed mass of regional nodes.
      N4 = Involvement of common iliac or para-aortic nodes.
Metastases: Mo = No evidence of distant metastases.
      M1 = Distant metastases.

Blood Tests.—It seems hardly necessary to justify measuring the haemoglobin. There may be leucoerythroblastic anaemia secondary to extensive marrow invasion or anaemia may be secondary to renal failure. When metastases are present, it is also worthwhile doing a platelet count as this is sometimes reduced. Basic tests of renal function are necessary because hydronephrosis may exist from chronic bladder outflow obstruction or from direct invasion of one or both of the ureters by the cancer.

Liver Function Tests.—These will be abnormal if there is extensive metastatic invasion of the liver. The alkaline phosphatase may be raised from either hepatic involvement or from secondaries in the bone. One can differentiate the source by measuring either iso-enzymes or gamma glutamyl transferase.

Acid Phosphatase.—Measurements of acid phosphatase have not been easy. Currently the prostatic fraction can be measured either by an enzyme technique or a radio-immuno assay. A raised value is strongly suggestive of prostate cancer but it is not a good screening test. 20% of patients with metastases will have a normal value. Currently its most important application is for following the pattern of disease when looking for a response to treatment. Serial estimations are also proving helpful to indicate relapse.

Radiological.—X-ray of the chest may reveal metastases either in the lung fields or the ribs. An abdominal x-ray may show the characteristic sclerotic metastases that occur only too commonly in the lumbar vertebrae and pelvic bones (fig. 1286). These metastases which are predominantly osteoblastic are quite unlike any others. The bone appears dense and coarse and sometimes difficulty is found distinguishing the change from that in Paget's disease of bone. Information will be required about the upper urinary tracts and this can be obtained either by excretion urography or by ultrasound of the kidneys and upper ureters.

Bone Scan.—Once the diagnosis has been established it would be normal to perform a bone scan as part of the staging procedure. This is achieved by the injection of 99 TC (Technetium), the isotope is then monitored using a gamma camera. It is important to remember that it is the distribution of the 'hotspots' that is important, as the isotope will go to any area of increased blood flow, *e.g.* arthritis, osteomyelitis, a healing fracture. Therefore if the hotspots are in the elbow and shoulder some sort of arthropathy is most likely whereas if they are in the ribs, the skull, the spine (in the absence of long-standing disc trouble) and the pelvic bones then metastases are far more likely.

Lymphangiography.—Assessment of the lymph nodes in the pelvis can be performed by lymphangiography. This is not a particularly easy test to perform and the results on the whole have proved disappointing. Certainly when one compares radiological evidence of disease with specimens removed at lymph node dissection there is a 30% inaccuracy in diagnosing involved nodes.

Bone Marrow Aspiration.—Sometimes examination of the bone marrow will reveal the presence of metastatic carcinoma cells. There has been a vogue for also measuring bone marrow acid phosphatase although its applicability in the clinical setting has yet to be established.

TREATMENT OF CARCINOMA OF THE PROSTATE ·

Surgery

Having had one's suspicions aroused the next question in one's mind should be; 'Is there significant bladder outflow obstruction?' If the answer is 'No', only trucut biopsy of the prostate is indicated to establish the diagnosis (fig. 1287). In the presence of outflow obstruction a transurethral resection should be performed. This will not only give material for diagnosis but should provide satisfactory symptomatic relief. This of course may not remove all the local cancer and it may be appropriate if the bone scan is normal to perform a 'second look TUR'.

Radical prostatectomy.—It has been the vogue particularly in the U.S.A. to perform radical prostatectomy for localised disease. This is a major surgical procedure which only too commonly results in total urinary incontinence and loss of potency. More recently, devices have been implanted to help the incontinence and Walsh has lately described a modification of the operation preserving the nerves responsible for erection.

Pelvic lymph node dissection and I¹³¹ seed implantation.—Many surgeons, again in the U.S.A., disillusioned by the complications of radical prostatectomy have chosen to implant radioactive iodine seeds into the prostate. A pelvic lymph node dissection with frozen section examination is performed. I¹³¹ seeds are then implanted into the prostate assuming the nodes are free of tumour. This technique delivers a high dose of radiotherapy with low penetration.

Orchidectomy.—In 1941 Huggins and Hodges described how prostate cancer could be responsive to a hormone change. Bilateral orchidectomy whether total or subcapsular will eliminate the major source of testosterone production.

Patrick C. Walsh, Contemporary. Professor of Urology, Johns Hopkins Hospital, Baltimore, Maryland, U.S.A.

Hypophysectomy and adrenalectomy.—In the past patients who had initially responded to hormone treatment but subsequently relapsed were thought to have a small chance of obtaining further relief if a hypophysectomy was performed. Fortunately this can now be done using drugs, thus saving the need for this unpleasant procedure.

Radiotherapy

Local.—Radical radiotherapy to the prostatic bed and pelvic lymph nodes has tended to be the treatment of choice in the United Kingdom rather than radical surgery. The treatment requires the patient to attend hospital on a daily basis for between four and six weeks. Some local complications are inevitable, namely irritation of the bladder, with urinary frequency, urgency and sometimes urge incontinence. There is often some upset to the rectum with diarrhoea and occasionally late radiation proctitis. The urinary frequency usually subsides a couple of months after the treatment although just occasionally continues to be a source of distress.

General.—Radiotherapy for symptomatic metastases is an excellent form of treatment often producing dramatic pain relief. More recently, interest has been shown in half body and now whole body irradiation but the place of this form of treatment has yet to be fully evaluated.

Drug Treatment

Hormonal.—Since the discovery that approximately two-thirds of patients with symptomatic disease will get relief of their symptoms whilst taking stilboestrol or following castration, there inevitably was great enthusiasm for this treatment. Patients were given stilboestrol in large doses whether orally or as a preparation called Honvan, (phosphorylated diethylstilboestrol), which can be given intravenously. Physicians accepted that gynaecomastia, loss of libido leading to impotence and some nausea were inevitable. Regrettably they lost sight of the other side effects, namely salt and water retention and an increased tendency to thrombosis. The result was these poor old men developed heart failure, became hypertensive, developed cerebrovascular accidents, had myocardial infarctions and deep venous thromboses. It seemed far too long before the lesson was learnt and the dose of stilboestrol was reduced to 1mg three times a day. Even on this dose complications can occur.

Other hormones that have been tried include the progestagens, and Provera has been shown to be of value. More recently cyproterone acetate has been introduced. Currently, interest has been shown in the use of aminoglutethimide which inhibits androgen production and Flutemide which interferes with androgen metabolism. Whether they will prove to have special advantages is at present uncertain. The most recent interest is in the LH RH analogues which cause suppression of testosterone at the level of the pituitary and therefore will hopefully avoid the unpleasant complications experienced with stilboestrol.

If hormone treatment is to be instituted gynaecomastia is inevitable. This is usually painful and it is possible to prevent the pain by giving a small dose of radiotherapy to the breast area. It does not prevent the swelling.

Cytotoxic.—Cytotoxic chemotherapy may be given using a single agent, combination of agents or the ingenious combination of oestrogen to a cytotoxic agent (Nitrogen Mustard-Estracyt). On the whole this approach has been disappointing.

Summary of Treatment. The patients seem to fall into three categories. (1) Incidentally diagnosed disease. (2) Localised disease. (3) Metastatic disease.

(1) *Incidentally diagnosed disease.* There is good evidence that the unsuspected cancer is being diagnosed with increasing frequency. *The majority of these patients do not exhibit disease progression and therefore these patients do not necessarily require any specific therapy other than a 'wait and watch' policy.* Unfortunately in a small proportion, the disease will progress but at present there is no way of detecting who they will be.

(2) *Localised disease.* This has been treated by radical prostatectomy, radical radiotherapy and transurethral resection with hormone therapy. In large well documented series a third of the patients survived fifteen years whichever treatment was chosen. Close inspection of some of this data suggests that the patients may have fared as well without any treatment at all. This is a hard policy to adopt. Complications are treated appropriately.

(3) *Metastatic disease.* Once metastases have developed the outlook is poor. For patients with symptoms there is no dilemma; hormonal manipulation of one's choice will provide symptomatic relief in over two-thirds of the patients. For the patient with asymptomatic metastases the need for treatment is less clear and still remains unanswered.

There are few hard and fast rules in the treatment of this cancer. The surgeon should be aware of all the possibilities for treating these patients but must be even more acutely sensitive to the side affects that they produce. It behoves one not to make the patients worse, through complications of treatment, than the disease process would have caused in its own right.

PROSTATITIS

In both acute and chronic prostatitis the seminal vesicles are usually infected, and when, as is often the case, the prostatic urethra is involved also, there is present a triad of pathological conditions, namely: posterior urethritis, prostatitis, and seminal vesiculitis. Symptoms due to infection of any one of these structures may predominate.

Acute Prostatitis

Aetiology.—Acute prostatitis is common.—The usual organism responsible is *Esch. coli*, but *Staphylococcus aureus* and *albus, Streptococcus faecalis*, and the *gonococcus* may be responsible. As a rule the infection is haematogenous from a distant focus, notably furunculosis, infected tonsils, carious teeth, or diverticulitis. In a minority of cases the infection ascends from the urethra or descends from the bladder or kidneys.

Clinical Features.—Infection in most cases seems to be blood-borne, as general manifestations overshadow the local: the patient feels ill, shivers, may have a rigor, has 'aches' all over, especially the back, and may easily be diagnosed as having influenza. The temperature may be up to 39°C. Pain on micturition is usual, but not invariable. The urine always contains threads in the first glass, and it is this initial specimen of urine which should be cultured. Perineal heaviness, rectal irritation and pain on defaecation can occur, and sitting may be uncomfortable. A urethral discharge is rare. Frequency occurs when the infection spreads up to the bladder. Rectal examination reveals a tender prostate, one lobe may be swollen more than the other, and the seminal vesicles may be involved. A frankly fluctuant abscess is uncommon.

Treatment.—Must be rigorous and prolonged or the infection will not be eradicated and recurrent attacks will ensue. Unless treated early, spread of the infection to the epididymes and testes is common. While awaiting the results of culture of the initial and a midstream specimen of urine, the patient is put to bed, given copious fluids, and started on a broad spectrum antibiotic. As soon as the culture result is available the most suitable drug can be chosen and continued for ten days. It should be followed by a month's treatment with one or two other drugs to which the organisms are sensitive. Avoidance of alcohol and sexual intercourse for six weeks is wise.

Prostatic Abscess.—In addition to the foregoing symptoms and signs, the advent of a prostatic abscess is heralded by the temperature rising steeply, rigors being not unusual. However, antibiotics disguise these leading features. Severe, unremitting perineal and rectal pain with occasional tenesmus often cause the condition to be confused with an anorectal abscess. Nevertheless, if a rectal examination is performed, the prostate will be felt to be enlarged, hot, extremely tender, and perhaps softened in one place. Retention of urine is likely to occur.

Treatment.—The abscess should be drained without delay. It is true that if a catheter is passed to relieve acute retention of urine, sometimes the abscess is ruptured into the prostatic urethra. However, in most cases such drainage is insufficient, and is followed by intractable chronic prostatitis or a residual abscess.

(a) The abscess can be drained by perurethral resection—unroofing the whole cavity.

(b) The perineal route is preferable when there is marked peri-prostatic spread.

Chronic Prostatitis

Aetiology.—This is a sequel of inadequately treated acute prostatitis. While pus is present in the prostatic secretion, often the responsible organism is difficult to find. Smears show bacteria in about 40% and cultures are positive in 70% of cases. The predominant organisms are E. coli, staphylococci, streptococci, and diphtheroids, in that order. Trichomonas has been found to be a cause of chronic prostatitis and may be common to both husband and wife. Clamydia is now believed to be the causative organism in many cases.

Pathology.—The lumina of the ducts become blocked with epithelial debris and pus. This causes a soft enlargement of the organ. Later fibrosis occurs, and the prostate becomes smaller and harder.

Clinical features are extremely varied.

1. Causing Chronic Posterior Urethritis.—Prostatitis should not be diagnosed unless, after irrigating the urethra and massaging the prostate, the resultant specimen shows fifteen or more pus cells per high power field.

2. Causing Epididymitis.—Acute or subacute non-tuberculous epididymitis rarely occurs unless prostatitis is present.

3. Pain: (a) Local pain is a dull ache in the perineum or rectum. It is increased

by sitting on a hard chair. (*b*) *Referred* Pain.—Particularly common is low back pain, sometimes extending down the legs; such pain is usually attributed to lumbago, and many sufferers from prostatitis receive orthopaedic treatment and physiotherapy without benefit.

4. *'Silent' Prostatitis.*—Arthritis, myositis, neuritis, and sometimes iritis and conjunctivitis are on occasions explained only when pus has been obtained from the prostate (see diagnosis).

5. *Recurring attacks of mild pyrexia*, lasting about three days and accompanied by malaise.

6. *Sexual Dysfunction.*—Premature ejaculations, prostatorrhoea, and impotence are sometimes due to prostatitis. Many patients with sexual dysfunction due to chronic prostatis become hypochondriacal.

Diagnosis: (*a*) *A three-glass urine test* is valuable. If the first glass shows urine containing prostatic threads, prostatitis is present.

(*b*) *Rectal examination* of the prostate may or may not confirm the diagnosis. If the organ is soft and boggy, it is obviously abnormal, as also it is if the prostate is smaller and harder than it should be. In mild chronic cases no change can be detected, and reliance must be placed on pathological examinations of the prostatic fluid.

(*c*) *Examination of the prostatic fluid* obtained by prostatic massage. Normal prostatic fluid is slightly opalescent and viscid. A stained specimen shows many pus cells and sometimes bacteria. Non-stained films, in addition to revealing normal epithelial cells, may show trichomonads, if present.

(*d*) *Urethroscopy* reveals inflammation of the prostatic urethra, and pus may be seen exuding from the prostatic ducts. The verumontanum is likely to be enlarged and oedematous.

Treatment.—*Antibiotic therapy* must be administered in accordance with bacteriological sensitivity tests. The blunderbuss administration of antibiotics in this condition is to be deprecated. It seems that the combination of trimethoprim and sulfamethoxazole (Septrin) is the most effective antibiotic. Where trichomonas is the responsible agent, a rapid response is obtained from administration of Flagyl (metronidazole) 200 mg by mouth three times daily, after meals, for seven days to both partners.

TUBERCULOSIS OF THE PROSTATE AND SEMINAL VESICLES

Tuberculosis of the prostate and seminal vesicles is associated with renal tuberculosis in at least 60% of cases. In 30% of cases there is a history of pulmonary tuberculosis within five years of the onset of genital tuberculosis.

Tuberculosis of one or both seminal vesicles is more common than tuberculosis of the prostate, and is often discovered when examining a patient with chronic tuberculous epididymitis, there being no symptoms referable to the internal genitalia. On rectal examination the affected vesicle is found to be nodular and tender. In process of time tuberculous seminal vesiculitis may lead to congestion and oedema of the base of the bladder, and later to basal cystitis.

When the Prostate is Involved.—Rectal examination reveals characteristically one or more well-defined nodules, most often near the upper or lower border of one or both lateral lobes. Less frequently a larger solitary mass is felt occupying a more central position. Nodules in the prostate lack the stony hardness of carcinoma.

A patient with tuberculous prostatitis usually presents with one or more of the following symptoms:

A urethral discharge is occasionally the first symptom. Then the diagnosis has to be made from gonorrhoea and abacterial urethritis entirely on bacteriological findings, for the prostate at this early stage is likely to feel normal.

Painful, sometimes blood-stained, ejaculations occur in 20% of cases.

A mild ache in the perineum is not uncommon.

Infertility.—In patients with tuberculous prostatitis and/or bilateral seminal vesiculitis, fertility is very much reduced; it is safe to say that 80% are sterile. In this connection, owing to the considerable interest in male fertility at the present time, a number of very early cases of tuberculous prostato-vesiculitis are being discovered by culture of the semen.

Urinary Symptoms.—In later cases, when the posterior urethra becomes involved from extension of tubercules from the prostate or by the discharge of a prostatic abscess, there is painful, frequent micturition and sometimes terminal haematuria.

Abscess Formation.—If a cold abscess forms in the prostate, it is felt as a slightly tender, soft swelling. Like other prostatic abscesses, it usually ruptures into the urethra, more rarely through the perineum or into the rectum. Occasionally an abscess of the prostate or seminal vesicle bursts into the bladder, and at cystoscopy a ragged, deep ulcer is seen alongside the trigone.

Special Forms of Investigation:

Even in cases without urinary symptoms a complete urological examination is necessary.

Radiography sometimes displays areas of calcification in the prostate and/or the seminal vesicles. Large scattered areas of calcification in the prostate suggest tuberculosis rather than endogenous prostatic calculi.

Bacteriological examination of the seminal fluid yields positive cultures for tubercle bacilli in most cases of tuberculous prostatitis.

Posterior urethrography often reveals one or more dilated prostatic ducts. Typically they are multiple and gaping. Dilated prostatic ducts are not specific for tuberculosis (they can occur in other forms of chronic prostatitis), but dilated ducts plus the findings of tubercle bacilli in the ejaculate establishes an absolute diagnosis.

Transmission of genital tuberculosis to the female partner is exceptional, but it does occasionally occur in the form of tuberculous cervicitis.

Treatment.—The general treatment given is as for tuberculosis (Chapter 4). On no account must a tuberculous prostate or seminal vesicle be subjected to massage. Urethral instrumentation should be avoided, or reduced to a minimum only to confirm the diagnosis.

If a prostatic abscess forms, it is better to evacuate it by the perineal route than to permit it to rupture spontaneously.

Considerable involvement of the prostate, which goes on to suppuration, is a comparatively unfavourable form of genito-urinary tuberculosis. On the other hand, tuberculous seminal vesiculitis and non-suppurative tuberculosis of the prostate usually heal after an associated lesion of the kidney or epididymis has been eradicated, but stricture of the prostatic urethra may occur.

AFFECTIONS OF THE SEMINAL VESICLES

Acute seminal vesiculitis always occurs in association with prostatitis. Prior to the antibiotic treatment of gonorrhoea, gonococcal vesiculitis was common. When a seminal vesicle is distended it can be palpated per rectum as an acutely tender swelling above and lateral to the prostate. The treatment is discussed in Chapter 60.

Abscess of a Seminal Vesicle.—In addition to the usual signs of acute prostatitis, pain is frequently referred to the suprapubic region. If on rectal examination the seminal vesicle is found to be greatly enlarged and tender, the abscess should be drained through an incision in the perineum. The incision is deepened until the swelling is palpated, and a haemostat is then thrust into the abscess cavity.

Chronic seminal vesiculitis is less frequently recognised than it should be, because the associated chronic prostatitis overshadows the symptoms of pain on coitus, haemospermia, aching in the sacral region, recurrent epididymitis, and, at times, associated disturbances of micturition and defaecation. The treatment is the same as for chronic prostatitis, except that in rebellious cases vasotomy and irrigation of the vesicle with isotonic saline is often rapidly curative.

Tuberculous Seminal Vesiculitis.—The clinical features and treatment have been discussed above.

Diverticulum of the seminal vesicle occurs occasionally. In such cases the kidney of that side is often absent, and the diverticulum represents an abortive ureteric bud. It is a cause of persistent infection of the urethra.

A cyst of the seminal vesicle is uncommon. It should be removed by dissection through an incision similar to that for perineal prostatectomy.

AFFECTIONS OF COWPER'S GLANDS

Cowperitis.—The diagnosis of Cowperitis is often wanting for lack of a simple examination. On passing the forefinger into the rectum and placing the thumb first on one side and then on the other of the median raphé of the perineum, Cowper's glands can be palpated. In acute cases the least pressure causes excruciating pain. In this way the condition is differentiated from an ischio-rectal or periurethral abscess. **Treatment.**—In acute cases antibiotic therapy, and rest in bed, often brings about resolution. Should suppuration occur, incision and drainage is necessary.

Fistula formation is the result of an abscess of the gland terminating in spontaneous rupture; it is necessary to excise the fistula and the remnants of the gland.

A cyst of Cowper's gland either bulges into the urethra and causes disturbances of micturition, or gives rise to a unilateral swelling in the anterior part of the perineum. The cyst should be excised.

William Cowper, 1666–1709. Surgeon and Anatomist, London.

CHAPTER 60

THE URETHRA AND PENIS

THE MALE URETHRA

CONGENITAL ABNORMALITIES OF THE URETHRA

Meatal Stenosis.—The external urinary meatus, normally the narrowest part of the male urethra, is occasionally the seat of congenital stenosis which is associated with phimosis. In the circumcised, meatal stenosis may also be acquired or increased by fibrosis following meatal ulceration. All degrees of narrowing are encountered. When the opening is reduced to a pin-hole, back-pressure affects the whole urinary system. Pin-hole meatus is occasionally a cause of enuresis, and at any age it may result in chronic retention of urine (fig. 1288).

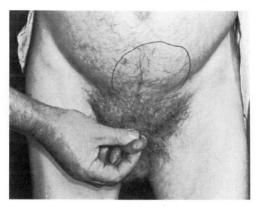

FIG. 1288.—Pin-hole meatus causing chronic retention of urine (distended bladder outlined) in a man of fifty-one. Cured by meatotomy.

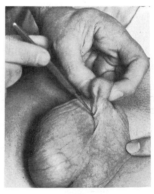

FIG. 1289.—Penile hypospadias. The patient passes urine through the orifice demonstrated by the probe.

Treatment.—Meatal stenosis, sufficient to (*a*) give rise to symptoms, (*b*) prevent free drainage of the discharge in cases of urethritis, or (*c*) obstruct the passage of full-sized urethral instruments or a cystoscope, should be treated by meatotomy. Lesser degrees of narrowing respond to dilatation with Hegar's dilators.

Meatotomy.—The narrowed section must be split back into normal urethra, and the mucosa stitched to the skin edge. Alternatively, a skin flap can be turned in from the underside of the skin behind the glans.

Congenital stricture of the urethra is very rare; some cases are due to reduplication of the urethra. Usually the symptoms are delayed until adolescence. Treatment by dilatation is effective.

Congenital valves of the posterior urethra are often symmetical and occur usually just below, but occasionally above, the verumontanum. They allow the ingress of a catheter but obstruct the outflow of urine. In a few instances the valves are incomplete and the patient may reach adolescent or adult life without symptoms; however, in such cases the prostatic urethra is greatly dilated and sacculation or diverticula of the bladder are present.

The valves are difficult to see at cysto-urethroscopy, because the irrigating fluid sweeps them into the open position. The most reliable method of confirming the diagnosis is

Alfred Hegar, 1830–1914. Professor of Obstretrics and Gynaecology, Freiburg, Germany.

voiding cysto-urethrography, by which is meant that radiographs are taken during attempts to micturate after the bladder has been filled with contrast medium. Alternatively, pressure above the pubes while the radiograph is taken achieves the same objective. In this way the dilated urethra above the valves is outlined, as well as the bladder.

Treatment.—Suprapubic drainage of the bladder is a life-saving measure; several weeks should intervene before attempting to remove the valves. This is done by transurethral resection.

Because of their importance in the differential diagnosis of congenital valves of the urethra, the following causes of chronic retention in childhood are included here:

Obstruction to the neck of the bladder (*syn.* **Marion's disease**) is analogous to hypertrophic pyloric stenosis of infants, and gives rise to symptoms identical with those of congenital valves. The diagnosis can often be appreciated cystoscopically as a hypertrophied inter-ureteric bar. Voiding cysto-urethrography demonstrates that the posterior urethra does not fill, and clarifies the differential diagnosis between the two conditions. Treatment consists in opening the bladder and performing a Y—V plasty (Chapter 59).

Neurogenic bladder must be excluded in both the above lesions. Spina bifida, and the accompanying lesions of the central nervous system, is the usual cause of retention of urine of neurological origin in childhood. As with obstruction due to congenital valves, cysto-urethrography shows the dilated prostatic urethra. In neurogenic obstruction, the ease with which the bladder can be emptied by manual pressure above the pubis serves as a ready means of distinguishing chronic retention of urine due to this cause from other varieties.

HYPOSPADIAS

Hypospadias is the commonest congenital malformation of the urethra, and it occurs once in every 350 males. The external meatus is situated at some point on the *under*-surface of the penis or in the perineum.

There are five degrees of the deformity, classified as follows:

1. **Glandular Hypospadias.**—There is an ectopic opening on the under-surface of the glans, separated from a blind depression at the normal site of the external urinary meatus. Sometimes a channel connects the ectopic to the normal meatus.

2. **Coronal Hypospadias.**—The meatus is situated at the junction of the under-surface of the glans with the body of the penis.

3. **Penile Hypospadias.**—The meatus opens at some part of the under-surface of the penis (fig. 1289).

4. **Peno-scrotal Hypospadias.**—The urethra opens at the junction of the penis with the scrotum.

5. **Perineal Hypospadias.**—The scrotum is split and the urethra opens between its two halves. This variety is sometimes associated with bilateral maldescended testes, in which event the sex of the child may be difficult to determine.

Glandular hypospadias is the most frequent variety, and is due to a failure of canalisation of the glans. The other varieties are looked upon as an absence of the urethra and corpus spongiosum distal to the ectopic orifice, the absent structures being represented by a fibrous cord. In all except the first variety the penis is curved in a downward direction (chordee). The farther away the opening is from the normal position, the more pronounced is the bowing. In all cases the inferior aspect of the prepuce is poorly developed ('hooded prepuce').

Treatment.—In glandular hypospadias no treatment is required, unless the opening is too small, in which case meatotomy is performed. In other varieties a plastic operation, of which there is a great variety, should be carried out. On this account circumcision during infancy should not be performed in these cases as the redundant skin will prove useful later.

Stage 1.— Preferably between one and a half and two years of age *straightening the penis* is undertaken. A transverse incision is made on the ventral surface 1·25 cm distal to the

Jean-Baptiste Camille-Georges Marion, 1869–1960. Emeritus Professor of Urology, Faculty of Medicine, Paris.

misplaced external urinary meatus, and the skin on either side of the urethra is undermined, exposing the fibrotic corpus spongiosum, which is detached from before backwards by severing its fibrous attachment to the corpora cavernosa. This accomplished, the urethral orifice recedes towards the perineum; thus a coronal hypospadias becomes penile, peno-scrotal, or perineal, and the penis is no longer tethered. The original transverse incision is further lengthened by carrying it into the under-surface of the prepuce on either side. The incision is then closed vertically, tension being relieved by making a longitudinal incision in the middle line through the skin of the dorsum of the penis and prepuce.

Stage 2.—Preferably between five and seven years of age. Diversion of all urine from the seat of operation can be accomplished only by *perineal urethrostomy*. A small catheter is passed into the bladder on an introducer. The introducer is withdrawn slightly, and rotated so that its beak can be felt in the perineum. Strictly in the middle line a small incision is made, and the catheter is seen within the urethra. The wall of the catheter is grasped in a haemostat while the assistant withdraws the introducer. The butt end of the catheter is then drawn along the urethra and made to emerge in the perineum. Two cotton sutures are tied around the catheter and utilised to anchor it to the edges of the perineal wound.

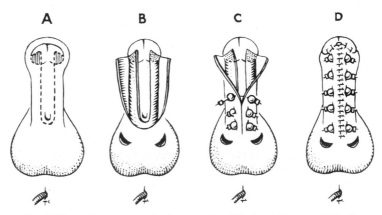

A   B   C   D

FIG. 1290.—Denis Browne's operation for hypospadias. The buried strip of skin forms the new urethra.

Fashioning a New Urethra (Denis Browne).—An incision is made as outlined in fig. 1290(A). The flaps are undermined, special attention being paid to freeing the skin in the direction of the perineum, so that when the flaps are united they lie well forward of the old urethral opening. When the undermining involves the scrotum, stab wounds should be made on either side to allow the ready escape of blood and serum. Next, with sharp scissors, a triangular area of glans is bared of skin on either side of the proposed new meatus (fig. 1290(B)). An incision is made through the skin along the whole length of the dorsum of the penis. This is to relieve tension, and the wound is allowed to epithelialise. The flaps are sutured, but not too tightly. Browne employed glass beads and small sections of soft aluminium tubing, which are crushed, and hold the sutures in place (fig. 1290(C)). No dressing is employed—only a spray of Nobecutane. An antibiotic such as trimethoprine is given for two weeks. The sutures are removed in a week, and the catheter is withdrawn on the tenth day. The perineal wound usually closes three to five days later.

Other operations have been devised to form a tube from the mucosal surface of the foreskin. The glans is tunnelled and a better anatomical appearance may be produced than with the Denis Browne operation.

EPISPADIAS

Unlike hypospadias, epispadias is very rare, occurring in one in 30,000 males and one in 400,000 females. The defect may be glandular (fig. 1291), penile, or total, the latter usually associated with ectopia vesicae. In the first two varieties the urethral orifice is situated on the dorsum, and in the second variety the penis curves upwards as well. The

Sir Denis John Wolko Browne, 1892–1967. Surgeon, Hospital for Sick Children, Great Ormond Street, London.

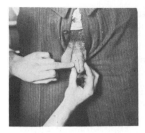

FIG. 1291.—Glandular Epispadias.

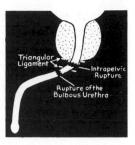

FIG. 1292.—Showing the two varieties of rupture of the urethra.

operative treatment is similar in principle to that of the hypospadias, and is somewhat less difficult to perform. The female variety is associated with many other abnormalities.

INJURIES OF THE URETHRA

Rupture of the urethra is divided into two distinct classes—rupture of the bulbous urethra, and rupture of the membranous urethra (*syn.* intrapelvic rupture) (fig. 1292). Each is again subdivided into complete and incomplete which relates to the circumferance of the urethral wall, and total and partial which relates to the thickness of the wall.

Rupture of the Bulbous Urethra

Rupture of the bulbous urethra is the more common accident. Almost without exception there is a history of a fall astride a projecting object. In the days of sailing-ships, the common cause was falling astride a spar from aloft. Today cycling accidents and a loose manhole cover (fig. 1293) account for a number of cases, as well as gymnasium accidents astride the 'beam'.

Clinical Features.—The triad of signs of a ruptured bulbous urethra is urethral haemorrhage, a perineal haematoma, and retention of urine.

Preliminary Treatment and Investigation.—If the condition is suspected, in order to diminish the possibility of extravasation, *the patient should be told not to try to pass urine.* No attempt should be made to catheterise him until he is fit to be taken to an operation theatre, where asepsis can be assured and operation can be undertaken in necessary cases. A suitable dose of morphine is given; a course of chemotherapy started. When circumstances are extenuating and the bladder

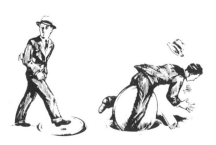

FIG. 1293.—The type of accident which results in rupture of the bulb of the urethra.
(After V. J. O'Connor.)

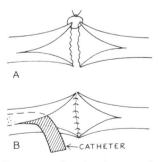

FIG. 1294.—Repair of ruptured bulbous urethra.

is full, it should be emptied by suprapubic puncture until the patient can be treated as above. If the patient has passed urine when first seen and there is no extravasation, then the rupture is partial and catheterisation should be avoided.

Treatment

1. Under strict aseptic precautions an attempt is made to pass a plastic coudé catheter (14–16 F). The roof of the urethra is the most likely part to be intact, so the beak of the catheter should be directed towards this.

2. If the catheter passes it should be left in position for forty-eight hours. A perineal haematoma must be drained, and the mid-line wound packed.

3. If the catheter fails to pass, the site of the obstruction is explored, with the patient in the lithotomy position, through a mid-line perineal incision. Should it be impossible to define the proximal end of the ruptured urethra, a suprapubic cystotomy is performed and a fully curved sound passed down from the internal meatus. The exposed ends of the urethra are trimmed and the ventral aspect split longitudinally for 1·5 cm. The circumference is then sutured as a flat ribbon, with fine catgut, the knots being left on the outside of the wall (fig. 1294). The bladder, if opened, is drained by a suprapubic catheter. If the repair has been accomplished without cystostomy the catheter can be passed into the bladder from the urethrostomy (fig. 1294 (B)). A small balloon Gibbon-type catheter (12 F) is very satisfactory. The perineal wound is packed, not stitched.

After-treatment.—A course of antibiotics is continued until healing is complete. The urine must be recultured after a week. The perineal wound is irrigated daily with a weak Eusol (hypochlorite) solution. The catheter is removed after eight to ten days. A perineal leak will persist for a few days. Sounds must be passed two weeks after healing to calibrate the urethra, and a urethrogram, performed two months later, will reveal the result.

Complications:

Subcutaneous extravasation of urine occurs in total rupture if the patient attempts to pass urine.

Stricture.—This common complication is due, for the most part, to infection.

Rupture of the Membranous Urethra
Extraperitoneal Rupture of the Bladder

Intrapelvic rupture of the urethra occurs in the membranous portion near the apex of the prostate (fig. 1292). Like extraperitoneal rupture of the bladder it may be due to penetrating wounds, but in civil life is more usually the result of fracture of the pelvis.

The prostate is firmly attached to the pubes by the puboprostatic ligaments and a displaced fracture of one ischiopubic ramus in front of the attachment of the corpus cavernosum usually ruptures the urethra. A 'butterfly' fracture of both pubic rami on each side usually springs back into place and the urethra remains intact.

Only about 10–15% of cases of fractured pelvis sustain either or both injuries.

Complete rupture with floating prostate	1–2%
Incomplete intrapelvic rupture of urethra	4–6%
Extraperitoneal rupture of bladder	4–6%
Combined urethra and bladder damage	1–2%

Clinical Features

The most common causes of pelvic fracture are road traffic accidents, severe crush injuries, and falls either from a building or a horse. One's attention intitially must be turned to the overall management of the patient remembering that these people have been involved in major trauma. Therefore there is often injury to the head, thorax, abdomen or fracture of the long bones. These patients are in a state of shock from blood loss and may be unconscious. A careful assessment of the whole patient must be made including radiographs of the head (if there is a history of head injury or loss of consciousness), the chest (to exclude a pneumothorax), the abdomen and pelvis and the appropriate long bones. An intravenous line should be inserted and blood replaced as appropriate.

The classic sign of urethral injury is blood at the external urinary meatus; this will be associated with gradual distension of the bladder assuming it is not injured. If there is an intraperitoneal rupture of the bladder signs of peritonitis will soon develop but if the rupture is extraperitoneal the diagnosis is often more difficult. Clinically with extraperitoneal rupture of the bladder there is some suprapubic tenderness and perhaps a little dullness to percussion. There will be blood in the urine and often clots. A plain x-ray to demonstrate pelvic or other bony injuries is essential. Likewise a blood count, blood grouping and cross-matching for blood transfusion (massive blood loss from ruptured pelvic veins can occur). Depending on one's view, cysto-urethrography may be attempted to aid diagnosis. A simple cystogram may not demonstrate the lesion and the diagnosis can only be confidently ruled out if voiding films do not show a leak.

Injury to the urethra with pelvic fracture occurs at the apex of the prostate in the area commonly known as the membranous urethra. One has to remember that this is in close association with the external sphincter mechanism. The injury may be *partial*, meaning that part of the urethral lining is in continuity, or *total*. The latter may be associated with complete disruption of the puboprostatic ligaments with the bladder and prostate floating up high in the pelvis (fig. 1295). A clue to this can be obtained clinically by the inability to feel the prostate, or a 'high prostate' felt on rectal examination.

Following the initial assessment craniotomy, thoracotomy, laparotomy and fixation of bones may be required. These of course may be life saving manoeuvres and therefore take preference over the urethra, although clearly drainage of the bladder must be achieved. This is best done with a suprapubic catheter in the emergency situation.

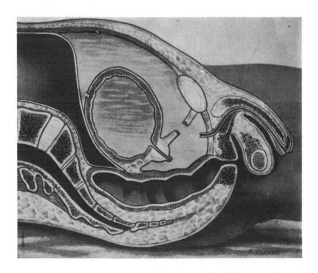

FIG. 1295.—Intrapelvic rupture of the urethra. Note the displacement of the bladder backwards, due to the tearing of the pubo-prostatic ligaments.

Treatment

Blood loss and shock are treated aggressively. Antibiotics are given. There are two schools of thought concerning the management of these injuries.

(1) The first proposed by Mitchell is based on the theory that the injury to the urethra is incomplete in the majority of these patients. He therefore feels that catheterisation via the urethra might result in further damage and cause the rupture to become complete. This school therefore believes that a suprapubic cystostomy should be performed and the bladder drained in this way. This allows the patient to recover from any other injuries and discourages young surgeons from attempting heroic primary repairs of the urethra on patients who have undergone severe trauma. The bladder is opened and by inserting two fingers it is possible to ascertain that the prostate is *not* floating so high that total rupture of the urethra neck is certain. Once reassured on this point the bladder is closed round a large (28F) Malécot catheter.

Careful endoscopy is then advocated approximately three weeks after the injury. If the rupture has been incomplete it will usually be possible to pass a cystoscope past an area of blood clot and granulation tissue into the urethra. In cases where the continuity of the urethra is not established with a combination of endoscopy from below and perhaps also from above, then an open procedure to re-establish continuity and the placement of a urethral catheter is advocated.

If the prostate is floating, and there is no doubt that the rupture is complete and total, then the older classical method, railroading a catheter across the gap, and drawing the prostate down on to the triangular ligament, should be adopted.

Railroad technique.—A metal bougie is passed from the bladder through the internal meatus into the retropubic space. A second metal bougie is passed from the external urinary meatus. The two bougies are manipulated until their tips touch (fig. 1296). By slowly withdrawing the first bougie and steadily advancing the second, while keeping their tips in contact, it is possible to guide the second bougie into the bladder past the seat of the rupture. The first bougie is withdrawn and a piece of plain rubber tubing of such a size as to fit tightly is threaded on to the beak of the second bougie, which is withdrawn, carrying with it the rubber tubing. Outside the external urinary meatus the bougie is

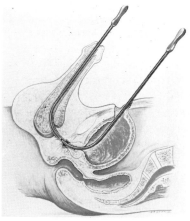

FIG. 1296.—Intrapelvic rupture of the urethra. Showing the tips of the metal bougies in contact.

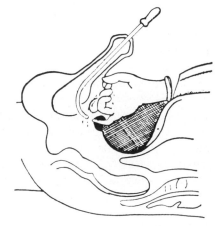

FIG. 1297.—Shahade and Shah procedure (see text).

John Phillimore Mitchell, Contemporary. Professor of Urology, United Bristol Hospitals.
Achille-Étienne Malécot, 1852–?. He invented his catheter while Interne des Hôpitaux de Paris, France.
M. G. Shahade, Contemporary. Formely Professor of Surgery, Govt. Medical College, Surat, Gujarat, India.
V. C. Shah, Contemporary. Surgeon, Rajkotwthin, Guiarat, India.

disengaged from the rubber tubing, and to the latter is fastened, by means of a stitch, the tip of a Foley's catheter. By pulling on the vesical end of the rubber tubing the tip of the Foley's catheter is drawn into the mouth of the suprapubic wound, where it is disconnected from the rubber tube.

At this stage it is advisable to tie a long piece of silk firmly to the tip of the Foley's catheter, and to wind the excess around a wooden spatula. (Thus, should the balloon burst, the Foley's catheter can be replaced by the rail-road method just described.) This completed, the balloon (30 ml) of the catheter is moderately distended with water and the side tube is ligated (fig. 1299).

The *Shahade and Shah procedure* (fig. 1297) employs the little finger instead of the first metal bougie as it makes the operation easier.

Concluding the Operation.—The catheter is drawn down so that the balloon rests upon the bladder neck. The bladder is closed around a Malécot catheter (fig. 1298), and the prevesical space is drained with corrugated rubber.

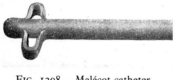

FIG. 1298.—Malécot catheter.

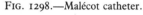

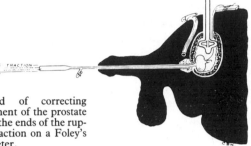

FIG. 1299.—Method of correcting backward displacement of the prostate and approximating the ends of the ruptured urethra by traction on a Foley's catheter.

(2) The alternative approach, advocated by Blandy, recommends a single attempt to pass a small soft urethral catheter. This should be done by an experienced surgeon using full aseptic technique. If this fails a suprapubic cystostomy should be performed and the bladder drained for a day or two until the patient is fit for management of the urethra to take priority. On the second or third day therefore the patient is taken to the operating room and urethroscopy performed under general anaesthetic. The patient should be given a broad spectrum antibiotic. If the cystoscope passes into the bladder a urethral catheter is inserted. If it fails a curved sound, a Hey Groves sound or a flexible cystoscope may be passed from above through the suprapubic site so one can find the upper end of the urethra from below. For patients with true floating prostate the deformity will be in the form of an S shaped bend. Once the line of the urethra is established a small silastic catheter is introduced and left in situ for approximately two weeks.

Whatever approach is adopted the placement of traction on the urethral catheter for patients with a dislocated prostate is not advised. The external sphincter mechanism is in close association with the area of urethral tear and is often rendered incompetent; this means the only zone of continence remaining is the bladder neck. Injury to this area from using traction may well result in total urinary incontinence. However, as a *temporary* measure to stabilise the bladder neck and reduce blood loss the method is still used in the immediate few days after injury by many surgeons who do not have sophisticated surgical circumstances.

Complications

The most taxing complication from the surgeons point of view is the ensuing urethral stricture. Advocates for the early placement of a urethral catheter claim that any sub-

Frederic Eugene Baisal Foley, 1891–1966. Urologist, Miller and Ancker Hospitals, St. Paul, U.S.A.
J. P. Blandy, Contemporary. Professor of Urology, The London Hospital and St. Peter's Hospital for Stone.

sequent stricture is easier to deal with and may even be managed endoscopically with an optical urethrotome or cautious resection of the posterior wedge of the 'step' in the urethra that develops. Should conservative measures fail, a complex urethroplasty will be necessary. The transpubic approach advocated by Waterhouse appears to allow a satisfactory end to end anastomosis to be performed.

Urinary incontinence.—As mentioned previously the external sphincter mechanism may be severely damaged by these injuries with continence solely relying on the competence of the bladder. Surgical manoeuvres that might affect bladderneck function should not be contemplated.

Impotence.—Erectile impotence is a common sequelae of this injury. It is assumed that it is secondary to the disruption of the nerve supply at the time of the fracture.

Orthopaedic.—For management of the fractured pelvis, see Chapter 17.

EXTRAVASATION OF URINE

Superficial extravasation occurs in neglected cases of complete rupture of the bulbous urethra, *i.e.* when operation is not undertaken within twelve to twenty-four hours, and in ruptured periurethral abscess.

The extravasated urine cannot pass (1) behind the mid-perineal point, because of the attachment of the perineal (Colles's) fascia to the triangular ligament; (2) into the thighs, for the deep layer of the superficial fascia of the abdominal wall (Scarpa's fascia) blends with the pubic portion of the fascia lata just distal to the inguinal ligament; (3) into the inguinal canals, because of the intercolumnar fibres and fascia of the external oblique (external spermatic fascia).

It therefore must pass (1) into the scrotum; (2) beneath the superficial fascia of the penis; (3) up the abdominal wall beneath the deep layer of the superficial fascia (fig. 1300).

Treatment.—Urgent operation is a necessity.

Multiple incisions are made in the infiltrated tissues of sufficient depth to penetrate the limiting fascia. By the time extravasation has occurred it is unlikely that the urethra can be repaired in the way described already (p. 1326), for the sutures would cut out of the oedematous inflamed tissues. It is therefore often advisable to adopt the sutureless operation of Rutherfurd. Suprapubic cystostomy is performed and a metal bougie is passed through the internal urinary meatus. The patient having been placed in the lithotomy position, another metal bougie is passed from the external urinary meatus to the perineum, and perineal section is carried out. A silastic tube with multiple holes is introduced from

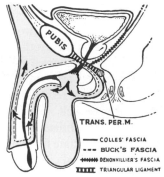

Fig. 1300.—The fascial planes concerned in superficial extravasation of urine. Trans. Per. M. = Transverse Perineal muscle.

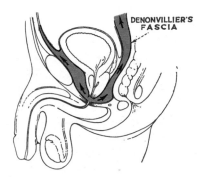

Fig. 1301.—Area occupied by extravasated blood and urine in the case of intrapelvic rupture of the urethra.

Antonio Scarpa, 1747–1832. Professor of Anatomy, Pavia, Italy.
Henry Rutherfurd, 1861–1929. Surgeon, Royal Infirmary, Glasgow, Scotland.

the external urinary meatus into the bladder in the same way as that described for intra-pelvic rupture of the urethra, and the bladder is closed around a de Pezzer catheter. The perineal wound is left widely open. The urethral catheter is removed after three or four days. In other respects the after-treatment is similar to that for complete rupture of the bulbous urethra.

Deep extravasation (fig. 1301) occurs in the case of extraperitoneal rupture of the bladder, intrapelvic rupture of the urethra, and after suprapubic puncture, when the bladder has been allowed to refill. It can also result from rupture or perforation of a ureter, or unnoticed damage to the bladder or prostatic capsule during perurethral resections. In these conditions urine extravasates in the layers of the pelvic fascia and in the retro-peritoneal tissues.

Treatment.—When extravasation is proceeding from the bladder, it is necessary to drain the prevesical space (cave of Retzius) and to perform suprapubic cystostomy. The treatment of the various conditions which give rise to deep extravasation of urine is considered in the appropriate sections.

INFLAMMATIONS OF URETHRA

Ulceration of the Urethral Meatus

Ulceration of the meatus in young male children is a common clinical entity. It is never found in the uncircumcised. It is common after circumcision, though an interval of three to eighteen months may elapse between the operation and the onset of symptoms. Lack of protection given by the prepuce is the initial cause. Friction of the clothing and ammoniacal urine are important secondary aetiological factors. The ulcer causes a scab to form which closes the meatus, and the child can only urinate by bursting this scab. This process is usually accompanied by pain and screaming, and a few drops of blood may be passed. Ulceration and scab formation alternate, and if neglected, cicatricial contracture of the meatus may result eventually in an acquired pin-hole meatus.

Treatment.—A simple regimen of washing the napkins in boric acid crystals after boiling and applying 5% boracic ointment (or Drapolene) locally is usually curative. These measures neutralise the alkaline urine. A few cases require meatotomy.

URETHRITIS

(1) **Gonorrhoea.**—A sexually transmitted disease due to *Neisseria gonorrhoeae* (gonococcus), a Gram-negative kidney shaped diplococcus which affects primarily the anterior urethra in the male, the urethra and cervix in the female and the oropharynx, rectum and anal canal of both sexes.

Gonorrhoea in the male.—Two to ten days after intercourse with an infected partner, there occurs some discomfort on micturition often progressing to a scalding pain. A urethral discharge ensues, seropurulent at first, then becoming purulent and yellowish. In chronic cases and male carriers (5% of the total) a slight purulent morning discharge, or some slight staining of the underclothes may be the only symptoms. There may be no signs at all.

Investigations.—The Gram-stained urethral smear will show numerous pus cells and both intra- and extra- cellular Gram-negative diplococci. *The two glass urine test*: the urine in the first glass is hazy, but clear in the second glass. Smears taken soon after micturition may show no organisms and in those from carriers and chronic cases, the diplococci may be scanty and predominantly extra-cellular. Urethral cultures should always be taken, but treatment need not await

Oscar Michel Benvenuto de Pezzer, 1853–1917. Assistant in the Urological Department, Necker Hospital, Paris.
Andreas Adolf Retzius, 1796–1860. Professor of Anatomy and Physiology, Carolina Institute, Stockholm.

confirmation when smear and history are typical. The Gonococcal Complement Fixation Test (GCFT) is obsolete. It is useless in early uncomplicated cases, frequently negative in chronic complicated cases, and sometimes positive in the absence of any gonococcal infection past or present.

Complications.—In the United Kingdom, but not in many third world countries, local complications are now comparatively rare and metastatic complications very rare. All can be prevented by effective early treatment followed by full tests of cure.

Local complications include posterior urethritis, prostatitis-acute or chronic, acute epididymo-orchitis, peri-urethral abscess, and urethral stricture.

The glands of Littré are frequently involved and Cowper's glands more rarely. Systemic (metastatic) complications include gonococcal arthritis, iridocyclitis, septicaemia and endocarditis. Blood culture is essential for diagnosis.

Treatment.—Over 90% cure rates should occur with the following schedules. Ampicillin 3g stat. with Probenecid 1g to delay excretion; Procaine Penicillin 1·2 to 4·8 mega units i.m. with Probenecid; Co-Trimoxazole (Septrin) 4 tablets b.d. for 5 days. Spectinomycin 2g stat.; Kanamycin 2g stat. and Cefuroxime 0·75g i.m. with oral Probenecid. Large dosages of penicillin are required to cure those patients infected with insensitive strains of gonococcus. Completely resistant β-lactamase producing strains, rare in the United Kingdom, will not respond to any penicillin dosage whatsoever.

Septrin and Kanamycin are non-treponemicidal and will not mask a concomitant syphilitic infection. The latter is ototoxic; the stated dose must not be exceeded and repeated dosage is cumulative in this respect.

Always every effort must be made to get *all* the sex partners to attend for investigation and, if necessary, treatment.

Gonorrhoea in the female.—Gonorrhoea affects primarily the urethra and the cervix in the female and is often symptomless. It can never be diagnosed on clinical grounds alone. Almost three quarters of all female cases attend initially as a result of the diagnosis of their male partners, and have no symptoms nor significant signs. These are completely absent in more than 50% of all cases or often only consist of a slight dysuria or a slight to moderate vaginal discharge unnoticed by the patient. The signs may include a bead of pus at the meatal orifice after emptying Skene's tubules by milking the urethra down against the posterior ramus of the pubis, some reddening or erosion of the cervix with a mucopurulent cervical plug. A copious vaginal discharge is more likely to be due to concomitant trichomonal vaginitis, except in the young prepubertal girl where a primary gonococcal vaginitis may occur. In the latter, infection readily occurs from a fomite, usually when her infected mother's towel is used by the child.

Complications.—Gonococcal proctitis occurs in at least 60–70% of cases. Usually symptomless, it is spread from the vaginal discharge. *Salpingitis.* Ten per cent of cases will present evidence of involvement of one or both tubes, acute or subacute. Lower abdominal pain and tenderness is present, with thickening and tenderness of the affected tube on bimanual palpation. Infertility due to bilateral gonococcal salpingitis is now rare. *Bartholinitis*, leading to an acutely tender Bartholin's abscess which should be aspirated. Systemic complications and treatment are as in the male. All known contacts must be investigated.

Alexis Littré, 1658–1726. Surgeon and Anatomist, Paris.
William Cowper, 1666–1709. Surgeon and Anatomist, London.
Alexander Johnston Chalmers Skene, 1828–1900. Professor of Gynaecology, Long Island College Hospital, New York.
Caspar Bartholin, 1655–1738. Professor of Medicine, Anatomy and Physics. Copenhagen.

Will all readers note that a high vaginal swab is an extremely unreliable method of diagnosis.

Gonorrhoea in the newborn (Gonococcal ophthalmia neonatorum).—Infection of the eye during birth, previously an important cause of blindness, is now fortunately rare. Unless rigorously treated the condition may progress rapidly disrupting the orbit. If unilateral, the unaffected eye should be covered, and the affected eye irrigated with isotonic saline as frequently as necessary to prevent accumulation of pus, followed by penicillin eye drops one mega-unit into each eye and i.m. penicillin. Smears and cultures for the gonococcus must always be taken before commencing treatment but treatment must not be delayed. The mother and her contact(s) must be treated. *Chlamydial ophthalmia neonatorum* must be treated with erythromycin systemically and tetracycline eye ointment locally. In such cases, the mother is *always* infected. Ophthalmia neonatorum from any cause described 'as a discharge from the eye of a neonate within 21 days of birth' is a notifiable disease by law (U.K.)—to the proper officer.

(2) Non-Gonococcal Urethritis (N.G.U.) or Non-specific Urethritis (N.S.U.)

A blunderbuss term used to describe especially in the male all forms of urethritis apart from gonorrhoea which have to be distinguished from physiological causes such as mucus from unrelieved sexual stimulation often associated with severe testicular pain, spermatorrhoea and prostatorrhoea (the last often following defaecation, the stool providing a physiological prostatic massage). Secondary urethritis follows trauma, accidents, iatrogenic insult (catheters) or foreign bodies deliberately inserted. Metabolic causes include oxaluria, urinary calculi or gout. Urinary tract or prostatic (non-venereal) infections from any cause are involved as well as malignant disease. Urethritis is a very rare complication of infectious diseases.

Organisms such as staphylococci or streptococci are rare causes of primary sexually acquired urethritis, as is also *Candida albicans*. *Trichomonas vaginalis* can cause male urethritis and is a very rare cause of painful prostatitis or of a reduced sperm count. *Diagnosis.*—A deep intraurethral specimen, the deposit from centrifuged urine or prostatic fluid may reveal the organism by hanging drop microscopy or culture.

Finally, by exclusion, this leaves a condition misleadingly known as non-specific urethritis, so called originally because of uncertain aetiology—or non-specific genital infection (NSGI) because in the female, it is commonly the hidden cervix that is infected. At present about 40% of all cases are known to be caused by *Chlamydia trachomatis* (Chlamydia A) types D – K which is also an important source of pelvic inflammatory disease. It is also a cause of ophthalmia neonatorum and chlamydial pneumonia which also occurs in the very young (about six weeks). *Contact tracing is therefore just as important as with syphilis and gonorrhoea.*

Ureaplasma urealytica (Mycoplasma T-strain) is also a proven cause of a number of cases of non-specific urethritis and seems more likely than Chlamydia to develop antibiotic resistance. This leaves a gap in our knowledge concerning the causation of more than half the cases, but organisms such as *Mycoplasma hominis* are being intensively investigated.

Clinical features.—Symptoms in the male from whatever cause are much the same and usually milder than those of gonorrhoea. Two to thirty days and even up to six weeks after sexual intercourse, a mucopurulent urethral discharge associated with dysuria appears. The urine is usually clear unless the discharge is excessive and contains shreds which on microscopy usually contain numerous pus cells. Gonococci are absent. Culture may grow Chlamydia or Ureaplasma or nothing at all. About 20% of males relapse—mostly due to reinfection but sometimes due to prostatitis. Epididymitis is not uncommon and urethral stricture rarely results. More commonly, a pre-existing stricture renders treatment ineffective.

Treatment.—Treatment consists usually of either oxytetracycline 500 mg b.d. or triple tetracycline (Detecло) 300 mg b.d. for 14 days. Alternatively, and in pregnant women, Erythromycin 500 mg b.d. for 14 days. Cotrimoxazole is a third string to the bow (tabs 2 b.d. for 14 days). Contacts must be seen and if from repeated treatment failure secondary urethritis is suspected, appropriate investigations done.

Non-specific Urethritis in the female.—As in the male, acute urethritis can be due to gonorrhoea or to non-gonococcal urethritis. Likewise, chronic urethritis may or may not be due to gonorrhoea, and in its severe forms is a urethrotrigonitis. The symptoms are increased frequency pain on micturition, urgency, terminal haematuria and low back pain. Urethral tenderness is an important sign of infection of Skene's tubules. Pressure on the urethra causes pus to exude from the orifices of the ducts surrounding the urethral opening. Incomplete cure of the infection in these tubules is a source of chronicity of anterior urethritis. In cases of posterior urethritis, urethral polypi are often present and can be seen on urethroscopy. Most cases of true NSGI involve the cervix rather than the urethra. The cervicitis caused rarely produces symptoms but pelvic inflammatory disease may supervene. Treatment is the same as for the male. Concentration on the woman offers the best hope of bringing this ubiquitous and troublesome infection under control.

Investigations.—Gram-stained smears of urethral and cervical secretions. Cultures are essential including rectal cultures from direct spread of infection. Wet film and culture of the vaginal secretion for *T. vaginalis* and *Candida albicans*. These investigations must be repeated three times with negative results to exclude the diagnosis or as tests of cure after treatment. In all married cases, sugar fermentations should be done to exclude other Neisseria species, especially *N. meningitidis*. Such infections usually result from orogenital sex. *N. gonorrhoeae* ferments glucose only and *N. meningitidis* glucose and maltose. This is the only medico-legal proof of these infections.

REITER'S DISEASE (SEXUALLY ACQUIRED REACTIVE ARTHRITIS)

This condition is venereal in the United Kingdom but abroad is more commonly dysenteric in origin. It commences as a subacute urethritis four to six weeks after contact. The discharge is usually devoid of organisms, being clear and viscid. A few days later conjunctivitis occurs, at first unilateral, and then bilateral in up to 50% of cases. In more severe cases, anterior uveitis may occur. Usually in ten days to two weeks arthritis supervenes, but genuine cases undoubtedly occur without arthritis. Another concurrent manifestation that often

Hans Reiter, 1861–1969. President of the Health Service and Honorary Professor of Hygiene, Berlin. Described Reiter's Disease in 1916. The syndrome had been noted previously by Sir Benjamin Brodie.

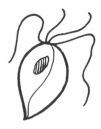

FIG. 1302.—*Trichomonas vaginalis.*

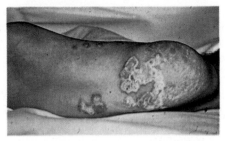

FIG. 1303.—Reiter's disease—keratoderma blennorrhagicum of the heel.

accompanies the onset of arthritis is keratoderma blennorrhagicum, consisting of nodules, vesicles and pustules frequently found on the soles of the feet (fig. 1303). In long standing cases, aortic regurgitation has occurred but in such cases syphilis must be excluded.

Differential Diagnosis.—In untreated gonorrhoea, arthritis and ophthalmic infection were not rare in the past. The absence of the gonococcus is of the highest importance in coming to the conclusion that the symptoms are due to Reiter's Disease, but *complete exclusion requires a blood culture.* In Reiter's disease the urethritis, as well as the arthritis, is milder and the incubation period is much longer than in gonorrhoea. Furthermore, the ocular manifestations of Reiter's disease are never as destructive as those of gonorrhoea, serious though they may be. The presence of sacro-iliitis confirmed radiologically appears to be correlated with the more severe eye symptoms, as does chronic prostatitis.

Prognosis.—The urethritis and conjunctivitis frequently subside in a few weeks, but more often than not the arthritis persists for many months. Severe anterior uveitis heralds a bad outlook as does the frequency of subsequent attack.

Treatment.—Clearly the ophthalmic complications must be treated thoroughly following the usual general lines (e.g. eye-baths and shades). Iritis will demand mydriatics and local steroids. Various antibiotics and fever-therapy indiced by graduated doses of triple typhoid vaccine (TAB) have been tried in the past (the last being given for the arthritis) but owing to occasional fatalities, such methods are now obsolete.

URETHRAL STRICTURE

Congenital.

Traumatic ———————— Bulbous.
——— Membranous.

Inflammatory ——— Post-gonorrhœal
——— Post-urethral chancre.
——— Tuberculous.

Instrumental ———————— Indwelling catheter.
——— Following the passage of a large calibre endoscope, notably a resectoscope.

Post-operative ——— Prostatectomy.
——— Amputation of the penis.

Post-gonorrhoeal stricture, which has become very much less common since the introduction of the antibiotic treatment of gonorrhoea, is situated most frequently (*a*) in the bulb (70%); (*b*) at the peno-scrotal junction; (*c*) in the distal part of the spongy urethra, in that order. The membranous and prostatic parts of the urethra are exempt.

Multiple strictures are relatively common. When there are two strictures, the deeper is the narrower; when there are three strictures, the deepest is the narrowest. If a stricture in the penile urethra has a very narrow orifice, there is seldom another stricture behind it.

Pathology.—Following inadequately treated gonorrhoea, infection persists in the periurethral glands, and spreads to the periglandular tissues, which become infiltrated with round cells and fibroblasts. Gradually the infiltrated periurethral tissues contract with the formation of scar tissue, localised thrombophlebitis of the corpus spongiosum playing a part in the more dense varieties. Whereas in the bulbous urethra the fibrosis is most in evidence in the roof, in the penile urethra it predominates in the floor. Most strictures develop during the first year after gonorrhoeal infection, but they may not give rise to difficulty in micturition for ten to fifteen years.

Clinical Features.—In a stricture of large calibre the only symptoms are the occasional passage of flakes (desquamated epithelium) in the urine and a varying amount of urethral discharge (gleet), most evident in the early morning (the morning 'dew-drop'). Often these symptoms are neglected until the diminished calibre of the urethra causes considerable difficulty in micturition. In contradistinction to obstruction due to an enlarged prostate, the patient finds he must strain to empty the bladder. Another distinguishing feature is the patient's age. He is often considerably younger than the prostatic sufferer, or the symptoms date back to some time prior to the fiftieth year. The stream becomes progressively narrower, micturition is prolonged, and after it has seemingly ended dribbling occurs. This is due to urine trickling from the dilated urethra above the stricture. Increasing frequency of micturition, at first during the day and then both by day and by night, is another common complaint, due either to incomplete emptying of the bladder at each act of micturition, or to cystitis, or to both. In long-standing cases it is often possible to palpate the stricture from without as an induration in the urethral floor. The evil effects of urethral obstruction upon the bladder, ureters, and kidneys are similar to those of prostatic obstruction (Chapter 59). Untreated, sooner or later retention of urine supervenes. Sometimes acute retention sets in while the stricture is still of moderate calibre; it is then due to superadded oedema of the urethral mucous membrane in the neighbourhood of the stricture, brought about by voluntary retention, alcoholic excess, or recrudescence of local infection. In other cases narrowness of the stricture results in increasing inability to expel residual urine, and acute-on-chronic retention, or retention-with-overflow, supervenes.

Urethroscopy renders the diagnosis of urethral stricture very precise.

The stricture can be seen as a white scar of fibrous tissue, and its position in the urethra, the size of its contained lumen, and its dilatability can be judged (fig. 1304).

Often a stricture encircles the whole urethra, and the lumen is more or less centrally placed, but from time to time a variety of urethroscopic appearances is noted in individual cases; for instance, the stricture may take the form of a crescent.

False passages may be seen. They are recent penetrations of the urethra in front of the stricture due to unskilful attempts to pass a bougie. False passages are particularly liable to bleed, and it is essential to abandon aero-urethroscopy if urethral haemorrhage occurs,

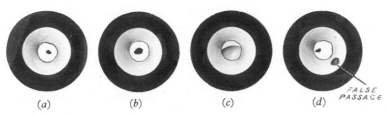

FIG. 1304.—Urethroscopic appearances. (*a*) Fine-bore stricture. (*b*) Moderate-bore stricture. (*c*) Crescentic stricture of the roof. (*d*) Stricture with false passage.

for fatal air embolism has resulted from air being pumped into the cavernous tissue through a urethral wound.

Urethrography supplies information concerning the length of a stricture, of dilatation or diverticulum formation above the stricture, or failure of the medium to pass a stricture (figs. 1305 and 1306).

Instrumental Treatment

Intermittent Dilatation.—Historically *urethral dilation* has been the traditional mode of treatment. Before each dilatation the patient should pass urine, the glans penis and urinary meatus are cleansed and the urethra is filled with a mild antiseptic solution, and local anaesthetic in a methyl cellulose base (Lidothesin). Dilatation must be carried out gently with bougies of increasing size.

On no account should the stricture be forcibly or over-dilated, both of which result in trauma that induces inflammatory oedema and subsequent formation of more fibrous tissue.

Strictures of very small calibre should be dilated twice a week at first. With this exception it is sufficient for the patient to attend for treatment at regular intervals, and an erstwhile reminder to the patient was that he must return for treatment 'once a week for a month, once a month for a year, and every year on his birthday'. A few strictures are cured by full dilatation, but in the majority the patient must be kept under supervision for the remainder of their lives.

Gum-elastic bougies (*syn*. French bougies) (fig. 1307) should be the standard instruments in the early stages of treatment of all but the very finest strictures. It is usual to commence with a No. 10 French, and if this cannot be passed, progressively smaller, or even filiform bougies are employed.

Filiform bougies are gum-elastic bougies varying in size from 1 to 3 French. If one fails to pass, it is often valuable to insert several as far as the stricture. By manipulating each

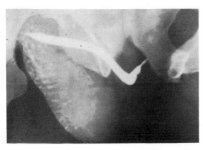

FIG. 1305.—Urethrogram showing a stricture of the membranous urethra following fracture of the pelvis.

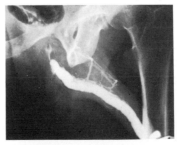

FIG. 1306.—Gonorrhoeal stricture of the bulbous urethra. Note that some contrast has entered the penile veins (Chapter 56).

back and forth, frequently one of them can be induced to negotiate the stricture (fig. 1308). If this method fails, it is sometimes possible to pass a filiform bougie through the stricture under the vision afforded by a urethroscope. If any bleeding has been occasioned by the attempt to pass bougies, urethroscopy should be postponed for several days. Very few urethral strictures are impassable, but it often requires patience to insinuate even the finest urethral guide: only when even a filiform bougie cannot be passed on three successive occasions is a stricture held to be impassable.

Filiform Bougies with Followers.—Filiform bougies furnished with threaded hollow mounts at their proximal ends are to be preferred, because screw-ended gum-elastic bougies of a larger size can be attached and guided by the filiform through the stricture. In this way many strictures of very small calibre can be dilated sufficiently to render subsequent dilatations less tedious.

By means of gum-elastic bougies a stricture is dilated up to the size of 14 French. Thereafter metal bougies are to be preferred.

Lister's metal bougies (*syn.* English bougies) (fig. 1310) are indicated after the second or third attendance of the patient, when it has been proved that the stricture is responding to dilatation by the French bougies. Metal bougies of a smaller size than 7/9 English should not be used, for fear of making a false passage.

Continuous dilatation necessitates some days of in-patient treatment, but it is of immense benefit in cases where little or very slow progress is made by intermittent dilatation. In a number of instances continuous dilatation obviates the necessity for operative treatment. After dilatation with gum-elastic bougies a catheter of corresponding size is tied into the urethra. On its removal two or three days later it will be found possible to pass much larger bougies.

Operative Treatment

1. External urethrotomy (Wheelhouse's operation) is the operation of choice if a full range of modern endoscopic equipment is unavailable when a patient presents with acute retention and the stricture proves impassable.

With the patient in the lithotomy position the Wheelhouse staff (fig. 1311) is passed down to the face of the stricture, and the urethra distal to the stricture opened by cutting down on to the groove in the staff. Stay sutures hold the edges open to display the face of the stricture. The mid-line incision is then carried backwards until the dilated proximal dilated urethra is opened. Urine will usually leak out under some pressure. A catheter is now passed from the external meatus across the opened urethra into the bladder, and the wound packed lightly. *Alternatively* the operation can be concluded formally as the first stage of a urethroplasty (see below) by stitching skin edge to mucosal edge.

2. Internal urethrotomy.—Used to be widely practised employing the Maisonneuve or Thompson Walker urethrotome as a blind procedure. These instruments have been superseded by the Sachse visual urethrotome. The stricture is seen through a zero degree end viewing lens and assessed. A fine ureteric catheter should then be carefully passed

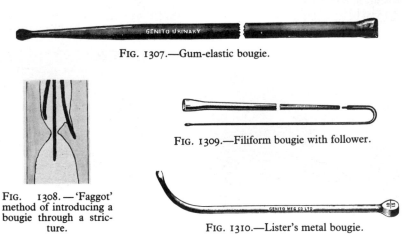

FIG. 1307.—Gum-elastic bougie.

FIG. 1309.—Filiform bougie with follower.

FIG. 1308. — 'Faggot' method of introducing a bougie through a stricture.

FIG. 1310.—Lister's metal bougie.

Lord Lister, 1827–1912. Professor of Surgery successively at Glasgow, Edinburgh, and King's College Hospital, London.
Claudius Galen Wheelhouse, 1826–1909. Surgeon, General Infirmary, Leeds, England.
Jules Germain Francois Maisonneuve, 1809–1897. Surgeon, France.
Sir John William Thomson-Walker, 1870–1937. Surgeon, St. Peter's Hospital for Stone, London.

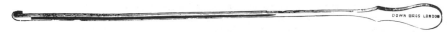

FIG. 1311.—The Wheelhouse staff.

through the stricture into the bladder. The stricture is then cut under vision with the sharp knife blade that can be projected from the tip of the instrument. The cut is normally performed in the 12 o'clock position but if unsatisfactory opening of the stricture is achieved a second cut can be performed at 6 o'clock. The instrument is gradually advanced along the line of the ureteric catheter with care being taken to ensure that the cut is not too deep, otherwise severe bleeding may occur. Once the instrument has reached the bladder a careful cystoscopy should be performed to rule out other pathology. A small urethral catheter should be left in situ for two or three days. There appears to be no advantage to leaving a catheter in situ for longer periods. The advantages of this method are that the procedure is done under direct vision minimising the chance of false passage formation; the stricture is cut in a single position so opening the fibrous band rather than causing generalised trauma throughout the circumference of the stricture as with the passage of a blind sound. For many surgeons this has become the first line of management for patients with a urethral stricture. A follow-up urethroscopy can be performed at some three months and procedure can be repeated if necessary.

3. Urethroplasty.—Urethroplasty is applicable to all strictures of the bulbar and penile portions, and is the treatment of choice if simple measures fail.

Johanson's Urethroplasty.—The urethra is exposed by a mid-line incision in the skin overlying the stricture. A Wheelhouse staff as described above is used to open the normal urethra for 2 cm distal to stricture (fig. 1312). 3–4 months after the procedure depicted when wound contraction is complete the urethra can be reconstructed by employing the principle of the Denis Browne repair of hypospadias, or constructing a urethra from the adjacent skin (fig. 1313). The skin outside the incision is mobilised to close in front of the reconstructed urethra, but a dorsal relieving incision may be necessary.

Where the stricture is in the bulb the first stage is similar. The urethral floor is divided up to and into normal urethra. In many cases this entails splitting the urethra through the external sphincter up into the wide prostatic urethra. In order to stitch skin between the

FIG. 1312.—Johanson's urethroplasty. In this case much of the urethra was strictured from the meatus. The urethra is cut clearly in the midline, through the stricture and 2 cm into proximal normal urethra. The cut edges of skin and urethra are stitched to each other, leaving a defect in the urethra through which urine will be passed while the stricture contracts.

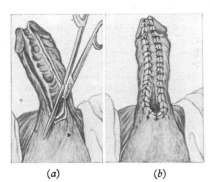

(a)   (b)

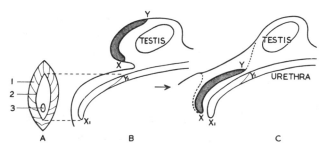

A   B   C

FIG. 1313. — Urethroplasty for the posterior part of the bulb using a funnel of scrotal skin.

1. Depressed funnel of skin.
2. Edge of urethra.
3. Membranous urethra opening.

Bengt Johanson, Contemporary. Associate Professor of Plastic Surgery, Gothenburg, Sweden.

edges, either a perineal skin flap has to be constructed at the time of skin incision (Blandy), or a scrotal funnel (Turner-Warwick) displaced backwards to be sutured to the open edges of the urethral defect (fig. 1314). Second stage closure is simple, a complete tube being reconstructed. A small catheter should be left in the urethra after these operations for 10–14 days.

For many patients staged urethroplasty has now been replaced by the 'island-flap technique' popularised by Orandi.

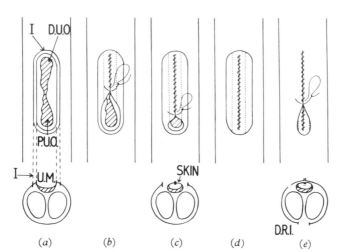

FIG. 1314.—Repair of urethral stricture. Diagrams show underside of shaft of the penis (a) Incisions (I) are made to encompass the whole area — D.U.O. = distal urethral opening, P.U.O. = proximal urethral opening, U.M. = urethral mucosa. (b), (c), (d) 3/0 chromic catgut suture of innermost skin edge to form a tube. (e) Covering skin sutured and tension avoided by a dorsal relieving incision (D.R.I.).

Other Causes of Urethral Stricture

Congenital stricture has been considered previously.

Traumatic stricture follows unskilful or delayed treatment of rupture of the urethra. If dilatation is unsatisfactory, a urethroplasty should be done.

The so-called stricture following neglected or untreated rupture of the membranous urethra is often not a stricture at all, but a complete loss of continuity of the urethra (fig. 1295). If, as frequently occurs, it proves impossible to keep a passage dilated by the usual methods, the only alternative to transplantation of the ureters is Badenoch's pull-through operation. With the patient in the lithotomy position, after the bladder has been opened suprapubically, a metal sound is passed up the urethra and when arrested by the stricture its tip is cut down upon in the perineum. The distal urethra is then freed as a tube for 4 to 6 cm. A large metal sound is passed suprapubically down the urethra and cut down upon from the perineum until it can be forced through the area of fibrosis. A rubber catheter is attached to it by the butt end and pulled back through the suprapubic opening. The freed distal urethra is threaded over the lower end of the catheter and its end stitched to the catheter some 10 cm from its tip with interrupted chromic catgut stitches. Traction on the catheter then guides the distal urethra into the prostatic urethra where it is held by attaching an artery forceps to the catheter as it emerges on to the abdominal wall. Finally, the perineum is closed and suprapubic cystostomy temporarily established.

Post-instrumental stricture can occur in any part of the urethra from trauma due to the passage of too large an endoscope, or from urethritis from an indwelling catheter. To avoid the former, some surgeons advise performing perineal urethrostomy in order to pass a resectoscope in patients with a narrow urethra, or an internal urethrotomy prior to all procedures where a large instrument is to be used over a period of more than ½ hour.

Post-operative Stricture.—A stricture develops in about 4% of cases after prostatectomy, irrespective of the method employed. The stricture is usually situated in the proximal end of the prostatic urethra. In many cases the stricture can be dilated by regular intermittent dilatation. When the stricture takes the form of a shelf at the junction of the bladder with the prostatic bed, it should be opened perurethrally with a urethrotome (or similar knife). The edges may need to be resected.

Post-operative stricture can also follow partial or complete amputation of the penis.

John Peter Blandy, Contemporary. Professor of Urology, London Hospital Medical College.
Richard Trevor Turner-Warwick, Contemporary. Urologist, The Middlesex Hospital, London.
Alec William Badenoch, Contemporary. Consulting Surgeon, St. Bartholomew's Hospital, London.
Ahmed Orandi, Contemporary. Fergus Falls, Minnesota, U.S.A.

Methods of avoiding this complication are described in the section dealing with these operations (p. 1350). Regular dilatation is satisfactory.

Complications of Urethral Stricture

1. Retention of urine (Chapter 58).
2. Urethral diverticulum.
3. Periurethral abscess.
4. Urethral fistula.
5. All the attendant evils of 'back pressure', culminating in bilateral hydronephrosis, combined with a susceptibility to urinary infection and an increased liability to urinary calculus.
6. Hernia, haemorrhoids, or rectal prolpase may be induced by the straining.

Diverticulum of the male urethra (*syn.* urethral pouch)
1. Congenital.
2. Due to increased intraurethral pressure behind a stricture.
3. Due to the long-standing presence of a urethral calculus.
4. Indwelling catheters in paraplegics.
In many cases the pouch can be seen and those which are not obvious at first become so when the patient interrupts the stream of urine.
Treatment is excision of the diverticulum and removal of the cause if possible.

PERIURETHRAL ABSCESS

There are two main varieties of acute abscess:

Penile periurethral abscess arises as an infection of one of the glands of Littré, and is usually a complication of acute gonococcal urethritis. A tender induration can be felt on the under-surface of the penis (fig. 1315). Left to nature, frequently the abscess bursts externally, and a urinary fistula is liable to result.
Treatment.—The passage of a bougie often causes the abscess to burst into the urethra. When this is unsuccessful, a ureteric meatotome is passed through a urethroscope and the abscess is opened by diathermy. When an abscess lies behind a stricture of the urethra it must be drained externally.

Bulbar periurethral abscess runs a variable course. Its most acute form, formerly termed periurethral abscess with extravasation of urine, is better termed periurethral phlegmon, because in 50% of cases there is no stricture of the urethra present. Of the remainder, the majority have a passable stricture, while in the minority the stricture is impermeable. Consequently, in the majority of cases there is no reason why urine should extravasate. The condition is due to a spreading cellulitis caused by streptococci and anaërobic organisms invading the same cellular plane as that of superficial extravasation of urine.

Clinical Features.—There is pain in the perineum, a high temperature, repeated rigors, and a rapid pulse-rate. In early cases the tenderness and swelling are limited to the perineum. Later, often in a matter of hours, the scrotum and then the penis becomes oedematous, and the infection spreads beneath the superficial fascia of the abdominal wall.

Treatment.—Antibiotics have greatly improved the prognosis.

Operation.—The perineal abscess should be opened. In addition, if spreading cellulitis is present, incisions deep enough to divide the superficial fascia are made into the infiltrated scrotum, penis, and abdominal wall, wherever considered necessary. When there is partial or complete retention of urine and if the infection is limited to the scrotum and the penis, after changing gloves and instruments, suprapubic cystostomy should be

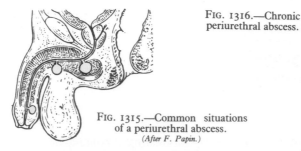

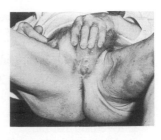

FIG. 1316.—Chronic periurethral abscess.

FIG. 1315.—Common situations of a periurethral abscess.
(After F. Papin.)

performed. If the superficial layer of the abdominal wall is implicated, it is best to drain the bladder by performing perineal urethrostomy. It should be noted that the abscess usually communicates with the urethra by a minute opening which cannot be found.

After-treatment.—After instilling hydrogen peroxide into them, the various incisions are irrigated with weak potassium permanganate solution. Later sitz baths[1] of the same solution are given. When the infection has been overcome, the stricture of the urethra, if present, is treated by one of the methods described already.

Chronic periurethral abscess is nearly always situated in the perineum (fig. 1316) and is associated with much periurethritis. It is almost invariably the result of a long-standing stricture of the bulbous urethra. The abscess should be opened, together with the various pockets that are often present. Later the associated stricture must receive adequate treatment. The condition is liable to be complicated by a urethral fistula which occurs either spontaneously or as a result of incision of the abscess.

URETHRAL FISTULA

The most frequent cause of an acquired external urethral fistula is bursting or incision of a periurethral abscess. When the opening is situated in the penile urethra or at the peno-scrotal junction, the amount of urine that escapes at each act of micturition is often small. A fistula following a periurethral abscess of the bulbous urethra can be either single or multiple. In the latter case the fistulas originate behind a tight stricture and the patient passes most or all of his urine through the various fistulas (watering-can perineum). A fistula can also follow external urethrotomy when there is a stricture situated more distally.

Treatment.—A small fistula often closes spontaneously after repeated dilatation of the urethra. Searing the track with the diathermy needle often encourages closure. Occasionally urethroplasty is indicated.

URETHRAL CALCULUS

Calculi occur less frequently in the urethra than in any other part of the urinary tract. A urethral calculus can arise primarily in the urethra behind a stricture or in an infected urethral diverticulum. The latter are composed of phosphates. Less rarely a calculus which has migrated from the ureter becomes arrested in the prostatic, bulbous, or penile portions of the urethra. Migratory calculi are arrested in the urethra relatively frequently in children under the age of two, the explanation being that the comparatively large vesical neck allows them to pass out of the bladder.

Clinical Features.—In the case of a migratory calculus arrested in the urethra, typically there is a history of an attack of ureteric colic two or three days previously. During micturition the patient experiences sudden pain in the urethra and the stream of urine ceases abruptly. A few drops of blood-stained urine follow, and then there is retention of urine. A stone can be palpated readily through the floor of the urethra. When the stone has been arrested in the prostatic urethra a rectal examination usually reveals a tender, hard nodule in the middle line of the prostate, generally near its apex. A calculus forming behind a urethral stricture often does so without causing much additional discomfort and

---

[1] Sitz bath = in which the patient sits in a bath-tub, bathing only the hips and the buttocks.

it sometimes attains a considerable size before giving rise to retention of urine or painful dysuria. In some cases such a stone can be felt easily; in others, owing to periurethral thickening, its presence is not suspected until it is seen at urethroscopy, or a grating sensation is experienced on passing a gum-elastic bougie or a characteristic click is heard if a metal bougie has been employed. In all but superficially placed calculi giving rise to acute symptoms, radiography is necessary to confirm the presence, and particularly to reveal the size of the calculus before commencing treatment.

Treatment:

(1) *Prostatic Urethra.*—When the stone is arrested in the prostatic urethra a general anaesthetic is given, and a metal bougie is inserted along the urethra as far as the calculus. In cases of recent impaction the stone can be pushed into the bladder, where it can be crushed by litholapaxy and the fragments evacuated. In cases of long-standing the stone is hour-glass shaped, and impacted firmly, in which event it is best approached through the bladder.

(2) *Membranous* and (3) *Bulbous Urethra.*—Occasionally a small stone can be removed from the deeper parts of the urethra by means of urethral forceps passed through a urethroscope. On no account must aero-urethroscopy be employed (danger of air embolism if bleeding occurs). A stone impacted in the proximal urethra sometimes can be manipulated forward if the urethra is distended with lotion. Another method is to pass a number of filiform bougies beyond the stone, twist them, and endeavour to dislodge the calculus by pulling all the bougies out together. A stone impacted in the fossa navicularis, or manipulated into this position, sometimes can be removed by urethral forceps, or by inserting a probe behind it.

Operative Measures (situations 2 and 3).—Meatotomy is often required to permit the stone to be withdrawn. When a stone cannot be removed by one of the expedients described above, an incision is made through the floor of the urethra on to the stone (external urethrotomy). After the stone has been extracted, in the absence of a stricture and gross infection, the urethra can be closed in layers.

NEOPLASMS OF THE MALE URETHRA

Polypi are usually multiple and occur most frequently in the region of the verumontanum. As seen at urethroscopy, each polypus is a pale, finger-like projection with blood vessels coursing over it. Polypi are never found without chronic infection. Sometimes, if the infection can be cured, the polypi disappear: conversely, if polypi are destroyed, chronic urethritis, which previously resisted treatment, often responds to it. Possibly this condition should be classified as a granuloma.

Papilloma.—From time to time a solitary papilloma occurs, most often within the fossa navicularis and, as it enlarges, it protrudes from the external urinary meatus. Multiple papillomas associated with penile papillomas sometimes arise from mucous membrane just within the external urinary meatus. Papillomatosis of the urethra is most often associated with papillomas of the bladder—the posterior urethra is considerably more often affected than the anterior urethra. The typical symptom of papilloma of the urethra is slight haematuria immediately preceding micturition.

Angioma is rare. The haematuria to which it gives rise is often profuse, and may occur independently of micturition.

Treatment of all the foregoing neoplasms is diathermy coagulation through a urethroscope. Exceptionally the neoplasm is so accessible that it can be fulgurated without employing a urethroscope.

Carcinoma is rare. Usually a urethral stricture is antecedent to the carcinoma. Spread to the inguinal lymph nodes often occurs. Blood-borne distant metastases are uncommon unless the cavernous tissue of the penis becomes implicated.

Clinical Features.—As a rule, the first and only symptom is a profuse urethral discharge. Carcinoma of the urethra is therefore one of the many causes of 'urethritis'. Later, the discharge becomes blood-stained and the symptoms of stricture of the urethra supervene. The chronic nature of the condition in a man past forty years of age, the presence of blood in the discharge or in the urine, a tendency to bleed easily during instrumentation, and above all palpable induration, are factors that lead to a suspicion of carcinoma. In the deeper parts of the urethra, sometimes the first manifestation is an indolent periurethral abscess that after incision not only fails to heal, but the periurethral induration increases.

Biopsy then establishes the diagnosis.

Treatment.—When the growth is in the anterior part of the penile urethra partial amputation of the penis can be carried out, and provided the growth had been diagnosed reasonably early, long survival can be expected. Complete amputation with the construction of a perineal meatus is required when the neoplasm is situated more posteriorly.

When the carcinoma is situated further back a still more extensive operation, which includes radical prostatectomy, is the only hope of eradicating the disease.

ABNORMALITIES AFFECTING THE FEMALE URETHRA

Prolapse of the Urethra.—Prolapse of the posterior margin of the urethra occurs in many women past the menopause, and is symptomless unless it is associated with senile urethritis when, on account of straining at micturition, the condition is progressive. Prolapse of the urethral mucous membrane occurs also as a congenital condition. When half or more of the circumference prolapses the local discomfort, especially on walking, is proportionate to the degree of the prolapse. The urinary meatus is examined while the patient strains: when the prolapse is complete the opening of the urethra is central; when it is partial, the opening is eccentric.

Treatment.—The associated urethritis, if present, must be treated first. Often lesser degrees of prolapse can be cured by making one or more linear grooves in the long axis of the mucous membrane of the urethra with a diathermy needle, employing the coagulating current. Subsequent contraction of the scar reduces or obliterates the prolapse. More advanced cases are treated by transfixing the whole thickness of the prolapse as far from its extremity as possible with four catgut sutures placed at equidistant intervals. Redundant urethral mucous membrane is excised distal to the sutures, which prevent retraction of the stump into the canal. The cut edges of the mucous membrane are then united.

Urethral Stricture.—An adult female urethra which fails to admit freely a No. 20 French bougie is the seat of a urethral stricture.

The causes are (a) urethritis, not necessarily gonococcal, and (b), trauma as the result of difficult labour. Inflammatory stricture is situated at the external meatus; traumatic stricture usually affects the middle or posterior part of the urethra.

Sometimes the stricture will only admit a guide, and in these cases acute retention of urine is particularly prone to occur. Dilatation of the stricture yields satisfactory results. The recognition and treatment of a stricture often clears up an obscure case of pain on micturition.

Urethral diverticulum (*syn.* urethrocele) is more common in women than in men. Arguments favour a congenital origin in one of Gärtner's ducts,[1] but some diverticula are acquired by (a) rupture of a distended urethral gland or (b) injury of the urethra during parturition. A small uninfected pouch may be symptomless. As the diverticulum enlarges, inability to pass all the urine at one time, or dribbling after micturition, occurs. Once infected—and infection is almost inevitable if the diverticulum is not evacuated completely at each micturition—recurrent attacks of cystitis perpetuated by reinfection from, the diverticulum continue in spite of antibiotics and chemotherapy. On digital examination a swelling can be felt on the anterior vaginal wall in the line of the urethra, and when it is compressed, urine, usually obviously purulent, is expressed. If the beak of a curved metal bougie is passed gently along the floor of the urethra, from time to time the orifice of the diverticulum is large enough for the beak to enter the sac. In 10% of cases a stone forms in the diverticulum, and haematuria may then occur.

Treatment.—The simplest method is to open the diverticulum through an incision in the vaginal wall. After irrigating the interior of the diverticulum, the mucous membrane is curetted, and the cavity is packed lightly with Oxycel. The incision in the diverticulum and vaginal wall is then closed by interrupted catgut sutures. An indwelling catheter remains in place for a week. It is presumed that fibrosis obliterates the sac (Lane). This procedure is so often successful that formal excision is seldom required, and is reserved for diverticula with wide mouths.

Calculus impacted in the female urethra is exceptional. When it occurs it can be removed by grasping it with forceps while a finger on the anterior vaginal wall presses it forward.

---

[1] The unobliterated distal end of the mesonephric duct.

Hermann Treschow Gärtner, 1785–1829. Surgeon and Anatomist, Copenhagen.
Daniel Francis Victor Lane, Contemporary. Surgeon, Meath Hospital, Dublin.

Urethral caruncle is common in middle-aged and elderly women. The condition presents as a soft, raspberry-like, pedunculated, granulomatous mass about the size of a pea, attached to the posterior urethral wall near the external urinary meatus. Histologically it is composed of highly vascular connective tissue stroma infiltrated with polymorpho-nuclear leucocytes and covered by squamous epithelium.

Clinical Features.—There is increased frequency of micturition, and often great pain during and after micturition. Terminal haematuria often occurs, and there may be a blood-stained discharge independent of micturition. The condition can be diagnosed on inspection, although it must be differentiated from prolapse of the mucous membrane. With a probe it can be determined that the protrusion arises from a pedicle attached to the posterior urethral wall. The mass is exquisitely tender and bleeds readily.

Treatment.—The pedicle should be divided flush with the floor of the urethra with a diathermy needle, using a cutting current, after which that portion of the urethra from which the pedicle arose is coagulated with the diathermy current. The chronic urethritis with which the condition is always associated should be treated by Furacin suppositories and intermittent urethral dilatation until the patient is symptom-free.

Papillomas acuminata occur on the external urinary meatus, and spread on to the labia minora. They differ in no respect from, are acquired in the same way as, and the treatment is similar to that of, papillomas acuminata of the penis. In female Africans papillomas acuminata are common, and they increase at an alarming rate during pregnancy. Towards term, so great does the neoplastic mass become that it may obstruct labour and necessitate Caesarean section (Bowesman).

Carcinoma of the urethra occurs twice as frequently in the female as in the male. Whether or not a caruncle can become malignant is disputed, but a visible bleeding protrusion is the commonest manifestation of a carcinoma of the urethra, and the most common site of the carcinoma in its early stages is the external urinary meatus. A carcinoma commencing within the urethra gives rise to dysuria, haematuria, and sometimes retention of urine. Usually induration distinguishes it from an innocent tumour.

Treatment.—Interstitial irradiation by gold grains or radium needles is the method of choice. If this fails to cure the condition, the advanced state of the disease necessitates total urethro-cystectomy. The prognosis tends to be poor.

THE PENIS

PHIMOSIS

While the condition can be acquired as a result of chronic or acute inflammation of the lining of the prepuce, usually it is due to congenital narrowing of the preputial orifice, often associated with an unduly long foreskin. In extreme examples of congenital phimosis, when the patient micturates the prepuce balloons out first, and a thin, weak stream or urine follows. Difficulty of micturition, with residual urine, hydroureters, and hydronephroses are rarely due to phimosis, but more often occur as a result of atresia meati which may lie hidden by the phimosis. The treatment is circumcision.

Circumcision[1]

Indications.—(a) *In infants and young boys*, because of a request by the parents (religious and personal); because of recurrent balanitis with inability to retract the prepuce; and, rarely, because of a very long prepuce. Except for the ritual operation most circumcisions are unnecessary: it is normal for the prepuce to be long and adherent to the glans within, for these parts become satisfactorily separ-

[1] Apparently circumcision did not originate among the Jews: they took the custom from either the Babylonians or the Negroes, probably the latter. It has been practised in West Africa for over 5000 years.

Charles Bowesman, Contemporary. Formerly Surgical Specialist, Colonial Medical Service, Kumasi, Ghana.

ated and the prepuce mobile in the first few years of life. Recurrent balanoposthitis and phimosis often follow attempts by the parents forcibly to retract the prepuce. (*b*) *In adults*, because of inability to retract for intercourse, a tight fraenum, balanitis, and sometimes prior to radiotherapy for carcinoma. A dorsal slit may suffice.

Technique in an infant

The much advocated method of applying a clamp or bone forceps across the redundant prepuce distal to the glans with blind division of the foreskin can no longer be condoned. To see one little boy with partial or total amputation of the glans is enough to realise the folly of this technique. It is far better to perform a proper circumcision under direct vision as in an adult.

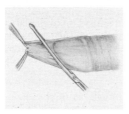

FIG. 1317.—Applying sinus forceps preparatory to excising the redundant skin.

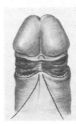

FIG. 1318. — The 'four-in-one' fraenal stitch.

In adolescents and adults the following method is preferable. The prepuce is retracted until its tense orifice is apparent, or until the tip of the glans comes into view, and on to the edge of the prepuce are placed three haemostats, one in the middle line ventrally and two either side of the middle line dorsally. The prepuce is then slit up in the middle line dorsally to within 1·25 cm of the corona. The under-surface of the prepuce having been completely separated from the glans and the corona, the layers of each flap are excised, keeping 1·25 cm distal to the corona. The superficial layer is retracted and bleeding-points are secured and ligated. The inner layer of the prepuce having been trimmed to 3 mm from the corona, the two cut edges are approximated accurately with fine interrupted catgut stitches. The cut edges in the immediate vicinity of the fraenum can be drawn together neatly by a mattress suture. It is best dressed by wrapping a thin layer of wool round and painting this with Tinct. Benz. Co. (Friar's Balsam).

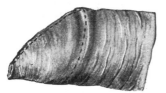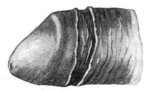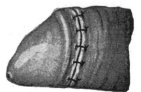

FIG. 1319.—Method of circumcision in an adult.

Perhaps an even better method is initially to stretch the phimosis allowing division of the glandular adhesions and then perform two circumferential incisions of the foreskin. First one marks out the cut to be made on the shaft skin at the level of the coronal sulcus. A circumferential incision is then made and the prepuce retracted. A second circumferential incision is then made just proximal to the coronal sulcus so as to leave an adequate 'mucosa'. The released redundant foreskin is removed, two transverse sutures are inserted to reconstruct the frenulum and the mucosa and skin then opposed with interrupted chromic sutures. This provides the best cosmetic result.

PREPUTIAL CALCULI

Late in life, chronic posthitis resulting in fibrosis constricts an already inadequate orifice of a preputial sac. When the prepuce has not been retracted nor its interior cleansed for many years, preputial calculi are wont to form. Three types are described: 1. Those resulting from inspissated smegma. 2. Those consisting of a mixture of smegma and urinary salts. 3. Those consisting entirely of urinary salts. The treatment is circumcision.

PARAPHIMOSIS

The tight prepuce has been retracted but cannot be returned, and it is constricting the glans which is engorged and oedematous. The diagnosis is apparent at a glance.

Treatment.—One ml of isotonic saline containing 150 turbidity units of hyaluronidase is injected into each lateral aspect of the swollen ring of prepuce. Fifteen minutes later the swelling is much reduced, and in early cases reduction (fig. 1320) can be accomplished with ease. If this is unsuccessful, a general anaesthetic must be given and the constricting band is incised, and the narrow cuff of skin which formed the constricting band excised (fig. 1321). There is now no obstruction to reduction, and it remains only to remove a broad cuff of normal skin on the proximal side of the gap and unite the cut free edges, thus performing circumcision.

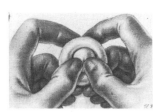

FIG. 1320.—Reducing a paraphimosis.

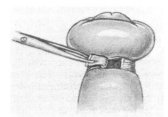

FIG. 1321.—Excising the constricting band.

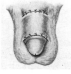

FIG. 1322. — Covering the denuded shaft of the penis by burying it in a scrotal tunnel.

Often the tissues are too oedematous to achieve a good cosmetic result and it is far better to simply perform a dorsal slit to relieve the constriction. A circumcision to trim the redundant skin is done at a later date.

INJURIES

Avulsion of the Skin of the Penis.—Entanglement of clothing in rotating machinery accounts for the majority of these injuries. Repair can be carried out by burying the shaft of the penis in the scrotum (fig. 1322), with subsequent surgical release at a propitious time.

The prepuce is also at risk in the zip fastening of pants, and freedom may only be achieved at the expense of emergency circumcision (Shah).

Fracture of the penis is a very uncommon accident due, most often, to the erect organ being bent forcibly downwards. Following trauma, the erect organ suddenly becomes flaccid. The extravasation of blood, which is considerable, causes great pain and swelling. In early cases incision, clearing out blood-clot, and suture of the ruptured corpus cavernosum has yielded good results.

STRANGULATION OF THE PENIS BY RINGS

Removal is prevented by venous engorgement. Consequently aspiration of the corpora cavernosa may assist in removal of the ring in early cases, otherwise a ring cutter or a hacksaw must be employed. If a tight ring is not removed within six hours, unless the bladder is drained suprapubically, or perineal urethrostomy performed, rupture of the urethra with extravasation may ensue.

Dr. Tushar J. Shah, Contemporary. Asst. Professor of Surgery, Ahmenabad, Gujarat, India.

INFLAMMATIONS

Balanoposthitis.—An inflammation of the prepuce is known as posthitis; an inflammation of the glans penis is called balanitis. Frequently the opposing surfaces of the prepuce and the glans are implicated in the inflammatory process—hence the term balanophosthitis. Local skin conditions often affect the penis and may be quite localised, for example lichen planus or psoriasis. Fixed drug reactions due to tetracycline or sulphonamides are not uncommon.

N.B.—It is imperative to bear in mind that cancer, chancre, or sugar in the urine may be the primary factor, and that the condition is nearly always associated with some degree of phimosis. In mild cases the only symptom is itching and some discharge. Acute cases show a red, swollen and tender foreskin with exuding pus. Monilial (candida) infections are quite common.

Treatment.—Every effort must be made to prevent drops of urine (which must be tested for glycosuria) from getting under the prepuce. For mild exudative eczemas local copper sulphate 0·2% is useful. Skin eruptions should receive appropriate treatment. If there is a phimosis with much purulent discharge, subpreputial washouts combined with a sulphonamide almost invariably produce resolution and operation is rarely required. Broad-spectrum antibiotics and penicillin which might mask a subjacent syphilitic sore should not be given.

GENITAL HERPES

Usually sexually transmitted, it is caused mainly by Herpes virus hominis [H.P.V.][1] type 2 but also by type 1. Recurrent attacks occur in fifty per cent of cases. Pain along the distribution of the sensory nerve, usually genito-femoral, precedes the eruption by two days, and around the perianal region may be exceptionally severe. Then appears a group of tiny vesicles which rapidly erode to form shallow red or yellow based ulcers which may coalesce forming a serpiginous outline. In the female the lesions often spread on to the thighs during the first attack. Involvement of the urethra may cause retention of urine for 2–3 days due to intense dysuria. If this lasts longer for ten to fourteen days, the cause is likely to be a radiculitis of the second and third sacral nerves. Syphilis must always be excluded by dark ground and blood tests and if possible, viral tests carried out to confirm the diagnosis.

Acyclovir (Acycloguanosine) marks an important advance in treatment seeing that all previous remedies were virtually useless. For very severe cases in women, it should be given by infusion taking one hour of 5 mg/kg 8 hourly for 15 doses. For less severe cases especially first attacks, tablets 200 mg—4 hourly (except at night) for 5 days is satisfactory and for mild recurrences, the cream applied similarly. Recurrences, however, are not prevented.

Owing to the risk of fatal generalised Herpes in the neonate, Caesarean section should be performed on any woman with genital herpes close to the time of delivery or who with a past history has a positive cervical culture for the virus four to six weeks prior to delivery but not otherwise. All such patients should have annual cytology tests for life due to the increased risk of carcinoma of the cervix. Close cooperation between departments of surgery and genito-urinary medicine facilitates this.

It is now established that not only does HPV infection in the patient predispose to carcinoma of the cervix, but also that in her husband or consort.

LYMPHOGRANULOMA VENEREUM

A sexually transmitted tropical disease caused by Chlamydia trachomatis (Chlamydia A) types L1 to 3. The primary lesion is a fleeting, painless, genital papule or ulcer often unnoticed by the patient.

After two to eight weeks, occasionally as long as sixteen, in both sexes the inguinal glands become enlarged, painful and matted together both above and

---

[1] H.P.V. = human papilloma virus.

below the inguinal ligament which produces the 'sign of the groove'. The overlying skin reddens and fluctuation develops. In the female, proctitis may develop after a few weeks which, if untreated, may produce a rectal stricture. The later stages are due to lymphatic spread and blockage leading to oedema of the genitals, vaginal stricture and esthiomene (vulval elephantiasis) in the female and even elephantiasm of the legs. Urethritis and urethral stricture occur in the male.

Confirmatory Tests.—Isolation of Chlamydia A from the lesions, the Frei skin test (if available) and the L.G.V. Complement Fixation Test (LGVCFT) in a titre of 1 in 40—or better still a rising titre. The modern micro-IF (micro-immunofluorescent) test, if available, should be performed.

Treatment.—A course of Sulphonamide 1 g four times a day, Oxytetracycline 500 mg four times daily, Erythromycin 500 mg or, if available, triacetyloeandomycin (Evramycin), all for fourteen days, may prevent abscess formation and cure the infection. On no account should the multilocular bubo be incised—aspiration is indicated.

GRANULOMA INGUINALE

A chronic slowly progressive ulcerative tropical disease affecting the genitalia and surrounding tissues but occasionally occurring on extra-genital sites. It is usually sexually transmitted and tends to occur in poor Negroes living in primitive conditions. The average incubation period is from 7 to 30 days but may be shorter and also very much longer.

Clinical course.—A painless vesicle or indurated papule usually on the external genitals but occasionally elsewhere on the skin gradually erodes into a slowly extending ulcer with a beefy red granulomatous base. More chronic lesions may assume a greyish colour especially at the edges where after months or years, malignant change may develop. The ulcerated area readily bleeds if touched but is surprisingly painless. Without treatment only partial healing occurs and keloid scars are liable to form. Metastases in bone occasionally occur, particularly in women.

Diagnosis.—Material from the edge of the lesion treated with Giemsa's stain will show Donovan bodies—short safety-pin Gram-negative rods within the cytoplasm of the large mononuclear cells.

Treatment is best with Oxytetracycline 500 mg q.d.s. for twenty days, or Streptomycin 4 g in divided dosage for 5 days or Cotrimoxazole (but not ordinary sulphonamides), 2 tablets b.d. for 10 days.

CONDYLOMATA ACUMINATA (GENITAL WARTS) (fig. 1323)

Are caused by varieties of the human papilloma virus (HPV) and are sexually transmitted. Ordinary cutaneous warts may also occur on the genitals by direct contact with finger lesions. Usually, the former are soft, moist and often pedunculated. Most commonly they occur under the prepuce in the coronal sulcus but may be found anywhere including the urinary meatus. In women, most commonly found on the vulva, they may line the vagina and occur on the cervix. Perianal warts are common.

Other sexually transmitted diseases should be excluded—candidiasis and trichomoniasis mainly in women, and in men, syphilis or gonorrhea particularly with

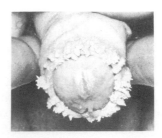

FIG. 1323.—Penile warts. Most commonly they occur under the prepuce, in the coronal sulcus, but may be found anywhere including the urinary meatus. In women, most commonly found on the vulva, they may line the vagina and occur on the cervix. Perianal warts are common.

perianal warts. HIV infection must be remembered in homosexual patients with genital warts.

Treatment is by chemical or physical means. For the former, podophyllin 25% in spirit is best used. It must be carefully applied to the wart with an orange stick and the area powdered to protect the surrounding surfaces. It should be washed off after 6 hours. For hard warts, trichloroacetic acid is more satisfactory and for intrameatal warts, both the acid and podophyllin applied together give much better results. On no account should patients be allowed to apply these substances themselves or take them home—serious burns may result. Several applications may be necessary.

If these methods fail, cryosurgery may be successful but electrocautery, particularly for perianal warts, is better. A local or general anaesthetic must be used. Infiltration of the perianal subcutaneous tissues with 1 in 300,000 adrenaline solution will allow the individual warts to be excised with scissors which results in little or no scarring. Following an operation, patients should be seen at least weekly so that possible recurrences can be dealt with as soon as they occur, and should not be discharged for one year (Thomson).

Syphilis, Yaws, Chancroid and Candidiasis.—See Chapter 4.

CHORDEE[1]

Chordee is a fixed bending or bowing of the penis due to (*a*) hypospadias or (*b*) acutely as a result of general urethritis. Erection is grotesque and very painful. The treatment is stilboestrol 6 mg daily, but surgical relief may be required (p. 1321).

INDURATIO-PENIS-PLASTICA (*syn.* PEYRONIE'S DISEASE)

Usually the patient is over forty years of age and seldom is there a history of venereal disease. At the onset pain and curving of the penis on erection cause the patient to seek advice, but after a few weeks the pain disappears. On palpation an indurated plaque can be felt on the dorsal surface of one corpus cavernosum. The condition is slowly progressive and sometimes extends across the middle line. Its aetiology is uncertain; bygone trauma is a possible explanation and it is sometimes associated with Dupuytren's contracture (Chapter 24).

Treatment has remained an unsolved problem for over 200 years. In some cases there is a tendency to slow resolution over three to five years. Steroids may assist.

PERSISTENT PRIAPISM

The penis remains erect, and is painful. The glans and the corpus spongiosum are not involved. Most often the erection is due to idiopathic thrombosis occurring in the prostatic venous plexus. Less frequently it is associated with leukaemia or sickle-celled anaemia. Secondary malignant deposits in the corpora cavernosa, or in the pelvis, account for about

---

[1] *Cordee* (Fr.) = corded.

J. P. S. Thomson, *Contemporary. Consultant Surgeon, St. Mark's Hospital, London.*
François de la Peyronie, 1678–1747. Surgeon to Louis XIV and Founder of the Royal Academy of Surgery, Paris.

7% of cases. In another completely different category are cases due to spinal injury or disease.

Diagnosis.—A low spinal anaesthetic will cause priapism of neurogenic origin to abate temporarily. A blood-count is essential to exclude leukaemia.

Treatment.—Local applications are useless. Anastomosis of the saphenous vein to one corpus cavernosum can be very effective if done within the first 48 hours. The corpora should be washed out with saline. Alternatively, the corpora cavernosa can be anastomosed to the corpus spongiosum. The use of heparin and streptokinase in late cases has not given very good results.

CARCINOMA OF THE PENIS

Aetiology.—For a reason that is only partially understood, circumcision correctly performed soon after birth confers almost total immunity against carcinoma of the penis. On the other hand (and this is difficult of explanation) circumcision after early infancy does not provide the same degree of protection. Mohammedans, who are circumcised between the ages of four and nine years, exemplify this. For practical purposes, then, carcinoma of the penis occurs in men who have not been circumcised in early infancy, and undoubtedly the development of this neoplasm is favoured by chronic balanophosthitis. Furthermore, there are definite pre-carcinomatous states, viz.:

(*a*) **Leukoplakia of the glans** is exactly comparable to the well-known condition of the tongue.

(*b*) Long-standing **genital warts** (above) due to H.P.V. infection.

(*c*) **Paget's Disease of the Penis** (*syn. Erythroplasia of Querat*).—'I have seen a persistent rawness of the glans like a long-standing balanitis followed by cancer of the substance of the penis' (Sir James Paget). It is possible that penile Paget's disease escapes detection until carcinoma has developed. Treatment is by radium or diathermy excision.

Pathology.—There are two types of squamous carcinoma of the penis—the flat or infiltrating, and the papilliferous. The former may be associated with leukoplakia; the latter commences in a papilloma of long standing. The growth remains purely local for months. The earliest spread is to the inguinal, and then to the iliac lymph nodes. Direct spread to the body of the penis is prevented for many months by the fascial sheath of the corpora cavernosa, but once this barrier becomes broken the growth extends more rapidly and the iliac lymph nodes (fig. 1324) become involved. Distant metastatic deposits are infrequent.

Clinical Features.—It is a mistake to believe that this is a disease confined to the elderly—40% of the sufferers are under forty years of age. The progress of the disease is slow; the first symptoms are a mild irritation and a purulent discharge from the prepuce. These symptoms are often neglected (fig. 1325), and by the time the patient reports, sometimes more than a year after symptoms have appeared, there is a blood-stained, foul discharge. Pain is singularly absent. The inguinal lymph nodes are enlarged in over 60% of cases, but in only half of these is the enlargement due to secondary deposits, the remainder being due to sepsis. In most cases the prepuce cannot be retracted, and in order to view the lesion the prepuce must be slit. In all cases a biopsy should be performed.

Untreated, the whole glans becomes a fungating and particularly foul-smelling mass. Later, the inguinal lymph nodes fungate through the skin of the groin, and often death relieves the victim by torrential haemorrhage following erosion of the femoral or external iliac artery.

Sir James Paget, 1814–1899. Surgeon, St. Bartholomew's Hospital, London.

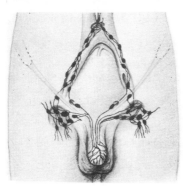

FIG. 1324.—The lymphatic drainage of the penis. Superficial lymphatics drain to the inguinal, and deep lymphatics to the iliac, lymph nodes.
(After Archie L. Dean.)

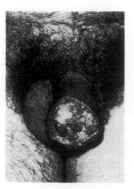

FIG. 1325.—Carcinoma of the penis.

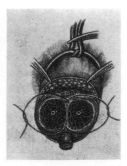

FIG. 1326.— Partial amputation of the penis.

Treatment:

Radiotherapy gives good results (60 to 70% five-year survival) with small well-differentiated tumours. **Surgery** is needed for large anaplastic growths; if there is infiltration of the shaft of the penis; when radiotherapy has failed; in elderly men who do not mind the mutilation as much as the pain to be expected from the extensive reaction to radiotherapy. *Partial amputation* is used for distal growths providing there is at least 2 cm of the dependant shaft which is not involved. With an advanced, infiltrating, or anaplastic lesion *total amputation* must be performed.

Radiotherapy methods are: implantation with flexible radio-active tantalum wires (total dose 6000 rad in five to seven days); medium or high-voltage x-rays (5000 to 6000 rad given in divided doses over five weeks); by radium mould applicators worn intermittently or continuously (not exceeding 6000 rad in seven to ten days). If not already performed, a dorsal slit is a prerequisite for treatment and nursing.

Partial Amputation Technique (guillotine amputation).—A tourniquet, in the form of a No. 6 French rubber catheter, is placed around the most proximal portion of the penis, being tied once, and the knot clipped in a haemostat. An abdominal pack is placed over the glans penis and with a piece of strong silk is tied tightly to the shaft of the penis at the proposed level of section. A ventral flap is fashioned and amputation is then performed, and the pack, with its contents, is dropped into a receptacle. The exposed cross-section of the penile stump is examined for extensions of the growth. If, as is usual, none is present, the dorsal vessels are ligated. The corpus spongiosum is dissected from the corpora cavernosa for 1 cm. A long straight needle carrying a double stout catgut suture is passed from the ventral to the dorsal aspect of the fibrous septum separating the two corpora cavernosa, the needle entering just distal to the attached portion of the corpus spongiosum. The needle having been removed (fig. 1326), each corpus cavernosum is ligated firmly. The free portion of the urethra and its surrounding corpus spongiosum is divided dorsally and ventrally for nearly 1 cm. The tourniquet is now removed. The split urethra is passed through a suitable opening made in the skin flap and affixed by interrupted stitches that pass through the whole thickness of the corporus spongiosum, thereby avoiding a post-operative stricture. Bleeding-points having been ligated, the remaining portions of the skin edges are approximated vertically over the cut corpora cavernosa. An indwelling catheter is employed until the dressings are dispensed with.

Complete amputation includes the removal of the corpora cavernosa from the pubic bones and division of the corpus spongiosum so as to leave at least 1·5 cm protruding from the perineum, as a perineal urethrostomy, via an incision behind the scrotum. Careful suture of the split urethra to the skin avoids a subsequent stricture.

The Treatment of Associated Enlarged Inguinal Lymph Nodes.—It is advisable to wait for at least three weeks after the local lesion has been dealt with by one of the methods described. If the enlargement is due to inflammation, the lymph nodes will decrease in size or disappear with antibiotic treatment. When these lymph nodes remain unaltered at the end of this period, block dissection of the more affected side should be undertaken, followed by contralateral block dissection at a later date. The five-year survival rate falls to some 35% in these cases.

If the enlarged lymph nodes are massive and fixed (inoperable), x-ray therapy causes some temporary regression.

Buschke-Loewenstein tumour is uncommon. It has the histological pattern of a verrucous carcinoma. It is locally destructive and invasive. but appears not to spread to lymph nodes, nor metastasise. Treatment is surgical excision.

Secondary carcinoma of the penis occurs from time to time, and about a hundred cases have been reported. The primary source of the disease is usually the bladder, rectum, or prostate.

The metastasis arrives in the penis in one of three ways: (*a*) by direct spread: (*b*) by retrograde lymphatic transport; (*c*) by retrograde venous embolism via the dorsal vein of the penis. The condition must be differentiated from Peyronie's disease. As would be expected, secondary carcinoma of the penis occurs only late in the course of the disease; nevertheless, in many instances active treatment is worth while.

CHAPTER 61

THE TESTES AND THE SCROTUM

CONGENITAL ABNORMALITIES

Anterior inversion is said to be present in one in every fifty males. The epididymis lies anteriorly, and the body of the testis and the tunica vaginalis posteriorly. When the organ is diseased this anomaly may cause confusion in diagnosis.

Polar inversion is less frequent. In some cases when there is complete inversion the globus major lies inferiorly. In other cases it lies horizontally. Both varieties predispose to torsion. Complete inversion, impossible to detect clinically, is an incidental finding at operation, when it is observed that the hydatid of Morgagni is situated at the lower, instead of the upper, pole.

IMPERFECT DESCENT OF THE TESTIS

Under this heading are included two conditions:

Incomplete Descent.—The testis is arrested in some part of its path to the scrotum.

Ectopic Testis.—The testis is abnormally placed outside this path.

Development of the Testes.—The testes develop from the genital fold, which lies medial to the mesonephros (Wolffian body), and therefore in early fetal life they lie in the coelomic cavity behind the peritoneum and below the developing kidneys. The primitive testis is attached to the posterior abdominal wall by a mesentery, the mesorchium, which contains the testicular blood-vessels and nerves, derived from the tenth and twelfth dorsal segments respectively. About the tenth week of intra-uterine life some of the transverse tubules of the mesonephros unite with the rete testis to form the vasa efferentia; others remain rudimentary. Most of the Wolffian body disappears, but the Wolffian duct becomes the epididymis and vas deferens. About this time tissue in a fold of peritoneum (plica inguinalis) develops, containing the precursor of the gubernaculum[1]; it is attached to the junction of the vas deferens and epididymis, and can be traced through the abdominal wall to end in the region of the developing phallus. The processus vaginalis appears as a dimple of peritoneum about the tenth week and precedes the testis through the layers of the abdominal wall down into the scrotum. Muscular fibres develop in the mesoderm of the plica inguinalis to form the gubernaculum but there is still no certainty as to the part this structure plays in regulating testicular descent.

Chorionic gonadotrophin from the maternal circulation stimulates the growth of the testis and may play some part in the migration of the organ. Undoubtedly imperfect development of a testis is a significant factor in incomplete descent of the organ.

Morphology.—Most of the misplacements of the testes in man are a counterpart of the varying normal placements of the testes in animals. In the whale and the elephant the testes remain in the undescended abdominal position throughout life. Rodents and hibernating animals, such as the hedgehog, the mole and the bat, maintain open inguinal canals, and the testes are housed in the abdomen, to descend into the scrotum only during the breeding season.

INCOMPLETELY DESCENDED TESTIS

Incidence:

In the Neonatal Period.—At birth, and for a variable number of weeks afterwards, the cremasteric reflex, which is so active in young boys, is absent. Scorer examined 2000

---

[1] Gubernaculum = a rudder. It was first described by John Hunter, who believed that its function was to guide the testis into the scrotum.

Giovanni Battista Morgagni, 1682–1771. Professor of Anatomy, Padua, Italy. He held the Chair for fifty-six years, and is regarded as the founder of Pathological Anatomy.
Kaspar Friedrich Wolff, 1733–1794. Professor of Anatomy and Physiology, St. Petersburg (now Leningrad), U.S.S.R.
John Hunter, 1728–1793. Surgeon, St. George's Hospital, London.
Charles Gordon Scorer, Contemporary. Surgeon, Hillingdon Hospital, Uxbridge, Middlesex, England.

newborn male infants and found that the incidence of incomplete descent on one or both sides was 4% in full-term infants and 30% in premature infants. A follow-up of all cases showed that in more than 50% the testis or testes reached the scrotum during the first month of life. More often than not incomplete descent of the testis is not detected during infancy.

In later childhood and puberty the incidence is 2%. Frequently the condition still remains unrecognised unless a routine examination is made by the school medical officer. In a few cases the presence of a hernia, pain in the region, or acute torsion, in that order of frequency, directs attention to the abnormality.

In Adult Life.—It is inconceivable that a man can fail to notice the absence of one or both testes in his scrotum, yet there must be many with this abnormality who do not seek advice about it unless symptoms develop. Sometimes the condition is first discovered at the medical examination for entrance to one of the Public Services. In an examination of 10,000 recruits during World War II the incidence was found to be 0·8%..In 10% of unilateral cases there is a familial history.

Pathology.—Up to the age of six years there are no microscopical differences between an incompletely descended testis and a normal testis. After that time, due, it is believed, to the higher temperature to which it is subjected, the development of the incompletely descended organ becomes progressively retarded.[1] By the time puberty has been reached the incompletely descended testis is flabby and hardly more than half the size of its intrascrotal counterpart. Histologically, the epithelial elements are grossly immature, and by the age of sixteen irreversible destructive changes have occurred in the germinal epithelium.

The *external secretory mechanism* of an incompletely descended testis functions but feebly and, often after a few months or years, ceases; thus its power of spermato-genesis may be negligible.

The internal secretory activity of an incompletely descended testis is reduced. In bilateral cryptorchism about half the normal amount of androgen is produced: notwithstanding, the secondary sexual attributes of a cryptorchid are seldom noticeably in abeyance.

If an incompletely descended testis is brought down satisfactorily *before puberty* it often develops and functions satisfactorily.

Clinical Features.—The right testis alone is affected in 50% of cases, the left alone in 30%, while double arrested descent occurs in 20%. Other abnormalities of the urinary tract may be present.

The testis may be:

1. *Retained within the abdomen* extraperitoneally, usually just above the internal abdominal ring.

2. *In the Inguinal Canal.*—Early in life the testis is a soft structure, and when, as in this instance, it is submerged in the non-resisting floor of the inguinal canal, and shielded by the overlying tendinous aponeurosis of the external oblique, it cannot be felt.

When both testes are in the abdomen or the inguinal canals and are consequently. impalpable, the condition is known as cryptorchidism (hidden testes) (fig. 1327).

3. *In the Superficial Subinguinal Pouch.*—Very frequently during childhood the testes are mobile, each being withdrawn by the contraction of the cremasters into the superficial subinguinal pouch (fig. 1328), a space lined by loose areolar

---

[1] The scrotum is a thermo-regulator to the testes, and keeps them at a temperature at least 1°C lower than that of the inguinal canals.

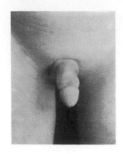

Fig. 1327.—A cryptorchid, aged 12. Note the retracted, underdeveloped scrotum. In cases of retractile testes the scrotum is comparatively well-developed.

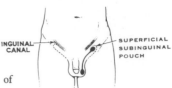

Fig. 1328.—Mechanism of retractile testes.

tissue superficial to the external oblique aponeurosis or into the inguinal canal. Reflex retraction occurs from a very slight stimulus such as touching the thigh or the abdomen, or even by exposure of the parts. Not infrequently this testicular mobility continues throughout childhood on both sides, or less frequently on one side. At all times it is liable to be mistaken for incomplete descent unless a special method of examination is undertaken, if necessary on more than one occasion. Retractile testes should be suspected if the scrotum is normal; in incomplete descent the corresponding side of the scrotum is undeveloped. This inspection completed, the pulps of two fingers are placed over the superficial inguinal pouch, exerting moderate pressure. By drawing the fingers towards the neck of the scrotum a testis of the retractile type can be pushed into the upper part of the scrotum, where it is grasped between the finger and thumb of the other hand. *Only if the testis cannot be made to touch the bottom of the scrotum[1] is it imperfectly descended.* When the testis *can* be placed in a normal position temporarily it is not truly an imperfectly descended testis, and it should be known by its fitting title '*retractile testis*'. Such testes require neither endocrine nor operative treatment. In course of time (it may be delayed until puberty), the testis will take up a normal position permanently. Another valuable method of encouraging the testes to drop down into the scrotum is to make the child squat, the thighs being brought up on to the abdomen.

In infancy 80% of non-apparent testes are retractile. In the remaining 20% true incomplete descent is present.

The Hazards of Incomplete Descent

1. *Sterility* in bilateral cases.

2. *Pain.* An inguinal testis is liable to oft-repeated trauma.

3. *An associated indirect inguinal or interstitial hernia* is present in 70% of cases, and in adolescent and adult patients it is frequently the hernia that causes the symptoms.

4. *Torsion.*

5. *Epididymo-orchitis.*—Right-sided epididymo-orchitis occurring in an incompletely descended organ is extremely difficult, if not impossible, to differentiate from an acute appendicitis. It is, however, very rare because the abnormal testis is less likely to become involved by descending infection.

---

[1] Only by applying the test carefully and correctly in every case will the extravagant claims of some of those who employ endocrine therapy be dissipated.

6. *Atrophy*, even before puberty, sometimes occurs when the testis is situated in the inguinal canal. This is attributed to recurrent trauma.

7. *Increased Liability to Malignant Disease.*—All types of malignant testicular tumour have been recorded as developing in undescended testes, and in those brought down surgically. It is definite that seminoma is more common possibly because the testis is frequently histologically abnormal. Some compute that 1 in 20 abdominal and 1 in 80 inguinal testes become malignant; others say this estimation is far too high. Reliable statistical evidence as to whether orchiopexy diminishes the liability to tumour formation later, is not available. However, at the worst it should improve the prospect of early diagnosis.

Treatment by Orchiopexy.—Most surgeons used to favour performing the operation between the ages of six and eight years. Many others now choose an even earlier age in order to reduce the incidence of thermal damage to the germinal epithelium. Providing safe anaesthetic services are available, it is now regarded as acceptable to operate in the child's fourth year, but the operation *is never performed in the first two years*. After the age of puberty the percentage of successful operations, which at the optimum age approaches 80%, falls considerably. In cryptorchidism one side should be operated upon at a time, with an interval of six months between the operations.

The operation consists of (1) mobilising the spermatic cord and testicular vessels; (2) retaining the mobilised testis in the descended position.

1. **Mobilising the Spermatic Cord.**—The inguinal canal is opened. The cord and testis are freed from surrounding structures and a concomitant inguinal hernial sac is dealt with. The dissection of the diaphanous sac from the cord is greatly facilitated by opening the sac and injecting a small amount of isotonic saline just underneath that part which is adherent. Near the internal inguinal ring all the coverings of the cord are divided; every muscle fibre and fibrous band is severed, leaving only the vas and its blood-vessels and the spermatic blood-vessels. Sometimes this provides sufficient length for the testis to be placed in the scrotum. If not, the spermatic vessels are dissected from the peritoneum to which they are adherent. This abolishes the wide, outward curve of the vessels, thereby gaining up to 2·5 cm. It is most exceptional for the above measures to fail to elongate the pedicle sufficiently for the testis to be placed in the scrotum, and even beyond it: the avoidance of vascular tension is the keystone of plastic surgery. The empty half of the scrotum is stretched thoroughly with the index finger passed into it through the inguinal incision.

2. **Retaining the testis in the scrotum** is effected by one of a number of ingenious methods, of which the following are popular:

(*a*) *Narrowing the neck of the scrotum and fixation of the testis to the bottom of the scrotum*, is all that is needed in many cases. The neck of the scrotum is narrowed with catgut sutures, and the testis is anchored below by an unabsorbable suture passed through the scrotal skin, this suture being removed after one week.

(*b*) *Dartos pouch.*—The testis is retained in the scrotum by placing it in a dartos pouch just under the scrotal skin.

(*c*) *Ombrédanne's operation* is similar, but the testis is passed through a gap in the scrotal septum, which is then narrowed round the cord. This is useful when the length of cord is short as the septum can be drawn across to the external ring. The weight of the opposite testis will supply gentle traction which will gradually draw the undescended one further down.

Failure to bring the testis down.—(1) Sometimes a two-stage procedure is successful: mobilisation as far as possible, and anchorage with an unabsorbable suture, followed six months later by further mobilisation. (2) *Orchiectomy*, if the other testis is normal, and the incompletely descended testis is hopelessly atrophic, or, after puberty.

Orchio-coelioplasty (abdominal replacement of the organ). This measure is justifiable when the contralateral organ has been removed previously and orchiopexy is found to be

Louis Ombrédanne, 1871–1956. Surgeon, Hôpital des Enfants Malades, Paris.

impossible. It is then the only method of preserving a supply of internal testicular secretion and protecting the organ from injury.

Hormone Treatment.—The only indications for hormone treatment are:

1. Cases of bilateral incomplete descent associated with hypogenitalism and obesity.

2. In cases of uncertainty as to whether the case is one of testes retracting into the inguinal canal or one of true incomplete descent.

Of many preparations having a gonadotrophic action, chorionic gonadotrophin extracted from the placenta (Pregnyl) is the one usually employed. It should be given at about eight years of age, and 1000 international units are given twice a week until the testes descend, the limit of the course being ten weeks, after which it must *never* be repeated, otherwise secondary male characteristics may develop prematurely.

ECTOPIC TESTIS

An ectopic testis may be found, in order of frequency:

1. Anchored in the superficial inguinal pouch. 2. In the perineum. 3. At the root of the penis. 4. In the femoral triangle.

Unlike the imperfectly descended testis, an ectopic organ often develops well, if not fully. Its main hazard is that it is liable to injury.

Aetiology.—To explain the appearance of the testis in these anomalous positions, Lockwood advanced the ingenious theory of many gubernacular tails. His theory postulates that in ectopic testis the scrotal tail becomes ruptured. As a consequence the testis, adrift from its usual mooring, follows one of the accessory rudders.

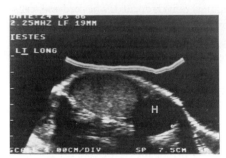

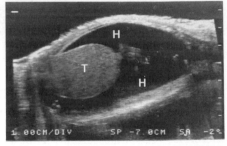

FIG. 1329.—Longitudinal scan of testicle with a haematocele (H) at the lower pole.
(Dr N. Barrett.)

FIG. 1330.—Longitudinal scan of testis (T) with a large hydrocele (H).
(Dr J. Boultbee.)

INJURIES OF THE TESTIS

Closed rupture of the testis from blows and the like is an uncommon accident owing to the extreme mobility of the organ within the scrotum. Severe contusion and rupture are each associated with a haematocele which surrounds the testis, rendering the differential diagnosis impossible without exploration. Operation is advisable in these cases in order to:

1. Evacuate the haematoma.

2. Repair the tunica albuginea, if split, excising only that part of the testicular tissue that extrudes. If the testis is severely damaged, orchiectomy should be performed.

Haematocele (p. 1362) fig. 1329.

Traumatic Displacement of the Testis.—As a result of a blow the testis occasionally becomes displaced and (by reason of blood-clot) anchored, usually in one of the positions described under ectopic testis. Unless the displacement is reduced early by manipulation, an operation is required to replace the organ in the scrotum.

Charles Barrett Lockwood, 1856–1914. Surgeon, St. Batholomew's Hospital, London.

TORSION OF THE TESTIS (*syn.* TORSION OF THE SPERMATIC CORD)

Predisposing Causes.—Torsion of the testis is uncommon. It does not occur in a normal fully descended testis: its anchorage prevents rotation. Therefore one of several anomalies must be present.

(*a*) *Inversion of the Testis.*—This appears to be the commonest predisposing cause. (*b*) *High investment of the tunica vaginalis* causes the testis to hang within the tunica like a clapper in a bell. Very occasionally torsion is extravaginal. (*c*) *In cases where the body of the testis is separated from the epididymis*, torsion of the body can occur without involving the cord. The twisting is confined to the mesentery that joins the testis to the epididymis.

Exciting Causes.—Normally the cremaster contracts *pari passu* with violent contraction of the abdominal musculature. Contractions of the spirally attached cremaster favour rotation around the vertical axis in relevant cases. Straining at stool, lifting a heavy weight, and coitus are all exciting causes, but often the history fails to reveal any one of them. Occasionally torsion develops during sleep.

Clinical Features.—The highest incidence is between ten and twenty-five years of age, and the second most common age period is during infancy. The symptoms vary with the degree of torsion present. Most commonly the patient experiences sudden and agonising pain in the groin and lower abdomen, and vomits. Upon theoretical grounds one might think that the diagnosis is simple, but sometimes it is practically impossible to distinguish *torsion of an imperfectly descended testis* from a strangulated inguinal hernia until the parts have been displayed by operation. The fact that the side of the scrotum is empty and oedematous is certainly in favour of the tender lump at the external abdominal ring being the testis with its twisted cord. *Torsion of a completely descended testis* is a less difficult problem. Sometimes the actual twists in the cord can be felt, thus establishing the diagnosis. At other times the condition can be mimicked exactly by a small, tense, strangulated inguinal hernia compressing the cord and causing congestion of the pampiniform plexus.

Torsion of the fully descended testis can also simulate closely acute epididymo-orchitis; after a lapse of six hours or so the skin of the scrotum becomes reddened and the temperature is raised slightly—37·2°C. Elevation of the scrotum usually relieves the pain in epididymitis, but increases it in torsion of the spermatic cord. Therefore in a boy (if mumps has been excluded) and in a man (if urethritis has been eliminated), a diagnosis of torsion of the testis should be *insisted* upon, and almost invariably when the testis is exposed the diagnosis will be substantiated.

Treatment.—In the first hour or so an attempt to untwist the testis may immediately relieve the pain and gentle twisting should be tried in one direction first. If this is the correct way, continue until relief is obtained. If one has chosen the wrong direction pain will increase. If untwisting can be achieved it removes the urgency, but operation and fixation should be performed as quickly as possible.

Urgent exploration of the scrotum is indicated if untwisting is not successful in relieving pain. If after undoing the torsion the testis is viable, then it must be fixed to prevent a recurrence. The opposite testis should also be fixed at the same time, as the anatomical variation responsible is likely to be bilateral. A totally infarcted testis should be removed. Should the patient not be operated upon, but only seen days or weeks later when pain has subsided little is to be gained by exploring the affected side; the testis will slowly become woody hard and shrink to a fibrous nodule. The opposite testis must be fixed at an early date.

Torsion of an Appendage of the Testis.—Vestigial structures related to the testis and epididymis are liable to undergo axial rotation. The most common of these structures to twist is the appendix of the epididymis (the pedunculated hydatid). The condition is often mistaken for acute epididymo-orchitis of unknown origin and cannot be distinguished with certainty from torsion of the testis. Immediate operation with ligation of the pedicle and amputation of the twisted appendage cures the condition.

Idiopathic Scrotal Oedema (4–12 years) (fig. 1331) may occur in childhood and has to be differentiated from torsion of testis or appendage. The scrotum is very swollen but has not the exquisite tenderness of torsion, and pain is slight. The swelling may extend to the perineum or groin and penis. The swelling subsides after 1–2 days. It may be a recurrent phenomenon. It might also be allergic in origin—occasionally an eosinophilia is present.

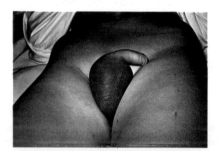

FIG. 1331.—Oedema of the scrotum.

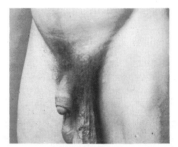

FIG. 1332.—A large varicocele.
Note the left inguinal hernia.

VARICOCELE

Varicocele is a state of varicosity of the testicular veins.

Surgical Anatomy.—The veins of the testis and epididymis form an anastomosing plexus—the pampiniform plexus—which is the most bulky constituent of the spermatic cord. As the veins pass upward through the inguinal canal they become reduced in number to between four and eight. Coalescence in the neighbourhood of the internal inguinal ring brings about further reduction in their number, and by the time the posterior abdominal wall is reached, a single, or a duplicated testicular vein pursues its cephalad course behind the peritoneum, to empty into the renal vein on the left, and the inferior vena cava on the right. Only near their terminations are the testicular veins provided with valves, and not infrequently even these valves are absent, in which case valves will be found nearby in the renal veins. The cremasteric veins anastomose with the testicular veins, so providing an alternative (collateral) venous return and draining mainly into the inferior epigastric veins.

Aetiology.—(1) Most varicoceles are noted in the 'teens' or early adult life. The left side is affected in 95% of cases. The left testicular vein joins the renal vein and reflux into this vein can be demonstrated by angiograms. Nathan found that the left testicular artery arches over the left renal vein in 16% of cases and may obstruct it.

(2) In many cases the dilated vessels are cremasteric veins, and not veins of the pampiniform plexus. The cremasteric veins drain into the inferior epigastric

Hilel Nathan (formerly Notkovich), Contemporary. Professor and Chairman, Department of Anatomy and Anthropology, Tel-Aviv University Medical School, Tel-Aviv, Israel.

veins mainly, but also communicate freely with the veins in the pampiniform plexus.

(3) Obstruction of the left testicular vein by growth of a hypernephroma along the left renal veins is a rare cause of a recent varicocele arising in middle life. *Characteristically this varicocele does not decompress in the supine position.*

Clinical Features.—Varicocele is more frequent and more troublesome in hot climates; in all parts of the world tall, thin, visceroptotic men are frequently affected, whereas short, fat individuals are seldom so. Usually symptoms are entirely absent, but in some cases the patient experiences a dragging pain in the affected side. Pain is due to the fact that the elongated scrotum no longer supports the testis, whose full weight is now borne by the cord. The scrotum, particularly the left side, hangs lower than normal (fig. 1332), and on palpation with the patient standing, the varicose plexus feels like a bag of worms. If, while lightly holding the varicocele between the fingers and thumb, the patient is instructed to bow, tension within the veins becomes appreciably less. An impulse is often felt when the patient coughs. When the patient lies down and the scrotum is elevated, the veins will be emptied by gravity and the opportunity of comparing the size of the left testis with its fellow should be taken. In longstanding cases the left testis is somewhat smaller and softer than the right, due to a minor degree of atrophy. Infertility can be caused by a varicocele.

Varicocele and Spermatogenesis.—The testis is supported in the scrotum by the cremaster and the dartos muscles. The main function of the cremaster is one of defence, for a fright or threat of trauma will cause reflex retraction of the testis towards the external inguinal ring, especially in the young. The dartos bears the weight of the testis and is reflexly controlled by temperature changes and acts as a kind of thermostat for efficient spermatogenesis at some 2·5°C lower than rectal temperature. On exposure to cold it raises the testis to the body so conserving heat, while a too warm environment causes relaxation of the dartos. An explanation for the characteristic elongation of the scrotum in this condition is that venous engorgement in the varicosities reduces the temperature differential (scrotum/rectum) to about 0·1°C which may seriously depress spermatogenesis. The dartos relaxes in a vain attempt to maintain the temperature differential. It also follows that the modern tendency to wear tight and poorly ventilated pants and scrotal supports is to be deprecated.

Treatment.—Operation for varicocele is not indicated unless there is (1): pain; (2) serious depression of spermatogenesis (oligospermia). The simplest procedure of ligating the testicular vein above the inguinal ligament is the best. Only occasionally, if this leaves a group of tortuous varicosities, is local excision necessary.

As a result of this operation the testis becomes cooler, and the dartos contracts, supports the testis, and relieves pain, while cases of oligospermia shows a 70 to 80% improvement with a conception rate of about 30%.

HYDROCELE

Congenital (fig. 1333).

Primary, or idiopathic.

Acquired < Secondary, due to disease of testis < Acute / Chronic.

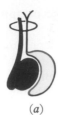 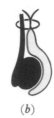 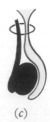 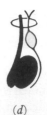

(a)   (b)   (c)   (d)

FIG. 1333.—(a) Vaginal hydrocele (very common); (b) 'infantile' hydrocele (unusual); (c) congenital
hydrocele; (d) encysted hydrocele of the cord.

A hydrocele is a collection of serous fluid in some part of the processus vaginalis, usually in the tunica. Four anatomical varieties of congenital hydrocele are
encountered.

Aetiology.—A hydrocele can be produced in four ways:
1. By excessive production of fluid within the sac, *e.g.* secondary hydrocele.
2. By defective absorption of hydrocele fluid by the tunica vaginalis.

Defective absorption appears to be the most common cause of the common variety of
primary hydrocele, but the reason for the defective absorption is obscure. Damage to the
endothelial wall by low-grade infection seems to be the probable explanation.
3. By interference with the drainage of fluid by the lymphatic vessels of the cord.
4. By connection with the peritoneal cavity, as in the congenital variety.

Hydrocele fluid is amber coloured, and registers a specific gravity of 1·022 to 1·024. It
contains water, inorganic salts, 6% of albumin, and a quantity of fibrinogen. The last
constituent confers upon the fluid a characteristic feature. If the contents of a hydrocele
are allowed to run through a cannula into a receptacle, the fluid does *not* clot, but if a few
drops of blood which have come into contact with cut tissues are stirred into even a
large quantity of hydrocele fluid, the whole clots firmly. In old-standing cases the fluid
sometimes contains so much cholesterol that it is irridescent, and occasionally tyrosine
crystals are found.

DIAGNOSTIC RULES FOR ALL HYDROCELES

*Ninety-nine out of every 100 hydroceles are translucent. On examination it is possible
'to get above the swelling'.*

(a) **Primary vaginal hydrocele** most often appears in middle-aged or elderly
men, but it is not uncommon in early childhood. The condition is particularly
common in tropical countries. The only complaint of the patient is the swelling,
and occasionally he does not seek relief until the sac has attained enormous
dimensions. *Beware of the acute hydrocele in a young man; there may be an underlying
testicular neoplasm. A scrotal ultrasound will show if the testis is normal* (fig. 1330).

About 5% of inguinal hernias are associated with a vaginal hydrocele of the
same side.[1] Often a large hydrocele obscures a small inguinal hernia, even if the
latter has been especially looked for.

(b) **Infantile hydrocele** does not necessarily appear in infants. The tunica and the
processus vaginalis are distended up to the internal abdominal ring, but the sac has no
connection with the general peritoneal cavity.

(c) **Congenital Hydrocele.**—The processus vaginalis communicates with the peritoneal cavity. Usually the communicating orifice is too small for the development of a hernia.

---

[1] Edward Gibbon, 1737–1794, the English historian, who is best known for his 'History of the
Decline and Fall of the Roman Empire', was greatly embarrassed by a large hydrocele. The second
time this was tapped the hydrocele became infected, and Gibbon died a few days after the operation.
The hydrocele was associated with a large scrotal hernia which, probably, was punctured.

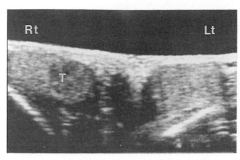

FIG. 1334.—Transverse scan showing both testicles. Right testicle has a well defined small mass. T = tumour (teratoma).
(Dr J. Boultbee.)

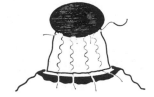

FIG. 1335.—Lord's operation. A series of 10–12 catgut or Dexon sutures are woven radially from the cut edge of the tunica to the reflection of the tunica from the testis and epididymis. When these are tied the whole tunica is bunched into a 'ruff' at the edge of the testis. (Peter Lord, FRCS, High Wycombe, England and Karger Verlag, Basel, Switzerland.)

When the patient is horizontal, *e.g.* at night, the fluid in the pouch disappears within the abdominal cavity, but it returns when the erect posture is resumed. The hydrocele cannot be emptied by digital pressure, as this results in an 'inverted ink bottle' effect at the internal ring. Especially in bilateral cases, ascites or ascitic tuberculous peritonitis should be suspected.

(*d*) **Encysted Hydrocele of the Cord.**—There is a smooth, oval swelling associated with the spermatic cord, which is liable to be mistaken for an irreducible inguinal hernia. If, with gentle traction upon the testis, the swelling moves downwards and becomes less mobile, the diagnosis of hydrocele of the cord is confirmed.

Hydrocele of the canal of Nuck is a condition comparable to the foregoing. It occurs in females, the cyst being in relationship to the round ligament. Unlike a hydrocele of the cord, a hydrocele of the canal of Nuck is always wholly, or partially, in the inguinal canal.

Hydrocele en Bisac.—A rare condition where the hydrocele has two intercommunicating sacs, one above and one below the neck of the scrotum. The upper lies superficial to or partly within the inguinal canal and it may insinuate itself in between the muscle layers.

Complications of a Hydrocele

1. *Rupture* is usually traumatic, but may possibly be spontaneous. On rare occasions a cure results after absorption of the fluid.
2. *Hernia of the hydrocele sac* sometimes occurs in old-standing cases. Tension of fluid within the tunica causes herniation through the dartos muscle.
3. *Transformation into a haematocele* occurs both spontaneously and as the result of trauma.
4. *Calcification* of the sac wall sometimes occurs in long-standing cases.

Treatment of a Hydrocele.—*Lord's Operation.*—This procedure has replaced subtotal excision when the tunica is not thickened. No tissue dissection is performed, no reactionary oedema occurs, bleeding is minimised and recurrence is unlikely as the tunica cannot surround the testis again.

A small incision in between the lines of scrotal blood vessels is made through all layers, including the tunica, well away from the testis. The testis is allowed to prolapse through the wound so that the tunica is totally everted (see fig. 1335 and legend).

Sharma and Jhawer's minimal dissection technique involves the minimal incision consistent with the delivery of the testis through the opening in the sac (no 'ruffing' with sutures), and they lodge the testis in a pocket created by blunt and finger dissection between the fascial layers of the scrotum.

Anton Nuck, 1650–1692. Professor of Anatomy and Medicine, Leiden, Netherlands.
Peter Herent Lord, Contemporary. Surgeon, High Wycombe General Hospital, High Wycombe, Bucks, England.
Laxman Sharma, Contemporary. Surgeon, Medical College, Indore, M.P., India.
Pramod Jhawer, Contemporary. Surgeon, Bombay Hospital, India.

Subtotal excision necessitates a larger incision, complete delivery of the hydrocele through the wound, excision of the major part of the tunica and the most scrupulous attention to haemostasis.

Tapping.—After transillumination, the swelling is made tense by manual compression. A fine trocar and cannula is inserted into an unquestionably translucent area and the fluid evacuated. The sac usually refills. Many patients are content to be relieved at regular intervals in this way. Repeated tapping is liable to be followed by a little oozing into the sac. Deposits of blood on the walls of the sac in time increase its thickness, and so diminish its translucency. *After tapping, the testis should always be examined.*

Secondary hydrocele is an effusion into the tunica vaginalis that accompanies certain affections of the testis. It is frequently associated with acute and chronic epididymo-orchitis. It is nearly always present in the syphilitic affections of the testis, and occasionally complicates malignant disease of the organ. A secondary hydrocele rarely attains a large size, and in most instances is lax and does not interfere unduly with the palpation of the testis and its epididymis. Occasionally the question as to whether a hydrocele is or is not secondary to some underlying disease of the testis can be settled only after the contents of the hydrocele have been aspirated.

In the case of acute epididymo-orchitis usually a secondary hydrocele subsides *pari passu* with the primary lesion.

Post-herniorrhaphy hydrocele is a secondary hydrocele that appears after an operation for inguinal hernia in 0·2% of cases in which there was no evidence of a hydrocele pre-operatively. Possibly this is due to damage of the lymphatic vessels of the tunica vaginalis, which pass with those of the testis, along the spermatic cord, mostly superficial to the blood-vessels.

Hydrocele of a Hernial Sac.—The neck of a hernial sac becomes plugged with omentum or occluded by adhesions, and a hydrocele results.

Filarial Hydroceles and Chyloceles.—As one proceeds from temperate climates towards the Equator, the incidence of vaginal hydrocele increases. Filariasis (p. 121) accounts for 80% of hydroceles in some tropical countries. In most instances neither are microfilariae discovered in nocturnal samples of blood, nor is a history of filariasis elicited. Usually filarial hydroceles follow repeated attacks of filarial epididymitis, and develop rapidly or gradually and can be large or small: frequently they are bilateral. In early cases the hydrocele fluid is similar to that found in the idiopathic variety. In cases of some standing, if the fluid is placed in a tall glass, after a few hours a film of liquid fat (chyle) will be floating on the surface. This is rich in cholesterol, and is derived from rupture of a lymph varix into the tunica. The presence of chyle is proof-positive of the filarial origin of a hydrocele. Adult worms of the *Wuchereria bancrofti* have been found in the epididymis removed by operation, or at necropsy on these cases. In long-standing chyloceles dense adhesions form between the scrotum and its contents. Filarial elephantiasis of the scrotum supervenes in a small proportion of cases.

Treatment.—Acute cases should be treated by rest and aspiration. The more usual chronic cases can be cured by excision of the sac.

Haematocele can be either recent, or present as the clinical entity 'old clotted haematocele' (see below).

Recent haematocele is usually the result of injury of a small blood-vessel during tapping or aspiration of a hydrocele. Prompt refilling of the sac with considerable pain and tenderness, and poor or absent transillumination, leave no doubt as to the diagnosis. The treatment should be urgent operation, with evacuation of blood and excision or eversion of the sac. If this course is not followed a clotted haematocele will almost certainly result.

Acute haemorrhage into a previously normal tunica vaginalis can result from a blow on the testis. The treatment should be similar to the above for the reasons given, and also because without exploration it is impossible to tell whether or not the testicle is ruptured. Furthermore, a neoplasm can sometimes present in this way.

Old Clotted Haematocele.—Curiously, slow haemorrhage into the tunica vaginalis can occur spontaneously, and apparently painlessly, for most of the patients presenting with an old clotted haematocele give neither a history of trauma to the testis nor of pain in the organ. An old clotted haematocele simulates a neoplasm of the testis so closely that pre-operative differential diagnosis is sometimes impossible.

Treatment.—Unless exposure of the organ leaves no doubt as to the innocent nature of the swelling, unquestionably orchiectomy should be performed. As a rule it is imposs-ible to be certain of the diagnosis until the mass has been bisected. As can be seen in fig. 1336, the testicle is often so compressed as to be virtually functionless, so the responsibilities of removing it unnecessarily are not great.

CYSTS CONNECTED WITH THE EPIDIDYMIS

1. Cysts of the Epididymis.—A cyst of the epididymis, filled with crystal-clear fluid (as opposed to the barley-water-like fluid of a spermatocele or the amber-coloured fluid of a vaginal hydrocele), is a common condition.

Aetiology.—A cyst of epididymis is due to cystic degeneration of:
(*a*) The paradidymis (or organ of Giraldes), which is the most likely cause.
(*b*) The appendix of the epididymis (pedunculated hydatid of Morgagni) (fig. 1337).
(*c*) The appendix of the testis (sessile hydatid of Morgagni).
(*d*) The vas aberrans (of Haller).

Clinical Features.—Cysts of the epididymis usually are found during middle life, and, due no doubt to their congenital origin, they are often bilateral. They are tense, as opposed to the softness of a spermatocele, and they consist of an aggregation of a number of small cysts which on careful palpation feel like a bunch of tiny grapes. Cysts of the epididymis are situated *behind* the body of the testis, and on transillumination, because of the numerous septa, their brilliant translucency is finely tesselated, giving an appearance like that of a Chinese lantern.

Treatment.—As epididymal cysts are multilocular, aspiration is useless. If causing discomfort, which is unusual, they must be excised. They should not be operated on without considering the fact that excision will almost certainly cause infertility from blockage.

Cyst of an appendage of the testis is a separate clinical entity. It forms a small globular swelling at the superior pole of the testis; it is usually unilateral, and when pedunculated (fig. 1337) it is liable to undergo axial rotation. The treatment of this variety of cyst is removal by ligation and severance of its pedicle.

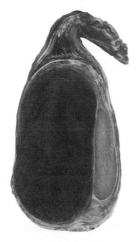

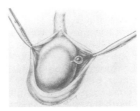

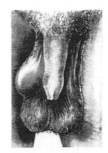

FIG. 1336.—An old clotted haematocele. The long-standing pressure has flat-tened the testis.

FIG. 1338.—A large spermatocele.

FIG. 1337.—Cyst of the pedunculated hydatid of Morgagni.

Joachim Albin Cardazo Cazado Giraldes, 1808–1875. Professor of Surgery, Paris.
Albrecht von Haller, 1708–1777. Professor of Anatomy, Physiology, Surgery, and Botany, Göttingen, Germany.

2. **Spermatocele** is a unilocular retention cyst derived from some portion of the sperm-conducting mechanism of the epididymis.

Clinical Features.—A spermatocele is nearly always situated in the head of the epididymis, and is therefore above and behind the body of the testis. Filled with fluid resembling barley water and containing spermatozoa, the swelling is typically softer than other cysts occurring within the scrotum but, like them, is translucent. Spermatoceles give rise to few symptoms, and are usually small and unobtrusive. Less frequently they are large enough to attract notice, and some patients imagine that they have three testicles (fig. 1338).

Treatment.—Small spermatoceles can be ignored. Larger ones, if causing symptoms, can be aspirated or excised via a scrotal incision. The thin coverings of the cyst are carefully peeled off, layer by layer, and any residual attachments are ligated and divided.

ACUTE EPIDIDYMO-ORCHITIS

In many instances inflammation remains confined to the epididymis, in which case it is referred to as epididymitis; when the infection spreads to the body of the testis the condition is known as epididymo-orchitis.

Mode of Infection.—As a rule infection reaches the epididymis via the lumen of the vas, and affects the globus minor first. It is secondary to infection of the urethra, prostate and seminal vesicles. Blood-borne infections affect the globus major of the testis primarily.

Clinical Features.—The initial symptoms are those of acute prostatitis. Some days later an ache in the groin with some increase in fever heralds the onset of epididymitis. Severe pain and swelling of the testis occurs rapidly: the scrotal wall becomes red, oedematous and shiny. The epididymis may become adherent to the scrotal skin and may soften and, later, discharge. Resolution is heralded by scaling of the scrotal skin. Complete resolution of the swelling in the epididymis may take 6–8 weeks.

Acute epididymitis due to *Esch. coli*, streptococcus, staphylococcus or proteus is a not uncommon clinical entity. As a rule there is no evidence of urethritis. Especially in *Esch. coli* infection, it is sometimes unaccompanied by infection of the urine (an initial specimen should be sent for bacteriological examination). In the absence of any local cause, the infection is assumed to be blood-borne.

Acute epididymitis can follow any form of urethral instrumentation. It usually occurs when there is an associated infection in the prostate. Indwelling catheters encourage organisms normally found in the distal urethra to migrate upwards.

Epididymitis complicating non-gonococcal urethritis is more frequent than it is in gonorrhoea, and unless correct antibiotic therapy is given early, suppuration is usual.

Acute gonococcal epididymitis is much less common than formerly, as a result of the antibiotic treatment of acute gonorrhoea. Epididymitis usually commences during the second or third week of gonococcal posterior urethritis. In 90% of cases the infection is unilateral. When the epididymis becomes involved the urethral discharge lessens and pain commences in the testis. On the following day the urethral discharge ceases, but the urine is hazy with pus cells. The temperature rises to $38 \cdot 9°$–$39 \cdot 5°C$, and the patient feels so ill that he goes to bed. About the third day the skin of the scrotum often becomes reddened and adherent to the globus minor, but in cases where the gonococcus is the sole infecting organism suppuration does not occur. After the fifth day the symptoms commence to abate, and by the eighth to tenth day the condition subsides. Induration of the globus minor sometimes persists for months. In cases of persistent infection of the corresponding vesicle, subacute attacks of recurrent epididymitis are not infrequent.

Epididymitis from Retrograde Passage of Urine.—Epididymitis can develop during an unusual exertion or violent strain while the bladder is full, and it is caused by the urine being forced along the vas deferens. The degree of inflammation that results depends upon whether the urine is infected, or if there is an active or latent infection in the prostate or seminal vesicles. This 'reflux' epididymitis can also occur due to the presence of a stricture in the urethra.

Acute Tuberculous Epididymitis.—In cases where the vas is thickened and there is little response to the usual treatment, the possibility of the infection being due to tuberculosis of the epididymis, which is not rare, must receive due consideration.

Acute epididymo-orchitis of mumps develops in about 18% of males suffering from mumps, usually as the parotid inflammation is waning. The testis becomes swollen and painful. Rarely, the testicular precede the salivary manifestations. Resolution or fibrosis, as opposed to suppuration, nearly always occurs, but in 55% of cases atrophy of the testis follows. It often takes many months for signs of testicular atrophy to become apparent. A small incision into the tunica vaginalis and drainage, if undertaken early in the attack, prevents this atrophy and relieves the intense pain. It is often stated that the body of the testis is alone involved, but the epididymis is also acutely inflamed, as has been witnessed at operation. Especially in infants, epididymo-orchitis of mumps can occur without parotitis.[1] Partial atrophy is commonly associated with a tendency to recurrent pain in the testis.

Acute post-operative epididymitis was a serious and frequent complication of prostatectomy. It can be abolished by prophylactic division of the vasa deferentia (Chapter 59), and has been greatly reduced by closed drainage, catheter care and antibiotics which have reduced the rate of post-operative urinary infection.

Other causes include Bornholm disease,[2] Brucellosis, and Lympho-granuloma venereum.

Treatment.—The patient must be kept in bed until the acute symptoms have abated. A broad spectrum antibiotic such as tetracycline should be given (500 mg q.d.s.) until the result of the urine culture is available. The scrotum is supported on a sling formed by broad adhesive plaster attached across the thighs. Upon the sling is placed a nest of cotton wool, and in this the inflamed organ rests and cooling lotions are applied. The urine is rendered alkaline, and a high fluid intake is necessary. Antibiotic treatment should be continued for two weeks or until the inflammation has subsided. If suppuration occurs, drainage is necessary. Atrophy of the testis may follow as a sequela in any case of epididymo-orchitis.

CHRONIC EPIDIDYMO-ORCHITIS

Chronic Tuberculous Epididymitis.—Nearly 90% of cases of chronic epididymo-orchitis are tuberculous, and the great majority commence insidiously.

Aetiology.—The frequency with which the globus minor is first attacked indicates that infection is commonly retrograde along the vas deferens from an infected seminal vesicle. Blood-borne infection commences in the globus major.

Clinical Features.—A slight ache in the testis or a trivial injury, calls the patient's attention to the swelling in relation to the testis. An early manifestation is a discrete, indurated, slightly tender nodule in the globus minor—rarely in the globus major. As the disease progresses other nodules appear, and eventually the entire epididymis becomes involved, and is felt as a firm, craggy, often painless, mass situated behind the testis, which feels normal. In 30% of cases a lax secondary hydrocele is present. When the testis is anteverted, these changes are found in front of the testis. The vas on the affected side sometimes becomes 'beaded' due to submucous tubercles. Rectal examination reveals a thickened, and later an irregular, indurated seminal vesicle of the corresponding side, and sometimes of the contralateral vesicle as well. The prostate in advanced cases contains one or more discrete nodules. In 20% of cases the patient first presents himself with a 'cold' abscess in the lower and posterior aspect of the scrotum or with a discharging sinus, which may have healed and reopened several times. Untreated, after a varying time (from a few

---

[1] A complement fixation test for the virus of mumps is sometimes positive.

[2] Epidemic myalgia. Bornholm is a Danish island in the Baltic Sea.

Sir David Bruce, 1855–1931. Major-General, Royal Army Medical Service.

months to a year or so), the contralateral epididymis becomes similarly diseased. The body of the testis remains uninvolved for a long period, often years.

In two-thirds of the cases there is either active tuberculosis in the renal tract or evidence of previous disease. In the remainder the patient is apparently healthy.

In all cases of chronic epididymitis the urine is examined for tubercle bacilli, if necessary on several occasions, and pyelography should be undertaken. The chest is x-rayed (evidence of disease in about 50%). Culture of the semen can also be a useful means of confirming the tuberculous nature of an epididymitis.

Treatment.—When tuberculous epididymitis is secondary, the primary lesion should receive priority. The epididymitis may well resolve during the treatment.

When renal tuberculosis is present, the renal lesion is treated as detailed in Chapter 57. Rarely active pulmonary tuberculosis will be present.

Treatment with anti-tuberculous drugs (Chapter 4) is less effective in genital tuberculosis than in urinary tuberculosis. If there is no sign of resolution within two months, epididymectomy or orchiectomy is advisable. Subsequently, in the absence of evidence of active tuberculosis elsewhere, a further course of anti-tuberculous drugs is necessary.

Chronic non-tuberculous epididymitis either follows an acute attack or is chronic from the commencement. The condition is difficult to distinguish from tuberculosis, but as a rule the epididymis in non-specific epididymitis is larger and smoother. It is essential to exclude a urethral stricture.

Treatment.—In most cases associated posterior urethritis, vesiculitis, or prostatitis must be eradicated. If the condition fails to resolve after six to eight weeks of conservative treatment and antibiotic therapy, epididymectomy or orchiectomy may be needed.

ORCHITIS

Syphilitic Orchitis.—Syphilis attacks the body of the testis, and like other late manifestations of the disease, all three varieties have become uncommon, interstitial fibrosis the least so. The three varieties of syphilitic orchitis are:

(*a*) *Bilateral orchitis* occurs in congenital syphilis (Chapter 4).

(*b*) *Interstitial fibrosis* is bilateral, symptomless, and leads to gradual destruction of the seminiferous tubules. The testes are not enlarged. They are firmer than normal, and there is a gradual loss of testicular sensation. In bisecting the testis, irregularly distributed streaks of fibrosis are seen traversing the parenchyma.

(*c*) *Gumma.*—The condition is nearly always unilateral. The body of the testis enlarges slowly and painlessly. It feels extremely hard. Testicular sensation is lost, and there is often a secondary hydrocele. Softening then occurs anteriorly and a gummatous ulcer forms. If the response to treatment is not rapid if is better to perform orchiectomy than risk the possibility of overlooking a neoplasm with purely coincidental positive serological tests.

Leprous Orchitis.—Over 25% of male lepers have testicular atrophy due to fibrosis engendered by the direct action of the *Mycobacterium leprae*, and in 20% of those so affected the orchitis is associated with gynaecomazia.

NEOPLASMS OF THE TESTIS

The lymphatics of the testis run upwards in the spermatic cord, and, passing through the internal inguinal ring, they branch fountain-wise (behind and adherent to the posterior peritoneum) towards the para-aortic lymph nodes in the region of the origin of the spermatic vessels. Above this level the lymph drains into the thoracic duct which extends through the mediastinum to the left supraclavicular fossa, where it drains into the left innominate vein. Lymphatics from the medial side of the testis may run with the artery to the vas and drain into a lymph node at the bifurcation of the common iliac artery (fig. 1339).

When lymphatic spread of a neoplasm occurs, contralateral lymph nodes can be affected. Inguinal lymph nodes are only affected if the scrotum is involved.

MALIGNANT NEOPLASMS OF THE TESTIS

About 99% of neoplasms of the testis are malignant, and though they only constitute about 1–2% of malignant tumours in the male, they are one of the commonest forms of cancer in young adult males. Maldescent undoubtedly predisposes to malignancy. It is curious that a testicle bearing such a tumour, contained as it is in a bag of skin bereft of fat, and thus more readily accessible to the examining fingers than a tumour of any other organ in the body, only too often escapes detection until it has metastasised. In this connection, perhaps the worst error is to plunge a trocar and cannula into the enlarged testis in the belief that it is a hydrocele, for want of applying the test of translucency. This has been done more often than the reader may be inclined to believe.

Types of Tumour.—Tumours of the testis are classified as follows:

(1)	Seminoma	40%
(2)	Teratoma	32%
(3)	Combined Seminoma and Teratoma	14%
(4)	Interstitial tumours	1·5%
(5)	Lymphoma	7%
(6)	Other tumours	5·5%

The percentage of the first two subdivisions varies in different series. Those series emanating from hospitals for Service personnel show a higher percentage of teratoma as patients in such hospitals are likely to be of a younger age-group than found in the community at large; **the peak incidence** of teratoma being between twenty and thirty-five years of age, while that of seminoma is between thirty-five and forty-five. Seminoma has only once been recorded before puberty.

Seminoma commences in the mediastinum of the testis, and as it increases in size the neighbouring testicular tissue is compressed (fig. 1340). Macroscopically the enlarged testis is firm and smooth, and on section homogeneous and pink or cream in colour. Occasionally fibrous septa give it a lobulated appearance. In rapidly growing tumours areas of necrosis are sometimes present, in which case the consistency is variable.

Histologically it is composed of rounded, slightly oval cells with clear cytoplasm and large rounded nuclei containing acidophile nucleoli. The cells are arranged in sheets separated by a fine fibrous stroma. Derived from the seminiferous tubules, the cells resemble spermatocytes. Stromal and tumour infiltration by lymphocytes suggest a good host reaction (? autoimmune reaction) and tends to improve the prognosis.

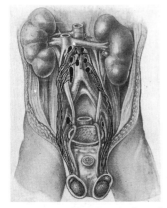

FIG. 1339.—The lymphatics of the testes.
(After Rouvier.)

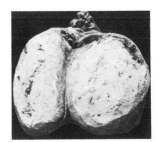

FIG. 1340.—Seminoma of the testis.

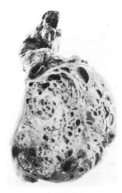

FIG. 1341.—Teratoma of the testis containing solid and cystic areas.
(Dr. Keith Simpson, London.)

A seminoma metastasises almost exclusively by the lymph vessels to lymph nodes; only occasionally does it disseminate by the blood-stream and give rise to secondary deposits in other situations.

Teratoma arises in the rete testis from toti-potent cells; accordingly, elements of ectoderm, mesoderm, or endoderm are often represented. Usually one of these predominates and attains malignancy. The tumour varies in size from that of a peanut to that of a coconut, and even when large, as it is moulded by the tunica vaginalis, the shape of the testis is more or less retained but the surface is usually slightly irregular.

The most usual variety[1] is yellowish in colour and shows cystic spaces (fig. 1341) containing gelatinous fluid. Cartilaginous nodules are often present.

Histology.—The Testicular Tumour Panel have classified teratomas as follows:

(1) **Teratoma Differentiated (T.D.)** (1%[2]).—The best-known variety of this type of tumour is a dermoid cyst. If a teratoma has no histologically recognisable malignant components, it is termed differentiated, but it cannot be considered to be benign, because such growths may have metastasised. This tumour may be made up of cartilage, muscle, bone and have glandular elements.

(2) **Malignant Teratoma Intermediate, Teratocarcinoma. (M.T.I.—A and B)** (30%), consisting of definitely malignant and incompletely differentiated tissues. In type A some mature tissues will be seen. Type B is more malignant and no fully differentiated tissue can be found.

(3) **Malignant Teratoma Anaplastic (M.T.A.) Embryonal carcinoma** (15%) is composed of quite undifferentiated cells of embryonal nature in parts, and also with cells presumed to be of yolk-sac origin. These latter are often responsible for elevated AFP (alpha-feto-protein) levels. It is not always radiosensitive.

(4) **Malignant Teratoma Trophoblastic (M.T.T.)** (1%) contains within the other tissue types a syncytial cell mass with malignant villous or papillary cytotrophoblast (chorio-carcinoma). It is associated with the production of chorionic gonadotrophin, elevated BHCG levels in the serum and occasionally gynaecomazia. Spread is by the blood-stream as well as by lymphatics while the primary tumour is small, and it is often described as the most malignant tumour known.

Interstitial Cell Tumour.—A tumour of the testis arising in the interstitial cells occurs at an early age or the prime of life, and arises either in the cells of Leydig or those of Sertoli.

A Leydig cell tumour masculinises; a Sertoli cell tumour feminises. For clinical reasons these tumours are classified as those occurring before or after puberty.

Prepubertal tumour is characterised by an excessive output of androgen, which is responsible for sexual precocity and extreme muscular development. This results in an infant Hercules, in all respects similar to the condition produced by an adrenal cortical tumour, except that on palpation a swelling of the testis can be elicited. Exceptionally the tumour is bilateral, but it must be noted that in this condition the contralateral normal testis frequently becomes hypertrophied. In so far as the neoplasm is concerned, removal of the testis is curative; in some cases the symptoms regress, in others (where the contralateral testis is hypertrophied) the regression is incomplete.

Post-Pubertal Tumour.—In a high percentage of cases the tumour arises in the cells of Sertoli, and consequently the output of feminising hormone becomes excessive. Gynaeco-mazia, loss of libido, and aspermia result; in such cases the Aschheim-Zondek test is positive. As a rule the tumour is innocent, and orchiectomy is curative.

Human Chorionic Gonadotrophin can be measured in blood and urine by a very sensitive radio-immune assay method. Normal levels are up to 100 iu HCG.

Clinical Features of Testicular Tumours.—Various clinical types are met with.

1. **Typical.**—The patient may not seek advice until four to six months after

---

[1] Formerly known as 'fibro-cystic' disease.
[2] The percentages given refer to all cases of testicular neoplasm.

Franz von Leydig, 1821–1908. Professor of Histology, Bonn, Germany.
Enrico Sertoli, 1842–1910. Professor of Experimental Physiology, Milan, Italy.
Selmar Aschheim, 1878–1965. Formerly Honorary Professor of Gynaecology, University of Berlin.
Bernhard Zondek, 1891–1966. Professor of Obstetrics and Gynaecology, Haddassah Medical School, Hebrew University, Jerusalem, Israel.

the first symptom, which is enlargement of the testicle. A sensation of heaviness is complained of when the testis has reached two to three times its normal size. Pain is complained of in only about 30% of cases (Fergusson). There is a history of trauma to the affected side in over 10%. It is generally conceded that injury merely calls attention to the testicular enlargement and in no way initiates the neoplasm.

On examination the body of the testis is found to be enlarged, firm, smooth, and heavy. Later one or more softer bosses may be palpable. In no other disease is testicular sensation lost so early or so completely, but the greatest gentleness must be exercised in eliciting this sign for fear of disseminating the neoplasm. A secondary hydrocele is present in 10% of cases; it is usually lax, and seldom obscures the enlarged testis. The epididymis is normal at first; later it becomes so flattened or incorporated in the growth that it is imperceptible. The spermatic cord remains normal for a considerable time. It then becomes thickened, due to cremasteric hypertrophy and enlargement of testicular vessels. The vas is never thickened. Rectal examination reveals no abnormality in the prostate or seminal vesicles.

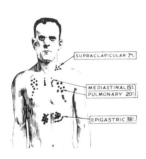

FIG. 1342.—Distribution of metastases in teratoma of the testis.

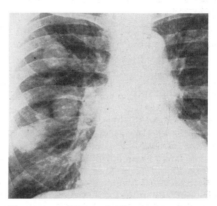

FIG. 1343.—'Cannon ball' metastases from a testicular tumour.

Next, the sites of possible metastases (fig. 1342) should be examined. The abdomen is palpated for secondary retroperitoneal deposits (their most usual situation being just *above the umbilicus* on the same side, the opposite side, or both sides) and for hepatic enlargement. The left supraclavicular region is examined, and occasionally the first presenting sign is an enlarged supra clavicular lymph node. An x-ray of the chest may show metastases in the lungs, particularly in cases of teratoma (fig. 1343).

2. **When the predominant symptoms are due to metastases:** (*a*) with a seminoma the patient complains of abdominal or lumbar pain, and on examination a mass is discovered in the epigastrium. (*b*) Pulmonary metastases from a teratoma of the testis give rise to few, if any, early symptoms. Later the patient may complain of pain in the chest, dyspnoea, and perhaps haemoptysis.

In either case the enlargement of the testis may not have been noticed by the

John Douglas Fergusson, 1910–1979. Surgeon, St. Paul's Hospital, London.

patient, and is discovered only by a thoughtful clinician. Sometimes the primary growth is tiny and will only be discovered by operative exploration.

3. **Atypical Cases.**—The variations are:

(*a*) Some cases (7%) simulate *epididymo-orchitis*; there may even be organisms in the urine. Failure to respond to a short sharp course of antibiotics should make one say 'this could be a tumour' and action must be taken. Rarely, patients will present with severe pain and acute swelling due to a haemorrhage. Between 1 to 5% of cases have gynaecomastia (mainly the teratomas).

(*b*) *The Hurricane Type.*—Metastases from a highly malignant tumour bring about a fatal termination in a matter of weeks.

(*c*) *The Slowly Growing Type.*—In a few cases of teratomas, the patient notices an increasing enlargement of the testis for two or three years.

Staging Testicular Tumours—Treatment

The action to be taken when the clinical diagnosis is made is aimed at staging the tumour in order to assist in planning treatment.

1. Collect a specimen of blood for radio-immune assay of BHCG, Alpha-feto-protein and lactic hydrogenase 'markers', which are essential to monitor response to treatment.

2. Chest x-ray to exclude secondary deposits.

3. Orchiectomy[1] (or exploration) by the inguinal route with high ligation of the cord as the first step.

4. Confirmation of pathology by serial histology.

5. Radiography.

Orchiectomy (Orchidectomy)[1].—This should be done at once. Through an inguinal incision the inguinal canal is opened to display the spermatic cord, which is divided and ligated at the level of the internal inguinal ring. The spermatic cord and the testis are then removed from above downwards by separating them from their attachments. Testicular tumours should never be removed via the scrotum.

The traditional treatment for these patients following orchidectomy has been a course of radiotherapy in the form of an inverted Y to the paraortic and external iliac lymphatic chains. Radical excision of the retroperitoneal lymph nodes has been the treatment of choice in the USA. In general terms seminomas respond well to radiotherapy and the teratomas less well. The debate as to which form of treatment is best has continued for many years.

Two diagnostic tools have been responsible for aiding the dramatic change in testicular cancer treatment. The first is the measurement of the tumour markers and the second has been the introduction of scanning (fig. 1344). Serial investigations using these aids have enabled not only more accurate tumour staging at the time of diagnosis but also a method for monitoring the course of the tumour and its response to treatment. Cytotoxic chemotherapy has largely replaced radiotherapy when facilities are available for using these highly toxic drugs.

Exploration.—On occasion when the clinical diagnosis is in doubt, delay is still dangerous, and nothing is lost by exposing the testis first, providing a 'soft' clamp is placed across the cord above to prevent dissemination. The testis may have to be split open and any doubtful material subjected to immediate frozen section. Wedge biopsy without frozen section and needling should not be attempted for fear of involving the scrotum and opening up an alternative way of lymphatic spread (to inguinal lymph nodes).

---

[1] Dispute continues as to the correct word to describe removal of the testis. Orchis (Lat.) and Orchos (Gk.) = the plant, and in Greek = the testicle. 'Orchotomy' was previously in use. 'Orchidectomy' is still in common usage.

Confirmation of Pathology.—The pathologist will report the type and grade of the tumour (p. 1368).

Radiography.—The radiologist's help is invaluable.

(*a*) *X-ray of the chest* to exclude metastases.

(*b*) *Excretory urography (I.V.P.).*—This has two purposes: (1) Protection of kidney from radiotherapy, for besides ascertaining the function of the kidneys, their position must be marked out so that they may be shielded during irradiation in order to prevent radiation nephritis and hypertension. (2) Detecting the presence and extent of retroperitoneal metastases by the displacement of the ureters or deformity of a renal pelvis. Changes in radiographs after irradiation may indicate the radio-sensitivity of the tumour.

(*c*) *Lymphangiography* can demonstrate secondary deposits in para-aortic lymph-nodes. Its greatest value lies in outlining enlarged nodes which can be observed during radiation for shrinkage.

(*d*) CT scan of whole body.

(*e*) Gallium scan for seminoma metastases.

(*f*) Ultra-sound and CT scans for both para-aortic lymph nodes and liver secondaries (fig. 1344).

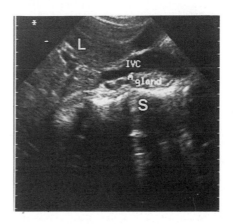

FIG. 1344.—Para-aortic glands in a case of seminoma testis. Longitudinal scan showing the IVC with glands lying posterior. S = spine; L = liver.

(*Dr. J. Boultbee.*)

Staging of Testicular Tumours

Stage 1 = Lesion in testis only—no evidence of spread.

Stage 2 = Nodes involved below diaphragm (*a*) less than 2 cm diameter, (*b*) 2·5 cm diameter, (*c*) more than 5 cm diameter.

Stage 3 = Nodes above diaphragm.

Stage 4 = Pulmonary or hepatic metastases.

Management after Staging and Histological Diagnosis

Seminomas.—It has been known for many years that seminomas are radiosensitive. Excellent results have been achieved by irradiating Stage 1 and Stage 2. More recently it has been found that this tumour is exquisitely sensitive to cisplatinum which is already being used for patients with metastatic disease. A question remaining unanswered at present is whether one should advise adjuvant treatment for patients with Stage 1 disease.

Teratomas are less sensitive to irradiation. Stage 1 is managed by watching the markers (above) afterwards, and by repeated CT scan. Stages 2–4 are managed with chemotherapy. Cisplatinum, methotrexate, bleomycin, vincristine in some combination have changed survival rates dramatically, and these drugs are the first line of treatment. Radiotherapy is still used occasionally.

Debulking operations to remove masses for histological examination are performed when all markers suggest no residual disease. These operations are less likely to produce impotence and sterility which often follow radical lymphadenectomy, a procedure which will be displaced completely by increasing successes with chemotherapy.

Prognosis of Testicular Tumours.—The histological appearance of the tumour and the presence or absence of metastases at the time of operation are the two main factors in assessing prognosis:
Seminoma.—No evidence of metastases; with orchiectomy and radiotherapy 95% survive five years. If metastases are present survival can still be excellent, but perhaps drops to 75%.
Teratoma.—In Stage 1 and 2 survival for five years is being achieved in over 85%. In Stage 3 and 4, the survival is about 60%, and increasing with improvements in chemotherapy.
Testicular tumours in children most commonly appear during the first year of life and are exceedingly rare after the third birthday. The tumours at this time of life are teratomas, many of these being anaplastic (T.A.) in which event, in spite of treatment, the patient dies within a few months. Now and then the tumour proves to be differentiated (T.D.) when, following orchiectomy alone, the prognosis is exceptionally good. On rarer occasions still, the tumour proves to be an interstitial cell tumour, in which case, following orchiectomy, the prognosis is also excellent.
Tumours of the Epididymis.—Mesothelioma is a unique innocent tumour that usually springs from the globus minor: most examples have been about the size of a cherry. Sarcoma, and very rarely carcinoma, arise in the epididymis, and those who put their trust in the aphorism that swellings of the epididymis are invariably inflammatory may one day rue it. If the swelling in question does not respond to rest and antibiotic therapy quickly, it should be treated by epididymectomy or, if obviously malignant, by orchiectomy.

THE SCROTUM

Prepenile scrotum is an exceedingly rare congenital condition. The scrotum, suspended from the mons pubis, is situated anterior to the penis.
Idiopathic Scrotal Oedema is described on page 1358.

Idiopathic gangrene of the scrotum (*syn.* Fournier's gangrene) is uncommon but fearful in effect. It is a vascular disaster of infective origin. The three cardinal characteristics of this disease are: (1) sudden appearance of scrotal inflammation in the midst of apparently good health; (2) rapid onset of gangrene (fig. 1345); (3) absence of any cause in over half the cases. It has been known to follow minor injuries or procedures in the perineum, such as a bruise, scratch, dilatation of stricture, injection of anal fissure or opening a periurethral abscess.

The haemolytic streptococcus (sometimes micro-aerophilic) associated with other organisms (staphylococci, *E. coli, Cl. welchii*) set up a fulminating inflammation within the scrotal subcutaneous tissues that results in obliterative arteritis of the arterioles supplying the overlying skin (*cf.* gangrene of the abdominal wall, Chapter 55).

The clinical features are: sudden pain in the scrotum, prostration, pallor, and pyrexia. At first only the scrotum is involved: still unchecked, if the patient

Jean Alfred Fournier, 1832–1914. Founder of the Venereal and Dermatological Clinic, Hôspital St. Louis, Paris.

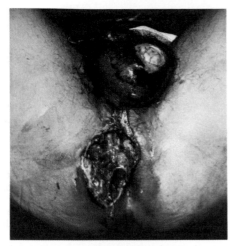

FIG. 1345.—Fournier's gangrene.

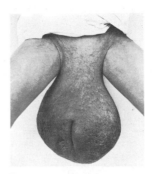

FIG. 1346.—Elephantiasis of the scrotum, burying the penis.
(*Professor M. Bahadur Khan, Hyderabad, India.*)

survives, the cellulitis spreads along those planes so well known in superficial extravasation of urine. Sometimes the entire scrotal coverings slough, leaving the testes hanging exposed, bared to their tunica, though, remarkably, free from gangrene.

Treatment.—Pending the bacteriological report, chloramphenicol or gentamycin and ceporin are the antibiotics of choice as the organisms are usually sensitive.

The scrotum should be incised. If gangrene has commenced, wide excision of all sloughing areas saves time, rids the patient of scrotal tissue that is doomed, provides the freest possible drainage, and stops the spread of gangrene.

Filarial elephantiasis of the scrotum is confined to those who dwell, or have dwelt, in tropical and subtropical countries, and is due to obstruction of the lymphatic vessels of the pelvis by *Wuchereria bancrofti* with superadded infection and lymphangitis. The earliest manifestation is an attack of funiculitis with the development of a secondary hydrocele. Repeated attacks cause the scrotum to remain oedematous and the scrotal skin and subcutaneous tissue greatly thicken. In long-standing cases the scrotum becomes immense, and the penis is buried within it (fig. 1346).

Treatment.—There is no medical treatment for the condition. The principle of operative treatment is the construction of new lymphatic pathways. This can be achieved by constructing cellular-cutaneous bridges of generous size uniting the scrotum to the thigh, for the purpose of permitting the scrotal lymph to be absorbed via the uninvolved thighs. In very advanced cases excision of all involved skin together with implantation of the testes into the thighs and skin grafting of the bared shaft of the penis, is the only curative treatment. It should be especially noted that the *inner layer* of the prepuce is rarely involved: it should therefore be spared and in many instances it can be utilised to cover the bare shaft of the penis (Bowesman). In all cases concomitant hydroceles are dealt with by excision of the sac at the time of the operation.

Non-filarial elephantiasis can be acquired in non-tropical as well as tropical climates, and it is consequent upon fibrosis of lymphatic vessels due to lymphogranuloma venereum. Non-filarial elephantiasis never reaches the extravagant proportions of tropical elephantiasis. There is no effective medical treatment: the scrotum-thigh cutaneous tunnel operation described above is recommended.

Sebaceous cysts are common in the skin of the scrotum. They are usually small and multiple (fig. 1347).

Carcinoma of the Scrotum.—In the last century squamous epithelioma of the

Charles Bowesman, Contemporary. Formerly Surgical Specialist, Colonial Medical Service, Kumasi, Ghana.

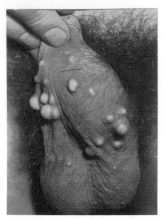

FIG. 1347.—Sebaceous cysts of the scrotum.

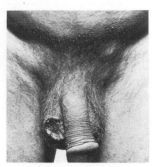

FIG. 1348.—Carcinoma of the scrotum with bilateral metastases in the inguinal nodes.
(*Department of Medical Photography, Cardiff Royal Infirmary.*)

scrotum was rife amongst chimney sweeps.[1] With improved working conditions, this occupational disease ceased to exist as far as chimney sweeps were concerned, but with the mechanisation of the cotton industry, lubricating oil from the spinning jenny soaked the crutch of the mule spinners' trousers, and proved more carcinogenic than soot. Now that a lubricating oil free from impurities has been substituted it is hoped that carcinoma of the scrotum will no longer attack[2] mule spinners in particular. A few cases still occur in tar and shale oil workers, but in the majority of cases encountered at the present time there is no known aetiological factor. It is remarkable that, in contradistinction to carcinoma of the penis, carcinoma of the scrotum is almost unknown in India and Asiatic countries.

Clinical Features.—The growth commences in a wart or an ulcer (fig. 1348). As it extends it may involve the underlying testis.

Treatment.—The growth, together with a considerable margin of healthy tissue, is excised by diathermy. If, as is often the case, the inguinal lymph nodes are enlarged and do not subside with antibiotic treatment, a block dissection of the nodes, and the external iliac nodes, should be carried out, usually on both sides.

MALE INFERTILITY

Causes.—These are as follows:

1. *Impotence* due to (*a*) malformations or loss of the penis; (*b*) psychic causes; (*c*) chromosome defects.

2. *Oligospermia or aspermia* due to small (fibrotic) or soft (partially atrophic) testes resulting from mumps (quarter of cases), varicocele, cryptorchism, over-exposure to x-rays, and occasionally bilateral epididymo-orchitis.

3. *Aspermia Due to a Faulty Sperm-conducting Mechanism.*—Leading examples are (*a*) urethral fistula, (*b*) tight urethral stricture, (*c*) obliteration by scar tissue of both common ejaculatory ducts or both vasa deferentia. 15% of all cases of infertility are due to gonorrhoea, (*d*) absent vasa and vesicles.

---

[1] This disease was first described in 1775 by Percivall Pott (1714–1788), Surgeon, St. Bartholomew's Hospital, London. In those days the chimney sweep's apprentice climbed up and down the chimney.

[2] As it may take up to twenty years for the result of exposure to carcinogens to become manifest, the outcome as yet is uncertain.

Investigation includes: (*a*) three semen analyses at weekly intervals, and an adjudication of the average, (*b*) plasma FSH, LH, prolactin, testosterone, and oestradiol when there is a low sperm count, (*c*) search for sperm antibodies when there is a normal count, (*d*) testicular biopsy and vasogram when there is azoospermia and normal sized testes, (*e*) chromosomal studies particularly when the testes are atrophic.

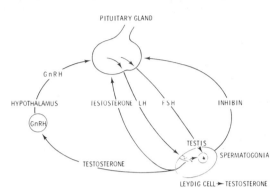

FIG. 1349.—Hormonal interrelationships between the pituitary gland, the hypothalamus and the testis.

Treatment.—(1) Avoid wearing tight pants. (2) Cold bathing of the scrotum. (3) Clomiphene in cases of low FSH levels and maturation defect. (4) Oral testosterone (mesterolone 100 mg daily) in patients with a low count, relatively normal semen and low plasma testosterone. Or fluoxymesterone (5 mg daily) where motility is reduced. (5) Vitamin B_{12} has been reported to improve semen morphology. (6) Operation for varicocele, if present, and if there is a low count and low motility. (7) Epididymovasostomy in cases of obstruction, when vas is proved patent, and testicular biopsy is normal, and the epididymes show dilated and congested tubules visible macroscopically.

Operation.—The vas is divided above the portion considered to be obliterated, and in order to make certain of its patency, the proximal end is catheterised with a suitably-sized piece of silkworm gut, and patency down to the urethra proved by the injection of a weak solution of methylene blue while observing the verumontanum with a urethroscope. The silkworm gut is removed and the free end of the vas is split (spatulated) for a short distance. The dilated epididymal tubules are opened by an incision as low as possible in the body of the epididymis and the spatulated vas sutured to the edges of the sheath over these cut ends in the hope that the opened tubule will drain into the vas. Overall success rates are low.

Vasectomy for Sterilization

Vasectomy for the purpose of sterilisation should be undertaken only after very careful counselling, and this is best done by the general practitioner who knows the family thoroughly. Many requests for reversal follow the break-up of a marriage within a year of vasectomy. Also it is unwise to give a 100% guarantee that natural rejunction cannot occur.

The operation should be performed carefully under general anaesthesia, the edges of the external spermatic fascia should be held on haemostats so that the lower cut end of the vas can be double-tied bent on itself and pushed back beneath this fascia while the upper end, similarly ligated, can be held outside this fascia, the edges of which are closed around it. The upper end therefore lies beneath the skin and dartos muscle.

Reanastomosis can be successful in up to 80% or more if carefully performed and sperm leak prevented. Results are best within the first 3–4 years of vasectomy—later the results are poorer. On this account little of the vas should be excised at vasectomy.

CHAPTER 62

ORGAN TRANSPLANTATION

Background.—The transplantation of tissues and organs has a venerable history. Skin transplantation dates back to about 1500 BC. Corneal and bone transplantation developed in the second half of the nineteenth century and whole organ transplantation was pioneered by Alexis Carrel early this century. Only with the advent of immunosuppressive drugs to prevent rejection in the early 1960's did successful kidney and other organ transplantation become a clinical reality. For organ failure which would otherwise result in the death of a person, the replacement of the diseased organ (in the recipient) is carried out by taking a healthy organ from another person (the donor). Where the organ is a single organ and non-regenerative (*e.g.* the heart, the liver) the donor is always a cadaver. The kidneys, however, are paired organs and, if healthy, one is capable of functioning as efficiently as two. Thus, living related donors are able to give a kidney to a person who has end-stage renal disease. In bone marrow transplants, the tissue which is donated is regenerative, and only a portion of it is given, so there is no risk to the health of the living donor.

There are two main factors which limit organ transplantation as a successful treatment. They are (1) *immunological*—the problem of rejection; and (2) '*supply and demand*'—the supply of organs continually falls behind the demand of increasing numbers of patients with end-stage organ disease.

Rejection of transplants.—Most tissue and organ transplants are rejected when the donor and recipient are genetically dissimilar. This rejection is an immunological phenomenon in which the recipient produces antibodies to antigens which the donor possesses but the recipient does not. Classically this rejection takes between 10–14 days to develop and to become fully effective. The result of this rejection is widespread infiltration of the transplant with lymphocytes, and microvascular changes which result in failure of the blood supply to the transplant. Any attempt, therefore, to make organ transplantation a clinically acceptable procedure, has to modify this rejection process.

KIDNEY TRANSPLANTATION

Dialysis or Transplantation?—In end stage renal disease regular *dialysis*, which may be *haemodialysis* or *peritoneal dialysis*, is an alternative treatment to transplantation. *Haemodialysis* may be carried out in the patient's own home where he maintains some measure of independence, the loss of which in hospital is a significant factor in the psychological adjustment for patients with end stage renal disease needing dialysis. *Peritoneal dialysis.*—During the 1980's C.A.P.D. (continuous ambulatory peritoneal dialysis), where a bag is worn under the clothing (dialysis continuing while the patient goes about his daily business), has allowed a new measure of freedom. However, dialysis by this method may not

Alexis Carrel, 1873–1944. Surgeon, Member of the Staff of the Rockefeller Institute for Medical Research, New York, U.S.A.

be as efficient as the more restricting methods of haemodialysis, and there is a risk of peritonitis due to the presence of an intra-peritoneal catheter.

Many patients on dialysis have anaemia, bone disease, hypertension, infertility, and many have a sense of poor health and loss of independence. There is an increased risk of blood-borne disease. Careful screening of blood donors for hepatitis B antigen has reduced the incidence of hepatitis in dialysis units, and the identification of HIV antibodies in potential blood donors has so far prevented AIDS from becoming a significant problem among the dialysis population.

Transplantation.—The recipient of a successful renal transplant returns to a normal life in most respects. The quality of life is much superior to that experienced on regular dialysis and this fact alone justifies organ transplantation, and, in addition, the cost of transplantation is considerably less than regular dialysis.

Haemodialysis: Access for Circulation. Shunt. Fistula

Shunt.—This is achieved by the insertion of Teflon cannulas either at the ankle or the wrist. The artery at the ankle is usually the posterior tibial artery while the vein may be the long or short saphenous vein. At the forearm, the radial artery and basilic or cephalic veins are used. These procedures can often be performed under local anaesthesia. The two Teflon cannulas are connected with a Silastic loop which is used for linkage to the dialysis unit. Thrombosis and infection of a shunt is frequent.

Internal Fistula.—For most patients, a Cimino fistula is made at the wrist by anastomosing the radial artery to the cephalic vein. It is wise to create an internal fistula before chronic haemodialysis becomes necessary, usually when the plasma creatinine approaches 900 μmol/litre. This then removes the need for a shunt. Surprisingly, distal gangrene as a result of fistula is rare. If the cephalic vein has been obliterated by previous intravenous infusion then an internal fistula can be made in the thigh by mobilising the long saphenous vein into a subcutaneous position and anastomosing its distal end to the femoral artery above the popliteal fossa.

It is important to place any fistula in a position which is accessible to the patient, *i.e.* a right-handed patient needs a fistula in the left arm.

If a patient is in incipient renal failure infusion should *never* be placed in a vessel likely to be used for an internal arteriovenous fistula.

While undergoing haemodialysis, any problems of congestive cardiac failure, tuberculosis, hypersecretion of gastric acid, secondary hyperparathyroidism, uraemic peripheral neuropathy and uraemic pericarditis can be corrected.

Preparation for Transplantation

The Recipient of a Donated Kidney.—It is preferable if the prospective recipient is prepared for transplantation by haemodialysis. Pretransplantation blood transfusion of at least 2 units of blood, during this period of haemodialysis, appears to produce better transplant results (and see DST below).

Donor Selection.—There are two sources of donated kidneys: (1) cadaver and (2) living related.

1. Cadaver Kidneys.—Most kidneys for transplantation come from people who have had been diagnosed as brain dead. These patients are usually victims of head injuries; some have had cerebrovascular accidents or primary brain tumours. They are maintained while there is still hope for life on a mechanical ventilator in an intensive care unit. When treatment has not been successful and brain death has been diagnosed, the doctors caring for the patient contact the transplant team, providing always that the patient's relatives have given permission for organs to be removed for transplantation. Many hospitals have renal

James E. Cimino, Contemporary, Chief, Renal Service Dialysis Unit, Veterans Administration Hospital, Bronx, N.Y., U.S.A.

transplant co-ordinators who organise the necessary preliminary tests including blood group and tissue typing so that possible suitable recipients will be identified in the local hospital or in hospitals elsewhere. These potential recipients may be dialysed while preparations are made to remove the donor organs.

Diagnosis of Death (brief guidelines).—Brain death occurs when brainstem reflexes are no longer present. It is diagnosed in a person, who must be normo-thermic and free of all types of sedative and anaesthetic drugs, when:

(1) There is no spontaneous respiratory movement for 3 minutes when the patient's pCO_2 is normal (this test should be repeated at regular intervals).
(2) There are no reflexes (gag, corneal, caloric).
(3) There are bilateral fixed dilated pupils.

These tests have to be repeated at least once over a period lasting several hours. The diagnosis of death must be made by physicians of some standing, who are not involved in the transplant. If the patient's death has been reported to the coroner then the coroner must give consent for removal of the organs. This will always be the case with an accident victim.

Ownership of the Body.—Permission for the use of organs must be obtained from the person who owns the body. This is usually the next of kin. If a 'reason-able search' fails to find a next of kin, then the hospital administration (in the U.K.) own the body and may give permission for the removal of organs. The finding of a 'donor card' does not over-rule the instructions of the owners of the body, but should guide them.

Potential donors must be free of malignant disease (although primary brain tumour is not a contraindication to transplant) and free of systemic infection. There should be no history of previous significant renal disease including hypertension and diabetes. In general it is preferable to have donors under 60 years of age. Kidneys from children are usually best transplanted into children of similar age. It is important that the urine output of potential donors should be maintained at 50 ml per hour or more so that no significant tubular damage is sustained. Intravenous isotonic saline, 10% mannitol, and inotropic drugs, *e.g.* dopamine, may be employed to maintain adequate renal function.

2. Living Related Donors.—An identical twin or immediate relative (brother or sister, father or mother, son or daughter) may offer a kidney to a patient on dialysis. A number of screening tests are carried out. They must be ABO blood group compatible. Blood biochemistry, haematology, urinalysis, 24-hour urine protein, glomerular filtration rate, must all be normal in the donor. Hepatitis B antigen and other infections must be excluded and there should be no significant medical disorder, *e.g.* hypertension. Chest x-ray and i.v. urogram are arranged and if these are normal a bilateral renal arteriogram is carried out to demonstrate the vascular patterns in the two kidneys. If the donor and potential recipient do not have identical tissue types, then a *mixed leucocyte culture* (MLC—see below) can be carried out and this is followed by *donor specific blood transfusion* (DST) which increases the chance of success of the transplant (when the matching is not perfect) to over 90%. DST involves taking about 250 ml of blood from the poten-tial donor and transfusing it on three separate occasions at two-weekly intervals to the recipient. Some surgeons consider MLC and DST unnecessary for success, and do not perform these procedures. A negative direct T-cell crossmatch (see below) on the day of transplant is essential.

Unrelated Donors.—In exceptional circumstances it may be acceptable to consider an unrelated living donor, *e.g.* husband or wife or first cousin. All live donors must be able to give adult, informed consent to the procedure. Thus children, young teenagers, and mentally handicapped people are unacceptable as potential live related donors.

Compatibility.—The principal histocompatibility antigens in man are those of the *Major Histocompatibility Complex* (MHC) and the *ABO blood group system*. The Human MHC is located on the short arm of Chromosome 6 and includes the genetic loci which code for antigen specificities inherited in simple Mendelian fashion from father and mother. These specificities are conveniently detected on peripheral blood lymphocytes and are known as *Human Leucocyte Antigens* (HLA).

Tissue Typing refers to the serological detection of the antigens of the A, B and C loci whilst those of the D locus are detected only by Mixed Leucocyte Culture (MLC). Recently it has become possible to detect D-related (DR) antigens serologically on the subpopulation of lymphocytes known as B cells, and matching of these is regarded by some as of major importance in graft survival (fig. 1350). MLC measures direct cell-to-cell reactions of lymphocytes from donor and recipient. The HLA D locus antigens are important in these reactions, and matching for MLC reactivity may be better correlated with graft survival than matching of other loci.

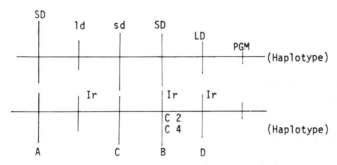

FIG. 1350.—Schematic HLA complex on chromosome 6. Serologically Loci A, B and C and lymphocyte defined D locus. Genes coding for phosphoglucomutase and complement components as well as immune response genes are located on the chromosome.
(After Charles Marks, FRCS, New Orleans.)

Sensitisation of the recipient to MHC antigens through multiple blood transfusions or a previous transplant is detected by antibody screening, and ultimately by the pre-transplant lymphocytotoxic crossmatch. Such presensitisation may produce accelerated rejection, but not all antibodies are considered detrimental; for instance a crossmatch positive against B cells but negative to T cells is not considered by some to be a contraindication to transplantation. In living related donor transplants there is a 1:4 chance that a sibling will be HLA identical, and a 2:4 chance that a sibling will be one haplotype identical. There is a 1:4 chance that a sibling will be a complete mismatch. Parents will have one haplotype identity with a child, and where parents have antigens in common with one another, the match between a parent and child may be even better than one haplotype. Identical, or one haplotype identical relatives, are suitable as potential donors, as the transplant would

Gregor Johann Mendel, 1822–1884. Austrian monk and naturalist, who became Abbot of the Augustinian Monastery at Brunn (Brno), Czechoslovakia.

have an excellent chance of success. It is a matter of current controversy whether or not HLA tissue matching for cadaver transplants is particularly important using modern immunosuppressive drugs, but there is no doubt that blood group ABO compatibility and a negative T cell direct crossmatch remain essential for successful renal transplantation.

Operations—The Donor Operation

(1) **Living Related Donor.**—The living donor operation is a nephrectomy performed by an experienced surgeon in an operating theatre adjacent to the transplant surgeon who prepares the recipient to receive the kidney. As much artery and vein as possible, and a reasonable length of ureter, are preserved on the donor organ. Subcutaneous heparin, 5000 units, is given to the donor every 12 hours for three days beginning at the time of the operation. This is to prevent the major post-operative calamity of a pulmonary embolus.

(2) **Cadaver Donor.**—As soon as possible after the confirmation of brain death the patient is taken to the operating theatre for removal of the transplant organs. In multiple organ donation the kidneys and the liver are prepared and mobilised while the heart is still beating and the patient's ventilation maintained. The portal circulation is cannulated and the aorta and vena cava are also cannulated, and the kidneys and liver perfused. When the abdominal organs have been fully prepared and cannulated (which may take two or three hours) the heart is removed; then the liver is removed together with aorta, coeliac axis, vena cava and portal vessels. The kidneys are removed en bloc with vena cava and aorta. Throughout these procedures the kidneys and liver have been perfused with icy perfusion fluid to minimise the warm ischaemic time (see below). Finally the kidneys are separated with the renal artery (or arteries) on a cuff of aorta, and a patch of vena cava with the veins. They are then packed in plastic bags surrounded by ice in an insulated box. The kidneys can be stored in this manner for up to 72 hours if necessary.

If only the kidneys are to be removed from the donor, they are usually removed en bloc with vena cava and aorta and perfused and packed in ice as described above. Although multiple organ donation is becoming more common, most donor operations are for the kidneys alone.

The warm ischaemic time is the time from when circulation ceases through the donor organ to the time of cold perfusion with Collin's solution[1] at 4°C. When in-situ perfusion is used the warm ischaemic time may be zero. However, kidneys with warm ischaemic times up to 30 minutes are suitable for transplantation. There will be variable degrees of acute tubular necrosis in the transplanted organ if there is warm ischaemic damage to the kidneys. This will cause delay in function of the transplant and the patient will need to be dialysed during this post-transplant oliguric phase.

The cold ischaemic time is the period from cold perfusion of the kidney until the new circulation is established in the transplant. This includes cold perfusion time, storage in ice, and cooling during transplant anastomosis. Providing the fluid used for perfusion has a high concentration of potassium (80 mmol/l) and a high osmolality (400 mosmol/kg) the cold ischaemic time can be up to 72 hours. Usually 24–30 hours is sufficient storage time for the kidney to be matched, a suitable donor found, the kidney transported and the operation performed.

Operations—The Recipient Operation

While the donor kidney is being excised, the recipient is anaesthetised, and a lower quadrant incision is made above and parallel to the inguinal ligament. The internal and external iliac vessels are cleared of lymph nodes and adipose tissue, and then clamped superiorly with bulldog clamps. The renal artery may be anastomosed end to end with the internal iliac artery or end to side with the external iliac arteries.

Post-Operative Management

(1) **Immunosuppression.**—*Cyclosporin A.*—This is a potent, relatively new immunosuppressant. It is a metabolite of a soil fungus. Various regimes are recommended. It may be given intravenously for 24 hours, 4 mg/kg in 500 ml of isotonic saline starting at the beginning of the transplant operation. On the first post-operative day the patient may start taking the medication orally in a dose of 12 mg/kg daily. The dose is reduced over

---

[1] Collin's solution = potassium chloride (K 1·5 mmol), potassium acid phosphate (K 1·5 mmol), potassium phosphate trihydrate (K 8·5 mmol), sodium bicarbonate (Na 1·0 mmol), procaine hydrochloride (10 mg), phenoxybenzamine (2·5 mg), magnesium sulphate (Mg 3·0 mmol), dextrose (2·5 g), heparin (500 iu) made up to 100 ml with water to a pH of 7·0.

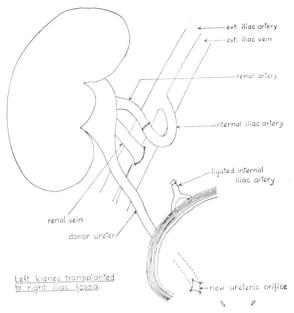

ext. iliac artery

ext. iliac vein

renal artery

internal iliac artery

ligated internal
iliac artery

renal vein

donor ureter

Left kidney transplanted
to right iliac fossa.

new ureteric orifice

FIG. 1351.—Renal transplantation (recipient operation).

subsequent weeks to a maintenance dose of 4 or 5 mg/kg orally. Plasma levels of cyclosporin are monitored twice weekly and high levels of cyclosporin may be nephrotoxic. The dose should be reduced if toxic levels occur.

Cyclosporin A may be used as the sole immunosuppressant, but frequently in addition to cyclosporin, prednisolone is given in a low dose of 2·5 mg three times daily.

Azathioprine and Prednisolone.—For nearly 20 years these were the standard immunosuppressants in renal transplantation. Although they have been superceded by cyclosporin A[1] in a significant number of transplant units, they are still commonly used. Various dosage regimes are popular but one is azathioprine 3 mg/kg intravenously for 24 hours and then 2·5 mg/kg orally. Prednisolone is given in a dose of 1 mg/kg per 24 hours and the dose is reduced every three days to a maintenance level of 5 mg t.d.s.

(2) **Fluid Balance.**—Urinary output is measured hourly and replaced ml for ml with dextrose saline up to a urinary output of 200 ml/hour. It should not be forgotten than an anephric patient needs 500 ml of fluid per day to replace insensible loss. This can be replaced at 20 ml/hour of isotonic saline at the same time as the dextrose-saline replacement of urinary output. It is convenient to add the immunosuppressive drugs into the isotonic saline for 24 hours, so that a steady administration of drugs is achieved. A central venous pressure line assists in fluid management especially in the first 24 hours after surgery.

Management of Post-operative Oliguria. Most live related donor transplant kidneys diurese immediately after the transplant because there has been a relatively short ischaemic time and therefore minimal acute tubular necrosis. Many cadaver renal transplants also diurese immediately but a significant proportion of cadaver renal transplants and a small number of live related donor transplants do not produce urine initially. There may be an anuric or oliguric period which lasts for days or even several weeks. During this time the patient must be dialysed at regular intervals. Acute tubular necrosis resolves spon-

---

[1] Cyclosporin A was introduced into clinical practice in 1979 by Calne. Its advantage has been an increased transplant success rate compared to transplant recipients immunosuppressed with azathioprine and prednisolone. Its main disadvantage is a tendency to produce nephrotoxicity and therefore elevated serum creatinine in the successfully functioning transplant. Multiple drug regimens have been tried, most of them including cyclosporin A. It is possible to achieve transplant success rates comparable with those seen with cyclosporin, using azathioprine and prednisolone as the sole primary immunosuppressant when antithymocyte globulin (ATG) is added for treatment of difficult rejection episodes. The advantage of this regime is the absence of nephrotoxicity. New forms of cyclosporin are being developed which may be less nephrotoxic.

Sir Roy Yorke Calne, FRS, Contemporary. Professor of Surgery, Cambridge University, England.

taneously and a diuresis will eventually occur. However, there are other possible causes of oliguria and these must be distinguished from ATN (acute tubular necrosis) as they may require treatment.

Differential Diagnosis of Causes of Oliguria.—1. Acute tubular necrosis, 2. Rejection, 3. Obstruction of the collecting system, 4. Infarction.

The commonest of these occurrences are ATN and rejection. Rejection may occur at any time but is more likely from the 5th post-operative day. Twice weekly DTPA (diethylene triamine penta acetic acid) isotope renography and gamma camera scan of the kidney confirms perfusion of the kidney when oliguria is present (figs. 1352 and 1353). A deterioration in the perfusion index may suggest rejection superimposed on ATN but is not diagnostic. Percutaneous needle biopsy which can be carried out under local anaesthetic in the transplant ward is necessary to confirm the presence of rejection. This is done on the 5th post-operative day if oliguria persists and is repeated when necessary. Ultrasonography is also performed twice weekly to detect peri-renal collections of lymph or blood and it is particularly useful to confirm or exclude the presence of urinary tract obstruction. ·

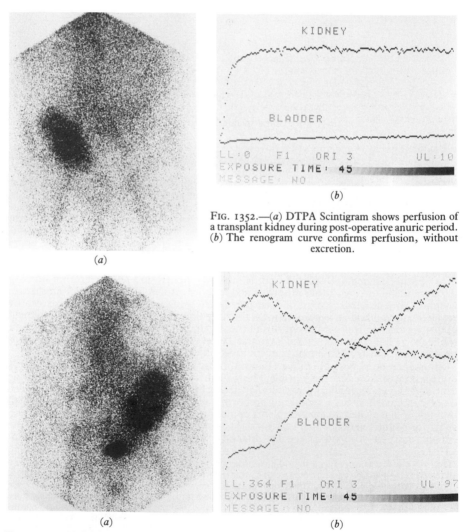

(b)

FIG. 1352.—(a) DTPA Scintigram shows perfusion of a transplant kidney during post-operative anuric period. (b) The renogram curve confirms perfusion, without excretion.

(a)

(a)   (b)

FIG. 1353.—(a) DTPA Scintigram in a transplant recipient shows good perfusion and excretion after onset of diuresis. (b) The renogram curves show excretion into the bladder.

Rejection

Diagnosis of Rejection.—In the oliguric kidney a percutaneous or open renal biopsy is essential for accurate diagnosis. In a diuresing kidney where renal function has been satisfactory the serum creatinine is a sensitive indicator of the onset of rejection. While function is good the serum creatinine will continue to fall; with the onset of rejection the creatinine will rise. Other possible causes of a rising serum creatinine are urinary tract obstruction or systemic infection. A high level of plasma cyclosporin A may also elevate the serum creatinine. Intravenous pyelography and certain drugs (*e.g.* cotrimoxazole; cimetidine) may also cause a rising serum creatinine in the transplanted patient. Ultrasonography will exclude obstruction and may demonstrate the 'fat pyramids' associated with rejection (fig. 1354). Two types of rejection may be seen on biopsy. Infiltration of the parenchyma with lymphocytes and plasma cells is known as cellular rejection. This usually responds satisfactorily to anti-rejection treatment. Vascular rejection consists of deposition of fibrin in arterioles and thickening of the intima. This form of rejection responds poorly to treatment and usually progresses to complete occlusion of the blood vessels with failure of the transplant.

Treatment of Rejection.—Rejection may occur at any time after transplantation. If there is ABO blood group incompatibility or if there are antibodies to T cells present in the serum, hyperacute rejection will occur within minutes of vascularisation of the transplant. The kidney, which is initially bright pink, becomes blotchy and dark blue. This occurrence should be rare if one observes the rules that transplants must be ABO compatible and the direct cross match must be negative. Acute rejection may occur within a few days of the transplant and is common during the first three months. It is unusual more than 12 months after the transplant. Acute rejection of the cellular type will usually respond to high doses of intravenous steroid. Chronic rejection may occur at any time after transplantation and often includes a vascular element. It responds poorly to high doses of steroids. Rejection which occurs 12 months or more after transplant, while not common, responds poorly to treatment.

Whether primary immunosuppression is with cyclosporin A or with prednisone and azathioprine, rejection is treated with high doses of steroids, *e.g.* 1 g of methylprednisolone intravenously daily for three days. This may be repeated on one or two further occasions if indicated. Excessive doses of steroids should be avoided to diminish steroid side effects. If there is an inadequate response to high dose steroid, then ATG (antithymocyte globulin) or ALG (antilymphocyte globulin) is often effective. A good response to anti-rejection treatment is evident when the serum creatinine decreases or when an adequate diuresis occurs after a period of oliguria. If there is no response within two or three days of anti-rejection treatment a further renal biopsy will confirm that rejection is still present. The decision to give further anti-rejection treatment is balanced against the possible dangers of cumulative high dose immunosuppressive therapy. It may be better to allow rejection of the kidney to avoid serious complications from over-treatment.

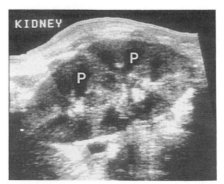

Fig. 1354.—Ultrasonogram of transplanted kidney. Transverse scan showing well defined medullary pyramids (P) (fat pyramids) in rejection.

(Dr. J. Boultbee.)

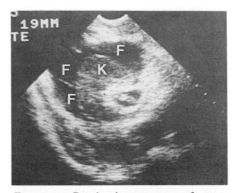

Fig. 1355.—Renal ultrasonogram of transplanted kidney. The transverse scan demonstrates the lower pole of the transplant (K) surrounded by fluid (F) (? haematoma, lymphocele, urinoma).

(Dr. J. Boultbee.)

Complications of Renal Transplantation

1. Hazards of Immunosuppression.—*Infection* is more common in immunosuppressed patients and may be with unusual organisms, *e.g.* Cytomegalovirus (CMV), Herpes, Pneumocystis, Varicella, Epstein Barr Virus, Monilia, etc.

Steroids.—High doses predispose to gastrointestinal bleeding, which can be prevented by giving ranitidine or cimetidine. With a high cumulative dose of steroid there is increasing incidence of steroid bone disease including necrosis of the femoral head. Cataracts are more common. Wound healing may be delayed. There is masking of intra-abdominal emergencies, *e.g.* perforated diverticular disease. The response to sepsis, *e.g.* pneumonia, may be abnormal.

Azathioprine.—Depression of the white cells and platelets may occur making infection particularly hazardous. Azathioprine must be stopped if the white cell count falls below $3 \times 10^9/l$ or if the platelet count falls below $100 \times 10^9/l$. Recovery may take several days and then azathioprine may be started again. Allopurinol potentiates the effect of azathioprine and should be avoided in transplant patients. There is an increased incidence of malignant disease in patients on azathioprine immunosuppression. Malignancies of the reticuloendothelial system, the central nervous system and the skin, in particular, are more common.

Cyclosporin A.—This immunosuppressant is nephrotoxic. This effect is more pronounced when there has been a period of oliguria. Transient paraesthesiae are not uncommon. Hirsutism is increased and the incidence of lymphomas is also increased, particularly if high doses of cyclosporin A have been used.

Antithymocyte globulin (ATG) *and antilymphocyte serum* (ALS).—There is an increased incidence of viral infection, particularly CMV (cytomegalovirus) after ATG or ALS treatment.

2. Surgical Complications of Renal Transplantation.—(*a*) *Urinary tract obstruction.*—This presents in the diuresing kidney with a sudden deterioration in renal function—a rising serum creatinine and a falling urine output. It may be due to an extra-renal collection of blood or of lymph (a lymphocele). It may be associated with a collection of urine due to extravasation from ureter or bladder. Diagnosis is greatly assisted by ultrasonography which will show dilatation of the calyces and pelvis and ureter, and any peri-renal collections (fig. 1355). Aspiration of the collections may be carried out under ultrasound control and the fluid sent for analysis. Extravasated urine will have a high concentration of potassium and urea (compared to serum concentrations) in the functioning transplant kidney. Where there is significant obstruction leading to oliguria and a rising serum creatinine, percutaneous nephrostomy will provide temporary drainage of the kidney and pyeloureterography will outline the upper urinary tract and define the site of obstruction and any leakage.

Treatment may involve re-implantation of the ureter in the bladder or if there is associated sloughing of ureter, the ureter can be anastomosed to the patient's own ureter on the side of the transplant. A nephrostomy is always left in place to prevent leakage of urine through the anastomosis line during the healing process which may be prolonged because of steroids and immunosuppressive drugs.

A recurring lymphocele causing obstruction may be treated initially by regular aspiration. If recurrence persists, then radioactive gold may be inserted percutaneously into the lymphocele and after one or two insertions recurrence of the collection is unusual.

(*b*) *Urinary Leakage.*—This may occur from the upper urinary tract, *e.g.* a calyx, the pelvis, the ureter. Because the renal arteries are end arteries, if one artery is occluded the associated calix may slough and leak. If there is damage to the blood supply of the ureter either during removal of the kidney or during the transplant operation, sloughing and leakage may occur one to two weeks after transplant. Treatment includes a nephrostomy and excision of sloughed tissue. The ureter may be re-anastomosed to the patient's own ureter if there is not sufficient length to reimplant in the bladder.

Leakage from the bladder may occur at the site of the ureter implant or at the site of the cystostomy. Urethral catheter drainage may empty the bladder sufficiently to allow the area to heal. If the defect does not heal, surgical exploration is necessary, with excision of the sloughed tissue, re-suturing of the defect, and patching with omentum. If necessary, the ureter should be re-implanted.

(*c*) *Vascular Complications.*—The commonest vascular complication is secondary haemorrhage occurring within two weeks of transplantation. An unusual emergency is spontaneous rupture of the transplanted kidney—which causes severe haemorrhage. These conditions require urgent resuscitation of the patient and immediate surgical exploration.

There is a significant risk of loss of the kidney in this situation and nephrectomy may have to be carried out if vascular repair is not possible. Renal infarction is usually due to faulty surgical technique. An isotope renal scan will show absence of perfusion. Nephrectomy must be carried out.

Results of Kidney Transplantation

It is important to differentiate between patient survival and transplant survival. When a kidney ceases to function the kidney can be removed and the patient returned to haemodialysis. There has been a considerable improvement in both patient survival and transplant survival in the last decade. A number of factors have been responsible:

(1) Blood transfusions in the preoperative months/years.
(2) HLA DR matching.
(3) The use of cyclosporin A.
(4) Lower doses of steroids.

The one year cadaver kidney transplant survival rate is now 75–80% and the patient survival rate after cadaver renal transplant has been improved to 95% at one year. The failure rate of cadaver kidneys in subsequent years is about 1–3% per annum. After live related transplantation, success rates of 95% at one year may be expected and patient survival rates approach 100%.

Over 50,000 renal transplants have been performed worldwide and the high success rate now expected represents a major achievement in the management of end stage renal disease—a disease which until 25 years ago was invariably fatal.

LIVER TRANSPLANTATION[1]

The indications for liver transplantation are primary biliary atresia, certain cirrhotic conditions and primary malignant disease of the liver. Children do particularly well after this type of surgery, but a limiting factor in obtaining suitable livers for children is the size of the donor liver. As the liver is placed orthotopically in the bed of the resected diseased liver, the only suitable donor is another child. There are a number of conditions which are not suitable for liver transplantation and these include chronic active hepatitis B, and secondary carcinomas of the liver. Primary carcinomas of the common bile duct are also unsuitable.

Tissue typing and crossmatching are unnecessary in liver transplantation and do not influence results.

The donor organ is retrieved at the same time as removal of the kidneys for transplant (see earlier). The liver is stored cold but must be transplanted within a few hours of removal. It is not yet possible to store the liver for more than six to ten hours, which is a disadvantage compared to the kidney. After removal of the recipient diseased liver, the donor vena cava is anastomosed end to end to the recipient vena cava above and below the liver. The portal vessels are anastomosed end to end. The donor coeliac artery is anastomosed to the recipient common hepatic artery. Finally the biliary tracts are anastomosed and a T-tube stent is used to allow drainage of the bile during the healing period. The recipient operation has been greatly facilitated in the 1980's, by the use of pump

---

[1] Three centres in the world have led the way in transplantation of the liver. These are Cambridge, where Professor Calne's team has pioneered this work in Europe, and Denver and Pittsburgh where Dr Thomas Starzl has been the main exponent of this procedure in the United States.

Thomas E. Starzl, Contemporary. Transplant Surgeon, University of Pittsburgh, Pittsburgh, U.S.A.

driven veno-venous by-pass to return portal and systemic venous blood to the systemic circulation during the procedure.

Although the liver is best transplanted into the normal orthotopic sub-diaphragmatic position—which requires recipient hepatectomy—there is an alternative method to this. It involves using the liver transplant as an auxilliary to the recipient's own liver. This is known as a heterotopic liver transplant.

Until five years ago the one year patient survival rate was 30%, but since the advent of cyclosporin A both Calne and Starzl have achieved 80% one year survival rates. There are now several patients who have had a successful liver transplant for more than 10 years. With these improved results, it is inevitable that there will be an increase in the number of surgical teams carrying out liver transplantation, and this procedure will become more generally available for patients with severe liver disease—patients who would otherwise die from their illness.

HEART TRANSPLANTATION AND HEART/LUNG
TRANSPLANTATION (See Chapter 41)

The heart is removed from the recipient at the same time as removal of other donor organs including liver and kidneys (see earlier). It is stored in cold saline at 4°C and it is used as soon as possible after removal from the donor. At the transplant operation the pulmonary veins are anastomosed to the left atrium of the donor heart. A cuff of recipient right atrium is anastomosed to a suitable cuff of donor right atrium. The donor and recipient aortas are anastomosed and the pulmonary artery of the donor heart is anastomosed to the recipient's pulmonary artery. Throughout the procedure the circulation to the patient is maintained by cardiopulmonary by-pass.

PANCREAS

Pancreas transplantation is still relatively uncommon, and the main reason for this is that results remain disappointing with a one year graft survival rate of 30–40%. The purpose of transplanting the pancreas is to provide a severe diabetic with endogenous insulin. The recipient is usually a diabetic with renal failure who receives a pancreas transplant after a successful kidney transplant. The pancreas may be transplanted as the tail alone or as a combined pancreas/duodenal segment. The advantage of the duodenal segment is that the exocrine secretion is drained into the bowel, whereas with a tail segment transplant the exocrine ducts must be occluded. This is usually achieved by ligating them or by injecting liquid polymers (e.g. neoprene) to block the ducts. Complications from fistulas, due to secretion of the pancreatic enzymes, are common. These technical complications continue to make pancreas transplantation a formidable problem. In addition, high doses of steroid, necessary to treat rejection, which is common, are diabetogenic.

BONE MARROW

Bone marrow transplantation is increasingly used for the treatment of some leukaemias, aplastic anaemia, and certain immune deficiency syndromes. The recipients are usually treated by total body irradiation prior to engraftment in order to increase graft acceptance.[1] HLA compatibility is essential in bone marrow transplant, as bone marrow is active immune tissue. Not only is it capable of being rejected, it is also capable of mounting a rejection process against the host (GVH—Graft Versus Host disease). Donor banks have been set up to record the tissue types of volunteers. Computer scanning of the lists of

---

[1] In 1986, the nuclear reactor disaster in Chernobyl, USSR, produced total body irradiation in many workers who automatically became candidates for bone marrow transplantation.

volunteers may produce compatible unrelated donors of a tissue type identical to patients who require the bone marrow graft.

The laboratory and clinical logistics of bone marrow transplantation are considerable. The surgical technique, however, is relatively minor. Bone marrow, aspirated from bone of the donor, is transplanted by intravenous injection to the recipient. Several weeks pass before haematological parameters will indicate whether or not the transplant has been successful. Immunosuppression is with cyclosporin A. GVH is treated with steroids.

CHAPTER 63

THE SURGICAL PATIENT

The conditions described in this book have all happened to real people, people who have had their private reactions to their misfortune and who have had to cope with the implications of being ill. In proper clinical management all these aspects are taken into account in order:

1. to understand the significance and the meaning of the illness for the patient;

2. to identify psychological and environmental factors which might have a bearing on the aetiology;

3. to plan treatment or the timing of operations in accordance with the patient's wishes, needs and personal or material circumstances;

4. to make realistic estimates of recovery times, return to activity and longer term prognosis.

Psychosocial Background

Patients lying quietly in hospital beds have as many responsibilities, anxieties and personal concerns as the doctors looking after them, plus all the problems associated with being ill, away from home and not earning; and there may also be social and environmental problems and psychiatric symptoms. The most important of these Psychosocial Factors can be assessed quite rapidly under the following headings:

1. *Bereavement*, from the death of any family member of close friend within the past 12 months. 2. *Serious Illness or Disability* in anyone living with the patient or having to be cared for by the patient. 3. *Previous Psychiatric History* or use of psychotropic drugs. 4. *Problems with Children (if any)*, dependant or adult. 5. *Work Problems*, actual or threatened, no sick pay, bad working conditions, difficult relations with superiors or subordinates, retirement. 6. *Home Problems*, the building itself, local environment, personal relationships in the home and with neighbours. 7. *General Level of Satisfaction with Life*.

Pre-operative Preparation

Levels of Anxiety.—An operation is a major event in anyone's life, and so a moderate degree of anxiety is expected in any patient who has an accurate grasp of what is going on. Some patients may display high anxiety and will benefit from explanation and reassurance (which may have to be repeated), and also from tranquillising medication. Others will appear as relaxed and uncomplaining 'good patients' but they may in fact be denying, ostrich-fashion, the realities and implications of the operation. They require special attention and explanation, to overcome their denial of the realities, otherwise they may become resentful and uncooperative in the postoperative period when the realities are unavoidable.

Any operation may be of particular importance to a patient if, for example, a relative died after an apparently similar one, or indeed died from some totally different cause in the same hospital or even in the same ward.

Special Organs and Procedures.—Operations on the heart, eye, uterus, and breast, are followed by a disproportionate number of psychological and social problems, as they pose a threat to life itself, to the individual's independence, or to personal or sexual identity. Furthermore, some of these patients will spend time in intensive care units or be blindfolded for a period. High levels of anxiety, disorientation and even hallucinations can develop which respond well to careful explanation of what is going on. If sedation is required it needs to be designed so as not disorientate the person further.

Colostomy, ileostomy, amputation and organ transplantation are of special importance because of the drastic effect they have on the individual's life and self-image. Specialised technical advice about appliances and facilities is available, but patients need the opportunity to discuss their fears, the future function of their bodies (particularly sexual function), and they need personal support while they adapt to their new style of life.

Post-operative Phase

Anxious post-operative patients lie rigid in bed, hold their muscles tight, fail to breathe freely or move their legs, and so predispose themselves to post-operative complications. Detailed pre-operative explanation (if relevant, with the partner present) is the best way to reduce post-operative anxiety. Patients with an accurate knowledge of what to expect—drains, dressings, intravenous infusions, how to breathe, how to move in bed, how much pain to expect and how long it will last—will require less post-operative analgesia and spend less time in hospital than patients who have no idea of what is involved.

Recovery

The self-employed man is the soonest back to work. Delayed recovery, no matter how good the clinical reason, calls for a psychosocial enquiry. There may be claims for compensation outstanding, problems at home or at work; or if there has been prolonged disability, the resumption of full health—with all the normal demands made on healthy people—may be a mixed blessing.

What to Tell the Patient

'I knew I was done for when the doctors didn't stop at the bed any more.' Patients lying in bed all day are minutely sensitive to every aspect of the doctor's behaviour. Surveys of patients with incurable diseases show that the majority want to know what is wrong with them, however bad the prognosis.

Anyone given the diagnosis of cancer or an incurable illness is bound to react emotionally. This is normal and must be accepted. After all, how would you take such news? People take time to adjust to the realities, and may go through periods of denial of the truth, depression, anger, and resentment against the staff. But with warm support and plenty of opportunity for frank expression of feelings, often involving family, chaplain, general practitioner and social worker as the case may be, most people can be brought through to a state where they can accept peacefully that there is no hope of recovery.

There will, of course, be a smaller number who really should not be confronted with the realities of fatal illness. Doctors who are sensitive to their patients (and who have overcome their own anxieties in dealing with the dying) will recognise who these are, but no one should ever be left in ignorance by default. All members of the team and the general practitioner must agree about what to tell the patient, but the most experienced member should be the one to do the telling.

Those Who Cannot be Cured

Real help for the terminally ill begins when that state is fully accepted, and there is no longer any pretence about curing the condition. The next step involves the reality of death. It can be difficult to allow dying people the time to talk about their anxieties or their dread of the process of dying. It can make you feel uncomfortable and want to withdraw. But you should stay there and share the person's fears.

At a practical level, the surgeon has many skills that can be used to help those for whom there can be no cure—procedures to reduce vomiting, appliances to lessen the distress and indignity of incontinence, measures to control diarrhoea and constipation. Patients should be out of bed, if possible, and given physio-therapy to assist breathing and limb movement.

Most important is the management of chronic pain, which is quite different from the management of acute pain. There is no standard dose of analgesic. The correct dose for someone with a painful terminal illness is that dose which the patient says relieves the pain. The drug is titrated against the patient's pain, and the next dose is administered before the effects of the previous one have worn off.

Benzodiazepines and phenothiazines can reduce anxiety and enhance the effects of analgesics, and so avoid excessive sedation. When the pain is severe there should never be any hesitation in using morphine or related alkaloids (such as diamorphine which is less likely to cause nausea). Questions of addiction or escalating dosage are irrelevant in terminal care. These drugs can bring a consol-ing sense of calm in the final stages.

Hospice Care

Hospice care can be used in many cases to assist with caring for and comforting the incurable patient. Even if such care is not available, doctors can and should learn from the experts who work in such centres. The control of pain and the maintenance of morale of dying patients has been brought to such a pitch of excellence in these institutions that it raises such skills beyond simple com-passion and into the sphere of established science.

INDEX

A

Abdomen, gunshot wounds of, 15
Abdomino-perineal excision, 1126
Abscess, acute, 26
  cold, 655, 748
  See under various organs and regions
Acanthosis nigricans, 139
Achilles tendonitis, 181
Achilles tendon, rupture of, 340
Achondroplasia, 394
Acid-base balance, 87–90
Acidosis, 89
Acoustic neuroma, 473, 479
Acrocyanosis, 233
Acromegaly, 481
Acromioclavicular dislocation, 270
Actinomycosis, 48
  of right iliac fossa, 1051
  See under various organs
Adamantinoma, 596, *See* Ameloblastoma
Adductor tenotomy, 429
Addison's disease, 702
Adenoids, 625–628
Adenolymphoma, 567
Adenoma, 103
Adiposis dolorosa, 103
Adrenal glands, 700–711
Adrenalectomy, 706
Aerocele, 458
AIDS, 50, 538, 578
Ainhum, 219
Albumin, human 4·5%, 71, 75
Aldosteronism, 706
Alkalosis, 88
Alveolar abscess, 600–603
Amaurosis fugax, 207
Amazia, 715
Ameloblastoma, 596
Amoebiasis, intestinal, 1119
  of liver, 911
Ampulla of Vater, carcinoma of,
  995–1000
Amputations, 219–224
Amyloid disease, 55
Anaemia, haemolytic, 945
  Mediterranean, 949
  sickle cell, 74, 940
Anal canal, 1131–1164
Analgesia, 75
Anaphylaxis, 62
Anastomoses, 814–826
Aneurysmal bone cysts, 373, 614
Aneurysms, 224–231
  abdominal aorta, 225–229
  arterio-venous, 230
  cirsoid, 435
  dissecting, 811
  femoral, 230
  iliac, 230
  intracranial, 484
  mycotic, 224

of renal artery, 1217
of splenic artery, 942
  thoracic aorta, 810
  ventricular, 810
Angiodysplasia (colon), 1031
Angiofibroma, laryngeal, 644
  nasopharyngeal, 632
Angioma, 137–139
  intracranial, 488
  plexiform, 139
  sclerosing, 136
  strawberry, 138
  venous, 138
Angioplasty, balloon, 204
Anion gap, 90
Ankle fractures, 333–339
Ankylosing spondylitis, 370
Ankylosis, positions for, 350
Anthrax, 48
Antibioma, 27, 718
Antibiotics, 21, 31, 36, 39, 46
Anticoagulant therapy, 184–185
Anti-sepsis, 19–32
Antrum, maxillary, 617
Anuria, 1202–1207
Anus and Anal canal, 1131–1164
  abscesses of, 1154
  anatomy, physiology, 1131–1134
  chancre, 1143
  condylomas of, 1347
  congenital abnormalities of, 1135–1139
  examination of, 1134
  fissure, 1142
  fistula, 1156–1161
  haemorrhoids, 1145–1153
  incontinence, 1141
  lymphatics, 1133
  malignant tumours, 1162–1164
  papilla, hypertrophied, 1145
  stricture, 1161
  valves and crypts, 1132
  warts, 1347
Aorta, aneurysms, 225
  coarctation of, 797
  rupture of, 812
  valve operations on, 806
Appendicectomy, 1102
Appendicitis, 1091–1106
  differential diagnosis of, 1097
Appendix, vermiform, 1090–1109
  abscess of, 1101, 1106
  carcinoid tumour of, 1109
  carcinoma of, 1109
  congenital abnormalities of, 1091
  diverticula of, 1108
  mass, 1000–1104
  mucocele of, 1108
Apudomas, 699
Argenaffinoma, 1053, *See* Carcinoid
Arnold- Chiari malformation, 482
Arrhenoblastoma, 705

Arterial investigations, 197–200
  management of stenosis, 200–207
  operations, 203–207, 212
  stenosis or occlusion, 193–213
Arteriography, 199
  renal, 1198
Arteritis, 231–232
Artery, injuries of, 212–213
  myxomatous degeneration of, 232
  stenosis or occlusion of, 193–213
Arthritis, See Osteo, Rheumatoid
  sexually acquired reactive, 1332
  suppurative, 347
  tuberculous, 351
Arthrodesis, 364
  triple, 425
Arthrogryphosis multiplex congenita, 394
Arthroplasty, 365
Ascariasis, 977
Ascites, 992, 1016–1018
Astrocytoma, 470–478
Atelectasis, 776
Atrial septal defect, 799
Atrophic scirrhous, 728
Autotransfusion, 72
Auriculo-temporal syndrome, 571
Avascular necrosis, femoral head, 310
Axonotmesis, 515

                    B

Bacteriaemia, 26
Baghdad sore, 116
Baker's cyst, 421
Balanoposthitis, 1346
Balloon angioplasty, 204
Bamboo spine, 371
Barlow's sign, 380, 381
Barrett's ulcer, 835
Barton's fracture, 294
Battered child, 262
Bazin's disease, 116
Behçet's syndrome, 576
Bedsores, 217
Bell's palsy, 512
Bennett's fracture, 299
Berry aneurysm, 485
Betel nut, 582, 586
Biceps brachii, rupture of, 417
Bile ducts and gall bladder, 953–979
Bile, limey, 962
  'white', 973
Bilharziasis, 1282–1285
Biliary atresia, 960
Billroth operations for peptic ulcer,
    876–878
Bisgaard treatment of venous ulcer, 191
Bites, 11, 166
Bladder, 1254–1297
  accidental wounding, 1258
  bilharziasis, of, 1282–1285
  calculus, 1269
  carcinoma of, 1286–1293
  clot retention, 1305
  diverticula of, 1273–1276
  exstrophy of, 1255
  foreign bodies in, 1272
  hernia of, 1275
  infection, 1278–1285
  in spinal injuries, 1261–1263

  neck contracture, 1308
  neoplasms, 1285–1293
  papilloma, 1285
  physiology, 1254, 1264, 1267
  rupture of, 1256, 1324
  'thimble', 1281
  trabeculation of, 1300
  tuberculosis, 1281
Blast injuries, 16
Blastomas, 102
Blind loop syndrome, 1032
Blood, coagulation failure (DIC), 74
  fractions, 70
  grouping and cross-matching, 71
  loss, measurement of, 57
  substitutes, 75
  transfusion, 69–75
  volume, 58
Boas's sign in gall stones, 967
Bochdalek, foramen of, hernia, 781
Boeck's sarcoidosis, 130
Boils, 132
Bolus obstruction, 1085
Bomb injuries, 12–18
Bones, diseases of, congenital, 391–394
  dysplasias (dystrophies), 392, 612
  See also under proper names for diseases
      named after them
  fractures of, See also Fractures and
      under names of bones
  secondary tumours in, 376
  tumours of, 372–379
Bowen's disease, 139
Bow-leg, 401
Brachial neuralgia, 522
  plexus lesions, 520–522
Brain injuries, 437–464
  stem injury, 457
  swelling, 440
  tumours of, 468–479
Branchial cyst and fistula, 648
Branchiogenic carcinoma, 649
Breast, 712–739
  abscess, 717–720
  Brodie's serocystic disease of, 725
  carcinoma, 725–739
  congenital abnormalities, 715
  cystosarcoma phylloides, 725
  cysts, 722
  drill (needle) biopsy of, 713
  duct ectasia, 715
    papilloma, 724
  dysplasia of, 721
  fat necrosis of, 717
  fibroadenoma, 724
  fibroadenosis of, 721
  galactocele of, 723
  hypertrophy of, diffuse, 716
  inflammations, 717
  injuries of, 716
  lipomatous carcinoma, 728
  lymphatics, 712
  lymphangiosarcoma, 731
  male, 738
  massive swellings of, 724
  mastitis carcinomatosa, 728
  milk (mamillary), fistula, 719
  Mondor's disease of, 720
  nipple, lesions of, 714
  sarcoma, 739

screening for cancer, 735
syphilis, 720
tuberculous, 720
Brodie's bone abscess, 348–349
Bronchial tree anatomy, 740
Bronchiectasis, 758
Bronchopneumonia, post-operative, 776
Bronchus, carcinoma of, 761–767
   foreign bodies in, 757
   fracture of, 748
   tumours of, benign, 760
   See also Lungs
Broomstick plaster, 407
Brown tumours, 414
Bubonocele, 1169
Budd-Chiari's syndrome, 924
Buerger's disease, 231
   exercises and position, 201
Bullet wounds, 11–16
Bunion and bunionette, 177
Burkitt tumour, 130
Burns and scalds, 147–156
   of eye, 535
   of mouth, 579
Burr holes, 452–478
Bursae, 420
Burst abdomen, 1188
'Burst' fractures, 493, 496
Buschke-Loewenstein tumour, 1351
Butcher's thigh, 7

C

CDH, 380–387
CT (brain) scanning, 455, 474, 475, 480, 487
Cachexia ovarica, 113
Caecostomy for intestinal obstruction, 1064
Caecum, carcinoma of, 1057–1059
   diverticulum of, 1039
   failure of descent of, 1028
   volvulus of, 1080
Caisson (decompression) disease, 212
Calcitonin, 695
Calcium, 83
Calculus anuria, 1205
Calculus, *See under organs*
Caldwell-Luc operation, 618
Callus, 236
Cancer. *See* Carcinoma *and under names of organs and regions*
Cancrum oris, 578
Candidiasis, 47, 577, 1331
Caput Medusae, 921
Carbuncle, 133
   of kidney, 1240
Carcinoid tumour, 1053
Carcinoma, 107–109, 760
   basal-celled, 140
   squamous-celled, 107, 141
   See also under names of organs and regions
Cardiac arrest, 790–792
   investigation, 787
   massage, 791
   surgery, scope of, 792–813
   tamponade, 794
   tumours, 807
   See also under Heart

Cardiospasm, 844
Carotid artery stenosis, 206
Carotid body tumour, 656
Carpal tunnel compression, 418
Carpus, injuries of, 295
Cartilage, necrosis of, 405
   normal healing of, 265
   of knee, 324–326
Cat-scratch fever, 125
Catheterisation, arterial, 199
   cardiac, 789
   suprapubic, 1259
   ureteric, 1197
   urethral, 1259
Cauda equina, conditions of, 503–509
Causalgia, 529
Cavernous sinus thrombosis, 558
Cellulitis, 25
   of abdominal wall, 1191
   of orbit, 26, 531
Central venous pressure, 66–67
Cerebellar tumours, 473
Cerebral abscess, 464–468
   injury, 437–440
   palsy, 428
   tumours, 468–479
Cervical disc protrusions, 507
   injuries, 494
   plexus, injuries to, 520
   rib, 650
   spondylosis, 508
Chancre, 42
Chancroid, 47
Charcot's biliary triad, 972
   joints, 431
Chauffeur's fracture, 294
Cheek, tumours of, 581
Cheilosis, 577
Chemodectoma, 656
Cherubism, 614
Chest, injuries to, 16, 743–747
Chimney sweep's cancer, 1374
Chlamydia, 1331–1333
Cholangiography, 955–959
Cholangiocarcinoma, 978
Cholangio-hepatitis-asiatic, 977
Cholangitis, 910
   sclerosing, 976
   suppurative, 973
Cholecystjejunostomy, 976
Cholecystectomy, 970–972
Cholecystitis, acalculous, 968
   acute, 966
   chronic, 965
   glandularis proliferans, 969
Cholecystography, 954
Cholecystotomy, 970, 971
Cholecystoses, 969
Choledochoduodenostomy, 975
Choledochoscopy, 974, 978
Choledochotomy, 971–973
Choledochal cyst, 961
Cholelithiasis, 962. *See also* Gallstones
Cholesterosis, 969
Chondroma, 373, 393, 749
Chondromatosis, multiple, 393
Chondromalacia patellae, 359
Chondrosarcoma, 375, 749
Chordee, 1348
Choroid, malignant melanoma of, 147

Christmas disease, 71
Chvostek's sign, 695
Chylocele filiarial, 122
Chylothorax, 753
Chylous reflux, in lymphoedema, 123
Circle of Willis, aneurysm of, 484
Circumcision, 1344
Clavicle fractures of, 269
Claw-foot and toes, 176, 179
Cleft lip and cleft palate, 540–545
Clonorchiasis, 977
Clostridium difficile, 35, 1119
Clot retention of urine, 1305
Club-foot, 387–391
Clutton's joints, 45
Coccydnia, 302
Coccyx, fractures of, 302
Cock's peculiar tumour, 134
Codman's triangle, 374
Colic, gall-stone, 965, 972
    renal, 1193
    ureteric, 1193
Colitis, ischaemic, 1088
    pseudomembranous, 35
    ulcerative, 1039–1045
Collar-stud abscess, 655–656
Colles' fracture, 291–294
Colon, angiodysplasia of, 1031
    carcinoma of, 1055–1061
    diverticula, 1033–1039
    familial adenomatous polyposis of, 1054
    redundant, 1030
    volvulus of, 1080
Colostomy, 1062–1064
Coma, hepatic, 904
    scale, 447
Compartmental syndrome, 213
Concussion, 439
Condylomata acuminata, 1347
Congenital heart disease, 795
Coning, 441, 472
Conjunctivitis, 535
Conn's syndrome, 708
Contre-coup, 441
Cooley's anaemia, 949
Cord injury syndrome, 497
Corneal injuries, 533
Corns, 135
Coronary artery, surgery of, 808–810
Corpora amylacea, 1310
Costo-clavicular syndrome, 522
Coup, 441
Courvoisier's law, 972
Cowper's glands, affections of, 1319
Cranio-cerebral injuries, 437–464
Craniopharyngioma, 481
Craniotomy, technique of, 452
Crepitus, 35, 238
Cretinism, 664
Crohn's disease, 1047–1050
Crush syndrome, 69
Crutch palsy, 523
Cryosurgery, 638
Crystalluria and anuria, 1207
Curling's ulcer, 866
Cushing's syndrome, 481, 704
Cut throat, 652
Cylindroma, 141
Cyst-basal cell naevus syndrome, 610
Cystic fibrosis, 986

Cystic Hygroma, 649
Cysticercosis, 112
Cystitis, 1278–1285
    acute haemorrhagic abacterial, 1280
    cystica, 1282
    interstitial, 1281
Cystography, 1199
Cystoscopy, 1201
Cysts, 110–113
    chylolymphatic, 1023
    dermoid, See Dermoid
    emphysematous, 771
    false, 110
    hydatid, See Hydatids
    in OA, 358
    sebaceous, 133
    See organs and regions

D

Death, diagnosis of, 1378
Deflected nasal septum, 619
Delayed primary suture, 7, 13–15
Delhi boil, 116
Dental caries, 600
Dental and dentigerous cysts, 609
Dental disease, complications, 604
Denture induced granuloma, 613
de Quervain's diseases, 418, 690
Dercum's disease, 103
Dermatitis, artefacta, 115
Dermatofibroma, 136
Dermoid, 102, 111, 112, 130, 786
    external angular, 130
    implantation, 102, 112
    lingual and sublingual, 580
    of scalp, 434
    of testis, 1368
    mediastinal, 786
    post-anal, 1138
    periauricular, 545
    sequestration, 102, 111
    tubulo-, 111
Desmoid, 1192
Dextran, 74
Dialysis, peritoneal, in anuria, 1205
    shunts for, 1376
Diaphragm, 780–783
Diaphyseal aclasis, 393
Dietl's crisis, 1220
Disappearing pulse, 196
Dislocation, 235, See under names of joints
Diuretics, osmotic, 456
Divarication of recti abdominis, 1190
Diverticula and diverticulum
    alimentary, 1033
    See under names of organs
Diverticulosis, -itis, 1035–1039
Doppler ultrasound, 184, 197–199
Dormia basket, 1232
Dornier lithotriptor, 1228
Ductus arteriosus, patent, 795
Duhamel's operation, 1029
Duke's staging, 1123
'Dumping syndrome', 889
Duodenography, 997
Duodenum and stomach, 855–901
    atresia and stenosis of, 865
    diverticula of, 901
    neoplasms of, 900

rupture of, 902
 ulcer, 866–892
Dupuytren's contracture, 419
Dwarfism 394
Dysentery, amoebic and bacillary, 1119
Dysphagia, 828
 lusoria, 812

E

Ear, afflictions of, 619–624
Ecchondroma, 373
Ectopia vesicae, 1255
Ectopic gestation, ruptured, 1099
Ectropion, 531
Elbow-joint, injuries to, 283–288
Electrolyte balance, 79–90
Elephantiasis, 122
 filarial, scrotal, 1373
 neuromatosa, 106
Embolectomy, 209, 779
Embolism, 207
 air, 210
 fat, 211, 458
 mesenteric, 210
 pulmonary, 778
 therapeutic, 212
Emphysema, mediastinal, 641, 833
 surgical, 746
Empyema, 753–757
 necessitatis, 749
Encephalocele, 436
Enchondroma, 373
Endothelioma, 110
Enuresis, in children, 1269
Ependymoma, intramedullary, 470–479
Epicondyle, medial, fracture of, 282
Epididymis, cysts of, 1363
 tumours of, 1372
Epididymo-orchitis, 1364
Epilepsy, 466, 470
 post-traumatic, 464
Epiphysis, disorders of, 402–408
Epiplocele, 1166
Episcleritis, 536
Epispadias, 1322
Epistaxis, 619
Epithelioma, 141
 benign calcifying, 137
Epulis, 607–609
Erb-Duchenne paralysis, 521
E.R.C.P., 957, 958, 976
Erysipelas, 48
Erythema induratum, 116
Erythroplasia of Querat, 1349
Eventration, 780
Ewing's tumour, 378
Exomphalos, 1179
Exophthalmos of thyrotoxicosis, 675
Exostoses, bony, of auditory meatus, 621
 ivory, 373
 multiple, 393
 subungual, 181
Extradural haematoma, 442–444, 451–454
Eye, 530–538
 excision, 537

F

Face, 539–558
Faecal impaction, 1089
Fallot's tetralogy, 800
Fanconi's syndrome, 413
Fat necrosis, 990
Felty's syndrome, 948
Femoral epiphysis, slipped, 402–404
Femur, absence of, 391
 fractures of, 306–318
Fibrinolysins, 209
Fibroids, recurrent, 109
Fibroma, 103
 of bone, 373
Fibrosarcoma, 109, 377
Fibrositis, 415
Fibula and tibia, fractures of, 329–339
 absence of, 391
Filariasis, 121–122, 1362, 1373
Fingers, 157–170
First aid, 9
 in burns, 147
Fissure-in-ano, 1142
Fistulas, 116
 arteriovenous, 230
 aortoduodenal, 229
 biliary, 979
 bladder, 1276–1278
 branchial, 648
 broncho-pleural, 771
 duodenal, 887, 902
 faecal, 1061
 gastro-jejuno-colic, 888
 hepato-bronchial, 773
 milk, 719
 pancreatic, 988
 recto-vaginal, 1042
 salivary, 565
 thyroglossal, 693
 tracheo-oesophageal, 830
 umbilical, 1186
 uretero-vaginal, 1277
 urethral, 1278, 1340
 urinary, 1276
 vesico-intestinal, 1276
 vesico-vaginal, 1276
Fistula-in-ano, 1156–1161
Flail chest, 745
Flat-foot, 174
Fluid and electrolyte balance, 76–90
Fluid levels, 1070
Foot, 171–181, 340–343
Foreign bodies in air passages, 639
 in bladder, 1272
 in bronchial tree, 757
 in ear, 620
 in larynx, 639
 in oesophagus, 830–832
 in rectum, 1114
 in stomach, 900
 in tissues, 10
Fournier's gangrene, 1372
Fovea coccygea, 1139
Fractures, principles of, 235–268
 clinical features of, 237
 comminuted, 235
 complications of, 256–261
 compound, 238
 compression, 236

Fractures—*contd.*
consolidated, 242
delayed union, 242
fatigue, 264
greenstick, 263
healing of, 236, 240, 243
malunion of, 260
march, 343
maxillo-facial, 552
non-union, 242, 260
operative treatment of, 253–255
pathological, 265
reduction of, 246–248
stabilisation (immobilisation) of,
248–253
'stress', 264
transchondral, 265
treatment of, 245–256
See also under names of bones
Framboesia, 46
Freiberg's disease, 408
Frey's syndrome, 571
Fröhlich's syndrome, causes of, 481
Froin syndrome, 505
Froment's sign for ulnar paresis, 526
Frostbite, 218
'Frozen shoulder', 417
Funnel chest, 748
Furuncle, 132

G

Galactocele, 723
Galeazzi fracture-dislocation, 290
Gall bladder and bile ducts, 953–979
abnormalities of, congenital, 959
carcinoma of, 977
empyema, 968
gas in, 968
injuries, 962
mucocele of, 968
perforation of, 966
polyposis, 969
physiology of, 954
porcelain, 954
strawberry, 969
torsion, 962
typhoid, 970
'Gallows' splint, 316
Gall-stones, 962
colic, 965
dissolving, 965
gas in, 962
in bile ducts, 972
silent, 964
Ganglion, simple, 420
compound palmar, 355
Ganglioneuroma, 105, 708–710, 750
Gangrene, 213–219
chemical, 219
diabetic, 216
dry, 214
ergot, 218
Fournier's, 1372
gas, 35
moist, 214
progressive post-operative, 1191
traumatic, 217
venous, 185
Gargoylism, 394

Gas cysts, intestinal, 1051
Gas infections, 35
Gastrectomy for carcinoma, 898
Gastric emptying, 859
function tests, 856–862
mucosa, 856
mucus, 857
neoplasms, 892–899
polypeptides, 857–858
polyposis, 892
secretion tests, 856–862
ulcer, 865–892
See also Stomach
Gastroduodenoscopy, 872
Gastro-intestinal suction, 1073
Gastro-jejunostomy, 879
Gastrostomy, 96
Gaucher's disease, 950
Gelatin, 75
Genital, herpes and warts, 1346
Giant cell tumour, 376, 377, 414, 613
Gingivitis, 607
Glandular fever, 125
Glasgow coma scale, 447
Glaucoma, 536
Gliomas, 470–479
Glomus tumour, 106, 624
Glossitis, 583
Glossodynia, 589
Glottis, acute oedema of, 639
Glue ear, 621
Goitres, 666
See also Thyroid gland
Golfer's elbow, 410
Gonorrhoea, 1329, 1330
Goodsall's rule, 1158
Granulation tissue, 3
Granuloma inguinale, 1347
intubation, 644
pyogenicum, 136
umbilical, 1185
Graves' disease, 673
Grawitz's tumour of kidney, 1248
Guinea worm, 117
Gums, diseases of, 607
Gynaecomazia, 738

H

Haemangioblastoma, 479
Haemangioma, 137
of liver, 933
of rectum, 1122
Haemarthrosis, 74
Haematemesis and melaena, 882–885
Haematocele of testis, 1362
Haematocrit, 58
Haematoma, acute extradural, 442–444
acute intracerebral, 445
acute subdural, 444
chronic subdural, 462
of scalp, 433
perianal, 1152
Haematuria, 1193
Haemolytic anaemia, 945
Haemophilia, 74
Haemorrhage, 56–61
Haemorrhoids, 1145–1153
Haemothorax, 746, 751

Hair-ball, 900
Hallux rigidus, 178
  valgus, 177
Hamartoma, 107, 760
Hammer-toes, 179
Hand, infections of, 157–166
  injuries of, 166–170
'Hangman' fracture, 496
Hansen's disease, 37–41
Hare-lip, 541
Harrington instrumentation, 399, 494
Hartmann's operation, 1129
Harvey's sign, 196
Hashimoto's disease, 690–692
Head, gunshot wounds of, 16
Head injuries, 437–464
Heart and pericardium, 787–813
  congenital disease of, 795–803
  disorders of rhythm, 807
    See also Cardiac
  transplantation, 812
  tumours of, 807
  valve operations, 803–807
Heller's operation for cardiospasm, 845
Hemi-colectomy, 1059
Hemi-hepatectomy, 936
Hemivertebrae, 400
Henoch-Schonlein purpura, 946
Hepatitis, amoebic, 911
  A Virus, 910
  B Virus, 49
Hepatocellular failure, 904
Hepatolenticular degeneration, 922
Hernia, 1165–1192
  diaphragmatic, 780
  epigastric (linea alba), 1182
  femoral, 1176–1179
  funicular, 1169, 1173
  gluteal and sciatic, 1184
  hiatus, 835–842
  incarcerated, 1166
  incisional (ventral), 1188
  inflamed, 1168
  inguinal, 1168–1175
  internal, 1084
  interparietal, interstitial, 1183
  in-W (Maydl's), 1175
  irreducible, 1166
  lumbar, 1184
  obstructed, 1166
  obturator, 1184
  of bladder, 1175, 1275
  operations, See types of hernia
  pantaloon (saddle-bag), 1173
  para-oesophageal ('rolling'), 841
  para-umbilical, 1180
  perineal, 1184
  reducible, 1166
  reduction-en-masse of, 1175
  Richter's, 1168
  sliding, 1175
  Spigelian, 1184
  strangulated, 1167, 1174, 1178, 1182
  umbilical, 1179–1182
  ventral, 1188
Herpes simplex infections, 576
Herpes, genital, 1346
Hip-joint, congenital dislocation, 380–387
  dislocation of, 304–306
  OA of, 358, 366

replacement, 366, 370
  tuberculosis of, 351–355
Hippocratic facies, 1006
Hirschsprung's disease, 1028
HIV infection, 50, 538, 578
Hodgkin's lymphoma, 125–129
Holism, 1388
Horner's syndrome, 224
Horns, 134, 137
Horseshoe kidney, 1208
Hospice care, 1390
Housemaid's knee, 421
Humerus, fractures of, 273–283
Hunner's ulcer of bladder, 1281
Hutchinson's melanotic freckle, 146
  teeth, 45
  triad, 45
  wart, 582
Hydatids, of kidney, 1212
  of liver, 915–918
  of lung, 772
Hydradenitis suppurativa, 132, 1159
Hydroceles, 1359
Hydrocephalus, 482
Hydronephrosis, 1218
Hygroma, cystic, 649
Hypercalcuria, idiopathic, 1229
Hypercatabolic, state, 91
Hypercorticism, 703
Hyperhidrosis, 529
Hypernatraemia, 81
Hypernephroma, 1248
Hyperparathyroidism, 696
Hypersplenism, 948
Hyperthyroidism, 673
Hypertrophic pyloric stenosis, 862
Hyphaema, 534
Hypocorticism, 701
Hypokalaemia, 82
Hypokalaemic alkalosis, 88
Hyponatraemia, 79
Hypoparathyroidism, 695
Hypospadias, 1321
Hypothyroidism, 664

I

Ileal loop conduit, 1294
Ileocystoplasty, 1281
Ileostomy, for ulcerative colitis, 1044
Ileum, atresia or stenosis of, 1074
Ileus, duodenal, chronic, 902
  meconium, 1075
  paralytic, 1086
Immunology, 51–55
Immunosuppression, 54, 1380–1387
Impetigo, 133
Incisions, 6
Incontinence, anal, 1141
  of urine, 1263
Induratio-penis-plastica, 1348
Infection, 19–30
Inferior epigastric artery tearing, 1190
Infertility, male, 1374
Inflammation, 3
Ingrowing toenail, 171
Insulinoma, 1001
Intermittent claudication, 193
Intervertebral disc, prolapse, 505–509

Intestinal obstruction, 1065–1089
  acute, 1067
    of newborn, 1074
  acute-on-chronic, 1069–1074
  adynamic, 1065, 1086, 1087
  chronic, 1089
  closed-loop, 1067
  due to adhesions and bands, 1082
  due to amoebiasis, 1045
  due to bolus, 1085
  due to faecal impaction, 1089
  due to food, 891, 1085
  due to gall-stones, 1085
  due to gastrectomy, 891
  due to ileus, 1086
  due to internal herniae, 1084
  due to Meckel's diverticulum, 1034
  due to mesenteric embolus, 210, 1087,
    thrombosis, 210, 1087
  due to stercolith, 1085
  due to strictures, 1084
  due to volvulus, 1080
  due to worms, 1085
  dynamic, 1065
  fluid levels in, 1070
  gas shadows in, 1070
  strangulation in, 1069
  treatment of, 1071–1074
Intestines,
  adenomatous, polyps of, 1052–1054
  amoebiasis of, 1045
  blindloop syndrome, 1032
  carcinoid tumour of, 1053
  carcinoma of, 1055
  congenital malformations of, 1027
  Crohn's disease of, 1047
  diverticula of, 1033–1039
  haemangioma of, 1055
  large, tumours of, 1053
  lipomas of, 1055
  lymphosarcoma of, 1052
  polyposis of, 1052–1054
  rupture of, traumatic, 1031
  small, obstruction of, 1071
    tumours of, 1052
  tuberculosis of, 1050
In-toeing, 401
Intussusception, 1076–1080
Involucrum, 344
Ischio-rectal abscess, 1155

J

Jarisch Herxheimer reaction, 45
Jaundice, acholuric familial, 945
  in carcinoma of pancreas, 996
  in newborn, 1185
  with cholelithiasis, 972
Jaws, bone tumours of, 612–617
  cysts of, 609–612
  osteomyelitis of, 605
Jejunum, diverticulum of, 1033
  stenosis of, atresia and, congenital,
    1074
Jod-Basedow thyrotoxicosis, 680
Joints, congenital diseases of, 380–395
  loose body in, 408
  neuropathic, 431
  position for immobilisation, 350

tuberculosis, 351
tumours of, classification of, 377

K

Kanavel's sign, 162
Kantor's 'string' sign, 1049
Kaposi's sarcoma, 130, 538
Kehr's sign in ruptured spleen, 941
Keller's operation, 178
Keloid, 6
Keratitis, 45, 536
Kerato-acanthoma, 136
Keratosis, senile (or solar), 139
Kernohan's notch, 441
Kidneys, 1208–1253
  aberrant renal vessels, 1212
  arteriography of, 1198
  artery stenosis, 193, 207
  calculus, 1222–1230
  carbuncle, of, 1240
  carcinoma of, 1248
  congenital abnormalities, 1208, 1212
  crossed dystrophia, 1209
  cysts of, 1209–1212
  ectopic, 1208
  function tests, 1195–1202
  horse-shoe, 1208
  hydatid cyst of, 1212
  hydronephrosis of, 1218–1222
  infections of, 1234–1246
  injuries of, 1215–1217
  neoplasms of, 1247–1253
  pelvis, duplication of, 1212
    papilloma of, 1251
  percutaneous stone removal, 1228
  removal of, 1252
  transplantation of, 1376–1385
  tuberculosis of, 1242–1246
  unilateral fusion, 1209, 1212
Kienböck's disease, 407
King's evil, 655
'Kiss cancer', 108
Klumpke's paralysis, 522
Knee-joint, 321
  injuries to, 321–328
  tuberculosis of, 351
Knock-knee, 401
Kocher's method for shoulder dislocation,
  272
Köhler's disease, 407
Kondeoleon's operation, 123
Krukenberg's tumour, 108, 894, 896
Küntscher intramedullary nail, 316
Kwashiorkor, 919
Kypho-scoliosis, 748
Kyphus, 352

L

Lachrymal swellings, 531
Laminectomy, 505, 507
Laryngeal paralysis, 642
Laryngectomy, speech after, 647
Laryngocele, 644
Laryngo-fissure, 646
Laryngopharynx, tumour of, 636

Larynx, 639–647
  carcinoma of, 645–647
  foreign body in, 639
  papilloma of, 644
Lateral condyle fracture, 281
Lateral rhinotomy, 633
Le Fort's classification, 552
Leishmania, 116
Lentigo, 142
Leprosy, 37–41
  orchitis, 1366
Leriche's syndrome, 196
Leucoplakia of tongue, 585–587
Leukaemia, 951
Leydig cell tumour, 1368
Lichen planus, 575, 587
Ligamentum patellae, ruptures of, 326
Linitis plastica, 896
Lip, 540–550
  carcinoma of, 548
  pigmented, 547
Lipoma, 103–105
Liposarcoma, 104
Lisfranc dislocation, 342
Litholapaxy, 1271
Lithotomy, suprapubic, 1272
Lithotriptor (Dornier), 1228
Little's area, 619
Littre's hernia, 1166
Liver, 903–936
  abscess of, 911–914
  actinomycosis of, 915
  amoebic infection, 911
  biopsy, 906
  carcinoid, secondary, 935
  carcinoma of, 933
  cirrhosis of, 919
  cysts of, non-parasitic, 919
  enlargements of, 909
  failure, 904
  function tests, 906
  hydatid disease of, 915–918
  injuries of, 908
  melanoma of, secondary, 532, 935
  neoplasms of, 933–936
  scanning of, 907, 917
  syphilis, 915
  tuberculosis, 915
  virus infections, 909
Loose bodies, in joints, 408
  in peritoneum, 1018
Lotheissen's operation, 1178
Lowsley's operation, 1297
Lucid interval, 443
Ludwig's angina, 584
Lumbar puncture, danger of, 467, 472,
  653
Lunate dislocation, 296
Lung function, 741
Lung, shock, 747
Lungs, abscess of, 767
  cysts, 770
  developmental anomalies, 741
  injury to, 743–747
  post-operative, 775
  transplantation of, 779
  tuberculosis of, 773
  tumours of, 760
Lupus vulgaris, 133
Luxatio in erecta, 271

Lymphadenitis, 124
  cervical, 654–656
  iliac, suppurative, 1102
  mesenteric, acute non-specific, 1021
  tuberculous, 124, 1022
Lymphangiography, 118
Lymphangioma, 123, 649
Lymphangiosarcoma, 731
Lymphangitis, 118
Lymphocytes in immunity, 51–54
Lymph nodes, 118–131
  tuberculous mesenteric, 1022
Lymphoedema, 120–123
Lympho-granuloma venereum, 1346
Lymphomas, 125–130

M

McBurney's point, 1091
Macrocheilia, 548
Macroglossia, 584
Madura foot, 173
Madura hand, 166
Magnesium, 83
Magnetic resonance imagining, (MRI),
  474, 790
Malar bone, fracture of, 555
Malherbe's epithelioma, 137
Mallet finger, 297
Mallory-Weiss syndrome, 883
Malnutrition, 91
Mammography, 713
Mandible, fractures of, 556
  neoplasms, 614
Mannitol, 69, 456, 477
March fracture, 343
Marion's disease, 1321
Marjolin's ulcer, 140
Mastitis carcinomatosa, 728
Mastoiditis, acute, 622
Maxilla, fractures of, 550–556
  tumours of, 615–617
Meckel's diverticulum, 1033
Meconium ileus, 1075
Medial epicondyle fracture, 282
Mediastinum, tumours of, 782
Medulloblastoma, 470–479
Megacolon, 1028
Megalo-ureter, congenital, 1214
Meibomian cyst, 530
Meig's syndrome, 1017
Melanoma, 142–147
  intraocular, 532
Melanosis coli, 1031
'Melon seed', bodies, 355
Menetrier's disease, 893
Menière's syndrome, 624
Meningioma, 469–479
Meningitis, infective, acute, 499
  in head injuries, 458
Meningocele, 435, 500
Meningomyelocele, 427, 500
Menisectomy, 326
Menisci, cysts of, 326
Meralgia paraesthetica, 528
Mercedes Benz sign, 962
Mesenteric adenitis, 1021–1023
  artery occlusion, 207, 210, 1087
  cysts, 1023
Mesentery, lesions of, 1021

Mesothelioma, 110, 1019
Metacarpal injuries, 299
Metaplasia, 101, 107
Metatarsalgia, Morton's, 181
Metatarsals, fractures of, 342
Metatarsus primus varus, 177
Microcephaly, 435
Micrognathism, 546
Micturition physiology, 1254
Mikulicz's disease, 573
Milroy's disease, 120
Milwaukee brace, 398
Missile injuries, 13–16
Mitral valve disease, 803
Molluscum fibrosum, and sebaceum, 135, 136
Mondor's disease, 720
Monilial stomatitis, 577
Monteggia's fracture-dislocation, 290
Montgomery, gland of, retention cyst of, 714
Moon's molars, 45
Morgani, foramen of, hernia through, 780
Mouth and tongue, 574–595
    to mouth ventilation, 791
Mucoviscidosis, see Cystic fibrosis, 986
MUGA scans, 789
Multiple endocrine syndromes, 699
Multiple sclerosis, 430
Mumps, acute epididymo-orchitis of, 1365
Murphy's (Naunyn's) sign, 965
Muscles, dysplasia of , 394
Myasthenia gravis, 784
Myelocele, 500
Mycosis fungoides, 130
Myositis ossificans, 283
Myringotomy, 627
Myxoedema, 664–666
    pretibial, 676

N

Naevus, 135–142
    blue, 142
    spider, 139, 921
    tardes, 139
Nail-patella syndrome, 394
Nasal polypi, 618
Naso-labial, -palatine cysts, 611
Nasopharynx, tumours of, 632
Neck, 648–659
    'block' dissection of, methods, 658
    carcinoma of, 657
Nephroblastoma, 1247
Nephrocalcinosis, 696
Nephrolithotomy, 1227
Nephroscopy, 1227
Nephrostomy, for calculus anuria, 1206
Nephro-ureterectomy, 1246
Nerves, 510–529
    axillary (circumflex), 523
    common peroneal, 528
    compression of, 517
    concussion, of, 514
    eighth, injuries of, 513
        tumours of, 473, 479
    eleventh, injuries of, 513
    entrapment, 517
    facial, 511, 559

fifth (trigeminal), 510
fourth, injuries of, 510
grafting of, 520, 522
laryngeal, 642
median, compression of, 418
    injuries of, 525
ninth, injuries of, 513
olfactory, injuries of, 510
operative procedures, for paralysis, 426
    repair, 518, 522
optic, injuries of, 510
peroneal, common, 528
phrenic, 520
radial, injuries of, 523
regeneration, rates of, 515, 517
sciatic, injuries of, 528
seventh, injuries of, 511–513
sixth, injuries of, 511
suture of, 519
tenth, injuries of, 513
third, injuries of, 510
tibial, 528
to serratus anterior, 523
twelfth, injuries of, 514
ulnar, anterior transposition of, 527
    injuries of, 526
vagus, 513
Neuralgia, brachial, 522
    glosso-pharyngeal, 513
    trigeminal, 510
Neurapraxia, 514
Neurilemmoma, 105, 473, 892
Neuroblastoma, 105, 709
Neurofibroma, 105
    macroglossia and, 584
    of chest wall, 750
    spinal, 502
Neurofibromatosis, 106
Neuroma, 105
    acoustic, 473, 479
Neuropathic joints, 431, 432
Neuropathy entrapment, 517
Neurotmesis, 517
Nipple, 714
Nissen operation, 839
Non-Hodgkin's lymphoma, 129
Nose, fractured, 552
Nutrition, 91–100

O

Ochsner- Sherren regimen, 1104
Odontomes and odontogenic tumours, 596
Oedema, lymphatic, 120
Oesophageal varices, 925–931
Oesophagectomy, for carcinoma, 852
Oesophagitis, 834
Oesophagoscopy, 829
Oesophagus, 827–854
    achalasia, of, 844
    burns and scalds, of, 847
    carcinoma of, 848–854
    congenital abnormalities of, 830
    diverticulum of, 834
    foreign bodies in, 832, 830
    hiatus hernia, 835–842
    injuries of, 832
    motility studies, 827
    perforation of, 832

rupture of, spontaneous, 833
scleroderma of, 846
'short', 832, 835
spasms of, 843
stricture of, 847
tumours of, 847–854
ulceration of, peptic, 834
varices of, 925
Olecranon, fractures of, 286
Oligodendro-glioma, 470–479
Omentocele, 1166
  strangulated, 1168
Omentum, conditions of, 1020
Onychogryphosis, 172
Ophthalmia neonatorum, 1331
Orbit, cellulitis, 26, 531
  swellings and tumours, 531, 532
Orchiectomy, for neoplasm of testis, 1370
Orchiopexy, 1355
Orchitis, leprous and syphilitic, 1366
Orf, 166
Oriental sore, 116
Oropharynx, neoplasms of, 635
Orthosis, 425
Os calcis, fracture of, 341
Osgood Schlatter's disease, 408
Osmotic diuretics, 456
Osteitis deformans, 410
Osteitis fibrosa cystica, 414
Osteitis pubis, 1307
Osteoarthritis and osteoarthrosis, 357–370
Osteochondritis, 404–409
  dissecans, 408
Osteochondromas, 372, 373, 393
Osteoclastoma (giant cell), 376, 377, 414
Osteogenesis imperfecta, 393
Osteoma, 372, 373
Osteomalacia, 413
Osteomyelitis, acute and chronic,
    344–349
  of jaws, 605
  of skull, 436
  of spine, 501
Osteopetrosis, 394
Osteoporosis, 412
Osteosarcoma, 374–378
Osteotomy, for CDH, 386
  for osteoarthrosis, 364
Otitis, external, 620
  media, 621
  serous, 623
Otosclerosis, 623
Ovary, arrhenoblastoma of, 705
Oxycephaly, 435
Oxygen therapy, 58
Oxyuris vermicularis, 1085, 1093

P

Paget's disease of bones, 410
  of jaws, 613
  of nipple, 728
  of penis, 1349
Pain, relief postoperatively, 75
  relief in terminal care, 1389
Painful arc syndrome, 416
Palate, lesions of, 547
Palm, infections of, 161
Pancoast tumours, 762

Pancreas, 980–1002
  annular, 987
  beta-cell tumour of, 1001
  calculi of, 994
  carcinoma of, 995
  cysts of, 992
  ectopic, 987
  fibro-cystic disease of, 986
  fistula of, 988
  function tests, 981, 997
  injuries, 987
  islet-cell tumours of, 1000
  scanning of, 982, 983, 992
Pancreatitis, 988–995
Pancreatoduodenectomy, 999
Pannus, synovial, 360
Papilloma, 103, 135
  acuminata, 1343
Paracentesis abdominis, 1017
Paralysis, 423–427
  laryngeal, 642
  in spinal cord lesions, 496
  'Saturday night', 524
  spastic, 428
Parapharyngeal abscess, 654
Paraphimosis, 1345
Parathyroids, 694–700
Parenteral nutrition, 96–100
Parona, space of, 163
Paronychia, 157, 172
Parotid, 559–573
  calculi, 565
  cysts of, 566
  neoplasms of, 566–571
  strictures and fistulas, 565
Parotidectomy, 570, 571
Parotitis, 561, 563
Patella, injuries to, 318–321, 326–328
  tendinitis, 417
Patent ductus arteriosus, 795
Paterson-Brown Kelly syndrome, 843
Patient, The Surgical, 1388–1390
Peau d'orange, 727
Pectus excavatum, 748
Pelvic abscess, 1008
Pelvis, cellutitis of cellular tissue, 26
  fractures, injuries of, 301–304
Pendred's syndrome, 666
Penis, 1343–1351
Peptic ulcer, 866–892
Perforated peptic ulcer, 880
Perianal abscess, 1155
Perianal haematoma, 1152
Pericardium, 794
Pericarditis, 794
Pericoronitis, 598
Perinephric abscess, 1241
Perithelioma, 110
Peritoneal adhesions and bands, 1016
  dialysis in anuria, 1205
  loose bodies (mice), 1018
  neoplasms, 1018
Peritoneo-venous shunts, 1018
Peritoneoscopy, 1020
Peritonitis, 1003–1018
  acute, 1003
  bile, 1012
  complications of, 1008
  meconium, 1012
  periodic, 1014

Peritonitis—*contd.*
  pneumococcal, 1013
  post-operative, 1011
  sclerosing, 1016
  starch, 1018
  streptococcal, 1014
  tuberculous, 1015
Perlèche, 577
Perthes' disease, 405–407
  test, 190
Pes calcaneus, 387
  cavus, 176
  equinus, 387
  planus, 174
Peutz-Jeger's syndrome, 1052
Peyronie's disease, 1348
Phaeochromocytoma, 709
Phagedaena, 47
Phalanx, fractures of, 297–299
Phantom pain, 224
Pharynx, 625–638
  diverticulum (pouch), 629–631
  neoplasms of, 631–638
Phimosis, 1343
Phocomelia, 391
Phrygian cap, 960
Piles, *See also* Haemorrhoids, 1145
'Pill', contraceptive,
  contraindications, pre-operative, 183
  sclerosant injections and, 189
Pilonidal sinus, 166, 1139–1141
Pineal gland, tumours of, 472
Pituitary disorders affecting skeleton, 414
  failure, 458
  tumours, 479–482
Plantar abscess, 172, 173
  fasciitis, 181
Plasma, 70, 71
Plaster-of-Paris splinting hazards, 249
Plethysmography, 198, 199
Pleura, diseases of, 750–757
Pleural effusion, 752
Plummer-Vinson syndrome, 843
Pneumatosis cystoides intestinales, 1051
Pneumaturia, 1037
Pneumothorax, 745, 750
Poliomyelitis, 429
Polymazia, 716
Polyposis, familial, 1054, 1121
Porphyria, 950
Porta-systemic encephalopathy, 905
Portal blood pressure, measurement of, 930
  hypertension, 923
  portal pyaemia, 910
  venography, 939
Port wine stain, 137
Positron Emission Tomography (PET), 475
Post-gastrectomy syndromes, 889
Post-splenectomy septicaemia, 952
Post-vagotomy syndromes, 891
Postural drainage, 759
Potassium balance, 81
Potato tumour, 656
Pott's disease, 351
  fracture, 333
  'puffy' tumour, 465
Pregangrene, 195
Presbyoesophagus, 846

Priapism, persistent, 1348
Primary suture, 1, 7
Proctalgia fugax, 1145
Proctitis, 1118
Profundaplasty, 204
Prognathism, mandibular, 546
Prolactin secreting adenomas, 481
Prostate, 1298–1319
  abscess of, 1316
  and bladder neck contracture, 1308
  calculi, 1309
  carcinoma of, 1310–1315
  enlargement of, benign, 1299
  operations, 1304–1309
  tuberculosis of, 1317
Prostatisme sans prostate, 1308
Prostatitis, 1315
Pruritus ani, 1153
Pseudarthrosis, 243
Pseudo-myxoma peritonei, 1019
Pseudoproptosis, 531
Psoas abscess, 352, 1177
Pulmonary capillary wedge pressure, 64
  embolism, 778
  function, 741
  oedema, 773
  postoperative complications, 775
  tuberculosis, treatment of, 36, 773
Pulp space infection, 158
Pulseless disease, 232
P.U.R.P., 1304
Purpura, 946
Pyelitis, 'honeymoon', 1234
Pyelography, retrograde, 1197
Pyelolithotomy, 1227
Pyelonephritis, 1234
Pylephlebitis, 910
Pyloric stenosis, hypertrophic, of adults, 865
  complicating peptic ulcer, 885
  of infants, 862
Pyloroplasty, 789
Pyogenic granuloma, 136
Pyonephrosis, 1240
Pyuria, abacterial, 1247

Q

Qat, 586
Quadriceps injury, 326–328
Quinsy, 628

R

Radial bursa, infection of, 162
Radiotherapy. *See under organs and conditions*
Radius, congenital absence of, 392
  fractures of, 287–295
Ramstedt's operation, 864
Randall's plaque, 1223
Ranula, 580
Raynaud's disease, and phenomena, 232–233
Rectal infusion, continuous, 86

Rectum 1110–1130
  bilharziasis of, 1119
  benign tumours of, 1120
  carcinoid, 1130
  carcinoma of, 1122–1130
  endometrioma, 1122
  fibroma, 1122
  foreign bodies, 1114
  haemangioma, 1122
  injuries of, 1114
  lymphatics, 1111, 1123
  lymphoma, 1122
  polyps of, 1121
  prolapse of, 1115
  strawberry lesion of, 1119
  stricture of, 1161
  tuberculosis of, 1119
  ulcer of, solitary, 1120
  villous adenoma of, 1121
Rectus femoris, rupture of, 327
Regional enteritis, 1047–1050
Reiter's disease, 1332
Renal function, tests of, 1195
Resuscitation, 790
Rest pain, 194
Retention of urine, 1258–1263
Retinoblastoma, 532
Retrograde pyelography, 1197
Retroperitoneal cysts and tumours, 1025
  fibrosis, idiopathic, 1233
Retropharyngeal abscesses, 629
Rhagades, 578
Rheumatism, non-articular, 415
Rheumatoid arthritis (RA), 360–370
Rhinophyma, 137
Rhinorrhoea, CSF, 458
Rib, cervical, 650
  fractured, 743–747
  tumours of, 749
Rickets, 413
Riedel's thyroiditis, 692
Ring, string method of removal, 168
Risser cast, 399
Risus sardonicus, 34
Rodent ulcer, 140

S

Sacrococcygeal tumour, 102, 1138
SAG-M blood, 71
Saint's triad, 964
Salivary calculi, 564, 565
Salmon patch, 137
Salmonella, 36
Salter and Harris epiphysis fractures, 263
Saphena varix, 188
Sarcoid, 130
Sarcoma, 109–110
  osteogenic, 374–378
  See also under names of organs and
    regions
Savage's intestinal decompressor, 1072
Scalds and burns, 147–156
Scalene syndrome and cervical rib, 650
Scalp, 433
Scaphoid fractures of, 295
Scapula, winging of, 523
  fractures of, 270

Scars, 4–6
Scheuermann's disease, 408
Schistosomiasis, 1282–1285
Schmorl's node, 506
Schneeberg cancer, 762
Scleritis, 536
Scleroderma, 233, 846
Scoliosis, 396–400
Screening for breast cancer, 735
Scrotum, 1372–1374
  idiopathic oedema of, 1358
Scurvy, 414
Sebaceous cysts, 133
Seminal vesicles, 1318
Seminoma, 1367
Sengstaken tube, 926
Sepsis, 19–30
Septicaemia, 26, 952
Sequestrum, 344
Sertoli cell tumour, 1368
Sever's disease, 408
Shenton's line, 385
Shock, 61–69
  in burns, 147–150
  lung, 747
  septic, 62
Shotgun injuries, 16
Shoulder injuries, 269–273
Shoveller's fracture, 490
Sialoadenitis, 563
Sialography, 561
Sialosis, 573
Sick cell syndrome, 63
Sinding-Larsen's disease, 408
Singer's nodules, 644
Sinus, 116
  frontal, compound fractures of, 458,
    460
  median mental, 603
  pilonidal, 1139–1141
  preauricular, 545
Sinusitis, maxillary, 617
Sister Joseph's nodule, 1188
Sistrunk's operation, 693
Sjögren's syndrome, 572
Skin, 132
  grafting, 154–156
  pre-malignant conditions of, 139
Skull, 435
  fractures of, 459–462
  traction, 495
Smith's fracture, 293
Sodium balance, 79
Spastic paralysis, 428
Spermatic cord, encysted hydrocele,
  1361
Spermatocele, 1364
Spherocytosis, hereditary, 944
Sphincterotomy, transduodenal, 974
Spina bifida, 427, 499
Spinal canal, tumours of, 502–505
  concussion (shock), 496
  cord, injury, 489–499
  rehabilitation, 498
Spinal epidural abscess, 499
Spine, congenital deformities of, 392
  fractures and dislocations of, 489–502
  osteomyelitis of, 501
  tuberculous disease of, 351
  tumours of, 501–505

Spleen, 937–952
  abscess of, 951
  congenital absence of, 940
  cysts of, 940
  enlargements of, 943
  functions of, 937
  infarction of, 942
  malarial, rupture of, 942
  neoplasms of, 949
  rupture of, 940–942
  scanning of, 938
  schistosomiasis of, 947
  tuberculosis of, 949
Splenectomy, 951
  effects of, 937, 988
Splenic artery, aneurysm of, 942
Splenomegaly, Egyptian, 947
  tropical, 948
Splenoportography, 939
Splenunculi, 940
Spondylolisthesis, 509
Spondylosis, cervical, 508
Spongioblastoma, 470–479
Sprengel's shoulder, 392
Stensen's duct, 560
Sterility, male, 1374
Sterno-clavicular joint, dislocation of, 270
Sternomastoid 'tumour', 395
Still's disease, 361
Stomach and duodenum, 855–902
  carcinoma of, 893–899
  colloid carcinoma, 896
  dilation of, acute, 900
  foreign bodies in, 900
  giant rugal hypertrophy of, 901
  handbag, 886
  hour-glass, 885
  leather-bottle, 896
  lymphatics, 896
  neoplasms of, benign, 892
  physiology of, 856–862
  sarcoma of, 899
  'teapot', 886
  ulcer of, 865–892
  volvulus of, 900
  See also Gastric.
Stomatitis, 574–580
Stones, See Calculus
'Stork bites', 137
Stove-in-chest, 745
Struma ovarii, 693
Student's elbow, 420
Stye, 132
Subarachnoid haemorrhage, 486
Subclavian artery stenosis and steal,
    206–207
Subdural haematoma, 444, 462
Submandibular gland, 560
  excision of, 564
Subphrenic abscess, 1009
Subtalar instability, 424
Subungual exostosis, 181
  infection, 159
  melanoma, 146
Sudeck's atrophy, 261
Supracondylar fracture, 277–281
Supraspinatus tendonitis and rupture,
    416, 417
Suture materials, 823
Swan Ganz catheter, 64

Sympathectomy, 201, 234
Syndactyly, 391
Synovectomy, 367, 369, 370
Synovial sarcoma, 110, 377, 378
Syphilis, 42–46
  See also under names of organs and
    regions
Syringomyelia, 432
Syringo-myelocele, 500

T

Takayasu's arteriopathy, 232
Talc granuloma, 1016
Talipes, 387–391
Talus, congenital vertical, 391
  fracture of, 340
Tarsal injuries, 340–343
Teeth, 596–604
Temporal arteritis, 232
Temporo mandibular joint, 607
Tendons, injuries and ruptures, 169, 340,
    417
  supraspinatus, calcification of, 416
  transfer, 426
Tennis elbow, 415
Tenosynovitis, 418
  suppurative, 162–164
  tuberculous, 355
Teno-vaginitis, stenosing, 418
Teratoma, 102, 786, 1138
Terminal care, 1389
Testis, abnormalities of descent,
    1352–1356
  abnormalities of, congenital, 1352
  injuries of, 1356
  lymphatics, 1366
  neoplasms of, 1366–1372
  retractile, 1354
  syphilis and leprosy of, 1366
  torsion of, 1357
Tetanus, 33
Tetany, gastric, 901
  parathyroid, 695
Thalassaemia, 949
Thermography, 713
Thiopentone, intra-arterial injection of,
    causing gangrene, 218
Thomas splint, 314
Thoracic duct, wounds of, 653
Thoracoplasty, 774
Thoracotomy, technique of, 741
Thrombo-angiitis obliterans, 231
Thrombophlebitis, 182
  migrans, 182
Thrombosis
  axillary vein, 185
  cavernous sinus, 558
  of mesenteric vessels, 1087
  venous, 182–185
Thrush, 47
Thymus, 783–786
Thyroglossal tract, anomalies of, 692
Thyroid gland, 660–693
  antibodies, 661, 691
  carcinoma of, 684–690
  ectopic and aberrant, 692
  function tests, 661
  lateral aberrant, 693
  lingual, 692

needle biopsy, 670
retrosternal 672, 782
scanning, 664
solitary nodule, 669
Thyroidectomy, 680–683
tetany after, 695
Thyroiditis, 690
Thyrotoxic crisis, post-operative, 683
Thyrotoxicosis, 673–684
factitia, 680
Jod-Basedow, 680
neonatal, 680
Tibia, fractures of, 328–333
pseudarthrosis (congenital), 391
vara, 394
Tibial tubercle, avulsion of, 328
Tibio-fibular joint, interior, diastasis of, 334–338
Tic douloureux, 511
Tietze's disease, 748
Tinel's sign, 517
TNM classification of carcinoma, 108
Toe-nail, ingrowing, 171
Toes, congenital abnormalities of, 391
Tongue, lesions of, 582–595
benign tumours of, 589
carcinoma of, 589–595
congenital fissure or furrowing, 583
geographical, 583
hairy, 588
inflammation of, 584
injuries of, 584
melanoma of, malignant, 595
nerve lesions of, 588
syphilis of, 585
tuberculosis of, 585
ulcers of, 588
Tongue-tie, 582
Tonsils, 625–628
tumours of, malignant, 628
Toothache, emergency treatment, 601
Torticollis, congenital, 394
Tourniquet, use of, 59
Toxoplasmosis, 125
Tracheal resection, 757
stenosis, 757
Tracheal wounds, 652
Tracheostomy, 639–642
Trachoma and urethritis, 1331–1333
Traction and counter traction, skull, 495
Transplantation of bone marrow, 1386
heart, 812, 1386
kidneys, 1376–1385
liver, 1385
lungs, 779, 812, 1386
pancreas, 1386
Transposition of great vessels, 802
Treacher Collins syndrome, 546
Trench foot, 218
Trendelenburg's embolectomy, 779
sign, 384
test, in varicose veins, 118
Trichobezoar, 900
Trichomonas vaginalis, 1331–1333
Trigeminal neuralgia, 510
Trigger finger, 418
Triple test (pancreas), 982
Trochanter, lesser, avulsion of, 312
Troisier's sign, 895
Tropical splenomegaly, 948

Trotter's triad, 635
Trousseau's sign, 695, 895
Truss, 1172
Tuberculosis, 36
See under names of organs and regions
Tumours, 101–110
turban, 141
See also under names of organs and regions
T.U.R.P., 1304
Typhoid fever, complications of surgical, 1046
osteomyelitis and, 347

U

Ulcer, 113–116
anastomotic, 888
aphthous, 576
decubitus, 217
oral, 579
peptic, 865–892
perforating, 114
rodent, 140
stress, 866
tongue, 588
trophic, 113
tuberculous, 115
venous, 190
Ulcerative colitis, 1039–1045
Ulna, fractures of, 286–291
Ulnar bursa, infection of, 162
Ultrasound, 184, 197, 956, 982
Umbilicus, 1185–1188
infection of cord, 1185
neoplasms of, 1187
Umbolith, 1186
Unconscious patient, care of, 450
Urachus, patent, 1187
Ureaplasma, 1331
Ureter, abnormalities of, 1212
accidental ligation of, 1207
calculus in, 1230–1233
injuries to, 1217
neoplasms of, primary, 1252
Ureterocele, 1214
Uretero-anastomoses, 1268, 1294
Uretero-lithotomy, 1233
Urethra, 1320–1343
abscess peri-, 1339
abnormalities of, congenital, 1320
calculus of, 1340
caruncle of, 1343
diverticula of, 1339, 1342
fistula of, 1340
inflammations of, 1329
injuries of, 1323
meatus of, ulceration, 1329
neoplasms of, 1341, 1343
papillomas, 1341
prolapse of, 1342
rupture of, 1323–1328
strictures of, 1333–1339, 1342
congenital, 1320
valves of, congenital, 1320
Urethral pressure profile, (UPP), 1264
Urethritis, 1329–1333
Urethrocele, 1342
Urethrography, 1335
Urethroplasty, 1337

Urethroscopy, anterior and posterior, 1202
Urethrotomy, 1336
Urethro-trigonitis, 1280
Urine, diversion operations, 1293
  extravasation of, 1328
  incontinence of, 1263–1269
  normal output, 77
  residual, 1301–1303
  retention of, 1258–1263
    after rectum excision, 1263
    due to drugs, 1261
      enlargement, 1303
    in spinal cord lesion, 1261
    post-operative, 1260
    with overflow, 1260
  suppression of, 1202
Urodynamic studies, 1264, 1267
Urography, 1196
Uveitis, 536

V

Vagotomy, 876–879, 891
Varices, oesophageal, 925–931
Varicocele, 1358
Vascular rings (Dysphagia lusoria), 812
Vasectomy, 1375
Veins, thrombosis of, 182–186
  varicose, 186–192
    ruptured, treatment of, 186
Venography, 191
Venous pump, 186
Vertebral column, 489–509
Ventriculoseptal defect, 799
Vincent's infection, angina, 578
Vitello-intestinal duct, 1186
Vocal cord, tumours, of, 643–647
Volkmann's ischaemic contracture, 249
Volvulus, 1080–1082
  neonatorum (midgut), 1075
  of stomach, 900

Von Recklinghausen's diseases, 106, 414, 696
Von Rosen sign, 380, 381
Von Willebrand's disease, 74

W

Waldenstrom's disease, 404
Waldeyer's rings, 625
Wallerian degeneration, 515
Warthin's tumour, 567
Warts, 135
  Hutchinson's 585
  venereal, 1347
Water balance, 76–78
Waterhouse-Friderichsen syndrome, 702
Wayne's clinical diagnostic index, 675
Webspace, infection, 160, 172
Wharton's duct, 561
Whipple's triad, 1001
Wilm's tumour of kidney, 1247
Worms, 977, 1085, 1093
Wounds, 1–18
Wound healing, factors influencing, 4, 815
Wound infection, 19–32
Wrist joint, tuberculosis of, 355

X

Xeromammography, 713

Y

Yaws, 46

Z

Zollinger-Ellison syndrome, 699, 867, 1002
Zygomatic arch, fracture of, 555

BAILEY & LOVE'S
SHORT PRACTICE
OF SURGERY

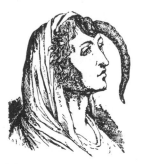

Sebaceous horn (page 134).
(The owner, the widow
Dimanche, sold water-cress in
Paris.)
  A favourite illustration of
Hamilton Bailey and McNeill
Love, well known to readers of
earlier editions of 'Short
Practice'.